Invitation to Health with Pretests

Merced College Edition

2nd Edition

Dianne Hales

CENGAGE
Learning™

Australia • Brazil • Japan • Korea • Mexico • Singapore • Spain • United Kingdom • United States

CENGAGE
Learning™

Invitation to Health with Pretests: Merced College Edition, 2nd Edition

Executive Editors:
Maureen Staudt
Michael Stranz

Senior Project Development Manager:
Linda deStefano

Marketing Specialist:
Courtney Sheldon

Senior Production/Manufacturing Manager:
Donna M. Brown

PreMedia Manager:
Joel Brennecke

Sr. Rights Acquisition Account Manager:
Todd Osborne

Cover Image:
Getty Images*

*Unless otherwise noted, all cover images used by Custom Solutions, a part of Cengage Learning, have been supplied courtesy of Getty Images with the exception of the Earthview cover image, which has been supplied by the National Aeronautics and Space Administration (NASA).

An Invitation to Health: Choosing to Change, 14th Edition
Dianne Hales

For product information and technology assistance, contact us at
Cengage Learning Customer & Sales Support, 1-800-354-9706

For permission to use material from this text or product,
submit all requests online at **cengage.com/permissions**
Further permissions questions can be emailed to
permissionrequest@cengage.com

This book contains select works from existing Cengage Learning resources and was produced by Cengage Learning Custom Solutions for collegiate use. As such, those adopting and/or contributing to this work are responsible for editorial content accuracy, continuity and completeness.

Compilation © 2010 Cengage Learning
ISBN-13: 978-1-111-46640-4

ISBN-10: 1-111-46640-8

Cengage Learning
5191 Natorp Boulevard
Mason, Ohio 45040
USA
Cengage Learning is a leading provider of customized learning solutions with office locations around the globe, including Singapore, the United Kingdom, Australia, Mexico, Brazil, and Japan. Locate your local office at:
international.cengage.com/region.

Cengage Learning products are represented in Canada by Nelson Education, Ltd.
For your lifelong learning solutions, visit **www.cengage.com/custom.**
Visit our corporate website at **www.cengage.com.**

Printed in the United States of America

To my husband, Bob, and my daugher Julia,
who make every day an invitation to joy.

BRIEF CONTENTS

CONTENTS

KEY FEATURES

PREFACE

To the Student

This textbook is an invitation to you—an invitation to a healthier, happier, fuller life. Every day you make choices that can affect both how long and how well you live. The knowledge you acquire in this course will help you make better choices, ones that will have a direct impact on how you look, feel, and function—now and for decades to come.

Perhaps you are in good health and think you know all you need to know about how to take care of yourself. If so, take a minute and ask yourself some questions:

- How well do you understand yourself? Are you able to cope with emotional upsets and crises? Do you often feel stressed out?
- How nutritiously do you eat? Are you always going on—and off—diets?
- Do you exercise regularly?
- How solid and supportive are your relationships with others? Are you conscientious about birth control and safe-sex practices?
- Do you occasionally get drunk or high? Do you smoke?
- What do you know about your risk for infectious diseases, heart problems, cancer, or other serious illnesses?
- Are you a savvy health-care consumer? Do you know how to evaluate medical products and health professionals?
- How much do you know about complementary and alternative medicine?
- If you needed health care, do you know where you'd turn or how you'd pay?
- Have you taken steps to ensure your personal safety at home, on campus, and on the streets?
- Can you improve your odds for living a long and healthy life?
- What are you doing today to prevent physical, psychological, social, and environmental problems in the future?

As you consider these questions, chances are there are some aspects of health you haven't considered before—and others you feel you don't have to worry about for years. Yet the choices you make and the actions you take now will have a dramatic impact on your future.

Your health is your personal responsibility. Over time, your priorities and needs will inevitably change, but the connections between various dimensions of your well-being will remain the same: The state of your mind will affect the state of your body, and vice versa. The values that guide you through today can keep you mentally, physically, and spiritually healthy throughout your lifetime. Your ability to cope with stress will influence your decisions about alcohol and drug use. Your commitment to honest, respectful relationships will affect the nature of your sexual involvements. Your eating and exercise habits will determine whether you develop a host of medical problems.

This edition of *An Invitation to Health: Choosing to Change* is packed with information, advice, recommendations, and research, and provides the first step in taking full charge of your own well-being. An important theme of this book is choosing to change. Ultimately, the power to implement healthy change belongs to you—and it's a lot easier than you might think. You could simply add a walk or workout to your daily routine. You could snack on fruit instead of high-fat foods. You could cut back on alcohol. You could buckle your seat belt whenever you get in a car. These are small changes and relatively easy ones to make. They may not seem like a big deal now, yet they could make a crucial difference in determining how active and fulfilling the rest of your life will be.

Knowledge alone can't assure you a lifetime of well-being. The rest depends on you. The skills you acquire, the habits you form, the choices you make, the ways you live day by day will all shape your health and your future. You cannot simply read this book and study health the way you study French or chemistry. You must decide to make it part of your daily life.

This is our invitation to you.

—*Dianne Hales*

To the Instructor

I am writing to invite you to something new. Yes, *An Invitation to Health* has been the leading college health textbook for years, and this new edition once again presents up-to-date, concise, research-based coverage of personal health. As has been true since the early editions, facts and concepts are presented in the context of implementing healthy change.

The emphasis on behavior change has grown steadily, and continues even stronger in this edition. The theme of this edition is *choosing* to change. This theme is important because it is not enough to know *how* to change; one must make the conscious *choice* to change in order to use the tools of change successfully.

In addition to "Your Strategies for Change" and "Your Health Action Plan"—features familiar from earlier editions—this edition introduces "Making Change Happen," which ties to our ground-breaking supplement *Invitation to Personal Change* and offers a four-step plan for creating sucessful change.

As always, this edition defines health in the broadest sense of the word—not as an entity in itself but as an integrated process for discovering, using, and protecting all possible resources within the individual, family, community, and environment.

New in *Invitation to Health: Choosing to Change*

Chapter 1 has been extensively revised to include coverage of pressing social issues like the toll of poverty as well as consumer health issues such as getting good medical advice online. New features in the chapters extend these themes. "Community Focus" provides a larger perspective on common health issues and suggests ways for students to become informed and involved with concerns such as homelessness (Chapter 3), feeding the world (Chapter 6), and creating a healthier environment (Chapter 19).

"Health on a Budget" appears in every chapter and provides practical suggestions for low- or no-cost strategies for making healthy choices. In most cases, the suggestions are not about how to be a better shopper but rather about how to be more resourceful in using what we already have or more creative about freeing and using internal resources.

In keeping with the theme of this edition—choosing to change—each chapter now offers "Making Change Happen," which gives students a practical four-step plan for making healthy changes such as low-cost fitness aids (Chapter 5), soul food (Chapter 2), and sleep power (Chapter 15). This feature is linked to the more extensive plans outlined in *Invitation to Personal Change,* the ground-breaking supplement coauthored with Dr. Kenneth W. Christian.

"Consumer Alert" replaces "Savvy Consumer" and provides Things to Know and Steps to Take to be a smart consumer of a wide range of products from sleeping pills (Chapter 2) to weight-loss products (Chapter 5) to online dating (Chapter 8).

Within chapters we've retained, updated, and enhanced popular features, including "Your Strategies for Change/Your Strategies for Prevention," "Reality Check," "Point/Counterpoint," and "Learn It/Live It."

At the end of each chapter is a Self Survey, followed by a Health Action Plan. Other end-of-chapter resources include Review Questions, Critical Thinking Questions, and Key Terms. At the end of the book is a full Glossary, and on the companion website, you will find the *Hales Health Almanac,* which includes a directory of resources, emergency procedures, and a guide to common medical tests.

 This edition includes gender-specific information in every chapter, flagged with icons representing men and women. As in previous editions, icons also indicate material related to students and campus life and to cultural or racial diversity.

Because the health sciences advance so rapidly, all of the chapters have been updated with the most current research, including many citations published in 2009 and incorporating the latest available statistics. The majority come from primary sources, including professional books, medical, health, and mental health journals, health education periodicals, scientific meetings, federal agencies and consensus panels, publications from research laboratories and universities, and personal interviews with specialists in a number of fields. In addition, "Internet Connections" presents reliable Internet addresses where students can turn for additional information.

As I tell students, *An Invitation to Health: Choosing to Change* can serve as an owner's manual to their bodies and minds. By using this book and taking your course, they can acquire a special type of power—the power to make good decisions, to assume responsibility, and to create and follow a healthy life-style. This textbook is our invitation to them to live what they learn and make the most of their health and of their lives.

This textbook also is an invitation to you as an instructor. I invite you to share your passion for education and to enter into a partnership with the editorial team at Wadsworth Cengage Learning. We welcome your feedback and suggestions. Please let us hear from you at **www.cengage.com/health.** I personally look forward to working with you toward our shared goal of preparing a new generation for a healthful future.

An Overview of Changes

Following is a chapter-by-chapter listing of some of the key topics that have been added, expanded, or revised for this edition:

Chapter 1: Your Invitation to Healthy Change
Updated Section: A Report Card on the Health of Americans
Updated Section: Healthy People 2010/2020
Updated Section: Health Disparities
Updated Section: The Toll of Poverty
New Section: Strategies for Prevention: If You Are at Risk
Updated Section: A Report Card on the Health of Young Adults
New Reality Check
New Health on a Budget: Invest in Your Future
Updated Section: Healthy Campus 2010/2020
New Point/Counterpoint: Who Is Responsible for Students' Health?
Updated Section: Make Quality Health-Care Decisions
New Section: Finding Good Advice Online
New Section: Getting Medical Facts Straight
New Section: Making Sense of Medical Research
New Section: Evidence-Based Medicine
New Consumer Alert: Too Good to Be True?
Updated Section: The Stages of Change
New Making Change Happen: Choosing Change

Chapter 2: Psychological and Spiritual Well-Being
New Making Change Happen: Soul Food
Updated Section: Practicing Positive Psychology
Updated Section: Boosting Emotional Intelligence
Updated Section: Pursuing Happiness
New Health on a Budget: Happiness for Free!
Updated Section: Spiritual Health
New Section: Spirituality and Physical Health
New Section: Deepening Spiritual Intelligence
Updated Section: Enriching Your Spiritual Life
Updated Section: Praying
Updated Section: Forgiving
New Community Focus: Volunteering on Campus
Updated Section: Sleepless on Campus
Updated Section: Sleep's Impact on Health
Updated Section: What Happens When We Sleep?
Updated Section: Sleep Disorders
Updated Section: How Much Sleep Do You Need?
New Section: Sleeping Pills
New Consumer Alert: Sleeping Pill Precautions

upplemental Resources

n Invitation to Personal Change

ey part of our integrated *An Invitation to Health: Choosing to
nge* approach to lifelong healthy choices is the supplement, *An
itation to Personal Change (IPC)*, coauthored by Dianne Hales
l Kenneth W. Christian, Ph.D., a psychologist with more than 30
rs of experience in personal change and maximum potential.
ed on decades of psychological research and clinical practice,
serves as a curriculum for change, inviting students to take
ropriate action in simple, compellingly straightforward ways.
The *IPC* icons throughout this book signal links to *Labs for An
itation to Personal Change*, which present step-by-step blue-
nts for creating healthier habits, eliminating harmful behaviors,
ximizing performance, and achieving greater physical, psycho-
ical, and spiritual well-being. The labs focus on key dimensions
)ersonal health, including:

sychological and spiritual well-being ("The Grateful Thread,"
Soul Food," "Your Psychological Self-Care Pyramid," "Defusing
est Stress," "Rx: Relax," "Taming a Toxic Temper," "Finity").
ealthy habits ("Excise Exercise Excuses," "Thinking Thinner,"
Mind over Platter," "Sleep Power").
ehavioral Choices ("Do It Now," "Don't Go There," "Your Alco-
ol Audit," "Butt Out," "The Seduction of Safer Sex," "To Have or
ave Not").
ommunication skills ("Listen Up," "Help Yourself," "What's
our Intimacy Quotient?").

• Social dimensions of health ("Health Assurance," "Your Guardian Angel," "YourSpace"). We invite you to sample *An Invitation
to Personal Change* by going to **servicedirect.cengage.com**.

CengageNOW™ Class-tested and student-praised, Cengage-
NOW™ offers a variety of features that support course objectives
and interactive learning. This online tutorial for students, available
with new texts, offers a Personalized Change Plan, pre- and post-
tests, a wellness journal, and a variety of activities, all designed to
get students involved in their learning progress and to be better
prepared for class participation and class quizzes and tests. Students log on to CengageNOW by using the access code available
with the text.

**PowerLecture for Health, Fitness, and Wellness: A Micro-
soft® PowerPoint® Link Tool** This teaching tool contains lecture presentations that feature more than 100 PowerPoint® slides,
including a text outline, art, ABC Videos, and resources such as the
Instructor's Manual with Test Bank, all on one convenient DVD.
PowerLecture also includes JoinIn® on TurningPoint™ content,
which allows you to enhance your students' interaction with you,
your lecture, and each other using JoinIn® content for Response
Systems tailored to the text.

Instructor's Manual and Test Bank These two essential ancil-
laries are bound together for your convenience. The Instructor's
Manual provides chapter outlines, learning objectives, classroom
handouts, discussion questions, a video list, a resource integration guide, and more. The Test Bank has been thoroughly revised
to include test questions that are linked to the book's Chapter
Objectives. Questions within the Test Bank has been categorized
according to Bloom's taxonomy, and are broken down by types:
remembering/fact recall, understanding, applying, and analyzing.

JoinIn® on Turning Point™ Enhance how your students interact with you, your lecture, and each other using JoinIn® content
for Response Systems tailored to this text. Cengage Learning's
exclusive agreement to offer TurningPoint™ software lets you pose
book-specific questions and display students' answers seamlessly
within the Microsoft® PowerPoint® slides of your own lecture, in
conjunction with the "clicker" hardware of your choice.

ExamView Computerized Testing Create, deliver, and cus-
tomize the thorough Test Bank in minutes with this easy-to-use
assessment and tutorial system. *ExamView* offers both a *Quick Test
Wizard* and an *Online Test Wizard* that guide you step-by-step
through the process of creating tests, while it allows you to see
the test you are creating on the screen exactly as it will print or
display online. You can build tests of up to 250 questions using up
to 12 question types. Using *ExamView*'s complete word-processing
capabilities, you can enter an unlimited number of new questions
or edit existing questions.

InfoTrac® College Edition Student Guide for Health This
24-page booklet offers detailed guidance for students on how to
use the *InfoTrac College Edition* database. Includes log-in help,
a complete search tips "cheat sheet," and a topic list of key word
search terms for health, fitness, and wellness. Available *free* when
packaged with the text.

Careers in Health, Physical Education, and Sport This is the essential manual for majors who are interested in pursuing a position in their chosen field. It guides them through the complicated process of picking the type of career they want to pursue, suggests how to prepare for the transition into the working world, and offers information about different career paths, education requirements, and reasonable salary expectations. The supplement also describes the differences in credentials found in the field and testing requirements for certain professions.

Diet Analysis Plus 9.0 This is the market-leading diet assessment program used by colleges and universities that allows students to create their own personal profiles based on height, weight, age, sex, and activity level. Its new dynamic interface makes it easy for students to track the types and serving sizes of the foods they consume, from one day to 365 days! Now including even more exciting features, the updated 9.0 version includes a 20,000+ food database, ten reports for analysis, a food recipe feature, the latest Dietary References, and goals and actual percentages of essential nutrients, vitamins, and minerals. New in 9.0 are assignments designed to guide students in using their personal information to analyze and improve their eating habits. Students can use this information to adjust their diet and gain a better understanding of how nutrition relates to their personal health goals. Thoroughly revised and updated, the software is available online or on a new Windows/Mac® compatible CD-ROM.

Behavior Change Workbook *The Behavior Change Workbook* includes a brief discussion of the current theories behind making positive lifestyle changes, along with exercises to help students effect those changes in their everyday lives.

Health and Wellness Resource Center at gale.cengage .com Gale's Health and Wellness Resource Center is a new comprehensive website that provides easy-to-find answers to health questions.

Walk4Life® Elite Model Pedometer This pedometer tracks steps, elapsed time, distance, and includes a calorie counter. Whether used as an activity in class or as a tool to encourage students to simply track their steps and walk toward better fitness awareness, this is a valuable item for everyone.

Readings in Healthy Living As a frequent author of health-related articles produced by Parade® Magazine, Dianne Hales has published numerous articles that students will find useful and interesting. This 12-article reader is a collection of key articles, including "Take Your Meds—The Right Way" and "You Can Think Yourself Thin."

ABC Videos for Health and Wellness These videos, available on the PowerLecture DVD, allow you to integrate the news-gathering and programming power of the ABC News networks into the classroom to show students the relevance of course topics to their everyday lives. The videos include news clips correlated directly with the text and can help you launch a lecture, spark a discussion, or demonstrate an application. Students can see first-hand how the principles they learn in the course apply to the stories they hear in the news.

Acknowledgments

One of the joys of writing *An Invitation to Health: Choosing Change* is the opportunity to work with a team I consider the ve best of the best in textbook publishing.

I thank Laura Pople, our fearless leader, for her unwavering s port. Nedah Rose, our Senior Development Editor, has been e lessly supportive and enthusiastic and has made every step of t process of creating this edition go smoothly.

I thank Kristina Chiapella, our editorial assistant, who provid endless help—with endless patience and good humor. Thanks Trudy Brown and Rita Jaramillo, Content Project Managers, expertly shepherding this edition from conception to producti to Brian Salisbury for his vibrant new design, and to Lachina Pu lishing Services for art. Terri Miller, our photo researcher, has p vided us with dazzling, dynamic images that capture the divers and energy of today's college students. I appreciate the skill a dedication of copy editor Amy Mayfield.

My thanks to Laura McGinn, Senior Marketing Manager, her enthusiastic support, to Belinda Krohmer for her work on promotional materials, to Samantha Arvin, who guided the an laries, and to Stephanie Thiel, my student intern.

Finally, I would like to thank the reviewers whose input been so valuable through these many editions. For the *Choosing Change* Edition, I thank the following for their comments a helpful assistance:

Elaine D. Bryan, *Georgia Perimeter College*
Robert Dollinger, *Florida International University College of Medicine*
Amy Hedman, *Mankato State University*
Terry Oehrtman, *Ohio University*
Lorraine Peniston, *Hartford Community College*

Thanks also to the reviewers who gave feedback about the s plements for this edition:

Elaine D. Bryan, *Georgia Perimeter College*
Amy Hedman, *Mankato State University*
Anthony E. Kiszewski, *Bentley University*
Kim H. Miller, *University of Kentucky*

For their help with earlier editions, I offer my gratitude to:

Ghulam Aasef, *Kaskaskia College*
Andrea Abercrombie, *Clemson University*
Daniel Adame, *Emory University*
Carol Allen, *Lone Community College*
Lana Arabas, *Truman State University*
Judy Baker, *East Carolina University*
Marcia Ball, *James Madison University*
Jeremy Barnes, *Southeast Missouri State University*
Rick Barnes, *East Carolina University*
Lois Beach, *SUNY-Plattsburg*
Liz Belyea, *Cosumnes River College*
Betsy Bergen, *Kansas State University*
Nancy Bessette, *Saddleback College*
Carol Biddington, *California University of Pennsylvania*
David Black, *Purdue University*

About the Author

Dianne Hales is one of the most widely published and honored freelance journalists in the country. She has written 14 trade books, including *La Bella Lingua, Think Thin, Just like a Woman,* and *Caring for the Mind,* as well as articles for many nationally publications such as *Family Circle, Fitness, Glamour, Good Housekeeping, Health, Mademoiselle, McCall's, New York Times, Psychology Today, Reader's Digest, Redbook, Science Digest, Self, Seventeen, Washington Post, Woman's Day,* and *World Book.* She has served as a contributing editor for *Parade, Ladies Home Journal, Working Mother,* and *American Health.*

Dianne Hales has received writing awards from the American Psychiatric Association, the American Psychological Association. an EMMA (Exceptional Media Merit Award) for health reporting from the National Women's Political Caucus and Radcliffe College, three "EDI" (Equality, Dignity, Independence) awards for print journalism from the National Easter Seal Society, the National Mature Media Award, Arthritis Foundation, California Psychiatric Society, CHADD (Children and Adults with Attention Deficit/ Hyperactivity), Council for the Advancement of Scientific Education, and the New York City Public Library.

Taking Charge of Your Health

HEALTH may be a science; living is an art. The principles that can help you understand the science and practice the art are simple and timeless and form the basic premise of this book: You have more control over your life and well-being than anything or anyone else does. Through the decisions you make and the habits you develop, you can influence how well—and perhaps how long—you will live. This section defines health and wellness and provides the information you need to take charge of your well-being now and in the years to come.

Chapter 1 - Taking Charge of Your Health

1) **A major goal of the Healthy People 2010/2020 Initiative is to (pg. 7)**
   ___ eliminate health disparities among minorities
   ___ provide universal health care to all citizens
   ___ get people to live to 95 years of age
   ___ increase more people to get checked for diabetes

2) **An important guideline to consider when evaluating the accuracy and reliability of a medical website should be : (pg. 17-18)**
   ___ products that are being promoted so you can purchase medicines immediately after you find out what   is wrong with you
   ___ information is based on scientific evidence and reported in peer reviewed medical journals
   ___ the use of personal testimonies as you can determine that the product truly does work for ordinary people like yourself
   ___ a commerical website as the facts are more reliable since the site is produced by professional web developers

3) **When Kate willingly took responsibility for her bad habit and made the effort to change this unhealthy habit, she was exhibiting: (pg. 26)**
   ___ self efficacy
   ___ reinforcement behavior
   ___ external locus of control
   ___ internal locus of control

4) **Wellness can be defined as: (pg. 4)**
   ___ one's personal responsibility to make the best of their situation in life
   ___ a decision that one makes toward their optimal health goals
   ___ the development of happiness and health in one's current situation
   ___ all of the above are a part of wellness

5) **All of the following are examples of reinforcing factors except (pg. 22)**
   ___ you buy yourself a new outfit for quitting smoking
   ___ your parent offers you money to earn good grades
   ___ after losing 10 pounds, your friends compliment how good you look
   ___ your family complains to you about your alcohol drinking

6) **A successful technique to help a person to make a positive behavioral change is to use: (pg. 25-26)**
   ___ affirmations
   ___ persistence and go all the way
   ___ set sights on the target
   ___ all of the above are good techniques to use

7) **All of the following are dimensions of health except: (pg. 4-6)**
   ___ physical
   ___ economic
   ___ psychological
   ___ social

8) **When one is judged to have good psychological health, this means that: (pg. 5)**
   ___ critical thinking skills are sharply defined
   ___ the absence of problems or illness in their life
   ___ their intellectual quotient is in the normal range
   ___ their emotional and mental state is healthy

9) **Health literacy is defined as (pg. 17)**
   ___ health materials developed on a sixth grade reading level
   ___ being able to read medical jargon and understand what is being said
   ___ ability to understand health information and make an informed decision about one's health
   ___ improving the intelligence of minority groups who may not be able to read

10) **As far as gender health issues go, women are more likely to suffer from which health condition that men will not ? (pg. 10)**
   ___ stroke
   ___ autoimmune disorder like rheumatoid arthritis
   ___ alcohol problems
   ___ attention deficit disorder

11) **Successful change depends on all of the following except:** (pg. 26)
___ locus of control
___ self efficacy
___ self talk
___ positive reinforcements only

12) **Judy and Jason are comfortable expressing their feelings to each other and they trust teach other in their relationship. This relates to which component of health?** (pg. 5)
___ intellectual
___ social
___ sexual
___ psychological

13) **Which stage of change is basically where one is in denial about an unhealthy behavior and has no intention of changing it?** (pg. 24)
___ precontemplation
___ preparation
___ termination
___ contemplation

14) **Which Healthy People 2010/2020 initiative has not been met so far to improve the health and wellbeing of Americans ?** (pg. 7)
___ improving physical fitness
___ reducing alcohol abuse
___ improving immunization rates
___ reducing obeseity

15) **Abby has a good spiritual life and believes in the power of prayer to help give her a sense of peace and inner strength. She is practicing which component of health?** (pg. 5)
___ emotional health
___ psychological health
___ spiritual health
___ social health

16) **When making a lifestyle behavioral change, it is suggested to use a 'step and stretch' goal technique. Which statement best describes this step and stretch process?** (pg. 22)
___ weighing the potential plusses and minuses before taking on the challenge
___ do something out of your comfort zone and take a risk to keep moving forward with your goal
___ do an anaerobic cardio kickboxing exercise program
___ go up one flight of stairs and then stretch for 5 minutes

17) **When one has a drinking problem and he decides that maybe he should try quitting and get some help, which stage of the behavioral change model is this describing?** (pg. 24)
___ contemplation
___ maintenance
___ action
___ precontemplation

18) **To view one's health in a holistic approach means to:** (pg. 4)
___ look at health and the individual as a 'whole' being
___ look at health in a spiritual or holy way
___ tear apart all the various components of health on the body
___ look at health and wellness in a scientific method

19. **All of the following are examples of reinforcing factors except:** (p. 22)
A. you buy yourself a new outfit for quitting smoking
B. after losing 10 pounds, your friends compliment how good you look
C. your family complains to you about your alcohol drinking
D. your parent offers you money to earn good grades

20. **Andrea's fitness center where she exercises is just across the street from her apartment. Which factor does this situation help Andrea to better maintain her fitness goals?** (p. 22)
A. enabling
B. endorsing
C. reinforcing
D. predisposing

A leesha always thought of health as something you worry about when you get older. Then her twin brother developed a health problem she'd never heard of: prediabetes (discussed in Chapter 14), which increases his risk of diabetes and heart disease. At a health fair on campus, she learned that her blood pressure was higher than normal. "Maybe I'm not too young to start thinking about my health," she concluded. Neither are you—whether you're a traditional-age college student or older, like an ever-increasing number of undergraduates.

Your Invitation to Healthy Change

An Invitation to Health asks you to go beyond thinking about your health to taking charge and making healthy choices for yourself and your future. This book is both *about* and *for* you: It includes material on your mind and your body, your spirit and your social ties, your needs and your wants, your past and your potential. It will help you explore options, discover possibilities, and find new ways to make your life worthwhile. If you don't make the most of what you are, you risk never discovering what you might become.

Being healthy, as you'll learn in this chapter, means more than not being sick or in pain. Health is a personal choice that you make every day when you decide on everything from what to eat to whether to exercise to how to handle stress. Sometimes making the best choices demands making healthy changes in your life. This chapter, along with the supplement *An Invitation to Personal Change (IPC)* will show you how.

This chapter also extends an invitation to live more fully, more happily, and more healthfully. It is an offer that you literally cannot afford to refuse. The quality of your life depends on it.

> **After studying the material in this chapter, you should be able to**
>
> - **Define** health and wellness.
> - **Name** three ways in which gender impacts health.
> - **Describe** the *Healthy People 2010/2020* initiative.
> - **List** three to five attributes of credible medical information websites.
> - **Describe** the stages of change and give an example of each.
> - **Make** a decision about a lifestyle behavior you want to change.

Log on to CengageNOW for Health at **www.cengage.com/sso** to find your Behavior Change Planner and to explore self-assessments, interactive tutorials, and practice quizzes.

3

Health and Wellness

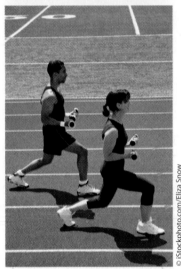

Health is the process of discovering, using, and protecting all the resources within our bodies, minds, spirits, families, communities, and environment.

By simplest definition, **health** means being sound in body, mind, and spirit. The World Health Organization defines health as "not merely the absence of disease or infirmity," but "a state of complete physical, mental, and social well-being."[1] Health is the process of discovering, using, and protecting all the resources within our bodies, minds, spirits, families, communities, and environment.

Health has many dimensions: physical, psychological, spiritual, social, intellectual, and environmental. This book integrates all these dimensions within a *holistic* approach that looks at health and the individual as a whole, rather than part by part. Your own definition of health may include different elements, but chances are you and your classmates agree that it includes at least some of the following:

- A positive, optimistic outlook.
- A sense of control over stress and worries; time to relax.
- Energy and vitality; freedom from pain or serious illness.
- Supportive friends and family and a nurturing intimate relationship with someone you love.
- A personally satisfying job.
- A clean environment.

Wellness can be defined as purposeful, enjoyable living or, more specifically, a deliberate lifestyle choice characterized by personal responsibility and optimal enhancement of physical, mental, and spiritual health. In the broadest sense, wellness is:

- A decision you make to move toward optimal health.
- A way of life you design to achieve your highest potential.
- A process of developing awareness that health and happiness are possible in the present.
- The integration of body, mind, and spirit.
- The belief that everything you do, think, and feel has an impact on your state of health and the health of the world.[2]

"The 'well' person is not necessarily the strong, the brave, the successful, the young, the whole, or even the illness-free being," notes John Travis, M.D., author of *The Wellness Workbook*. "No matter what your current state of health, you can begin to appreciate yourself as a growing, changing person and allow yourself to move toward a happier life and positive health."[3] (See Self Survey: "Wellness Inventory" on page 28.)

In wellness, health, and sickness, there is considerable overlap of the functions of the mind, body, and spirit. As scientists have shown again and again in recent decades, psychological factors play a major role in enhancing physical well-being and preventing illness, but they also can trigger, worsen, or prolong physical symptoms. Similarly, almost every medical illness affects people psychologically as well as physically.

The Dimensions of Health

By learning more about the six dimensions of health, you gain insight into the complex interplay of factors that determine your level of wellness.

Physical Health

The various states of health can be viewed as points on a continuum (Figure 1.1). At one end is early and needless death; at the other is optimal wellness, in which you feel and

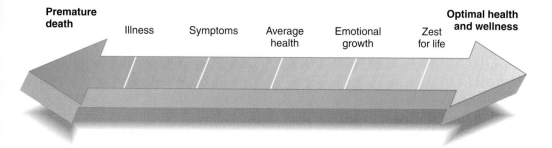

perform at your very best. In the middle, individuals are neither sick enough to need medical attention nor well enough to live each day with zest and vigor.

What matters even more than your place on the continuum is the direction in which you are moving: toward high-level wellness or toward premature death. Individuals in physical good health who are always worrying or not working to develop more fully may be on the right of the neutral point but facing toward illness. Others who may be disabled or have a chronic health problem may have a positive outlook and a network of mutually supportive relationships that keep them focused toward wellness.[4]

For the sake of optimal physical health, we must take positive steps away from illness and toward well-being. We must feed our bodies nutritiously, exercise them regularly, avoid harmful behaviors and substances, watch for early signs of sickness, and protect ourselves from accidents.

Psychological Health

Like physical well-being, psychological health is more than the absence of problems or illness. Psychological health refers to both our emotional and mental states—that is, to our feelings and our thoughts. It involves awareness and acceptance of a wide range of feelings in oneself and others, the ability to express emotions, to function independently, and to cope with the challenges of daily stressors.

Spiritual Health

Spiritually healthy individuals identify their own basic purpose in life; learn how to experience love, joy, peace, and fulfillment; and help themselves and others achieve their full potential. As they devote themselves to others' needs more than their own, their spiritual development produces a sense of

greater meaning in their lives. (See Chapter 2 for an in-depth discussion of spiritual and emotional well-being.)

Many studies have confirmed health benefits for individuals who pray, attend religious services, and engage in spiritual practices. However, the largest-ever study of "intercessory" prayer (praying for other individuals) found no benefits for coronary bypass patients. In fact, the patients who knew strangers were praying for them fared significantly worse than those who received no prayers.

Social Health

Social health refers to the ability to interact effectively with other people and the social environment, to develop satisfying interpersonal relationships, and to fulfill social roles. It involves participating in and contributing to your community, living in harmony with fellow human beings, developing positive interdependent relationships (discussed in Chapter 8), and practicing healthy sexual behaviors.

In times of crisis, social connections provide comfort and support. Even in tranquil times, social isolation increases the risk of sickness and mortality. People with spouses, friends, and a rich social network may outlive isolated loners by as much as 30 years.

Health educators are placing greater emphasis on social health in its broadest sense as they expand the traditional individualistic concept of health to include the complex interrelationships between one person's health and the health of the community and environment. This change in perspective has given rise to a new emphasis on **health promotion,** which educators define as "any planned combination of educational, political, regulatory, and organizational supports for actions and conditions of living conducive to the health

health A state of complete well-being, including physical, psychological, spiritual, social, intellectual, and environmental dimensions.

wellness A deliberate lifestyle choice characterized by personal responsibility and optimal enhancement of physical, mental, and spiritual health.

health promotion Any planned combination of educational, political, regulatory, and organizational supports for actions and conditions of living conducive to the health of individuals, groups, or communities.

of individuals, groups, or communities." Examples on campus include establishing smoke-free policies for all college buildings, residences, and dining areas; prohibiting tobacco advertising and sponsorship of campus social events; promoting safety at parties; and enforcing alcohol laws and policies.

Intellectual Health

Your brain is the only one of your organs capable of self-awareness. Every day you use your mind to gather, process, and act on information; to think through your values; to make decisions, set goals, and figure out how to handle a problem or challenge. Intellectual health refers to your ability to think and learn from life experience, your openness to new ideas, and your capacity to question and evaluate information. Throughout your life, you'll use your critical thinking skills, including your ability to evaluate health information, to safeguard your well-being.

Environmental Health

You live in a physical and social setting that can affect every aspect of your health. Environmental health refers to the impact your world has on your well-being. It means protecting yourself from dangers in the air, water, and soil, and in products you use—and working to preserve the environment itself. (Chapter 19 offers a thorough discussion of environmental health.)

A Report Card on the Health of Americans

 The United States spends more than any other nation on health care: a whopping $2.2 trillion total, or $7,421 per person per year.[5] However, Americans rank twenty-third in life expectancy for men and twenty-fifth for women. Men in Hong Kong, with a life expectancy of 79 years, and women in Japan, with a life expectancy of 85.6 years, are at the top of the ratings. The Russian federation has the lowest life expectancy for both men (59.1 years) and women (72.4 years).

Yet Americans are living longer. Life expectancy at birth in 2007 reached a record high of 78.1 years, up from 75.4 years in 1975. This represents an increase of 3.6 years for men and 1.9 years for women. The gender gap in longevity has narrowed from 7 years in 1990 to 5.3 years in 2007. The racial longevity gap also has shrunk, from a difference of 7 years between whites and blacks in 1990 to 4.9 years in 2007.[6]

Are we also living well? Here is a summary of the latest findings on Americans' health and health behaviors from the U.S. Centers for Disease Control and Prevention (CDC):

- **Fitness.** Americans have not become more active over the last 30 years. About one in three adults over age 18 engages in regular physical activity; about a fifth do strength-training exercises.

- **Weight.** The percentage of obese adults has more than doubled in the last 40 years, rising from 13 percent to 34 percent.

- **Smoking.** About one in five (21 percent) of adults currently smoke cigarettes, the same percentage as in the last two years. More men (24 percent) than women (18 percent) smoke.

- **Alcohol use.** Twenty percent of all adults over age 18 reported having five or more drinks on at least one day in the last year; 9 percent reported five or more drinks on at least 12 days last year.

- **Drug use.** Six percent of all adults over age 12 used marijuana in the last month; 3 percent reported nonmedical use of prescription drugs.

• **Health conditions.** The percentage of Americans who describe their health as fair or poor increases with age, from 6 percent of those between 18 and 44 to 28 percent of those older than 75. More African Americans and Hispanics report poor health than white Americans. Many conditions, including hypertension and high cholesterol, increase with age. Although the incidence of vaccine-preventable diseases like measles has declined, the rate of infections such as *Chlamydia* has increased.

• **Mental disorders.** Three percent of adults report serious psychological distress. Those living in poverty have four times the rate of mental problems as others.

• **Health care.** According to federal statistics, there are 1.1 billion visits to doctors' offices, hospital emergency rooms, and outpatient care departments every year. More than eight in ten (83 percent) of the population visited a physician or hospital at least once. About half of Americans (47 percent) received at least one drug prescription in the last month; 20 percent received three or more.

 • **Health insurance.** Some 17 percent of people under age 65 did not have health insurance coverage at some point in time, including 10 percent of children under age 18. More than a third of Hispanics, American Indians, and Alaska Natives were uninsured at some time, compared with less than a fifth of those in other racial and ethnic groups.

 • **Mortality.** Deaths from heart disease have declined 38 percent overall since 1990, while cancer deaths are down 16 percent. Although mortality rates for African Americans have dropped, they remain significantly higher than those of whites, particularly for stroke, heart disease, diabetes, and HIV/AIDS. Homicide continues to be the leading cause of death for young African American men between the ages of 18 and 44.

The Healthy People Project

Since 1979 the federal Healthy People project has set science-based, 10-year national objectives for promoting health and preventing disease. In 2000 the *Healthy People 2010* program set two overarching goals: to increase the quality and quantity of years of healthy life and to eliminate health disparities (discussed in the next section).

As you read in the preceding section, Americans are indeed living longer. However, many of the goals in specific focus areas have not been met. For instance, the percentage of obese Americans—34 percent—remains more than twice the target goal of 15 percent. Despite intensive public education campaigns, seven in ten Americans do not exercise regularly—far fewer than the 50 percent objective. Smoking rates also remain stubbornly high: 21 percent rather than the target of 12 percent.[7] However, progress is being made on other fronts, and the lessons from *Healthy People 2010* may lead to greater success in meeting the objectives of *Healthy People 2020*.

Your choices and behaviors during your college years can influence how healthy you will be in the future.

Health Disparities

 Despite great improvements in the overall health of the nation, Americans who are members of racial and ethnic groups—including black or African Americans, American Indians, Alaska Natives, Asian Americans, Hispanics, Latinos, and Pacific Islanders—are more likely than whites to suffer poor health and die prematurely. Many factors, including genetic variations, environmental influences, and specific health behaviors, contribute to these disparities. Inequities in health, such as those between black and white and rich and poor, shrank from 1966 to 1980 but have since widened for some groups.

The Toll of Poverty

The primary reason for the health problems faced by minorities in the United States is poverty. Without adequate insurance or the ability to pay, many cannot afford the tests and treatments that could prevent illness or overcome it at the earliest possible stages. According to public health experts, low income may account for one-third of the racial differences in death rates for middle-aged African American adults.

Both genetic and environmental factors have contributed to the increase in diabetes among the Pima tribe. Half of all Pima adults in the United States have diabetes.

© Lawrence Migdale/Stone/Getty Images

In some cases, both genetic and environmental factors may play a role. Take, for example, the high rates of diabetes among the Pima Indians. Until 50 years ago, these American Indians were not notably obese or prone to diabetes. After World War II, the tribe started trading handmade baskets for lard and flour. Their lifestyle became more sedentary and their diet higher in fats. In addition, researchers have discovered that many Pima Indians have an inherited resistance to insulin that increases their susceptibility to diabetes. The combination of a hereditary predisposition and environmental factors may explain why the Pimas now have epidemic levels of diabetes.

Why Race Matters

We live in the most diverse nation on Earth, one that is becoming increasingly diverse. For society, this variety can be both enriching and divisive. Tolerance and acceptance of others have always been part of the American creed. By working together, Americans have created a country that remains, to those outside our borders, a symbol of opportunity.

This racial diversity also means varying susceptivity to disease. However, in defining race as a risk factor for certain health conditions, classifications such as "black" or "Hispanic" may be overly broad. Among Hispanics, for instance, Puerto Ricans suffer disproportionately from asthma, HIV/AIDS, and high infant mortality, while Mexican Americans have higher rates for diabetes. If, like many Americans, you come from a racially mixed background, your health profile may be complex.

Black Americans lose substantially more years of potential life to homicide (nine times as many), stroke (three times as many), and diabetes (three times as many) as whites. Hispanics suffer more fatal injuries, chronic liver disease, and cirrhosis of the liver. Compared with whites, blacks have more new AIDS cases. American Indian and Alaska Native women are less likely to receive prenatal care, and Asian American women have significantly lower rates of mammography.[8] A number of studies have documented racial and ethnic disparities in pain control and management. In emergency departments, for instance, white patients are more likely to be given painkillers than are minority ones.[9]

Caucasians are prone to osteoporosis (progressive weakening of bone tissue); cystic fibrosis; skin cancer; and phenylketonuria (PKU), a metabolic disorder that can lead to mental retardation.

Native Americans, including those indigenous to Alaska, are more likely to die young than the population as a whole, primarily as a result of accidental injuries, cirrhosis of the liver, homicide, pneumonia, and the complications of diabetes. The suicide rate among American Indians and Alaska Natives is 50 percent higher than the national rate. The rates of co-occurring mental illness and substance abuse (especially alcohol) are also higher among Native American youth and adults.

If you do face greater health threats because of your race or ethnicity, it is up to you to educate yourself, take responsibility for the risks within your control, and become a savvy, assertive consumer of health-care services. The federal Office of Minority Health (**www.cdc.gov/omh**), which provides general information and the latest research and recommendations, is a good place to start.

The Department of Health and Human Services has identified several areas in which racial and ethnic minorities experience significant disparities in health access and outcomes. These include the following.

Cancer Screening and Management
Overall, black Americans are more likely to develop cancer than persons of any other racial or ethnic group. Black women have higher rates of colon, pancreatic, and stomach cancer. Black men have higher rates of prostate, colon, and stomach cancer.

African Americans have the highest death rates for lung cancer of any racial or ethnic group in the United States. Medical scientists have debated whether the reason might be that treatments are less effective in blacks or whether many are not diagnosed early enough nor treated rigorously enough.

African American women are more than twice as likely to die of cervical cancer than are white women and are more likely to die of breast cancer than are women of any other racial or ethnic group. Native Hawaiian women have the highest rates of breast cancer. Women from many racial minorities, including those of Filipino, Pakistani, Mexican, and Puerto Rican descent, are more likely to be diagnosed with late-stage breast cancer than white women.[10]

Cardiovascular Disease Heart disease and stroke are the leading causes of death for all racial and ethnic groups in the United States, but rates of death from heart disease and from stroke are higher among African American adults than among white adults. African Americans also have higher rates of high blood pressure (hypertension), develop this problem earlier in life, suffer more severe hypertension, and have higher rates of stroke.

Diabetes American Indians and Alaska Natives, African Americans, and Hispanics are twice as likely to be diagnosed with diabetes compared with non-Hispanic whites. American Indians have the highest rate of diabetes in the world.

Infant Mortality African American, American Indian, and Puerto Rican infants have higher death rates than white infants.

Mental Health American Indians and Alaska Natives suffer disproportionately from depression and substance abuse. Minorities have less access to mental health services and are less likely to receive needed high-quality mental health services.

Infectious Disease Asian Americans and Pacific Islanders have much higher rates of hepatitis B. Black teenagers and young adults become infected with hepatitis B three to four times more often than those who are white. Black people also have a higher incidence of hepatitis C infection than white people. Almost 80 percent of reported cases affect racial and ethnic minorities.

HIV and Sexually Transmitted Infections
Although African Americans and Hispanics represent only about a quarter of the U.S.

YOUR STRATEGIES FOR PREVENTION
If You Are at Risk

Certain health risks may be genetic, but behavior influences their impact. Here are specific steps you can take to protect your health:

- Ask if you are at risk for any medical conditions or disorders based on your family history or racial or ethnic background.

- Find out if there are tests that could determine your risks. Discuss the advantages and disadvantages of such testing.

- If you or a family member require treatment for a chronic illness, ask your doctor whether any medications have proved particularly effective for your racial or ethnic background.

- If you are African American, you are significantly more likely to develop high blood pressure, diabetes, and kidney disease. Being overweight or obese adds to the danger. The information in Chapters 5, 6, and 7 can help you lower your risk by keeping in shape, making healthy food choices, and managing your weight.

- Hispanics and Latinos have disproportionately high rates of respiratory problems, such as asthma, chronic obstructive lung disease, and tuberculosis. To protect your lungs, stop smoking and avoid secondary smoke. Learn as much as you can about the factors that can trigger or worsen lung diseases.

population, they account for about two-thirds of adult AIDS cases and more than 80 percent of pediatric AIDS cases. The rate of syphilis infection for African Americans is nearly 30 times the rate for whites.

Why Gender Matters

"Sex does matter. It matters in ways that we did not expect. Undoubtedly, it also matters in ways that we have not begun to imagine." This was the conclusion of the Institute of Medicine Committee on Understanding the Biology of Sex and Gender Differences in a landmark review of the status of sex and gender differences in biomedical research.

Sex, the committee stated, is "a classification, generally as male or female, according to the reproductive organs and functions that derive from the chromosomal complement." *Gender* refers to "a person's self-representation as male or female or how that person is responded to by social institutions on the basis of the individual's gender presentation." Rooted in biology, gender is shaped by environment and experience.

The experience of being male or female in a particular culture and society can and does have an effect on physical and psychological well-being. In fact, sex and gender may have a greater impact than any other variable on how our bodies function, how long we live, and the symptoms, course, and treatment of the diseases that strike us.

This realization is both new and revolutionary. For centuries, scientists based biological theories solely on a male model and viewed women as shorter, smaller, and rounder versions of men. Even modern medicine is based on the assumption that, except for their reproductive organs, both sexes are biologically interchangeable. We now know that this simply isn't so (Figure 1.2). Sex begins in the womb, but sex and gender differences affect behavior, perception, and health throughout life.

As you will see throughout this text, gender affects many aspects of health. Women, for instance, are far more susceptible to autoimmune disorders such as rheumatoid arthritis,[11] and both sexes may respond differently to various treatments. Men are less likely to suffer strokes as a complication of heart valve surgery, but women's overall survival rates are better.[12]

He:

- averages 12 breaths a minute
- has lower core body temperature
- has a slower heart rate
- has more oxygen-rich hemoglobin in his blood
- is more sensitive to sound
- produces twice as much saliva
- has a 10 percent larger brain
- is 10 times more likely to have attention deficit disorder
- as a teen, has an attention span of 5 minutes
- is more likely to be physically active
- is more prone to lethal diseases, including heart attacks, cancer, and liver failure
- is five times more likely to become an alcoholic
- has a life expectancy of 75.2 years

She:

- averages 9 breaths a minute
- has higher core body temperature
- has a faster heart rate
- has higher levels of protective immunoglobulin in her blood
- is more sensitive to light
- takes twice as long to process food
- has more neurons in certain brain regions
- is twice as likely to have an eating disorder
- as a teen, has an attention span of 20 minutes
- is more likely to be overweight
- is more vulnerable to chronic diseases, like arthritis and autoimmune disorders, and age-related conditions like osteoporosis
- is twice as likely to develop depression
- has a life expectancy of 80.4 years

Figure 1.2 Some of the Many Ways Men and Women Are Different

A Report Card on the Health of Young Adults

The years between ages 18 and 29 represent a major life transition. During this time young people become legally and emotionally independent. With less oversight by parents and others, young adults become increasingly responsible for decisions that directly affect their current and future health.

In their late teens and twenties, young adults pursue higher education, begin working, and may choose to marry or to have children. More young adults are completing high school and going on to college or other types of education. The age at marriage is going up, and birth rates for some (but not all) unmarried young women are going down.

According to a recent analysis by the CDC, most young adults are in good health, but these "young invincibles," as they are sometimes called, are not immune to illness, injury, or death (see Figure 1.3). Here are the key findings on their health and health behaviors:

- **Fitness.** During their leisure time, 39 percent of young men and 32 percent of young women engage in regular physical activity. About a third of young men and a fifth of young women report strength training.

- **Weight.** About one in four (24 percent) are obese. This is triple the percentage of obese young adults 30 years ago.

- **Smoking.** More than a quarter of young adult men and a fifth of young women smoke. This represents a decline for women, but not for men.

- **Alcohol use.** About a quarter of young men report having five or more drinks a day on at least 12 days during the past year. Nine percent of women engaged in comparable levels of binge drinking.

- **Drug use.** Almost 40 percent of young people ages 18 to 20 said they had used an illicit drug in the past year, compared to a third of 21- to 25-year-olds and a quarter of 26- to 29-year-olds. The most commonly reported drugs were marijuana or hashish, followed by prescription drugs.

- **Health conditions.** Four to five percent of young adults described their health as fair or poor or had to limit their activity because of a health condition. Eighteen percent of young women and 12 percent of young men have been diagnosed with a specific health condition, such as asthma or hypertension (see Figure 1.3). Human papillomavirus (HPV) is widespread in this age group, affecting 45 percent of women from 20 to 24 years of age and 27 percent of women from 25 to 29.

- **Mental disorders.** Almost 9 percent of young adults suffered a mental disorder in the previous 12 months. Young women (11 percent) were almost twice as likely as young men (6 percent) to have major depression, generalized anxiety disorder, or a panic disorder. Almost 7 percent of young adults were

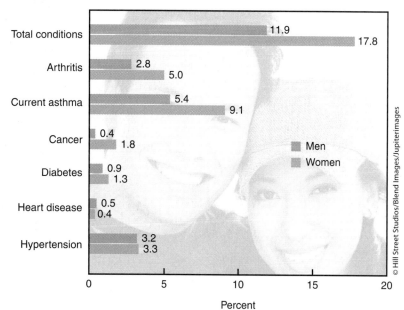

Figure 1.3 Young Adults 18–29 Years: Health Status

(Chart data, Percent)

Condition	Men	Women
Total conditions	11.9	17.8
Arthritis	2.8	5.0
Current asthma	5.4	9.1
Cancer	0.4	1.8
Diabetes	0.9	1.3
Heart disease	0.5	0.4
Hypertension	3.2	3.3

© Hill Street Studios/Blend Images/Jupiterimages

Undergraduates often switch from participating in sports in high school to watching them on television.

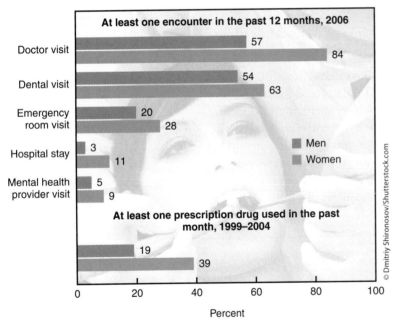

At least one encounter in the past 12 months, 2006

	Men	Women
Doctor visit	57	84
Dental visit	54	63
Emergency room visit	20	28
Hospital stay	3	11
Mental health provider visit	5	9

At least one prescription drug used in the past month, 1999–2004

	Men	Women
	19	39

Percent

Figure 1.4 Young Adults 18–29 Years: Health Care Utilization

diagnosed with depression in the past year.

- **Health care.** Eighty-four percent of young women and 57 percent of young men visited a doctor in the past year (see Figure 1.4). Young women were almost four times as likely to report a hospital stay in the past year (11 percent) as young men (3 percent) and twice as likely to report taking a prescription drug in the past month (39 percent versus 19 percent). Young adults have the highest rate of emergency department visits related to injuries of all age groups. The three most common causes are motor vehicle accidents, being struck by objects or people, and falls.

- **Health insurance.** Both young men and women are equally likely to be covered by private health insurance. However, young adults ages 20 to 24 are more than twice as likely to be uninsured as those 45 to 64 years of age. Some put off needed medical and dental care because they can't afford it. (See Reality Check, p. 15.)

- **Mortality.** More than 47,000 young adults, three-quarters of them male, die every year. The most common cause by far is unintentional injury, followed by murder, suicide, cancer, and heart disease.

As you review these findings, what grades would you give America's young adults in each of these categories? How do you compare?

Remember, at any age, health problems are not inevitable. The choices you make as a young adult have an enormous impact on the way you look and feel today and the way you will look and feel in the future.

Staying Healthy on Campus

As one of almost 15 million college students in the United States, you are part of a remarkably diverse group. Today's undergraduates come from every age group and social, racial, ethnic, economic, political, and religious background. You may have served in the military, started a family, or immigrated from another country. You might be enrolled in a two-year college, a four-year university, or a technical school. Your classrooms might be in a busy city or a small town—or exist solely as a virtual campus. Although most undergraduates are "traditional" age—between 18 and 24 years old—more and more of you are over age 25.

The health of college students is as varied as their demographic makeup. In the American College Health Association National College Health Assessment, based on surveys of more than 30,000 students, 58 percent (62 percent of men and 56 percent of women) rated their health as very good or excellent. The most common health problems students experienced in the previous 12 months were allergies (51 percent) and lower back pain (49 percent). The most common impediments to academic performance were stress (33 percent), sleep difficulties (25 percent), and cold/flu/sore throat (25 percent). Almost 90 percent said they had felt exhausted (not from physical activity) within the last 12 months.[13]

The health habits of college students also vary. About one in five reported smoking in the last month; a third had consumed five or more drinks in a single setting within the prior two weeks. About half said they had used a condom (mostly or always) during vaginal intercourse in the last 30 days. More than a quarter reported no vigorous or moderate exercise in the prior week.

Many students simply don't get enough sleep or keep irregular schedules that throw their sleep patterns off. Often it seems that there aren't enough hours in the day for all the things undergraduates need or want to do—study, socialize, pursue extracurricular activities, surf the Internet, care for families and homes, work at part- or full-time jobs, participate in community service. Sleeping less and juggling more, students can quickly end up exhausted—and at greater risk for colds, flus, digestive problems, and other maladies.

Students also become more sedentary in college, as they log more hours in classes and in front of computers. The combination of a high-fat diet and a sedentary lifestyle in college can set the stage for the development of health problems that include obesity, diabetes, metabolic syndrome, heart disease, and certain cancers.

Your personal health depends on many factors, including your age, gender, race,

Invest in Your Future

As the economy has declined, visits to doctors have dropped, and millions of people are not taking prescribed medications. However, trying to save money in the short term by doing without needed health care can cost you a great deal—financially and physically—in the long term. Here are some ways to keep medical costs down without sacrificing your good health:

- **Stay healthy.** Use this book to learn the basics of a healthy lifestyle, then live accordingly. By eating nutritiously, exercising, getting enough sleep, not smoking, and getting regular immunizations you'll reduce your risk of conditions that require expensive treatments.
- **Build a good relationship** with a primary care physician. Although your choices may be limited, try to schedule appointments with the same doctor. A physician who knows you, your history, and your concerns can give the best advice on staying healthy.
- **Don't go to a specialist** without consulting your primary care provider, who can help you avoid overtesting and duplicate treatments.
- **If you need a prescription,** ask if a generic form is available. Brand names cost more, and most insurers charge higher co-payments for them.
- **Take medications as prescribed.** Skipping doses or cutting pills in two may seem an easy way to save money, but you may end up spending more for additional care because the treatment won't be as effective.
- **Don't go to an emergency department** unless absolutely necessary. Call your doctor for advice, or go to the student health service. Emergency departments are overburdened with caring for the very ill and injured, and their services are expensive.

and ethnic background. If you're in your late teens or early twenties, you are in a potentially risky transition. According to a longitudinal study that followed 10,000 young Americans from adolescence into adulthood, health risks increased significantly as they came of age. Young men and women of every race and ethnic group are more likely to eat fast food, not exercise, be obese, and smoke cigarettes. Many do not have health insurance, do not get regular physical or dental examinations, and do not receive health care when they need it. (See Health on a Budget.) Drug abuse and sexually transmitted infections (STIs) are widespread in this age group.

No single race or ethnic group leads or falters in health across all of the health indicators studied. White Americans, who have the best health in adolescence, experience the greatest decline in early adulthood. American Indians face higher health risks both as teens and adults. Individuals in minority groups are most likely to need care but to be unable to pay for it.

Preventing Health Problems

College students often think they are too young to worry about serious health conditions. Yet many chronic problems begin early in life. Two percent of college-age women already have osteoporosis, a bone-weakening disease; another 15 percent have osteopenia, low bone densities that put them at risk of osteoporosis. Many college students have several risk factors for heart disease, including high blood pressure and high cholesterol. Others increase their risk by eating a high-fat diet and not exercising regularly. The time to change is now.

No medical treatment, however successful or sophisticated, can compare with the power of **prevention.** Two out of every three deaths and one in three hospitalizations in the United States could be prevented by changes in six main risk factors: tobacco use, alcohol abuse, accidents, high blood pressure, obesity, and gaps in screening and primary health care. Prevention remains the best weapon against cancer and heart disease.

Prevention can take many forms. Primary, or before-the-fact, prevention efforts might seek to reduce stressors and increase support to prevent problems in healthy people. Consumer education, for instance, provides guidance about how to change our lifestyles to prevent problems and enhance well-being. Other preventive programs identify people at risk and empower them with information and support so they can avoid potential problems. Prevention efforts may target an entire community and try to educate all of its members about the dangers of alcohol abuse or environmental hazards, or they may zero in on a particular group (for instance, seminars on safer sex practices offered to teens) or an individual (such as one-on-one counseling about substance abuse).

Simply by acquiring more years of schooling, you increase your chance of a long and healthful life. Many risk factors for disease—including high blood pressure, elevated cholesterol, and cigarette smoking—decline steadily as education increases, regardless of how much money people make. Education may be good for the body as well as the mind by influencing lifestyle behaviors, problem-solving abilities, and values. People who earn college degrees acquire positive attitudes about the benefits of healthy living, learn how to gain access to preventive health services, join peer groups that promote healthy behavior, and develop higher self-esteem and greater control over their lives.

This course in itself may be good for your health. In studies on the impact of health and wellness courses, students reported that they not only learned about the many dimensions of health but also made changes to improve their health. Many changed their

prevention Information and support offered to help healthy people identify their health risks, reduce stressors, prevent potential medical problems, and enhance their well-being.

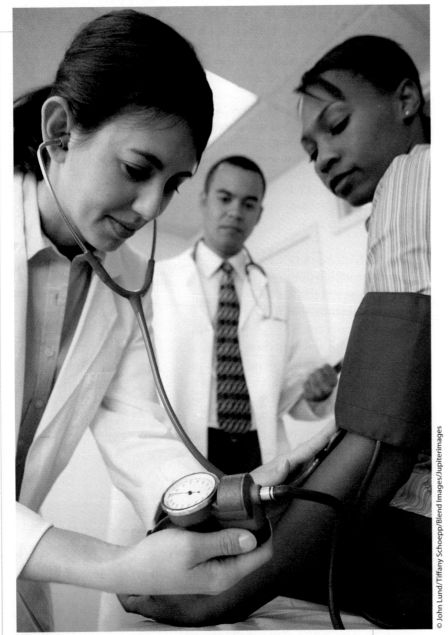

Regular screening of vital signs, such as blood pressure, can lead to early detection of a potentially serious health problem.

© John Lund/Tiffany Schoepp/Blend Images/Jupiterimages

diet and eating habits, began exercising at a campus gym, developed schedules for better time management, engaged in stress-releasing activities, or altered a dangerous habit, such as smoking or drinking.

Protecting Yourself

There is a great deal of overlap between prevention and **protection.** Some people might think of immunizations (discussed in Chapter 15) as a way of preventing illness; others see them as a form of protection against dangerous diseases. In many ways, protection picks up where prevention leaves off. You can prevent STIs or unwanted pregnancy by abstaining from sex. But if you decide to engage in sexual activities, you can protect yourself with condoms and spermicides (discussed in Chapter 15). Similarly, you can prevent many automobile accidents by not driving when road conditions are hazardous. But if you do have to drive, you can protect yourself by wearing a seat belt and using defensive driving techniques (discussed in Chapter 18). For additional suggestions, see Your Strategies for Prevention.

The very concept of protection implies some degree of risk—immediate and direct (for instance, the risk of intentional injury from an assailant or unintentional harm from a fire) or long-term and indirect (such as the risk of heart disease and cancer as a result of smoking). To know how best to protect yourself, you have to be able to realistically assess risks.

Understanding Risky Behaviors

Risky behaviors are not new or unusual on campus, but today's students face different—and potentially deadlier—risks than undergraduates did a generation or two ago. The problem is not that students who engage in risky behavior do not know the danger or feel invulnerable. Young people, according to recent research, actually overestimate the risk of some outcomes. However, they also overestimate the benefit of immediate pleasure when, for instance, engaging in unsafe sex, and underestimate the negative consequences, such as a sexually transmitted infection.[14]

College-age men are more likely than women to engage in risky behaviors—to use drugs and alcohol, to have unprotected sex,

☑ **REALITYCHECK** ··

• *How many young adults did not seek needed medical care, prescription medicines, mental health care, or eyeglasses because they could not afford it? _____%*
• *How many did not seek needed dental care because they couldn't afford it? _____%*

Answers on next page.

and to drive dangerously. Men also are more likely to be hospitalized for injuries and to commit suicide. Three-fourths of the deaths in the 15- to 24-year age range are men.

Drinking has long been part of college life and, despite the efforts across U.S. college campuses to curb alcohol abuse, two out of five students engage in binge drinking—consumption of five or more drinks at a single session for men, four for women. Heavy drinking increases the likelihood of other risky behaviors, such as smoking cigarettes, using drugs, or having multiple sexual partners. (See "Don't Go There" in *Labs for IPC.*)

Some behaviors are riskier than students realize. "Body art"—piercings and tattoos—may seem harmless, but health officials warn of hidden risks, including hepatitis B and C infection and transmission of HIV (see Chapter 15).

Student Health Norms

Psychologists use the term *norm, or* **social norm**, to refer to a behavior or attitude that a particular group expects, values, and enforces. Norms influence a wide variety of human activities, including health habits. However, perceptions of social norms are often inaccurate. Only anonymous responses to a scientifically designed questionnaire can reveal what individuals really do—the actual social norms—as compared to what they may say they do to gain social approval.

Undergraduates are particularly likely to misjudge what their peers are—and aren't—doing. In recent years colleges have found that publicizing research data on behaviors such as drinking, smoking, and drug use helps students get a more accurate sense of the real health norms on campus.[15]

The gap between students' misperceptions and accurate health norms can be

---

YOUR STRATEGIES FOR PREVENTION
Smart Steps to Take Now

• To lower your risk of heart disease, get your blood pressure and cholesterol checked. Don't smoke. Stay at a healthy weight. Exercise regularly.

• To lower your risks of major diseases, get regular checkups. Make sure you are immunized against infectious illnesses.

• To lower your risks of substance abuse and related illnesses and injuries, don't drink, or limit how much you drink. Avoid illegal drugs.

• To lower your risk of sexually transmitted infections (STIs) or unwanted pregnancy, abstain from sex. If you engage in sexual activities, protect yourself with contraceptives, condoms, and spermicides.

• To prevent car accidents, stay off the road in hazardous circumstances, such as bad weather. Wear a seat belt when you drive, and use defensive driving techniques.

protection Measures that an individual can take when participating in risky behavior to prevent injury or unwanted risks.

social norm A behavior or attitude that a particular group expects, values, and enforces.

enormous. For example, undergraduates in the ACHA-NCHA survey estimated that 42 percent of students had smoked cigarettes daily in the previous month. In fact, only 6 percent had. Similarly, students guessed that 41 percent of their peers drank alcohol every day. In reality, only .07 percent did.[16] Providing accurate information on drinking norms on campus has proven effective in changing students' perceptions and in reducing alcohol consumption by both men and women.

A feature in every chapter of this book, Reality Check, tests the accuracy of your perceptions of health norms by asking what you think is normal for college students and then providing findings from recent research. You saw the first one on page 15.

The Healthy Campus Project

The American College Health Association has adapted the federal *Healthy People* project goals for college and universities. Its *Healthy Campus* initiative has identified focus areas and objectives particularly relevant for students. Schools that participate in the program can compare data on their students to national norms and identify the key targets that would most improve health on their campuses.

Find out if your college has a similar set of priorities. What do you think they should include? What are your personal priorities for your health during your college career? (See Point/Counterpoint, p. 17.)

© iStockphoto.com/saluha

Although popular, tattoos and piercing can pose serious health risks, including infection and hepatitis.

Making Quality Health-Care Decisions

Although you may not realize it, you make crucial decisions that affect your health every day. You choose what you eat, whether you exercise, if you smoke or drink, when to fasten your seat belt. You determine when to see a doctor, what kind of doctor, and with what sense of urgency. You decide what to tell the physician and whether to follow his or her advice, take a prescribed medication as directed, or seek further help or a second opinion. The entire process of maintaining or restoring health depends on your decisions. It cannot start or continue without them. The following sections can help you make better choices about your health and health care.

POINT

Many colleges are taking steps to promote student health. These range from requiring vaccination against meningitis, to banning alcohol at athletic and social events, to eliminating vending machines for soft drinks, to constructing more trails for hiking and biking.

COUNTERPOINT

Health is a personal responsibility, and students should be treated as adults with the right to make their own choices. Rather than acting as health "police," colleges should focus on their educational mission.

YOUR VIEW

Do you think that communities, including campuses, bear some responsibility for the health of their members? Find out what your school is doing to encourage healthy choices and behaviors. Would you like to see more programs and policies to safeguard your well-being?

Improving Your Health Literacy

According to federal estimates, about one-third of the population in the United States has limited ability to understand health information and to use that information to make good decisions about health and medical care. Because of poor **health literacy,** more than 90 million Americans may not understand how to take medication, monitor cholesterol levels or blood sugar, manage a chronic disease, find health providers and services, or fill out necessary forms. According to research studies, people with limited health literacy are more likely to report poor health, to skip important preventive measures such as regular Pap smears, to have chronic conditions such as diabetes or asthma, and to have higher rates of preventable hospitalizations.[17]

Even people with advanced literacy skills may have difficulty understanding the specialized language that doctors use and the complexity of many treatments—particularly when in stressful or unfamiliar situations. Health professionals also may not communicate clearly or provide adequate information. In one study, a quarter of doctors did not state the name of the medication they were prescribing, almost half did not specify the number of pills to take, and two-thirds did not discuss adverse side effects or explain how long to take the drug.

Regardless of their literacy skills, college students often do not seek out information on health concerns. In one study that tracked college students' communications for a two-week period, they sought health-related advice and information in a little more than one-fourth of their communications about health. When they did seek help, they were most likely to turn to family and friends.[18] About half of students also turn to health educators for information, and most rank them and health center medical staff as believable. Although students regularly get information from flyers, pamphlets, magazines, and television, they are less likely to consider these as authoritative, believable sources.

Finding Good Advice Online

Three in four Internet users are "e-health" consumers who seek information or support, communicate with health-care providers, or buy medical products online. "They use the Internet as an adjunct to physicians, who remain their primary source of health advice," says Mark Bard, president of Manhattan Research, a health-care marketing firm. About three in four college students have used the Internet to get health information, but many are skeptical of what they find.

If you go to websites for medical information, here are some guidelines for evaluating them:

- **Check the creator.** Websites are produced by health agencies, health support groups, school health programs, health-product advertisers, health educators, and health-education organizations. Read site headers and footers carefully to distinguish biased commercial advertisements from unbiased sites created by scientists and health agencies.

YOUR STRATEGIES FOR PREVENTION

How to Boost Health Understanding

- Always ask these three questions of your doctor, nurse, or pharmacist:
  - What is my main problem?
  - What do I need to do?
  - Why is it important for me to do this?
- If you don't understand, say, "This is new to me. Can you explain it one more time?"
- If you don't know the meaning of a medical term, don't hesitate to ask what it means. Health professionals sometimes forget they're using technical terms, such as "myocardial infarction" for heart attack.
- Write down a list of your health concerns, and bring it with you whenever you seek health care.

See "Health Assurance" in *Labs for IPC* for more advice on taking charge of your health care.

health literacy Ability to understand health information and use it to make good decisions about health and medical care.

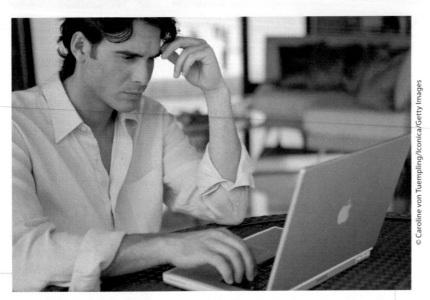
Millions of Americans go online to learn about medical problems and treatments and to chat with others who have similar conditions.

- **If you are looking for the most recent research,** check the date the page was created and last updated as well as the links. Several nonworking links signal that the site isn't carefully maintained or updated.
- **Check the references.** As with other health-education materials, web documents should provide the reader with references. Unreferenced suggestions may be scientifically unsound and possibly unsafe.
- **Consider the author.** Is he or she recognized in the field of health education or otherwise qualified to publish a health-information web document? Does the author list his or her occupation, experience, and education?
- **Look for possible bias.** Websites may be attempting to provide health information to consumers, but they also may be attempting to sell a product. Many sites are merely disguised advertisements. (See Table 1.1 for some doctor-endorsed websites.)

Getting Medical Facts Straight

Cure! Breakthrough! Medical miracle! These words make headlines. Remember that although medical breakthroughs and cures

do occur, most scientific progress is made one small step at a time. Rather than putting your faith in the most recent report or the hottest trend, try to gather as much background information and as many opinions as you can. (See Consumer Alert, p. 21.)

When reading a newspaper or magazine story or listening to a radio or television report about a medical advance, look for answers to the following questions:

- **Who are the scientists involved?** Are they recognized, legitimate health professionals? What are their credentials? Are they affiliated with respected medical or scientific institutions? Be wary of individuals whose degrees or affiliations are from institutions you've never heard of, and be sure that the person's educational background is in a discipline related to the area of research reported.
- **Where did the scientists report their findings?** The best research is published in peer-reviewed professional journals, such as the *New England Journal of Medicine*. Research developments also may be reported at meetings of professional societies.
- **Is the information based on personal observations?** Does the report include testimonials from cured patients or satisfied customers? If the answer to either question is yes, be wary.
- **Does the article, report, or advertisement include words like** *amazing, secret,* **or** *quick*? Does it claim to be something the public has never seen or been offered before? Such sensationalized language is often a tip-off to a dubious treatment.
- **Is someone trying to sell you something?** Manufacturers who cite studies to sell a product have been known to embellish the truth.
- **Does the information defy all common sense?** Be skeptical. If something sounds too good to be true, it probably is.

Making Sense of Medical Research

Medical research is the only way that anyone, physician or consumer, can assess the quality of diagnostic methods, medications, or

TABLE 1.1

Doctor Recommended Websites

National Library of Medicine: MedlinePlus　　　　　　　　　　　　　　http://medlineplus.gov

MedlinePlus contains links to information on hundreds of health conditions and issues. The site also includes a medical dictionary, an encyclopedia with pictures and diagrams, and links to physician directories.

FDA Center for Drug Evaluation and Research　　　　　　　　　　　　　www.fda.gov

Click on Drugs@FDA for information on approved prescription drugs and some over-the-counter medications.

WebMD　　　　　　　　　　　　　　　　　　　　　　　　　　　　　　www.webmd.com

WebMD is full of information to help you manage your health. The site's quizzes and calculators are a fun way to test your medical knowledge. Get diet tips, information on drugs and herbs, and check out special sections on men's and women's health.

Mayo Clinic　　　　　　　　　　　　　　　　　　　　　　　　　　　http://mayoclinic.com

The renowned Mayo Clinic offers a one-stop health resource website. Use the site's Health Decision Guides to make decisions about prevention and treatment. Learn more about complementary and alternative medicine, sports medicine, and senior health in the Healthy Living Centers.

Centers for Disease Control　　　　　　　　　　　　　　　　　　　　www.cdc.gov

Stay up to date on the latest public health news and get the CDC's recommendations on travelers' health, vaccines and immunizations, and protecting your health in case of a disaster.

Medscape　　　　　　　　　　　　　　　　　　　　　　　　　　　　www.medscape.com

Medscape delivers news and research specifically tailored to your medical interests. The site requires (free) registration.

---

surgical treatments. The principal rule of science is that nothing works until it's been proved.

Researchers rely on a variety of studies to determine whether a new approach to prevention, diagnosis, or treatment works. These include:

- **Epidemiological studies**, in which scientists assess the health status of a large, defined group of people, such as the population of a country or region. They may look at various health habits, such as alcohol consumption, to determine whether those who practice these habits have a higher likelihood of developing certain diseases.

- **Animal studies, or preclinical trials,** in which scientists administer a drug or try a procedure on various laboratory animals to assess its safety and determine its effects.

- **Clinical trials,** in which volunteers agree to act as test subjects—"human guinea pigs," as it were. Patients must give written permission in order to participate. Clinical trials generate data for the purpose of evaluating one or more diagnostic or therapeutic approaches in a population. Well-designed clinical trials, which must have strict eligibility criteria, a standardized intervention, follow-up, and measures of outcome, set the "gold standard" for new diagnostic tests or medical or surgical treatments.

In *controlled studies,* the group receiving an experimental drug or treatment is compared with a group receiving no treatment or standard therapy. In *single-blind studies,* the subjects don't know whether they're receiving the experimental drug or treatment, or an inactive substance. In *double-blind studies,* neither the subjects nor the researchers have this information. In *prospective studies,* patients are selected, assessed, participate in the trial, and are then followed for a preset period. In *retrospective studies,* investigators look back at their past experiences with a certain group of patients.

The results of even the most careful studies aren't considered conclusive in and of themselves. The FDA reviews every new drug, as well as the research methods used to test it, before it's allowed on the market. And a new therapy is widely accepted (or rejected) only after publication of study results in a *peer-reviewed* journal (one in which scientists in the same field critique the research methods before accepting the paper) and after *replication* (the repetition of the same investigation by other researchers with similar results). In recent years,

meta-analysis Summarization and review of research in a particular area to evaluate the results of several large clinical trials in a uniform manner.

evidence, or scientific proof, that a particular treatment is effective. **Evidence-based medicine,** which emerged in the 1990s, is a way of improving and evaluating patient care by combining the best research evidence with the patient's personal values.[19]

Reviewing all available medical studies pertaining to an individual patient or group of patients helps doctors to diagnose illnesses more precisely, to choose the best tests, and to select the best treatments or methods of disease prevention. By using evidence-based medical techniques for large groups of patients with the same illness, doctors can develop **practice guidelines** for evaluating and treating particular illnesses. Practice guidelines help improve treatment and provide a way for doctors and hospitals to evaluate their performance. Evidence-based practice guidelines have proven beneficial in reducing mortality (chance of dying) from heart attacks and improved care for diabetes and other common conditions.

Look online for evidence-based medical guidelines for any health problems that you or your family develops. The best places to start are: National Institutes of Health, www.nih.gov; The Cochrane Collection, www.cochrane.org; and Centre for Evidence-Based Medicine, www.cebm.net. Talk with your doctor about the best evaluation and treatment plans based on available medical evidence. Understanding why your doctor recommends a certain test or treatment can help you make better health-care and lifestyle choices.

a technique called **meta-analysis,** which summarizes and reviews research in a particular area, has been used to evaluate the results of several large trials in a uniform manner.

One reason why study results must be confirmed is that, no matter what treatment patients receive, one-third to one-half of all patients improve temporarily. This well-documented but little-understood phenomenon is called the *placebo effect.* Scientific trials of a new treatment must show that the patients receiving the experimental medication or therapy improve *more* than those receiving a sugar pill or mock procedure (the placebo).

Evidence-Based Medicine

Large randomized controlled trials and large prospective studies provide the best

Making Healthy Changes

In terms of human health, the 1800s were the century of hygiene, with life-saving advances in sanitation and clean drinking water. The 1900s were the century of medicine, with breakthroughs in diagnosing and treating major illnesses. The 2000s, medical experts predict, will be the century of

behavioral change, when individuals take charge of their health by breaking unhealthy habits and creating new healthier ones.

The stakes for modifying student behavior are high. Four in ten students are binge drinkers; one in four smokes. Among those who are sexually

Too Good to Be True?

Almost every week you're likely to see a commercial or an ad for a new health product that promises better sleep, more energy, clearer skin, firmer muscles, lower weight, brighter moods, longer life—or all of these combined. As the Consumer Alerts throughout this book point out, you can't believe every promise you read or hear. Keep these general guidelines in mind the next time you come across a health claim.

Facts to Know

- **Do your own research.** Check with your doctor or with the student health center. Go to the library or do some online research to gather as much information as you can.

- **Check credentials.** Anyone can claim to be a scientist or a health expert. Find out if advocates of any type of therapy have legitimate degrees from recognized institutions and are fully licensed in their fields.

Steps to Take

- **Look for objective evaluations.** If you're watching an infomercial for a treatment or technique, you can be sure that the enthusiastic endorsements have been skillfully scripted and rehearsed. Even ads that claim to be presenting the science behind a new breakthrough are really sales pitches in disguise.

- **Consider the sources.** Research findings from carefully controlled scientific studies are reviewed by leading experts in the field and published in scholarly journals. Just because someone has conducted a study doesn't mean it was a valid scientific investigation.

- **If it sounds too good to be true,** it probably is. If a magic pill could really trim off excess pounds or banish wrinkles, the world would be filled with thin people with unlined skin. Look around and you'll realize that's not the case.

---

active, almost three in four say they've engaged in unprotected sex. Only about a third of undergraduates exercise regularly. Their nutrition is notoriously poor. Weights—and weight problems—are rising on campus. By graduation, one in four students has at least one major risk factor for diabetes, metabolic syndrome, or heart disease. Yet even students who recognize the risks and want to change their behavior often have no idea how to begin.

If you would like to improve your health behavior, you have to realize that change isn't easy. Between 40 and 80 percent of those who try to kick bad health habits lapse back into their unhealthy ways within six weeks.

Yet even simple behavioral changes could have a significant impact. A study that tracked about 20,000 adults in the United Kingdom found that those who adopted just four healthy habits lived an average of 14 years longer than the others. These life-extending behaviors are:

- Not smoking.
- Eating lots of fruits and vegetables.
- Exercising regularly.
- Drinking alcohol in moderation.[20]

Participants got a point for each of these healthy habits, and those who scored four points were four times less likely to die than those who scored zero.

Fortunately, our understanding of change has itself changed. Thanks to decades of research, we now know what sets the stage for change, the way change progresses, and the keys to lasting change. We also know that personal change is neither mysterious nor magical but a methodical science that anyone can master. (See "Part I: The New Science of Personal Change" in *IPC* for a comprehensive review.)[21]

Understanding Health Behavior

Three types of influences shape behavior: predisposing, enabling, and reinforcing factors (Figure 1.5).

Predisposing Factors **Predisposing factors** include knowledge, attitudes, beliefs, values, and perceptions. Unfortunately, knowledge isn't enough to cause most people to change their behavior; for example, people fully aware of the grim consequences of smoking often continue to puff away. Nor is attitude—one's likes and dislikes—sufficient; an individual may dislike the smell and taste of cigarettes but continue to smoke regardless.

Beliefs are more powerful than knowledge and attitudes, and researchers report that people are most likely to change health behavior if they hold three beliefs:

evidence-based medicine The choice of a medical treatment on the basis of large randomized controlled research trials and large prospective studies.

practice guidelines Recommendations for diagnosis and treatment of various health problems based on evidence from scientific research.

predisposing factors The beliefs, values, attitudes, knowledge, and perceptions that influence our behavior.

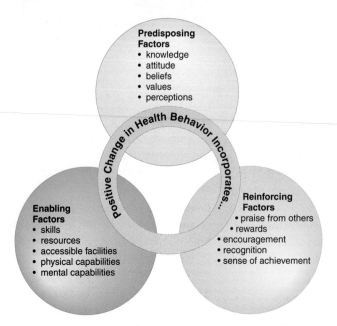

Predisposing Factors
- knowledge
- attitude
- beliefs
- values
- perceptions

Positive Change in Health Behavior Incorporates...

Enabling Factors
- skills
- resources
- accessible facilities
- physical capabilities
- mental capabilities

Reinforcing Factors
- praise from others
- rewards
- encouragement
- recognition
- sense of achievement

Figure 1.5 Factors That Shape Positive Behavior

- **Susceptibility.** They acknowledge that they are at risk for the negative consequences of their behavior.
- **Severity.** They believe that they may pay a very high price if they don't make a change.
- **Benefits.** They believe that the proposed change will be advantageous to their health.

There can be a gap between stated and actual beliefs, however. Young adults may say they recognize the very real dangers of casual, careless sex in this day and age. Yet, rather than act in accordance with these statements, they may impulsively engage in unprotected sex with individuals whose health status and histories they do not know. The reason: Like young people everywhere and in every time, they feel invulnerable, that nothing bad can or will happen to them, that if there were a real danger, they would somehow know it. Often it's not until something happens—a former lover may admit to having a sexually transmitted infection—that their behaviors become consistent with their stated beliefs.

Enabling Factors Enabling factors include skills, resources, accessible facilities, and physical and mental capacities. Before you initiate a change, assess the means available

to reach your goal. No matter how motivated you are, you'll become frustrated if you keep encountering obstacles. That's why breaking a task or goal down into step-by-step strategies is so important in behavioral change.

Reinforcing Factor Reinforcing factors may be praise from family and friends, rewards from teachers or parents, or encouragement and recognition for meeting a goal. Although these help a great deal in the short run, lasting change depends not on external rewards but on an internal commitment and sense of achievement. To make a difference, reinforcement must come from within.

A decision to change a health behavior should stem from a permanent, personal goal, not from a desire to please or impress someone else. If you lose weight for the homecoming dance, you're almost sure to regain pounds afterward. But if you shed extra pounds because you want to feel better about yourself or get into shape, you're far more likely to keep off the weight.

How and Why People Change

Change can simply happen. You get older. You put on or lose weight. You have an accident. Intentional change is different: A person consciously, deliberately sets out either to change a negative behavior, such as chronic procrastination, or to initiate a healthy behavior, such as daily exercise. For decades psychologists have studied how people intentionally change and have developed various models that reveal the anatomy of change.

In the *moral model*, you take responsibility for a problem (such as smoking) and its solution; success depends on adequate motivation, while failure is seen as a sign of character weakness. In the *enlightenment model*, you submit to strict discipline to correct a problem; this is the approach used in Alcoholics Anonymous. The *behavioral model* involves rewarding yourself when you make positive changes. The *medical model* sees the behavior as caused by forces beyond your control (a genetic predisposition to being overweight, for example) and employs an expert to provide advice or treatment. For many people, the most effective approach is the *compensatory model*, which doesn't assign blame but puts responsibility on individuals to acquire whatever skills or power they need to overcome their problems.

The Health Belief Model Psychologists developed the **health belief model (HBM)** about 50 years ago to explain and predict health behaviors by focusing on the attitudes and beliefs of individuals. (Remember that your attitudes and beliefs are predisposing influences on your capacity for change.) According to this model, people will take a health-related action (e.g., use condoms) if they:

- **Feel that they can avoid a negative consequence,** such as a sexually transmitted infection (STI).
- **Expect a positive outcome** if they take the recommended advice, for instance, that condoms will protect them from STIs.
- **Believe that they can successfully take action,** for example, use condoms comfortably and confidently.

Readiness to act on health beliefs, in this model, depends on how vulnerable individuals feel, how severe they perceive the danger to be, the benefits they expect to gain, and the barriers they think they will encounter. Another key factor is self-efficacy, their confidence in their ability to take action.

Over the years the health belief model has been used to help people change unhealthy behaviors, such as smoking, overeating, and inactivity, or to encourage them to take positive health actions, such as using condoms and getting needed vaccinations and medical checkups.

Self-Determination Theory This approach, developed several decades ago by psychologists Edward Deci and Richard Ryan, focuses on whether an individual lacks motivation, is externally motivated, or is intrinsically motivated. Someone who is "amotivated" does not value an activity, such as exercise, or does not believe it will lead to a desired outcome, such as more energy or lower weight. Individuals who are externally motivated may engage in an activity like exercise to gain a reward or avoid a negative consequence (such as a loved one's nagging). Some people are motivated by a desired

Your *stated* knowledge-based belief may be that unsafe driving can cause accidents. Your *actual* belief is that it won't happen to you.

outcome; for instance, they might exercise for the sake of better health or longer life. Behavior becomes self-determined when someone engages in it for its own sake, such as exercising because it's fun.

Numerous studies have evaluated self-determination as it relates to health behavior. In research on exercise, individuals with greater self-determined motivation are less likely to stop exercising and have stronger intentions to continue exercise, higher physical self-worth, and lower social anxiety related to their physique.

Motivational Interviewing Health professionals, counselors, and coaches use motivational interviewing, developed by psychologists William Miller and Stephen Rollnick, to inspire individuals, regardless of their enthusiasm for change, to move toward improvements that could make their lives better. Building a collaborative partnership, the therapist does not persuade directly but uses empathy and respect for the patient's perspective to evoke recognition of the desirability of change.[22]

The Transtheoretical Model
Psychologist James Prochaska and his colleagues, by tracking what they considered to

enabling factors The skills, resources, and physical and mental capabilities that shape our behavior.

reinforcing factors Rewards, encouragement, and recognition that influence our behavior in the short run.

health belief model (HBM) A model of behavioral change that focuses on the individual's attitudes and beliefs.

be universal stages in the successful recovery of drug addicts and alcoholics, developed a way of thinking about change that cuts across psychological theories. Their **transtheoretical model** focuses on universal aspects of an individual's decision-making process rather than on social or biological influences on behavior.[23]

The transtheoretical model has become the foundation of programs for smoking cessation, exercise, healthy food choices, alcohol cessation, weight control, condom use, drug use cessation, mammography screening, and stress management. However, conclusive scientific evidence for its usefulness in lifestyle change remains limited.

The following sections describe these key components of the transtheoretical model:

- **Stages of change.**

- **Processes of change**—cognitive and behavioral activities that facilitate change.

- **Self-efficacy**—the confidence people have in their ability to cope with challenge.

The Stages of Change   According to the transtheoretical model of change, individuals progress through a sequence of stages as they make a change (Figure 1.6). No one stage is more important than another, and people often move back and forth between them. Most "spiral" from stage to stage, slipping from maintenance to contemplation or from action to precontemplation before moving forward again.

People usually cycle and recycle through the stages several times. Smokers, for instance, report making three or four serious efforts to quit before they succeed.

The six stages of change are:

1. **Precontemplation.** You are at this stage if you, as yet, have no intention of making a change. You are vaguely uncomfortable, but this is where your grasp of what is going on ends. If you feel healthy and are busy with your classes and activities, for instance, you may never think about exercise. Then you notice that it's harder to zip your jeans or that you get winded walking up stairs. Still you don't quite register the need to do anything about it.

   During precontemplation, change remains hypothetical, distant, and vague. Yet you may speak of something bugging you and wish that things were somehow different.

2. **Contemplation.** In this stage you begin to get it. You acknowledge that something is amiss and begin to consider what it is and whether you can do anything about it. You still prefer not to

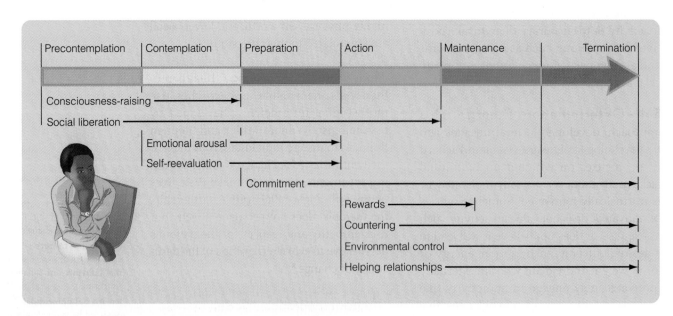

Figure 1.6 The Stages of Change and Some Change Processes
These change processes can help you progress through the stages of change. Each may be most useful at particular stages.

have to change, but you start to realize that you can't avoid reality. Maybe none of your jeans fit anymore, or you feel sluggish and listless. As you begin to weigh the trade-offs of standing pat versus acting, you may alternate between wanting to take action and resisting it.

The way you talk to yourself expresses your feeling that change is necessary but demonstrates your lack of commitment to taking action. Here are some examples of how the contemplation stage sounds:

- "I hate it that I keep . . . "
- "I should . . . "
- "Maybe I'll do it someday—not tomorrow, but someday."

3. **Peparation.** At some point you stop waffling, make a clear decision, and feel a burst of energy. This decision heralds the preparation stage. You gather information, make phone calls, do research online, and look into exercise classes at the gym. You begin to think and act with change specifically in mind even if you hold something back.

If you eavesdrop on what you're saying to yourself, you would hear statements such as, "I am going to do this," and you set a date, such as, "I will begin on New Year's Day." Yet you may not share your plans with others, despite all the internal progress you've made.

4. **Action.** This is the stage of actively modifying your behavior according to your plan. Your resolve is strong, and you know you're on your way to a better you. You no longer keep your plan under wraps—not that you could. Change produces signs that are visible to others. You may be getting up to 15 minutes earlier to make time for a healthy breakfast or to walk to class rather than taking the shuttle. In a relatively short time you acquire a sense of comfort and ease with the change in your life.

5. **Maintenance.** Maintenance is about locking in and consolidating gains. This stabilizing stage, which follows the flurry of specific steps taken in the action stage, is absolutely necessary to retain what you've worked for and to make change permanent. In this stage, you strengthen, enhance, and extend the changes you've initiated. You bring the rest of what you do into line with the change to support it. By securing the progress you've made, even if you hit a plateau or slip backward, you can regain your footing and keep moving forward.

6. **Termination.** At this stage, your "change" has become status quo. While it may take two to five years, the behavior has become so deeply ingrained that you can't imagine abandoning it. More than eight in ten college seniors who exercised regularly remain as active, or even more active, after graduation.

As research on college students has shown, attitudes and feelings are related to stages of change. Smokers who believe that continuing to smoke would have only a minor or no impact on their health remain in the precontemplation stage; those with respiratory symptoms move on to contemplation and preparation. In a study at Ohio State University, researchers classified student heavy drinkers according to the stages of change: Nearly two-thirds of the "precontemplators" continued to drink heavily and had no intention of changing their behavior. In the maintenance stage, students drank an average of one alcoholic drink a month even though they felt that heavy drinking was the norm on their campus.

The Processes of Change Anything you do to modify your thinking, feeling, or behavior can be called a change process. The nine included in the transtheoretical model are shown in Figure 1.6 in their corresponding stages.

- **Consciousness-raising.** The most widely used change process involves increasing knowledge about yourself or the nature of your problem. As you learn more, you gain understanding and feedback about your behavior.

  Example: Reading Chapter 6 on making healthy food choices.

- **Social liberation.** This process takes advantage of alternatives in the external environment that can help you begin or continue your efforts to change.

  Example: Spending as much time as possible in nonsmoking areas.

transtheoretical model A model of behavioral change that focuses on the individual's decision making; it states that an individual progresses through a sequence of six stages as he or she makes a change in behavior.

Do you picture yourself as master of your own destiny? You are more likely to achieve your health goals if you do.

- **Emotional arousal.** This process, also known as dramatic relief, works on a deeper level than consciousness-raising and is equally important in the early stages of change. Emotional arousal means experiencing and expressing feelings about a problem behavior and its potential solutions.

    Example: Resolving never to drink and drive after the death of a friend in a car accident.

- **Self-reevaluation.** This process requires a thoughtful reappraisal of your problem, including an assessment of the person you might be once you have changed the behavior.

    Example: Recognizing that you have a gambling problem and imagining yourself as a nongambler.

- **Commitment.** This process acknowledges—first privately and then publicly—that you are responsible for your behavior and the only one who can change it.

    Example: Joining a self-help or support group.

- **Rewards.** This process reinforces positive behavioral changes with self-praise or small gifts.

    Example: Getting a massage after a month of consistent exercise.

- **Countering.** Countering, or counterconditioning, substitutes healthy behaviors for unhealthy ones.

    Example: Chewing gum rather than smoking.

- **Environmental control.** This action-oriented process restructures your environment so you are less likely to engage in a problem behavior.

    Example: Getting rid of your stash of sweets.

- **Helping relationships.** This process recruits individuals—family, friends, therapist, coach—to provide support, caring, understanding, and acceptance.

    Example: Finding an exercise buddy.

Researchers are zeroing in on the optimal stages to address certain behaviors. A study of college students, for instance, indicated that precontemplation might be the best time to address alcohol consumption, healthy eating, and managing depression (by means of Prochaska's recommended processes of consciousness-raising, dramatic relief, and environmental reevaluation). The contemplation stage might be a better time to address smoking by helping students minimize what they see as the drawbacks of quitting (such as awkwardness around friends who smoke).[24]

Self-Efficacy and Locus of Control Do you see yourself as master of your fate, asserting control over your destiny? Or do so many things happen in your life that you just hang on and hope for the best? The answers to these questions reveal two important characteristics that affect your health: your sense of **self-efficacy** (the belief in your ability to change and to reach a goal) and your **locus of control** (the sense of being in control of your life). See Chapter 2 in *IPC* for a detailed discussion and assessment of your locus of control.

Your confidence in your ability to cope with challenge can determine whether you can and will succeed in making a change. In his research on self-efficacy, psychologist Albert Bandura of Stanford University found that the individuals most likely to reach a goal are those who believe that they can. The stronger their faith in themselves, the more energy and persistence they put into making a change. The opposite is also true, especially for health behaviors. Among people who begin an exercise program, those with lower self-efficacy are more likely to drop out.

If you believe that your actions will make a difference in your health, your locus of control is internal. If you believe that external forces or factors play a greater role, your locus of control is external. Hundreds of studies have compared people who have these different perceptions of control. "Internals," who believe that their actions largely determine what happens to them, act more independently, enjoy better health, and are more optimistic about their future. "Externals," who perceive that chance or outside forces determine their fate, find it harder to cope with stress, and feel increasingly helpless over time. When it comes to weight, for instance, they see themselves as destined to be fat.

self-efficacy Belief in one's ability to accomplish a goal or change a behavior.

locus of control An individual's belief about the sources of power and influence over his or her life.

Choosing Change

An Invitation to Personal Change (IPC), the supplement to this text, provides a minicourse in how to make a change, based on the stages of change we have just discussed. The *Labs for An Invitation to Personal Change* offer an opportunity to practice what you've learned. Each lab contains step-by-step instructions that are precise blueprints for change. All follow a similar pattern, with sections called **Get Real, Get Ready, Get Going,** and **Lock It In.** You can use this four-part pattern as a template to create your own personal change maps for *any* personal change you want to make—now or in the future.

In "Get Real," you take a realistic audit of where you are so you can determine where to go. The "Get Ready" section provides instructions and exercises designed to prepare you for making the actual behavioral change, such as identifying and gathering support and resources. "Get Going" involves initiating and beginning to practice new, more effective thoughts and behaviors that will replace old, ineffective, self-defeating ones. "Lock It In" ensures enduring change by showing you how to deal with setbacks and how to integrate the change permanently into your life.

We recommend that all students complete the one-week introductory lab "Choosing to Change, Choosing a Change" to identify the behavioral changes that are most relevant and compelling for them as they begin the class. Here is a preview.

Choosing a Change

Having choice means having freedom. Having to choose, on the other hand, brings a burden: You become responsible for the choices you make.

If you clutch at the prospect of taking responsibility, remember this: Not choosing is also a choice—in our opinion, not a very good one because it represents another attempt to escape the burden freedom bestows. When you do not choose for yourself or even appear not to be taking control of your life, you create a vacuum that someone else will try to fill.

Own your choices and embrace responsibility for them. Choose to change, and choose your changes as responsibly and brilliantly as possible. Your life is your own, and you can choose how to use it. Your current habits may seem like a safe place to hide out—a fortress. But if you stay locked inside, what really is the difference between a fortress and a prison?

You will make many more choices over the course of your life. Making mistakes goes with the territory of learning any new skill. And knowing how to choose is a skill. As with anything, practice makes perfect. The more choices you make for yourself, the stronger your sense of control over your life will become.

Perhaps you feel you have never made many, or any, significant choices. Maybe others have advised you or even made decisions for you. Or perhaps you feel hesitant to choose because you have made some bad choices in the past. Either way, help is here. The other *IPC* change labs provide blueprints for developing new skills. The "Choosing a Change" lab provides a series of exercises to help you choose the best change to go for first. This too is a skill.

Get Real

In order to choose a change, start by appraising where you are now in relation to making a choice. Here are four of the six steps in the lab that will help you get real about where you are in the process.

- **How close are you to making a choice?**

    In your *IPC Journal,* write a number between 0 to 100 to describe how ready or close you are to making a choice, with 0 representing that you are not ready at all and 100 representing that you are completely ready to choose.

- **What is your usual approach to choosing?**

    Observe how you make choices now and survey how you have made choices in the past. Respond to each of the following questions. Be honest. You have no one to fool. Do not show your answers to anyone else.
    - Do you usually avoid choosing?
    - Would you ordinarily look for what would appear to be the easiest lab to knock out without any effort?
    - Are you afraid to choose because you feel you could choose incorrectly?
    - Do you wonder what you "should" choose in the sense of how others will think?

- **Evaluate past decisions.**

    For five important decisions you have made in your life to date, write down:
    - how the decision turned out.
    - whether you consulted anyone for advice and, if so, whom.
    - your appraisal of the benefits of the decision.
    - your appraisal of any drawbacks of the decision.

Get Ready

Some changes and some skills create a basis for many others. For example, mastery of swimming is a good basis for playing water polo. For that reason, it may make sense to make changes in one particular area before making others.

- **Assess your greatest change needs.**

    Most people know some areas they need to change. For you it could be order, diet, exercise, or finding balance in your life. List the changes you would like to make if only you knew how in your *IPC Journal.* Then rate which one is the most pressing, most important need to deal with first.

Get Going

This task is straightforward: Get started working on your goal.

Lock It In

- **Check out the available labs.**

    Stay with the lab you chose. You may hit flat spots of disinterest. Even if you become discouraged, however, we *strongly* urge you to keep going. Do not entertain for a second the notion that you chose poorly or that you should start over on another lab.

Ultimately you have more control over your health than any-one else. Use this course as an opportunity to zero in on at least one less-than-healthful behavior and improve it. Here are some suggestions for small steps that can have a big payoff:

- **Use seat belts.** In the last decade, seat belts have saved more than 40,000 lives and prevented millions of injuries.

- **Eat an extra fruit or vegetable every day.** Adding more fruit and vegetables to your diet can improve your diges-tion and lower your risk of several cancers.

- **Get enough sleep.** A good night's rest provides the en-ergy you need to make it through the following day.

- **Take regular stress breaks.** A few quiet minutes spent stretching, looking out the window, or simply letting yourself unwind are good for body and soul.

- **Lose a pound.** If you're overweight, you may not think a pound will make a difference, but it's a step in the right direction.

- **If you're a woman, examine your breasts regularly.** Get in the habit of performing a breast self-examination ev-ery month after your period (when breasts are least swol-len or tender).

- **If you're a man, examine your testicles regularly.** These simple self-exams can spot the signs of cancer early, when it is most likely to be cured.

- **Get physical.** Just a little exercise will do some good. A regular workout schedule will be good for your heart, lungs, muscles, bones—even your mood.

- **Drink more water.** Eight glasses a day are what you need to replenish lost fluids, prevent constipation, and keep your digestive system working efficiently.

- **Do a good deed.** Caring for others is a wonderful way to care for your own soul and connect with others.

Ask yourself these questions:

- What healthy change can I make in my life today?

- This week?

- This month?

- This term?

SELF SURVEY   Wellness Inventory

What Is Wellness?* by John W. Travis, M.D.

CENGAGENOW™ Go to HealthNow for more activities.

Most of us think in terms of illness and assume that the absence of ill-ness indicates wellness. There are actually many degrees of wellness, just as there are many degrees of illness. The Wellness Inventory is designed to stir up your thinking about many areas of wellness.

While people often lack physical symptoms, they may still be bored, depressed, tense, anxious, or generally unhappy with their lives. Such emotional states often set the stage for physical and mental disease. Even cancer may be brought on through the lowering of the body's resis-tance from excessive stress. These same emotional states can also lead to abuse of the body through smoking, overdrinking, and overeating. Such behaviors are usually substitutes for other, more basic human needs such as recognition from others, a more stimulating environment, caring and affection from friends, and greater self-acceptance.

Wellness is not a static state. High-level wellness involves giving good care to your physical self, using your mind constructively, expressing your emotions effectively, being creatively involved with those around you, and being concerned about your physical, psychological, and spiritual environments.

Instructions

Set aside a half hour for yourself in a quiet place where you will not be disturbed while taking the Inventory. Record your responses to each statement in the columns to the right where:

    2 = Yes, usually

    1 = Sometimes, maybe

    0 = No, rarely

Select the answer that best indicates how true the statement is for you presently.

After you have responded to all the appropriate statements in each section, compute your average score for that section and transfer it to the corresponding box provided around the Wellness Inventory Wheel on page 29. Your completed Wheel will give you a clear presentation of the balance you have given to the many dimensions of your life.

You will find some of the statements are really two in one. We do this to show an important relationship between the two parts—usually an awareness of an issue, combined with an action based on that aware-ness. Mentally average your score for the two parts of the question.

Each statement describes what we believe to be a wellness attribute. Because much wellness information is subjective and "unprovable" by current scientific methods, you (and possibly other authorities as well) may not agree with our conclusions. Many of the statements have further explanation in a footnote. We ask only that you keep an open mind until you have studied available information, then decide.

This questionnaire was designed to educate more than to test. All statements are worded so that you can easily tell what we think are well-ness attributes (which also makes it easy to "cheat" on your score). This means there can be no trick questions to test your honesty or consis-tency—the higher your score, the greater you believe your wellness to be. Full responsibility is placed on you to answer each statement as honestly as possible. It's not your score but what you learn about yourself that is most important.

If you decide that a statement does not apply to you, or you don't want to answer it, you can skip it and not be penalized in your score.

Transfer your average score from each section to the correspond-ing box around the Wheel. Then graph your score by drawing a curved line between the "spokes" that define each segment. (Use the scale provided—beginning at the center with 0.0 and reaching 2.0 at the circumference.) Last, fill in the corresponding amount of each wedge-shaped segment, using different colors if possible.

*Reprinted with permission of the author from *The Wellness Workbook*, 3rd ed., John W. Travis, M.D. and Regina Sara Ryan, Celestial Arts, Berkeley, CA. © 1981, 1988, 2004 by John W. Travis, www.wellnessworkbook.com.

SAMPLE QUESTIONS

	Yes, usually: 2	Sometimes, maybe: 1	No, rarely: 0
1. I am an adventurous thinker.	✓		
2. I have no expectations, yet look to the future optimistically.		✓	
3. I am a nonsmoker.	✓		
4. I love long, hot baths.			✓
	4	+ 1	+ 0

Total points for this section = 5

Divided by 4 (number of statements answered) = 1.3 Average score for this section.

Section 1 WELLNESS AND SENSING

Yes, usually: 2   Sometimes, maybe: 1   No, rarely: 0

1. My place of work has mostly natural lighting or full-spectrum fluorescent lighting.[1]   _____   _____   _____
2. I avoid extremely noisy areas or wear protective ear covers.[2]   _____   _____   _____
3. I take long walks, hikes, or other outings to actively explore my surroundings.   _____   _____   _____
4. I give myself presents, treats, or nurture myself in other ways.   _____   _____   _____
5. I enjoy getting, and can acknowledge, compliments and recognition from others.   _____   _____   _____
6. It is easy for me to give sincere compliments and recognition to other people.   _____   _____   _____
7. At times I like to be alone.   _____   _____   _____
8. I enjoy touching or hugging other people.[3]   _____   _____   _____
9. I enjoy being touched or hugged by others.[4]   _____   _____   _____
10. I get and enjoy backrubs or massages.   _____   _____   _____

Total points for this section = ☐   _____ + _____ + _____

Divided by _____ (number of statements answered) = _____ Average score for this section.
(Transfer to the Wellness Inventory Wheel on p. 29.)

Section 2 WELLNESS AND EATING

Yes, usually: 2   Sometimes, maybe: 1   No, rarely: 0

1. I am aware of the difference between refined carbohydrates and complex carbohydrates and eat a majority of the latter.[5]   _____   _____   _____
2. I think my diet is well balanced and wholesome.   _____   _____   _____
3. I drink fewer than five alcoholic drinks per week.   _____   _____   _____
4. I drink fewer than two cups of coffee or black (nonherbal) tea per day.[6]   _____   _____   _____
5. I drink fewer than five soft drinks per week.[7]   _____   _____   _____
6. I add little or no salt to my food.[8]   _____   _____   _____
7. I read the labels for the ingredients of all processed foods I buy and I inquire as to the level of toxic chemicals used in production of fresh foods—choosing the purest available to me.   _____   _____   _____
8. I eat at least two raw fruits or vegetables each day.   _____   _____   _____
9. I have a good appetite and am within 15 percent of my ideal weight.   _____   _____   _____
10. I can tell the difference between "stomach hunger" and "mouth hunger," and I don't stuff myself when I am experiencing only "mouth hunger."[9]   _____   _____   _____

Total points for this section = ☐   _____ + _____ + _____

Divided by _____ (number of statements answered) = _____ Average score for this section.
(Transfer to the Wellness Inventory Wheel on p. 29.)

---

[1] Full-spectrum light, like sunlight, contains many different wavelengths. Most eyeglasses, and the glass windows in your home or car, block the "near" ultraviolet light needed by your body. Special bulbs and lenses are available.

[2] Loud noises that leave your ears ringing cause irreversible and cumulative nerve damage over time. Ear plugs/muffs, obtained in sporting goods stores, should be worn around power saws, heavy equipment, and rock concerts!

[3,4] Long recognized by hospitals as therapeutic, touch can be a powerful preventative as well.

[5] Refined carbohydrates (white flour, sugar, white rice, alcohol, and others) are burned up by the body very quickly and contain no minerals or vitamins. Complex carbohydrates (fruits and vegetables) burn evenly and provide the bulk of dietary nutrients.

[6] Coffee and nonherbal teas contain stimulants that, when overused, abuse your body's adrenal glands.

[7] Besides caffeine, the empty calories in these chemical brews may cause a sugar "crash" shortly after drinking. Artificially sweetened ones may be worse. Consider the other nutrients you won't be getting, and the prices!

[8] In addition to having a presumed connection with high blood pressure, the salting of foods during cooking draws out minerals, which are lost when the water is poured off.

[9] Stomach hunger is a signal that your body needs food. Mouth hunger is a signal that it needs something else (attention/acknowledgment), which you are not getting, so it asks for food, a readily available "substitute."

Section 3 WELLNESS AND THINKING

Yes, usually: 2   **Sometimes, maybe: 1**   **No, rarely: 0**

1. I am in charge of the subject matter and the emotional content of my thoughts and am satisfied with what I choose to think about.[10]   _____ _____ _____

2. I am aware that I make judgments wherein I think I am "right" and others are "wrong."[11]   _____ _____ _____

3. It is easy for me to concentrate.   _____ _____ _____

4. I am conscious of changes (such as breathing pattern, muscle tension, skin moisture, and so on) in my body in response to certain thoughts.[12]   _____ _____ _____

5. I notice my perceptions of the world are colored by my thoughts at the time.[13]   _____ _____ _____

6. I am aware that my thoughts are influenced by my environment.   _____ _____ _____

7. I use my thoughts and attitudes to make my reality more life-affirming.[14]   _____ _____ _____

8. Rather than worry about a problem when I can do nothing about it, I temporarily shelve it and get on with the matters at hand.   _____ _____ _____

9. I approach life with the attitude that no problem is too big to confront, and some mysteries aren't meant to be solved.   _____ _____ _____

10. I use my creative powers in many aspects of my life.   _____ _____ _____

Total points for this section = ☐   _____ + _____ + _____

Divided by _____ (number of statements answered) = _____ Average score for this section.
(Transfer to the Wellness Inventory Wheel on p 29.)

Section 4 WELLNESS AND PLAYING/WORKING

Yes, usually: 2   **Sometimes, maybe: 1**   **No, rarely: 0**

1. I enjoy expressing myself through art, dance, music, drama, sports, or other activities and make time to do so.   _____ _____ _____

2. I regularly exercise my creativity "muscles."   _____ _____ _____

3. I enjoy spending time without planned or structured activities and make the effort to do so.   _____ _____ _____

4. I can make much of my work into play.   _____ _____ _____

5. At times I allow myself to do nothing.[15]   _____ _____ _____

6. At times I can sleep late without feeling guilty.   _____ _____ _____

7. The work I do is rewarding to me.   _____ _____ _____

8. I am proud of my accomplishments.   _____ _____ _____

9. I am playful and the people around me support my playfulness.   _____ _____ _____

10. I have at least one activity, hobby, or sport that I enjoy regularly but do not feel compelled to do.   _____ _____ _____

Total points for this section = ☐   _____ + _____ + _____

Divided by _____ (number of statements answered) = _____ Average score for this section.
(Transfer to the Wellness Inventory Wheel on p. 29.)

---

[10] When you are unconscious of the content of your thoughts, they are more likely to control you. Observing them objectively develops self-awareness and strengthens your ability to take charge.

[11] Rather than trying to completely stop yourself from judging, you can observe your judgments as efforts by your ego to avoid getting on with life and hiding behind "right/wrong" game playing.

[12] Both biofeedback and the field of psycho-neuro-immunology have shown the connections between the mind, nervous system, and body. The more you become consciously aware of that connection, the greater responsibility you can take for your health.

[13] Being aware of your internal distortion of perceptions can allow you to step back and reassess a situation more objectively.

[14] Honesty, tempered with care and concern, clears out many negative thoughts that can clutter up your mind, thus making your reality more fun. "Positive thinking" without honesty and truthfulness can backfire by suppressing valid concerns that must be addressed.

[15] Doing "nothing" can give us access to the more creative and nonverbal aspects of our being, so from another perspective, doing nothing becomes doing much more.

Section 5 WELLNESS AND FINDING MEANING

	Yes, usually: 2	Sometimes, maybe: 1	No, rarely: 0
1. I believe my life has direction and meaning.	_____	_____	_____
2. My life is exciting and challenging.	_____	_____	_____
3. I have goals in my life.	_____	_____	_____
4. I am achieving my goals.	_____	_____	_____
5. I look forward to the future as an opportunity for further growth.	_____	_____	_____
6. I am able to talk about the death of someone close to me.	_____	_____	_____
7. I am able to talk about my own death with family and friends.	_____	_____	_____
8. I am prepared for my death.	_____	_____	_____
9. I see my death as a step in my evolution.[16]	_____	_____	_____
10. My daily life is a source of pleasure to me.	_____	_____	_____

Total points for this section = ☐   _____ + _____   _____ + _____   _____

Divided by _____ (number of statements answered) = _____ Average score for this section.
(Transfer to the Wellness Inventory Wheel on p. 29.)

Section 6 of the Inventory goes beyond the scope of most generally accepted "scientific" principles and expresses the values and beliefs of the authors. It is intended to stimulate interest in these areas. If you have strong beliefs to the contrary, you can skip the questions or make up your own.

Section 6 WELLNESS AND TRANSCENDING

	Yes, usually: 2	Sometimes, maybe: 1	No, rarely: 0
1. I perceive problems as opportunities for growth.	_____	_____	_____
2. I experience synchronistic events in my life (frequent "coincidences" seeming to have no cause-effect relationship).[17]	_____	_____	_____
3. I believe there are dimensions of reality beyond verbal description or human comprehension.	_____	_____	_____
4. At times I experience confusion and paradox in my search for understanding of the dimensions referred to above.	_____	_____	_____
5. The concept of God has personal definition and meaning to me.	_____	_____	_____
6. I experience a sense of wonder when I contemplate the universe.	_____	_____	_____
7. I have abundant expectancy rather than specific expectations.	_____	_____	_____
8. I allow others their beliefs without pressuring them to accept mine.	_____	_____	_____
9. I use the messages interpreted from my dreams.	_____	_____	_____
10. I enjoy practicing a spiritual discipline or allowing time to sense the presence of a greater force in guiding my passage through life.	_____	_____	_____

Total points for this section = ☐   _____ + _____   _____ + _____   _____

Divided by _____ (number of statements answered) = _____ Average score for this section.
(Transfer to the Wellness Inventory Wheel on p. 29.)

Section 7 WELLNESS, SELF-RESPONSIBILITY, AND LOVE

	Yes, usually: 2	Sometimes, maybe: 1	No, rarely: 0
1. I believe how I live my life is an important factor in determining my state of health, and I live it in a manner consistent with that belief.	_____	_____	_____
2. I vote regularly.[18]	_____	_____	_____
3. I feel financially secure.	_____	_____	_____

[16] Seeing your death as a stage of growth and preparing yourself consciously is an important part of finding meaning in your life.
[17] Modern physics reveals that the idea of cause and effect may be as limited as Newton's theory of a mechanical universe. It suggests that we must expand our view to see that everything in the universe is connected to everything else. (Synchronicity describes that experience.)
[18] Voting is a simple measure of your willingness to participate in the social system, which ultimately impacts your state of health.

4. I conserve materials/energy at home and at work.[19]   ____   ____   ____

5. I protect my living area from fire and safety hazards.   ____   ____   ____

6. I use dental floss and a soft toothbrush daily.   ____   ____   ____

7. I am a nonsmoker.   ____   ____   ____

8. I am always sober when driving or operating dangerous machinery.   ____   ____   ____

9. I wear a safety belt when I ride in a vehicle.   ____   ____   ____

10. I understand the difference between blaming myself for a problem and simply taking responsibility (ability to respond) for that problem.   ____   ____   ____

Total points for this section = ☐   ____ + ____ + ____

Divided by ____ (number of statements answered) = ____ Average score for this section. (Transfer to the Wellness Inventory Wheel on p. 29.)

....

Section 8 WELLNESS AND BREATHING

Yes, usually: 2   Sometimes, maybe: 1   No, rarely: 0

1. I stop during the day to become aware of the way I am breathing.   ____   ____   ____

2. I meditate or relax myself for at least 15 to 20 minutes each day.   ____   ____   ____

3. I can easily touch my hands to my toes when standing with knees straight.[20]   ____   ____   ____

4. In temperatures over 70°F (21°C), my fingers feel warm when I touch my lips.[21]   ____   ____   ____

5. My nails are healthy and I do not bite or pick at them.   ____   ____   ____

6. I enjoy my work and do not find it overly stressful.   ____   ____   ____

7. My personal relationships are satisfying.   ____   ____   ____

8. I take time out for deep breathing several times a day.   ____   ____   ____

9. I have plenty of energy.   ____   ____   ____

10. I am at peace with myself.   ____   ____   ____

Total points for this section = ☐   ____ + ____ + ____

Divided by ____ (number of statements answered) = ____ Average score for this section. (Transfer to the Wellness Inventory Wheel on p. 29.)

....

Section 9 WELLNESS AND MOVING

Yes, usually: 2   Sometimes, maybe: 1   No, rarely: 0

1. I climb stairs rather than ride elevators.[22]   ____   ____   ____

2. My daily activities include moderate physical effort.[23]   ____   ____   ____

3. My daily activities include vigorous physical effort.[24]   ____   ____   ____

4. I run at least 1 mile three times a week (or do equivalent aerobic exercise).[25]   ____   ____   ____

5. I run at least 3 miles three times a week (or do equivalent aerobic exercise).   ____   ____   ____

6. I do some form of stretching/limbering exercise for 10 to 20 minutes at least three times per week.[26]   ____   ____   ____

[19] Besides recycling glass, paper, aluminum, and other recyclables, if you purchase products that are reusable rather than disposable, and are packaged with a minimum of material, you will reduce the drain of resources and the toxic load on the environment caused by the disposal of wastes.

[20] A lack of spinal flexibility is usually a symptom of chronic muscle tension as well as indicative of a poor balance of physical activities.

[21] If your hand temperature is below 85°F (30°C) in a warm room, you're cutting off circulation to your hands via an overactive sympathetic nervous system. You can learn to warm your hands with biofeedback and to thereby better relax.

[22] If a long elevator ride is necessary, try getting off five flights below your destination. Urge building managers to keep stair doors unlocked.

[23] Moderate = rearing young children, gardening, scrubbing floors, brisk walking, and so on.

[24] Vigorous = heavy construction work, farming, moving heavy objects by hand, and so on.

[25] Aerobic exercise (like running) should keep your heart rate at about 60 percent of its maximum (120–150 bpm) for 12–20 minutes. Brisk walking for 20 minutes every day can produce effects similar to aerobic exercise.

[26] The stretching of muscles is important for maintaining maximum flexibility of joints and ligaments. It feels good, too.

7. I do some form of stretching/limbering exercise for 10 to 20 minutes at least six times per week.   _____   _____   _____

8. I enjoy exploring new and effective ways of caring for myself through the movement of my body.   _____   _____   _____

9. I enjoy stretching, moving, and exerting my body.   _____   _____   _____

10. I am aware of and respond to messages from my body about its needs for movement.   _____   _____   _____

Total points for this section = ☐   _____   +   _____   +   _____

Divided by _____ (number of statements answered) = _____ Average score for this section.
(Transfer to the Wellness Inventory Wheel on p. 29.)

· ·

Section 10 WELLNESS AND FEELING

	Yes, usually: 2	Sometimes, maybe: 1	No, rarely: 0
1. I am able to feel and express my anger in ways that solve problems, rather than swallow anger or store it up.[27]	_____	_____	_____
2. I allow myself to experience a full range of emotions and find constructive ways to express them.	_____	_____	_____
3. I am able to say "no" to people without feeling guilty.	_____	_____	_____
4. I laugh often and easily.	_____	_____	_____
5. I feel OK about crying and allow myself to do so when appropriate.[28]	_____	_____	_____
6. I listen to and consider others' criticisms of me rather than react defensively.	_____	_____	_____
7. I have at least five close friends.	_____	_____	_____
8. I like myself and look forward to the rest of my life.	_____	_____	_____
9. I easily express concern, love, and warmth to those I care about.	_____	_____	_____
10. I can ask for help when needed.	_____	_____	_____

Total points for this section = ☐   _____   +   _____   +   _____

Divided by _____ (number of statements answered) = _____ Average score for this section.
(Transfer to the Wellness Inventory Wheel on p. 29.)

· ·

Section 11 WELLNESS AND COMMUNICATING

	Yes, usually: 2	Sometimes, maybe: 1	No, rarely: 0
1. In conversation I can introduce a difficult topic and stay with it until I've gotten a satisfactory response from the other person.	_____	_____	_____
2. I enjoy silence.	_____	_____	_____
3. I am truthful and caring in my communications with others.	_____	_____	_____
4. I assert myself (in a nonattacking manner) in an effort to be heard, rather than be passively resentful of others with whom I don't agree.[29]	_____	_____	_____
5. I readily acknowledge my mistakes, apologizing for them if appropriate.	_____	_____	_____
6. I am aware of my negative judgments of others and accept them as simply judgments—not necessarily truth.[30]	_____	_____	_____
7. I am a good listener.	_____	_____	_____
8. I am able to listen to people without interrupting them or finishing their sentences for them.	_____	_____	_____

[27] Learning to take charge of your emotions and using them to solve problems can prevent disease, improve communications, and increase your self-awareness. Suppressing emotions or using them to manipulate others is destructive to all.
[28] Crying over a loss relieves the body of pent-up feelings. In our culture males often have a difficult time allowing themselves to cry, while females may have learned to cry when angry, using tears as a means of manipulation.

[29] Attacking others rarely accomplishes your goals in the long run. Persisting in your convictions without using force is more effective and usually solves the problem without creating new ones.
[30] It is important to recognize that our internal judgments of others are based on personal biases that often have little objective basis.

9. I can let go of my mental "labels" (for example, this is good, that is wrong) and judgmental attitudes about events in my life and see them in light of what they offer me.

_____   _____   _____

10. I am aware when I play psychological "games" with those around me and work to be truthful and direct in my communications.[31]

_____   _____   _____

Total points for this section = ☐

_____ + _____ + _____

Divided by _____ (number of statements answered) = _____ Average score for this section.
(Transfer to the Wellness Inventory Wheel on p. 29.)

....

Section 12 WELLNESS AND SEX

	Yes, usually: 2	Sometimes, maybe: 1	No, rarely: 0
1. I feel comfortable touching and exploring my body.	_____	_____	_____
2. I think it's OK to masturbate if one chooses to do so.	_____	_____	_____
3. My sexual education is adequate.	_____	_____	_____
4. I feel good about the degree of closeness I have with men.	_____	_____	_____
5. I feel good about the degree of closeness I have with women.	_____	_____	_____
6. I am content with my level of sexual activity.[32]	_____	_____	_____
7. I fully experience the many stages of lovemaking rather than focus only on orgasm.[33]	_____	_____	_____
8. I desire to grow closer to some other people.	_____	_____	_____
9. I am aware of the difference between needing someone and loving someone.	_____	_____	_____
10. I am able to love others without dominating or being dominated by them.	_____	_____	_____

Total points for this section = ☐

_____ + _____ + _____

Divided by _____ (number of statements answered) = _____ Average score for this section.
(Transfer to the Wellness Inventory Wheel on p. 29.)

Your Health Action Plan for Maximum Wellness

When you have completed the Wellness Inventory, study your wheel's shape and balance. How smoothly would it roll? What does it tell you? Are there any surprises in it? How does it feel to you? What don't you like about it? What do you like about it?

We recommend that you use colored pens to go back over the questions, noting the ones on which your scores were low and choosing some areas on which you are interested in working. It is easy to overwhelm yourself by taking on too many areas at once. Ignore, for now, those of lower priority to you. Remember, if you don't enjoy at least some aspects of the changes you are making, they probably won't last.

Here are some guidelines to help you:

- **Get support from friends,** but don't expect them to supply all the reinforcement you need. You may join a group of overweight individuals and rely on their encouragement to stick to your diet. That's a great way to get going, but in the long run your own commitment to losing weight has got to be strong enough to help you keep eating right and light.

- **Focus on the immediate rewards** of your new behavior. You may stop smoking so that you'll live longer, but take note of

every other benefit it brings you—more stamina, less coughing, more spending money, no more stale tobacco taste in your mouth.

- **Remind yourself of past successes** you've had in making changes. Give yourself pep talks, commending yourself on how well you've done so far and how well you'll continue to do. This will boost your self-confidence.

- **Reward yourself regularly.** Plan a pleasant reward as an incentive for every week you stick to your new behavior—sleeping in on a Saturday morning, going out with some friends, or spending a sunny afternoon outdoors. Small, regular rewards are more effective in keeping up motivation than one big reward that won't come for many months.

- **Expect and accept some relapses.** The greatest rate of relapse occurs in the first few weeks after making a behavior change. During this critical time, get as much support as you can. In addition, work hard on self-motivation, reminding yourself daily of what you have to gain by sticking with your new health habit.

---

[31] Psychological games, as defined by Eric Berne in *Games People Play*, are complex unconscious manipulations that result in the players' getting negative attention and feeling bad about themselves.
[32] Including the choice to have no sexual activity.

[33] A common problem for many people is an overemphasis on performance and orgasm, rather than on enjoying a close sensual feeling with their partner whether or not they experience orgasm.

MAKING THIS CHAPTER WORK FOR YOU

Review Questions

1. The development of health behaviors is influenced by all of the following *except*
   a. reinforcing factors, which involve external recognition for achieving a goal.
   b. preexisting health factors, which take into account the individual's current position on the wellness continuum.
   c. predisposing factors, which include knowledge, attitudes, and beliefs.
   d. enabling factors, which are related to an individual's skills and capabilities to make behavioral changes.

2. A group of students is discussing the differences between the sexes. Whose statement is *incorrect?*
   a. Matt: "Men breathe faster but have a slower heart rate—and have a larger brain."
   b. Elena: "But women have more neurons in certain brain regions."
   c. Kristin: "And women *are* less likely to get arthritis."
   d. Rick: "Got me there—Men *are* more likely to have heart attacks and to get cancer."

3. Which of the following statements about health information on the Internet is true?
   a. Chat rooms are the most reliable source of accurate medical information.
   b. Physicians who have websites must adhere to a strict set of standards set by the American Medical Association.
   c. Government-sponsored sites such as that of the Centers for Disease Control and Prevention are excellent sources of accurate health-care information.
   d. The Internet is a safe and cost-effective source of prescription drugs.

4. The term for a behavior or attitude that a particular group expects is
   a. social health.
   b. self-efficacy.
   c. social norm.
   d. reinforcement.

5. Which of the following is *not* a question you must ask your doctor to understand your health condition and what to do about it?
   a. What is my main problem?
   b. Why do I have this problem?
   c. What do I need to do?
   d. Why is it important for me to do this?

6. According to the stages of change in the transtheoretical model of change, which statement is *incorrect?*
   a. In the maintenance stage, individuals have avoided relapse for six months.
   b. In the contemplation stage, individuals are considering changing a problem behavior in the next six months.
   c. In the action stage, individuals are actually modifying their behavior according to their plan.
   d. In the preparation stage, individuals intend to change a problem behavior in the next six months.

7. Relapses are common (you're human, aren't you?), but don't let them keep you from your goal. Which of these strategies might help you recover from a relapse?
   a. Have a hot fudge sundae.
   b. Decide to think about it after finals.
   c. Analyze what went wrong and why.
   d. Put yourself back into contemplation stage.

8. Which of the following statements about the dimensions of health is true?
   a. Spirituality provides solace and comfort for those who are severely ill, but it has no health benefits.
   b. The people who reflect the highest levels of social health are usually among the most popular individuals in a group and are often thought of as the life of the party.
   c. Intellectual health refers to one's academic abilities.
   d. Optimal physical health requires a nutritious diet, regular exercise, avoidance of harmful behaviors and substances, and self-protection from accidents.

9. Change processes—cognitive and behavioral activities that facilitate change—include all of these *except*
   a. consciousness-raising.
   b. health awareness.
   c. countering.
   d. helping relationships.

10. If you want to change unhealthy behavior, which of the following strategies is *least* likely to promote success?
    a. Believe that you can make the change.
    b. Reward yourself regularly.
    c. Remind yourself about all your faults.
    d. Accept that you are in control of your health.

    Answers to these questions can be found on page 650.

Critical Thinking

1. Where are you on the wellness–illness continuum? What variables might affect your place on the scale? What do you consider your optimum state of health to be?

2. Talk to classmates from different racial or ethnic backgrounds than yours about their culture's health attitudes. Ask them what is considered healthy behavior in their cultures. For example, is having a good appetite a sign of health? What kinds of self-care practices did their parents and grandparents use to treat colds, fevers, rashes, and other health problems? What are their attitudes about the health-care system?

3. Jocelyn has been experiencing a great deal of fatigue and frequent headaches for the past couple of months. She doesn't have health insurance and doesn't want to spend

money on a doctor visit. So she did some research on the Internet about ways to relieve her symptoms and was considering taking a couple of herbal supplements that were touted as potential treatments. If she asked you for your advice, what would you tell her? Do you think that self-care is appropriate in this situation?

Media Menu

CENGAGENOW™ Go to the CengageNOW for Health website at **www .cengage.com/sso** that will:
- Help you evaluate your knowledge of the material.
- Allow you to take an exam-prep quiz.
- Provide a Personalized Learning Plan targeting resources that address areas you should study.
- Coach you through identifying target goals for behavioral change and creating and monitoring your personal change plan throughout the semester.

Internet Connections

www.goaskalice.columbia.edu/index.html
Sponsored by Columbia University, this site offers questions and answers as well as an interactive service on a wide variety of health-related topics.

http://wellness.uwsp.edu/Other/lifescan
This site, created by Bill Hettler, M.D., of the National Wellness Institute, helps you identify specific lifestyle factors that can impair your health and longevity. Take the health questionnaire to determine your personal lifestyle risks. Your results provide a score for general results, nutrition results, and height/weight results. Your ranking among the top ten causes of death is provided, as well as suggestions on how to improve.

www.uri.edu/research/cprc/TTM/detailedoverview.htm
This site describes the transtheoretical model of change, including descriptions of effective interventions to promote health behavior change, focusing on the individual's decision-making strategies.

Key Terms

The terms listed are used on the page indicated. Definitions of the terms are in the Glossary at the end of the book.

enabling factors 23
evidence-based medicine 21
health 5
health belief model (HBM) 23
health literacy 17
health promotion 5
locus of control 26
meta-analysis 19
practice guidelines 21
predisposing factors 21
prevention 14
protection 15
reinforcing factors 23
self-efficacy 26
social norms 15
transtheoretical model 25
wellness 5

Chapter 2 - Psychological and Spiritual Well-Being

1. The ability to perceive reality as it really is, to respond to its challenges and to develop rational coping strategies defines: (Pg. 40)
   A. emotional health
   B. mental health
   C. spiritual health
   D. social health

2. A mentally healthy student who receives a 'D' on an exam will likely be very disappointed with the grade, but will: (Pg. 40)
   A. reassess the course options and drop from the class
   B. try to assess the reasons for the low grade and resolve to work harder
   C. make an appointment with the instructor and insist the instructor reevaluate the test results to get more points
   D. become cynical about passing the class and stop trying to get an 'A'

3. An emotionally healthy person will likely exhibit all but which of the following traits: (Pg. 40)
   A. makes an effort to be healthy
   B. has compassion and empathy for others
   C. that the self should be the center of the universe
   D. can adapt to a variety of circumstances

4. Which of the following statements does not define 'emotional intelligence'. (Pg. 41)
   A. the ability to monitor and use emotions to guide thinking and actions
   B. a higher emotional quotient person is usually more productive at work
   C. is more likely to experience stress and be anxious
   D. identifying emotions and not relying on gut feelings

5. If Madelyn wants to boost her self esteem, which technique would be most productive? (Pg. 42)
   A. provide constructive criticism to herself
   B. provide positive self talk to herself
   C. obtain feedback from her friends
   D. be willing to take risks

6. Which of the following best describes optimism? (Pg. 46)
   A. doing something nice for someone else
   B. using assertive communications with your colleagues
   C. an inclination to expect the best possible outcome
   D. developing realistic goals and expectations

7. Which of the following is an example of Tom's internal locus of control. (Pg. 48)
   A. Tom blames the heavy traffic for being late getting to class on time
   B. Staying at a party later than Tom expected made him not get a homework assignment completed on time
   C. Tom admitted his procrastination on writing a research paper resulted in a poorly written paper which received a lower grade than he expected
   D. Tom's roommate accidentally threw away Tom's pile of papers he needed for class and Tom blamed the roommate for the poor grade he received.

8. Having lower mental stress and enhanced psychological well-being are benefits of: (Pg. 47)
   A. happiness
   B. optimism
   C. altruism
   D. assertiveness

9. One method to shake off a bad mood which resulted from a bad experience you had would be to: (Pg. 47)
   A. have a few beers to shake off the funky bad mood you are in
   B. use a process called reframing to analyze what went wrong and how can you improve on that situation
   C. analyze why you are feeling bad and continue to beat yourself up until your head clears up
   D. sleep it off for a few days

10. To experience true happiness in life, one needs to: (Pg. 45)
    A. look for it in the right places
    B. be genetically predisposed to happiness
    C. do things that will make yourself happy
    D. make more money to become happy

11. **A sustained emotional condition that can make our thoughts and feelings very unclear for a few hours or days is known as:** (Pg. 46)
    A. sad feelings
    B. negative thoughts
    C. negative ideas
    D. mood

12. **It is reported that people who regularly pray experience which of the following health benefits:** (Pg. 53)
    A. lower blood pressure
    B. stronger immune system
    C. often hospitalized less
    D. all of the above

13. **Which person is exemplifying their spirituality in everyday life?** (Pg. 50)
    A. Mary goes to her church service early and meditates before the service begins
    B. Matt spends an hour every day doing yoga poses and deep breathing
    C. Connor goes for long walks 3 times a week and focuses on deep breathing
    D. all are examples of spirituality in action

14. **The criteria one uses to evaluate things, people, events, and even yourself make up:** (Pg. 51)
    A. values
    B. beliefs
    C. religion
    D. expectations

15. **Religiosity refers to which of the following statements:** (Pg. 50)
    A. various religious practices that one may engage in
    B. religiosity and spirituality mean the same thing
    C. religiosity is attending weekly church services
    D. religious people are more happy and less judgmental

16. **Which of the following examples explains altruism?** (Pg. 54)
    A. Kyle grudgingly did his chores because his Dad made him to them
    B. John spent a month volunteering in Africa working with HIV patients
    C. Annmarie spent the entire day staying focused and completing all her homework
    D. Tim blamed the icy roads for causing his car accident while trying to rush to work on time

17. **All of the following except one are essential for functioning well with a good night's sleep :** (Pg. 56)
    A. your brain and memory work better to retain information
    B. more weight is gained with too much sleep
    C. less sleep will likely weaken your immune system
    D. quality of life is enhanced with adequate sleep

18. **Which of the following suggestions would not be recommended if you are trying to develop better sleeping patterns in your life?** (Pg. 58)
    A. develop a sleeping ritual before going to sleep, such as reading or praying
    B. keep regular hours for going to bed and for awaking to set a pattern
    C. take long naps in the daytime so you will be more tired late at night to fall asleep
    D. Don't drink coffee or use nicotine later in the evening

19. **In which non-REM sleep stage is the brain in its most profound unconsciousness?** (Pg. 57)
    A. stage 1 twilight zone
    B. stage 2 brain slow down
    C. stage 3-4 deep slow sleep
    D. REM sleep dreaming phase

20. **Circadian rhythm sleep disorders are more likely to occur with people in which example:** (Pg. 58)
    A. people traveling from across the globe and dealing with many time changes   through the air flights
    B. sleeping in a room with the lights on instead of it being darkened
    C. going to a late night party and having drank too much alcohol
    D. none of the above

Adam never considered himself a spiritual person until he enrolled in a class on the science of personal well-being. For a homework assignment he had to pursue different paths to happiness. As part of his experiment, he went to a Mardi Gras celebration and partied all night to see if having fun made him happier. To test whether doing good makes a person happy, Adam volunteered to help build a house for a homeless family. "I can't remember the name of a single person I met at the party," he says. "But I'll never forget the look on the family's faces when we handed them the keys to their new home."

Psychological and Spiritual Well-Being

For his final project, Adam, who did not have a religious upbringing, focused on developing a richer spiritual life. "The spirituality didn't end with the term," he says. "I continue to meditate, do yoga, and read religious texts because I believe a more spiritual life will help me in the long run with happiness and health."

The quest for a more fulfilling and meaningful life is attracting more people of all ages. The reason? As the burgeoning field of positive psychology has resoundingly proved, people who achieve emotional and spiritual health are more creative and productive, earn more money, attract more friends, enjoy better marriages, develop fewer illnesses, and live longer.

This chapter reports the latest findings on making the most of psychological strengths, enhancing happiness, and developing the spiritual dimension of your health and your life. (See Making Change Happen, p. 44, and *IPC*.) It also explores an often overlooked dimension of physical and emotional well-being: sleep.

> **After studying the material in this chapter, you should be able to**
>
> - **Identify** the characteristics of emotionally healthy persons.
> - **Name** the two pillars of authentic happiness.
> - **Discuss** some of the health benefits of prayer.
> - **Describe** four ways that sleep affects well-being.

Log on to CengageNOW for Health at **www.cengage.com/sso** to find your Behavior Change Planner and to explore self-assessments, interactive tutorials, and practice quizzes.

39

Psychological Well-Being

Unlike physical health, psychological well-being cannot be measured, tested, X-rayed, or dissected. Yet psychologically healthy men and women generally share certain characteristics: They value themselves and strive toward happiness and fulfillment. They establish and maintain close relationships with others. They accept the limitations as well as the possibilities that life has to offer. And they feel a sense of meaning and purpose that makes the gestures of living worth the effort required.

Psychological health encompasses both our emotional and mental states—that is, our feelings and our thoughts. **Emotional health** generally refers to feelings and moods, both of which are discussed later in this chapter. Characteristics of emotionally healthy persons, identified in an analysis of major studies of emotional wellness, include the following:

- Determination and effort to be healthy.
- Flexibility and adaptability to a variety of circumstances.
- Development of a sense of meaning and affirmation of life.
- An understanding that the self is not the center of the universe.
- Compassion for others.
- The ability to be unselfish in serving or relating to others.
- Increased depth and satisfaction in intimate relationships.
- A sense of control over the mind and body that enables the person to make health-enhancing choices and decisions.

"Emotional vitality," a sense of positive energy and engagement in life, correlates with physical vitality. In a recent study the individuals who ranked highest in this state of heightened emotional well-being had the lowest risk of cardiovascular disease.[1]

Mental health describes our ability to perceive reality as it is, to respond to its challenges, and to develop rational strategies for living. The mentally healthy person doesn't try to avoid conflicts and distress but can cope with life's transitions, traumas, and losses in a way that allows for emotional stability and growth. The characteristics of mental health include:

- The ability to function and carry out responsibilities.
- The ability to form relationships.
- Realistic perceptions of the motivations of others.
- Rational, logical thought processes.
- The ability to adapt to change and to cope with adversity.

Culture also helps to define psychological health. In one culture, men and women may express feelings with great intensity, shouting in joy or wailing in grief, while in another culture such behavior might be considered abnormal or unhealthy. In our diverse society, many cultural influences affect Americans' sense of who they are, where they came from, and what they believe. Cultural rituals help bring people together, strengthen their bonds, reinforce the values and beliefs they share, and provide a sense of belonging, meaning, and purpose.

To find out where are you on the psychological well-being scale, take the Self Survey on p. 61.

Practicing Positive Psychology

Psychology, a field that traditionally concentrated on what goes wrong in our lives and in our minds, has shifted its focus to the study of human strengths, virtues, and positive emotions. The three major areas of positive psychology are the study of positive emotions, such as hope and trust; positive traits, such as wisdom and courage; and positive institutions, such as strong families and democracy.

According to psychologist Martin Seligman, Ph.D., who started the positive psychology movement more than a decade ago, everyone, regardless of genes or fate, can achieve a happy, gratifying, meaningful life. The goal is not simply to feel good momentarily or to avoid bad experiences,

© Tom Stewart/Corbis

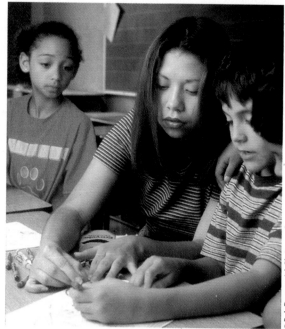

© Bob Daemmrich Photography

Psychologically healthy people have compassion for others and form strong and deep relationships. They adapt to a variety of circumstances, overcome challenges, and strive to achieve their full potential.

but to build positive strengths and virtues that enable us to find meaning and purpose in life. The core philosophy is to add a "build what's strong" approach to the "fix what's wrong" focus of traditional psychotherapy. The traits that may well protect us from physical and mental illness include courage, optimism, hope, interpersonal skills, a work ethic, responsibility, future-mindedness, honesty, and perseverance.

Research on positive psychology has mainly focused on healthy people who did not have mental disorders. In the limited number of studies of individuals diagnosed with depression, those using positive psychology practices, such as identifying three good things that happen every day, rated as happier and less depressed than those who did not.[2] Many of the exercises and labs in *An Invitation to Personal Change (IPC)* apply the principles of positive psychology.

You can start practicing positive psychology right away. The next time you think, "I've never tried that before," also say to yourself, "This is an opportunity to learn something new." When something seems too complicated, remind yourself to tackle it from another angle. If you get discouraged and feel that you're never going to get better at some new skill, tell yourself to give it another try.

Boosting Emotional Intelligence

A person's "IQ"—or intelligence quotient—was once considered the leading predictor of achievement. However, psychologists have determined that another "way of knowing," dubbed **emotional intelligence,** makes an even greater difference in a person's personal and professional success.

"EQ" (for emotional quotient) is the ability to monitor and use emotions to guide thinking and actions. Strong social or interpersonal skills are one measure of EQ. As more than a decade of research has shown, people with high EQ are more productive at work and happier at home. They're also less prone to stress, depression, and anxiety and bounce back more quickly from serious illnesses.

According to recent research, females score slightly higher in emotional intelligence than males, but in both sexes, individuals who are outgoing, dependable, and independent-minded tend to have higher EQs.[3] Both sexes are equally capable of cultivating greater emotional intelligence. Emotional intelligence isn't fixed at birth, nor is it the same as intuition. Among the emotional competencies that most benefit students are focusing on clear, manageable goals and identifying and understanding emotions rather than relying on "gut" feelings.

emotional health The ability to express and acknowledge one's feelings and moods and exhibit adaptability and compassion for others.

mental health The ability to perceive reality as it is, respond to its challenges, and develop rational strategies for living.

culture The set of shared attitudes, values, goals, and practices of a group that are internalized by an individual within the group.

emotional intelligence A term used by some psychologists to evaluate the capacity of people to understand themselves and relate well with others.

Knowing Your Needs

Newborns are unable to survive on their own. They depend on others for the satisfaction of their physical needs for food, shelter, warmth, and protection, as well as their less tangible emotional needs. In growing to maturity, children take on more responsibility and become more independent. No one, however, becomes totally self-sufficient. As adults, we easily recognize our basic physical needs, but we often fail to acknowledge our emotional needs. Yet they, too, must be met if we are to be as fulfilled as possible.

The humanist theorist Abraham Maslow believed that human needs are the motivating factors in personality development. First, we must satisfy basic physiological needs, such as those for food, shelter, and sleep. Only then can we pursue fulfillment of our higher needs—for safety and security, love and affection, and self-esteem. Few individuals reach the state of **self-actualization**, in which one functions at the highest possible level and derives the greatest possible satisfaction from life (Figure 2.1). (See Making Change Happen, p. 44.)

Feeling the Power of Self-Esteem

Each of us wants and needs to feel significant as a human being with unique talents, abilities, and roles in life. A sense of **self-esteem,** of belief or pride in ourselves, gives us confidence to dare to attempt to achieve at school or work and to reach out to others to form friendships and close relationships. Self-esteem is the little voice that whispers, "You're worth it. You can do it. You're okay."

Health and wealth don't equal happiness. People with disabilities report almost the same level of life satisfaction as people who do not have disabilities.

© Altrendo Images/ Getty Images

Self-esteem is based not on external factors like wealth or beauty, but on what you believe about yourself. It's not something you're born with; self-esteem develops over time. It's also not something anyone else can give to you, although those around you can either help boost or diminish your self-esteem.

The seeds of self-esteem are planted in childhood when parents provide the assurance and appreciation youngsters need to push themselves toward new accomplishments: crawling, walking, forming words and sentences, learning control over their bladder and bowels.

Adults, too, must consider themselves worthy of love, friendship, and success if they are to be loved, to make friends, and to achieve their goals. Low self-esteem is more common in people who have been abused as children and in those with psychiatric disorders, including depression, anxiety, alcoholism, and drug dependence. Feeling a lack of love and encouragement as a child can also lead to poor self-esteem. Adults with poor self-esteem may unconsciously enter relationships that reinforce their self-perceptions and may prefer and even seek out people who think poorly of them.

One of the most useful techniques for bolstering self-esteem and achieving your goals is developing the habit of positive thinking and talking. While negative observations—such as constant criticisms or reminders of the most minor faults—can undermine self-image, positive affirmations—compliments, kudos, encouragements—have proved effective in enhancing self-esteem and psychological well-being. Individuals who fight off negative thoughts fare better psychologically than those who collapse when a setback occurs or who rely on others to make them feel better.

Self-esteem has proved to be one of the best predictors of college adjustment. Students with high self-esteem report better personal, emotional, social, and academic adjustment.

Pursuing Happiness

"Imagine a drug that causes you to live eight or nine years longer, to make $15,000 more a year, to be less likely to get divorced," says Martin Seligman, the "father" of positive

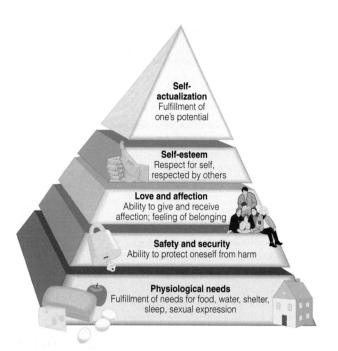

Figure 2.1 The Maslow Pyramid

To attain the highest level of psychological health, you must first satisfy your needs for safety and security, love and affection, and self-esteem.

Source: From A. Maslow, R. Frager (ed.), J. Fadiman (ed.), *Motivation and Personality*, 3rd ed., © 1987. Electronically reproduced by permission of Pearson Education, Inc., Upper Saddle River NJ.

psychology. "Happiness seems to be that drug."[4] But even if just about everyone might benefit by smiling more and scowling less, can almost anyone learn to live on the brighter side of life?

Skeptics who dismiss "happichondria" as the latest feel-good fad are dubious. (See Point/Counterpoint, p. 45.) "The notion that behavior modification can bring about true happiness is as bogus as can be," says psychiatrist Charles Goodstein, M.D., of New York University. "Happiness enhancement correlates with a sort of smug self-satisfaction because people think they're doing something real, but they're not."[5]

Happiness researchers, now backed by thousands of scientific studies, cite mounting evidence to the contrary. "Happiness is measurable, and it's buildable," says Seligman. "We're not talking about just feeling good but about something more substantial and durable. The newest finding of positive psychology is that simple, proven strategies can make you lastingly happier. However, it's not easy, and it's not obvious how to go about it."

As researchers and therapists agree, happiness is more than a smiley face. Rather

self-actualization A state of wellness and fulfillment that can be achieved once certain human needs are satisfied; living to one's full potential.

self-esteem Confidence and satisfaction in oneself.

Soul Food

There is more to you than intellect and passion, more than what resides between your ears or below your waist. Sometimes overshadowed by the speed and loud talk that surround you is the quieter, feeling part of you. Although immaterial, it is no less real. Tied to your spiritual self, it can be seen as your essence—what is always there and what is most essentially you.

If you feel you have been running too hard, need more down time, are close to burnout, or are in some way seeking to make better contact with your deeper self, "Soul Food" in *Labs for IPC* will help you provide the nourishment that your spirit needs. Here is a preview:

Get Real

To provide sound nutrition for the soul, you need to know what makes up such a diet. Here is the first step:

Assess your soul food diet.

For each of thirteen items, you will put a + (if you meet this daily requirement) or a – (if you don't) in the space provided. Here are three examples:

- **Movement:** _____

   You consciously and intentionally pay disciplined attention to the movement of your body, be it in some slow, mindful exercise like yoga or tai chi, or in dance, or in stretching or walking.

- **Being:** _____

   You set aside a time when you are not multitasking—or tasking at all. It is one thing to *do,* and there is much to do. It is another thing to focus on *being.* Being there, being you—not working, worrying, or calculating. In this sitting-on-the-stoop or front-porch mode, you attune yourself to being alive in the moment.

- **Creating:** _____

   You daily take time to express your creative nature through painting, drawing, writing, composing music, choreographing dance, solving a problem, cooking—the possibilities are inexhaustible.

If you did not mark a plus by many activities listed in the lab, your soul food diet is insufficient. Progressing through the stages of change by completing the lab will help you correct this. We guarantee you are going to love the results.

Get Ready

We know that as a college student you are busy. You may need to cut or trim activities or reclaim time that currently goes to activities that do not feed your deeper, quieter self. Start with this step:

- **Examine your schedule.** When are you going to fit in, on a daily basis, time for soul food? Will your schedule require fine-tuning?

Get Going

In this stage your task is to provide yourself with soul food by completing each of thirteen activities a minimum of four times per week. Here are three examples of the minimum dietary requirements for feeding your soul:

- Movement: 5 minutes
- Being: 10 minutes
- Creating: 10 minutes

Lock It In

It will take time and practice to lock in the habit of feeding your soul on a regular basis. This is why we offer the following advice:

- Regardless of how often you have or have not done the activities in this lab, most of them are likely to seem completely natural. But some may present a challenge. Do not be concerned about whether you are moving, being, creating, or doing any of the other activities correctly. Just relax . . .

---

than a superficial sense of glee, true happiness "has depth and deliberation to it," as one writer put it. "It encompasses living a meaningful life, utilizing your gifts and your time, living with thought and purpose. It's maximized when you also feel part of a community and when you confront annoyances and crises with grace. It involves a willingness to learn and stretch and grow, which sometimes involves discomfort. It requires acting on life, not merely taking it in. It's not joy, a temporary exhilaration, or even pleasure, that sensual rush—although

a steady supply of those feelings course through those who seize the day."[6]

Why pursue happiness? The answer goes beyond the psychological benefits. As a meta-analysis of long-term studies has shown, happiness reduces the risk of dying—both in healthy people and in those with diagnosed diseases. "Happiness is beneficial over and above the absence of misery," researchers have concluded. The reason may be that happiness induces changes in the brain or encourages stronger social connections.[7]

The Keys to Happiness Genetics, as research on thousands of sets of twins has demonstrated, accounts for about 50 percent of your happiness quotient and for related personality traits, such as extraversion and conscientiousness.[8] But even if you inherited the family frown rather than its joy genes, you're not fated to a life of gloom. Just don't pin your hopes on advantages like fitness, fortune, education, or good looks. The healthy, the wealthy, the bookish, and the beautiful report only somewhat greater happiness than those who are less blessed. Unless you're extremely poor or gravely ill, life circumstances account for only about 10 percent of happiness. The other 40 percent depends on what you do to make yourself happy.[9] (See Health on a Budget, p. 46.)

Unfortunately, most of us look for happiness in all the wrong places. We assume that external things—a bigger house, a better job, a winning lottery ticket—will gladden our lives. While they do bring temporary delight, the thrill invariably fades.

In one study, more than 150 older college students rated a recent purchase—either of an object or of a life experience—that they invested in to make themselves happy. Those who spent their money on a pleasurable experience reported feeling more alive and invigorated than those who bought material things. The reason, according to the researchers, is that life experiences bring people closer, satisfy a natural human need for connection, and create memories that can be savored again and again.[10]

"After 18 years studying happiness, I fell into the same trap as everyone else," says psychologist Sonja Lyubomirsky, Ph.D., author of *The How of Happiness: A Scientific Approach to Getting the Life You Want.* "I was so excited to get a new car, a hybrid I'd wanted for a long time, but within two months driving it became routine. Happiness is like weight loss. We all know how to take off a few pounds but the trick is maintaining it."[11]

In cutting-edge research, Lyubomirsky and her colleagues have fine-tuned proven strategies into practical prescriptions to enhance happiness. "Different methods are a better 'fit' for different people," she explains. "Keeping a daily gratitude journal

POINT COUNTERPOINT *"Learning" Happiness*

POINT
Happiness, the subject of countless articles, talk shows, and books, has morphed into a big business. Even colleges and universities are offering highly popular courses devoted to the quest for happiness and personal satisfaction. Positive psychologists argue that learning how to live a joyful, fulfilling life is as important, if not more so, than anything else in the undergraduate curriculum.

COUNTERPOINT
Some skeptics view the happiness bandwagon as a pop trend. Self-styled "joyologists" and laughter workshops, they contend, may amuse but have no significant impact on an individual's personality and outlook on life. Colleges should focus on educating students' minds, some argue, rather than trying to help them feel good about themselves and their lives.

YOUR VIEW
Do you think happiness can be taught and learned? Should colleges and universities offer courses in personal happiness and fulfillment? Would you enroll in such a class? Why or why not?

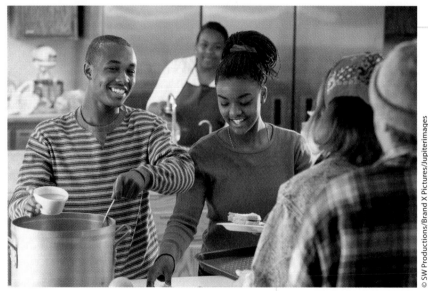

© SW Productions/Brand X Pictures/Jupiterimages

Volunteering to help others, like these students serving meals to the homeless, can contribute to a profound sense of life happiness.

seems hokey to some people, but writing a letter of gratitude may be very meaningful." Timing and "doses" also matter. Performing five acts of kindness on a single day, she's found, yields a greater halo effect than a single daily altruistic gesture. "But to sustain happiness you have to make the effort and commitment every day for the rest of your life," she emphasizes. For enduring joy, the key is looking beyond fleeting pleasures to the two pillars of "authentic" happiness: engagement with family, work, or a passionate pursuit and finding meaning from some higher purpose.

Happiness for Free!

Money can't buy happiness. As long as you have enough money to cover the basics, you don't need more wealth or more possessions for greater joy. Even people who win a fortune in a lottery return to their baseline of happiness within months. So rather than spending money on lottery tickets, try these ways to put a smile on your face:

- **Make time for yourself.** It's impossible to meet the needs of others without recognizing and fulfilling your own.
- **Invest yourself in closeness.** Give your loved ones the gift of your time and caring.
- **Work hard at what you like.** Search for challenges that satisfy your need to do something meaningful.
- **Be upbeat.** If you always look for what's wrong about yourself or your life, you'll find it—and feel even worse.
- **Organize but stay loose.** Be ready to seize an unexpected opportunity to try something different.

Education, intelligence, gender, and race do not matter much for happiness. African Americans and Hispanics have lower rates of depression than white Americans, but they do not report greater happiness. Neither gender is clearly happier, but in different studies women are both happier and sadder than men.

In a recent study of college students, possessions mattered less to their personal satisfaction than how much they valued them. "The American undergraduates who are happiest in this life are not necessarily those who amass great numbers of things," the researchers concluded. "Rather they are those who both have the things they want and want the things they have."[12]

In another survey of 222 college students, psychologists found that the "happiest" 10 percent, as determined by six different rating scales, shared one distinctive characteristic: a rich and fulfilling social life. Almost all were involved in a romantic relationship as well as in rewarding friendships. The happiest students spent the least time alone, and their friends rated them as highest on good relationships.

Even people we don't know may make us happy. By analyzing 20 years of data on the social ties of almost 5,000 participants in the Framingham Heart Study, researchers found that happy people spread happiness to others.[13] Spouses, neighbors, relatives, and friends benefit most, but so did more distant contacts. The more happy people you surround yourself with, the happier you—and your social network—are likely to be in the future.[14]

Becoming Optimistic

The dictionary defines **optimism** as "an inclination to anticipate the best possible outcome." For various reasons—because they believe in themselves, because they trust in a higher power, because they feel lucky—optimists expect positive experiences from life. When bad things happen, they tend to see setbacks or losses as specific, temporary incidents. In their eyes, a disappointment is "one of those things" that happens every once in a while, rather than the latest in a long string of disasters. And rather than blaming themselves ("I always mess things up," pessimists might say), optimists look at all the different factors that may have caused the problem.

Individuals aren't born optimistic or pessimistic; in fact, researchers have documented changes over time in the ways that individuals view the world and what they expect to experience in the future. The key is disputing the automatic negative thoughts that flood our brains and choosing to believe in our own possibilities.

Managing Your Moods

Feelings come and go within minutes. A **mood** is a more sustained emotional state that colors our view of the world for hours or days. According to surveys by psychologist Randy Larsen of the University of Michigan, bad moods descend upon us an average of three out of every ten days. "A few people—about 2 percent—are happy just about every day," he says. "About 5 percent report bad moods four out of every five days."[15]

 There are gender differences in mood management: Men typically try to distract themselves (a partially successful strategy) or use alcohol or drugs (an ineffective tactic). Women are more likely to talk to someone (which can help) or to ruminate on why they feel bad (which doesn't help). Learning effective mood-boosting, mood-regulating strategies can help both men and women pull themselves up and out of an emotional slump.

The most effective way to banish a sad or bad mood is by changing what caused it in the first place—if you can figure out what made you upset and why. "Most bad moods are caused by loss or failure in work or intimate relationships," says Larsen. "The questions to ask are: What can I do to fix the failure? What can I do to remedy the loss? Is there anything under my control that I can change? If there is, take action and solve it." Rewrite the report. Ask to take a makeup exam. Apologize to the friend whose feelings you hurt. Tell your parents you feel bad about the argument you had.

If there's nothing you can do, accept what happened and focus on doing things differently next time. "In our studies, resolving to try harder actually was as effective in improving mood as taking action in the present," says Larsen. You also can try to think about what happened in a different way and put a positive spin on it. This technique, known as *cognitive reappraisal, or reframing,* helps you look at a setback in a new light: What lessons did it teach you? What would you have done differently? Could there be a silver lining or hidden benefit?

If you can't identify or resolve the problem responsible for your emotional funk, the next-best solution is to concentrate on altering your negative feelings. For example, try setting a quick, achievable goal that can boost your spirits with a small success. Clean out a drawer; sort through the piles of paper on your desk; send an e-mail or text message to an old friend.

Another good option is to get moving. In studies of mood regulation, exercise consistently ranks as the single most effective strategy for banishing bad feelings. Numerous studies have confirmed that aerobic workouts, such as walking or jogging, significantly improve mood. Even nonaerobic exercise, such as weight lifting, can boost

©Robert W. Ginn/PhotoEdit

You may not have complete control over your destiny, but you can control how you respond to challenges.

spirits; improve sleep and appetite; reduce anxiety, irritability, and anger; and produce feelings of mastery and accomplishment.

Looking on the Light Side

Humor, which enables us to express fears and negative feelings without causing distress to ourselves or others, is one of the healthiest ways of coping with life's ups and downs. Laughter stimulates the heart, alters brain wave patterns and breathing rhythms, reduces perceptions of pain, decreases stress-related hormones, and strengthens the immune system. In psychotherapy, humor helps channel negative emotions toward a positive effect. Even in cases of critical or fatal illnesses, humor can relieve pain and help people live with greater joy until they die.

Joking and laughing are ways of expressing honest emotions, of overcoming dread and doubt, and of connecting with others. They also can defuse rage. After all, it's almost impossible to stay angry when you're laughing. To tickle your funny bone, try keeping a file of favorite cartoons or jokes. Go to a comedy club instead of a movie. If you get an e-mail joke that makes you laugh out loud, don't keep it to yourself—multiply the mirth by sharing it with a friend.

optimism The tendency to seek out, remember, and expect pleasurable experiences.

mood A sustained emotional state that colors one's view of the world for hours or days.

Feeling in Control

Although no one has absolute control over destiny, we can do a great deal to control how we think, feel, and behave. By assessing our life situations realistically, we can make plans and preparations that allow us to make the most of our circumstances. By doing so, we gain a sense of mastery. In nationwide surveys, Americans who feel in control of their lives report greater psychological well-being than those who do not, as well as extraordinarily positive feelings of happiness.

Developing Autonomy

One goal that many people strive for is **autonomy,** or independence. Both family and society influence our ability to grow toward independence. Autonomous individuals are true to themselves. As they weigh the pros and cons of any decision, whether it's using or refusing drugs or choosing a major or career, they base their judgment on their own values, not those of others. Their ability to draw on internal resources and cope with challenges has a positive impact on both their psychological well-being and their physical health, including recovery from illness.

Those who've achieved autonomy may seek the opinions of others, but they do not allow their decisions to be dictated by external influences. For autonomous individuals, their **locus of control**—that is, where they view control as originating—is *internal* (from within themselves) rather than *external* (from others). (See Chapter 1.)

Asserting Yourself

Being **assertive** means recognizing your feelings and making your needs and desires clear to others. Unlike aggression, a far less healthy means of expression, assertiveness usually works. You can change a situation you don't like by communicating your feelings and thoughts in nonprovocative words, by focusing on specifics, and by making sure you're talking with the person who is directly responsible.

Becoming assertive isn't always easy. Many people have learned to cope by being passive and not communicating their feelings or opinions. Sooner or later they become so irritated, frustrated, or overwhelmed that they explode in an outburst—which they think of as being assertive. However, such behavior is so distasteful to them that they'd rather be passive. But assertiveness doesn't mean screaming or telling someone off. You can communicate your wishes calmly and clearly. Assertiveness is a behavior that respects your rights and the rights of other people even when you disagree.

Even at its mildest, assertiveness can make you feel better about yourself and your life. The reason: When you speak up or take action, you're in the pilot seat. And that's always much less stressful than taking a backseat and trying to hang on for dear life.

Connecting with Others

 At every age, people who feel connected to others tend to be healthier physically and psychologically. This is certainly true in college when young adults, often living independently for the first time, need to form new relationships—and not just online. (See Chapter 8 for a discussion of social networking and virtual communities.) In a study at a large Midwestern university, the students—particularly the women—who felt the greatest sense of belonging reported fewer physical symptoms than those who had not forged close friendships.

Giving and getting support from others is fundamental to good psychological health and emotional well-being.

© iStockphoto.com/Aldo Murillo

The research also revealed a gender difference: Female students seek out, forge, and maintain more supportive ties than men, rely on friends more in times of stress, and provide more support than men.

The opposite of *connectedness* is **social isolation**, a major risk factor for illness and early death. Individuals with few social contacts face two to four times the mortality rate of others. The reason may be that their social isolation weakens the body's ability to ward off disease. Medical students with higher-than-average scores on a loneliness scale had lower levels of protective immune cells. The end of a long-term relationship—through separation, divorce, or death—also dampens immunity.

It is part of our nature as mammals and as human beings to crave relationships. But invariably we end up alone at times. Solitude is not without its own quiet joys—time for introspection, self-assessment, learning from the past, and looking toward the future. Each of us can cultivate the joy of our own company, of being alone without crossing the line and becoming lonely.

Overcoming Loneliness

More so than many other countries, ours is a nation of loners. Recent trends—longer work hours, busy family schedules, frequent moves, high divorce rates—have created even more lonely people. Only about a quarter of Americans say they're never lonely. Loneliest of all are those who are divorced, separated, or widowed and those who live alone or solely with children. Loneliness is most likely to cause emotional distress when it is chronic rather than episodic.

To combat loneliness, people may join groups, fling themselves into projects and activities, or surround themselves with superficial acquaintances. Others avoid the effort of trying to connect, sometimes limiting most of their personal interactions to chat groups on the Internet.

The true keys to overcoming loneliness are developing resources to fulfill our own potential and learning to reach out to others. In this way, loneliness can become a means to personal growth and discovery.

Facing Shyness and Social Anxiety

Many people are uncomfortable meeting strangers or speaking or performing in public. In some surveys, as many as 40 percent of people describe themselves as shy or socially anxious. Some shy people—an estimated 10 to 15 percent of children—are born with a predisposition to shyness. Others become shy because they don't learn proper social responses or because they experience rejection or shame.

Some people are "fearfully" shy; that is, they withdraw and avoid contact with others and experience a high degree of anxiety and fear in social situations. Others are "self-consciously" shy. They enjoy the company of others but become highly self-aware and anxious in social situations.

 In studies of college students, men have reported somewhat more shyness than women. Students may develop symptoms of shyness or social anxiety when they go to a party or are called on in class. Some experience symptoms when they try to perform any sort of action in the presence of others, even such everyday activities as eating in public, using a public restroom, or writing a check.

About 7 percent of the population could be diagnosed with a severe form of social anxiety, called **social phobia,** in which individuals typically fear and avoid various social situations. Childhood shyness, as reported by parents, and chronic illness increase the likelihood of this problem. Adolescents and young adults with severe social anxiety are at increased risk of major depression.

autonomy The ability to draw on internal resources; independence from familial and societal influences.

locus of control An individual's belief about the sources of power and influence over his or her life.

assertive Behaving in a confident manner to make your needs and desires clear to others in a nonhostile way.

social isolation A feeling of unconnectedness with others caused by and reinforced by infrequency of social contacts.

social phobia A severe form of social anxiety marked by extreme fears and avoidance of social situations.

Phobias are discussed later in this chapter. The key difference between these problems and normal shyness and self-consciousness is the degree of distress and impairment that individuals experience.

If you're shy, you can overcome much of your social apprehensiveness on your own, in much the same way as you might set out to stop smoking or lose weight. For example, you can improve your social skills by pushing yourself to introduce yourself to a stranger at a party or to chat about the weather or the food selections with the person next to you in a cafeteria line. Gradually, you'll acquire a sense of social timing and a verbal ease that will take the worry out of close encounters with others. Those with more disabling social anxiety may do best with psychotherapy and medication, which have proved highly effective.

Loving and Being Loved

"One can live magnificently in this world if one knows how to work and how to love, to work for the person one loves and to love one's work," Leo Tolstoy wrote. You may not think of love as a basic need like food and rest, but it is essential for both physical and psychological well-being.

Mounting evidence suggests that people who lack love and commitment are at high risk for a host of illnesses, including infections, heart disease, and cancer. "Love and intimacy are at the root of what makes us sick and what makes us well," says cardiologist Dean Ornish, author of *Love & Survival: The Scientific Basis for the Healing Power of Intimacy*. "No other factor in medicine—not diet, not smoking, not exercise—has a greater impact." (See Chapter 8 for more on relationships.)[16]

Spiritual Health

Whatever your faith, whether or not you belong to any formal religion, you are more than a body of a certain height and weight occupying space on the planet. You have a mind that equips you to learn and question. And you have a spirit that animates everything you say and do. **Spiritual health** refers to this breath of life and to our ability to identify our basic purpose in life and to experience the fulfillment of achieving our full potential. Spiritual readings or practices can increase calmness, inner strength, and meaning; improve self-awareness; and enhance your sense of well-being. Religious support has also been shown to help lower depression and increase life satisfaction beyond the benefits of social support from friends and family.

Spirituality is a belief in what some call a higher power, in someone or something that transcends the boundaries of self. It gives rise to a strong sense of purpose, values, morals, and ethics. Throughout life you make choices and decide to behave in one way rather than another because your spirituality serves as both a compass and a guide.

The term *religiosity* refers to various spiritual practices. That definition may seem vague, but one thing is clear. According to thousands of studies on the relationship between religious beliefs and practices and health, religious individuals are less depressed, less anxious, and better able to cope with crises such as illness or divorce than are nonreligious ones. The more that a believer incorporates spiritual practices—such as prayer, meditation, or attending services—into daily life, the greater his or her sense of satisfaction with life.

Spirituality and Physical Health

A growing body of scientific evidence indicates that faith and spirituality can enhance health—and perhaps even extend life. Individuals who pray and report greater spiritual well-being consistently describe themselves as enjoying greater psychological and overall well-being.[17]

Church attendance may account for an additional two to three years of life (by comparison, exercise may add three to five extra years), according to researchers' calculations. According to data on nearly

95,000 participants in the landmark Women's Health Initiative, attending a weekly church service, regardless of an individual's faith, lowers the risk of death by 20 percent, compared with those who don't attend at all. Attending less frequently also reduces the risk, but by a smaller percentage. How does going to church add years to a life? Researchers speculate that the reason may be the sense of community or support or that people feel less depressed when they join in religious services.[18]

Prayer and other religious experiences, including meditation, may actually change the brain—for the better. Using neuroimaging techniques, scientists have documented alterations in various parts of the brain that are associated with stress and anxiety. This effect may slow down the aging process, reduce psychological symptoms, and increase feelings of security, compassion, and love.[19]

Deepening Spiritual Intelligence

Mental health professionals have recognized the power of **spiritual intelligence,** which some define as "the capacity to sense, understand, and tap into the highest parts of ourselves, others, and the world around us." Spiritual intelligence, unlike spirituality, does not center on the worship of a God above, but on the discovery of a wisdom within.

All of us are born with the potential to develop spiritual intelligence, but most of us aren't even aware of it—and do little or nothing to nurture it. Part of the reason is that we confuse spiritual intelligence with religion, dogma, or old-fashioned morality. "You don't have to go to church to be spiritually intelligent; you don't even have to believe in God," says Reverend Paul Edwards, a retired Episcopalian minister and therapist in Fullerton, California. "It is a scientific fact that when you are feeling secure, at peace, loved, and happy, you see, hear, and act differently than when you're feeling insecure, unhappy, and unloved. Spiritual intelligence allows you to use the wisdom you have when you're in a state of inner peace. And you get there by changing the way you think, basically by listening less to what's in your head and more to what's in your heart."[20]

Clarifying Your Values

Your **values** are the criteria by which you evaluate things, people, events, and yourself; they represent what's most important to you. In a world of almost dizzying complexity, values can provide guidelines for making decisions that are right for you. If understood and applied, they help give life meaning and structure.

There can be a large discrepancy between what people say they value and what their actions indicate about their values. That's why it's important to clarify your own values, making sure you understand what you believe so that you can live in accordance with your beliefs.

When you confront a situation in which you must choose different paths or behaviors, follow these steps:

1. Carefully consider the consequences of each choice.
2. Choose freely from among all the options.
3. Publicly affirm your values by sharing them with others.
4. Act out your values.

Values clarification is not a once-in-a-lifetime task, but an ongoing process of sorting out what matters most to you. If you believe in protecting the environment, do you shut off lights, or walk rather than drive, in order to conserve energy? Do you vote for political candidates who support environmental protection? Do you recycle newspapers, bottles, and cans? Values are more than ideals we'd like to attain; they should be reflected in the way we live day by day.

Enriching Your Spiritual Life

Do you attend religious services? Pray or meditate on a weekly basis? In a national survey, a majority of the members of the Class of 2011 answered yes: Eight in ten went to religious services frequently or occasionally, while a third prayed or meditated every week. These percentages are somewhat lower than in the past, but a growing number of students report frequent discussions of religion.

Whatever role religion plays in your life, you have the capacity for deep, meaningful

Prayer, a spiritual practice of millions, is the most widely used form of complementary and alternative medicine.

spiritual health The ability to identify one's basic purpose in life and to achieve one's full potential.

spirituality A belief in someone or something that transcends the boundaries of self.

spiritual intelligence The capacity to sense, understand, and tap into ourselves, others, and the world around us.

values The criteria by which one makes choices about one's thoughts, actions, goals, and ideals.

- Take the tombstone test: What would you like to have written on your tombstone? In other words, how would you like to be remembered? Your honest answer should tell you, very succinctly, what you value most.

- Describe yourself, as you are today, in a brief sentence. Ask friends or family members for their descriptions of you. How would you have to change to become the person you want to be remembered as?

- Try the adjective test: Choose three adjectives that you'd like to see associated with your reputation. Then list what you've done or can do to earn such descriptions.

spiritual experiences that can add great meaning to everyday existence. You don't need to enroll in theology classes or commit to a certain religious preference. The following simple steps can start you on an inner journey to a new level of understanding:

- **Sit quietly.** The process of cultivating spiritual intelligence begins in solitude and silence. "There is an inner wisdom," says Dr. Dean Ornish, the pioneering cardiologist who incorporates spiritual health into his mind-body therapies, "but it speaks very, very softly." To tune into its whisper, you have to turn down the volume in your busy, noisy, complicated life and force yourself to do nothing at all. This may sound easy; it's anything but.

    Start small. Create islands of silence in your day. Don't reach for the radio dial as soon as you get in the car. Leave your earpods on as you walk across campus but turn off the music. Shut the door to your room, take a few huge deep breaths, and let them out very, very slowly. Don't worry if you're too busy to carve out half an hour for quiet contemplation. Even ten minutes every day can make a difference.

- **Step outside.** For many people, nature sets their spirit free. Being outdoors, walking by the ocean, or looking at the hills gives us a sense of timelessness and puts the little hassles of daily living into perspective. As you wait for the bus or for a traffic light to change, let your gaze linger on silvery ice glazing a branch or an azalea bush in wild bloom. Follow the flight of a bird; watch clouds float overhead. Gaze into the night sky and think of the stars as holes in the darkness letting the light of heaven shine through.

- **Use activity to tune into your spirit.** Spirituality exists in every cell of the body, not just in the brain. As a student, mental labor takes up much of your day. To tap into your spirit, try a less cerebral activity, such as singing, chanting, dancing, or drumming. Alternative ways of quieting your mind and tuning into your spirit include gardening, walking, arranging flowers, listening to music

that touches your soul, or immersing yourself in a simple process like preparing a meal.

- **Ask questions of yourself.** Some people use their contemplative time to focus on a line of scripture or poetry. Others ask open-ended questions, such as What am I feeling? What are my choices? Where am I heading? Dr. Ornish ends his own daily meditations by asking, "What am I not paying attention to that's important?"

    In her meditations, one minister often paints a lush scene with a golden meadow, a shade tree, and a gentle brook and invites the divine spirit to enter. "Rarely do I get an immediate answer or solution, but later that day something may happen—often just a random conversation—-and I suddenly find myself thinking about a problem from a perspective I never considered before."

- **Trust your spirit.** While most of us rely on gut feelings to alert us to danger, our inner spirit usually nudges us, not away from, but toward some action that will somehow lead to a greater good—even if we can't see it at the time. You may suddenly feel the urge to call or e-mail a friend you've lost touch with—only to discover that he just lost a loved one and needed the comfort of your caring. If you ignore such silent signals, you may look back and regret the consequences. Pay a little more attention the next time you feel an unexpected need to say or do something for someone.

- **Develop a spiritual practice.**

    - **If you are religious:** Deepen your spiritual commitment through prayer, more frequent church attendance, or joining a prayer group.

    - **If you are not religious:** Keep an open mind about the value of religion or spirituality. Consider visiting a church or synagogue. Read the writings of inspired people of deep faith, such as Rabbi Harold Kushner and Rev. Martin Luther King, Jr.

    - **If you are not ready to consider religion:** Try nonreligious meditation or relaxation training. Research has shown that focusing the mind on a single sound or image can slow heart rate, respiration, and brain waves; relax muscles; and lower stress-related hormones—responses similar to those induced by prayer.

Praying

Prayer, a spiritual practice of millions, is the most commonly used form of complementary and alternative medicine. However, only in recent years has science launched rigorous investigations of the healing power of prayer.

Petitionary prayer—praying directly to a higher power—affects both the quality and quantity of life, says Dr. Harold Koenig, director of Duke University's Center for the Study of Religion/Spirituality and Health. "It boosts morale; lowers agitation, loneliness, and life dissatisfaction; and enhances ability to cope in men, women, the elderly, the young, the healthy, and the sick."[21]

People who pray regularly have significantly lower blood pressure and stronger immune systems than the less religious, says Dr. Koenig. They're also less prone to alcoholism and less likely to smoke heavily, and are hospitalized less often. Science cannot explain the physiological mechanisms for what happens in human beings when they pray, but in cultures around the world throughout recorded history when people or their loved ones are sick, they pray.

Some scientists speculate that prayer may foster a state of peace and calm that could lead to beneficial changes in the cardiovascular and immune systems. Sophisticated brain imaging techniques have shown that prayer and meditation cause changes in blood flow in particular regions of the brain that may lead to lower blood pressure, slower heart rate, decreased anxiety, and an enhanced sense of well-being. Membership in a faith community provides an identity as well as support, although individuals vary in their religious practices and observances.

In recent research, praying for others has not improved their symptoms or recovery. In a study of patients undergoing heart procedures, prayers (whether by Christian, Muslim, Jewish, or Buddhist groups) and other complementary bedside therapies,

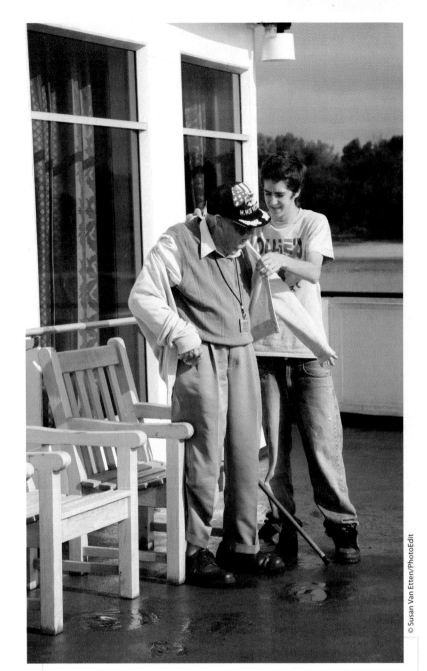

Helping or giving to others enhances self-esteem, relieves stress, and protects psychological well-being.

such as imaging and therapeutic touching, did not measurably improve their outcome.

Will science ever be able to prove the power of prayer? No one is certain. "While I personally believe that God heals people in supernatural ways, I don't think science can shape a study to prove it," says Duke's Dr. Koenig. "But we now know enough, based on solid scientific research, to recommend prayer, much like exercise and diet, as one of the best and most cost-effective ways of protecting and enhancing health."

- Compose an apology letter. Address it to yourself, and write it from someone who's hurt you. This simple task enables you to get a new perspective on a painful experience.
- Leap forward in time. In a visualization exercise imagine that you are very old, meet a person who hurt you long ago, and sit down together on a park bench on a beautiful spring day. You both talk until everything that needs to be said finally is. This allows you to benefit from the perspective time brings without having to wait for years to achieve it.
- Talk with "safe" people. Vent your anger or disappointment with a trusted friend or a counselor without the danger of saying or doing anything you'll regret later. And if you can laugh about what happened with a friend, the laughter helps dissolve the rage.
- Forgive the person, not the deed. In themselves, abuse, rape, murder, or betrayal are beyond forgiveness. But you can forgive people who couldn't manage to handle their own suffering, misery, confusion, and desperation.

Expressing Gratitude

A grateful spirit brightens mood, boosts energy, and infuses daily living with a sense of glad abundance. Although giving thanks is an ancient virtue, only recently have researchers focused on the "trait" of gratitude—appreciation, not just for a special gift, but for everything that makes life a bit better.

"Gratitude is an emotional and intellectual phenomenon that rises out of recognition that someone has treated you benevolently," says psychologist Michael McCullough of Southern Methodist University, a pioneer in gratitude research. "It's not feeling happy because something good happens, but realizing that someone who didn't have to deliberately did something of value to you."[22]

Since gratitude is not just a feeling but a mental outlook, we can consciously become more grateful—with practice. "Volunteers on college campuses who are asked to list things they're grateful for every day report more positive feelings," says McCullough. "They have more energy. They sleep better. They feel richer, regardless of how much money they have. Even their families notice visible, positive changes." For ways to help your gratitude grow, see "Grateful Thread" in *Labs for IPC*.

Forgiving

While "I forgive you" may be three of the most difficult words to say, they are also three of the most powerful—and the most beneficial for the body as well as the soul. Being angry, harboring resentments, or reliving hurts over and over again is bad for your health in general and your heart in particular. The word *forgive* comes from the Greek for letting go, and that's what happens when you forgive: You let go of all the anger and pain that have been demanding your time and wasting your energy.

To some people, forgiveness seems a sign of weakness or submission. People may feel more in control, more powerful, when they're filled with anger, but forgiving instills a much greater sense of power.

When you forgive, you reclaim your power to choose. It doesn't matter whether someone deserves to be forgiven; you deserve to be free. However, forgiveness isn't easy. It's not a one-time thing but a process that takes a lot of time and work. Most people pass through several stages in their journey to forgiveness. The initial response may involve anger, sadness, shame, or other negative feelings. Later, there's a reevaluation of what happened, then reframing to try to make sense of it or to take mitigating circumstances into account. This may lead to a reduction in negative feelings, especially if the initial hurt turns out to be accidental rather than intentional.

Doing Good

Altruism—helping or giving to others—enhances self-esteem, relieves physical and mental stress, and protects psychological well-being.[23] Hans Selye, the father of stress research, described cooperation with others for the self's sake as altruistic egotism, whereby we satisfy our own needs while helping others satisfy theirs. This concept is essentially an updated version of the golden rule: Do unto others as you would have them do unto you. The important difference is that you earn your neighbor's love and help by offering him or her love and help. (See the Community Focus features such as the one on page 55 and throughout this text for ideas on how to put your good intention into action.)

Volunteerism helps those who give as well as those who receive. People involved in community organizations, for instance, consistently report a surge of well-being called *helper's high*, which they describe as a unique sense of calmness, warmth, and enhanced self-worth. College students who provided community service as part of a semester-long course reported changes in attitude (including a decreased tendency to blame people for their misfortunes), self-esteem (primarily a belief that they can make a difference), and behavior (a greater commitment to do more volunteer work).

Sleepless on Campus

You stay up late cramming for a final. You drive through the night to visit a friend at another campus. You get up for an early class during the week but stay in bed until noon on weekends. And you wonder: "Why am I so tired?" The answer: You're not getting enough sleep.

You're hardly alone. In the course of a year, 30 to 40 percent of the population suffers symptoms of insomnia.[24] The cumulative long-term effects of sleep loss and sleep disorders include an increased risk of hypertension, diabetes, obesity, depression, heart attack, and stroke. Drowsy drivers are responsible for almost 20 percent of all serious car crash injuries.

 Sleep problems start young. Nearly one-half of adolescents sleep less than eight hours on school nights; more than half report feeling sleepy during the day.[25] College students are notorious for staying up late to study and socialize during the week and sleeping in on weekends. Only 11 percent of college students report good quality sleep, while 30 percent suffer chronic sleep difficulties.

COMMUNITY FOCUS *Volunteering on Campus*

PROBLEM High school students often volunteer because they're required to do so or they know that community service adds value to their college applications. Volunteering is voluntary in college, although federal officials are considering offering tuition breaks of up to $4,000 for college students who perform 100 hours of community service. But even without that financial incentive, volunteering provides the opportunity to do good for your community and feel good about yourself. How can you get started?

BECOME INFORMED

- Look around campus bulletin boards, newspapers, posters, and websites to learn more about groups looking for volunteers. Think through which would be a good match for your interests and skills.
- Go into the community to see what the needs are. Do children at a shelter need tutoring? Is the library looking for volunteer readers? Would an assisted living center want someone to take elderly residents for walks or to local gardens or museums?
- Websites such as Volunteer Match (**http://www.volunteeringinameria.gov/**) provide listings of volunteer opportunities in every zip code. You can find other sites on social networks such as Facebook, MySpace, and ning.
- Find out about extended and international volunteer opportunities. Through groups such as International Student Volunteers, **http://www.isvonline.com/**, you can join with others to save endangered species or restore forest habitats around the world.

BECOME INVOLVED

- Evaluate your schedule and current commitments. Be realistic in assessing how much time you have available to give to others. If you have only an hour or two a week, that's enough to serve a meal at a center for the homeless or read to children at a library.
- Organize your friends. If your campus is sponsoring a beach clean-up or your community is organizing a diabetes research walkathon, get your friends to join with you to make an even bigger difference— and have more fun!
- If you attend a church regularly, ask about its volunteer programs. Even singing in the choir is a way of giving of yourself and contributing to the congregation.
- If you're interested in health, volunteer to assist at screening days on campus or in the community. Check the schedule of upcoming local events sponsored by groups such as the American Cancer Society, American Heart Association, and American Lung Association.
- Check out programs like AmeriCorps and the Peace Corps as post-graduation options. You'll learn a lot about life, the world, and yourself while providing help to people who need it most.

altruism Acts of helping or giving to others without thought of self-benefit.

On average college students go to bed 1 to 2 hours later and sleep 1 to 1.6 hours less than students of a generation ago. When compared to exhaustion levels reported by workers in various occupations, college students score extremely high.

In one study, about 60 percent of the undergraduates surveyed had pulled at least one all-nighter in college. Those who had done so typically felt more energetic in the evening than in the morning, went to bed later (by an average of 40 minutes), and had somewhat lower (0.2) grade point averages (GPAs) than the others.[26]

Fortunately, college students can learn to sleep better. In an experiment with introductory psychology students—mostly freshmen—those who learned basic sleep skills significantly improved their overall sleep quality compared with students who did not receive such training.

In a study of 200 college students, those who learned how to play a video game in the morning or evening performed better the next day after a night's rest, apparently because their brains were actively absorbing what they'd learned as they slept. The researchers' conclusion: "People who are pulling all-nighters are not doing themselves a favor."[27]

In another recent study undergraduates who recorded their sleep times and learned the basics of good sleep hygiene increased their average sleep by over 50 minutes per night.[28] Commonsense steps, such as cutting back on caffeine, can make a difference. In a recent study, abstaining from caffeine all day improved the participants' quality of sleep, while those who drank decaffeinated coffee had less trouble falling asleep.[29]

Sleep's Impact on Health

Sleep is essential for functioning at your best—physically and psychologically. The following are some of the key ways in which your nighttime sleep affects your daytime well-being.

- **Learning and memory.** When you sleep, your brain helps "consolidate" new information so you are more likely to retain it in your memory.
- **Metabolism and weight.** The less you sleep, the more weight you may gain. Chronic sleep deprivation may cause weight gain by altering metabolism (for example, changing the way individuals process and store carbohydrates) and by stimulating excess stress hormones. Loss of sleep also reduces levels of the hormones that regulate appetite (discussed in Chapter 7), which may encourage eating.
- **Safety.** People who don't get adequate nighttime sleep are more likely to fall asleep during the daytime. Daytime sleepiness can cause falls, medical errors, air traffic mishaps, and road accidents.
- **Mood/quality of life.** Too little sleep—whether just for a night or two or for longer periods—can cause psychological symptoms, such as irritability, impatience, inability to concentrate, moodiness, and lowered long-term life satisfaction.[30] Poor sleep also affects motivation and ability to work effectively. Growing evidence suggests that disturbed sleep is associated with increased risk of psychiatric disorders.
- **Life satisfaction.** Sleep-deprived university students score lower on life-satisfaction scales. Students who get eight hours of sleep but shift their sleep schedules by as little as two hours suffer more depressive symptoms, lower sociability, and more frequent attention and concentration problems. They even get lower grades.
- **Cardiovascular health.** In a five-year study of middle-aged men and women, an extra hour of shut-eye was linked with healthier arteries and less build-up of calcium.[31] Serious sleep disorders such as insomnia and sleep apnea have been linked to hypertension, increased stress hormone levels, irregular heartbeats, and increased inflammation (which, as discussed in Chapter 14, may play a role in heart attacks).
- **Immunity/cancer prevention.** If you get less than seven hours of sleep a night, you're three times more likely to catch a cold. And if you sleep poorly, you're five times more susceptible.[32] Sleep deprivation alters immune function, including the activity of the body's killer cells. For example, inadequate sleep at the time of a flu vaccination can

reduce the production of flu-fighting antibodies. Keeping up with sleep may also help fight cancer. Harvard researchers have shown that women who work at night are at increased risk for breast and colon cancer, possibly because light at night alters production of melatonin, a hormone that helps put us to sleep.[33]

What Happens When We Sleep?

A normal night of sleep consists of several distinct stages of sleep, divided into two major types: an active state, characterized by **rapid eye movement (REM)** and called **REM sleep** (or dream sleep), and a quiet state, referred to as non-REM or NREM sleep, that consists of four stages:

- **In Stage 1,** a twilight zone between full wakefulness and sleep, the brain produces small, irregular, rapid electrical waves. The muscles of the body relax, and breathing is smooth and even.

- **In Stage 2,** brain waves are larger and punctuated with occasional sudden bursts of electrical activity. The eyes are no longer responsive to light. Bodily functions slow still more.

- **Stages 3 and 4** constitute the most profound state of unconsciousness. The brain produces slower, larger waves, and this is sometimes referred to as "delta" or slow-wave sleep (Figure 2.2).

After about an hour in the four stages of non-REM sleep, sleepers enter the time of vivid dreaming called REM sleep, when brain waves resemble those of waking more than those of quiet sleep. The large muscles of the torso, arms, and legs are paralyzed and cannot move—possibly to prevent sleepers from acting out their dreams. The fingers and toes may twitch; breathing is quick and shallow; blood flow through the brain speeds up; men may have partial or full erections.

Sleep Disorders

Three of four Americans struggle to get a good night's sleep at least a few nights a week. According to the National Commission on Sleep Disorders Research, 40 million adults suffer from a specific sleep disorder, such as chronic insomnia or sleep apnea; an additional 20 to 30 million have occasional sleep difficulties. The estimated economic

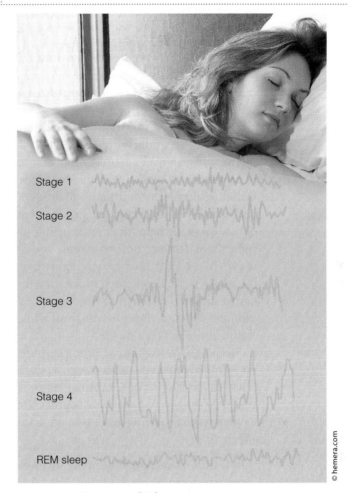

Figure 2.2 Stages of Sleep
Differences in brain wave patterns characterize the various stages of sleep.

cost of sleeplessness may be higher than $300 million a year.[34]

Insomnia Individuals with insomnia—a lack of sleep so severe that it interferes with functioning during the day—may toss and turn for an hour or more when they get into bed, wake frequently in the night, wake up too early, or not be able to sleep long enough to feel alert and energetic the next day. Most often insomnia is transient, typically occurring before or after a major life event (such as a job interview) and lasting for three or four nights. During periods of prolonged stress (such as a marriage breakup), short-term insomnia may continue for several weeks. Chronic or long-term insomnia,

rapid eye movement (REM) sleep
Regularly occurring periods of sleep during which the most active dreaming takes place.

PART 2: *Just the Facts*
- *Young adults need about* **8 to 8.5 hours** *of sleep a night.*
- *College students average about* **6 to 6.98 hours** *a night.*
- **30 percent** *of college students report chronic sleep problems.*

Source: Sleep: "Snooze or Lose," University of Michigan Health Service, www.uhs.umich.edu/wellness/other/sleep.html.

which can begin at any age, may persist for long periods. About three-fourths of insomniacs struggle to sleep more for at least a year; almost half, for three years.[35]

For about a third of those with chronic insomnia, the underlying problem is a mental disorder, most often depression or an anxiety disorder. Many substances, including alcohol, medications, and drugs of abuse, often disrupt sleep. About 15 percent of those seeking help for chronic insomnia suffer from "learned" or "behavioral" insomnia. While a life crisis may trigger their initial sleep problems, each night they try harder and harder to get to sleep, but they cannot—although they often doze off while reading or watching a movie.

Sleeping pills may be used for a specific, time-limited problem—always with a physician's supervision. (See Consumer Alert, p. 59.) In the long term, behavioral approaches, including the following, have proved more effective:

- **Relaxation therapy,** which may involve progressive muscle relaxation, diaphragmatic breathing, hypnosis, or meditation.

- **Cognitive therapy,** which challenges misconceptions about sleep and helps shift a poor sleeper's mind away from anxiety-inducing thoughts.

- **Stimulus control therapy,** in which individuals who do not fall asleep quickly must get up and leave their beds until they are very sleepy.

- **Sleep restriction therapy,** in which sleep times are sharply curtailed in order to improve the quality of sleep.

Breathing Disorders (Snoring and Sleep Apnea)
Although most people snore in certain positions or when they have stuffed-up noses, snoring can be a sign of a serious problem. Caused by the vibration in tissues in the mouth and throat as a sleeper tries to suck air into the lungs, snoring can be so loud that it disrupts a bed partner or others in the same house. In young people, the cause is most likely to be enlarged tonsils or adenoids. In adults, extreme snoring may be a symptom of sleep apnea, which may itself be harmful to health.

Translated from the Greek words meaning "no" and "breath," apnea is exactly that: the absence of breathing for a brief period. People with sleep apnea may briefly stop breathing dozens or even hundreds of times during the night. As they struggle for breath, they may gasp for air, snore extremely loudly, or thrash about.

Although apnea, which can lead to high blood pressure, stroke, and heart attack, may affect as many as 10 million Americans, most are unaware of the problem. More physical activity and fewer hours sitting can lead to improvements.[36] Effective treatments include weight loss (if obesity is contributing to the problem), a nasal mask that provides continuous positive airway pressure (CPAP) to ensure a steady flow of air into the lungs and, in severe cases, surgery to enlarge the upper airway.

Movement Disorders
Restless legs syndrome, which may affect 12 million Americans, is a movement disorder characterized by symptoms that patients describe as pulling, burning, tingling, creepy-crawly, grabbing, buzzing, jitteriness, or gnawing. Many people with these symptoms have difficulty falling or staying asleep but do not realize that the cause is a medical disorder that can be treated with regular physical activity.[37] Medications also are available.

Circadian Rhythm Sleep Disorders
Problems involving the timing of sleep are called circadian rhythm disorders because they affect the basic circadian ("about a day") rhythm that influences many biological processes. The most common causes are jet lag and shift work. Jet lag generally improves on its own within two to seven days, depending on the length of the trip and the individual's response. Avoiding caffeine and alcohol and immediately switching to the new time zone's schedule can help in overcoming jet lag.

A "shift work" circadian rhythm disorder consists of any inability to sleep when one wants or to stay alert when needed because of frequently changing work shifts. Behavioral strategies and good sleep habits can help. In addition, phototherapy—exposure to bright light for periods ranging from 30 minutes to two hours—has shown promise as an experimental treatment to help shift workers adjust to their changing schedules.

How Much Sleep Do You Need?

Over the last century, we have cut our average nightly sleep time by 20 percent. More than half of us try to get by with less than seven hours of shut-eye a night. College students are no exception, with an average sleep time slightly less than seven hours, with little difference between men and women.

No formula can say how long a good night's sleep should be. Normal sleep times range from five to ten hours; the average is seven and a half. About one or two people in a hundred can get by with just five hours; another small minority needs twice that amount. Each of us seems to have an innate sleep *appetite* that is as much a part of our genetic programming as hair color and skin tone.

To figure out your sleep needs, keep your wake-up time the same every morning and vary your bedtime. Are you groggy after six hours of shut-eye? Does an extra hour give you more stamina? What about an extra two hours? Since too much sleep can make you feel sluggish, don't assume that more is always better. Listen to your body's signals, and adjust your sleep schedule to suit them.

Are you better off pulling an all-nighter before a big test or closing the books and getting a good night's sleep? According to researchers, that depends on the nature of the exam. If it's a test of facts—Civil War battles, for instance—cramming all night works. However, if you will have to write analytical essays in which you compare, contrast, and make connections, you need to sleep to make the most of your reasoning abilities.

Sleeping Pills

The use of prescription sleeping pills has more than doubled since 2000, and increasing numbers of teenagers and young adults use these medications either occasionally or regularly. An even greater number buy nonprescription or over-the-counter (OTC) sleep inducers. Others rely on herbal remedies, antihistamines, and other medications to get to sleep.

In the long run, good sleep habits, regular exercise, and a tranquil sleep environment are the cornerstones of high-quality sleep. But if circumstances, travel, injury, or illness have disrupted your sleep, you may consider sleep medications. Here is what you need to know about them.

- **Over-the-counter medications.** Various over-the-counter sleeping pills, sold in any pharmacy or supermarket, contain antihistamines, which induce drowsiness by working against the central

Sleeping Pill Precautions

Chances are you've taken some form of sleep medication. After aspirin, they are the most widely used drugs in the United States. If sleeping pills seem the best option at a certain time in your life, use them with caution.

Facts to Know

- **Sleeping pills** are not a long-term solution to a sleep problem, but they can be helpful if travel, injury, or illness interfere with your nightly rest.

- **Prescription and over-the-counter sleep aids** can interact with other medications or a medical condition, so always check with your doctor before taking them.

- **If taken too often** or for more than several nights, some sleeping pills may cause rebound insomnia—sleeplessness that returns in full force when you stop taking the medication.

Steps to Take

- **Read carefully.** Take time to read through the informational materials and warnings on pill containers. Make sure you understand the potential risks and the behaviors to avoid.

- **Avoid alcohol.** Never mix alcohol and sleeping pills. Alcohol increases the sedative effects of the pills. Even a small amount of alcohol combined with sleeping pills can make you feel dizzy, confused, or faint.

- **Quit carefully.** When you're ready to stop taking sleeping pills, follow your doctor's instructions or the directions on the label. Some medications must be stopped gradually.

- **Watch for side effects.** If you feel sleepy or dizzy during the day, talk to your doctor about changing the dosage or discontinuing the pills.

nervous system chemical histamine. They may help for an occasional sleepless night, but the more often you take them, the less effective they become.

- **Dietary supplements.** The most widely publicized dietary supplement is the hormone melatonin, which may help control your body's internal clock. The melatonin supplements most often found in health food stores and pharmacies are synthetic versions of the natural hormone. Although these supplements may help some people fall asleep or stay asleep and may sometimes help prevent jet lag, there are many unanswered questions about melatonin. Reported side effects include drowsiness, headaches, stomach discomfort, confusion, decreased body temperature, seizures, and drug interactions. The optimal dose isn't certain, and the long-term effects are unknown. Other supplements—such as valerian, chamomile, and kava—have yet to be fully studied for safety or effectiveness in relieving insomnia.

- **Prescription medications.** The newest sleep drugs—nonbenzodiazepine hypnotic medications such as Lunesta (eszopiclone), Ambien/Ambien CR (zolpidem), and Sonata (zaleplon)—quiet the nervous system, which helps induce sleep. They're metabolized quickly, which helps reduce the risk of side effects the next day. These medications are mainly intended for short-term or intermittent use.

- Benzodiazepines, such as Halcion (triazolam) and Restoril (temazepam), belong to an older class of sleeping pills that are more likely to cause drowsiness or headaches the next morning. They also may become habit forming.

The FDA has required stronger language about the potential risks of both nonbenzodiazepine and benzodiazepine sleeping pills. These include severe allergic reactions and complex sleep-related behaviors, including sleep-driving (driving while not fully awake after taking a sleeping pill with no memory of the driving).

LEARN IT LIVE IT Keys to a Fulfilling Life

Just like physical health, psychological well-being involves more than an absence of problems. By developing your inner strengths and resources, you become the author of your life, capable of confronting challenges and learning from them. As positive psychologists have discovered, you have greater control over how happy, optimistic, upbeat, and lovable you are than anyone or anything else. But only by consciously taking charge of your life can you find happiness and fulfillment. (See "Your Perfect Balance Point" in *IPC*.)

- **Up your appreciation quotient.** Regularly take stock of all the things for which you are grateful. To deepen the impact, write a letter of gratitude to someone who's helped you along the way.

- **String beads.** Think of every positive experience during the day as a bead on a necklace. This simple exercise focuses you on positive experiences, such as a cheery greeting from a cashier or a funny e-mail from a friend, and encourages you to act more kindly toward others.

- **Cultivate memories.** If you have to choose between buying a new car and studying abroad, pack your bags. Cars inevitably break down. International study pays the dividend of memories you can cherish for decades.

- **Look on the lighter side.** "Humor is like salt on meat," observes psychologist Martin Seligman. "It amplifies everything." Watch reruns of the classic shows that never fail to make you laugh. Smile at the absurdities of daily nuisances.

- **Create a virtual DVD.** Visualize several of your happiest memories with as much detail as possible. Smell the air. Feel the sun. Hear the sea. Play this video in your mind when your spirits slump.

- **Fortify optimism.** Whenever possible, see the glass as half-full. Keep track of what's going right in your life. Imagine and write down your vision for your best possible future and track your progress toward it.

- **Immerse yourself.** Find activities that delight and engage you so much that you lose track of time. Experiment with creative outlets. Look for ways to build these passions into your life.

- **Do good.** Acts of kindness, however small, bring as much pleasure to the giver as the recipient. Give time, money, or both to worthy causes. At the least, offer a smile or a prayer.

- **Don't isolate yourself.** Even spending time with strangers bolsters your sense of well-being. You laugh much harder when you're with other people in a theatre than when you watch a movie at home.

- **Seize the moment.** Rather than waiting to celebrate big birthday-cake moments, savor a bite of cupcake every day. Delight in a child's cuddle, a glorious sunset, a lively conversation. Cry at movies. Cheer at football games. This life is your gift to yourself. Open it!

Well-Being Scale

Part I

The following questions contain statements and their opposites. Notice that the statements extend from one extreme to the other. Where would you place yourself on this scale? Place a circle on the number that is most true for you at this time. Do not put your circles between numbers.

Life Purpose and Satisfaction

1. During most of the day, my energy level is	very low	1 2 3 4 5 6 7	very high
2. As a whole, my life seems	dull	1 2 3 4 5 6 7	vibrant
3. My daily activities are	not a source of satisfaction	1 2 3 4 5 6 7	a source of satisfaction
4. I have come to expect that every day will be	exactly the same	1 2 3 4 5 6 7	new and different
5. When I think deeply about life	I do not feel there is any purpose to it	1 2 3 4 5 6 7	I feel there is a purpose to it
6. I feel that my life so far has	not been productive	1 2 3 4 5 6 7	been productive
7. I feel that the work* I am doing	is of no value	1 2 3 4 5 6 7	is of great value
8. I wish I were different than who I am.	agree strongly	1 2 3 4 5 6 7	disagree strongly
9. At this time, I have	no clearly defined goals for my life	1 2 3 4 5 6 7	clearly defined goals for my life
10. When sad things happen to me or other people	I cannot feel positive about life	1 2 3 4 5 6 7	I continue to feel positive about life
11. When I think about what I have done with my life, I feel	worthless	1 2 3 4 5 6 7	worthwhile
12. My present life	does not satisfy me	1 2 3 4 5 6 7	satisfies me
13. I feel joy in my heart	never	1 2 3 4 5 6 7	all the time
14. I feel trapped by the circumstances of my life.	agree strongly	1 2 3 4 5 6 7	disagree strongly
15. When I think about my past	I feel many regrets	1 2 3 4 5 6 7	I feel no regrets
16. Deep inside myself	I do not feel loved	1 2 3 4 5 6 7	I feel loved
17. When I think about the problems that I have	I do not feel hopeful about solving them	1 2 3 4 5 6 7	I feel very hopeful about solving them

Part II

Self-Confidence During Stress (Answer according to how you feel during stressful times.)

1. When there is a great deal of pressure being placed on me	I get tense	1 2 3 4 5 6 7	I remain calm
2. I react to problems and difficulties	with a great deal of frustration	1 2 3 4 5 6 7	with no frustration
3. In a difficult situation, I am confident that I will receive the help that I need.	disagree strongly	1 2 3 4 5 6 7	agree strongly
4. I experience anxiety	all the time	1 2 3 4 5 6 7	never
5. When I have made a mistake	I feel extreme dislike for myself	1 2 3 4 5 6 7	I continue to like myself
6. I find myself worrying that something bad is going to happen to me or those I love	all the time	1 2 3 4 5 6 7	never
7. In a stressful situation	I cannot concentrate easily	1 2 3 4 5 6 7	I can concentrate easily
8. I am fearful	all the time	1 2 3 4 5 6 7	never
9. When I need to stand up for myself	I cannot do it	1 2 3 4 5 6 7	I can do it easily
10. I feel less than adequate in most situations.	agree strongly	1 2 3 4 5 6 7	disagree strongly
11. During times of stress, I feel isolated and alone.	agree strongly	1 2 3 4 5 6 7	disagree strongly
12. In really difficult situations	I feel unable to respond in positive ways	1 2 3 4 5 6 7	I feel able to respond in positive ways
13. When I need to relax	I experience no peace—only thoughts and worries	1 2 3 4 5 6 7	I experience a peacefulness— free of thoughts and worries
14. When I am frightened	I panic	1 2 3 4 5 6 7	I remain calm
15. I worry about the future	all the time	1 2 3 4 5 6 7	never

*The definition of work is not limited to income-producing jobs. It includes childcare, housework, studies, and volunteer services.

Scoring

The number you circled is your score for that question. Add your scores in each of the two sections and divide each sum by the number of questions in the section.

- Life Purpose and Satisfaction: _____ x 17 = _____.___
- Self-Confidence During Stress: _____ x 15 = _____.___
- Combined Well-Being:
  (add scores for both) _____ x 32 = _____.___

Each score should range between 1.00 and 7.00 and may include decimals (for example 5.15).

Intepretation

VERY LOW: 1.00 TO 2.49
MEDIUM LOW: 2.50 TO 3.99
MEDIUM HIGH: 4.00 TO 5.49
VERY HIGH: 5.50 TO 7.00

These scores reflect the strength with which you feel these positive emotions. Do they make sense to you? Review each scale and each question in each scale. Your score on each item gives you information about the emotions and areas in your life where your psychological resources are strong, as well as the areas where strength needs to be developed.

If you notice a large difference between the LPS and SCDS scores, use this information to recognize which central attitudes and aspects of your life most need strengthening. If your scores on both scales are very low, talk with a counselor or a friend about how you are feeling about yourself and your life.

Your Health Action Plan for Psychological Well-Being

Just as you can improve your physical well-being, you can enhance the state of your mind. Here are some suggestions:

- **Recognize and express your feelings.** Pent-up emotions tend to fester inside, building into anger or depression.

- **Don't brood.** Rather than merely mulling over a problem, try to find solutions that are positive and useful.

- **Take one step at a time.** As long as you're taking some action to solve a problem, you can take pride in your ability to cope.

- **Spend more time doing those activities you know you do best.** For example, if you are a good cook, prepare a meal for someone.

- **Separate what you do, especially any mistakes you make, from who you are.** Instead of saying, "I'm so stupid," tell yourself, "That wasn't the smartest move I ever made, but I'll learn from it."

- **Use affirmations**, positive statements that help reinforce the most positive aspects of your personality and experience. Every day, you might say, "I am a loving, caring person," or "I am honest and open in expressing my feelings." Write some affirmations of your own on index cards and flip through them occasionally.

- **List the things you would like to have or experience.** Construct the statements as if you were already enjoying the situations you list, beginning each sentence with "I am." For example, "I am feeling great about doing well in my classes."

- **When your internal critic**—the negative inner voice we all have—starts putting you down, force yourself to think of a situation that you handled well.

- **Set a limit on self-pity.** Tell yourself, "I'm going to feel sorry for myself this morning, but this afternoon, I've got to get on with my life."

- **Volunteer.** A third of Americans—some 89 million people—give of themselves through volunteer work. By doing the same, you may feel better too.

- **Exercise.** In various studies around the world, physical exertion ranks as one of the best ways to change a bad mood, raise energy, and reduce tension.

CENGAGENOW If you want to write your own goals to enhance your state of mind, go to the Wellness Journal at HealthNow: **www.cengage .com/sso**

MAKING THIS CHAPTER WORK FOR YOU

Review Questions

1. Lack of sleep
   a. improves memory and concentration.
   b. may cause irritability.
   c. may cause weight loss.
   d. enhances the immune system.

2. Which statement about sleep is correct?
   a. People cannot learn to sleep better.
   b. People dream during REM sleep.
   c. Drinking alcohol helps most people sleep better.
   d. Snoring may be a symptom of insomnia.

3. Normal shyness can usually be overcome by
   a. medication.
   b. psychotherapy.
   c. retail therapy.
   d. working at improving social skills.

4. Psychological health is influenced by all of the following *except*
   a. emotional health.
   b. physical agility.
   c. culture.
   d. a firm grasp on reality.

5. Which of the following activities can contribute to fulfillment?
   a. being a Big Sister or Big Brother to a child from a single-parent home
   b. being accepted by your first choice sorority or fraternity
   c. being a regular participant in an Internet chat room
   d. negotiating the price on a new car

6. Enduring happiness is most likely to come from
   a. winning a sweepstakes.
   b. work you love.
   c. a trip to the place of your dreams.
   d. having more money than your friends and neighbors.

7. Which activity is probably enriching the student's spiritual life?
   a. Claire goes dancing with her friends.
   b. James takes a 15-minute walk along the river trail with a group of friends every day.
   c. Kate keeps a gratitude journal.
   d. Charlie goes to a taize music group with friends.

8. Which of these statements about self-esteem is *true*?
   a. Self-esteem is determined by genetics.
   b. Parents have little influence on a child's self-esteem.
   c. A person's sense of self-esteem can change over time.
   d. Self-esteem is seldom boosted by achievement.

9. People who pray regularly
   a. are less likely to get cancer.
   b. never get sick.
   c. recover from heart attacks more quickly.
   d. get better grades.

10. Individuals who have developed a sense of mastery over their lives are
    a. aware that their locus of control is internal, not external.
    b. skilled at controlling the actions of others.
    c. usually passive and silent when faced with a situation they don't like.
    d. aware that their locus of control is external, not internal.

    Answers to these questions can be found on page 650.

Critical Thinking

1. Would you say that you view life positively or negatively? Would your friends and family agree with your assessment? Ask two of your closest friends for feedback about what they perceive are your typical responses to a problematic situation. Are these indicative of positive attitudes? If not, what could you do to become more psychologically positive?

2. Were you raised in a religious family? If yes, have you continued the same religious practices from your childhood? Why or why not? If no, have you been to places of worship to explore religious practices? Why or why not?

3. What is your personal experience with lack of sleep? Have you suffered effects described in the text? Has cramming all night ever worked for you? Why or why not?

Media Menu

CENGAGENOW™ Go to the CengageNOW for Health website at **www.cengage.com/sso** that will:
- Help you evaluate your knowledge of the material.
- Allow you to take an exam-prep quiz.
- Provide a Personalized Learning Plan targeting resources that address areas you should study.
- Coach you through identifying target goals for behavioral change and creating and monitoring your personal change plan throughout the semester.

Internet Connections

www.ppc.sas.upenn.edu
This positive psychology website at the University of Pennsylvania has questionnaires on authentic happiness and gratitude.

www.apa.org
The APA is the scientific and professional organization for psychology in the United States. Its website provides up-to-date information on psychological issues.

www.spiritualityhealth.org
Developed by the Publishing Group of Trinity Church, Wall Street in New York City, this website offers self-tests, guidance on spiritual practices, resources for people on spiritual journeys, and subscriptions to a bimonthly print magazine.

www.newvision-psychic.com/bookshelf/wottenspirit.html
A comprehensive list of books dealing with women and spirituality.

www.beliefnet.com
An eclectic, informative guide to different forms of religion and spirituality.

Key Terms

The terms listed are used on the page indicated. Definitions of the terms are in the Glossary at the end of the book.

altruism 55
assertive 49
autonomy 49
culture 41
emotional health 41
emotional intelligence 41
locus of control 49
mental health 41
mood 47
optimism 47
rapid-eye-movement (REM) sleep 57
self-actualization 43
self-esteem 43
social isolation 49
social phobia 49
spiritual health 51
spiritual intelligence 51
spirituality 51
values 51

Chapter 3 - Personal Stress Management

1) **When our body is trying to create an adaptive response, this means that:**   (pg. 67)
   ___ the body is resisting the bad things happening to us
   ___ the body is trying to restore homeostasis
   ___ the body is attempting to adapt to stressors
   ___ the body is gearing up for the flight or fight response

2) **The following is true about stress:**   (pg. 67)
   ___ Stress does not affect our general health condition.
   ___ We can usually eliminate all stressors in our lives if we try hard enough.
   ___ Stress produces a physical response of our bodies to the changes and challenges of life.
   ___ Stress is only produced by externally imposed factors

3) **Which of the following is likely to cause a posttraumatic stress disorder?** (pg. 82)
   ___ a woman who was raped
   ___ a child who was brutally sexually abused
   ___ soldiers fighting and killing in a combat war zone
   ___ all of the above

4) **A state of physical and mental exhaustion caused by excessive stress is called:**   (pg. 67)
   ___ hassled   ___ burntnout
   ___ conflicted   ___ wiped out

5) **During which phase of the general adaptation syndrome has the physical and psychological energy used to fight the stressors been depleted?**   (pg. 68)
   ___ endurance phase
   ___ alarm phase
   ___ exhaustion phase
   ___ resistance phase

6) **Which of the following is a time management tip to reduce stress?**   (pg. 85)
   ___ let your mail pile up and only look at it once a week
   ___ don't bother to clean up messes and clutter until you have time to do it right
   ___ make a list of tasks, prioritize them, and budget extra time to get the work done
   ___ take an extra day off to relax, even if you have assignments due immediately

7) **Which stress reduction technique employs the use of breathing as part of the routine?** (pg. 80)
   ___ guided imagery
   ___ visualization
   ___ mindfulness
   ___ meditation

8) **Hearing unknown footsteps following you late at night on campus would likely trigger the _____ phase of GAS.** (pg. 68)
   ___ alarm
   ___ defensive
   ___ recovery
   ___ exhaustion

9) **Homeostasis means that our body is:**   (pg. 67)
   ___ in a steadily increasing state of euphoria
   ___ in an unstable physical state
   ___ in a constant state of exhaustion
   ___ stable and consistent physical condition

10) **One of the best techniques a college student can use to minimize procrastination is to:** (pg. 85- 86)
   ___ do the least enjoyable task or homework first
   ___ establish ground rules for meeting your own needs
   ___ think of alternative ways to get the work done
   ___ all of the above can be good techniques to avoid procrastination

11) Which of the following is not a result of severe stress on the cardio system of the body?   (pg. 69)

___ increased risk for blood clotting in the arteries
___ persistently elevated blood pressure
___ greater risk for stroke
___ lowered blood pressure

12) An example of a student who is said to be resilient means that: (pg. 83)

___ their attitude has been strengthen to become a stronger person
___ positive changes can result from the horrible experience they may have had
___ they can bounce back from a stressful or traumatic experience
___ all of the above are examples of resiliency

13) Which is an example of a eustress situation?   (pg. 66)

___ you and your boyfriend are getting engaged
___ you have 3 exams in one day to prepare for
___ someone in your family dies
___ your father has a heart attack and you must leave college to care for him

14) Shelly wants to de-stress her life and take stock on what the stressors are in her life. She plans to use a technique that utilizes a mental inventory of her physical 'hot' spots or tightness in her body. This technique is known as: (pg. 79)

___ focusing
___ reconstruction of stressors
___ mental hypnotics
___ self improvement

15) How does chronic stress create physical breakdown in the human body?   (pg. 9)

___ fat and protein are not broken down properly and causes the cells to age more
___ it forces change in the DNA of the body cells which then atrophy and break down the cells
___ cells begin to crack up from the body stress, thus leaking fluid and die
___ bombards the brain cells to admitting failure and stress and weakens the immune system

16) All of the following may be warning signs of stress overload except: (pg. 69)

___ having frequent illnesses
___ committing violent crimes
___ becoming accident prone
___ feeling irritable

17) The nonspecific response of the body to any demand made upon it is known as: (pg. 66)

___ adaptive response
___ homeostasis
___ resistance
___ stress

18) Defense mechanisms are a tool to help one to reduce stress and anxiety. Which one of the following is not a defense mechanism?   (pg. 79)

___ denial of one's reality to a painful situation
___ drinking alcohol to numb the pain or grief
___ repression of bad things to try to forget them
___ true projection of your anger to the source of the problem

19) Distress refers to: (pg. 66)

___ alarm reactions to the brain
___ adaptation of harmful effects
___ negative effects on the body
___ happy events in one's life

20) Which of the following best describes the technique of meditation. (pg. 80- 81)

___ creating mental pictures
___ maintaining awareness in the present moment
___ sitting quietly and concentrating on a word or image
___ increasing and decreasing muscle tension

Tasha, a single mother who recently went back to college to finish her degree, wishes she had an extra arm to hold her baby and an extra hour every day to fit in all she needs to do. She wakes up before dawn to finish her homework before Kylie wakes up. All day long she rushes—to the day care center, to class, to the computer lab, to the supermarket, to her part-time job at the mall. "The evenings are a whirl of feeding Kylie, bathing her, and settling her down to sleep," says Tasha. "Stress? It's just a way of life."

Personal Stress Management

Like Tasha, you live with stress every day, whether you're studying for exams, meeting people, facing new experiences, or figuring out how to live on a budget. You're not alone. College students rank stress as the top impediment to their academic performance.[1] Everyone, regardless of age, gender, race, or income, has to deal with stress—as an individual and as a member of society.

As researchers have demonstrated time and again, stress has profound effects, both immediate and long-term, on our bodies and minds. While stress alone doesn't cause disease, it triggers molecular changes throughout the body that make us more susceptible to many illnesses. Its impact on the mind is no less significant. The burden of chronic stress can undermine one's ability to cope with day-to-day hassles and can exacerbate psychological problems like depression and anxiety disorders.

Yet stress in itself isn't necessarily bad. What matters most is not the stressful situation itself, but an individual's response to it. This chapter will help you learn to anticipate stressful events, to manage day-to-day hassles, to prevent stress overload, and to find alternatives to running endlessly on a treadmill of alarm, panic, and exhaustion. As you organize your schedule, find ways to release tension, and build up coping skills, you will begin to experience the sense of control and confidence that makes stress a challenge rather than an ordeal.

After studying the material in this chapter, you should be able to

- **Define** stress and stressors and **describe** how the body responds to stress according to the general adaptation syndrome theory.
- **List** the physical changes associated with frequent or severe stress and **discuss** how stress can affect the cardiovascular, immune, and digestive systems.
- **Describe** some personal stressors, especially those experienced by students, and **discuss** how their effects can be prevented or minimized.
- **Describe** some techniques to help cope with stress.
- **Explain** how stressful events can affect psychological health and **describe** the factors contributing to posttraumatic stress disorder.
- **Identify** ways of managing time more efficiently.
- **List** the main causes of stress in your life, and **name** a strategy for managing each of them.

Log on to CengageNOW for Health at **www.cengage.com/sso** to find your Behavior Change Planner and to explore self-assessments, interactive tutorials, and practice quizzes.

What Is Stress?

People use the word *stress* in different ways: as an external force that causes a person to become tense or upset, as the internal state of arousal, and as the physical response of the body to various demands. Dr. Hans Selye, a pioneer in studying physiological responses to challenge, defined **stress** as "the nonspecific response of the body to any demand made upon it." In other words, the body reacts to **stressors**—the things that upset or excite us—in the same way, regardless of whether they are positive or negative.

Based on nearly 300 studies over four decades, researchers have distinguished five categories of stressors:

- **Acute time-limited stressors** include anxiety-provoking situations such as having to give a talk in public or work out a math problem, such as calculating a tip or dividing a bill, under pressure.

- **Brief naturalistic stressors** are more serious challenges such as taking SATs or meeting a deadline for a big project.

- **Stressful event sequences** are the difficult consequences of a natural disaster or another traumatic occurrence, such as the death of a spouse. The individuals involved recognize that these difficulties will end at some point in the future.

- **Chronic stressors** are ongoing demands caused by life-changing circumstances, such as permanent disability following an accident or caregiving for a parent with dementia, that do not have any clear end point.

- **Distant stressors** are traumatic experiences that occurred long ago, such as child abuse or combat, yet continue to have an emotional and psychological impact.

Not all stressors are negative. Some of life's happiest moments—births, reunions, weddings—are enormously stressful. We weep with the stress of frustration or loss; we weep, too, with the stress of love and joy. Selye coined the term **eustress** for positive stress in our lives (*eu* is a Greek prefix meaning "good"). Eustress challenges us to grow, adapt, and find creative solutions in our lives. **Distress** refers to the negative effects of stress that can deplete or even destroy

© Corbis

© BananaStock/Jupiterimages

An automobile accident is an acute negative stressor. A wedding is an example of a positive stressor that triggers both joy and anxiety.

life energy. Ideally, the level of stress in our lives should be just high enough to motivate us to satisfy our needs and not so high that it interferes with our ability to reach our fullest potential.

What Causes Stress?

Of the many biological theories of stress, the best known may be the **general adaptation syndrome (GAS),** developed by Hans Selye. He postulated that our bodies constantly strive to maintain a stable and consistent physiological state, called **homeostasis.** Stressors, whether in the form of physical illness or a demanding job, disturb this state and trigger a nonspecific physiological response. The body attempts to restore homeostasis by means of an **adaptive response.**

General Adaptation Syndrome

Selye's general adaptation syndrome, which describes the body's response to a stressor—whether threatening or exhilarating—consists of three distinct stages:

1. **Alarm.** When a stressor first occurs, the body responds with changes that temporarily lower resistance. Levels of certain hormones may rise; blood pressure may increase (Figure 3.1). The body quickly makes internal adjustments to cope with the stressor and return to normal activity.

2. **Resistance.** If the stressor continues, the body mobilizes its internal resources to try to sustain homeostasis. For example, if a loved one is seriously hurt in an accident, we initially respond intensely and feel great anxiety. During the subsequent stressful period of recuperation, we struggle to carry on as normally as possible, but this requires considerable effort.

3. **Exhaustion.** If the stress continues long enough, we cannot keep up our normal functioning. Even a small amount of additional stress at this point can cause a breakdown.

Among the nonbiological theories is the cognitive-transactional model of stress, developed by Richard Lazarus, which looks at the relation between stress and health. As he sees it, stress can have a powerful impact on health. Conversely, health can affect a person's resistance or coping ability. Stress, according to Lazarus, is "neither an environmental stimulus, a characteristic of the person, nor a response, but a relationship between demands and the power to deal with them without unreasonable or destructive costs."[2] Thus, an event may be stressful for one person but not for another, or it may seem stressful on one occasion but not on another. For instance, one student may think of speaking in front of the class as extremely stressful, while another relishes the chance to do so—except on days when he's not well-prepared.

At any age, some of us are more vulnerable to life changes and crises than are others. The stress of growing up in families troubled by alcoholism, drug dependence, or physical, sexual, or psychological abuse may have a lifelong impact—particularly if these problems are not recognized and dealt with. Other early experiences, positive and negative, also can affect our attitude toward stress—and our resilience to it.

Stressful experiences in childhood, as recent studies have shown, have long-lasting effects on immunity and health. Years after they were physically abused or placed in orphanages as children, adolescents continued to show impaired immune function.[3] A large-scale, multinational study documented an increased risk of developing asthma in stressed youngsters who suffered abuse, the death of a parent, parental criminal behavior or substance abuse, and other types of adversity.[4] Living in a stressful household, regardless of whether the cause was an accident, illness, death, divorce, unemployment, or violence, can increase a child's risk of becoming obese.[5] Our general outlook on life, whether we're optimistic or pessimistic, can determine whether we expect the

stress The nonspecific response of the body to any demands made upon it; may be characterized by muscle tension and acute anxiety, or may be a positive force of action.

stressors Specific or nonspecific agents or situations that cause the stress response in a body.

eustress Positive stress, which stimulates a person to function properly.

distress A negative stress that may result in illness.

general adaptation syndrome (GAS) An anxiety disorder characterized as chronic distress.

homeostasis The body's natural state of balance or stability.

adaptive response The body's attempt to reestablish homeostasis or stability.

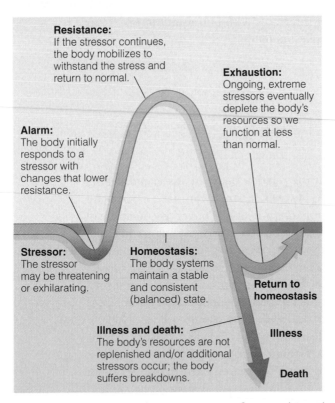

Figure 3.1 General Adaptation Syndrome (GAS)
The three stages of Selye's GAS are alarm, resistance, and exhaustion.

Resistance:
If the stressor continues, the body mobilizes to withstand the stress and return to normal.

Exhaustion:
Ongoing, extreme stressors eventually deplete the body's resources so we function at less than normal.

Alarm:
The body initially responds to a stressor with changes that lower resistance.

Stressor:
The stressor may be threatening or exhilarating.

Homeostasis:
The body systems maintain a stable and consistent (balanced) state.

Return to homeostasis

Illness and death:
The body's resources are not replenished and/or additional stressors occur; the body suffers breakdowns.

Illness

Death

units that estimate each change's impact. The death of a partner or parent ranks high on the list, but even changing apartments is considered a stressor. People who accumulate more than 300 life-change units in a year are more likely to suffer serious health problems. Scores on the scale, however, represent "potential stress"; the actual impact of the life change depends on the individual's response. (See Self Survey: "Student Stress Scale," p. 87.)

If you score high on the Student Stress Scale, think about the reasons your life has been in such turmoil. Of course, some events, such as your or your parents' divorce or a friend's accident, are beyond your control. Even then, you can respond in ways that may protect you from disease, such as those listed in Your Health Action Plan at the end of this chapter.

The Diathesis Stress Model

The **diathesis stress model** is a psychological theory that explains behavior as a result of both nature (biological factors such as genetics) and nurture (early life experiences). Originally developed to explain the causes of psychiatric disorders such as schizophrenia, this model has stimulated research on the impact of many common stressors.

According to this model, particular stressors have different effects on different people because individuals vary in their vulnerabilities or predispositions—called diatheses—to psychological problems and mental disorders. Biological and psychological factors, including genetics, put certain people at greater risk but do not in themselves trigger illness. Interaction with stressful life events (whether social, psychological, or biological) must occur to precipitate symptoms.

The greater one's inherent vulnerability, the less environmental stress is required to cause problems. In someone with a diathesis for depression, for instance, a job layoff, a breakup, or even normal milestones such as puberty can be powerful enough to create depressive symptoms. Similar events might not faze other individuals that much. Research is continuing on identifying hidden or latent diatheses and developing protective strategies in times of stress.

worst and feel stressed or anticipate a challenge and feel confident. The when, where, what, how, and why of stressors also affect our reactions. The number and frequency of changes in our lives, along with the time and setting in which they occur, have a great impact on how we'll respond.

"Perceived" stress—an individual's view of how challenging life is—undermines a sense of well-being in people of all ages and circumstances. However, good self-esteem, social support, and internal resources buffer the impact of perceived stress.

Our level of ongoing stress affects our ability to respond to a new day's stressors. Each of us has a breaking point for dealing with stress. A series of too-intense pressures or too-rapid changes can push us closer and closer to that point. That's why it's important to anticipate potential stressors and plan how to deal with them.

Stress experts Thomas Holmes, M.D., and Richard Rahe, M.D., devised a scale to evaluate individual levels of stress and potential for coping, based on *life-change*

Stress and Physical Health

These days we've grown accustomed to warning labels advising us of the health risks of substances like alcohol and cigarettes. Medical researchers speculate that another component of twenty-first-century living also warrants a warning: stress. In recent years, an ever-growing number of studies has implicated stress as a culprit in a range of medical problems. While stress itself may not kill, it clearly undermines our ability to stay well.

While stress alone doesn't cause disease, it triggers molecular changes throughout the body that make us more susceptible to many illnesses. Severe emotional distress—whether caused by a divorce, the loss of a job, or caring for an ill child or parent—can have such a powerful effect on the DNA in body cells that it speeds up aging, adding the equivalent of a decade to biological age. This occurs because of a shortening of structures called telomeres in the chromosomes of cells. An enzyme called telomerase maintains these structures but declines with age. Every time a cell divides, which is a continuous process, the telomeres shorten. The shorter your telomeres, the more likely you are to die.

Stress also triggers complex changes in the body's endocrine, or hormone-secreting, system. When you confront a stressor, the adrenal glands, two triangle-shaped glands that sit atop the kidneys, respond by producing stress hormones, including catecholamines, cortisol (hydrocortisone), and epinephrine (adrenaline), that speed up heart rate and raise blood pressure and prepare the body to deal with the threat. This "fight-or-flight" response prepares you for quick action: Your heart works harder to pump more blood to your legs and arms. Your muscles tense, your breathing quickens, and your brain becomes extra alert. Because it's nonessential in a crisis, your digestive system practically shuts down (Figure 3.2).

diathesis stress model A psychological theory that explains behavior as a result of both nature and nurture.

Brain becomes more alert.
- Stress hormones can affect memory and cause neurons to atrophy and die.
- Headaches, anxiety, and depression
- Disrupted sleep

Digestive system slows down.
- Mouth ulcers or cold sores

Heart rate increases and blood pressure rises.
- Persistently elevated blood pressure and heart rate can increase potential for blood clotting and risk of stroke or heart attack.
- Weakening of the heart muscle and symptoms that mimic a heart attack

Adrenal glands produce stress hormones.
- Cortisol and other stress hormones can increase central or abdominal fat.
- Cortisol increases glucose production in the liver, causing renal hypertension.

Skin problems such as eczema and psoriasis

■ = Immediate response to stress
■ = Effects of chronic or prolonged stress
■ = Other possible effects of chronic stress

Breathing quickens.
- Increased susceptibility to colds and respiratory infections

Immune system is depressed.
- Increased susceptibility to infection
- Slower healing

Digestive system slows down.
- Upset stomach

Reproductive system
- Menstrual disorders in women
- Impotence and premature ejaculation in men

Muscles tense.
- Muscular twitches or nervous tics

Figure 3.2 The Effects of Stress on the Body

Cortisol speeds the conversion of proteins and fats into carbohydrates, the body's basic fuel, so we have the energy to fight or flee from a threat. However, stress increases the amount of time required to clear triglycerides, a type of fat linked to heart disease, from the bloodstream.

Cortisol can cause excessive central or abdominal fat, which heightens the risk of diseases such as diabetes, high blood pressure, and stroke. Even slender, premenopausal women faced with increased stress and lacking good coping skills are more likely to accumulate excess weight around their waists, thereby increasing their risk of heart disease and other health problems.

 In one study, African American college students who scored low in coping skills had higher levels of cortisol than those better equipped to cope with stress. Challenges that seem uncontrollable or unpredictable have a greater impact on cortisol than others.

Figure 3.2 illustrates how persistent or repeated increases in the stress hormones can be hazardous throughout the body. Prolonged or severe stress can damage the brain's ability to remember and can actually cause brain cells, or neurons, to atrophy and die. Recent research has implicated stress in both contributing to the development of cancer and reducing the effectiveness of cancer treatment. The stress hormone epinephrine makes prostate and breast cancer cells more resistant to cell death.

Stress and the Heart

 The links between stress, behavior, and the heart are complex. Scientists continue to explore the impact of acute and chronic stress, gender, race, and socioeconomic status.[6] One way in which stress increases the risk of heart attack and other cardiovascular problems is by pushing people toward bad habits. In a study that followed about 6,500 men and women for seven years, those with the highest stress levels smoked more and exercised less—and had a 50 percent higher rate of heart attacks, strokes, and bypass surgeries.[7] The stress of social isolation also has emerged as a risk factor for cardiovascular disease.[8] Stress may be the most significant

inherited risk factor in people who develop heart disease at a young age. According to behavioral researchers, family transmission of emotional and psychosocial stress, specifically anger in males, greatly increases the likelihood of early heart disease. Young adults whose blood pressure spikes in response to stress may be at risk of hypertension as they get older.

In the 1970s, cardiologists Meyer Friedman, M.D., and Ray Rosenman, M.D., compared their patients to individuals of the same age with healthy hearts and developed two general categories of personality: Type A and Type B. Hardworking, aggressive, and competitive, Type As never have time for all they want to accomplish, even though they usually try to do several tasks at once. Type Bs are more relaxed, though not necessarily less ambitious or successful.

The degree of danger associated with Type-A behavior remains controversial. Of all the personality traits linked with Type-A behavior, the most sinister are anger and chronic hostility. People who are always mistrustful, cynical, and suspicious are twice as likely to suffer blockages of their coronary arteries. Social isolation, depression, and stress may be even stronger risk factors for men.

Stress and Immunity

The immune system is the network of organs, tissues, and white blood cells that defend against disease. Impaired immunity makes the body more susceptible to many diseases, including infections (from the common cold to tuberculosis) and disorders of the immune system itself. In the short term, stress "revs up" the immune system, a way of preparing for injury or infection. Acute time-limited stressors, the type that produce a fight-or-flight response, prompt the immune system to ready itself for the possibility of infections resulting from bites, punctures, or other wounds.

However, long-term, or chronic, stress creates excessive wear and tear, and the system breaks down. Chronic stressors, so profound and persistent that they seem endless and beyond a person's control, suppress immune responses the most. The longer the stress, the more the immune system shifts from potentially adaptive changes to potentially harmful ones, first in cellular immunity and then in broader immune function. Traumatic stress, such as losing a loved one through death or divorce, can impair immunity for as long as a year.

Even minor hassles that aren't related to trauma take a toll. Under exam stress, students experience a dip in immune function and a higher rate of infections. Researchers have documented a significant drop in the immune cells that normally ward off infection and cancer in medical students during exams.

Age and overall health also affect immune response. The immune systems of individuals who are elderly or ill are more vulnerable to acute and chronic stressors, possibly because their bodies find it more difficult to regulate their reactions. However, stress intensifies the symptoms and lowers the quality of life even for young adults with asthma and other chronic conditions.[9]

Stress and Digestion

Do you ever get butterflies in your stomach before giving a speech in class or before a big game? The digestive system is, as one psychologist quips, "an important stop on the tension trail." No studies have ever demonstrated that stress alone causes ulcers, but it may make people more vulnerable to infection with *Helicobacter pylori bacteria*, a known culprit in many cases. To avoid problems, pay attention to how you eat. Eating on the run, gulping food, or overeating results in poorly chewed foods, an overworked stomach, and increased abdominal pressure.

Some simple strategies can help you avoid stress-related stomachaches. Many people experience dry mouth or sweat more under stress. By drinking plenty of water, you replenish lost fluids and prevent dehydration. Fiber-rich foods counteract common stress-related problems, such as cramps and constipation. Do not skip meals. If you do, you're more likely to feel fatigued and irritable.

Be wary of overeating under stress. Some people eat more because they scarf down meals too quickly. Others reach for snacks to calm their nerves or comfort themselves. Watch out for caffeine. Coffee, tea, and cola drinks can make your strained nerves jangle even more. Also avoid sugary snacks. They'll send your blood sugar levels on a roller coaster ride—up one minute, down the next.

Other Stress Symptoms

The first signs of stress include muscle tightness, tension headaches, backaches, upset stomach, and sleep disruptions (caused by stress-altered brain-wave activity). Some people feel fatigued, their hearts may race or beat faster than usual at rest, and they may feel tense all the time, easily frustrated and often irritable. Others feel sad; lose their energy, appetite, or sex drive; and develop psychological problems, including depression, anxiety, and panic attacks (Chapter 4).

Stress also is closely linked to skin conditions. If you break out the week before an exam, you know firsthand that skin can be extremely sensitive to stress. Skin conditions worsened by stress include acne, psoriasis, herpes, hives, and eczema. With acne, increased touching of the face, perhaps while cramming for a test, may be partly responsible. Other factors, such as temperature, humidity, and cosmetics and toiletries, may also play a role.

Stress on Campus

 Being a student—full-time or part-time, in your late teens, early twenties, or later in life—can be extremely stressful. You may feel pressure to perform well to qualify for a good job or graduate school. To meet steep tuition payments, you may have to juggle part-time work and coursework. You may feel stressed about choosing a major, getting along with a difficult roommate, passing a particularly hard course, or living up to your parents' and teachers' expectations. If you're an older student, you may have children, jobs, housework, and homework to balance. Your days may seem so busy and your life so full that you worry about coming apart at the seams.

Today's students, according to a recent analysis, report more sources of stress (and of happiness) than undergraduates did 20 years ago. However, the sources of stress remain essentially the same. Then, as now, poor grades and worry about exams and grades produced the greatest stress, followed by concerns about money and not being able to complete assignments. (See Table 3.1.)

Other common stressors reported by students around the world include test pressures; financial problems; frustrations, such as delays in reaching goals; problems in friendships and dating relationships; and daily hassles.

Students under Stress

In college, as in life, stress seems to come with the territory. In a 2008 national survey of more than 2,000 undergraduates at 40 randomly chosen four-year schools, about four in ten said they frequently experience stress; a similar percentage said they sometimes feel stressed. (See Reality Check, p. 73.) About one in five felt too stressed to do schoolwork or be with friends; a similar number said stress had been so intense in the previous three months that they considered dropping out of school. Even though most students say the Internet is so important in their life that they can't imagine living without it, most feel very little or no stress from keeping up with instant messages or networking sites like MySpace or Facebook.[10]

Incoming freshmen often report the most stress. In a national poll of the class of 2011, 28 percent reported feeling overwhelmed by all they had to do.[11]

First-generation college students—those whose parents never experienced at least one full year of college—encounter more difficulties with social adjustment than freshmen whose parents attended college. Second-generation students may have several advantages: more knowledge of college life, greater social support, more preparation for college in high school, a greater focus on college activities, and more financial resources.

Students say they react to stress in various ways: physiologically (by sweating, stuttering, trembling, or developing physical symptoms); emotionally (by becoming anxious, fearful, angry, guilty, or depressed); behaviorally (by crying, eating, smoking, being irritable or abusive); or cognitively (by thinking about and analyzing stressful situations and strategies that might be useful in dealing with them).

Does stress increase drinking among college students? Many assume so, since life stress is a recognized risk for alcohol use, particularly for people with a family history of alcoholism. The relationship between drinking and stress is more complex. For some, drinking occasions were times to discuss problems with friends, regardless of the day's stress. On average, students tended to drink more on days when they were feeling good—possibly because of what researchers call the "celebratory and social" nature of college drinking. Drinking—and positive emotions—also peaked on weekends. (See Chapter 12 for more on student drinking.)

In a national poll, three-quarters of students said they turn to friends when stressed; nearly two-thirds, to their parents; and half to siblings. About a quarter of the survey participants said they had considered talking to a counselor or another professional; just 15 percent had actually done so. Only one in seven undergraduates said they were familiar with the counseling offered at their schools.[12]

Campuses are providing more frontline services than they have in the past, including career-guidance workshops, telephone hotlines, and special social programs for lonely, homesick freshmen. Undergraduates who learn relaxation and stress-reduction techniques report less stress, anxiety, and psychological distress than other students.

Coping with Test Stress

For many students, midterms and final exams are the most stressful times of the year. Studies

TABLE 3.1

What Stresses Students

- Schoolwork
- School grades
- Financial worries
- Family issues
- Relationships/dating

These are the factors students cite, in descending order, as having "a lot of impact" on their stress levels.

Source: mtvU/Associated Press Survey, March 2008. Edison Media Research. www.edisonresearch.com.

at various colleges and universities found that the incidence of colds and flu soared during finals. Some students feel the impact of test stress in other ways—headaches, upset stomachs, skin flare-ups, or insomnia.

Because of stress's impact on memory, students with advanced skills may perform worse under exam pressure than their less skilled peers. Sometimes students become so preoccupied with the possibility of failing that they can't concentrate on studying. Others, including many of the best and brightest students, freeze up during tests and can't comprehend multiple-choice questions or write essay answers, even if they know the material.

The students most susceptible to exam stress are those who believe they'll do poorly and who see tests as extremely threatening. Unfortunately, such negative thoughts often become a self-fulfilling prophecy. As they study, these students keep wondering: What good will studying do? I never do well on tests. As their fear increases, they try harder, pulling all-nighters. Fueled by caffeine, munching on sugary snacks, they become edgy and find it harder and harder to concentrate. By the time of the test, they're nervous wrecks, scarcely able to sit still and focus on the exam.

Can you do anything to reduce test stress and feel more in control? Absolutely. (See "Defusing Test Stress" in the *Labs for IPC.*) One way is through relaxation. Students taught relaxation techniques—such as controlled breathing, meditation, progressive relaxation, and guided imagery (visualization)—a month before finals tend to have higher levels of immune cells during the exam period and feel in better control during their tests.

Minority Students under Stress

Regardless of your race or ethnic background, college may bring culture shock. You may never have encountered such a degree of diversity in one setting. You probably will meet students with different values, unfamiliar customs, entirely new ways of looking at the world—experiences you may find both stimulating and stressful.

Minority students may face a greater stress burden because of the demands of

✓ **REALITYCHECK** ·······················

• *What percentage of students report experiencing stress "frequently"?*
• *What percentage of college women say they're often stressed?*
• *What percentage of college men say they're often stressed?*

Answers on next page.

acculturation, a complex psychosocial process in which an ethnic minority changes, both as individuals and as a group, as a consequence of contact with the ethnic majority. Minority students often confront widespread stereotypes—for instance, that Asian Americans are quiet and passive or that Latinos entered the country illegally. Such racist attitudes can affect students' sense of individual and collective self-esteem.

Acculturative stress has been linked to various psychological symptoms in African American, Asian, and Hispanic college students. In both African American and European American undergraduates, for instance, acculturative stress contributes to an increase in self-reported symptoms of depression and suicidal thoughts.[13]

acculturation The process of psychosocial change by which an ethnic minority changes as a consequence of contact with the ethnic majority.

The first year of college can seem overwhelming as you learn your way around the campus, meet new people, and strive to succeed.

© Bill Aaron/PhotoEdit

PART 2: *Just the Facts*
• **39** *percent of undergraduates report frequent stress.*
• **45** *percent of college women say they're often stressed.*
• **34** *percent of college men say they're often stressed.*

Source: mtvU/Associated Press Survey, March 2008. Edison Media Research. www.edisonresearch.com.

Racism and Discrimination Racism has indeed been shown to be a source of stress that can affect health and well-being. In the past, some African American students have described predominately white campuses as hostile, alienating, and socially isolating and have reported greater estrangement from the campus community and heightened estrangement in interactions with faculty and peers. However, the generalization that all minority students are more stressed may not be valid. Some coping mechanisms, especially spirituality, can buffer the negative effects of racism.[14]

All minority students do share some common stressors. In one study of minority freshmen entering a large, competitive university, Asian, Filipino, African American, and Native American students all felt more sensitive and vulnerable to the college social climate, to interpersonal tensions between themselves and nonminority students and faculty, to experiences of actual or perceived racism, and to racist attitudes and discrimination. Despite scoring above the national average on the SAT, the minority students in this study did not feel accepted as legitimate students and sensed that others viewed them as unworthy beneficiaries of affirmative action initiatives. While most said that overt racism was rare and relatively easy to deal with, they reported subtle pressures that undermined their academic confidence and their ability to bond with the university. Balancing these stressors, however, was a strong sense of ethnic identity, which helped buffer some stressful effects.

African American students at historically black colleges identified their top five sources of stress as:

• Important decisions about education.

• Respect of peers for what you have to say.

• Too many things to do at once.

• A lot of responsibilities.

• Financial burdens.

Women scored higher than men in feeling stressed about having too many things to do at once, being separated from people they care about, financial burdens, and important decisions about their education.[15]

Hispanic students have identified three major types of stressors in their college experiences: academic (related to exam preparation and faculty interaction), social (related to ethnicity and interpersonal competence), and financial (related to their economic situation). Some students who recently immigrated to the United States report feeling ostracized by students of similar ancestry who are second- or third-generation Americans.

African American women may develop chronic illnesses at an earlier age because

YOUR STRATEGIES FOR PREVENTION
How to Handle Test Stress

• **Plan ahead.** A month before finals, map out a study schedule for each course. Set aside a small amount of time every day or every other day to review the course materials.

• **Be positive.** Picture yourself taking your final exam. Imagine yourself walking into the exam room feeling confident, opening up the test booklet, and seeing questions for which you know the answers.

• **Take regular breaks.** Get up from your desk, breathe deeply, stretch, and visualize a pleasant scene. You'll feel more refreshed than you would if you chugged another cup of coffee.

• **Practice.** Some teachers are willing to give practice finals to prepare students for test situations, or you and your friends can test each other.

• **Talk to other students.** Chances are that many of them share your fears about test taking and may have discovered some helpful techniques of their own. Sometimes talking to your adviser or a counselor can also help.

• **Be satisfied with doing your best.** You can't expect to ace every test; all you can and should expect is your best effort. Once you've completed the exam, allow yourself the sweet pleasure of relief that it's over.

of their lifetime exposure to social and economic stressors. Chronic powerlessness and anger, researchers speculate, may explain why more African American than white women—47 percent compared with 35 percent—are affected by cardiovascular disease.[16]

Colleges Respond Because racism and discrimination can be hard to deal with individually, they are particularly sinister forms of stress. By banding together, however, those who experience discrimination can take action to protect themselves, challenge the ignorance and hateful assumptions that fuel bigotry, and promote a healthier environment for all.

In the last decade, there have been reports of increased intolerance among young people and greater tolerance of expressions and acts of hate on college campuses. To counteract this trend, many schools have set up programs and classes to educate students about each other's backgrounds and to acknowledge and celebrate the richness diversity brings to campus life. Educators have called on universities to make campuses less alienating and more culturally and emotionally accessible, with programs and policies targeted not only at minority students but also at the university as a whole. (See Point/Counterpoint.)

POINT COUNTERPOINT

POINT

Many students identify stress as the number-one barrier to better academic performance. Colleges have been trying to help students cope by providing more mental health services, training students to be peer counselors, and providing on-campus relaxation and stress management programs.

COUNTERPOINT

Some view today's students as overly pampered and argue that stress is a personal challenge, not a university problem. While students should have access to support and counseling, they should assume primary responsibility for meeting the demands of their classes and finding balance in their lives.

YOUR VIEW

Do you think colleges should do more to address the stress of undergraduates? Do you feel stressed out? What could your school do to help you cope with stress in your life? What are you doing on your own to manage stress?

Campus clubs and organizations provide an opportunity for individuals from different ethnic backgrounds to celebrate their culture and educate others about it. These undergraduates are preparing to perform an Indian dance at a special evening sponsored by Asian Students in America.

Men, Women, and Stress

Women, who make up 56 percent of today's college students, also shoulder the majority of the stress load. In a recent survey of incoming freshmen, 37 percent of female students but just 17 percent of the males reported feeling overwhelmed by all they had to do. More women than men also reported feeling depressed, insecure about their physical and mental health, and worried about paying for college. More men than women considered themselves above

average or in the top 10 percent of people their age in terms of emotional health.[17]

The immune and hormonal systems of men and women may respond differently to stressors. In psychological experiments men under stress display higher aggression (for example, delivering more shocks to another volunteer) than do women.

Gender differences in lifestyle also may explain why women feel so stressed. College men spend significantly more time doing things that are fun and relaxing: exercising, partying, watching TV, and playing video games. Women, on the other hand, tend to study more, do more volunteer work, and handle more household and child-care chores.

Where can stressed-out college women turn for support? The best source, according to University of California research, is other women. In general, the social support women offer their friends and relatives seems more effective in reducing the blood-pressure response to stress than that provided by men.

At all ages, women and men tend to respond to stress differently. While males (human and those of other species) react with the classic fight-or-flight response, females under attack try to protect their children and seek help from other females—a strategy dubbed *tend and befriend.* When exposed to experimental stress (such as a loud, harsh noise), women show more affection for friends and relatives; men show less. When working mothers studied by psychologists had a bad day, they coped by concentrating on their children when they got home. Stressed-out fathers were more likely to withdraw.

Other Personal Stressors

At every stage of life, you will encounter challenges and stressors. Among the most common are those related to money, anger, work, and illness.

Economic Stress

With the recent economic slump, millions of Americans have confronted a serious new stressor: unemployment. Workers who are laid off must deal with multiple losses: the loss of a job; the possible loss of the financial ability to support themselves; the loss of self-respect, security, and a daily routine; and—for some people—the loss of identity.[18]

Even those whose jobs seem secure may feel anxious. As their coworkers depart, many of those who remain feel "survivor's guilt." According to surveys by the American Psychological Association, nearly half of Americans say they are more stressed than a year ago. One-third rate their stress level as "extreme."[19] (See Health on a Budget, p. 77.)

The Anger Epidemic

In recent years, violent aggressive driving—which some dub *road rage*—has exploded. Sideline rage at amateur and professional sporting events has become so widespread that a Pennsylvania midget football game ended in a brawl involving more than 100 coaches, players, parents, and fans.

No one seems immune. Women fly off the handle just as often as men, although they're less likely to get physical. The young and the infamous, including several rappers and musicians sentenced to anger management classes for violent outbursts, may seem more volatile. However, ordinary senior citizens have erupted into "line rage" and pushed ahead of others simply because they feel they've "waited long enough" in their lives.

Experts single out three primary culprits for the anger epidemic: time, technology, and tension. Americans are working longer hours than anyone else in the world. The cell phones and pagers that were supposed to make our lives easier have put us on call 24–7–365. People are tense and low on patience, and the less patience they have, the less they monitor how they treat other people.

Getting a Grip For years therapists encouraged people to "vent" their anger. However, research now shows that letting anger out only makes it worse. "Catharsis is worse than useless," says psychology professor Brad Bushman of Iowa State University, whose research has shown that letting anger out makes people more aggressive, not less. "Many people think of anger as the psychological equivalent of the steam in a pressure cooker that has to be released or it will explode. That's not true. People who react by hitting, kicking, screaming, and swearing aren't dealing with the underlying cause of their anger. They just feel more angry."[20]

Over time, temper tantrums sabotage physical health as well as psychological equanimity. By churning out stress hormones, chronic anger revs the body into a state of combat readiness, multiplying the risk for stroke and heart attack—even in healthy individuals.

To deal with anger, you have to figure out what's really making you mad. Usually the jammed soda machine is the final straw that unleashes bottled-up fury over a more difficult issue, such as a recent breakup or a domineering parent or boss. Also monitor yourself for early signs of exhaustion and overload. While stress alone doesn't cause a blowup, it makes you more vulnerable to overreacting. (See "Taming a Toxic Temper" in *Labs for IPC*.)

Job Stress

More so than ever, many people find that they are working more and enjoying it less. Many people, including working parents, spend 55 to 60 hours a week on the job. More people are caught up in an exhausting cycle of overwork, which causes stress, which makes work harder, which leads to more stress. Even the workplace itself can contribute to stress. A noisy, open-office environment can increase levels of stress without workers realizing it.

High job strain—defined as high psychological demands combined with low control or decision-making ability over one's job—may increase blood pressure, particularly among men. People who become obsessed by their work and careers can turn into workaholics, so caught up in racing toward the top that they forget what they're racing toward and why. In some cases they throw themselves into their work to mask or avoid painful feelings or difficulties in their own lives.

Burnout Burnout is a state of physical, emotional, and mental exhaustion brought on by constant or repeated emotional pressure. No one—regardless of age, gender, or job—is immune. Mothers and managers, fire fighters

How to Handle Economic Stress

Whether or not you have a job—or lost one—the recent economic downturn has probably affected you or those close to you. But as always, what matters most isn't how stressful circumstances may be, but how you react to them:

- Pause but don't panic. Pay attention to what's happening around you, but refrain from getting caught up in doom-and-gloom hype, which can lead to high levels of anxiety and bad decision making.
- Avoid the tendency to overreact or to become passive. Remain calm and stay focused.
- Identify your financial stressors and make a plan. Although this can be anxiety-provoking in the short term, putting things down on paper can reduce stress. Write down specific ways you can reduce expenses or manage your finances more efficiently.
- If you are having trouble paying bills or staying on top of debt, reach out for help by calling your bank or credit card company. Credit counseling services and financial planners can help you take control over your money situation.
- Recognize how you deal with stress related to money. In tough economic times some people turn to unhealthy activities like smoking, drinking, gambling, or emotional eating. If these behaviors are causing you trouble, seek help from a campus counselor before the problem gets worse.

(Adapted from materials from the American Psychological Association.)

Stressed by tough economic times, people may overreact to unexpected bad news.

© Pixland/Jupiterimages

burnout A state of physical, emotional, and mental exhaustion resulting from constant or repeated emotional pressure.

- **Become an impartial observer.** Act as if you were watching someone else's two-year-old have a temper tantrum at the supermarket.
- **Stay calm.** Letting your emotions loose only adds fuel to fury. Talk quietly and slowly; let the person know you understand that he or she is angry.
- **Refuse to engage.** Step back to avoid invading his or her space. Retreat farther if need be until the person is back in control.
- **Find something to agree upon.** Look for common ground, if only to acknowledge that you're both in a difficult situation.

COMMUNITY FOCUS *The Stress of Homelessness*

PROBLEM Each year, according to the National Law Center on Homelessness and Poverty, more than 3 million people experience homelessness, including 1.3 million children. These numbers are expected to grow as the economy falters, home foreclosures increase, and more people lose their jobs. Even people who thought they were secure a few years ago may find themselves entering shelters or sleeping on the streets or in their cars.

A significant proportion of the homeless suffer from physical and psychological problems, including substance abuse, mental illnesses, and chronic medical conditions such as high blood pressure or diabetes. More than half have no health insurance. All struggle with the enormous stress of finding food and shelter for themselves and their families.

Communities around the country are trying different ways to help the homeless. Some provide for the day-to-day needs of the homeless with free meals, blankets, and beds. Others offer work opportunities that allow homeless people to earn some pocket money and to increase their personal dignity. What can you do?

BECOME INFORMED

- Are there homeless people in your community? Find out more about them. Approximately how many local residents are homeless? How many are families with children? Where do they stay? What keeps them on the street?
- What programs or shelters are available to the homeless in your community?
- What is your community doing to decrease the stressors that contribute to the problem of homelessness? Are any advocacy groups working on behalf of the homeless?

BECOME INVOLVED
Rather than thinking that homelessness is someone else's problem, you and others in your class can work together to become part of the solution. Start by discussing the following questions:

- How well do you think your community is meeting the needs of its homeless?
- What types of action could your community take to reduce homelessness?
- If there are homeless students on campus, how might they be helped?
- How can you and others in your class help the homeless? Could you relate differently to homeless people when you meet them on the street? Could you collect and donate canned goods and other staples to a local soup kitchen? Could you volunteer at a shelter or for an advocacy group? Could you tutor children of homeless families?

and flight attendants, teachers and telemarketers feel the flames of too much stress and not enough satisfaction. Many people, especially those caring for others at work or at home, get to a point where there's an imbalance between their own feelings and dealing with difficult, distressful issues on a day-to-day basis. If they don't recognize what's going on and make some changes, their health and the quality of their work suffer.

"Burnout doesn't stem from the job or the person but from both," says psychologist Christina Maslach, Ph.D., author of *Banishing Burnout.* "What matters is the relationship you have with work rather than with the work that you do."[21] As with other long-term commitments, it takes time, attention, and effort to keep this relationship healthy—and to repair it if it breaks down.

Early signs of burnout include exhaustion; sleep problems or nightmares; increased anxiety or nervousness; muscular tension (headaches, backaches, and the like); increased use of alcohol or medication; digestive problems (such as nausea, vomiting, or diarrhea); loss of interest in sex; frequent body aches or pain; quarrels with family or friends; negative feelings about everything; problems concentrating; job mistakes and accidents; and feelings of depression, hopelessness, or helplessness.

Age is the one variable most consistently associated with burnout: Younger employees between ages 30 and 40 report the highest rates. Both men and women are susceptible to burnout. Unmarried individuals, particularly men, seem more prone to burnout than married workers. Single employees who've never been married have higher burnout rates than those who are divorced.

Illness and Disability

Just as the mind can have profound effects on the body, the body can have an enormous impact on our emotions. Whenever we come down with the flu or pull a muscle, we feel under par. When the problem is more serious or persistent—a chronic disease like diabetes, for instance, or a lifelong hearing impairment—the emotional stress of constantly coping with it is even greater.

 A common source of stress for college students is a learning disability, which may affect one of every ten Americans. Most people with learning disabilities have average or above-average intelligence, but they rarely live up to their ability in school. Some have only one area of difficulty, such as reading or math. Others have problems with attention, writing, communicating, reasoning, coordination, and social skills.

Not all students with learning disabilities experience greater stress. In one in-depth study comparing 34 undergraduates with and without learning disabilities, the students with learning disabilities (LD) reported significantly fewer college stressors and demonstrated a higher need for achievement. The LD students also scored significantly higher in resiliency and initiative in solving problems and working toward goals.

Societal Stressors

Centuries ago the poet John Donne observed that no man is an island. Today, on an increasingly crowded and troubled planet, these words seem truer than ever. Problems such as discrimination and terrorism can no longer be viewed only as economic or political issues. Directly or indirectly, they affect the well-being of all who inhabit Earth—now and in the future.

The deliberate use of physical force to abuse or injure is a leading killer of young people in the United States—and a potential source of stress in all our lives. If you or someone you know has been a victim of a violent crime, a sense of vulnerability may add to the stress of daily living. See "Your Strategies for Change" on page 80 and "Your Guardian Angel" in *Labs for IPC.*

Responses to Stress

It may be tempting to look for a "quick fix" for stress. (See Consumer Alert, p. 81.) Sometimes we respond to stress or challenge with self-destructive behaviors, such as drinking or using drugs. These responses can lead to psychological problems, such as anxiety or depression, and physical problems, including psychosomatic illnesses.

Defense Mechanisms

Defense mechanisms, such as those described in Table 3.2, are another response to stress. These psychological devices are mental processes that help us cope with personal problems. Such responses also are not the answer to stress—and learning to recognize them in yourself will enable you to deal with your stress in a healthier way.

Cognitive Restructuring

Every day about 60,000 thoughts pass through our brains as we plan, evaluate, judge, interpret, and remember. Some of these thoughts are as precise as a mathematical equation, but others are misleading or inappropriate. These inaccurate or self-defeating thoughts are the target of cognitive-behavioral therapy (CBT), a highly effective psychological treatment describe in Chapter 4.

Cognitive restructuring, one of the techniques of CBT, can reduce stress by helping people examine unhappy, negative thoughts that are making them anxious, challenging these thoughts, and in many cases rewriting the negative thinking that lies behind them. Because thoughts create feelings and drive

defense mechanism A psychological process that alleviates anxiety and eliminates mental conflict; includes denial, displacement, projection, rationalization, reaction formation, and repression.

YOUR STRATEGIES
FOR CHANGE
*How to Cope with
Distress after a Trauma*

Senseless acts of violence
or terrorism can trigger
a variety of emotions,
including shock, sorrow,
fear, anger, and grief.
You may have problems
sleeping, concentrating,
or going about simple
chores. Because the world
seems more dangerous, it
may take a while for you
to regain your sense of
equilibrium. The following
recommendations from the
American Psychological
Association can help.

- **Talk about it.** Ask for
  support from people
  who will listen to your
  concerns. It often helps
  to speak with others who
  have shared your experience so you do not feel
  so different or alone.
- **Strive for balance.**
  Remind yourself of peo-
  ple and events that are
  meaningful and comfort-
  ing, even encouraging.
- **Take a break.** Schedule
  breaks to focus on something you enjoy.
- **Take care of yourself.**
  Engage in healthy
  behaviors, such as exercise, that will enhance
  your ability to cope.
  Avoid alcohol and drugs
  because they can sup-
  press your feelings rather
  than help you to manage
  your distress.
- **Help others or do
  something productive.**
  Helping someone else
  often helps you feel better too.

> **TABLE 3.2**

Common Defense Mechanisms Used to Alleviate Anxiety and Eliminate Conflict

Defense Mechanism	Example
Denial: the refusal to accept a painful reality.	You don't accept as true the news that a loved one is seriously ill.
Displacement: the redirection of feelings from their true object to a more acceptable or safer substitute.	Instead of lashing out at a coach or a teacher, you snap at your best friend.
Projection: the attribution of unacceptable feelings or impulses to someone else.	When you want to end a relationship, you protect your unhappiness onto your partner.
Rationalization: the substitution of "good," acceptable reasons for the real motivations of our behavior.	You report a classmate who has been mean to you for cheating on an exam and explain that cheating is unfair to other students.
Reaction formation: adopting attitudes and behaviors that are the opposite of what we feel.	You lavishly compliment an acquaintance whom you really despise.
Repression: the way we keep threatening impulses, fantasies, memories, feelings, or wishes from becoming conscious.	You don't "hear" the alarm after the late night, or you "forget" to take out the trash.

behavior, this approach enables people to approach stressful situations in a positive frame of mind.

The first step is becoming aware of automatic thoughts that enter your brain, for instance, "I will never understand this material." "I'm going to flunk this test." "No one wants to talk with me." Then you challenge these negative assumptions with counter-arguments such as "I felt the same way in chemistry class, and eventually I figured it out," "If I focus on the questions I do know, I'll be okay," or "I can try smiling and striking up a conversation." You can also develop specific action techniques to blunt negative thoughts and lessen stress. For instance, you could master some of the relaxation and test-taking techniques described in this chapter and in *Labs for IPC.*

Routes to Relaxation

A more positive response to stress is relaxation—the physical and mental state opposite that of stress. Rather than gearing up for fight or flight, our bodies and minds grow calmer and work more smoothly. We're less likely to become frazzled and more capable of staying in control. The most effective relaxation techniques include progressive relaxation, visualization, meditation, mindfulness, and biofeedback. (Also see "Rx: Relax" in the *Labs for IPC.*)

Progressive relaxation works by intentionally increasing and then decreasing tension in the muscles. While sitting or lying down in a quiet, comfortable setting, you tense and release various muscles, beginning with those of the hand, for instance, and then proceeding to the arms, shoulders, neck, face, scalp, chest, stomach, buttocks, genitals, and so on, down each leg to the toes. Relaxing the muscles can quiet the mind and restore internal balance.

Visualization, or **guided imagery**, involves creating mental pictures that calm you down and focus your mind. Some people use this technique to promote healing when they are ill. Visualization skills require practice and, in some cases, instruction by qualified health professionals.

Meditation has been practiced in many forms over the ages, from the yogic techniques of the Far East to the Quaker silence of more modern times. Brain scans have shown that meditation activates the sections of the brain in charge of the autonomic nervous system, which governs bodily functions, such as digestion and blood pressure, that we cannot consciously control. Research with a group of Tibetan monks and lay practitioners with extensive experience in meditation has demonstrated that meditation produces changes in various regions of the brain and can actually cause people to be more compassionate.[22] Although many studies have documented the benefits of meditation for overall health, it may be particularly helpful for people

Stress Scams

Aromatic candles. Gurgling fountains. Squeezable foam balls. Incense burners. Soothing gels. Everywhere you turn you can find something that promises to relieve stress. Do they work? Most don't cause any harm, but they don't necessarily do much good either.

Facts to Know

- "Natural" products, such as herbs and enzymes, claim to have psychological effects. However, because they are not classified as drugs, these products have not undergone the rigorous scientific testing required of psychiatric medications, and little is known about their safety or efficacy. "Natural" doesn't mean risk-free. Opium and cocaine are "natural" substances that have dramatic and potentially deadly effects on the mind.

- Don't make matters worse by smoking (the chemicals in cigarettes increase heart rate, blood pressure, and stress hormones), consuming too much caffeine (it speeds up your system for hours), eating snacks high in sugar (it produces a quick high followed by a sudden slump), or turning to drugs or alcohol (they can only add to your stress when their effects wear off).

Steps to Take

- Be wary of instant cures. Regardless of the promises on the label, it's unrealistic to expect any magic ingredient or product to make all your problems disappear.

- Focus on stress-reducing behavior, rather than a product. An aromatic candle may not bring instant serenity, but if you light a candle and meditate, you may indeed feel more at peace.

- Experiment with physical ways to work out stress. Exercise is one of the best ways to lower your stress levels. Try walking, running, swimming, cycling, kickboxing—anything physical that helps you release tension.

---

dealing with stress-related medical conditions such as high blood pressure and heart problems and for preventing stress-induced changes in the immune system.[23]

Meditation helps a person reach a state of relaxation, but with the goal of achieving inner peace and harmony. There is no one right way to meditate, and many people have discovered how to meditate on their own, without even knowing what it is they are doing.

Increasing numbers of college students are turning to meditation as a way of coping with stress. Most forms of meditation have common elements: sitting quietly for 15 to 20 minutes once or twice a day, concentrating on a word or image, and breathing slowly and rhythmically. If you wish to try meditation, it often helps to have someone guide you through your first sessions. Or try tape recording your own voice (with or without favorite music in the background) and playing it back to yourself, freeing yourself to concentrate on the goal of turning the attention within.

Mindfulness is a modern form of an ancient Asian technique that involves maintaining awareness in the present moment. You tune in to each part of your body, scanning from head to toe, noting the slightest sensation. You allow whatever you experience—an itch, an ache, a feeling of warmth—to enter your awareness. Then you open yourself to focus on all the thoughts, sensations, sounds, and feelings that enter your awareness. Mindfulness keeps you in the here and now, thinking about *what* is rather than about *what if* or *if only.*

Biofeedback is a method of obtaining feedback, or information, about some physiological activity occurring in the body. An electronic monitoring device attached to the body detects a change in an internal function and communicates it back to the person through a tone, light, or meter. By paying attention to this feedback, most people can gain some control over functions previously thought to be beyond conscious control, such as body temperature, heart rate, muscle tension, and brain waves. Biofeedback training consists of three stages:

1. Developing increased awareness of a body state or function.

2. Gaining control over it.

3. Transferring this control to everyday living without use of the electronic instrument.

The goal of biofeedback for stress reduction is a state of tranquility, usually associated with the brain's production of alpha waves (which are slower and more regular than normal waking waves). After

progressive relaxation A method of reducing muscle tension by contracting, then relaxing, certain areas of the body.

visualization, or guided imagery An approach to stress control, self-healing, or motivating life changes by means of seeing oneself in the state of calmness, wellness, or change.

meditation A group of approaches that use quiet sitting, breathing techniques, and/or chanting to relax, improve concentration, and become attuned to one's inner self.

mindfulness A method of stress reduction that involves experiencing the physical and mental sensations of the present moment.

biofeedback A technique of becoming aware, with the aid of external monitoring devices, of internal physiological activities in order to develop the capability of altering them.

Writing in your journal about feelings and difficulties is a simple and effective way to help control your stress. You don't need to be a journalist. Just write about *you*.

several training sessions, most people can produce alpha waves more or less at will.

Exercise

Regular physical activity can relieve stress, boost energy, lift mood, and keep stress under control. Young adults who adopt and continue regular aerobic exercise show less intense cardiovascular responses to stress, which may protect them against coronary heart disease as they age. Strength training may have similar benefits.

Various studies have examined the correlation between physical activity and stress in college students. Students who report higher levels of leisure-time exercise, along with a good social network and time management skills, generally enjoy better mental health.[24] Other researchers have found that active students report as much stress as inactive ones.[25] Try an experiment with yourself: Keep track of the days when you work out in some way and those you don't. Rate your stress level every day, and see if exercise makes a difference for you.

Journaling

One of the simplest, yet most effective, ways to work through stress is by putting your feelings into words that only you will read. The more honest and open you are as you write, the better. College students who wrote in their journals about traumatic events felt much better afterward than those who wrote about superficial topics. Focus on intense emotional experiences and "autopsy" them to try to understand why they affected you the way they did. Rereading and thinking about your notes may reveal the underlying reasons for your response. See the chapter on "Power Journaling" in *IPC*.

Traumatic Life Events and Stress

Bad things happen. Cars crash. Close friends and relatives die. Floods, tornadoes, and earthquakes wreak havoc on communities. Armed students shoot senselessly at classmates and professors. According to epidemiological studies, about half of all people experience at least one potentially traumatic event—natural or man-made, large-scale or small—during the course of their lives.[26] As profoundly disturbing as such experiences can be, recent research has shown that after a trauma the vast majority of people, including children, cope well, continue to meet the demands of their daily lives, and recover fully.[27]

Traumatic experiences, as one researcher puts it, are like the common cold, "experienced at some time by nearly all."[28] In a recent study of college women, nine in ten reported having directly experienced at least one traumatic event, usually involving a threat to their own lives or to others. The most frequently reported trauma was a motor vehicle accident.[29]

Many people develop a temporary "acute stress reaction," characterized by symptoms such as reexperiencing the trauma, avoiding certain places or situations, and feeling a sense of arousal or hypersensitivity. But just as the common cold can lead to pneumonia and other serious complications, traumatic experiences can provoke more serious reactions in about 20 to 30 percent of trauma survivors. Of these, about half recover over time even without treatment.[30]

Posttraumatic Stress Disorder (PTSD)

In the past, **posttraumatic stress disorder (PTSD)** was viewed as a psychological response to out-of-the-ordinary stressors, such as captivity or combat. However, other experiences can also forever change the way people view themselves and their world. Individuals with PTSD often suffer cognitive impairments, including memory problems.[31]

An estimated 7.7 million American adults have PTSD.[32] Women are, on average, twice as vulnerable as men to PTSD, but not because they experience more traumatic events. Childhood traumas occur equally in both sexes. Adult men encounter more traumas—accidents, violence, combat, terrorism, disasters, injuries—than adult women. Women experience more sexual assaults and abuse. PTSD is especially high in women who have served in the military. Sexual trauma ranks as the most distressing for female veterans, followed by physical assault and war zone experience.

Veterans of combat in Iraq and Afghanistan have high rates of PTSD, along with other problems such as substance abuse. Many have experienced high-intensity guerilla warfare as well as the chronic threat of roadside bombs and improvised explosive devices; some have suffered traumatic brain injuries.[33] In the long term, veterans with PTSD face an increased chance of developing metabolic syndrome and coronary heart disease and of exhibiting greater risk-taking behavior.[34]

Some people may be especially vulnerable to PTSD. Scientists have identified certain genes that increase susceptibility.[35] Exposure to traumatic experience in childhood along with poverty, difficult temperament, and low IQ also increase the risk.

PTSD can cause a range of symptoms, including fear, worry, insomnia, and drug and alcohol abuse. Some individuals reexperience their terror and helplessness again and again in their dreams or intrusive thoughts. To avoid this psychic pain, they may try to avoid anything associated with the trauma. Some enter a state of emotional numbness and no longer can respond to people and experiences the way they once did, especially when it comes to showing tenderness or affection. Those who've been mugged or raped may be afraid to venture out by themselves.

Mental health professionals have found that no single approach to treatment works for all trauma victims. Some approaches, such as immediate "debriefing" to release emotions or treatment with anxiety-reducing medications, may not help and may even hinder long-term recovery.[36] But behavioral, cognitive, and psychodynamic therapy, sometimes along with psychiatric medication (described in Chapter 4), can usually help individuals suffering with PTSD.

Resilience

Adversity—whether in the form of a traumatic event or chronic stress—has different effects on individuals. Some people never recover and continue on a downward slide that may ultimately prove fatal. Others return, though at different rates, to their prior level of functioning. In recent years researchers have focused their attention on a particularly intriguing group: those people who not only survive stressful experiences but also thrive, that is, who actually surpass their previous level of functioning. See the chapter on "Shock Absorption" in *IPC*.

Resilience can take many forms. A father whose child is kidnapped and killed may become a nationwide advocate for victims' rights. A student whose roommate dies in a car crash after a party may campaign for tougher laws against drunk driving. A couple whose premature baby spends weeks in a neonatal intensive care unit may find that their marriage has grown closer and stronger. Even though their experiences were painful, the individuals often look back at them as bringing positive changes into their lives.

Researchers have studied various factors that enable individuals to thrive in the face of adversity. These include:

- **An optimistic attitude.** Rather than reacting to a stressor simply as a threat, these men and women view stress as a challenge—one they believe they can and will overcome. Researchers have documented that individuals facing various stressors, including serious illness and bereavement, are more likely to report experiencing growth if they have high levels of hope and optimism.

- **Self-efficacy.** A sense of being in control of one's life can boost health, even in times of great stress.

- **Stress inoculation.** People who deal well with adversity often have had previous experiences with stress that toughened them in various ways, such as teaching them skills that enhanced their ability to cope and boosting their confidence in their ability to weather a rough patch.

YOUR STRATEGIES FOR PREVENTION

How to Avoid Stress Overload

To avoid stress overload, watch for the following warning signals:

- You are experiencing physical symptoms, including chronic fatigue, headaches, indigestion, diarrhea, and sleep problems.
- You are having frequent illness or worrying about illness.
- You are self-medicating, including nonprescription drugs.
- You are having problems concentrating on studies or work.
- You are feeling irritable, anxious, or apathetic.
- You are working or studying longer and harder than usual.
- You are exaggerating, to yourself and others, the importance of what you do.
- You are becoming accident-prone.
- You are breaking rules, whether it's a curfew at the dorm or a speed limit on the highway.
- You are going to extremes, such as drinking too much, overspending, or gambling.

posttraumatic stress disorder (PTSD) The repeated reliving of a trauma through nightmares or recollection.

- **Secure personal relationships.** Individuals who know they can count on the support of their loved ones are more likely to be resilient.

- **Spirituality or religiosity.** Religious coping may be particularly related to growth and resilience. In particular, two types seem most beneficial: spiritually based religious coping (receiving emotional reassurance and guidance from God) and good-deeds coping (living a better, more spiritual life that includes altruistic acts).

Resilience sometimes means developing new skills simply because, in order to get through the stressful experience, people had to learn something they hadn't known how to do before—for instance, wrangling with insurance companies or other bureaucracies. By mastering such skills, they become more fit to deal with an unpredictable world and develop new flexibility in facing the unknown.

Individuals who engage in proactive coping, a concept based on the principles of positive psychology discussed in Chapter 2, perceive stressful situations as challenges instead of threats. In a study of college women who had experienced traumas, those who saw these events as learning experiences and who felt gratitude for what they had learned reported posttraumatic emotional growth, rather than distress, in the form of increased strength, confidence, and maturity.[37]

Along with new abilities comes the psychological sense of mastery. "I survived this," an individual may say. "I'll be able to deal with other hard things in the future." Such confidence keeps people actively engaged in the effort to cope and is itself a predictor of eventual success. Stress also can make individuals more aware of the fulfilling aspects of life, and they may become more interested in spiritual pursuits. Certain kinds of stressful experiences also have social consequences. If a person experiencing a traumatic event finds that the significant others in his or her life can be counted on, the result can be a strengthening of their relationship.

Organizing Your Time

We live in what some sociologists call hyperculture, a society that moves at warp speed. Information bombards us constantly. The rate of change seems to accelerate every year. Our "time-saving" devices—pagers, cell phones, modems, faxes, palm-size organizers, laptop computers—have simply extended the boundaries of where and how we work.

As a result, more and more people are suffering from "timesickness," a nerve-racking feeling that life has become little more than an endless to-do list. The best antidote is time management, and hundreds of books, seminars, and experts offer training in making the most of the hours in the day. Yet these well-intentioned methods often fail, and sooner or later most of us find ourselves caught in a time trap. (See the chapter on "Time Control" in *IPC.*)

Are You Running Out of Time?

Every day you make dozens of decisions, and the choices you make about how to use your time directly affect your stress level. If you have a big test on Monday and a term paper due Tuesday, you may plan to study all weekend. Then, when you're invited to a party Saturday night, you go. Although you set the alarm for 7:00 a.m. on Sunday, you don't pull yourself out of bed until noon. By the time you start studying, it's 4:00 p.m., and anxiety is building inside you.

How can you tell if you've lost control of your time? The following are telltale symptoms of poor time management:

- Rushing.
- Chronic inability to make choices or decisions.
- Fatigue or listlessness.
- Constantly missed deadlines.
- Not enough time for rest or personal relationships.
- A sense of being overwhelmed by demands and details and having to do

what you don't want to do most of the time.

One of the hard lessons of being on your own is that your choices and your actions have consequences. Stress is just one of them. But by thinking ahead, being realistic about your workload, and sticking to your plans, you can gain better control over your time and your stress levels.

Managing Your Time

Time management involves skills that anyone can learn, but they require commitment and practice to make a difference in your life. It may help to know the techniques that other students have found most useful:

- **Schedule your time.** Use a calendar or planner. Beginning the first week of class, mark down deadlines for each assignment, paper, project, and test scheduled that semester. Develop a daily schedule, listing very specifically what you will do the next day, along with the times. Block out times for working out, eating dinner, calling home, and talking with friends as well as for studying.

- **Develop a game plan.** Allow at least two nights to study for any major exam. Set aside more time for researching and writing papers. Make sure to allow time to revise and print out a paper—and to deal with emergencies like a computer breakdown. Set daily and weekly goals for every class. When working on a big project, don't neglect your other courses. Whenever possible, try to work ahead in all your classes.

- **Identify time robbers.** For several days keep a log of what you do and how much time you spend doing it. You may discover that disorganization is eating away at your time or that you have a problem getting started. (See the following section on "Overcoming Procrastination.")

- **Make the most of classes.** Read the assignments before class rather than waiting until just before you have a test. By reading ahead of time, you'll make it easier to understand the lectures. Go to class yourself. Your own notes will

be more helpful than a friend's or those from a note-taking service. Read your lecture notes at the end of each day or at least at the end of each week.

- **Develop an efficient study style.** Some experts recommend studying for 50 minutes, then breaking for 10 minutes. Small incentives, such as allowing yourself to call or visit a friend during those 10 minutes, can provide the motivation to keep you at the books longer. When you're reading, don't just highlight passages. Instead, write notes or questions to yourself in the margins, which will help you retain more information. Even if you're racing to start a paper, take a few extra minutes to prepare a workable outline. It will be easier to structure your paper when you start writing.

- **Focus on the task at hand.** Rather than worrying about how you did on yesterday's test or how you'll ever finish next week's project, focus intently on whatever you're doing at any given moment. If your mind starts to wander, use any distraction—the sound of the phone ringing or a noise from the hall—as a reminder to stay in the moment.

- **Turn elephants into hors d'oeuvres.** Cut a huge task into smaller chunks so it seems less enormous. For instance, break down your term paper into a series of steps, such as selecting a topic, identifying sources of research information, taking notes, developing an outline, and so on.

- **Keep your workspace in order.** Even if the rest of your room is a shambles, try to keep your desk clear. Piles of papers are distracting, and you can end up wasting lots of time looking for notes you misplaced or an article you have to read by morning. Try to spend the last ten minutes of the day getting your desk in order so you get a fresh start on the new day.

Overcoming Procrastination

Putting off until tomorrow what should be done today is a habit that creates a great deal of stress for many students. It also takes a surprising toll. In studies with students taking a health psychology course, researchers found that although procrastinating

MAKING CHANGE HAPPEN

Do It Now!

Chronic procrastination can trip you up, slow you down, stress you out, and sabotage your best efforts. You know that. But you may not realize that procrastination isn't a character flaw. All delay stems from a certain degree of fear—fear of failure, fear of success, fear of not being in control. People who procrastinate simply haven't yet developed good habits for getting work done, or they have bad habits they need to unlearn and replace. "Do It Now" in *Labs for IPC* will show you how to do both. Here's a preview.

Get Real

In this section you get a clear fix on when and how you procrastinate by checking yes for each of ten statements that describe your behavior, including these three examples:

- I put off studying subjects I find difficult.
- I put off studying subjects I find easy because I don't think they will demand much time.
- I wait to have a big block of time before starting a project.

The more checks, the greater your problem with procrastination.

Get Ready

At this stage you set aside time for various exercises, including writing refutations of excuses you have used for procrastinating and keeping a simple chart of dates assignments are given and dates they are due for each class.

Get Going

In this stage you engage in seven exercises, each designed to preempt procrastination. Here are two examples:

- **Complete the incompletes.** Every day find one thing that you began at some point but have not yet finished. It might be making the bed, replying to an e-mail, buying a birthday card for your grandfather, replacing the bulb in your bedside lamp . . .
- **Eavesdrop on your excuses.** Every time you balk at writing the first sentence of a report or reading the first page of the assigned novel, stop and listen to what you're telling yourself. Here are three of the excuses you're likely to hear:
  - I'm too tired. I'll rest first.
  - There's no point in starting. I've got to meet my friend Ravi in ten minutes.
  - "Why do it on Friday? The instructor won't get it until Monday?"

Write rebuttals to yourself. For instance, you might say, "Yes, I'm tired. I'll just work for half and hour, and then I'll go to bed." Or you might tell yourself, "I'll see how much I can get done in ten minutes."

Lock It In

Keep doing the exercises, including completing your incompletes. Don't let a day go by when you don't cross something off your to-do list—even if it's making a to-do list.

---

provided short-term benefits, including periods of low stress, the tendency to dawdle had long-term costs, including poorer health and lower grades. Early in the semester, the procrastinators reported less stress and fewer health problems than students who scored low on procrastination. However, by the end of the semester, procrastinators reported more health-related symptoms, more stress, and more visits to health-care professionals than nonprocrastinators. Students who procrastinate also get poorer grades in courses with many deadlines.

The three most common types of procrastination are putting off unpleasant things, putting off difficult tasks, and putting off tough decisions. Procrastinators are most likely to delay by wishing they didn't have to do what they must or by telling themselves they "just can't get started," which means they never do.

To get out of the procrastination trap, keep track of the tasks you're most likely to put off, and try to figure out why you don't want to tackle them. Think of alternative ways to get tasks done. If you put off library readings, for instance, is the problem getting to the library or the reading itself? If it's the trip to the library, arrange to walk over with a friend whose company you enjoy.

Do what you like least first. Once you have it out of the way, you can concentrate on the tasks you enjoy. Build time into your schedule for interruptions, unforeseen problems, and unexpected events, so you aren't constantly racing around. Establish ground rules for meeting your own needs (including getting enough sleep and making time for friends) before saying yes to any activity. Learn to live according to a three-word motto: Just do it! (See Making Change Happen, above, and Do It Now in *Labs for IPC*.)

LEARN IT / LIVE IT Coping with Stress

The key to coping with stress is realizing that your perception of and response to a stressor are crucial. Changing the way you interpret events or situations—a skill called reframing—makes all the difference. An event, such as a move to a new city, is not stressful in itself. A move becomes stressful if you see it as a traumatic upheaval rather than an exciting beginning of a new chapter in your life.

In times of stress, the following simple exercises can stop the stress buildup inside your body and help you regain a sense of calm and control.

- **Breathing.** Deep breathing relaxes the body and quiets the mind. Draw air deeply into your lungs, allowing your chest to fill with air and your belly to rise and fall. You will feel the muscle tension and stress begin to melt away. When you're feeling extremely stressed, try this calming breath: Sit or lie with your back straight and place the tip of your tongue on the roof of your mouth behind your teeth. Exhale completely through the mouth, then inhale through the nose for 4 seconds. Hold the breath for 7 seconds, then exhale audibly through the mouth for 8 seconds. Repeat four times.

- **Refocusing.** Thinking about a situation you can't change or control only increases the stress you feel. Force your mind to focus on other subjects. If you're stuck in a long line, distract yourself. Check out what other people are buying or imagine what they do for a living. Or imagine that you're in a hot shower and a wave of relaxation is washing your stress down the drain.

- **Serenity breaks.** Build moments of tranquility into your day. For instance, while waiting for your computer to start up or a file to download, look at a photograph of someone you love or a poster of a tropical island. If none is available, close your eyes and visualize a soothing scene, such as walking in a meadow or along a beach.

- **Stress signals.** Learn to recognize the first signs that your stress load is getting out of hand: Is your back bothering you? Do you have a headache? Do you find yourself speeding or misplacing things? Whenever you spot these early warnings, force yourself to stop and say, I'm under stress. I need to do something about it.

- **Reality checks.** To put things into proper perspective, ask yourself: Will I remember what's made me so upset a month from now? If I had to rank this problem on a scale of 1 to 10, with worldwide catastrophe as 10, where would it rate?

- **Stress inoculation.** Rehearse everyday situations that you find stressful, such as speaking in class. Think of how you might make the situation less tense, for instance, by breathing deeply before you talk or jotting down notes beforehand. Think of these small "doses" of stress as the psychological equivalent of allergy shots: They immunize you so you feel less stressed when bigger challenges come along.

- **Rx: Laughter.** Humor counters stress by focusing on comic aspects of difficult situations and may, as various studies have shown, lessen harmful effects on the immune system and overall health.

SELF SURVEY Student Stress Scale

The Student Stress Scale, an adaptation of Holmes and Rahe's Life Events Scale for college-age adults, provides a rough indication of stress levels and possible health consequences.

In the Student Stress Scale, each event, such as beginning or ending school, is given a score that represents the amount of readjustment a person has to make as a result of the change. In some studies, using similar scales, people with serious illnesses have been found to have high scores.

To determine your stress score, add up the number of points corresponding to the events you have experienced in the past 12 months.

1. Death of a close family member	100	
2. Death of a close friend	73	
3. Divorce of parents	65	
4. Jail term	63	
5. Major personal injury or illness	63	
6. Marriage	58	
7. Getting fired from a job	50	
8. Failing an important course	47	
9. Change in the health of a family member	45	
10. Pregnancy	45	
11. Sex problems	44	
12. Serious argument with a close friend	40	
13. Change in financial status	39	
14. Change of academic major	39	
15. Trouble with parents	39	
16. New girlfriend or boyfriend	37	
17. Increase in workload at school	37	
18. Outstanding personal achievement	36	
19. First quarter/semester in college	36	
20. Change in living conditions	31	
21. Serious argument with an instructor	30	
22. Getting lower grades than expected	29	
23. Change in sleeping habits	29	
24. Change in social activities	29	
25. Change in eating habits	28	
26. Chronic car trouble	26	
27. Change in number of family get-togethers	26	
28. Too many missed classes	25	
29. Changing colleges	24	
30. Dropping more than one class	23	
31. Minor traffic violations	20	
	Total Stress Score	_____

Here's how to interpret your score: If your score is 300 or higher, you're at high risk for developing a health problem. If your score is between 150 and 300, you have a 50–50 chance of experiencing a serious health change within two years. If your score is below 150, you have a 1 in 3 chance of a serious health change.

Source: Mullen, Kathleen, and Gerald Costello. *Health Awareness Through Discovery.* Minneapolis: Burgess Publishing Company, 1981.

Your Health Action Plan for Physical Fitness

College is a perfect time to learn and practice the art of stress reduction. You can start applying the techniques and concepts outlined in this chapter immediately. You may want to begin by doing some relaxation or awareness exercises. They can give you the peace of mind you need to focus more effectively on larger issues, goals, and decisions.

You needn't see stress as a problem to solve on your own. Reach out to others. As you build friendships and intimate relationships, you may find that some irritating problems are easier to put into perspective. Don't be afraid to laugh at yourself and to look for the comic or absurd aspects of a situation. In addition, you might try some simple approaches that can help boost your stress resistance and resilence, including the following:

- **Focusing.** Take a strain inventory of your body every day to determine where things aren't feeling quite right. Ask yourself, What's keeping me from feeling terrific today? Focusing on problem spots, such as stomach knots or neck tightness, increases your sense of control over stress.

- **Reconstructing stressful situations.** Think about a recent episode of distress; then write down three ways it could have gone better and three ways it could have gone worse. This should help you see that the situation wasn't as disastrous as it might have been and help you find ways to cope better in the future.

- **Self-improvement.** When your life feels out of control, turn to a new challenge. You might try volunteering at a nursing home, going for a long-distance bike trip, or learning a foreign language. As you work toward your new goal, you'll realize that you still can cope and achieve.

If stress continues to be a problem in your life, you may be able to find help through support groups or counseling. Your school may provide counseling services or referrals to mental health professionals; ask your health instructor or the campus health department for this information. Remember that each day of distress robs you of energy, distracts you from life's pleasures, and interferes with achieving your full potential.

MAKING THIS CHAPTER WORK FOR YOU

Review Questions

1. In this text we define stress as
   a. a negative emotional state related to fatigue and similar to depression.
   b. the physiological and psychological response to any event or situation that either upsets or excites us.
   c. the end result of the general adaptation syndrome.
   d. a motivational strategy for making life changes.

2. Which of the following illustrates the defense mechanism of displacement?
   a. You have a beer in the evening after a tough day.
   b. You act as if nothing has happened after you have been laid off from your job.
   c. You start an argument with your sister after being laid off from your job.
   d. You argue with your boss after he lays you off from your job.

3. An effective technique for dealing with test stress is
   a. planning ahead.
   b. going on a study blitz the night before the test.
   c. going out for a few beers with friends the night before the test.
   d. talking with friends about everything but the test.

4. A person suffering from posttraumatic stress disorder may experience which of the following symptoms?
   a. procrastination
   b. constant thirst
   c. drowsiness
   d. terror-filled dreams

5. According to the general adaptation syndrome theory, how does the body typically respond to an acute stressor?
   a. The heart rate slows, blood pressure declines, and eye movement increases.
   b. The body enters a physical state called eustress and then moves into the physical state referred to as distress.
   c. If the stressor is viewed as a positive event, there are no physical changes.
   d. The body demonstrates three stages of change: alarm, resistance, and exhaustion.

6. Burnout is
   a. the aftermath of extreme anger triggered by stress.
   b. a feeling of complete defeat.
   c. the feeling that comes after a long evening of partying.
   d. a state of exhaustion brought on by constant or repeated emotional pressure.

7. To develop an efficient studying style:
   a. Schedule your study time on a calendar or planner, have a friend go to class and take notes for you, and join the chess club.
   b. Schedule your study time on a calendar or planner, write notes or questions about the material in the margins of the book, and give yourself a small break after every study hour.
   c. Read assignments before class, call a friend before studying, and plan on working for four continuous hours.
   d. Read assignments before class, skip class when studying for an exam, and have snacks on hand.

8. Over time, increased levels of stress hormones have been shown to increase a person's risk for which of the following conditions?
   a. high blood pressure, memory loss, and skin disorders
   b. stress fractures, male pattern baldness, and hypothyroidism
   c. hemophilia, AIDS, and hay fever
   d. none of the above

9. A relaxed peaceful state of being can be achieved with which of the following activities?
   a. an aerobic exercise class
   b. playing a computer game
   c. meditating for 15 minutes
   d. attending a rap concert

10. Stress levels in college students
   a. may be high due to stressors such as academic pressures, financial concerns, learning disabilities, and relationship problems.
   b. are usually low because students feel empowered living independently of their parents.
   c. are typically highest in seniors because their self-esteem diminishes during the college years.
   d. are lower in minority students because they are used to stressors such as a hostile social climate and actual or perceived discrimination.

Answers to these questions can be found on page 650.

Critical Thinking

1. Identify three stressful situations in your life and determine whether they are examples of eustress or distress. Describe both the positive and negative aspects of each situation.

2. Can you think of any ways in which your behavior or attitudes might create stress for others? What changes could you make to avoid doing so?

3. What advice might you give an incoming freshman at your school about managing stress in college? What techniques have been most helpful for you in dealing with stress? Suppose that this student is from a different ethnic group than you. What additional suggestions would you have for this student?

Media Menu

CENGAGENOW™ Go to the CengageNOW for Health website at **www .cengage.com/sso** that will:
- Help you evaluate your knowledge of the material.
- Allow you to take an exam-prep quiz.
- Provide a Personalized Learning Plan targeting resources that address areas you should study.
- Coach you through identifying target goals for behavioral change and creating and monitoring your personal change plan throughout the semester.

Internet Connections

http://cehs.unl.edu/stress/resources.html
This online series of lectures on stress management is presented by Wesley E. Sime, Ph.D., M.P.H., Professor of Health and Human Performance at the University of Nebraska–Lincoln. It features information on the psychobiology of stress and relaxation, as well as the pathophysiology of stress.

www.teachhealth.com
This comprehensive website is written specifically for college students by Steven Burns, M.D. It features the following topics: signs of how to recognize stress, two stress surveys for adults and college students, information on the pathophysiology of stress, the genetics of stress and stress tolerance, and information on how to best manage and treat stress.

www.mindtools.com/smpage.html
This site covers a variety of topics on stress management, including recognizing stress, exercise, time management, coping mechanisms, and more. The site also features a free comprehensive personal self-assessment with questions pertaining to work and home stressors, physical and behavioral signs and symptoms, as well as personal coping skills and resources.

Key Terms

The terms listed are used on the page indicated. Definitions of the terms are in the Glossary at the end of the book.

acculturation 73
adaptive response 67
biofeedback 81
burnout 77
defense mechanisms 79
diathesis stress model 69
distress 67
eustress 67
general adaptation syndrome (GAS) 67
homeostasis 67
meditation 81
mindfulness 81
posttraumatic stress disorder (PTSD) 83
progressive relaxation 81
stress 67
stressor 67
visualization, or guided imagery 81

Chapter 4 - Taking Care of Your Mind

1. **Basically all human functions and activities are regulated by the: (Pg. 92)**
   A. heart
   B. brain
   C. nerves
   D. enzymes

2. **The neurons are considered to be the: (Pg. 92)**
   A. highway of information in the brain
   B. heart of the brain cells
   C. basic working units of the brain
   D. container for the neurotransmitters

3. **Electrochemical impulses travel along a fiber called the: (Pg. 92)**
   A. dendrite
   B. glia
   C. synapse
   D. axon

4. **Nerve impulses must cross a gap called the _____ to traverse from one neuron to another. (Pg. 93)**
   A. nucleus
   B. synapse
   C. receptor
   D. axon

5. **The neurotransmitter most responsible for affecting behavior, mood, and sexuality is: (Pg. 94)**
   A. dopamine
   B. serotonin
   C. adrenaline
   D. GABA

6. **A mentally healthy individual will possess which of the following traits? (Pg. 94)**
   A. values his/her self as a worthy and good person
   B. accepts their own limitations
   C. perceives reality as it really is
   D. all of the above are mentally healthy traits

7. **As defined by the American Psychiatric Association, a mental disorder is one that: (Pg. 98)**
   A. has present distress
   B. impaired dysfunction
   C. has significant risk for death or serious injury
   D. all of the above

8. **The most common psychological problem that college students seek counseling for is: (Pg. 98)**
   A. depression
   B. alcohol and drugs
   C. sexual dysfunction
   D. adjustment disorders

9. **Having feelings of emptiness, hopelessness, and a sadness that does not go away describes: (Pg. 100)**
   A. a panic disorder
   B. phobia
   C. anxiety attacks
   D. major depression

10. **Which of the following is not a key contributor to college students suffering from depression? (Pg. 100)**
    A. substance abuse
    B. sleep deprivation
    C. lack of friends
    D. stress

11. **The biggest danger for depression patients under the age of 20 years is that of: (Pg. 102)**
   A. depression in the adult years
   B. addiction to antidepressant drugs
   C. stunted growth from using antidepressants for too long
   D. higher risk of suicide

12. **Which of the following factors is not considered to be a reason why people attempt suicide? (Pg. 107)**
   A. having a mental disorder
   B. being on antidepressants
   C. family history of suicide
   D. none of the above

13. **What is considered to be the single greatest risk for teenage suicide? (Pg. 106)**
   A. lack of friends for emotional support
   B. depression
   C. body image problems
   D. ambivalent sexuality

14. **A useful strategy to provide to a friend who has shared with you that she is contemplating suicide is to:**
   (Pg. 111)
   A. offer trite reassurance such as living is much better than being dead
   B. listen attentively and ask questions to help her sort through her feelings
   C. challenge her on her motives for wanting to die
   D. not ask if she really is thinking of killing herself

15. **Which type of mental health therapy utilizes looking at negative thought patterns and implementing positive thought therapy.**
   (Pg. 113)
   A. solution focused therapy
   B. psychodynamic therapy
   C. interpersonal therapy
   D. cognitive behavioral therapy

16. **If one is experiencing a mental health problem, it is crucial to get professional help. In addition, the individual should work on their thriving and surviving in society by doing which of the following: (Pg. 115)**
   A. learning to love and accept themselves for who they are
   B. take as many psychotic-reducing pills as they can tolerate to get a handle on their life
   C. see only a psychiatrist for therapy
   D. none of the above

17. **Which of the following mental health professionals is legally allowed to prescribe medications to a patient?**
   (Pg. 112)
   A. psychologist
   B. licensed clinical social worker
   C. psychiatrist
   D. psychiatric nurse

18. **Which type of psychotherapy utilizes the assessment of the patient's earlier childhood experiences and those unconscious influences? (Pg. 113)**
   A. psychodynamic therapy
   B. cognitive behavioral therapy
   C. behavioral therapy
   D. interpersonal therapy

19. **You should consider all of the following options for psychological help except: (Pg. 116)**
   A. feeling overwhelmed and helpless
   B. asking your physician to recommend a therapist or to price medication for you
   C. if feeling compulsive about your alcohol drinking, that is considered normal
   college student life and does not require assistance
   D. struggling with homework and school commitments

For years, Travis put on his "happy face" around his friends and family. Popular and athletic in high school, he never let anyone know how desperately unhappy he actually felt. "Whatever I was doing during the day, nothing was on my mind more than wanting to die," he recalls. On a perfectly ordinary day in his senior year, Travis tried to kill himself with an overdose of pills. Rushed to a hospital, Travis recovered, resumed his studies, and entered college. By the middle of his freshman year, he was struggling once more with feelings of hopelessness. This time he realized what was

Taking Care of Your Mind

happening and sought help from a therapist. "I thought college was supposed to be the happiest time of your life," he said. "What went wrong?"

This is a question many young people might ask. Although youth can seem a golden time, when body and mind glow with potential, the process of becoming an adult is a challenging one in every culture and country. Psychological health can make the difference between facing this challenge with optimism and confidence or feeling overwhelmed by expectations and responsibilities. (To enhance your psychological health, see Making Change Happen, p. 96, and "Your Psychological Self-Care Pyramid" in *Labs for IPC*.)

This isn't always easy. At some point in life almost half of Americans develop an emotional disorder. Young adulthood—the years from the late teens to the mid-twenties—is a time when many serious disorders, including bipolar illness (manic depression) and schizophrenia, often develop. The saddest fact is not that so many feel so bad, but that so few realize they can feel better. Only a third of those with a mental disorder receive any treatment at all. Yet 80 to 90 percent of those treated for psychological problems recover, most within a few months.

By learning about psychological disorders covered in this chapter, you may be able to recognize early warning signals in yourself or your loved ones so you can deal with potential difficulties or seek professional help for more serious problems.

After studying the material in this chapter, you should be able to

- **List** the key structures of the brain and **describe** the role of neurons in communication within the brain.
- **Explain** the differences between mental health and mental illness and **list** some effects of mental illness on physical health.
- **List** some of the symptoms of depression and **discuss** the pros and cons of using antidepressants.
- **Discuss** some of the factors that may lead to suicide, as well as strategies for prevention.
- **Describe** the treatment options available for those with psychological problems.
- **Name** the option you will consider if you have a mental health problem, and **describe** the reasons for your choice.

The Brain: The Last Frontier

The brain has intrigued scientists for centuries, but only recently have its explorers made dramatic progress in unraveling its mysteries. Leaders in **neuropsychiatry**—the field that brings together the study of the brain and the mind—remind us that 95 percent of what is known about brain anatomy, chemistry, and physiology has been learned in the last 25 years. These discoveries have reshaped our understanding of the organ that is central to our identity and well-being and have fostered great hope for more effective therapies for the more than 1,000 disorders—psychiatric and neurologic—that affect the brain and nervous system.

Inside the Brain

The human brain, the most complex organ in the body, controls the central nervous system (CNS) and regulates virtually all our activities, including involuntary, or "lower," actions like heart rate, respiration, and digestion, and conscious, or "higher," mental activity like thought, reason, and abstraction. More than one hundred billion **neurons**, or nerve cells, within the brain are capable of electrical and chemical communication with tens of thousands of other nerve cells. (The basic anatomy of the brain is shown in Figure 4.1.)

The neurons are the basic working units of the brain. Like snowflakes, no two are exactly the same. Each consists of a cell body containing the **nucleus;** a long fiber called the **axon**, which can range from less than an inch to several feet in length; an **axon terminal,** or ending; and multiple branching fibers called **dendrites** (Figure 4.2). The **glia** serve as the scaffolding for the brain, separate the brain from the bloodstream,

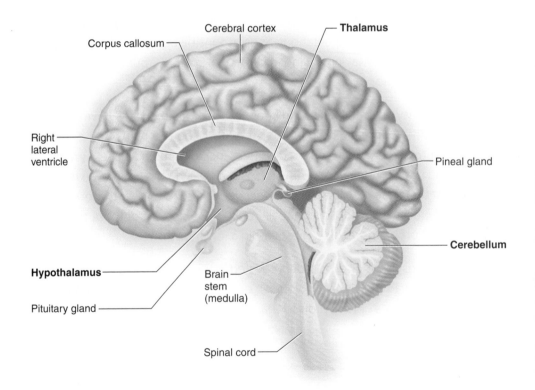

Figure 4.1   The Brain

The three major parts of the brain are the cerebrum, cerebellum, and brainstem (medulla). The cerebrum is divided into two hemispheres—the left, which regulates the right side of the body, and the right, which regulates the left side of the body. The cerebellum plays the major role in coordinating movement, balance, and posture. The brainstem contains centers that control breathing, blood pressure, heart rate, and other physiological functions.

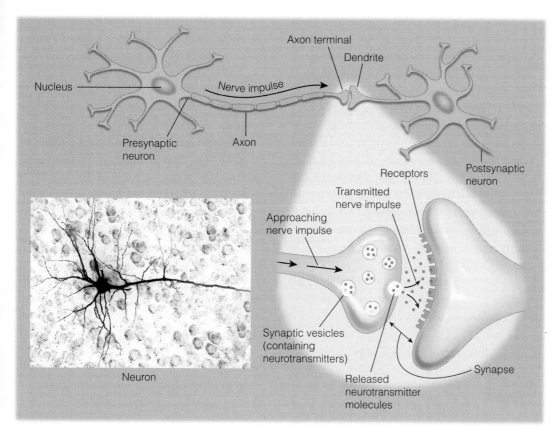

Figure 4.2 Brain Messaging: Anatomy of a Neuron

This figure shows how nerve impulses are transmitted from one neuron to another within the brain.

assist in the growth of neurons, speed up the transmission of nerve impulses, and engulf and digest damaged neurons.

Until quite recently scientists believed no new neurons or synapses formed in the brain after birth. This theory has been soundly disproved. The brain and spinal cord contain stem cells, which turn into thousands of new neurons a day. The process of creating new brain cells and synapses occurs most rapidly in childhood but continues throughout life, even into old age. Whenever you learn and change, you establish new neural networks.

Anatomically, the brain consists of three parts: the forebrain, midbrain, and hindbrain. The forebrain includes the several lobes of the cerebral cortex that control higher functions, while the mid- and hindbrain are more involved with unconscious, autonomic functions. The normal adult human brain typically weighs about three pounds.

Communication Within the Brain

Neurons "talk" with each other by means of electrical and chemical processes (see Figure 4.2). An electric charge, or impulse, travels along an axon to the terminal, where packets of chemicals called **neurotransmitters** are stored. When released, these messengers flow out of the axon terminal and cross a **synapse,** a specialized site at which the axon terminal of one neuron comes extremely close to a dendrite from another neuron. On the surface of the dendrite are **receptors,** protein molecules designed to bind with neurotransmitters. It takes only about a ten-thousandth of a second for a neurotransmitter and a receptor to come together. Neurotransmitters that do not connect with receptors may remain in the synapse until they are reabsorbed by the cell that produced them—a process called **reuptake**—or broken down by enzymes.

neuropsychiatry The study of the brain and mind.

neuron A nerve cell; the basic working unit of the brain, which transmits information from the senses to the brain and from the brain to specific body parts; each neuron consists of a cell body, an axon terminal, and dendrites.

nucleus The central part of a cell, contained in the cell body of a neuron.

axon The long fiber that conducts impulses from the neuron's nucleus to its dendrites.

axon terminal The ending of an axon, from which impulses are transmitted to a dendrite of another neuron.

dendrites Branching fibers of a neuron that receive impulses from axon terminals of other neurons and conduct these impulses toward the nucleus.

glia Support cells for neurons in the brain and spinal cord that separate the brain from the bloodstream, assist in the growth of neurons, speed transmission of nerve impulses, and eliminate damaged neurons.

neurotransmitters Chemicals released by neurons that stimulate or inhibit the action of other neurons.

synapse A specialized site at which electrical impulses are transmitted from the axon terminal of one neuron to a dendrite of another.

receptors Molecules on the surface of neurons on which neurotransmitters bind after their release from other neurons.

reuptake Reabsorption by the originating cell of neurotransmitters that have not connected with receptors and have been left in synapses.

antidepressant A drug used primarily to treat symptoms of depression.

A malfunction in the release of a neurotransmitter, in its reuptake or elimination, or in the receptors or secondary messengers may result in abnormalities in thinking, feeling, or behavior. Some of the most promising and exciting research in neuropsychiatry is focusing on correcting such malfunctions. The neurotransmitter serotonin and its receptors have been shown to affect mood, sleep, behavior, appetite, memory, learning, sexuality, and aggression and to play a role in several mental disorders. The discovery of a possible link between low levels of serotonin and some cases of major depression has led to the development of more precisely targeted **antidepressant** medications that boost serotonin to normal levels. (See "Psychiatric Drugs" later in the chapter.)

Sex Differences in the Brain

From birth, male and female brains differ in a variety of ways. Overall, a woman's brain, like her body, is 10 to 15 percent smaller than a man's, yet the regions dedicated to higher cognitive functions such as language are more densely packed with neurons—and women use more of them. When a male puts his mind to work, neurons turn on in highly specific areas. When females set their minds on similar tasks, cells light up all over the brain.

Male and female brains perceive light and sound differently. A man's eyes are more sensitive to bright light and retain their ability to see well at long distances longer in life. A woman hears a much broader range of sounds, and her hearing remains sharper longer.

The female brain responds more intensely to emotion. According to neuroimaging studies, the genders respond differently to emotions, especially sadness, which activates, or turns on, neurons in an area eight times larger in women than men.

Neither gender's brain is "better." Intelligence per se appears equal in both. The greatest gender differences appear both at the top and bottom of the intelligence scales. Nevertheless, more than half the time, regardless of the type of test, most women and men perform more or less equally—even though they may well take different routes to arrive at the same answers. Cognitive skills show greater variability both among women and among men than between the genders. The best evaluation may have come from essayist Samuel Johnson. When asked whether women or men are more intelligent, he responded, "Which man? Which woman?"

Understanding Mental Health

Mentally healthy individuals value themselves, perceive reality as it is, accept their limitations and possibilities, carry out their responsibilities, establish and maintain close relationships, pursue work that suits their talent and training, and feel a sense of fulfillment that makes the efforts of daily living worthwhile (Figure 4.3).

The state of mental health around the world is far from ideal. Psychiatric illness and substance abuse cause more premature deaths than any other factor, according to a recent report by the World Health Organization (WHO). These conditions also account for about a third of years lost to disability among people older than 14. The most

common psychiatric conditions worldwide are depression, alcohol dependence and abuse, bipolar disorder, schizophrenia, Alzheimer's and other forms of dementia, panic disorder, and drug dependence and abuse.[1]

Across the globe, depression is the leading cause of years of health lost to disease in both men and women. The worldwide rate of depression among women is 50 percent higher than in men, and women and girls have higher rates of anxiety disorders, migraine, and Alzheimer's disease. Men's rates of alcohol and substance abuse are nearly seven times higher than women's.[2]

Preventive steps can help maintain and enhance your psychological health, just as similar actions boost physical health. (See Making Change Happen, p. 96.)

What Is a Mental Disorder?

While lay people may speak of "nervous breakdowns" or "insanity," these are not scientific terms. The U.S. government's official definition states that a serious mental illness is "a diagnosable mental, behavioral, or emotional disorder that interferes with one or more major activities in life, like dressing, eating, or working."

The mental health profession's standard for diagnosing a mental disorder is the pattern of symptoms, or diagnostic criteria, spelled out for the almost 300 disorders in the American Psychiatric Association's *Diagnostic and Statistical Manual,* 4th edition (DSM-IV). Psychiatrists define a **mental disorder** as a clinically significant behavioral or psychological syndrome or pattern that is associated with present distress (a painful symptom) or disability (impairment in one or more important areas of functioning) or with a significantly increased risk of suffering death, pain, disability, or an important loss of freedom.[3]

Who Develops Mental Disorders?

In the course of their lifetime, almost half of all Americans experience a diagnosable psychological problem. The most common mental disorders are substance abuse (discussed in Chapters 11 and 12), mood disorders such as depression and bipolar disorder, and anxiety disorders such as phobias and panic disorder.

In a community survey, almost 30 percent of individuals needed mental health services, but less than a third received adequate treatment. In the past, many people did not seek help for mental disorders because of widespread stigma about these disorders. Attitudes toward mental health treatment have changed over the last decade, particularly among younger adults. However, the majority of Americans surveyed in a recent poll did not feel very comfortable talking with a professional about personal problems and said they would feel embarrassed if others found out about it.

Unlike most disabling physical diseases, mental illness starts early in life. Half of all lifetime cases begin by age 14; three-quarters

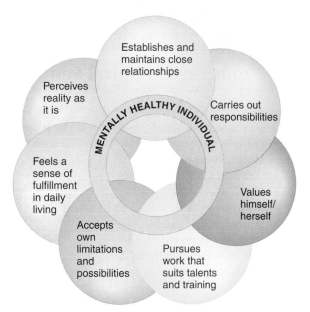

Figure 4.3 The Mentally Healthy Individual
Mental well-being is a combination of many factors.

by age 24. Adverse childhood experiences, such as abuse, increase the risk.

Anxiety disorders often begin in late childhood, mood disorders in late adolescence, and substance abuse in the early twenties. Researchers describe such problems as "the chronic diseases of the young," striking when men and women are in their prime. The prevalence of mental disorders increases from early adulthood (ages 18 to 29) to the next-oldest age group (ages 30 to 44) and then declines. Women have higher rates of depressive and anxiety disorders; men have higher rates of substance abuse and impulse disorders.

About 80 percent of those with mental disorders eventually seek treatment, but many suffer for years, even decades. As discussed later in this chapter, college students are especially likely to delay getting help for a psychological problem.[4] The median delay for all disorders is nearly 10 years. Those with social phobia and separation anxiety disorders may not get help for more than 20 years. The earlier in life that a disorder begins, the longer that individuals tend to delay treatment.

Without treatment, mental disorders take a toll on every aspect of life, including academics, relationships, careers, and risk-taking. Symptoms or episodes of a disorder typically become more frequent or severe. Individuals with one mental disorder are

mental disorder Behavioral or psychological syndrome associated with distress or disability or with a significantly increased risk of suffering death, pain, disability, or loss of freedom.

Your Psychological Self-Care Pyramid

Your physical well-being and psychological health are so intimately related that to a significant degree they are expressions of each other. Yes, grave diseases can occur despite a healthy mental outlook, and physically healthy people can experience psychological difficulties. But overwhelming evidence demonstrates that physical health affects mood and thoughts, and mood and thoughts affect physical health.

"Your Psychological Self-Care Pyramid" from *Labs for IPC* deals with optimizing your psychological health to benefit body, mind, and spirit. It will teach you how to infuse your life with mentally rewarding and stimulating activities that not only provide balance, prevent the blahs, and add zest but also, if continued, form a lifelong foundation for optimal mental health. Here's a preview.

Get Real

In this stage you rate yourself from 0 to 10, with zero being the low end and 10 the high end, on the degree to which you now include or exhibit in your weekly life the thirteen elements of Your Psychological Self-Care Pyramid shown in *Labs for IPC*. Here are three examples:

- **Self-knowledge and self-control.** _____ You make your inner world of feelings and thoughts and your relationship to the outer world a source of ongoing contemplation. You seek self-understanding and systematically develop your ability to consider and weigh actions before taking them.
- **Community.** _____ You have a circle of trusted friends and participate in a larger social milieu. You look out for and assist the interests of the community as a whole, not merely those of your circle of immediate friends.
- **Generosity.** _____ You are giving of your time and your self both toward others and toward yourself. You give materially when this is advisable but more than that when asked you give that which is most precious, that is, who you are.

You will then examine your self-ratings. Are some unacceptably lower than you would like them to be? Completing this lab will address this concern for the short run and, if you continue the activities, for the future.

Get Ready

In this stage you examine your schedule and create pockets of time for the activities that serve as building blocks of your psychological self-care pyramid and for journaling about your experiences doing so.

Get Going

In this stage you begin the exercises related to each of the areas you want to bolster by engaging in related activities for at least five minutes four times per week. *Immediately after* completing the exercise or at some other point the *same* day, you will make an entry of at least five lines in your *IPC Journal* and reflect on your experiences . . .

Lock It In

Just as you can use the USDA Food Pyramid to guide your eating choices every day, pay attention to Your Psychological Self-Care Pyramid. Here is one of the steps that can assure that you are providing adequate daily nourishment for your mind and spirit.

- **Rate yourself.** Every four weeks rate yourself between 0 to 10, with 0 being the low end and 10 the high end, on each element of Your Psychological Self-Care Pyramid. Record your scores.

at high risk of having a second one (this is called comorbidity).

About 6 percent of Americans have a "severe" mental disorder, one that significantly limits their ability to work or carry out daily activities or that has led to a suicide attempt or psychosis (a gross impairment of a person's perception of reality). On average, they are unable to function for nearly three months of the year.

The Mind–Body Connection

According to a growing number of studies, mental attitude may be just as important a risk factor for certain diseases as age, race, gender, education, habits, and health history. Positive states like happiness and optimism have been linked with longer lifespans as well as lower risk of cardiovascular and lung disease, stroke, diabetes, colds, and upper respiratory infections. Gratitude, in particular, has proven health benefits. (See "Health on a Budget.")

Mental disorders, on the other hand, can undermine physical well-being. Anxiety can lead to intensified asthmatic reactions, skin conditions, and digestive disorders. Stress can play a role in hypertension, heart attacks, sudden cardiac death, and immune disorders in the young as well as in older individuals. People who suffer from migraine headaches are at increased risk of depression, anxiety, and neurological disorders.[5]

The brain and the heart—and the health of each—are linked in complex ways. Heart disease increases the likelihood of depression, and depression increases the likelihood of heart disease. For people with heart disease, depression can be fatal. It may contribute to sudden cardiac death and increase all causes of cardiac mortality.[6] For depressed individuals, their risk of heart attacks, strokes, and other cardiovascular problems may be 50 percent greater. The reason may be that depressed people are less likely to practice good health habits, such as exercising regularly and eating healthful foods.[7] (See Chapter 14 for more on heart disease.)

Diabetes and depression also overlap. In a recent survey, the prevalence rate of major depression in adults with diabetes averaged 8 percent nationwide, but rose to a high of 29 percent in Alaska. American Indians/Alaska Natives reported the highest incidence.[8]

Major depression is associated with lower bone density in young men and in adolescent girls.[9] A history of depression increases the risk of physical problems such as headache and shoulder and neck pain in women as they reach middle age.

The Exercise Prescription Imagine a drug so powerful it can alter brain chemistry, so versatile it can help prevent or treat many common mental disorders, so safe that moderate doses cause few, if any, side effects, and so inexpensive that anyone can afford it. This wonder drug, proved in years of research, is exercise.

In addition to its head-to-toe physical benefits, discussed in Chapter 5, exercise may be, as one therapist puts it, the single most effective way to lift a person's spirits and to restore feelings of potency about all aspects of life. People who exercise regularly report a more cheerful mood, higher self-esteem, and less stress. Their sleep and appetite also tend to improve. In clinical studies, exercise has proved effective as a treatment for depression and anxiety disorders. But remember: Although exercise can help prevent and ease problems for many people, it's no substitute for professional treatment of serious psychiatric disorders.

Physical exercise not only produces psychological benefits, but the more you exercise, the greater the benefit. (See Figure

4.4.) In research that followed 14,000 people without mental illness for 15 years, those who were fittest at the start of the study were significantly less likely to develop depression than the less fit—regardless of their weight, general health, and smoking or drinking habits. In fact, for each additional minute they spent on an exercise treadmill during their initial evaluation, their odds of reporting depression symptoms in the subsequent years dropped 5 percent.[10]

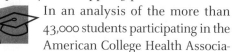 In an analysis of the more than 43,000 students participating in the American College Health Association National College Health Assessment, men and women who engaged in some aerobic or toning activity every week were less likely to feel hopeless or depressed compared with their inactive peers. Men and women who engaged in aerobic exercise also decreased their risk of suicide, with greater benefits the more often they exercised.[11]

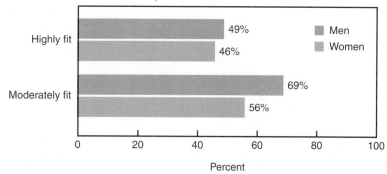

Figure 4.4 Can Exercise Chase the Blues Away?
Odds of reporting depressive symptoms compared with people who aren't fit.

Mental Health on Campus

The emotional difficulties of college students have become more complex and more severe than in the past. (Eating disorders, which are common among college students, are discussed in Chapter 7.) In one national survey, more than 80 percent of directors of counseling centers reported an increase in the number of students with serious psychological disorders. Some schools are setting up screening programs to identify students who may be a risk to themselves or others. (See Point/Counterpoint.)

Campus shootings in recent years focused national attention on the state of students' minds. In a national survey of more than 5,000 men and women between the ages of 19 and 25—the traditional age range for undergraduates—almost half reported some type of mental health problem in the past year. Alcohol abuse was slightly more common among college students, while nonstudents had higher rates of drug abuse. Depressive disorders and anxiety disorders affected almost equal percentages of students and nonstudents: about 12 percent.[12]

Among the strongest factors that put college students at risk for mental problems is a romantic breakup or loss. In the survey, about one in eight individuals reported a breakup in the previous year. Their odds of having a psychiatric disorder were more than 2.5 times higher than those who hadn't been through a breakup.[13] Some psychiatric symptoms increase the risk of developing other disorders. College women who reported symptoms of depression, for example, are at higher risk for alcohol problems.[14]

The few studies that have looked into ethnic differences in psychological health have yielded conflicting or inconclusive results: Some found no differences; others suggested higher rates of depression among Korean and South Asian students.

Hopelessness and feelings of depression are common on campus. In recent surveys, about 4 in 10 college students reported feeling that things are hopeless, and more than a quarter attributed trouble functioning during the academic year to depressive symptoms.[15] (See Table 4.1.)

In a recent study, only one quarter of young adults with a mental disorder sought professional help. Depressed students were the most likely to seek help, those with substance abuse disorders the least. Only about

POINT COUNTERPOINT

POINT

Concerned about identifying and treating students who might pose a danger to themselves or others, some campuses have set up websites or phone lines students can use to report their concerns about a classmate who seems troubled. Teachers and counselors are being urged to look for signs of mental disorders such as depression as well as signs of aggression and violence.

COUNTERPOINT

Programs that encourage observation and reporting of odd behaviors could violate a student's privacy. They also might lead to discrimination, overt or subtle, against individuals who do not conform to certain standards of acceptable behavior. Until and unless a student threatens harm to himself or others, campuses should encourage a live-and-let-live tolerance of others.

YOUR VIEW

Should colleges do more to identify potentially troubled students? Or should individual privacy and confidentiality be the top priority? How would you respond if a classmate or friend shows signs of a serious mental disorder? How do you think campus authorities should respond?

TABLE 4.1

Most Common Mental Disorders

Depression	13%
Anxiety	7%
Eating disorders	19%
Self-injury	14%
Suicide	6%
Any of the above mental problems	37%
Receiving any treatment	25%
Medicine	14%
Therapy	22%

Source: Zivin, K., et al. "Persistence of Mental Health Problems and Needs in a College Student Population." *Journal of Affective Disorders*, January 27, 2009.

© Jim Dandy/Stock Illustration Source/Getty Images

1 in 20 students with a drug or alcohol problem reported receiving any treatment for their condition in the preceding twelve months—half as many as nonstudents with similar problems.[16]

Why don't distressed students seek professional care? Many feel they don't need help. Others worry about the stigma of admitting there's something wrong or of seeing a therapist. When researchers assessed students' mental health and then checked back in two years later, more than a third of those surveyed had a mental health problem. Of the students with a disorder when the study began, 60 percent also had a problem two years later—although this varied with the type of disorder. More than half of those with eating disorders still had symptoms two years later compared to somewhat more than a quarter of those with probable depression. Yet many of the students with persistent disorders still did not think they needed help and did not seek treatment.[17]

Depressive Disorders

Depression, the world's most common mental ailment, affects the brain, the mind, and the body in complex ways. An estimated 8 to 17 percent of adults experience depression at some point in their lives.[18] The relationship between depression and race is complex. Rates of depression are higher among whites than African American and Caribbean blacks. However, depression is more likely to be unrecognized, untreated, severe, and disabling among blacks. After a single episode, the risk of a recurrence, or second episode, is about 50 percent. After a third, the risk of a fourth is about 90 percent. Stress-related events may trigger half of all depressive episodes; great trauma in childhood can increase vulnerability to depression later in life.

In a study of young adults ages 18 to 23, those who'd experienced the most adversity were at greatest risk of depression or an anxiety disorder. An estimated 15 to 40 percent of college-age men and women (18- to 24-year-olds) may develop depression. (See Self Survey: "Recognizing Depression," p. 115.)

Depression in Students

Once young people were considered immune to sadness. Now mental health professionals know better. An estimated 5 to 10 percent of American teenagers suffer from a serious depressive disorder; girls are twice as susceptible as boys. Prior to puberty, girls and boys are equally likely to develop depression.

According to the American College Health Association National College Health Assessment, the percentage of students diagnosed with depression has risen from 10 percent in 2000 to 16 percent in 2007, and the percentage seeking campus counseling has increased to 23 percent. More than one-third of today's undergraduates report that they have felt too depressed to function.[19]

Researchers at the University of Michigan have identified three key contributors to depression in college students: stress, substance abuse, and sleep loss. As they adjust to campus life, undergraduates face the ongoing stress of forging a new identity

Factors that can contribute to the development of depression in college include stressful events, poor academic performance, loneliness, and relationship problems.

© Randald Mackechnie/The Image Bank/Getty Images

and finding a place for themselves in various social hierarchies. This triggers the release of the so-called stress hormones (discussed in Chapter 3), which can change brain activity. Drugs and alcohol, widely used on campus, also affect the brain in ways that make stress even harder to manage. Too little sleep adds another ingredient to this dangerous brew. Computers, the Internet, around-the-clock television, and the college tradition of pulling all-nighters can conspire to sabotage rest and increase vulnerability to depression. Among the most vulnerable students are those being treated for mental disorders.

  According to a survey of more than 2,000 young women ages 16 to 23, white girls become less depressed as they age while black girls continue feeling the same. The reason may be that white girls tend to be unhappy with their bodies in their teens and may develop symptoms of depression as a result. Over time they become more satisfied with their shapes and sizes and less depressed. African American girls tend to accept their bodies from early adolescence into adulthood.

The risks of depression in the young are high. Four in ten depressed adolescents think about killing themselves; two in ten actually try to do so. Every year an estimated 11 to 13 in every 100,000 teens take their own lives, twice as many as the number who die from all natural causes combined.

No one knows the reason for this steady surge in sadness, but experts point to the breakdown of families, the pressures of the information age, and increased isolation. A family history of depression greatly increases a young person's vulnerability. A mother's anxiety and depression during early childhood can increase the risk that adolescents will develop symptoms of anxiety and depression. Racial and ethnic factors also contribute. Among Asian American college students, for instance, perfectionism has been linked to depressive symptoms.[20]

Teens who spend many hours watching television are at higher risk of depression as adults, according to a new study. With each hour in front of the tube, the odds of becoming depressed rise. No one knows the reason for this association, but researchers speculate that television bombards viewers with negative images and information and that television-watching might replace social, athletic, or intellectual activities that can ward off depression.[21]

The strongest predictor of depression is cigarette smoking. Depressed teens may smoke because they think smoking will make them feel better, but nicotine alters brain chemistry and actually worsens symptoms of depression. The link between tobacco and depression continues during college. Students diagnosed with or treated for depression are 7.5 times as likely as other students to use tobacco, possibly because of nicotine's stimulating effects, and to smoke more cigarettes per week. Young women with symptoms of depression and those who do not feel connected with a peer group are more likely to smoke. Individuals with other mental illnesses also are more likely to smoke.

Gender and Depression

 Female Depression Depression is twice as common in women as men, a gender gap found through most of the world. Some have argued that women are simply more willing than men to admit to being depressed or more likely to seek help. But even when these factors are accounted for, the sex difference persists. Others contend that men in distress drown their problems in alcohol rather than becoming sad, tearful, and hopeless. In studies of the Amish, who prohibit alcohol use, and of Jewish Americans, who also drink less than other groups, women and men are equally likely to develop depression. Yet these data do not mean that fewer women among teetotalers become depressed but that more men do.

Genes may make both men and women more vulnerable to depression. Brain chemistry and sex hormones also may play a role. Women produce less of certain metabolites of serotonin, a messenger chemical that helps regulate mood. Their brains also register sadness much more intensely than men's, and they are more sensitive to changes in light and temperature. Women are at least four times more likely than men to develop seasonal affective disorder (SAD) and to become depressed in the dark winter months.

Some women also seem more sensitive to their own hormones or to the changes in them that occur at puberty, during the menstrual cycle, after childbirth, or during perimenopause and menopause. Pregnancy, contrary to what many people assume, does not "protect" a woman from depression, and women who discontinue treatment when they become pregnant are at risk of a relapse. Women and their psychiatrists must carefully weigh the risks and benefits of psychiatric medications during pregnancy.

Childhood abuse also contributes to female vulnerability. In epidemiological studies, 60 percent of women diagnosed with depression—compared with 39 percent of men—were abused as children. In adulthood, relationships may protect women from depression, while a lack of social support increases vulnerability to depression. Women with at least one "confiding relationship," as researchers put it, are physically and psychologically more resilient.

Male Depression   More than six million men in the United States—1 in every 14—suffer from this insidious disorder, many without recognizing what's wrong. Experts describe male depression as an "under" disease: underdiscussed, underrecognized, underdiagnosed, and undertreated.

Depression "looks" different in men than women. Rather than becoming sad, men may be irritable or tremendously fatigued. They feel a sense of being dead inside, of worthlessness, hopelessness, helplessness, of losing their life force. Physical symptoms, such as headaches, pain, and insomnia, are common, as are attempts to "self-medicate" with alcohol or drugs.

Genes may make some men more vulnerable, but chronic stress of any sort plays a major role in male depression, possibly by raising levels of the stress hormone cortisol, and lowering testosterone. Men also are more likely than women to become depressed following divorce, job loss, or a career setback. Whatever its roots, depression alters brain chemistry in potentially deadly ways. Four times as many men as women kill themselves; depressed men are two to four times more likely to take their own lives than depressed women.

Minor Depression

Minor depression is a common disorder that is often unrecognized and untreated, affecting about 7.5 percent of Americans during their lifetime. Its symptoms are the same as those of major depression, but less severe and fewer in number. They include either a depressed mood most of the day, nearly every day, or diminished interest or pleasure in daily activities.

Psychotherapy is remarkably effective for mild depression. In more serious cases, antidepressant medication can lead to dramatic improvement in 40 to 80 percent of depressed patients. Exercise also works—several studies have shown that exercise effectively lifts mild to moderate depression.

Dysthymic Disorder   **Dysthymia** is a depressive disorder characterized by a chronically depressed mood. Symptoms include feelings of inadequacy, hopelessness, and guilt; low self-esteem; low energy; fatigue; indecisiveness; and an inability to enjoy pleasurable activities.

Major Depression

The simplest definition of **major depression** is sadness that does not end. The incidence of major depression has soared over the last two decades, especially among young adults. Major depression can destroy a person's joy for living. Food, friends, sex, or any form of pleasure no longer appeals. It is impossible to concentrate on work and responsibilities. Unable to escape a sense of utter hopelessness, depressed individuals may fight back tears throughout the day and toss and turn through long, empty nights. Thoughts of death or suicide may push into their minds.

The characteristic symptoms of major depression include:

- **Feeling depressed,** sad, empty, discouraged, tearful.

- **Loss of interest** or pleasure in once-enjoyable activities.

- **Eating more or less** than usual and either gaining or losing weight.

- **Having trouble sleeping** or sleeping much more than usual.

dysthymia   Frequent, prolonged mild depression.

major depression   Sadness that does not end; ongoing feelings of utter helplessness.

- **Feeling slowed down** or restless and unable to sit still.
- **Lack of energy.**
- **Feeling helpless,** hopeless, worthless, inadequate.
- **Difficulty concentrating,** forgetfulness.
- **Difficulty thinking clearly** or making decisions.
- **Persistent thoughts of death** or suicide.
- **Withdrawal from others,** lack of interest in sex.
- **Physical symptoms** (headaches, digestive problems, aches and pains).

As many as half of major depressive episodes are not recognized because the symptoms are "masked." Rather than feeling sad or depressed, individuals may experience low energy, insomnia, difficulty concentrating, and physical symptoms. An episode of major depression can trigger a relapse in individuals with substance abuse problems.

Treating Depression

Psychotherapy and drug therapy have both proven effective in treating depression.[22] Treatment with psychotherapy, medication, or both relieves depression for 80 percent of sufferers—yet only half of those with depression seek help and only 10 to 15 percent get optimal care.

Psychotherapy helps individuals pinpoint the life problems that contribute to their depression, identify negative or distorted thinking patterns, explore behaviors that contribute to depression, and regain a sense of control and pleasure in life. Two specific psychotherapies—cognitive-behavioral therapy and interpersonal therapy (described later in this chapter)—have proved as helpful as **antidepressant** drugs, although they take longer than medication to achieve results.

Antidepressants help about 70 percent of individuals feel better within six to ten weeks. According to long-term studies, treatment should continue for at least nine months after a single acute episode of depression, longer for chronic or recurrent depression.

Although antidepressants raise the suicide risk in children, they have the opposite effect in adults. (See Consumer Alert.) In a review of eight large studies that included more than 200,000 patients, SSRIs (a class of antidepressant) reduced the suicide risk by more than 40 percent among adults and more than 50 percent in the elderly.[23]

The Pros and Cons of Antidepressants

Millions of individuals have benefited from the category of antidepressant drugs called selective serotonin reuptake inhibitors (SSRIs). However, like all drugs, they can cause side effects that range from temporary physical symptoms, such as stomach upset and headaches, to more persistent problems, such as sexual dysfunction. The most serious—and controversial—risk is suicide.

Facts to Know
- The FDA has issued a "black box" warning about the risk of suicidal thoughts, hostility, and aggression in both children and young adults. The danger is greatest just after pill use begins.
- This risk of suicide while taking an antidepressant is about 1 in 3,000; the risk of a serious attempt is 1 in 1,000.
- Recent reviews of antidepressant use have found that the risk of suicide for both children and adults was *higher* in the month *before* starting treatment, dropped sharply in the month after it began, and tapered off in the following months.

Steps to Take
- If you are younger than age 20, be aware of the increased suicide risk with the use of SSRIs. Talk these over carefully with a psychiatrist. Discuss alternative treatments, such as psychotherapy.
- For individuals older than age 20, the benefits of antidepressants have proved to outweigh their risks in most cases. Adults treated with SSRIs are 40 percent less likely to commit suicide than depressed individuals who do not receive this therapy.
- Whatever your age, arrange for careful monitoring and follow-up with a psychiatrist when you start taking an antidepressant. Familiarize yourself with possible side effects, and seek help immediately if you begin to think about taking your own life.

When either medication or psychotherapy fails to lift depression, switching from one to the other or adding a second antidepressant can be highly effective. Medications have proved effective for patients who did not recover with psychotherapy alone, and psychotherapy can help those who do not benefit from medication alone.

Exercise also has proved beneficial in both the short and long term for both men and women. Although walking and jogging have been studied most extensively, all forms of exercise decrease depression to some degree. The greater the length of the exercise program and the larger the total number of sessions, the greater the decrease in depression.

For individuals who cannot take antidepressant medications because of medical problems, or who do not improve with psychotherapy or drugs, *electroconvulsive therapy* (ECT)—the administration of a controlled electrical current through electrodes attached to the scalp—remains the safest and most effective treatment. About 70 to 90 percent of depressed individuals improve after ECT. Experimental new techniques are using electrical and magnetic stimulation to treat depression.

Even without treatment, depression generally lifts after six to nine months. However, in more than 80 percent of people, it recurs, with each episode lasting longer and becoming more severe and difficult to treat. "All the while the depression goes untreated, it is causing ongoing damage that shrivels important regions of the brain," says John Greden, M.D., director of the University of Michigan Depression Center. "The exciting news is that, as brain scans show, treatment turns the destructive process around and stops depression in its tracks."[24]

Bipolar Disorder

Bipolar disorder, known as manic depression in the past, consists of mood swings that may take individuals from manic states of feeling euphoric and energetic to depressive states of utter despair. In episodes of full mania, they may become so impulsive and out of touch with reality that they endanger their careers, relationships, health, or even survival. Psychiatrists view bipolar symptoms on a spectrum that includes depression and states of acute irritability and distress.[25]

 One percent of the population—about 2 million American adults—suffer from this serious but treatable disorder. Men tend to develop bipolar disorder earlier in life (between ages 16 to 25), but women have higher rates overall. About 50 percent of patients with bipolar illness have a family history of the disorder.

The characteristic symptoms of bipolar disorder include:

- **Mood swings** (from happy to miserable, optimistic to despairing, and so on).
- **Changes in thinking** (thoughts speeding through one's mind, unrealistic self-confidence, difficulty concentrating, delusions, hallucinations).
- **Changes in behavio**r (sudden immersion in plans and projects, talking very rapidly and much more than usual, excessive spending, impaired judgment, impulsive sexual involvement).
- **Changes in physical condition** (less need for sleep, increased energy, fewer health complaints than usual).

During manic periods, individuals may make grandiose plans or take dangerous risks. But they often plunge from this highest of highs to a horrible, low depressive episode, in which they may feel sad, hopeless, and helpless and develop other symptoms of major depression.

Professional therapy is essential in treating bipolar disorders. An estimated 25 to 50 percent of bipolar patients attempt suicide at least once. About 1 percent take their own lives every year.[26] Mood-stabilizing medications are the keystone of treatment, although psychotherapy plays a critical role in helping individuals understand their illness and rebuild their lives. Most individuals continue taking medication indefinitely after remission of their symptoms because the risk of recurrence is high.

antidepressant A drug used primarily to treat symptoms of depression.

bipolar disorder Severe depression alternating with periods of manic activity and elation.

Anxiety Disorders

Anxiety disorders are as common as depression but are often undetected and untreated.[27] They may involve inordinate fears of certain objects or situations (**phobias**), episodes of sudden, inexplicable terror (**panic attacks**), chronic distress (**generalized anxiety disorder,** or **GAD**), or persistent, disturbing thoughts and behaviors (**obsessive–compulsive disorder,** or **OCD**). These disorders can increase the risk of developing depression. Over a lifetime, as many as one in four Americans may experience an anxiety disorder. More than 40 percent are never correctly diagnosed and treated. Yet most individuals who do get treatment, even for severe and disabling problems, improve dramatically.

Phobias

Phobias—the most prevalent type of anxiety disorder—are out-of-the-ordinary, irrational, intense, persistent fears of certain objects or situations. About two million Americans develop such acute terror that they go to extremes to avoid whatever it is that they fear, even though they realize that these feelings are excessive or unreasonable. The most common phobias involve animals, particularly dogs, snakes, insects, and mice; the sight of blood; closed spaces (*claustrophobia)*; heights (*acrophobia*); air travel and being in open or public places or situations from which one perceives it would be difficult or embarrassing to escape (*agoraphobia).*

Although various medications have been tried, none is effective by itself in relieving phobias. The best approach is behavioral therapy, which consists of gradual, systematic exposure to the feared object (a process called *systematic desensitization).* Numerous studies have proved that exposure—especially in vivo exposure, in which individuals are exposed to the actual source of their fear rather than simply imagining it—is highly effective. Medical hypnosis—the use of induction of an altered state of consciousness—also can help.

Panic Attacks and Panic Disorder

Individuals who have had panic attacks describe them as the most frightening experiences of their lives. Without reason or warning, their hearts race wildly. They may become light-headed or dizzy. Because they can't catch their breath, they may start breathing rapidly and hyperventilate. Parts of their bodies, such as their fingers or toes, may tingle or feel numb. Worst of all is the terrible sense that something horrible is about to happen: that they will die, lose their minds, or have a heart attack. Most attacks reach peak intensity within ten minutes. Afterward, individuals live in dread of another one. In the course of a lifetime, your risk of having a single panic attack is 7 percent.

Panic disorder develops when attacks recur or apprehension about them becomes so intense that individuals cannot function normally. Full-blown panic disorder occurs in about 2 percent of all adults in the course of a

Systematic desensitization is one behavioral approach to treating a fear of spiders and other phobias.

lifetime and usually develops before age 30. Women are more than twice as likely as men to experience panic attacks, although no one knows why. Parents, siblings, and children of individuals with panic disorders also are more likely to develop them than are others.

The two primary treatments for panic disorder are (1) cognitive-behavioral therapy (CBT), which teaches specific strategies for coping with symptoms like rapid breathing, and (2) medication. Treatment helps as many as 90 percent of those with panic disorder either improve significantly or recover completely, usually within six to eight weeks. Individuals with a greater internal locus of control (discussed in Chapter 1) may respond better to CBT.

Generalized Anxiety Disorder

About 10 million adults in the United States suffer from a generalized anxiety disorder (GAD), excessive or unrealistic apprehension that causes physical symptoms and lasts for six months or longer. It usually starts when people are in their twenties. Unlike fear, which helps us recognize and avoid real danger, GAD is an irrational or unwarranted response to harmless objects or situations of exaggerated danger. The most common symptoms are faster heart rate, sweating, increased blood pressure, muscle aches, intestinal pains, irritability, sleep problems, and difficulty concentrating.

Chronically anxious individuals worry—not just some of the time, and not just about the stresses and strains of ordinary life—but constantly, about almost everything: their health, families, finances, marriages, potential dangers. Treatment for GAD may consist of a combination of psychotherapy, behavioral therapy, and antianxiety drugs.

Obsessive-Compulsive Disorder

As many as 1 in 40 Americans has a type of anxiety called obsessive-compulsive disorder (OCD). Some of these individuals suffer only from an *obsession,* a recurring idea, thought, or image that they realize, at least initially, is senseless. The most common obsessions are repetitive thoughts of violence (for example, killing a child), contamination (becoming infected by shaking hands), and doubt (wondering whether one has performed some act, such as having hurt someone in a

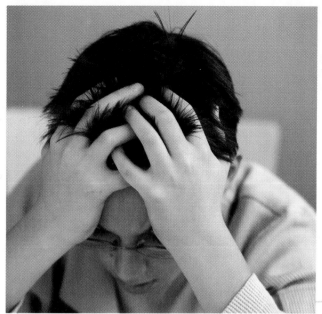

Worry is a normal part of daily life, but individuals with generalized anxiety disorder worry constantly about everything and anything that might go wrong.

© CORBIS/Photolibrary

traffic accident). Most people with OCD also suffer from a *compulsion,* a repetitive behavior performed according to certain rules or in a stereotyped fashion. The most common compulsions involve handwashing, cleaning, hoarding useless items, counting, or checking (for example, making sure dozens of times that a door is locked).

Individuals with OCD realize that their thoughts or behaviors are bizarre, but they cannot resist or control them. Eventually, the obsessions or compulsions consume a great deal of time and significantly interfere with normal routines, job functioning, or usual social activities or relationships with others. A young woman who must follow a very rigid dressing routine may always be late for class, for example; a student who must count each letter of the alphabet as he types may not be able to complete a term paper.

Treatment may consist of cognitive therapy to correct irrational assumptions, behavioral techniques such as progressively limiting the amount of time someone obsessed with cleanliness can spend washing and scrubbing, and medication. Using neuro-imaging techniques, researchers have found significant changes in activity in certain regions of the brain after four weeks of daily therapy in patients with obsessive-compulsive disorder.[28]

anxiety disorders A group of psychological disorders involving episodes of apprehension, tension, or uneasiness, stemming from the anticipation of danger and sometimes accompanied by physical symptoms, which cause significant distress and impairment to an individual.

phobia An anxiety disorder marked by an inordinate fear of an object, a class of objects, or a situation, resulting in extreme avoidance behaviors.

panic attack A short episode characterized by physical sensations of light-headedness, dizziness, hyperventilation, and numbness of extremities, accompanied by an inexplicable terror, usually of a physical disaster such as death.

generalized anxiety disorder (GAD) An anxiety disorder characterized as chronic distress.

obsessive-compulsive disorder (OCD) An anxiety disorder characterized by obsessions and/or compulsions that impair one's ability to function and form relationships.

panic disorder An anxiety disorder in which the apprehension or experience of recurring panic attacks is so intense that normal functioning is impaired.

Attention Disorders

Attention-deficit/hyperactivity disorder (ADHD) is the most common mental disorder in childhood. An estimated 3 to 7 percent of school-age children suffer from ADHD. Contrary to previous beliefs, most children do not outgrow it. For as many as two-thirds of youngsters, ADHD persists into adolescence and young adulthood. About 4 percent of college students have ADHD.[29]

ADHD looks and feels different in adults. Hyperactivity is more subtle, an internal fidgety feeling rather than a physical restlessness. As youngsters with ADHD mature, academic difficulties become much more of a problem. Students with ADHD may find it hard to concentrate, read, make decisions, complete complex projects, and meet deadlines. The academic performance and standardized test scores of college students with ADHD are significantly lower than those of their peers.

Relationships with peers also can become more challenging. Young people with ADHD may become frustrated easily, have a short fuse, and erupt into angry outbursts. Some become more argumentative, negative, and defiant than most other teens. Sleep problems, including sleeping much more or less than normal, are common. The likelihood of developing other emotional problems, including depression and anxiety disorders, is higher. As many as 20 percent of those diagnosed with depression, anxiety, or substance abuse also have ADHD.

The risk of substance use disorders for individuals with ADHD is twice that of the general population. According to several reports, between 15 and 25 percent of adults with substance use disorders have ADHD. In addition, individuals with ADHD start smoking at a younger age and have higher rates of smoking and drinking. (The use of stimulant medication to treat ADHD does not increase the risk of substance abuse.)

The medications used for this disorder include stimulants (such as Ritalin), which improve behavior and cognition for about 70 percent of adolescents. Extended-release preparations (including a skin patch) are longer acting, so individuals do not have to take these medications as often as in the past. As discussed in Chapter 11, misuse of prescription stimulants by students without ADHD is a growing problem on college campuses. An estimated 10 percent of students reported using prescription stimulants at some point in their college years. Their primary motivations were to stay awake or feel more energetic or to get high. ADHD medications do not have the same effects on individuals with the disorder. Although many students take stimulants to improve performance, they generally get poorer grades, perhaps because they fall behind and then take stimulants in order to cram and catch up.

An alternative nonstimulant treatment is Strattera (atomoxetine), which treats ADHD and coexisting problems such as depression and anxiety. Its effects are more gradual, and it does not seem to have any known potential for abuse. Adverse effects include drowsiness, loss of appetite, nausea, vomiting, and headaches. Its long-term effects are not known. A promising new approach is transcendental meditation (TM), which may calm anxiety and improve ability to concentrate.[30]

An estimated 1 percent of college students have an attention disorder that can have a significant impact on their academic performance and their personal lives. Undergraduates with ADHD are at higher risk of becoming smokers, abusing alcohol and drugs, and having automobile accidents. The normal challenges of college—navigating the complexities of scheduling, planning courses, and honing study skills—may be especially daunting.

Psychological therapies have not been studied extensively in adolescents and young adults with ADHD. However, if you have ADHD, check with your student health or counseling center to see if any special services are available. College health services may provide support, but health insurance coverage for ADHD treatment is limited and costly.

Schizophrenia

Schizophrenia, one of the most debilitating mental disorders, profoundly impairs an individual's sense of reality. As the National Institute of Mental Health (NIMH) puts it, schizophrenia, which is characterized by abnormalities in brain structure and chemistry, destroys "the inner unity of the mind" and weakens "the will and drive that constitute our essential character." It affects every aspect of psychological functioning, including the ways in which people think, feel, view themselves, and relate to others.

The symptoms of schizophrenia include:

- **Hallucinations.**
- **Delusions.**
- **Inability to think** in a logical manner.
- **Talking** in rambling or incoherent ways.
- **Making odd or purposeless movements** or not moving at all.
- **Repeating others' words** or mimicking their gestures.
- **Showing few, if any, feelings;** responding with inappropriate emotions.

- **Lacking will or motivation** to complete a task or accomplish something.
- **Functioning at a much lower level** than in the past at work, in interpersonal relations, or in taking care of themselves.

Schizophrenia is one of the leading causes of disability among young adults. The mean age for schizophrenia to develop is 21.4 years for men and 26.8 years for women. Although symptoms do not occur until then, they are almost certainly the result of a failure in brain development that occurs very early in life. The underlying defect is probably present before birth. Schizophrenia has a strong genetic basis and is not the result of upbringing, social conditions, or traumatic experiences.

For the vast majority of individuals with schizophrenia, antipsychotic drugs are the foundation of treatment. Newer agents are more effective in making most people with schizophrenia feel more comfortable and in control of themselves, helping organize chaotic thinking, and reducing or eliminating delusions or hallucinations, allowing fuller participation in normal activities.

Suicide

Suicide is not in itself a psychiatric disorder, but it is often the tragic consequence of emotional and psychological problems. Every year 30,000 Americans—among them many young people who seem to have "everything to live for"—commit suicide, and an estimated 811,000 attempt to take their own lives. There may be 4.5 million suicide "survivors" in the United States.[31]

 The suicide rate for African American and Caucasian men peaks between ages 20 and 40. It rises again after age 65 among white men and after age 75 among blacks. In general, whites are at highest risk for suicide,

followed by American Indians, African Americans, Hispanic Americans, and Asian Americans. Internationally, suicide rates are highest in Germany, Scandinavia, Eastern Europe, and Japan; average in the United States, Canada, and Great Britain; and low in Italy, Spain, and Ireland.

 At all ages, men *commit* suicide three to four times more frequently than women, but women *attempt* suicide much more often than men (Table 4.2). Elderly men are ten times more likely to take their own lives than elderly women. (See Chapter 20 for more on depression and suicide in older men and women.)

attention-deficit/hyperactivity disorder (ADHD) A spectrum of difficulties in controlling motion and sustaining attention, including hyperactivity, impulsivity, and distractibility.

schizophrenia A general term for a group of mental disorders with characteristic psychotic symptoms, such as delusions, hallucinations, and disordered thought patterns during the active phase of the illness, and a duration of at least six months.

TABLE 4.2

Suicide Risk

	Who Attempts Suicide?	Who Commits Suicide?
Sex	Female	Male
Age	Under 35	Under 20 or over 60
Means	Less deadly, such as a wrist slashing	More deadly, such as a gun
Circumstances	High chance of rescue	Low chance of rescue

Campus hot lines provide peer support to students who may be feeling overwhelmed but don't know where to turn for help.

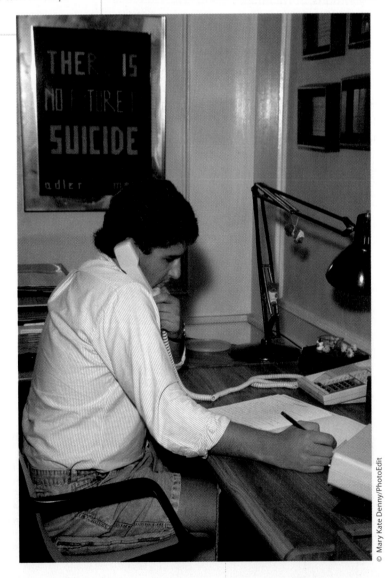

© Mary Kate Denny/PhotoEdit

Suicide in the Young

Suicide rates among youths between ages 10 and 19 in the United States have risen after a decade-long decline. In a national survey, an estimated 15 percent of high school students seriously considered suicide, and 7 percent attempted suicide at least once. Girls and black and Hispanic students wee most likely to attempt suicide. Up to 50 percent of adolescents who attempt suicide try again to take their own lives. An estimated 11 percent of those who attempt suicide eventually die by suicide.[32]

The controversy about the use of antidepressants in children and teens may play a role in the spike in youth suicide. Although several re-analyses and reviews have confirmed that these medications can themselves increase the likelihood of suicide in individuals younger than age 20, this risk is small.[33] In many cases, the benefits may well outweigh the risk, but there is a need for careful monitoring for warning signs of suicide whenever a child or teen begins antidepressant therapy.[34]

 Native American communities have especially high rates of suicide among both young men and women. Young African American men, historically at low suicide risk, are narrowing the gap with their white peers, while suicide by Hispanic young men has declined. The lowest rates are for Asian Pacific males and African American females.[35]

Firearms and suffocation (mainly by hanging) are the most common methods of suicide among young people. In recent years, deaths with firearms have decreased, in part because of laws restricting access to guns by youngsters.

 Researchers also have identified factors that protect young people from suicide. Number one for both boys and girls was feeling connected to their parents and family. For girls, emotional well-being was also protective; grade point average was an additional protective factor for boys. High parental expectations for their child's school achievement, more people living in the household, and religiosity were protective for some of the boys, but not for the girls. Availability of counseling services at school and parental presence at key times during the day were protective for some of the girls, but not for the boys.

Suicide on Campus

 More than a thousand college students take their own lives every year; 1.5 percent attempt to do so. As many as one in ten seriously consider suicide; 8 percent make a plan. (See Reality Check.) The reasons that students consider or attempt suicide vary, but the most significant is untreated depression. Two thirds of individuals who kill themselves experienced depressive symptoms at the time of their deaths.[36] However, rates of suicide attempts and completions are consistently lower than among college-age peers who are not in college.

Suicide rarely stems from a single cause. Researchers have identified several common ones for college students, including the following:

- Depression or depressive symptoms.
- Family history of mental illness.
- Personality traits, such as hopelessness, helplessness, impulsivity, and aggression.
- Alcohol use and binge drinking. Among college students, binge drinkers are significantly more likely to contemplate suicide, to have attempted suicide in the past, and to believe they would make a future suicide attempt than non-binge drinkers.
- Ineffective problem solving and coping skills.
- Recent sexual or physical victimization; being in an emotionally or physically abusive relationship; family problems; or a family history of mental illness.
- Exposure to trauma or stress.
- Feelings of loneliness or social isolation.
- Troubled or abusive relationships.

 The stress of acculturation (the psychosocial adjustments that occur when an ethnic minority interacts with the ethnic majority, discussed in Chapter 3) may also play a role. Blacks who take their own lives tend to be younger, less likely to have been depressed, and less likely to have financial problems, chronic illness, or substance abuse problems. While alcohol or cocaine play a role in more than 40 percent of suicides by European American youths, they are involved in less than 18 percent of suicides of African Americans. A recent study linked acculturative stress to increased thoughts of suicide by African American students who were depressed but not to others.[39]

Although many schools offer counseling and crisis services, students often don't

☑ **REALITYCHECK**
- *What percent of college students have seriously considered attempting suicide?*
- *What percent have developed a suicide plan?*
- *What percent have actually attempted suicide?*

Answers on next page.

know where to turn when they feel hopeless or are thinking about suicide. (See Community Focus.)

Factors That Lead to Suicide

Researchers have looked for explanations for suicide by studying everything from phases of the moon to seasons (suicides peak in the spring and early summer) to birth order in the family. They have found no conclusive

COMMUNITY FOCUS *Preventing Suicide*

PROBLEM Suicide claims more than the lives of the victims. It shatters families, dismays friends and loved ones, and shakes a community to its core. Yet by joining forces, all the members of a campus community can work together to protect each other and prevent the terrible losses suicide brings. Here's how you can get started.

BECOME INFORMED

- Read pages 107–111 of this chapter and 642–643 of Chapter 20 carefully. Make sure you are familiar with the warning signs of suicide.
- Get more information on student suicide at authoritative websites such as:
  http://suicidehotlines.com/national.html
  http://www.suicide.org/college-student-suicide.html http://www.sprc.org/ featured_resources/
  customized/college_student.asp
  http://suicideandmentalhealthassociationinternational.org/CollStud.html
- In one survey, only about a quarter of students were aware of any resources on campus for dealing with suicide. Find out if your school has a suicide prevention program in place. Are hot lines available? Are national numbers such as 1-800-SUICIDE (1-800-784-2433) posted or included in campus directories? Does the counseling service provide information on suicide prevention and student suicide during orientation?

BECOME INVOLVED

- Go to a meeting of a student group such as Active Minds (**http://www .activeminds.org/**) and participate in events such as National Stress Out Day.
- Volunteer as a peer counselor or at a local hotline for students in crisis.
- If you want to help a friend who is depressed, ask your school heath facility for assistance or call the National Suicide Prevention Lifeline at 1-800-273-TALK (1-800-273-8255) to be connected to a trained counselor at a suicide crisis center, or visit **http:// suicidehotlines.com/national.html**. The toll-free numbers are available 24 hours a day.

answers. A constellation of influences—mental disorders, personality traits, biologic and genetic vulnerability, medical illness, and psychosocial stressors—may combine in ways that lower an individual's threshold of vulnerability. The risk of suicide is higher in people who live in cities, are single, have a low income, or are unemployed. No one factor in itself may ever explain fully why a person chooses death.

Mental Disorders More than 95 percent of those who commit suicide have a mental disorder. Two in particular—depression and alcoholism—account for two-thirds of all suicides. Suicide also is a risk for those with other disorders, including schizophrenia, posttraumatic stress disorder, personality disorders, and untreated depression: The lifetime suicide rate for people with major depression is 15 percent.

Substance Abuse Many of those who commit suicide drink beforehand, and their use of alcohol may lower their inhibitions. Since alcohol itself is a depressant, it can intensify the despondency suicidal individuals are already feeling. Alcoholics who attempt suicide often have other risk factors, including major depression, poor social support, serious medical illness, and unemployment. Drugs of abuse also can alter thinking and lower inhibitions against suicide.

Hopelessness The sense of utter hopelessness and helplessness may be the most common contributing factor in suicide. When hope dies, individuals view every experience in negative terms and come to expect the worst possible outcomes for their problems. Given this way of thinking, suicide often seems a reasonable response to a life seen as not worth living. Optimism, on the other hand, correlates with fewer thoughts of suicide by college students.

Combat Stress According to a congressional report, veterans who have been exposed to the violence and trauma of combat or deployment in a war zone may account for as many as 20 percent of suicides. Conditions that may increase a veteran's risk of suicide include depression, PTSD, traumatic brain injury, and lack of social support.[40] In response to this, the Veterans Administration has set up a Suicide Prevention Hotline number: 1-800-274-TALK.

Family History One of every four people who attempt suicide has a family member who also tried to commit suicide. While a family history of suicide is not in itself considered a predictor of suicide, two mental disorders that can lead to suicide—depression and bipolar disorder (manic depression)—do run in families.

Physical Illness People who commit suicide are likely to be ill or to believe that they are. About 5 percent actually have a serious physical disorder, such as AIDS or cancer. While suicide may seem to be a decision rationally arrived at in persons with serious or fatal illness, this may not be the case. Depression, not uncommon in such instances, can warp judgment. When the depression is treated, the person may no longer have suicidal intentions.

Brain Chemistry Investigators have found abnormalities in the brain chemistry of individuals who complete suicide, especially low levels of a metabolite of the neurotransmitter serotonin. There are indications that individuals with a deficiency in this substance may have as much as a ten times greater risk of committing suicide than those with higher levels.

Access to Guns For individuals already facing a combination of predisposing factors, access to a means of committing suicide, particularly to guns, can add to the risk. Unlike other methods of suicide, guns almost always work. Suicide rates among children, women, and men of all ages are higher in states where more households have guns. Although only 5 percent of suicide attempts involve firearms, more than 90 percent of

If you worry that someone you know may be contemplating suicide, express your concern. Here are some specific guidelines:

- **Ask concerned questions.** Listen attentively. Show that you take the person's feelings seriously and truly care.

- **Don't offer trite reassurances.** Don't list reasons to go on living, try to analyze the person's motives, or try to shock or challenge him or her.

- **Suggest solutions or alternatives to problems.** Make plans. Encourage positive action, such as getting away for a while to gain a better perspective on a problem.

- **Don't be afraid to ask whether your friend has considered suicide.** The opportunity to talk about thoughts of suicide may be an enormous relief and--contrary to a long-standing myth--will not fix the idea of suicide more firmly in a person's mind.

- **Don't think that people who talk about killing themselves never carry out their threat.** Most individuals who commit suicide give definite indications of their intent to die.

- **Watch out for behavioral clues.** If your friend begins to behave unpredictably or suddenly emerges from a severe depression into a calm, settled state of mind, these could signal increased danger of suicide. Don't leave your friend alone. Call a suicide hotline, or get in touch with a mental health professional.

If you are thinking about suicide . . .

- **Talk to a mental health professional.** If you have a therapist, call immediately. If not, call a suicide hotline.

- **Find someone you can trust and talk honestly about what you're feeling.** If you suffer from depression or another mental disorder, educate trusted friends or relatives about your condition so they are prepared if called upon to help.

- **Write down your more uplifting thoughts.** Even if you are despondent, you can help yourself by taking the time to retrieve some more positive thoughts or memories. A simple record of your hopes for the future and the people you value in your life can remind you of why your own life is worth continuing.

- **Avoid drugs and alcohol.** Most suicides are the results of sudden, uncontrolled impulses, and drugs and alcohol can make it harder to resist these destructive urges.

- **Go to the hospital.** Hospitalization can sometimes be the best way to protect your health and safety.

these attempts are fatal. By comparison, 75 percent of all suicide attempts involve drugs and result in death less than 3 percent of the time.[41] States with stricter gun-control laws have much lower rates of suicide than states with more lenient laws. Health professionals are urging parents whose children undergo psychological treatment or assessment to remove all weapons from their homes and to make sure their youngsters do not have access to potentially lethal medications or to alcohol.

Other Factors   Individuals who kill themselves often have gone through more major life crises—job changes, births, financial reversals, divorce, retirement—in the previous six months, compared with others. Long-standing, intense conflict with family members or other important people may add to the danger. In some cases, suicide may be an act of revenge that offers the person a sense of control—however temporary or illusory. For example, some may feel that, by rejecting life, they are rejecting a partner or parent who abandoned or betrayed them.

Overcoming Problems of the Mind

Mental illness costs our society an estimated $150 billion a year in lost work time and productivity, employee turnover, disability payments, and death. Yet many Americans do not have access to mental health services, nor do they have insurance for such services. Despite the fact that treatments for mental disorders have a higher success rate than those for many other diseases, employers often restrict mental health benefits. HMOs and health insurance plans are much more likely to limit psychotherapy visits and psychiatric hospitalizations than treatments for medical illnesses.

Even when cost is not a barrier, many people do not seek treatment because they see psychological problems as a sign of weakness rather than illness. They also may

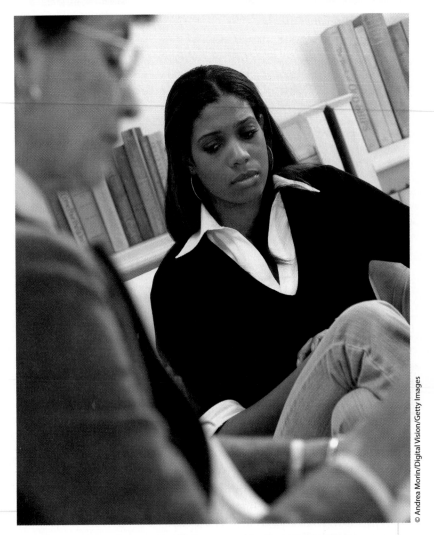

When choosing a therapist, you should always consider the individual's education, degree, and qualifications. Also important are qualities such as compassion and caring.

clinics and services; and there are usually local branches of national service organizations, such as United Way or Alcoholics Anonymous, other 12-step programs, and various support groups. You can call the psychiatric or psychological association in your city or state for the names of licensed professionals. (Check the telephone directory for listings.) Your primary physician may also be able to help.

The telephone book and the Internet are also good resources for special programs, found either by the nature of the service, by the name of the neighborhood or city, or by the name of the sponsoring group. In addition to suicide-prevention programs, look for crisis intervention, violence prevention, and child-abuse prevention programs; drug-treatment information; shelters for battered women; senior citizen centers; and self-help and counseling services. Many services have special hotlines for coping with emergencies. Others provide information as well as counseling over the phone.

Types of Therapists

Only professionally trained individuals who have met state licensing requirements are certified as psychiatrists, psychologists, or social workers. Before selecting any of these mental health professionals, be sure to check the person's background and credentials.

Psychiatrists are licensed medical doctors (M.D.) who complete medical school; a year-long internship; and a three-year residency that provides training in various forms of psychotherapy, psychopharmacology, and both outpatient and inpatient treatment of mental disorders. They can prescribe medications and make medical decisions. *Board-certified* psychiatrists have passed oral and written examinations following completion of residency training.

Psychologists complete a graduate program (including clinical training and internships) in human psychology but do not study medicine and cannot prescribe medication. They must be licensed in most states in order to practice independently.

Certified social workers or **licensed clinical social workers (LCSWs)** usually complete a two-year graduate program and have specialized training in helping people with mental problems in addition to conventional social work.

not realize that scientifically proven therapies can bring relief, often in a matter of weeks or months.

Where to Turn for Help

As a student, your best contact for identifying local services may be your health education instructor or department. The health instructors can tell you about general and mental health counseling available on campus, school-based support groups, community-based programs, and special emergency services. On campus, you can also turn to the student health services or the office of the dean of student services or student affairs. (See "Help Yourself" in *Labs for IPC.)*

Within the community, you may be able to get help through the city or county health department and neighborhood health centers. Local hospitals often have special

© Andrea Morin/Digital Vision/Getty Images

Psychiatric nurses have nursing degrees and have passed a state examination. They usually have special training and experience in mental health care, although no specialty licensing or certification is required.

Marriage and family therapists, licensed in some but not all states, usually have a graduate degree, often in psychology, and at least two years of supervised clinical training in dealing with relationship problems.

Other therapists include pastoral counselors, members of the clergy who offer psychological counseling; hypnotherapists, who use hypnosis for problems such as smoking and obesity; stress-management counselors, who teach relaxation methods; and alcohol and drug counselors, who help individuals with substance abuse problems. Anyone can use these terms to describe themselves professionally, and there are no licensing requirements.

Types of Therapy

The term **psychotherapy** refers to any type of counseling based on the exchange of words in the context of the unique relationship that develops between a mental health professional and a person seeking help. The process of talking and listening can lead to new insight, relief from distressing psychological symptoms, changes in unhealthy or maladaptive behaviors, and more effective ways of dealing with the world. "Spirituality oriented" psychotherapy pays particular attention to the roles that religion and spiritual and religious beliefs play in an individual's psychological life.[42]

Landmark research has shown that psychotherapy does not just benefit the mind but actually changes the brain. In studies comparing psychotherapy and psychiatric medications as treatments for depression, both proved about equally effective. But a particular group of patients—those who has lost a parent at an early age or had experienced childhood trauma, including physical or sexual abuse—gained greater benefits with talk therapy.[43]

The most common goal of psychotherapy is to improve quality of life.[44] Most mental health professionals today are trained in a variety of psychotherapeutic techniques and tailor their approach to the problem, personality, and needs of each person seeking their help. Because skilled therapists may combine different techniques in the course of therapy, the lines between the various approaches often blur.

Because insurance companies and health-care plans often limit the duration of psychotherapy, many mental health professionals are adopting a *time-limited* format in order to make the most of every session, regardless of the length of treatment. Brief or short-term psychotherapy typically focuses on a central theme, problem, or topic and may continue for several weeks to several months. The individuals most likely to benefit are those who are interested in solving immediate problems rather than changing their characters, who can think in psychological terms, and who are motivated to change.

Psychodynamic Psychotherapy For the most part, today's mental health professionals base their assessment of individuals on a **psychodynamic** understanding that takes into account the role of early experiences and unconscious influences in *actively* shaping behavior. (This is the *dynamic* in psychodynamic.) Psychodynamic treatments work toward the goal of providing greater insight into problems and bringing about behavioral change. Therapy may be brief, consisting of 12 to 25 sessions, or may continue for several years.

Cognitive–Behavioral Therapy (CBT) Cognitive-behavioral therapy (CBT) focuses on inappropriate or inaccurate thoughts or beliefs to help individuals break out of a distorted way of thinking. The techniques of **cognitive therapy** include identification of an individual's beliefs and attitudes, recognition of negative thought patterns, and education in alternative ways of thinking. Individuals with major depression or anxiety disorders are most likely to benefit, usually in 15 to 25 sessions. However, many of the positive messages used in cognitive therapy can help anyone improve a bad mood or negative outlook.[45]

Behavioral therapy strives to substitute healthier ways of behaving for maladaptive patterns used in the past. Its premise is that distressing psychological symptoms, like all behaviors, are learned responses that can be modified or unlearned. Some therapists believe that changing behavior also

psychiatrist Licensed medical doctor with additional training in psychotherapy, psychopharmacology, and treatment of mental disorders.

psychologist Mental health-care professional who has completed doctoral or graduate program in psychology and is trained in psychotherapeutic techniques, but who is not medically trained and does not prescribe medications.

certified social worker or licensed clinical social worker (LCSW) A person who has completed a two-year graduate program in counseling people with mental problems.

psychiatric nurse A nurse with special training and experience in mental health care.

marriage and family therapist A psychiatrist, psychologist, or social worker who specializes in marriage and family counseling.

psychotherapy Treatment designed to produce a response by psychological rather than physical means, such as suggestion, persuasion, reassurance, and support.

psychodynamic Interpreting behaviors in terms of early experiences and unconscious influences.

cognitive therapy A technique used to identify an individual's beliefs and attitudes, recognize negative thought patterns, and educate in alternative ways of thinking.

behavioral therapy A technique that emphasizes application of the principles of learning to substitute desirable responses and behavior patterns for undesirable ones.

Before taking any psychoactive drug (one that affects the brain), talk to a qualified health professional. Here are some points to raise:

- What can this medication do for me? What specific symptoms will it relieve? Are there other possible benefits?
- When will I notice a difference? How long does it take for the medicine to have an effect?
- Are there any risks? What about side effects? Do I have to take it before or after eating? Will it affect my ability to study, work, drive, or operate machinery?
- Is there a risk of suicide or increased aggression? What should I do if I start thinking about taking my own life or of harming others?

changes how people think and feel. As they put it, "Change the behavior, and the feelings will follow." Behavioral therapies work best for disorders characterized by specific, abnormal patterns of acting—such as alcohol and drug abuse, anxiety disorders, and phobias—and for individuals who want to change bad habits.

Interpersonal Therapy (IPT)
Interpersonal therapy (IPT), originally developed for research into the treatment of major depression, focuses on relationships in order to help individuals deal with unrecognized feelings and needs and improve their communication skills. IPT does not deal with the psychological origins of symptoms but rather concentrates on current problems of getting along with others. The supportive, empathic relationship that is developed with the therapist, who takes an even more active role than in psychodynamic psychotherapy, is the most crucial component of this therapy. The emphasis is on the here and now and on interpersonal—rather than intrapsychic—issues. Individuals with major depression, chronic difficulties developing relationships, and chronic mild depression are most likely to benefit. IPT usually consists of 12 to 16 sessions.[46]

Other Treatment Options

Psychiatric Drugs Medications that alter brain chemistry and relieve psychiatric symptoms have brought great hope and help to millions of people. Thanks to the recent development of a new generation of more precise and effective **psychiatric drugs,** success rates for treating many common and disabling disorders—depression, panic disorder, schizophrenia, and others—have soared. Often used in conjunction with psychotherapy, sometimes used as the primary treatment, these medications have revolutionized mental health care.

At some point in their lives, about half of all Americans will take a psychiatric drug. The reason may be depression, anxiety, a sleep difficulty, an eating disorder, alcohol or drug dependence, impaired memory, or another disorder that disrupts the intricate chemistry of the brain.

Psychiatric drugs are now among the most widely prescribed drugs in the United States. Serotonin-boosting medications (SSRIs) have become the drugs of choice in treating depression. They also are effective in treating obsessive compulsive disorder, panic disorder, social phobia, posttraumatic stress disorder, premenstrual dysphoric disorder, and generalized anxiety disorder. In patients who don't respond, psychiatrists may add another drug to boost the efficacy of the treatment.

According to various studies, 5 to 7 percent of college students take antidepressant medications. Direct-to-consumer advertisements for antidepressant drugs can influence students' perceptions of what is wrong with them. In one study, college women were more likely to rate themselves as having mild-to-moderate depression as a result of reading pharmaceutical company information for popular antidepressants. (See Your Strategies for Prevention: "Before Taking a Psychiatric Drug.")

Alternative Mind–Mood Products
People with serious mental illnesses, including depression and bipolar disorder, often use at least one alternative health-care practice, such as yoga or meditation. In a recent survey of women with depression, about half (54 percent) reported trying herbs, vitamins, and manual therapies such as massage and acupressure. Some "natural" products, such as herbs and enzymes, claim to have psychological effects. However, they have not undergone rigorous scientific testing.

St. John's wort has been used to treat anxiety and depression in Europe for many years. Data from clinical studies in the United States do not support the efficacy of St. John's wort for moderate to severe depression. In ten carefully controlled studies, the herb did not prove more effective than a placebo. However, more than two dozen studies have found that St. John's wort was similar in efficacy to standard antidepressants. Side effects include dizziness, abdominal pain and bloating, constipation, nausea, fatigue, and dry mouth. St. John's wort should not be taken in combination with other prescription antidepressants. St. John's wort can lower the efficacy of oral contraceptives and increase the risk of an unwanted pregnancy.

interpersonal therapy (IPT) A technique used to develop communication skills and relationships.

psychiatric drugs Medications that regulate a person's mental, emotional, and physical functions to facilitate normal functioning.

Like physical health, psychological well-being is not a fixed state of being, but a process. The way you live every day affects how you feel about yourself and your world. Here are some basic guidelines that you can rely on to make the most of the process of living:

- **Accept yourself.** As a human being, you are, by definition, imperfect. Come to terms with the fact that you are a worthwhile person despite your mistakes.

- **Respect yourself.** Recognize your abilities and talents. Acknowledge your competence and achievements, and take pride in them.

- **Trust yourself.** Learn to listen to the voice within you, and let your intuition be your guide.

- **Love yourself.** Be happy to spend time by yourself. Learn to appreciate your own company and to be glad you're you.

- **Stretch yourself.** Be willing to change and grow, to try something new and dare to be vulnerable.

- **Look at challenges as opportunities for personal growth.** "Every problem brings the possibility of a widening of consciousness," psychologist Carl Jung once noted. Put his words to the test.

- **Think of not only where but also who you want to be a decade from now.** The goals you set, the decisions you make, the values you adopt now will determine how you feel about yourself and your life in the future.

SELF SURVEY | Recognizing Depression

Depression comes in different forms, just like other illnesses such as heart disease. Not everyone with a depressive disorder experiences every symptom. The number and severity of symptoms may vary among individuals and also over time.

Read through the following list, and check all the descriptions that apply.

- ☐ I am often restless and irritable.
- ☐ I am having irregular sleep patterns—either too much or not enough.
- ☐ I don't enjoy hobbies, my friends, family or leisure activities any more.
- ☐ I am having trouble managing my diabetes, hypertension, or other chronic illness.
- ☐ I have nagging aches and pains that do not get better no matter what I do.
- ☐ Specifically, I often experience:
  - ☐ Digestive problems
  - ☐ Headache or backache
  - ☐ Vague aches and pains like joint or muscle pains
  - ☐ Chest pains
  - ☐ Dizziness
- ☐ I have trouble concentrating or making simple decisions.
- ☐ Others have commented on my mood or attitude lately.
- ☐ My weight has changed a considerable amount.
- ☐ I have had several of the symptoms I checked above for more than two weeks.
- ☐ I feel that my functioning in my everyday life (work, family, friends) is suffering because of these problems.
- ☐ I have a family history of depression.
- ☐ I have thought about suicide.*

Checking several items on this list does not mean that you have a depressive disorder because many conditions can cause similar symptoms. However, you should take this list with you to discuss with your health care provider or mental health therapist. Even though it can be difficult to talk about certain things, your health care provider is knowledgeable, trained, and committed to helping you.

If you can't think of what to say, try these conversation starters:

"I just don't feel like myself lately."

"My friend (parent, roommate, spouse) thinks I might be depressed."

"I haven't been sleeping well lately."

"Everything seems harder than before."

"Nothing's fun anymore."

If you are diagnosed with depression, remember that it is a common and highly treatable illness with medical causes. Your habits or personality did not cause your depression, and you do not have to face it alone.

*University of Michigan Depression Center, 800-475-MICH, www.med.umich.edu/depression

Your Health Action Plan for Getting Help for a Psychological Problem

Sometimes we all need outside help from a trained, licensed professional to work through personal problems. Here is what you need to know if you are experiencing psychological difficulties.

Consider Therapy If You . . .

- Feel an overwhelming and prolonged sense of helplessness and sadness, which does not lift despite your efforts and help from family and friends.
- Find it difficult to carry out everyday activities such as homework, and your academic performance is suffering.
- Worry excessively, expect the worst, or are constantly on edge.
- Are finding it hard to resist or are engaging in behaviors that are harmful to you or others, such as drinking too much alcohol, abusing drugs, or becoming aggressive or violent.
- Have persistent thoughts or fantasies of harming yourself or others.

Most people who have at least several sessions of psychotherapy are far better off than individuals with emotional difficulties who do not get treatment. According to the American Psychological Association, 50 percent of patients noticeably improve after eight sessions, while 75 percent of individuals in therapy improved by the end of six months.

Choosing a Therapist

Ask your physician or another health professional. Call your local or state psychological association. Consult your university or college department of psychology or health center. Contact your area community mental health center. Inquire at your church or synagogue.

- A good rapport with your psychotherapist is critical. Choose someone with whom you feel comfortable and at ease.

- Ask the following questions:
  - Are you licensed?
  - How long have you been practicing?
  - I have been feeling (anxious, tense, depressed, etc.), and I'm having problems (with school, relationships, eating, sleeping, etc.). What experience do you have helping people with these types of problems?
  - What are your areas of expertise—phobias? ADHD? depression?
  - What kinds of treatments do you use? Have they proved effective for dealing with my kind of problem or issue?
  - What are your fees? (Fees are usually based on a 45-minute to 50-minute session.) Do you have a sliding-scale fee policy?
  - How much therapy would you recommend?
  - What types of insurance do you accept?

Is Therapy Working?

As you begin therapy, establish clear goals with your therapist. Some goals require more time to reach than others. You and your therapist should decide at what point you might expect to begin to see progress.

As they begin therapy, some people may have difficulty discussing painful and troubling experiences. Feelings of relief or hope are positive signs indicating that you are starting to explore your thoughts and behaviors.

CENGAGENOW If you want to write your own goals for avoiding mood slumps or getting psychological help, go to the Wellness Journal at HealthNow at **www.cengage.com/sso.**

MAKING THIS CHAPTER WORK FOR YOU

Review Questions

1. Depression
   a. is not likely to occur in young adults.
   b. is twice as common in men as women.
   c. has the same symptoms in men and women.
   d. is more likely to occur again in those who suffer a first episode.

2. Which statement about depression treatment is true?
   a. Psychotherapy and drug therapy are effective in treating depression, but only about 50 percent of people seek treatment.
   b. Antidepressants help about 90 percent of individuals feel better within four weeks.
   c. Jogging has only a small benefit for most depressed individuals.
   d. With the right therapy, depression will not reoccur.

3. Neurons
   a. transmit information within the brain and throughout the body by means of electrical impulses and chemical messengers.
   b. are specialized support cells that travel through the spinal cord, carrying signals related to movement.
   c. are protein molecules designed to bind with neurotransmitters.
   d. cross a synapse before reuptake.

4. Students with attention-deficit/hyperactivity disorder
   a. perform as well on standardized tests as students without ADHD.
   b. have an increased risk of substance use disorders.
   c. have a decreased risk of developing depression or anxiety disorders.
   d. constitute 10 percent of the student population.

5. Some characteristic symptoms of major depression are
   a. difficulty concentrating, lack of energy, and eating more than usual.
   b. exaggerated sense of euphoria and energy.
   c. palpitations, sweating, numbness, and tingling sensations.
   d. talking in rambling ways, inability to think in a logical manner, and delusions.

6. Which of the following statements is true?
   a. Individuals with phobias are most likely to benefit from psychiatric medications.
   b. Antidepressant medications now require a warning label about the increased risk of suicidal thoughts.
   c. Only children have attention disorders.
   d. Interpersonal therapy focuses on the role of early experiences and unconscious influences in shaping patterns of behavior, such as repeated failed relationships.

7. Which of the following statements about anxiety disorders is true?
   a. Anxiety disorders are the least prevalent type of mental illness.
   b. An individual suffering from a panic attack may mistake her symptoms for a heart attack.
   c. The primary symptom of obsessive-compulsive disorder is irrational, intense, and persistent fear of a specific object or situation.
   d. Generalized anxiety disorders respond to systematic desensitization behavior therapy.

8. A mental disorder can be described as
   a. a condition associated with migraine headaches and narcolepsy.
   b. a condition that is usually caused by severe trauma to the brain.
   c. a behavioral or psychological disorder that impairs an individual's ability to conduct one or more important activities of daily life.
   d. a psychological disorder that is easily controlled with medication and a change in diet.

9. A person may be at higher risk of committing suicide if
   a. he is taking blood pressure medication.
   b. he lives in a rural environment and is married.
   c. he has been diagnosed with hyperactivity disorder.
   d. he has lost his job because of alcoholism.

10. Which of these therapies focuses on recognizing negative thought patterns and changing those patterns?
    a. psychodynamic psychotherapy
    b. behavioral activation
    c. interpersonal therapy
    d. cognitive therapy

Answers to these questions can be found on page 650.

Critical Thinking

1. Jake, who took antidepressants to recover from depression in high school, began feeling the same troubling symptoms. A physician at the student health center prescribed the same medication that had helped him in the past, but this time Jake noticed the warning about an increased risk of suicide. He has had thoughts of killing himself, and he worries whether or not to start the medication. When he did some online research, he learned that the risk of suicide is greater if depression is untreated than it is with medication. How would you counsel Jake? How would you weigh the risks and benefits of taking an antidepressant? Do you know someone who might benefit from taking antidepressants but is afraid to take them because of the possible risk of suicide? What might you say to this person based on what you have read in this chapter?

2. Research has indicated that many homeless men and women are in need of outpatient psychiatric care, often because they suffer from chronic mental illnesses or alcoholism. Yet government funding for the mentally ill is inadequate, and homelessness itself can make it difficult, if not impossible, for people to gain access to the care they need. How do you feel when you pass homeless individuals who seem disoriented or out of touch with reality? Who should take responsibility for their welfare? Should they be forced to undergo treatment at psychiatric institutions?

CENGAGENOW™ Go to the CengageNOW for Health website at **www.cengage.com/sso** that will:
- Help you evaluate your knowledge of the material.
- Allow you to take an exam-prep quiz.
- Provide a Personalized Learning Plan targeting resources that address areas you should study.
- Coach you through identifying target goals for behavioral change and creating and monitoring your personal change plan throughout the semester.

Internet Connections

www.save.org
This site (formerly American Foundation for Suicide Prevention) offers research, facts, survivor support, and more.

www.nimh.nih.gov
The National Institute of Mental Health is a federally sponsored organization that provides useful information on a variety of mental health topics including current mental health research.

www.apa.org
The APA is the scientific and professional organization for psychology in the United States. Its website provides up-to-date information on psychological issues and disorders.

www.nmha.org
This site features fact sheets on a variety of mental health topics, including depression screening, college initiative, substance abuse prevention, and information for families. Also available are current mental health articles, an e-mail newsletter, and a bookstore.

www.afsp.org
This site provides facts and statistics about suicide and depression, as well as information about current research and educational projects. It also provides support information for survivors.

www.activeminds.org
This provides fact sheets on mental illness and information about starting an Active Minds chapter and planning events at your campus to create awareness about mental health.

Key Terms

The terms listed are used on the page indicated. Definitions of the terms are in the Glossary at the end of the book.

© Workbook Stock/Jupiterimages

Healthy Lifestyles

Y OU have enormous influence over your health and vitality. This section provides information about the tools you have at hand to become healthier and feel more energetic throughout your lifetime. By learning how to eat a balanced and varied diet, how to manage your weight, and how to become physically fit, you can get started on a lifelong journey of becoming all you can be. As you take better care of your body today, you'll build the foundation for feeling your best for many tomorrows to come.

Chapter 5 - The Joy of Fitness

1. **All but one are components of physical fitness:** (Pg. 122)
   - A. body composition
   - B. cardiorespiratory fitness
   - C. body mass index
   - D. muscle strength

2. **To prevent our body joints from locking up, the physical fitness activity we should use would be:** (Pg. 145)
   - A. muscular strength exercises
   - B. bench pressing weight
   - C. cardio breathing exercises
   - D. flexibility stretching routines

3. **Exercising makes people feel better with their moods and disposition by increasing the levels of a brain mood-elevating chemical known as:** (Pg. 127)
   - A. adrenaline
   - B. endorphins
   - C. dopamine
   - D. serotonin

4. **What component of physical fitness is defined as the ability to sustain moderate intensity whole body activity for extended time periods?** (Pg. 133)
   - A. flexibility
   - B. body composition
   - C. cardiorespiratory fitness
   - D. muscular strength and endurance

5. **Cardiorespiratory fitness is usually accomplished by doing:** (Pg. 135)
   - A. anaerobic exercises
   - B. aerobic exercises
   - C. flexibility training
   - D. weight lifting exercises

6. **To achieve optimal cardiorespiratory fitness, it is recommended to improve our heart rate. This concept is known as:** (Pg. 134)
   - A. resting heart rate
   - B. target heart rate
   - C. aerobic exercise
   - D. anaerobic exercise

7. **What is the primary category of physical activity known to improve cardiovascular fitness?** (Pg. 135)
   - A. aerobic exercises
   - B. anaerobic exercises
   - C. body building
   - D. flexibility

8. **What is the result when one is able to perform repeated muscular efforts with larger amounts of weights?** (Pg. 140)
   - A. stamina
   - B. flexibility
   - C. strength
   - D. endurance

9. **All of the following are benefits of regular exercise except:** (Pg. 127- 128)
   - A. better bones
   - B. improved complexion
   - C. longer life
   - D. better mental health

10. **In order for any group of muscles to become stronger, one needs to practice a concept known as:** (Pg. 140)
    - A. anaerobic exercise
    - B. progressive overloading
    - C. sports doping
    - D. specificity principle

11. **Which aspect of the FITT principle does one work the muscles and cardio much harder?** (Pg. 132)
    - A. frequency
    - B. time
    - C. intensity
    - D. specific activity

12. **Jordan wants to increase his muscular endurance. Which plan should he follow to do this?** (Pg. 139)
    - A. more repetitions with lighter loads
    - B. more repetitions with heavier loads
    - C. progressive overloading with weights
    - D. fewer repetitions with heavier weights

13. **Core strength conditioning refers to:** (Pg. 142)
    - A. the ability of your leg muscles to hold your body up
    - B. the ability of your muscles to support your spine and keep your body balanced
    - C. the overall conditioning of all muscles in the body
    - D. upper body muscle coordination

14. **The fullest extent of possible movement in a particular joint is known as:** (Pg. 140)
    - A. static flexibility
    - B. dynamic flexibility
    - C. range of motion
    - D. isokinetic contractions

15. **When stretching a muscle during exercising, you should be careful not to pull the connective tissue. To avoid damaging your connective tissue, you should:** (Pg. 142)
    - A. don't force body parts beyond their normal range of motion
    - B. don't make quick or jerking movements while stretching
    - C. stretch individual muscles before doing groups of muscles
    - D. all of the above

16. **All but one of the following are risks when using anabolic steroids:** (Pg. 143)
    - A. shrinkage of the testicles in men
    - B. mellowed personality
    - C. baldness in both men and women
    - D. severe acne

17. **Good flexibility depends on all but which factor?** (Pg. 145)
    - A. blood type
    - B. joint structure
    - C. body composition
    - D. age

18. **Using the P.R.I.C.E. prescription plan is to help with:** (Pg. 159)
    - A. prevention of overtraining for sports
    - B. prevention of repetitive strains
    - C. coping with an exercise injury
    - D. calculating the costs for an exercise program

19. **All of these considerations except one are important to determine your success in a physical fitness program:** (Pg. 16)
    - A. your readiness to make a health change
    - B. determining what your fitness goals will be
    - C. scheduling the exercise into your daily routine
    - D. having all new gym clothes and shoes

20. **Which one of the following is not a health-related component of physical fitness?** (Pg. 122)
    - A. functional fitness
    - B. aerobic endurance
    - C. muscular strength
    - D. body composition

As a boy, Derek never thought about doing anything special to stay physically fit. He loved sports so much that he spent every free moment on a softball field or basketball court. He could sprint faster, jump higher, and hit a ball harder than any of his friends. In high school Derek's life revolved around practices and games. He was a varsity athlete and a regional all-star.

Early in his first year in college, an injury sidelined Derek. Frustrated that he had to sit out the season, he gave up his rigorous training routine. As he became im-

The Joy of Fitness

mersed in academics and other activities, Derek stopped going to the gym or working out on his own. Yet he continued to think of himself as an athlete in excellent physical condition. When Derek went home for spring break, he joined his younger brothers on a neighborhood basketball court. While he wasn't surprised that his long shots were off, Derek was amazed by how quickly he got winded. In 15 minutes, he was panting for breath. "Getting old," one of his brothers joked. "Getting soft," the other teased.

Often the college years represent a turning point in physical fitness. Like Derek, many students, busy with classes and other commitments, devote less time to physical activity. However, the choices you make and the habits you develop now can affect how long and how well you'll live. As you'll see in this chapter, exercise yields immediate rewards: It boosts energy, improves mood, soothes stress, improves sleep, and makes you look and feel better. In the long term, physical activity slows many of the changes associated with chronological aging such as loss of calcium and bone density, lowers the risk of serious chronic illnesses, and extends the lifespan. To motivate yourself to get moving, see "Making Change Happen," p. 126, and "Excise Exercise Excuses" in *Labs for IPC*.

This chapter can help you reap these rewards. It presents the latest activity recommendations, documents the benefits of exercise, describes types of exercise, and provides guidelines for getting into shape and exercising safely.

After studying the material in this chapter, you should be able to

- **Describe** the health benefits of regular physical activity.
- **List** the different forms of cardiorespiratory activities and **describe** their potential health benefits and risks.
- **Explain** the benefits of a muscle training program and **describe** how to design a workout.
- **List** the potential health risks of strength-enhancing drugs and supplements.
- **Define** flexibility and **describe** the different types of stretching exercises.
- **Describe** the PRICE plan for handling an exercise injury.
- **Assess** yourself in the five components of health-related fitness, and **develop** a strategy to improve in at least two of them.

Log on to HealthNow at **www.cengage.com/sso** to find your Behavior Change Planner and to explore self-assessments, interactive tutorials, and practice quizzes.

What Is Physical Fitness?

The simplest, most practical definition of **physical fitness** is the ability to respond to routine physical demands, with enough reserve energy to cope with a sudden challenge. You can consider yourself fit if you meet your daily energy needs; can handle unexpected extra demands; and are protecting yourself against potential health problems, such as heart disease. Fitness is important both for health and for athletic performance.

Health-Related Fitness

The five health-related components of physical fitness include aerobic or cardiorespiratory endurance, muscular strength, muscular endurance, flexibility, and body composition (the ratio of fat and lean body tissue).

Cardiorespiratory fitness refers to the ability of the heart to pump blood through the body efficiently. It is achieved through aerobic exercise—any activity, such as brisk walking or swimming, in which sufficient or excess oxygen is continually supplied to the body. In other words, aerobic exercise involves working out strenuously without pushing to the point of breathlessness.

Muscular strength refers to the force within muscles; it is measured by the absolute maximum weight that you can lift, push, or press in one effort. Strong muscles help keep the skeleton in proper alignment, improve posture, prevent back and leg aches, help in everyday lifting, and enhance athletic performance. Muscle mass increases along with strength, which makes for a healthier body composition and a higher metabolic rate.

Muscular endurance is the ability to perform repeated muscular effort; it is measured by counting how many times you can lift, push, or press a given weight. Important for posture, muscular endurance helps in everyday work as well as in athletics and sports.

Flexibility is the range of motion around specific joints—for example, the stretching you do to touch your toes or twist your torso. Flexibility depends on many factors: your age, gender, and posture; how muscular you are; and how much body fat you have. As children develop, their flexibility increases until adolescence. Then a gradual loss of joint mobility begins and continues throughout adult life. Both muscles and connective tissue, such as tendons and ligaments, shorten and become tighter if not consistently used through their full range of motion.

Body composition refers to the relative amounts of fat and lean tissue (bone, muscle, organs, water) in the body. As discussed in detail in Chapter 7, a high proportion of body fat has serious health implications, including increased incidence of heart disease, high blood pressure, diabetes, stroke, gallbladder problems, back and joint problems, and some forms of cancer.

Physical conditioning (or training) refers to the gradual building up of the body to enhance cardiorespiratory, or aerobic, fitness; muscular strength; muscular endurance; flexibility; and a healthy body composition.

Functional fitness, which is gaining greater emphasis among professional trainers, refers to the performance of activities of daily living. Exercises that mimic job tasks or everyday movements can improve an individual's balance, coordination, strength, and endurance.

Athletic, or Performance-Related, Fitness

You may jog five miles, work out with weights, and start each day with a stretching routine. This doesn't qualify you for the soccer team. Most sports, such as softball, tennis, and basketball, require additional skills, including:

- **Agility,** the ability to change direction rapidly.
- **Balance,** or equilibrium, the ability to maintain a certain body position.
- **Coordination,** the ability to integrate the movement of body parts to produce smooth, fluid movements.

© Lori Adamski Peek/Stone/Getty Images

Fitness can enhance every dimension of your health—improving your mood and your mind as well as your body. Go for the joy!

- **Power,** the product of force and speed.
- **Reaction time,** the time required to respond to a stimulus.
- **Speed,** or velocity, the ability to move rapidly.

While many amateur and professional athletes are in superb overall condition, you do not need athletic skills to keep your body operating at maximum capacity throughout life.

Fitness and the Dimensions of Health

The concept of fitness is evolving. Rather than focusing only on miles run or weight lifted, instructors, coaches, and consumers are pursuing a broader vision of total fitness that encompasses every dimension of health:

- **Physical.** As described later in this chapter, becoming fit reduces your risk of major diseases, increases energy and stamina, and may prolong your life.
- **Emotional.** Fitness lowers tension and anxiety, lifts depression, relieves stress, improves mood, and promotes a positive self-image.
- **Social.** Physical activities provide opportunities to meet new people and to work out with friends or family.
- **Intellectual.** Fit individuals report greater alertness, better concentration, more creativity, and improved personal health habits.
- **Occupational.** Fit employees miss fewer days of work, are more productive, and incur fewer medical costs.
- **Spiritual.** Fitness fosters appreciation for the relationship between body and mind and may lead to greater realization of your potential.
- **Environmental.** Fit individuals often become more aware of their need for healthy air and food and develop a deeper appreciation of the physical world.

Gender, Race, and Fitness

Men and women of all racial backgrounds benefit equally from fitness. However, there are some

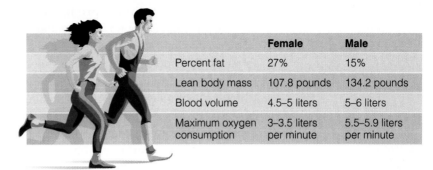

	Female	Male
Percent fat	27%	15%
Lean body mass	107.8 pounds	134.2 pounds
Blood volume	4.5–5 liters	5–6 liters
Maximum oxygen consumption	3–3.5 liters per minute	5.5–5.9 liters per minute

Figure 5.1 Physiological Differences Between Men and Women

physiological differences between men and women, many of which are related to size. On average, men are 10 to 15 percent bigger than women, with roughly twice the percentage of muscle mass and half the percentage of body fat. They have more sweat glands and a greater maximum oxygen uptake. A man's bigger heart pumps more blood with each beat. His larger lungs take in 10 to 20 percent more oxygen (Figure 5.1). His longer legs cover more distance with each stride. If a man jogs along at 50 percent of his capacity, a woman has to push to 73 percent of hers to keep up.

Women have a higher percentage of body fat than men, and more is distributed around the hips and thighs; men carry more body fat around the waist and stomach.

College-age men average 15 percent body fat; college-age women, 23 percent. On average, women have 11 percent more body fat and 8 percent less muscle mass than men.

Women are generally less active than men. Fewer than 12 percent of white women, 25 percent of African American women, and 27 percent of Hispanic women are active enough to improve their fitness levels. Among women who do exercise, most choose aerobic activities, and relatively few do any strength training. Yet women may benefit more from strength training than men because they typically have more body fat and face greater risk of osteoporosis.[1]

The average woman has a smaller heart and blood volume than a man. Because women have a lower concentration of red blood cells, their bodies are less effective at transporting oxygen to their working muscles during exercise.

physical fitness The ability to respond to routine physical demands, with enough reserve energy to cope with a sudden challenge.

cardiorespiratory fitness The ability of the heart and blood vessels to circulate blood through the body efficiently.

muscular strength Physical power; the maximum weight one can lift, push, or press in one effort.

muscular endurance The ability to withstand the stress of continued physical exertion.

flexibility The range of motion allowed by one's joints; determined by the length of muscles, tendons, and ligaments attached to the joints.

body composition The relative amounts of fat and lean tissue (bone, muscle, organs, water) in the body.

functional fitness The ability to perform real-life activities, such as lifting a heavy suitcase.

Even though training produces the same relative increases for both genders, a woman's maximum oxygen intake remains about 25 to 30 percent lower than that of an equally well-conditioned man. In elite athletes, the gender difference is smaller. Because the angle of the upper leg bone (femur) to the pelvis is greater in a woman, she is less efficient at running. Intense exercise provokes a rise in the stress hormone cortisol in men, but not women.

In some endurance events, such as ultramarathon running and long-distance swimming, female anatomy and physiology may have some aerobic advantages. The longer a race—on land, water, or ice—the better women perform.

In absolute terms, men are 30 percent stronger, but gender differences in absolute strength do not apply to all muscle groups.

Women have about 40 to 60 percent of the upper-body strength of men but 70 to 75 percent of the lower-body strength.

Exercise capacity, an indicator of how much your body can do and how much oxygen it needs to do it, is the most accurate predictor of a person's potential lifespan. This holds true for both men and women, for healthy individuals and those with cardiovascular disease, and, as the largest study ever of exercise capacity and mortality recently showed, for African Americans and whites. African Americans, whose mortality rates from all causes are as much as 60 percent higher than those of whites, benefit just as much from increased fitness as other racial groups.[2] Yet in one recent sampling, only 22 percent of African Americans reported getting the recommended levels of exercise.[3]

The Inactivity Epidemic

One in four Americans reports no physical activity at all, according to the Centers for Disease Control and Prevention (CDC). About half exercise occasionally, but not at the levels recommended by the National Center for Chronic Disease Prevention and Health Promotion. Fewer than one in four adults meets the levels of physical activity recommended by federal health officials.

According to a national survey, about a third of adolescents and 14 percent of adults between ages 20 and 49 fall into the category of "low fitness" because they engage in little or no physical activity. They are significantly more likely to develop diabetes, hypertension, and metabolic syndrome (discussed in Chapter 14) than those with higher fitness levels. Fit children are less likely to be obese or to have high blood pressure as young adults.[4]

Many factors affect physical activity levels, including geographic location, gender, education, and income. According to the CDC, city dwellers are more active than country folks, westerners more active than those in other regions. Men, people

with higher education levels, and high-income earners work out more often.

Neighborhoods have a major influence on how much people exercise. Those who live in places with higher levels of poverty (regardless of how much they earn), lower education, and more families headed by women are less likely to work out. Among the neighborhood-related factors that influence exercise levels are the amount of trust within the community, perceived violence, and beliefs that neighbors help each other. These qualities had more of an impact on women's exercise levels than on men's.[5]

 Where you live as a student also has an impact on your weight, eating, and exercise patterns. In a study of Texas undergraduate women, those who lived on campus were significantly more physically active than those who lived off campus. As measured by pedometers, they walked an average of 90,000 steps per week, compared to 42,000 steps for off-campus students. The reasons may be the greater distance from classrooms to dormitories than to bus stops or parking lots and higher levels of participation in intramural sports.[6]

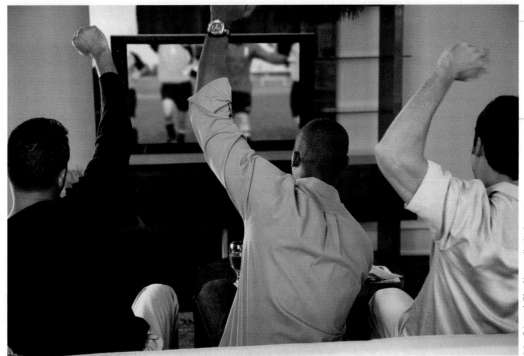

Watching sports often replaces participating in them when students enter college. Many exercise less with each succeeding year.

© Jon Feingersh/Blend Images/Jupiterimages

Regardless of where they live, Americans spend most of their leisure time watching television: on average, more than 30 hours a week. Yet the more time spent in front of the TV, the greater the risk of obesity and related chronic diseases. Compared with other sedentary activities, such as reading, writing, or driving, watching TV lowers metabolic rate, so people burn fewer calories.

The Toll of Sedentary Living

Physical inactivity, along with smoking, high body mass index, and low levels of income and education, may accelerate the aging process. A recent study found a significant difference in one biological indicator of human aging—the length of the telomeres (segments of DNA at the end of chromosomes) of white blood cells—between active and inactive twins. The most active individuals, regardless of age and sex, had telomeres the same length as sedentary individuals up to ten years younger. This means that sedentary individuals may be biologically ten years older.[7]

Sedentary living claims some 250,000 lives, accounting for 10 percent of all deaths in America every year, and contributes to four of the six leading causes of death: heart disease, cancer, stroke, and diabetes. Inactivity doubles the risk of cardiorespiratory diseases, diabetes, and obesity and increases the risk of colon cancer, high blood pressure, osteoporosis, depression, and anxiety. As a risk factor for heart disease, physical inactivity ranks as high as elevated cholesterol, high blood pressure, or cigarette smoking.

Working Out on Campus: Student Bodies in Motion

 By various estimates, only 15 to 30 percent of college students meet the recommended amount of physical activity for health benefits.[8] (See Reality Check, p. 127.)

College men are generally more active than women; full-time students and those without jobs exercise more than part-time or employed students. Undergraduates living on campus are more active than those living off campus; students living in fraternity or sorority housing engage in more exercise than those living in a house or an apartment. Single students report more days of vigorous workouts than married, divorced, or separated ones. Only 16 percent of students who are parents get the recommended levels of physical activity, compared with about half of those without children.[9] How do you compare?

Motivating Yourself to Get Moving

When was the last time you worked out? This means real exercise—a 30-minute run, not a three-minute sprint for the bus; a full circuit of the weight machines at the gym, not toting boxes to help a friend move. Was it yesterday, last week, last month, last summer? If you're already exercising most days of the week, great! If you'd like to exercise more but something always gets in the way, "Excise Exercise Excuses" in *Labs for IPC* can get—and keep—you moving. Here's a preview.

Get Real

In this stage you will ask yourself three crucial questions, starting with this one:
- **What was the best shape you've ever been in?**

Was it when you ran track in high school? When you worked as a lifeguard? When you were taking cardio kick-boxing classes? Right before you got married? When you were chasing after your two-year-old all day long? How did you feel about your body then?

Get Ready

At this point you will evaluate your readiness for change. Have you never even thought about becoming fit? You're in precontemplation. Is your exercise plan all thought and no action? You've reached contemplation. Have you become a bit more active but would like to do more? You will find specific advice based on your level of readiness. For example, if you're thinking about revving up the activity level in your life but haven't done so yet, you would:

- Think back to activities you found enjoyable in the past. Did you ever do karate? Play softball? Row? Check campus bulletin boards and blogs . . .
- Determine the types of activity you can realistically fit into your daily schedule. Can you find a gym with child care in the morning? What about signing up for an evening "butts-and-guts" fitness class?
- Find an image of the trimmer, fitter body you'd like to have— from a gym advertisement, for example—and post it where you can see it often.

Get Going

In this stage, you put powerful tools of personal change, such as visualization, to work to get you working out. Here's an example of how to use the language of change to make change happen:

- **Don't order yourself around.** If you have a voice inside that issues orders and barks criticisms like a drill sergeant, shut it off. Telling yourself, "I should work out," invites you to feel more over-whelmed and anxious. In your *IPC Journal*, write out a "have to" list of things you tell yourself about exercise. For example, "I have to run at least three miles." Next rewrite your list, but instead of using the words "I have to," use the words "I choose to." Replacing the words "I have to" with "I choose to" moves you from helplessness to a position of power.

Lock it In

Starting an exercise program is the easy part. Sticking with it is the hard part. That's why the skills of this stage, which include techniques to block sabotaging thoughts and to banish boredom, are so important. But what do you do if you fall off the exercise wagon?

- **Reboot.** Maybe you came down with the flu, or sprained your ankle, or visited a friend at another school. For whatever reasons, you stopped exercising. How do you get back on track? Here are some strategies to try:
  - Visualize yourself back in the gym, on the bike path, in yoga class, doing whatever activity you love most. Focus on the aspects of exercise you enjoy.
  - Line up exercise buddies for the first few weeks.
  - Rather than committing to your whole exercise routine, divide it into smaller parts. Tell yourself you have the option of stopping at the end of each one.

While two in three high school seniors engaged in regular vigorous physical activity (defined in one study as at least 20 minutes of an activity, such as basketball, soccer, running, swimming laps, or bicycling, that made them sweat), fewer than half of college students report the same level of exercise.

 Asian males were more active than whites, while Asian females were less active. Hispanic men and women were more active than their white peers.

As students progress from their first to fourth year of studies, they exercise less. The most drastic drop in physical activity occurs in the freshman year. In a recent study, physical fitness declined, and levels of total cholesterol, harmful LDL (low-density lipoprotein) cholesterol, and fasting glucose (blood sugar) levels increased over undergraduates' first 14-week school term. (See Chapter 14 for a complete discussion of these risk factors for heart disease.)

Students are somewhat more active on exercise-friendly campuses that rank high in characteristics such as bikeability, an appealing neighborhood, perceived safety from traffic, and proximity to local shops. However, even when campuses offer recreational facilities such as hiking trails and tennis courts, many students—particularly freshmen—are unaware of them.

✓ **REALITY**CHECK

• *What percentage of college students report exercising—either vigorously for at least 20 minutes or moderately for at least 30 minutes—on three or more of the last seven days?*
• *How many students report exercising to strengthen or tone their muscles at least three of the last seven days?*
• *How many students exercise to lose weight? How do men and women compare?*

Answers on next page.

Physical Activity and Health

Why Exercise?

If exercise could be packed into a pill, it would be the single most widely prescribed and beneficial medicine in the nation. Why? Because nothing can do more to help your body function at its best—a fact that not all students know. In a survey, eight in ten undergraduates realized that physical activity can prevent heart disease and prevent and treat obesity. However, fewer than half knew that it maintains bone density and can help prevent diabetes.

As Figure 5.2 illustrates, exercise provides head-to-toe benefits. With regular activity, your heart muscles become stronger and pump blood more efficiently. Your heart rate and resting pulse slow down. Your blood pressure may drop slightly from its normal level.

Exercise thickens the bones and can slow the loss of calcium that normally occurs with age. Physical activity increases flexibility in the joints and improves digestion and elimination. It speeds up metabolism and builds lean body mass, so the body burns more calories and body fat decreases. It heightens sensitivity to insulin (a great benefit for diabetics) and may lower the risk of developing diabetes. In addition, exercise enhances clot-dissolving substances in the blood, helping to prevent strokes, heart attacks, and pulmonary embolisms (clots in the lungs), and it helps lower the risk of certain cancers. Regular exercise can actually extend your lifespan and sharpen your memory and mind.

Even your eyes benefit from physical activity. Individuals who exercise three or more times a week may reduce their risk of age-related macular degeneration, which destroys the sharp central vision needed for tasks such as reading and driving.

Healthier Heart and Lungs Regular physical activity makes blood less likely to clot and cause a stroke or heart attack. Sedentary people are about twice as likely to die of a heart attack as people who are physically active. Although rigorous exercise somewhat increases the risk of sudden cardiac death for men, regular physical activity lowers the overall danger, especially in women. (See Chapter 14 for a discussion of heart disease.)

Vigorous exercise—such as cycling, running, swimming, and resistance training—may prevent or lessen chronic systemic low-grade inflammation, a recently recognized risk factor for several chronic conditions, including diabetes and heart disease. Studies have not shown similar benefits from more moderate activities such as walking.

Exercise also lowers levels of the indicators of increased risk of heart disease, such as high cholesterol and C-reactive protein, which are discussed in Chapter 14. Exercise itself, even without weight loss, may reduce the risk of developing the prediabetic condition called metabolic syndrome, which if untreated can lead to type 2 diabetes and increase the risk of heart disease.

In addition to its effects on the heart, exercise makes the lungs more efficient. The lungs take in more oxygen, and their vital capacity (the maximum amount of air volume the lungs can take in and expel)

PART 2: *Just the Facts*

• **40** *percent of college students exercised—either vigorously for at least 20 minutes or moderately for at least 30 minutes—on three or more of the last seven days.*

• **29** *percent of students exercised to strengthen or tone their muscles at least three of the last seven days.*

• **53** *percent of students—44 percent of men and 59 percent of women— exercise to lose weight.*

Source: American College Health Association. *American College Health Association National College Health Assessment: Reference Group Executive Summary Fall 2008. Baltimore: American College Health Association, 2008.*

pressure and the makeup of blood fats, including cholesterol and triglycerides. Exercise, along with a healthy weight, keeps blood fats at healthy levels over time. Prolonged, sustained endurance training prevents the stiffening of the heart muscle once thought to be an inevitable consequence of aging.

Protection Against Cancer Physical activity lowers the likelihood of getting some forms of cancer and, according to preliminary research, may lessen the risk of recurrence or a second cancer. According to the American Institute for Cancer Research, physical activity may lower the risk of colon cancer by 40

increases, providing more energy for you to use.

Even in young men, physical fitness is associated with improvements in blood

Figure 5.2 The Benefits of Exercise

Regular physical activity enhances your overall physical and mental health and helps prevent disease.

Health Benefits of Physical Activity—A Review of the Strength of the Scientific Evidence

Adults and Older Adults

Strong Evidence

Lower risk of:
  Early death
  Heart disease
  Stroke
  Type 2 diabetes
  High blood pressure
  Adverse blood lipid profile
  Metabolic syndrome
  Colon and breast cancers
Prevention of weight gain
Weight loss when combined with diet
Improved cardiorespiratory and muscular fitness
Prevention of falls
Reduced depression
Better cognitive function (older adults)

Moderate to Strong Evidence

Better functional health (older adults)
Reduced abdominal obesity

Moderate Evidence

Weight maintenance after weight loss
Lower risk of hip fracture
Increased bone density
Improved sleep quality
Lower risk of lung and endometrial cancers

Source:
http://www.health.gov/paguidelines/factSheetProf.aspx

Improves your mood, reduces psychological symptoms, and sharpens your thinking

Reduces your risk of heart disease

Increases your respiratory capacity

Improves your digestion and your fat metabolism

Lowers your body fat and reduces your weight

Strengthens your bones and increases joint flexibility

Improves your circulation

Reduces the risk of breast, ovarian, and colon cancer

Increases your muscle strength and tone

to 50 percent, the risk of breast, endometrial, and lung cancers by 30 to 40 percent, and the risk of prostate cancer by 10 to 30 percent.

The combination of excess weight and physical inactivity may account for a quarter to a third of all breast cancer cases. Regular, lifelong exercise may lower a woman's breast cancer risk by 20 percent, possibly by reducing weight and body mass and preventing metabolic syndrome and chronic inflammation (discussed in Chapter 14).[10] It is not clear whether exercise can prevent a recurrence in women who have had breast cancer, but it does improve their overall survival rates.[11] Women who exercised regularly in the year before a diagnosis of breast cancer have higher survival rates than sedentary women. Exercise also lowers the risk of recurrence in colon cancer, perhaps by lowering levels of substances such as insulin and insulin-like growth factor that drive the growth of cancer cells.

Less Risk of Disease Exercise may enhance immune function by reducing stress hormones like cortisol that can dampen resistance to disease. Women who walk briskly for 35 to 45 minutes five days a week experience half the number of sick days with cold symptoms as inactive women. While moderate exercise seems to bolster a person's immune system, heavy training may increase the risk of upper respiratory tract infections for endurance athletes.

An increase in physical activity can prevent type 2 diabetes even in those at high risk of developing the disease. In studies of high-risk individuals who exercised, took medication, or did nothing, those who became more active had the lowest incidence of diabetes

Brighter Mood and Less Stress Exercise makes people feel good from the inside out. Exercise boosts mood, elevates self-esteem, increases energy, reduces anxiety, improves concentration and alertness, and may help ward off dementia. During long workouts, some people experience what is called "runner's high," which may be the result of increased levels of mood-elevating brain chemicals called **endorphins.**

A highly effective stress reducer, exercise reduces muscle tension and cortisol secretion.[12] According to a recent study, psychological improvements occur even after a 20-minute bout of exercise, regardless of how intensely you exercise.[13] Physical activity also may boost memory and other cognitive abilities in certain individuals.

Better Mental Health and Functioning

Exercise is an effective—but underused—treatment for mild to moderate depression and may help in treating other mental disorders. Regular, moderate exercise, such as walking, running, or lifting weights, three times a week has proved helpful for depression and anxiety disorders, including panic attacks. Exercise is as effective as medication in improving mood and also helps prevent relapse.

Lifelong fitness may protect the brain as we age. According to numerous long-term studies, physically fit adults perform better on cognitive tests than their less fit peers. Improving cardiorespiratory fitness reduces the harmful effects of aging on brain structures as well as on memory and other functions. In a recent study, men and women with early-stage Alzheimer disease who were more physically fit had larger brains compared to their less-fit counterparts.

Better Bones By 2020, one in two Americans over age 50 may suffer from **osteoporosis**—a condition in which bones lose their mineral density and become susceptible to injury. Most are unaware that their bone health is in jeopardy. Four times as many men and almost three times as many women actually have osteoporosis than those that realize they do. (See Chapter 20 for more on osteoporosis and aging.)

You may think that weak, brittle bones are a problem only for the elderly. However, 2 percent of college-age women have osteoporosis; another 15 percent have already sustained significant losses in bone density and are at high risk of osteoporosis.

Exercise during adolescence and young adulthood may prevent bone weakening and fractures in old age. Women who did not participate in high school sports are seven times more likely to have low bone density than those who did. The college women at greatest risk often are extremely

endorphins Mood-elevating, pain-killing chemicals produced by the brain.

osteoporosis A condition in which the bones become increasingly soft and porous, making them susceptible to injury.

skinny and maintain their low weights and slim looks by dieting and by avoiding exercise so as not to increase their muscle mass. Some eliminate dairy products, an important source of calcium, from their diets. Depo-Provera, a method of birth control that consists of hormone injections every three months, also is associated with low bone density, especially with long-term use. (See Chapter 10 on contraception.)

What are the best exercises to boost bone density? According to a study of college women, high-impact aerobics, such as step exercising, "may offer the quickest route to building bone in young women." Resistance exercises such as squats, leg presses, and calf presses strengthened leg muscles but had no effect on bone density. The American College of Sports Medicine recommends moderate- to high-intensity weight-bearing activities to maintain bone mass in adults.

Lower Weight   For individuals on a diet, exercise provides extra benefits: A combination of dietary change and moderate- to high-level intensity exercise leads to greater weight loss than either alone. Dieters who work out lose more fat than lean muscle tissue, which improves their body composition. Exercise also may help to control weight by suppressing appetite. Aerobic activity, such as a vigorous 60-minute workout on a treadmill, affects the release of two key appetite hormones. Resistance training, such as 90 minutes of weightlifting, affects only one of these hormones.[14]

 College-age men who start exercising lose abdominal fat, which poses the greatest risk to health. (See Chapter 7 for information on exercise and weight control.)

Sexuality   By improving physical endurance, muscle tone, blood flow, and body composition, exercise improves sexual functioning. Simply burning 200 extra calories a day can significantly lower the risk of erectile dysfunction in sedentary men. Exercise also may increase sexual drive, activity, and sexual satisfaction in people of all ages.

Benefits for Students   Unlike middle-aged and older individuals, traditional-age college students cite

improved fitness as the number one advantage that exercise offers, followed by improved appearance and muscle tone. Undergraduates who recognize the benefits of exercise are more likely to be physically active than those who focus on barriers to working out.

Will exercise improve your grades? Not necessarily. A study at two Texas universities found that the fittest students didn't necessarily have higher GPAs. However, increasing their level of physical fitness did have a positive impact on the GPAs of the female students.

A More Active and Fulfilling Old Age
Exercise slows the changes that are associated with advancing age: loss of lean muscle tissue, increase in body fat, and decrease in work capacity. In addition to lowering the risk of heart disease and stroke, exercise helps older men and women retain the strength and mobility needed to live independently. In a study of overweight, post-menopausal women, exercise improved both physical and mental well-being—and the more the women exercised, the greater the improvements in their quality of life.[15] Even in old age, exercise boosts strength and stamina, lessens time in wheelchairs, and improves outlook and sense of control.

Longer Life   People who exercise regularly enjoy 3.7 years of additional life expectancy when compared with sedentary individuals. Formerly sedentary people, even the elderly, who begin to exercise live longer, on average, than those who remain inactive. However, for active people, light to moderate exercise won't do it—only vigorous exercise reduces the risk of dying of heart disease and of premature death from other causes.

Physical Activity Guidelines for Americans
In 2008 the U.S. Department of Health and Human Services issued *Physical Activity Guidelines for Americans,* based on the most significant research findings on the health benefits of physical activity. While recognizing that some activity is better than none, the *Guidelines* emphasize that more activity—consisting of both aerobic (endurance) and

muscle-strengthening (resistance) physical activity—is most beneficial. People of every age—children, adolescents, adults, seniors—and those in every racial and ethnic group, along with those with disabilities, can benefit from physical activity.[16]

Here are the government's key recommendations:

- All adults should avoid inactivity. Some physical activity is better than none, and adults who participate in any amount of physical activity gain some health benefits.

- For substantial health benefits, adults should do at least 150 minutes (2 hours and 30 minutes) a week of moderate-intensity, or 75 minutes (1 hour and 15 minutes) a week of vigorous-intensity aerobic physical activity, or an equivalent combination of moderate- and vigorous-intensity aerobic activity. Aerobic activity should be performed in episodes of at least 10 minutes, and, preferably, it should be spread throughout the week.

- For additional and more extensive health benefits, adults should increase their aerobic physical activity to 300 minutes (5 hours) a week of moderate-intensity, or 150 minutes a week of vigorous-intensity aerobic physical activity, or an equivalent combination of moderate- and vigorous-intensity activity. Additional health benefits are gained by engaging in physical activity beyond this amount.

- Adults should also do muscle-strengthening activities that are moderate or high intensity and involve all major muscle groups on two or more days a week, as these activities provide additional health benefits.

The American College of Sports Medicine (ACSM) and the American Heart Association (AHA) have released similar guidelines that call for:

Moderately intense cardiorespiratory exercise 30 minutes a day, 5 days a week

or

Vigorously intense cardiorespiratory exercise 20 minutes a day, 3 days a week *and*

8 to 10 strength-training exercises, with 8 to 12 repetitions of each exercise, twice a week.

According to the ACSM, moderate-intensity physical activity means working hard enough to raise your heart rate and break a sweat, yet still being able to carry on a conversation. The 30-minute recommendation is for the average healthy adult to maintain health and reduce the risk for chronic disease.

If you need to lose weight or want to keep off pounds you lost, you will need to exercise more. According to the ACSM's 2009 statement on "appropriate physical activity intervention strategies for weight loss and prevention of weight regain," long-term weight loss requires 250 or more minutes (2 hours and 30 minutes) of moderately intense physical activity per week.[17] Less exercise can prevent a gain greater than 3 percent of current weight but provides what the ACSM describes as "only modest" weight loss. In addition to aerobic workouts, the ACSM recommends resistance training to increase lean tissue and decrease fat.[18] (See Chapter 7 for more on exercise and weight.)

The Principles of Exercise

Your body is literally what you make of it. Superbly designed for multiple uses, it adjusts to meet physical demands. If you need to sprint for a bus, your heart will speed up and pump more blood. Beyond such immediate, short-term adaptations, physical training can produce long-term changes in heart rate, oxygen consumption, and muscle strength and endurance. Although there are limits on the maximum levels of physical fitness and performance that any individual can achieve, regular exercise can produce improvements in everyone's baseline wellness and fitness.

Figure 5.3 The Overload Principle

By increasing frequency, intensity, or duration, you will improve your level of fitness. Once your body adapts to (becomes comfortable with) the demands, you can again apply the overload principle to achieve a higher level of fitness.

State of fitness after adaptation to overload

Increased exercise overload

State of fitness after adaptation to overload

Exercise overload

Current fitness state

The following principles of exercise are fundamental to any physical activity plan.

Overload Principle

The **overload principle** requires a person exercising to provide a greater stress or demand on the body than it's usually accustomed to handling. For any muscle, including the heart, to get stronger, it must work against a greater-than-normal resistance or challenge. To continue to improve, you need further increases in the demands—but not too much too quickly. **Progressive overloading**—gradually increasing physical challenges—provides the benefits of exercise without the risk of injuries (Figure 5.3).

Overloading is specific to each body part and to each component of fitness. Leg exercises develop only the lower limbs; arm exercises, only the upper limbs. This is why you need a comprehensive fitness plan that includes a variety of exercises to develop different parts of the body. If you play a particular sport, you also need training to develop sports-specific skills, such as a strong, efficient stroke in swimming.

FITT

Although low-intensity activity can enhance basic health, you need to work harder—that is, at a greater intensity—to improve fitness. Whatever exercise you do, there is a level, or threshold, at which fitness begins to improve; a target zone, where you can achieve maximum benefits; and an upper limit, at which potential risks outweigh any further benefits. The acronym **FITT** sums up the four dimensions of progressive overload: *frequency* (how often you exercise), *intensity* (how hard), *time* (how long), and *type* (specific activity).

Frequency To attain and maintain physical fitness, you need to exercise regularly, but the recommended frequency varies with different types of exercise and with an individual's fitness goals. Health officials urge Americans to engage in moderate-intensity aerobic activity most days and in resistance and flexibility training two or three days a week.

Intensity Exercise intensity varies with the type of exercise and with personal goals. To improve cardiorespiratory fitness, you need at a minimum to increase your heart rate to a target zone (the level that produces benefits). To develop muscular strength and endurance, you need to increase the amount of weight you lift or the resistance you work against and/or the number of repetitions. For enhanced flexibility, you need to stretch muscles beyond their normal length.

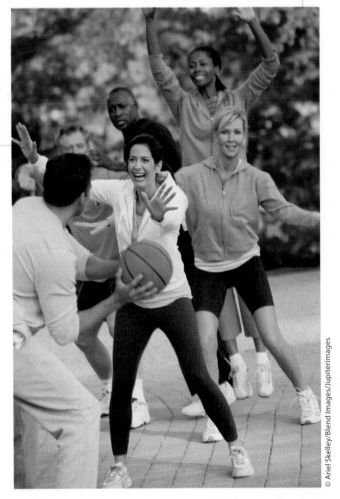

Group sports provide a fun alternative way to exercise, but an occasional game is no substitute for regular physical activity.

© Ariel Skelley/Blend Images/Jupiterimages

Time (Duration) The amount of time, or duration, of your workouts is also important, particularly for cardiorespiratory exercise. The American College of Sports Medicine recommends 30 to 45 minutes of aerobic exercise, preceded by 5 to 10 minutes of warm-up and followed by 5 to 10 minutes of stretching. However, experts have found similar health benefits from a single 30-minute session of moderate exercise as from several shorter sessions throughout the day. Duration and intensity are interlinked. If you're exercising at high intensity (biking or running at a brisk pace, for instance), you don't need to exercise as long as when you're working at lower intensity (walking or swimming at a moderate pace). For muscular strength and endurance and for flexibility, duration is defined by the number of sets or repetitions rather than total time.

Type (Specificity) The **specificity principle** refers to the body's adaptation to a particular type of activity or amount of stress placed upon it. Jogging, for instance, trains the heart and lungs to work more efficiently and strengthens certain leg muscles. However, it does not build upper body strength or enhance flexibility.

Reversibility Principle

The **reversibility principle** is the opposite of the overload principle. Just as the body adapts to greater physical demands, it also adjusts to lower levels. If you stop exercising, you can lose as much as 50 percent of your fitness improvements within two months. If you have to curtail your usual exercise routine because of a busy schedule, you can best maintain your fitness by keeping the intensity constant and reducing frequency or duration. The principle of reversibility is aptly summed up by the phrase, "Use it or lose it."

Improving Cardiorespiratory Fitness

Cardiorespiratory endurance refers to the ability of the heart, lungs, and circulatory system to deliver oxygen to muscles working rhythmically over an extended period of time. Unlike muscular endurance (discussed later in this chapter), which is specific to individual muscles, cardiorespiratory endurance involves the entire body. **Aerobic exercise,** which improves cardiorespiratory endurance, can take many forms, but all involve working strenuously without pushing to the point of breathlessness. A person who builds up good aerobic capacity can maintain long periods of physical activity without great fatigue.

In **anaerobic exercise,** the amount of oxygen taken in by the body cannot meet the demands of the activity. This quickly creates an oxygen deficit that must be made up later. Anaerobic activities are high in intensity but short in duration, usually lasting only about ten seconds to two minutes. An example is sprinting the quarter-mile, which leaves even the best-trained athletes gasping for air. In *nonaerobic exercise*, such as bowling, softball, or doubles tennis, there is frequent rest between activities. Because the body can take in all the oxygen it needs, the heart and lungs don't get much of a workout.

Are You Working Hard Enough?

A variety of methods can indicate if you're exercising hard enough to condition your heart and lungs, but not overdoing it.

Target Heart Rate To use your pulse, or heart rate, as a guide, feel your pulse in the carotid artery in your neck. Slightly tilt your head back and to one side. Use your middle finger or forefinger, or both, to feel for your pulse. (Do not use your thumb; it has a beat of its own.) To determine your heart rate, count the number of pulses you feel for 10 seconds and multiply that number by six, or count for 30 seconds and multiply that number by two. Learn to recognize the pulsing of your heart when you're sitting or lying down. This is your **resting heart rate.**

overload principle Providing a greater stress or demand on the body than it is normally accustomed to handling.

progressive overloading Gradually increasing physical challenges once the body adapts to the stress placed upon it to produce maximum benefits.

FITT A formula that describes the frequency, intensity, type, and length of time for physical activity.

specificity principle Each part of the body adapts to a particular type and amount of stress placed upon it.

reversibility principle The physical benefits of exercise are lost through disuse or inactivity.

aerobic exercise Physical activity in which sufficient or excess oxygen is continually supplied to the body.

anaerobic exercise Physical activity in which the body develops an oxygen deficit.

resting heart rate The number of heartbeats per minute during inactivity.

Figure 5.4 Target Heart Rates for Different Ages and Various Levels of Activity

Your maximum heart rate is 220 minus your age.

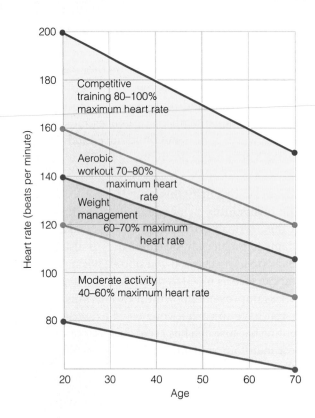

You can also use the following steps to determine your maximum heart rate and target heart rate (in beats per minute):

1. Maximum heart rate: Subtract your age from 220. So if you are 20, your maximum heart rate is $220 - 20 = 200$ beats per minute.

2. Lower-limit target heart rate: Multiply your maximum heart rate by 0.6. So if you are 20, your lower-limit target heart rate is $200 \times 0.6 = 120$ beats per minute.

3. Upper-limit target heart rate: Multiply your maximum heart rate by 0.65. If you are 20, your upper-limit target heart rate is $200 \times 0.65 = 130$.

Your target heart rate range is between your lower and upper limits.

According to the American College of Sports Medicine, for most people, exercising at the lower end of the target heart rate range for a long time is more beneficial than exercising at the higher end of the range for a short time. If your goal is losing weight, exercise at 60 to 70 percent of your maximum heart rate in order to burn fat calories. To improve aerobic endurance and strengthen your heart, work at 70 to 80 percent of your maximum heart rate. Competitive athletes may train at 80 to 100 percent of their maximum heart rate (Figure 5.4).

Start taking your pulse during, or immediately after, exercise, when it's much more pronounced than when you're at rest. Three minutes after heavy exercise, take your pulse again. The closer that reading is to your resting heart rate, the better your condition. If it takes a long time for your pulse to recover and return to its resting level, your body's ability to handle physical stress is poor. As you continue working out, however, your pulse will return to normal much more quickly.

You don't want to push yourself to your maximum heart rate. The ACSM recommends working at 55 to 65 percent of that maximum to get cardiorespiratory benefits from your training. This range is called your **target heart rate.** If you don't exercise intensely enough to raise your heart rate at least this high, your heart and lungs won't reap the most benefit from the workout. If you push too hard, and exercise at or near your absolute maximum heart rate, you run the risk of placing too great a burden on your heart. Figure 5.4 shows the target heart rate for various ages and activities. Find your age at the bottom of the figure and move up the grid to find your target heart rate for "aerobic workout."

Rating of Perceived Exertion (RPE)

Another option besides heart rate for monitoring your exercise intensity is the **Rating of Perceived Exertion (RPE),** a self-assessment scale that rates symptoms of breathlessness and fatigue. You can use the RPE scale to describe your sensation of effort when exercising and gauge how hard you are working. The ACSM revised the original RPE scale to a range of 0 to 10 (Figure 5.5). Most exercisers should aim for a perceived exertion of "somewhat strong" or "strong," the equivalent of 4 or 5 on the RPE scale.

RPE is considered fairly reliable, but about 10 percent of the population tends to over- or underestimate their exertion. Your health or physical education instructor can help you learn to match what your body is feeling to the RPE scale By paying attention to how you feel at different exercise intensities, you can learn to challenge yourself without risking your safety.

You can also experiment with alternative ways for determining exercise intensity. One of the easiest follows.

"Talk Test"   During "aerobic" exercise you should be able to carry on a somewhat stilted conversation if you are indeed "with oxygen"—which is what the word "aerobic" means.

If you are gasping for air and unable to talk, you are most likely working at or beyond the anaerobic "without oxygen" threshold—a very, very, very hard intensity level at or beyond the high end of the aerobic zone.

If you can sing the entire "Star Spangled Banner," you are probably not exerting much effort. If you can sing "Row Row Row Your Boat," but have to take a breath after every other word, you are probably working pretty hard—and just where you should be.

Designing an Aerobic Workout

Whatever activity you choose, your aerobic workout should consist of several stages: a warm-up, an aerobic activity, and a cool-down.

Warm-Up   Just as you don't get in your car and immediately gun your engine to 60 miles per hour, you shouldn't do the same with your body. You need to prepare your cardiorespiratory system for a workout, speed up the blood flow to your lungs, and increase the temperature and elasticity of your muscles and connective tissue to avoid injury.

After reviewing more than 350 scientific studies, the ACSM concluded that preparing for sports or exercise should involve a variety of activities and not be limited to stretching alone. They found little to no relationship between stretching and injuries or postexercise pain. A better option is a combination of warm-up, strength training, and balance exercises.

Aerobic Activity   The two key components of this part of your workout are intensity and duration. As described in the previous section, you can use your target heart rate range to make sure you are working at the proper intensity. The current recommendation is to

Figure 5.5   Revised Scale for Rating of Perceived Exertion (RPE)

You can learn to rate your exertion based on this scale.
Source: Original scale from Borg, G. "Psychophysical Bases of Perceived Exertion." *Medicine and Science in Sports and Exercise*, Vol. 14, No. 5, 2003, pp. 377–381.

keep moving for 30 to 60 minutes, either in one session or several briefer sessions, each lasting at least 10 minutes.

Cool-Down   After you've pushed your heart rate up to its target level and kept it there for a while, the worst thing you can do is slam on the brakes. If you come to a sudden stop, you put your heart at risk. When you stand or sit immediately after vigorous exercise, blood can pool in your legs. You need to keep moving at a slower pace to ensure an adequate supply of blood to your heart. Ideally, you should walk for 5 to 10 minutes at a comfortable pace before you end your workout session.

Your Long-Term Fitness Plan

One of the most common mistakes people make is to push too hard too fast. Often they end up injured or discouraged and quit entirely. If you are just starting an aerobic program, think of it as a series of phases: beginning, progression, and maintenance:

- **Beginning (4–6 weeks).** Start slow and low (in intensity). If you're walking, monitor your heart rate and aim for 55

target heart rate   Sixty to eighty-five percent of the maximum heart rate; the heart rate at which one derives maximum cardiovascular benefit from aerobic exercise.

Rating of Perceived Exertion (RPE)   A self-assessment scale that rates symptoms of breathlessness and fatigue.

percent of your maximum heart rate. Another good rule of thumb to make sure you're moving at the right pace: If you can sing as you walk, you're going too slow; if you can't talk, you're going too fast.

- **Progression (16–20 weeks).** Gradually increase the duration and/or intensity of your workouts. For instance, you might add 5 minutes every two weeks to your walking time. You also can gradually pick up your pace, using your target heart rate as your guide. Keep a log of your workouts so you can chart your progress until you reach your goal.

- **Maintenance (lifelong).** Once you've reached the stage of exercising for an hour every day, you may want to develop a repertoire of aerobic activities you enjoy. Combine or alternate activities to avoid monotony and keep up your enthusiasm (cross-training).

Aerobic Options

You have lots of choices for aerobic exercise, so experiment. Focus on one for a few weeks; alternate different activities on different days; try something new every month.

Stepping Out: Walk the Walk More men and women are taking to their feet. Some are casualties of high-intensity sports and can no longer withstand the wear and tear of rigorous workouts. Others want to shape up, slim down, or ward off heart disease and other health problems. The good news for all is that walking is good exercise.[19] Walking may reduce the risk factors for cardiorespiratory disease, such as insulin resistance, as much as vigorous activity does.[20]

Why Walk? One major study of women, the Nurses Health Study, found that women who walk briskly three hours a week are as well protected from heart disease as women who spend an hour and a half a week in more vigorous activities, such as aerobics or running. Women engaged in either form of exercise had a rate of heart attacks 30 to 40 percent lower than that of sedentary women.

Walking also protects men's hearts, whether they're healthy or have had heart problems.[21] Men who regularly engage in light exercise, including walking, have a significantly lower risk of death than their sedentary counterparts.

Walking has proved to be one of the safest and most effective ways of preventing bone and joint disorders in obese individuals. In a study that followed healthy men and women between the ages of 18 and 30 for fifteen years, the regular walkers gained less weight over time and were more likely to lose weight and keep pounds off.[22]

America on the Move How many steps do you walk every day? The typical adult averages about 5,310 steps; a child from 11,000 to 13,000. According to the American College of Sports Medicine, college students who used a pedometer to count their daily steps took an average of 7,700 steps per day. This falls short of the 10,000 steps recommended as part of the national "America on the Move" program.

How far is 10,000 steps? The average person's stride length is approximately 2.5 feet long. That means it takes just over 2,000 steps to walk 1 mile, and 10,000 steps is close to 5 miles. Wearing a pedometer is an easy way to track your steps each day. Start by wearing the pedometer every day for one week. Put it on when you get up in the morning and wear it until bedtime. Record your daily steps in a log or diary. By the end of the week, you can calculate your average daily steps. To increase your steps, add 500 daily steps every week until you reach 10,000.

Why 10,000 steps? According to researchers' estimates, you take about 5,000 steps just to accomplish your daily tasks. Adding about 2,000 steps brings you to a level that can improve your health and wellness. Another 3,000 steps can help you lose excess pounds and prevent weight gain. People who walk at least 10,000 steps a day are more likely to have healthy weights. In addition, 10,000 steps generally translates into 30 minutes of activity, the minimum recommended by the U.S. Surgeon General.

Over a year, individuals in a pedometer-based walking program can expect to lose about five pounds even without changing their diets, according to a review of nine studies. They lose more weight the longer they stick with the program.[23]

Treadmills are a good alternative to outdoor walks—and not just in bad weather. They keep you moving at a certain pace, they're easier on the knees, and they allow you to exercise in a climate-controlled, pollution-free environment—a definite plus for many city dwellers. Holding onto the handrails while walking on a treadmill reduces both heart rate and oxygen consumption, so you burn fewer calories. Experts advise slowing the pace if necessary so you can let go of the handrails while working out.

Jogging and Running The difference between jogging and running is speed. You should be able to carry on a conversation with someone on a long jog or run; if you're too breathless to talk, you're pushing too hard.

If your goal is to enhance aerobic fitness, long, slow, distance running is best. If you want to improve your speed, try *interval training*—repeated hard runs over a certain distance, with intervals of relaxed jogging in between. Depending on what suits you and what your training goals are, you can vary the distance, duration, and number of fast runs, as well as the time and activity between them.

If you have been sedentary, it's best to launch a walking program before attempting to jog or run. Start by walking for 15 to 20 minutes three times a week at a comfortable pace. Continue at this same level until you no longer feel sore or unduly fatigued the day after exercising. Then increase your walking time to 20 to 25 minutes, speeding up your pace as well.

When you can handle a brisk 25-minute walk, alternate fast walking with slow jogging. Begin each session walking, and gradually increase the amount of time you spend jogging. If you feel breathless while jogging, slow down and walk. Continue to alternate in this manner until you can jog for ten minutes without stopping. If you gradually increase your jogging time by one or two minutes with each workout, you'll slowly build up to 20 or 25 minutes per session. For optimal fitness, you should jog at least three times a week.

Other Aerobic Activities Because variety is the spice of an active life, many people prefer different forms of aerobic exercise.

All can provide many health benefits. Among the popular options:

- **Swimming.** For aerobic conditioning, you have to swim laps using the freestyle, butterfly, breaststroke, or backstroke. (The sidestroke is too easy.) You must also be a good enough swimmer to keep churning through the water for at least 20 minutes. Your heart will beat more slowly in water than on land, so your heart rate while swimming is not an accurate guide to exercise intensity. Try to keep up a steady pace that's fast enough to make you feel pleasantly tired, but not completely exhausted, by the time you get out of the pool.

- **Cycling.** Bicycling, indoors and out, can be an excellent cardiovascular conditioner, as well as an effective way to control weight—provided you aren't just along for the ride. If you coast down too many hills, you'll have to ride longer up hills or on level ground to get a good workout. An 18-speed bike can make pedaling too easy unless you choose gears carefully. To gain aerobic benefits, mountain bikers have to work hard enough to raise their heart rates to their target zone and keep up that intensity for at least 20 minutes.

- **Spinning™.** Spinning is a cardiovascular workout for the whole body that utilizes a special stationary bicycle. Led by an instructor, a group of bikers listens to music, and modifies their individual bike's resistance and their own pace according to the rhythm. An average spinning class lasts 45 minutes.

- **Cardio kick-boxing.** Also referred to as kick-boxing or boxing aerobics, this hybrid of boxing, martial arts, and aerobics offers an intense total-body workout. An hour of kick-boxing burns an average of 500 to 800 calories, compared to 300 to 400 calories in a typical step aerobics class.

- **Rowing.** Whether on water or a rowing machine, rowing provides excellent aerobic exercise as well as working the upper and lower body and toning the shoulders, back, arms, and legs. Correct rowing techniques are important to avoid back injury.

YOUR STRATEGIES FOR CHANGE
The Right Way to Walk and Run

Here are some guidelines for putting your best foot forward, whether you are walking or running:

- Take time to warm up.
- Maintain good posture. Keep your back straight, your head up, and your eyes looking straight ahead. Hold your arms slightly away from your body—your elbows should be bent slightly so that your forearms are almost parallel to the ground.
- Use the heel-to-toe method. The heel of your leading foot should touch the ground before the ball or toes of that foot do. Push off the ball of your foot, and bend your knee as you raise your heel. You should be able to feel the action in your calf muscles.
- Pump your arms back and forth. This burns more calories and gives you an upper-body workout as well.
- Do not walk or run on the balls of your feet. This produces soreness in the calves because the muscles must contract for a longer time. Avoid running on hard surfaces and making sudden stops and turns.
- End your walk or run with a cool-down period. Let your pace become more leisurely for the last five minutes.

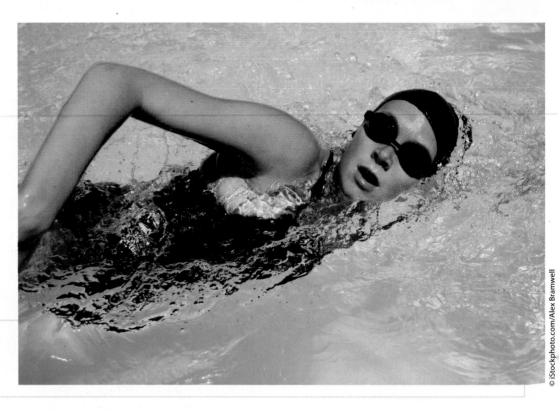

Swimming laps for 20 minutes or longer at a steady pace is a good option for aerobic exercise.

- **Skipping rope.** Essentially a form of stationary jogging with some extra arm action thrown in, skipping rope is excellent as both a heart conditioner and a way of losing weight. Always warm up before starting and cool down afterward.

- **Aerobic dancing.** This activity combines music with kicking, bending, and jumping. A typical class (you can also dance at home to a video or TV program) consists of stretching exercises and sit-ups, followed by aerobic dances and cool-down exercises. "Soft," or low-impact, aerobic dancing doesn't put as much strain on the joints as "hard," or high-impact, routines.

- **Step training, or bench aerobics.** "Stepping" combines step, or bench, climbing with music and choreographed movements. Basic equipment consists of a bench 4 to 12 inches high. The fitter you are, the higher the bench—but the higher the bench, the greater the risk of knee injury.

- **Stair climbing.** You could run up the stairs in an office building or dormitory, but most people use stair-climbing machines available in home models and at gyms and health clubs.

- **Inline skating.** Inline skating can increase aerobic endurance and muscular strength and is less stressful on joints and bones than running or high-impact aerobics. Skaters can adjust the intensity of their workout by varying the terrain.

- **Tennis.** As with other sports, tennis can be an aerobic activity—depending on the number of players and their skill level. In general, a singles match requires more continuous exertion than playing doubles.

Building Muscular Fitness

Although aerobic workouts condition your insides (heart, blood vessels, and lungs), they don't exercise many of the muscles that shape your outsides and provide power when you need it. Strength workouts are important because they enable muscles to work more efficiently and reliably. Conditioned muscles function more smoothly and contract somewhat more vigorously and with less effort. With exercise, muscle tissue becomes firmer and can withstand much more strain—the result of toughening the sheath protecting the muscle and developing more connective tissue within it (Figure 5.6).

The two dimensions of muscular fitness are strength and endurance. Muscular strength is the maximal force that a muscle or group of muscles can generate for one movement. Muscular endurance is the capacity to sustain repeated muscle actions. Both are important. You need strength to hoist a shovelful of snow—and endurance so you can keep shoveling the entire driveway.

The latest research on fat-burning shows that the best way to reduce your body fat is to add muscle-strengthening exercise to your workouts. Muscle tissue is your very best calorie-burning tissue, and the more you have, the more calories you burn, even when you are resting. You don't have to become a serious body-builder. Using hand-held weights (also called *free weights*) two or three times a week is enough. Just be sure you learn how to use them properly, because you can tear or strain muscles if you don't practice the proper weight-lifting techniques. As more people have begun to lift weights, injuries have soared.

A balanced workout regimen of muscle building and aerobic exercise does more for you than just burn fat. It gives you more endurance by promoting better distribution of oxygen to your tissues and increasing the blood flow to your heart.

Strength workouts increase circulation

The heart's right half pumps oxygen-poor blood to capillary beds in lungs. There, O_2 diffuses into blood and CO_2 diffuses out. The oxygenated blood flows into the heart's left half where it is then pumped to capillary beds throughout the body.

Heart

Capillary bed before strength workouts

Capillary bed after 8–12 weeks of strength workouts (extra capillaries develop, circulation increases)

Strength workouts build muscles

Outer sheath of connective tissue around muscle (toughened by strength workouts)

Bundles of muscle cells surrounded by connective tissue (more connective tissue develops from strength workouts)

Figure 5.6 Benefits of Strength Training on the Body
Strength training increases blood circulation and oxygen supply to body tissues and develops muscles.

Strength training has particular benefits for women: As numerous studies have documented, it makes their muscles stronger, their bodies leaner, and their bones more resistant to falls. In young women, it boosts self-esteem, body image, and emotional well-being. In middle-aged and older women, it enhances self-concept, boosts psychological health, and prevents weight gain.

Muscles at Work

Your muscles never stay the same. If you don't use them, they atrophy, weaken, or break down. If you use them rigorously and regularly, they grow stronger. The only way to develop muscles is by demanding more of them than you usually do. This is called **overloading.** (Remember the overload principle?) As you train, you have to gradually increase the number of repetitions or the amount of resistance and work the muscle to temporary fatigue. That's why it's important not to quit when your muscles start to tire. Progressive overload—steadily increasing the stress placed on the body—builds stronger muscles.

You need to exercise differently for strength than for endurance. *To develop strength,* do a few repetitions with heavy loads. As you increase the weight your muscles must move, you increase your strength. *To increase endurance,* do many more repetitions with lighter loads. If your muscles are weak and you need to gain strength in your upper body, you may have to work for weeks to do a half-dozen regular push-ups. Then you can start building endurance by doing as many push-ups as you can before collapsing in exhaustion.

Muscles can do only two things: contract or relax. As they do so, skeletal muscles either pull on bones or stop pulling on bones. All exercise involves muscles pulling on bones across a joint. The movement that takes place depends on the structure of the joint and the position of the muscle attachments involved.

In an **isometric** contraction, the muscle applies force while maintaining an equal length. The muscle contracts and tries to shorten but cannot overcome the resistance. An example is pushing against an immovable object, like a wall, or tightening an abdominal muscle while sitting. The muscle contracts, but there is no movement. Push or pull against the immovable object, with each muscle contraction held for five to eight seconds; repeat five to ten times daily.

An **isotonic** contraction involves movement, but the muscle tension remains the same. In an isotonic exercise, the muscle moves a moderate load several times, as in weight lifting or calisthenics. The best isotonic exercise for producing muscular strength involves high resistance and a low number of repetitions. On the other hand, you can develop the greatest flexibility, coordination, and endurance with isotonic exercises that incorporate lower resistance and frequent repetitions.

True **isokinetic** contraction is a constant speed contraction. Isokinetic exercises require special machines that provide resistance to overload muscles throughout the entire range of motion.

Designing a Muscle Workout

A workout with weights should exercise your body's primary muscle groups: the *deltoids* (shoulders), *pectorals* (chest), *triceps and biceps* (back and front of upper arms), *quadriceps* and *hamstrings* (front and back of thighs), *gluteus maximus* (buttocks), *trapezius* and *rhomboids* (back), and *abdomen* (Figure 5.7). Various machines and free-weight routines focus on each muscle group, but the principle is always the same: Muscles contract as you raise and lower a weight, and you repeat the lift-and-lower routine until the muscle group is tired.

A weight-training program is made up of **reps** (the single performance, or **repetition,** of an exercise, such as lifting 50 pounds one time) and **sets** (a *set* number of repetitions of the same movement, such as a set of 20 push-ups). You should allow your breath to return to normal before moving on to each new set. Pushing yourself to the limit builds strength. Although the ideal number of sets in a resistance-training program remains controversial, recent evidence suggests that multiple sets lead to additional benefits in short- and long-term training in young and middle-aged adults.

Maintaining proper breathing during weight training is crucial. To breathe correctly, inhale when muscles are relaxed and

overloading Method of physical training involving increasing the number of repetitions or the amount of resistance gradually to work the muscle to temporary fatigue.

isometric Of the same length; exercise in which muscles increase their tension without shortening in length, such as when pushing an immovable object.

isotonic Having the same tension or tone; exercise requiring the repetition of an action that creates tension, such as weight lifting or calisthenics.

isokinetic Having the same force; exercise with specialized equipment that provides resistance equal to the force applied by the user throughout the entire range of motion.

rep (or repetition) In weight training, a single performance of a movement or exercise.

set In weight training, the number of repetitions of the same movement or exercise.

Trapezius

Deltoid

Pectoralis major

Serratus anterior

Biceps brachii

External oblique

Pectoralis minor

Rectus abdominus

Internal oblique

Sartorius

Quadriceps femoris

Trapezius

Rhomboid minor

Rhomboid major

Erector spinae

Serratus posterior

Triceps

Latissimus dorsi

Gluteus maximus

Hamstrings

Gastrocnemius

Muscle Group	Exercise
Quadriceps, gluteals	Leg press
Hamstrings	Leg curl
Pectorals	Chest press
Latissimus dorsi	Lat pull down
Deltoids	Lateral raise
Triceps	Triceps press
Biceps	Biceps curl
Abdominals	Curl-up
Erector spinae	Back extension

Figure 5.7 Primary Muscle Groups
Different exercises can strengthen and stretch different muscle groups.

exhale when you push or lift. Don't ever hold your breath, because oxygen flow helps prevent muscle fatigue and injury.

No one type of equipment—free weight or machine—has a clear advantage in terms of building fat-free body mass, enhancing strength and endurance, or improving a sport-specific skill. Each type offers benefits but also has drawbacks.

Free weights offer great versatility for strength training. With dumbbells, for example, you can perform a variety of exercises to work specific muscle groups, such as the chest and shoulders. Machines,

in contrast, are much more limited; most allow only one exercise.

Strength-training machines have several advantages. They ensure correct movement for a lift, which helps protect against injury and prevent cheating when fatigue sets in. They isolate specific muscles, which is good for rehabilitating an injury or strengthening a specific body part. Because they offer high-tech options like varying resistance during the lifting motion, they can tax muscles in ways that a traditional barbell cannot.

The use of strength-training machines as well as free weights can build muscular strength and endurance.

© iStockphoto.com/Brian Pamphilon

from the workout and you avoid overtraining. Workouts on consecutive days do more harm than good because the body can't recover that quickly. Strength training twice a week at greater intensity and for a longer duration can be as effective as working out three times a week. However, your muscles will begin to atrophy if you let more than three or four days pass without exercising them.

Core Strength Conditioning

"Core strength," a popular trend in exercise and fitness, refers to the ability of the muscles to support your spine and keep your body stable and balanced. When you have good core stability, the muscles in your pelvis, lower back, hips, and abdomen work in harmony. This improves your posture, breathing, appearance, and performance in sports, while reducing your risk of muscle strain. When your core is weak, you become more susceptible to lower back pain and injury.

The major muscles of your core include the transverse abdominis, the deepest of the abdominal muscles; the external and internal obliques on the side and front of the abdomen around your waist; and the rectus abdominis, a long muscle that extends along the front of the abdomen. Strengthening all of your core muscles provides stability, improves balance, and protects you from injury.

Recovery

The American College of Sports Medicine recommends a minimum of eight to ten exercises involving the major muscle groups two to three days a week. Remember that your muscles need sufficient time to recover from a weight-training session. Never work a sore muscle, because soreness may indicate that too-heavy weights have caused tiny tears in the fibers. Allow no less than 48 hours, but no more than 96 hours, between training sessions, so your body can recover

Drugs Used to Boost Athletic Performance

In recent years, revelations that many athletes have used performance-enhancing drugs have shaken the sports profession. Some sports stars have served time in prison. Others have had to end their careers and see their reputations forever tarnished. Fiercely competitive and driven by the pursuit of fame and fortune, some professional athletes continue to use steroids and other

agents despite the threat of cancer, liver disease, blood diseases, severe arthritis, or sexual dysfunction. The number of college athletes using or at least checking into performance-enhancing drugs is believed to be growing. Some feel the stakes are high enough to outweigh the risks: being even a little faster and stronger and finding that extra edge can be worth millions. (See Consumer Alert, p. 143.)

Public attitudes about sports doping vary. Some blame team owners, who want to sell tickets and bring in revenues at any cost. Others criticize the athletes for letting down fans and acting as bad role models for children. In a study of college students' attitudes, more women than men felt that sports doping was unacceptable, but not at statistically significant levels.[24] (See Point/Counterpoint, p. 144.)

Despite the hype, in a review of more than 7,500 scientific investigations all but two found that performance-enhancing drugs do not provide strength benefits. The drugs have been shown to increase lean body mass, heart rate, and metabolic rate but these do not translate into improved performance.[25]

Here's what we know—and don't know—about the most widely used performance boosters.

- **Anabolic steroids** are synthetic derivatives of the male hormone testosterone that promote the growth of skeletal muscle and increase lean body mass. Taking them to improve athletic performance is illegal.

  Anabolic steroids have been reported to increase lean muscle mass, strength, and ability to train longer and harder, but they pose serious health hazards, including liver tumors, jaundice (yellowish pigmentation of skin, tissues, and body fluids), fluid retention, high blood

YOUR STRATEGIES FOR PREVENTION
How to Work with Free Weights

If you plan to work with free weights, here are some guidelines for using them safely and effectively:

- Don't train alone—for safety's sake. Work with a partner so you can serve as spotters for each other and help motivate each other as well.
- Always warm up before weight training; also be sure to stretch after training.
- Breathe! Holding your breath during exertion can produce a dangerous rise in blood pressure.
- Begin with relatively light weights (50 percent of the maximum you can lift), and increase the load slowly until you find the weight that will cause muscle failure at anywhere from eight to twelve repetitions. (Muscle failure is the point during a workout at which you can no longer perform or complete a repetition through the entire range of motion.)
- In the beginning, don't work at maximum intensity. Increase your level of exertion gradually over two to six weeks to allow your body to adapt to new stress without soreness.
- Always train your entire body, starting with the larger muscle groups. Don't focus only on specific areas, although you may want to concentrate on your weakest muscles.
- Always use proper form. Unnecessary twisting, lurching, lunging, or arching can cause serious injury. Remember, quality matters more than quantity. One properly performed set of lifts can produce a greater increase in strength and muscle mass than many sets of improperly performed lifts.
- Work through the full range of motion. Be careful not to hyperextend or overextend.

pressure, decreased immune function, and severe acne. Men may experience shrinking of the testicles, reduced sperm count, infertility, baldness, and development of breasts. Women may experience growth of facial hair, acne, changes in or cessation of the menstrual cycle, enlargement of the clitoris, and deepened voice. In women, these changes are irreversible. In men, side effects may be

CONSUMER**ALERT**

Watch Out for "Pump Fiction"

Shape up in seven days! Burn calories without breaking a sweat! A brand-new body in minutes a day!

Too good to be true? Absolutely. Advertisers promise no-sweat, no-effort ways to fitness with pills, potions, flab-melting belts, and thigh-slimming paddles. These claims amount to nothing more than what the American Council on Exercise calls "pump fiction." The benefits of fitness are real and well documented, but the only way to reap them is through regular exercise.

Facts to Know

- **Be wary** of any program or product that promises "easy" or "effortless" results. Athletes in peak condition might use them without breaking a sweat. Chances are that you, like most people, won't.
- **Watch out for "spot" reducers.** You can't lose a "spare tire" or firm flabby thighs by targeting only that area of your body. You need to lose weight and tone your entire body.

- **Don't believe testimonials** or celebrity endorsements. Slim, trim, smiling celebrities are paid well for their enthusiasm.

Steps to Take

- **Read the fine print.** Often it states that the results are based not just on the device but on dieting and exercise as well.
- **Be skeptical** of dramatic "before and after" photos. With today's technology, you never know if photos were doctored or if the results lasted.
- **Check the details** on warranties, guarantees, and return policies. The ads may promise a "30-day money-back guarantee" but fail to mention hefty shipping costs.

POINT COUNTERPOINT *Sports Doping on Campus*

POINT

College athletes are among the groups most likely to use performance-enhancing drugs. To stop sports doping on campus, some suggest more rigorous drug testing and immediate suspension from a team if athletes test positive. However, school officials may not want to jeopardize the success of a team, since winning can affect a college's ability to attract talented athletes and to solicit contributions from alumni.

COUNTERPOINT

The penalties for use of performance-enhancing drugs should be steeper, including dismissal of coaches who turn a blind eye on athletes' drug use. Rather than trying to win at any cost, schools should set and enforce a zero-tolerance standard for drug use in sports.

YOUR VIEW

Should college athletic departments focus on low-profile approaches to identifying and punishing students who test positive for performance-enhancing drug use? Do you think they should hold coaches and trainers who tolerate or endorse this practice responsible?

reversible once abuse stops. In adolescents, steroids may bring about a premature halt in skeletal maturation.

Anabolic steroid abuse may lead to aggression and other psychiatric side effects. Many users report feeling good about themselves while on anabolic steroids, but researchers report that anabolic steroid abuse can cause wild mood swings including maniclike symptoms leading to "'roid rage," or violent, even homicidal, episodes. Researchers have reported that users may suffer from paranoid jealousy, extreme irritability, delusions, and impaired judgment stemming from feelings of invincibility. Stopping the drugs abruptly can lead to depression.

- **Androstenedione ("andro").** This testosterone precursor is normally produced by the adrenal glands and gonads. Manufacturers claim that androstenedione improves testosterone concentration, increases muscular strength and mass, helps reduce body fat, enhances mood, and improves sexual performance. Studies have shown that supplemental androstenedione doesn't increase testosterone and muscles don't get stronger with andro use. Andro has been classified as a controlled substance, making its use illegal.

- **Creatine.** This amino acid is made by the body and stored predominantly in skeletal muscle. Creatine serves as a reservoir to replenish adenosine triphosphate (ATP), a substance involved in energy production. Some studies show creatine may increase strength and endurance. Other effects on the body remain unknown.

The Food and Drug Administration has warned consumers to consult a physician before taking creatine supplements. Creatine may cause dehydration and heat-related illnesses, reduced blood volume, and electrolyte imbalances. Some athletes drink quantities of water hoping to avoid such effects. However, many coaches forbid or discourage creatine use because its long-term effects remain unknown.

- **GBL (gamma butyrolactone).** This unapproved drug is being studied as a treatment for narcolepsy, a disabling sleep disorder. Nevertheless, it is marketed on the Internet and in some professional gyms as a muscle-builder and performance-enhancer.

The Food and Drug Administration has warned consumers to avoid any products containing GBL, noting that they have been associated with at least one death and several incidents in which users became comatose or unconscious.

- **Ergogenic aids.** These are substances used to enhance energy and provide athletes with a competitive advantage. These include everyday substances. *Caffeine,* for instance, may boost alertness in some people but cause jitteriness in others. *Baking soda* (sodium bicarbonate) is believed to delay fatigue by neutralizing lactic acid in the muscles, but its potential drawbacks include explosive diarrhea, abdominal cramps, bloating, and nausea.

  Glycerol is a natural element derived from fats. Some sports-drink manufacturers are testing formulations that include glycerol, which they claim can lower heart rate and stave off exhaustion in marathon events. Glycerol-induced hyperhydration (holding too much water in the blood) can have a negative impact on performance, however, and may be hazardous to health.

- **Human growth hormone.** According to an analysis of all existing research, human growth hormone increases lean body mass but does not affect exercise capacity or aerobic endurance.[26]

Previous studies found no beneficial effect on aging in healthy older people. Congress is considering legislation to make human growth hormone a controlled substance.

Becoming More Flexible

Flexibility is the characteristic of body tissues that determines the **range of motion** achievable without injury at a joint or group of joints. There are two types of flexibility: static and dynamic. **Static flexibility**—the type most people think of as flexibility—refers to the ability to assume and maintain an extended position at one end point in a joint's range of motion. **Dynamic flexibility,** by comparison, involves movement. It is the ability to move a joint quickly and fluidly through its entire range of motion with little resistance. The static flexibility in the hip joint determines whether you can do a split; dynamic flexibility is what would enable you to perform a split leap.

Static flexibility depends on many factors, including the structure of a joint and the tightness of the muscles, tendons, and ligaments attached to it. Dynamic flexibility is influenced by static flexibility but also depends on additional factors, such as strength, coordination, and resistance to movement.

Genetics, age, gender, and body composition all influence how flexible you are. Girls and women tend to be more flexible than boys and men to a certain extent because of hormonal and anatomical differences. The way females and males use their muscles and the activities they engage in can also have an effect. Over time, the natural elasticity of muscles, tendons, and joints decreases in both genders, resulting in stiffness.

The Benefits of Flexibility

Just as cardiorespiratory fitness benefits the heart and lungs and muscular fitness builds endurance and strength, a stretching program produces unique benefits, including enhancement of the ability of the respiratory, circulatory, and neuromuscular systems to cope with the stress and demands of our high-pressure world (Figure 5.8). Among the other benefits of flexibility are:

- **Prevention of injuries.** Flexibility training stretches muscles and increases the elasticity of joints. Strong, flexible muscles resist stress better than weak or inflexible ones. Adding flexibility to a training program for sports such as soccer, football, or tennis can reduce the rate of injuries by as much as 75 percent. In one study of competitive runners, weekly stretching sessions significantly reduced the incidence of low-back pain.

- **Relief of muscle strain.** Muscles tighten as a result of stress or prolonged sitting. If you study or work in one position for several hours, you'll often feel stiffness in your back or neck. Stretching helps relieve this tension and enables you to work more effectively.

- **Relaxation.** Flexibility exercises are great stress-busters that reduce mental strain, slow the rate of breathing, and reduce blood pressure.

- **Relief of soreness after exercise.** Many people develop delayed-onset muscle soreness (DOMS) one or two days after they work out. This may be the result of damage to the muscle fibers and supporting connective tissue.

- **Improved posture.** Bad posture can create tight, stressed muscles. If you slump in your chair, for instance, the muscles in the front of your chest may tighten, causing those in the upper spine to overstretch and become loose.

Stretching

When you stretch a muscle, you are primarily stretching the connective tissue. The

range of motion The fullest extent of possible movement in a particular joint.

static flexibility The ability to assume and maintain an extended position at one end point in a joint's range of motion.

dynamic flexibility The ability to move a joint quickly and fluidly through its entire range of motion with little resistance.

(a) Foot pull for the groin and thigh muscles

(b) Lateral head tilt

(c) Wall stretch for Achilles tendon

(d) Triceps stretch for the upper arm and shoulder

(e) Knee chest pull for lower back muscles

Figure 5.8 Some Simple Stretching Exercises

(a) Sit on the ground and bend your legs so that the soles of your feet touch. Pull your feet closer as you press on your knees with your elbows. Hold for 10 seconds; repeat. **(b)** Gently tilt your head to each side. Repeat several times. **(c)** Stand 3 feet from a wall or post with your feet slightly apart. Keeping your heels on the ground lean into the wall. Hold for 10 seconds; repeat. **(d)** Place your right hand behind your neck and grasp above the elbow with your left hand. Gently pull the elbow back. Repeat with the left elbow. **(e)** Lying on your back, clasp one knee and pull it toward your chest. Hold for 15–30 seconds; repeat with the other knee.

stretch must be intense enough to increase the length of the connective tissue without tearing it.

Static stretching involves a gradual stretch held for a short time (10 to 30 seconds). A shorter stretch provides little benefit; a longer stretch does not provide additional benefits. Since a slow stretch provokes less of a reaction from the stretch receptors, the muscles can safely stretch farther than usual. Fitness experts most often recommend static stretching because it is both safe and effective. An example of such a stretch is letting your hands slowly slide down the front of your legs (keeping your knees in a soft, unlocked position) until you reach your toes and holding this final position for several seconds before slowly straightening up. You should feel a pull, but not pain, during this stretch.

In **passive stretching,** your own body, a partner, gravity, or a weight serves as an external force or resistance to help your joints move through their range of motion. You can achieve a more intense stretch and a greater range of motion with passive stretching. There is a greater risk of injury, however, because the muscles themselves are not controlling the stretch.

Active stretching involves stretching a muscle by contracting the opposing muscle (the muscle on the opposite side of the limb). This method allows the muscle to be stretched farther with a low risk of injury.

Ballistic stretching is characterized by rapid bouncing movements, such as a series of up-and-down bobs as you try again and again to touch your toes with your hands. These bounces can stretch the muscle fibers too far, causing the muscle to contract rather than stretch. They also can tear ligaments and weaken or rupture tendons, the strong fibrous cords that connect muscles to bones. The heightened activity to stretch receptors caused by the rapid stretches can continue for some time, possibly causing injuries during any physical activities that follow. Because of its potential dangers, fitness experts generally recommend against ballistic stretching.

Stretching and Warming Up Warming up means getting the heart beating, breaking a sweat, and readying the body for more vigorous activity. Stretching is a specific activity intended to elongate the muscles and keep joints limber, not simply a prelude to a game of tennis or a three-mile run. According to a review of recent studies, the value of stretching varies with different activities. While it does not prevent injuries from jogging, cycling, or swimming, stretching may be beneficial in sports, like soccer and football, that involve bouncing and jumping.

For aerobic activities, one of the best times to stretch is after an aerobic workout. Your muscles will be warm, more flexible, and less prone to injury. In addition, stretching after aerobic activity can help a fatigued muscle return to its normal resting length and possibly helps reduce delayed-onset muscle soreness.

Stretching and Athletic Performance

Conventional wisdom holds that stretching improves athletic performance, but a review of the research finds that this isn't necessarily so. In some cases, active stretching can impede rather than improve performance in terms of muscle force and jumping height. Passive stretching prior to a sprint—a common practice—also has proved to reduce runners' speed. On the other hand, regular stretching can improve athletic performance in a variety of sports.

Mind–Body Approaches

Yoga, Pilates, and t'ai chi—increasingly popular on campuses and throughout the country, can help reduce stress, enhance health and wellness, and improve physical fitness, including balance.[27]

Yoga   One of the most ancient of mind-body practices, *yoga* comes from the Sanskrit word meaning "union." Traditionally associated with religion, yoga consists of various breathing and stretching exercises that unite all aspects of a person.

Once considered an exotic pursuit, yoga has gained acceptance as part of a comprehensive stress management and fitness program. Scientific studies have demonstrated its benefits, which include:

- **Improved flexibility**, which may offer protection from back pain and injuries.
- **Protection of joints** because yoga postures take joints through their full range of motion, providing a fresh supply of nutrients to joint cartilage.
- **Stronger, denser bones** from yoga's weight-bearing postures.

- **Enhanced circulation**, which also boosts the supply of oxygen throughout the body.
- **Lower blood pressure.**
- **Lower levels of the stress hormone cortisol**, which (as discussed in Chapter 3) can affect the immune system, interfere with memory, and increase the risk of depression and osteoporosis.
- **Lower blood sugar** in people with diabetes, which reduces the risk of complications.
- **Reduced pain** in people with back problems, arthritis, carpal tunnel syndrome, fibromyalgia, and other chronic problems.

The best way to get started is to find a class that appeals to you and learn a few yoga moves and breathing techniques. Once you have mastered these, you can easily integrate yoga into your total fitness program.

The ACSM cautions that yoga should help, not hurt. To prevent injuries to your knees, back, neck, shoulders, wrists, or ankles, avoid forcing your body into difficult postures. Proper technique is essential to safety.

Pilates   Used by dancers for deep-body conditioning and injury rehabilitation, Pilates (pronounced Pilah-teez) was developed more than seven decades ago by German

static stretching
A gradual stretch held for a short time of 10 to 30 seconds.

passive stretching   A stretching technique in which an external force or resistance (your body, a partner, gravity, or a weight) helps the joints move through their range of motion.

active stretching   A technique that involves stretching a muscle by contracting the opposing muscle.

ballistic stretching   Rapid bouncing movements.

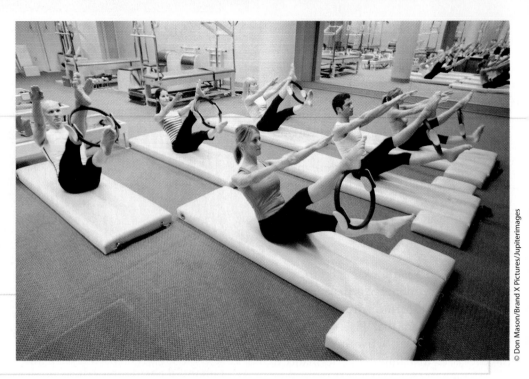

Pilates and similar exercises strengthen the core muscles while also improving flexibility and joint mobility.

© Don Mason/Brand X Pictures/Jupiterimages

immigrant Joseph Pilates. Increasingly used to complement aerobics and weight training, Pilates exercises improve flexibility and joint mobility and strengthen the core by developing pelvic stability and abdominal control.

Pilates-trained instructors offer "mat" or "floor" classes that stress the stabilization and strengthening of the back and abdominal muscles. Fitness centers also may offer training on Pilates equipment, primarily a device called the Reformer, a wooden contraption with various cables, pulleys, springs, and sliding boards attached that is used for a series of progressive, range-of-motion exercises. Instructors typically work one on one or with small groups of two or three participants and tailor exercise sessions to individual flexibility and strength limitations. Unlike exercise techniques that emphasize numerous repetitions in a single direction, Pilates exercises involve very few, but extremely precise, repetitions in several planes of motion.

According to research from the ACSM, Pilates enhances flexibility and muscular endurance, particularly for intermediate and advanced practitioners, but its potential to increase cardiorespiratory fitness and reduce body weight is limited. The intensity of a Pilates workout increases from basic to intermediate to advanced levels, as does the number of calories burned. For intermediate practitioners, a 30-minute session burns 180 calories, with each additional quarter-hour burning another 90 calories. A single weekly session enhances flexibility but has little impact on body composition.

T'ai Chi This ancient Chinese practice, designed to exercise body, mind, and spirit, gently works muscles, focuses concentration, and improves the flow of "qi" (often spelled "chi"), the vital life energy that sustains health. Popular with all ages, from children to seniors, t'ai chi is easy to learn and perform. Because of its focus on breathing and flowing gestures, t'ai chi is sometimes described as "meditation in motion."

Classes are available on campuses, in fitness centers, community centers, and some martial arts schools. Physicians may recommend t'ai chi for those with musculoskeletal disorders like arthritis to improve flexibility and build muscle strength gently and gradually. The ACSM reports that t'ai chi has proved effective in reducing falls in the elderly and those with balance disorders.

Keeping Your Back Healthy

The average person has an 80 percent chance of experiencing low-back pain in the course of a lifetime. Back pain strikes slightly more women than men and is most common between the ages of 20 and 55. You are at greater risk if you smoke or if you're overstressed, overweight, or out of shape. Back pain, which accounts for 40 percent of sickness absences, causes more lost workdays and costs the country more than any other malady.

In most cases the most effective treatment for low back pain, which usually is caused by degeneration of the lumbar spinal disks, is a combination of physical therapy and anti-inflammatory medication. According to a review of research on this common problem, 90 percent of patients with low back pain recover within three months, most within six weeks. One of the most effective ways to prevent or recover from back problems is to strengthen the core muscles.[28]

Once bedrest was the primary treatment for back pain, but now doctors urge patients to avoid it. Even two to seven days of bedrest may provide little, if any, benefit. Acetaminophen (Tylenol) is the first-line therapy for pain relief. If it is not effective, doctors recommend nonsteroidal anti-inflammatory drugs, such as ibuprofen (Motrin or Advil). Muscle relaxants seem to be effective for a spasm in the lower back. The sooner that back patients return to normal activity, the less pain medication they require and the less long-term disability they suffer. Fewer than 1 percent of patients with chronic low-back pain benefit from surgery.

Body Composition

Body composition, the fifth component of fitness, can tell you a lot about risk for cardiorespiratory disease and diabetes.

A combination of regular exercise and good nutrition is the best way to maintain a healthy body composition. Aerobic exercise helps by burning calories and increasing metabolic rate (the rate at which the body uses calories) for several hours after a workout. Strength training increases the proportion of lean body tissue by building muscle mass, which also increases the metabolic rate.

Experts debate which measure of body composition—body mass index (BMI), waist circumference, or waist-to-hip ratio—is the best indicator of central or visceral obesity, which increases the risk of heart disease, metabolic syndrome, diabetes, and other illnesses.

Body Mass Index (BMI)

Body mass index (BMI), a ratio between weight and height, is a mathematical formula that correlates with body fat. You can determine your BMI from Figure 5.9. A healthy BMI ranges from 18.5 to 24.9.

A BMI of 25 or greater defines **overweight** and marks the point at which excess weight increases the risk of disease. If your BMI is between 25 (23.4 for Asians) and 29.9, your weight is undermining the quality of your life. You suffer more aches and pains. You find it harder to perform everyday tasks. You run a greater risk of serious health problems.

A BMI of 30 or greater defines **obesity** and marks the point at which excess weight increases the risk of death. If your BMI is between 30 and 34.9 (class 1 obesity), you face all the preceding dangers plus one more: dying. The risk of premature death increases even more if your BMI is between 35 and 39.9 (class 2 obesity). A BMI of 40 or higher indicates class 3 or severe obesity.

Doctors use BMI to determine whether a person is at risk for weight-related diseases like diabetes. However, using BMI as an

body mass index (BMI) A mathematical formula that correlates with body fat; the ratio of weight to height squared.

overweight A condition of having a BMI between 25.0 and 29.9.

obesity The excessive accumulation of fat in the body; class 1 obesity is defined by a BMI between 30 and 34.9; class 2 obesity is defined by a BMI between 35 and 39.9; class 3, or severe obesity, is a BMI of 40 or higher.

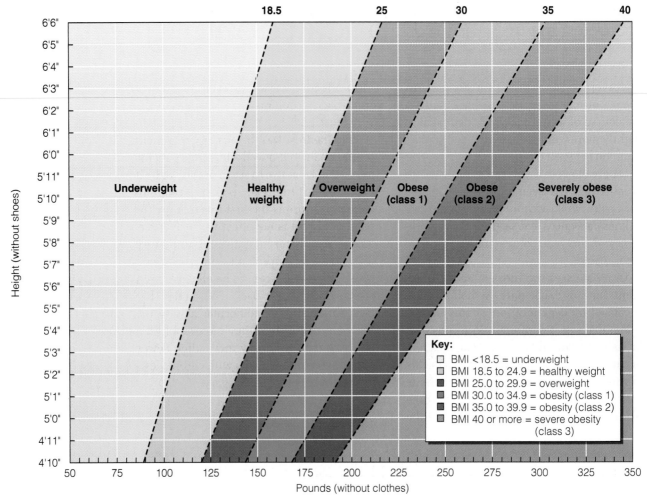

Figure 5.9 BMI Values Used to Assess Weight for Adults

assessment tool has limitations. Muscular individuals, including athletes and body builders, may be miscategorized as overweight or obese because they have greater lean muscle mass. BMI also does not reliably reflect body fat, an independent predictor of health risk, and is not useful for growing children, women who are pregnant or nursing, or the elderly. In addition, BMI, which was developed in Western nations, may not accurately indicate the risk of obesity-related diseases in Asian men and women.

Waist Circumference

Even if your scale shows that you haven't gained a lot of weight, your waist may widen—particularly if you've been under stress. Because of the physiological impact of stress hormones, fat accumulates around your midsection in times of tension and turmoil.

A widening waist or "apple" shape is a warning signal. In women, a wider waist correlates with high levels of harmful blood fats, such as LDL cholesterol and triglycerides. In both sexes, abdominal fat, unlike fat in the thighs or hips, increases the risk of high blood pressure, type 2 diabetes, high cholesterol, and metabolic syndrome (a perilous combination of overweight, high blood pressure, and high levels of cholesterol and blood sugar, discussed in Chapter 14).

To measure your waist circumference, place a tape measure around your bare abdomen just above your hip bone. Be sure that the tape is snug but does not compress your skin. Relax, exhale, and measure.

When is a waist too wide? Various studies have produced different results, but the general guideline is that a waist measuring more than 35 inches in a woman or more than 40 inches in a man signals greater health risks. These waist circumferences indicate "central" obesity, which is characterized by fat deposited deep within the central abdominal area of the body. Such "visceral" fat is more dangerous than "subcutaneous" fat just below the skin because it moves more readily into the bloodstream and directly raises levels of harmful cholesterol. Individuals with a large belly at midlife also are at increased risk of dementia later in life.[29]

 Body composition varies with race and ethnicity. Asians, for instance, may be more likely and African Americans less likely to accumulate visceral fat than Caucasians.

Waist-to-Hip Ratio

Another way of determining your health risk is your **waist-to-hip ratio (WHR).** In addition to measuring your waist, measure your hips at the widest part. Divide your waist measurement by your hip measurement. For women, a ratio of 0.80 or less is considered safe; for men, the recommended ratio is 0.90 or less. For both men and women, a 1.0 or higher is considered "at risk" or in the danger zone for undesirable health consequences, such as heart disease and other ailments associated with being overweight.

Men of all ages are more prone to develop the "apple" shape characteristic of central obesity; women in their reproductive years are more likely to accumulate fat around the hips and thighs and acquire a pear shape (Figure 5.10).

Measuring Body Fat

Knowing your specific body composition can provide useful information about body fat and health. Ideal body fat percentages for men range from 7 to 25 percent and for women from 16 to 35 percent. Methods of assessing body composition range from skin calipers to more high-tech methods.

Skinfold Measurement   *Skinfold measurement is* determined using a caliper to measure the amount of skinfold. The usual sites include the chest, abdomen, and thigh for men, and the tricep, hip, and thigh for women. Various equations determine body fat percentage, including calculations that take into account age, gender, race, and other factors. This relatively simple and low-cost method requires considerable technical skill for an accurate reading.

Home Body Fat Analyzers   Handheld devices and stand-on monitors sold online and in specialty stores promise to make measuring your body fat percentage as easy as finding your weight. None has been extensively tested.

Laboratory Methods

- **Bioelectrical Impedance Analysis (BIA).** This noninvasive method is based on the principle that electrical current applied to the body meets greater resistance with different types of tissue. Lean tissue, which contains large amounts of water and electrolytes, is a good electrical conductor; fat, which does not, is a poor conductor. In theory, the easier the electrical conduction, the greater an individual's lean body mass.

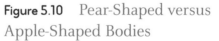

Figure 5.10   Pear-Shaped versus Apple-Shaped Bodies

PEAR
Fat stores around hips predominate

APPLE
Fat stores around waist predominate

- When standing, shift your weight from one foot to the other. If possible, place one foot on a stool, step, or railing four to six inches off the ground. Hold in your stomach, tilt your pelvis toward your back, and tuck in your buttocks to provide crucial support for the lower back.

- Because sitting places more stress on the lower back than standing, try to get up from your seat at least once an hour to stretch or walk around. Whenever possible, sit in a straight chair with a firm back. Avoid slouching in overstuffed chairs or dangling your legs in midair. When driving, keep the seat forward so that your knees are raised to hip level; your right leg should not be fully extended. A small pillow or towel can help support your lower back.

- Sleep on a flat, firm mattress. The best sleep position is on your side, with one or both knees bent at right angles to your torso. The pillow should keep your head in line with your body so that your neck isn't bent forward or to the side.

- When lifting, bend at the knees, not from the waist. Get close to the load. Tighten your stomach muscles, but don't hold your breath. Let your leg muscles do the work.

waist-to-hip ratio (WHR)   The proportion of one's waist circumference to one's hip circumference.

Skinfold measure accuracy depends on the technician's skill; laboratory methods such as DXA don't have that subjective component.

- **Hydrostatic (underwater) weighing.** According to the Archimedes Principle, a body immersed in a fluid is buoyed by a force equal to the weight of the displaced fluid. Since muscle has a higher density than water and fat has a lower density, fat people tend to displace less water than lean people.
- **Dual-energy X-ray absorptiometry (DXA).** X-rays are used to quantify the skeletal and soft tissue components of body mass. The test requires just 10 to 20 minutes, and radiation dosage is low (800 to 2,000 times lower than a typical chest X-ray). Some researchers believe that DXA will supplant hydrostatic testing as the standard for body composition assessment.
- **The Bod Pod®.** This large, egg-shaped fiberglass chamber uses an approach based on air displacement plethysmography, that is, the calculation of the relationship between pressure and volume to derive body volume.

Evaluating Fitness Products and Programs

As fitness has become a major industry in the United States, consumers have been bombarded with pitches for products that promise to do everything from whittle a waistline to build up biceps. As always, you have to ask questions and do your own research—whether you're buying basic exercise aids or joining a health club. Beware of any promise that sounds too good to be true. And keep in mind that nothing matters more than your own commitment.

Exercise Equipment

Always try out equipment before buying it. If you decide to purchase a stationary bicycle, for instance, read all the product information. Ask someone in your physical education department or at a local gym for recommendations. Try out a bicycle at the gym. Any equipment you purchase should be safe and durable, but not necessarily expensive (see Health on a Budget, p. 154).

Well-padded tongue prevents extensor tendinitis and irritation of dorsum of foot

Laces not too long so they stay tied longer

High, rounded toe box (at least 1 1/2 in. high) prevents subungual hematomas ("black toes")

Studded sole absorbs shock and provides traction in mud and snow

Well-molded Achilles pad prevents irritation of Achilles tendon

Firm heel counter for hindfoot stability

Flared heel for stability and beveled or rounded heel for quick roll-off

Soft, raised heel wedge to absorb impact at heel strike

Flexible midsole helps prevent Achilles tendon problems

Figure 5.11 What to Look For When You Buy Running Shoes

Athletic Shoes Footwear has come a long way from the days of canvas sneakers. With so many new materials and high-tech options, choosing the right shoe for working out can be confusing. The best shoes aren't necessarily the most expensive but the ones that fit you best. (See Figure 5.11.) Here are some basic guidelines:

- **Choose the right shoe for your sport.** If you're a walker or runner, you want maximum overall shock absorption for the foot, with extra cushioning in the heel and under the ball of the foot (the metatarsal area) to prevent pain, burning, and tenderness. If you also participate in other types of exercise, consider "cross-trainers," shoes that are flexible enough in the front for running but provide the side-to-side, or lateral, control you need for aerobics or tennis.

- **Check out the shoe.** A "slip-lasted" shoe, made by sewing together the upper like a moccasin and gluing it to the sole, is lightweight and flexible. A "board-lasted" shoe has a leather, nylon mesh, or canvas upper sewn to a cardboardlike material, which provides more support and control. A "combination-lasted"

shoe offers the advantages of both and works well for a variety of foot types.

- **Shop late.** Try on shoes at the end of the day or after a workout, when your foot size is at its maximum (sometimes half a shoe size larger than in the morning). Wear socks similar to those you'll wear for workouts.

- **Give your toes room.** Allow a half-inch, or the width of your index finger, between the end of your longest toe and the tip of the shoe. Try on both shoes. If one foot is larger than the other, buy the larger size.

- **Check the width.** A shoe should be as wide as possible across the forefoot without allowing the heel to slip. Lace up the shoe completely and walk or jog a few steps to make sure the shoes are comfortable.

- **Replace shoes when they lose their cushioning.** After about 300 to 500 miles of running or 300 hours of aerobic activity, your shoes are no longer absorbing the pounding and jarring of your sport. Don't put yourself at increased risk of knee and ankle injuries.

Build your core strength and improve your balance inexpensively with a stability ball. Maintaining appropriate air pressure is important—the exercise will become more difficult as pressure increases.

© Polka Dot Images/Jupiterimages

HEALTH ON A BUDGET $

Low-Cost Fitness Aids

Not all fitness equipment comes with a big price tag. Here are some affordable ways to expand and enhance a home workout:

- **Dumbbells.** You can purchase light weights to carry when walking and jogging to build and firm arm muscles. Training with heavier weights increases muscle strength and endurance, improves balance and body composition, and may reverse some bone loss. An adjustable dumbbell set allows you to add more weight as you build strength.
- **Stability balls.** A large inflatable rubber ball can be a fun, effective way of building core strength, improving posture, and increasing balance. When performing standard exercises like crunches and abdominal curls, the ball provides an additional challenge: maintaining a stable trunk throughout each exercise. You also can sit on the ball while working with hand weights to build core strength and balance. Introductory videos and DVDs are available for rental or purchase.
- **Resistance tubing.** Developed by physical therapists for rehabilitation after injuries, elastic bands and tubing come in different strengths, based on the thickness of the plastic. If you're a beginner, start with a thin band, particularly for the upper body. The lightweight, inexpensive, and easy-to-carry bands aren't particularly risky, but you should check for holes or worn spots, choose a smooth surface, maintain good posture, and perform the exercises in a slow, controlled manner.

Fitness Centers

Begin by checking out the recreational facilities on your own campus. Is there a gym, running track, pool, basketball court, athletic fields? Are they crowded at certain times? Are they convenient? Are classes in spinning or Pilates available?

If you decide to join a private gym or health club, find out exactly what facilities and programs it offers. The club should be located close to home, campus, or work and should be open at convenient hours. Think about your schedule and when you'll have time to work out. Visit the club at the times you're most likely to use it.

A club should have facilities for a complete workout, including both aerobic and muscle workouts: exercycles, rowing machines, treadmills, stair-climbing machines, stationary bicycles, a running track, aerobics classes, a swimming pool, strength-training equipment, and, if it's what you're looking for, racquetball courts and a large gym for basketball and volleyball.

Find out whether all facilities are available to all members at all times. Some clubs reserve the pool for families only or kids' lessons at certain times. Ask if you can try out the club before joining. Find out what the membership includes. Will you end up paying extra for lockers, towels, classes, and the like? Are student discounts offered? Beware of long-term memberships; many clubs go out of business or change ownership often. Do the members seem to be significantly older or younger, or in much better or worse shape, than you are? Remember: You're more likely to work out regularly in a place, and with people, you like. In a study of undergraduates in university physical activity classes (such as spinning, aerobic water exercise, kickboxing, and aerobics), students reported greater effort, enjoyment, and commitment to future exercise and lower tension and anxiety about their physiques when they perceived the atmosphere in the class as caring and positive.[30]

Sports Nutrition

In general, active people need the same basic nutrients as others and should follow the recommendations in Chapter 6. However, athletes in competitive sports—amateur as well as professional—may have increased energy requirements.

Contrary to a common misconception, athletes generally do not need more protein; the exception may be those engaged in intense strength training. Like most Americans, athletes typically consume more than the Recommended Daily Allowance for protein and do not need increased protein. A high-protein diet can be high in fat and low in the nutrients supplied by fruits, vegetables, and grains and can put a strain on the liver and kidneys. However, in a recent study of undergraduates, college men and women who engaged in vigorous exercise ate more fruits and vegetables than their less active classmates.

Although complex carbohydrates are essential in an athlete's diet, fat also plays a role. Including the right types of fat in the daily diet can actually improve athletic performance—not just by providing calories, but by replenishing intramuscular fat stores (fat stored within the muscle and used to fuel extended exercise).

Not just *what* you eat but *when* you eat can affect your exercise performance. If you eat immediately prior to a workout, you may feel sluggish or develop nausea, cramping, or diarrhea. If you don't eat, you may feel weak, faint, or tired.

Time your meals so that you exercise three to four hours after a large meal and one to two hours after a small one. Most people can eat a snack right before exercise. After a workout, eat a meal containing both protein and carbohydrates within two hours to help your muscles recover and to replace fuel stores.

Water

Water, which we need more than any other nutrient, is even more important during exercise and exertion. Thirst, the body's way of telling you to replace lost fluids, is not a good way for athletes to monitor their fluid needs. Rather than waiting until you're already somewhat dehydrated, you should be fully hydrated when you begin your activity or exercise and, depending on the duration and intensity of your workout, continue to replace fluids both during and afterward.

The American College of Sports Medicine (ACSM) recommends fluid intake before, during, and after exercise to regulate body temperature and replace body fluids lost through sweating. The failure to replace fluids during exercise can lead to dehydration, which can cause muscle fatigue, loss of coordination, heat exhaustion, and an elevation of body-core temperature to dangerously high levels. To avoid this danger, the ACSM advises:

- **Consume a nutritionally balanced diet and drink adequate fluids** in the 24 hours before an exercise event.
- **Drink about 17 ounces of fluid** about two hours before.
- **During exercise, start drinking early** and at regular intervals to replace all the water lost through sweating (i.e., body weight loss).
- **Drink fluids with carbohydrates and/or electrolytes** for exercise lasting more than an hour. For shorter periods, there is little evidence of differences between drinking a carbohydrate–electrolyte drink and plain water.

Too much water during prolonged bouts of exercise, such as a marathon, can lead to *hyponatremia*, or water intoxication. This condition occurs when the body's sodium level falls below normal as a result of salt loss from sweat and dilution of sodium in the bloodstream by overdrinking. Symptoms of hyponatremia include nausea, vomiting, weakness, and in severe cases, seizures, coma, and death.

Sports Drinks

More than twenty "power" beverages compete for the $1 billion market of drinks for active people. As noted above, water best meets the fluid needs of most athletes, but you have other choices. According to a recent study, non-fat milk is more effective than even a soy protein beverage or sports drink such as Gatorade at burning fat and building lean muscle mass. Young men who consistently drank fat-free milk after resistance training gained 40 percent more muscle mass than those who consumed soy drinks, and 60 percent more than those consuming carbohydrate-based sport drinks.

What you are actually consuming in a sports drink is a mixture of simple sugars, sodium, and other electrolytes. Sugars help maintain hydration and blood glucose and may be especially beneficial for strenuous endurance workouts that last longer than 45 minutes or during prolonged competitive games that demand repeated intermittent activity.

Most sports drinks contain about 7 percent carbohydrate (about half the sugar of ordinary soft drinks). Less than 6 percent may not enhance performance; more than 8 percent could cause abdominal cramping, nausea, and diarrhea.

Sodium and other electrolytes in sports drinks help replace those lost during physical activity. However, most exercisers do not have to replace minerals lost in sweat immediately. A meal eaten within several hours does so soon enough.

If you exercise to lose weight, sports drinks may be counterproductive since you take in 50 to 100 calories with every 8-ounce drink. Water, on the other hand, replenishes lost fluids without adding empty calories. (See Chapter 6 for a discussion of sodas and energy drinks.)

Dietary Supplements

Athletes and active individuals of all ages take dietary supplements, sometimes to ensure that they're getting the nutrients they need and sometimes to enhance their performance. Vitamin and mineral supplements, as discussed in Chapter 6, are safe when taken at recommended doses. Excess amounts can contribute to serious health problems. Vitamin supplements marketed for athletes are poorly regulated, and some may be adulterated with banned substances, such as ephedrine. Always look for the USP (United States Pharmacopeias) certification on the label when buying vitamins.

Athletes involved in heavy training may need more of several vitamins, such

as thiamin, riboflavin, and B_6, which are involved in energy production. The best source, nutritionists advise, is vitamin-rich foods, such as fruits and vegetables.

Mineral deficiencies, such as too little iron in female athletes, can impair athletic performance. Women who exercise rigorously should undergo regular blood testing and, if needed, take iron supplements. In general, calcium, magnesium, iron, zinc, and copper supplements do not enhance sport performance in well-nourished athletes. Chromium, boron, and vanadium have been studied as possible performance boosters, but researchers have not reported any beneficial effects on body composition or muscular strength and endurance.

Energy Bars

Sold as snacks, meal substitutes, or performance enhancers, energy bars come in different forms. High-carbohydrate bars derive more than 70 percent of their calories from carbohydrates (such as corn syrup, grape and pear juice concentrate, oat bran, and brown rice) and are low in protein and fat. Another type gets 40 percent of its energy from carbohydrate, 30 percent from protein, and 30 percent from fat.

Little scientific research has studied the actual benefits of the various types of energy bars, including their effects on blood glucose levels and athletic performance. According to one nutritional analysis, high-carbohydrate energy bars are similar to candy bars in their impact on glucose—even though sugars composed 31 percent of the high-carbohydrate energy bar and 86 percent of the candy bar. In fact, the high-carbohydrate energy bar caused a more rapid peak in blood glucose followed by a sharper decline than did the candy bar. This effect may be desirable for athletes involved in short-duration events who want a quick increase in blood glucose.

Energy bars with a lower carbohydrate level produce a more moderate, sustained increase in blood glucose level, possibly because the protein and fat in a 40–30–30 bar diminish blood glucose response. These bars would be a better choice for athletes involved in endurance events. As an alternative, try fiber-rich whole foods, like nuts and fruit, that provide a steady release of energy.

Safe and Healthy Workouts

Whenever you work out, you don't want to risk becoming sore or injured. Starting slowly when you begin any new fitness activity is the smartest strategy. Keep a simple diary to record the time and duration of each workout. Get accustomed to an activity first and then begin to work harder or longer. In this way, you strengthen your musculoskeletal system so you're less likely to be injured, you lower the cardiorespiratory risk, and you build the exercise habit into your schedule.

To prevent exercise-related problems before they happen, use common sense and take appropriate precautions, including the following:

- **Get proper instruction** and, if necessary, advanced training from knowledgeable instructors.

- **Make sure you have good equipment** and keep it in good condition. Know how to check and do at least basic maintenance on the equipment yourself. Always check your equipment prior to each use (especially if you're renting it).

- **Always warm up before and cool down** after a workout.

- Rather than being sedentary all week and then training hard on weekends, **try to stay active throughout the week** and not overdo on weekends.

- **Use reasonable protective measures,** including wearing a helmet when cycling or skating.

- For some sports, such as boating, **always go with a buddy.**

- **Take each outing seriously**—even if you've dived into this river a hundred times before, even if you know this mountain like you know your own backyard. Avoid the unknown under adverse conditions (for example, hiking unfamiliar terrain during poor weather or kayaking a new river when water levels are unusually high or low) or when accompanied by a beginner whose skills may not be as strong as yours.

- **Never combine alcohol or drugs with any workout or sport.**

Temperature

Prevention is the wisest approach to heat and cold problems. And knowing what can go wrong is part of that preventive approach.

Heat Cramps These muscle cramps are caused by profuse sweating and the consequent loss of electrolytes (salts). They occur most often during exercise in hot weather. Salty snacks and sports beverages like Gatorade can help, but be aware that sports drinks can be very high in calories. Salt tablets usually aren't necessary except in cases of extreme sweating.

Heat Syndromes More serious temperature-related conditions include heat exhaustion and heat stroke. These are most likely to occur when both temperature and humidity are high, because sweat does not evaporate as quickly, preventing the body from releasing heat quickly. Other conditions that limit the body's ability to regulate temperature are old age, fever, obesity, dehydration, heart disease, poor circulation, sunburn, and drug and alcohol use. Some medicines that increase the risk include allergy medicines (antihistamines), some cough and cold medicines, blood pressure and heart medicines, diet pills, laxatives, and psychiatric medications.

Heat Exhaustion Heat exhaustion is a mild from of heat-related illness that can be caused by exercise or hot weather. The signs of heat exhaustion are heavy sweating, paleness, muscle cramps, tiredness, weakness, dizziness, headache, nausea or vomiting, and/or fainting. Your pulse rate or heart rate may be fast and weak, and your breathing fast and shallow.

If you think you may have heat exhaustion, get out of the heat quickly. Rest in a cool, shady place and drink plenty of water or other fluids. Do *not* drink alcohol, which

Heeding Heat

- Increase your fluid intake during hot temperatures by two to four glasses of cool fluids each hour. Cold beverages can cause stomach cramps; alcoholic beverages can cause you to lose more fluid.
- Cool off with a cool shower or sponge bath.
- Move into an air-conditioned environment.
- Wear lightweight clothing.
- Check weather conditions. The National Weather Service has produced a Heat Index chart that can be accessed online at **www.crh.noaa.gov/pub/heat.php.**

Handling Cold

- Dress appropriately. Choose several layers of loose clothing made of wool, cotton, down, or synthetic down. Make sure your head, feet, and hands are well protected. A pair of cotton socks inside a pair of wool socks will keep your feet warm.
- Don't go out in the cold after drinking. Alcohol can make you more susceptible to cold and can impair your judgment and sense of time.
- When snowshoeing or cross-country skiing, always let a responsible person know where you're heading and when you expect to be back. Stick to marked trails.
- Carry a small emergency kit that includes waterproof matches, a compass, a map, high-energy food, and water.
- Don't eat snow; it could lower your body temperature.

can make heat exhaustion worse. If you do not feel better within 30 minutes, see your doctor. If left untreated, heat exhaustion may lead to a heat stroke.

Heat Stroke   A heat stroke can occur when the body temperature rises to 106 degrees Fahrenheit or higher within 10 to 15 minutes. A heat stroke is a medical emergency that can be fatal. The warning signs are extremely high temperature; red, hot, and dry skin; rapid, strong pulse; throbbing headache; dizziness; nausea; confusion or unconsciousness.

If you think someone might have heat stroke, you should take him or her to a cool, shady place quickly, and call a doctor. Remove unnecessary clothing and bathe or spray the victim with cool water. People with heat stroke may seem confused. They may have seizures or go into a coma.

Protecting Yourself from the Cold   The tips of the toes, fingers, ears, nose, and chin and the cheeks are most vulnerable to exposure to high wind speeds and low temperatures, which can result in *frostnip.*

Because frostnip is painless, you may not even be aware that it is occurring. Watch for a sudden blanching or lightening of your skin. The best early treatment is warming the area by firm, steady pressure with a warm hand; blowing on it with hot breath; holding it against your body; or immersing it in warm (not hot) water. As the skin thaws, it becomes red and starts to tingle. Be careful to protect it from further damage. Don't rub the skin vigorously or with snow, as you could damage the tissue.

More severe is *frostbite.* There are two types of frostbite: *superficial* and *deep.* Superficial frostbite, the freezing of the skin and tissues just below the skin, is characterized by a waxy look and firmness of the skin, although the tissue below is soft. Initial treatment should be to slowly rewarm the area. As the area thaws, it will be numb and bluish or purple, and blisters may form. Cover the area with a dry, sterile dressing, and protect the skin from further exposure to cold. See a doctor for further treatment. Deep frostbite, the freezing of skin, muscle, and even bone, requires medical treatment. It usually involves the tissues of the hands

and feet, which appear pale and feel frozen. Keep the victim dry and as warm as possible on the way to a medical facility. Cover the frostbitten area with a dry, sterile dressing.

The center of the body may gradually cool at temperatures above, as well as below, freezing—usually in wet, windy weather. When body temperature falls below 95 degrees Fahrenheit, the body is incapable of rewarming itself because of the breakdown of the internal system that regulates its temperature. This state is known as **hypothermia**. The first sign of hypothermia is severe shivering. Then the victim becomes uncoordinated, drowsy, listless, and confused and is unable to speak properly. Symptoms become more severe as body temperature continues to drop, and coma or death can result.

Hypothermia requires emergency medical treatment. Try to prevent any further heat loss. Move the victim to a warm place, cover him or her with blankets, remove wet clothing, and replace it with dry garments. If the victim is conscious, administer warm liquids, not alcohol.

Protect yourself in cold weather (or cold indoor gyms) by covering as much of your body as possible, but don't overdress. Wear one layer less than you would if you were outside but not exercising. Don't use warm-up clothes made of waterproof material, because they tend to trap heat and keep perspiration from evaporating. Make sure your clothes are loose enough to allow movement and exercise of the hands, feet, and other body parts, thereby maintaining proper circulation. Choose dark colors that absorb heat. And because 40 percent or more of your body heat is lost through your head and neck, wear a hat, turtleneck, or scarf. Make sure you cover your hands and feet as well; mittens provide more warmth and protection than gloves.

Warm up and cool down. Cold weather constricts muscles, so you need to allow enough time for proper stretching to warm up muscles before you exercise.[31]

Types of Injuries

According to the American Physical Therapy Association, the most common exercise-related injury sites are the knees, feet, back, and shoulders, followed by the ankles and hips. **Acute injuries**—sprains, bruises, and pulled muscles—are the result of sudden trauma, such as a fall or collision. **Overuse injuries,** on the other hand, are the result of overdoing a repetitive activity, such as running. When one particular joint is overstressed—such as a tennis player's elbow or a swimmer's shoulder—tendinitis, an inflammation at the point where the tendon meets the bone, can develop. Other overuse injuries include muscle strains and aches and stress fractures, which are hairline breaks in a bone, usually in the leg or foot.

Men and women may be vulnerable to different types of injuries. Studies of male and female college basketball and soccer players have shown that gender differences in the neuromuscular control of the knee places female athletes at higher risk for knee injuries. Balance training may reduce the risk.

Taking Care of Injuries

Sooner or later most active people suffer an injury. Although most are minor, they all require attention. Ignoring a problem or trying to push through the pain can lead to more serious complications.

PRICE If you develop aches and pains beyond what you might expect from an activity, stop. Never push to the point of fatigue. If you do, you could end up with sprained or torn muscles. Figure 5.12 gives the PRICE prescription for coping with an exercise injury.

Overtraining About half of all people who start an exercise program drop out within six months. One common reason is that they **overtrain,** pushing themselves to work too intensely too frequently. Signs of overdoing it include persistent muscle soreness, frequent injuries, unintended weight loss, nervousness, and an inability to relax. Overtraining for endurance sports like marathon running can damage the lungs and intensify asthma symptoms. You may find yourself unable to complete a normal workout or to recover after a normal workout.

If you develop any of the symptoms of overtraining, reduce or stop your workout sessions temporarily. Make gradual increases in the intensity of your workouts. Allow 24 to 48 hours for recovery between workouts. Make sure you get adequate rest. Check with a physical education instructor, coach, or trainer to make sure your exercise program fits your individual needs.

Exercise Addiction Excessive exercise can become a form of addiction, and "exercise dependence" is not uncommon among young men and women. Although most physically active college students work out at healthy levels, some exercise to an extent that could signal dependence. In a study of undergraduates, the most common symptoms of exercise dependence were interference with family and social life, withdrawal, and exercising for social as well as health reasons. However, men and women may exhibit different symptoms.

hypothermia An abnormally low body temperature; if not treated appropriately, coma or death could result.

acute injuries Physical injuries, such as sprains, bruises, and pulled muscles, which result from sudden traumas, such as falls or collisions.

overuse injuries Physical injuries to joints or muscles, such as strains, fractures, and tendinitis, which result from overdoing a repetitive activity.

overtrain Working muscles too intensely or too frequently, resulting in persistent muscle soreness, injuries, unintended weight loss, nervousness, and an inability to relax.

Figure 5.12 PRICE: How to Cope with an Exercise Injury

- **P**rotect the area with an elastic wrap, a sling, splint, cane, crutches, or an air cast.
- **R**est to promote tissue healing. Avoid activities that cause pain, swelling, or discomfort.
- **I**ce the area immediately, even if you're seeking medical help (don't put the ice pack directly on the skin). Repeat every two or three hours while you're awake for the first 48 to 72 hours. Cold reduces pain, swelling, and inflammation in injured muscles, joints, and connecting tissues and may slow bleeding if a tear has occurred.
- **C**ompress the area with an elastic bandage until the swelling stops. Begin wrapping at the end farthest from your heart. Loosen the wrap if the pain increases, the area becomes numb, or swelling is occurring below the wrapped area.
- **E**levate the area above your heart, especially at night. Gravity helps reduce swelling by draining excess fluid.
- After 48 hours, if the swelling is gone, you may apply warmth or gentle heat, which improves the blood flow and speeds healing.

This chapter has given you the basic information you need to launch a fitness program. However, you're more likely to succeed if you create a plan and follow it. These basic steps can help you determine where you are now and how to get to where you want to be.

- **Evaluate your readiness for change.** Use this chapter's Self Survey to determine your stage of behavioral change. Don't expect to progress directly from one stage to another just once. Most people "recycle" several times before a change becomes permanent.

- **Consider your fitness goals.** Do you have an overall conditioning goal, such as losing weight? Or do you have a training goal, such as preparing for a 5K race or trying out for the volleyball team? Break down your goal into smaller "step" goals that lead you toward it.

- **Think through your personal preferences.** What are your physical strengths and weaknesses? Do you have good upper body strength but easily get winded? Do you have a stiff back? Do your allergies flare up when you exercise outdoors? By paying attention to your needs, likes, and dislikes, you can choose activities you enjoy—and are more likely to continue.

- **Schedule exercise into your daily routine.** If you can, block out a half-hour for working out at the beginning of the day, between classes, or in the evening. Write it into your schedule as if it were a class or doctor's appointment. If you can't find 30 minutes, look for two 15-minute or three 10-minute slots that you can use for "mini-work-outs." Once you've worked out a schedule, write it down. A written plan encourages you to stay on track.

- **Assemble your gear.** Make sure you put your athletic shoes in your car or in the locker at the gym. Lay out the clothes you'll need to shoot hoops or play racquetball.

- **Start slowly.** If you are just beginning regular activity or exercise, begin at a low level. If you have an injury, disability, or chronic health problem, be sure you get medical clearance from a physician.

- **Progress gradually.** If you have not been physically active, begin by incorporating a few minutes of physical activity into each day, building up to 30 minutes or more of moderate-intensity activities. If you have been active but not as often or as intensely as recommended, become more consistent. Continue to increase the frequency, intensity, and duration of your workouts.

- **Take stock.** After a few months of leading a more active life, take stock. Think of how much more energy you have at the end of the day. Ask yourself if you're feeling any less stressed, despite the push and pull of daily pressures. Focus on the unanticipated rewards of exercise. Savor the exhilaration of an autumn morning's walk; the thrill of feeling newly toughened muscles bend to your will; or the satisfaction of a long, smooth stretch after a stressful day. Enjoy the pure pleasure of living in the body you deserve.

SELF SURVEY Are You Ready to Become More Active?

Physical Activity Stages of Change Questionnaire

For each of the following questions, please circle Yes or No. Please be sure to read the questions carefully.

Physical activity or exercise includes activities such as walking briskly, jogging, bicycling, swimming, or any other activity in which the exertion is at least as intense as these activities.

1. I am currently physically active.   NO   YES

2. I intend to become more physically active in the next 6 months.   NO   YES

For activity to be regular, it must add up to a total of 30 minutes or more per day and be done at least 5 days per week. For example, you could take one 30-minute walk or take three 10-minute walks for a daily total of 30 minutes.

3. I currently engage in regular physical activity.   NO   YES

4. I have been regularly physically active for the past 6 months.   NO   YES

Scoring Algorithm

	Question			
	1	**2**	**3**	**4**
Precontemplation	No	No		
Contemplation	No	Yes		
Preparation	Yes		No	
Action	Yes		Yes	No
Maintenance	Yes		Yes	Yes

Sources: From B. H. Marcus & L. H. Forsyth, 2003, *Motivating People to be Physically Active,* page 21. © 2003 by Bess H. Marcus and Leigh Ann H. Fosyth. Reprinted with permission from Human Kinetics (Champaign, IL).

Your Health Action Plan for Physical Fitness

Physical Activity Stages of Change Questionnaire

Once you know your stage of motivational readiness, you can employ the cognitive and behavioral strategies most likely to work for you now. As you progress through the stages of change, you can shift to other approaches. Here are some suggestions:

Precontemplation (not active and not thinking about becoming active)

- Use this course as an opportunity to learn about the benefits of physical activity, including better mood, lower stress, stronger bones, and a lower risk of cardiovascular disease.

- Set a small, reasonable goal that does not involve working up a sweat, such as looking up "exercise, benefits of" in the index of this book and reading the pages cited.

- List what you see as the cons of physical activity. For example, do you fear it would take time you need for your studies? Think of small changes that don't require time, for instance, standing rather than sitting when talking on the phone, doing stretches while watching television, or taking a quick walk down the hall or up the stairs while waiting for a friend or a class.

- Identify barriers to physical activity, such as lack of money. Take advantage of your student status, and check out facilities, such as the swimming pool at the athletic center, or opportunities, such as an intramural soccer team, available to you free (or almost).

Contemplation (not active but thinking about becoming active)

- Think back to activities you found enjoyable in the past. You might consider inline skating to class or around campus, or plan a hike for a weekend or school break.

- Determine the types of activity you can realistically fit into your daily schedule. You might join friends for softball every Saturday, or sign up for an evening body-sculpting class.

- Visualize success. Focus on the person you want to become: How would you look? What would you do differently? Find an image—from a magazine advertisement, for example—and post it where you can see it often.

- Plan your rewards. Use a technique called shaping, which reinforces progress on the way to a goal. For instance, initially you might reward yourself once you engage in physical activity for 15 minutes a day. After a week, you get the reward only after 20 minutes a day. Over time you increase the number of days you are physically active as well as the number of minutes of activity per day.

- Reach out for support. Find a friend, family member, or classmate who is willing or able to provide support for being active. Or join an organized martial arts class or an informal team.

Preparation (active but not at recommended levels)

- Identify specific barriers that limit your activity. If your daily jogs are rained or snowed out, develop a list of indoor alternatives, such as walking stairs or working out to an exercise video.

- Set specific daily and weekly goals. Your daily goal might begin with 10 or 15 minutes of activity. Your weekly goal might be to try a new activity, such as spinning or a dance class.

- Divide physical activity over the course of the day with a 10 or 15 minute walk in the morning, another at lunch, and a third at the end of the day.

- Document your progress. You could use a monthly calendar to keep track of the number of days you've exercised as well as the length of each workout. Or you can keep a more detailed record, noting the types of exercise you do every day, the intensity you work at, the duration of each workout, and so forth.

Action and Maintenance (active at recommended levels for less than six months)

- Identify risk factors that might lead to relapse. If vacations or holiday breaks disrupt your routine, make a plan for alternative ways to remain active before you leave campus.

- Stress-proof your fitness program. In crunch times, you may feel you don't have time to spare for exercise. Multiple 10-minute walks during the day may be particularly useful both to keep up your fitness and to relieve stress buildup.

- Avoid boredom. Think through ways to vary your exercise routine. Take different routes on your walks. Invite different friends to join you. Alternate working with free weights and resistance machines at the gym.

- Set secondary goals. Once you've reached and maintained your goal for physical activity, set goals related to secondary benefits of exercise, for instance, losing weight or changing your body composition.

CENGAGENOW If you want to write your own goals for improved fitness, go to the Wellness Journal at CengageNow for Health: **www.cengage .com/sso.**

MAKING THIS CHAPTER WORK FOR YOU

Review Questions

1. The benefits of regular physical activity include
   a. decreased bone mass.
   b. lowered risk of shin splints.
   c. enhanced immune response.
   d. altered sleep patterns.

2. Which of the following precautions could help to prevent a serious sports injury from occurring?
   a. Wear swimming goggles when doing laps to decrease the irritating effects of chlorine.
   b. Wear knee pads when cycling to prevent knee gashes if you fall off your bicycle.
   c. To eliminate persistent muscle soreness, increase the frequency and/or time period of your workout.
   d. Wear a helmet, wrist guards, and knee pads when inline skating to help prevent fractures and head injuries.

3. Michael started a walking program two weeks ago. Which of these workouts would you recommend to him for aerobic exercise?
   a. 5 minutes of brisk walking, 30 minutes of flexibility exercises, 5 minutes of brisk walking
   b. 5 minutes of stretching, 15 minutes of slow walking, 5 minutes of brisk walking, 15 minutes of slow walking
   c. 10 minutes of slow walking, 35 minutes of brisk walking, 5 minutes of slow walking
   d. 10 minutes of stretching, 45 minutes of brisk walking

4. Which of the following statements is true?
   a. Inactivity does not affect health until middle age.
   b. Total fitness includes emotional and social dimensions of health besides the physical.
   c. Men and women have the same physiological capacities.
   d. Total fitness is one dimension of physical fitness.

5. A regular flexibility program provides which of the following benefits?
   a. stronger heart and lungs
   b. relief of muscle strain and soreness
   c. increased strength and endurance
   d. increased bone mass and leaner muscles

6. To motivate yourself to stick to an exercise program:
   a. Watch professional athletic competitions.
   b. Set a long-term goal, then break it down into short-term goals that can be achieved in a few months.
   c. Keep a detailed record of all the times that you avoided working out.
   d. Join an expensive health club so that you feel pressured to get your money's worth.

7. For any muscle to get stronger, it must work against a greater-than-normal resistance. This is called the
   a. reversibility principle.
   b. overload principle.
   c. FITT principle.
   d. principle of compound interest.

8. Jessica takes a step aerobics class three times a week. Which component of physical fitness does her exercise routine emphasize?
   a. muscular strength and endurance
   b. flexibility
   c. cardiorespiratory fitness
   d. body composition

9. If you are a healthy weight,
   a. you are always hungry.
   b. your BMI is between 18.5 and 24.9.
   c. your waist measurement is 25 to 28 inches.
   d. your waist-to-hip ratio is greater than 1.0.

10. Which nutrient is the most important during exercise and exertion?
    a. water
    b. carbohydrates
    c. fat
    d. protein

Answers to these questions can be found on page 650.

Critical Thinking

1. Allison knows that exercise is good for her health, but she figures she can keep her weight down by dieting and worry about her heart and health when she gets older. "I look good. I feel okay. Why should I bother exercising?" she asks. What would you reply?

2. College athletes have died unexpectedly from heart-related problems. The American Heart Association has identified guidelines to screen competitive athletes. Does your school follow these guidelines? If not, what precautions are taken to protect young athletes?

3. Your younger brother Andre is hoping to get a starting position on his high school football team. Practices began in July. You are aware that a couple of other players have suffered heat-related incidents, but according to Andre, these players just weren't tough enough. What can you do to help your brother protect his health?

4. Research is mixed on whether stretching can decrease delayed-onset muscle soreness. Do you think a placebo effect can occur in studies on exercise and training as it does in research on medications? Why or why not?

Media Menu

CENGAGENOW™ Go to the CengageNOW for Health website at **www .cengage.com/sso** that will:
- Help you evaluate your knowledge of the material.
- Allow you to take an exam-prep quiz.
- Provide a personalized Learning Plan targeting resources that address areas you should study.
- Coach you through identifying target goals for behavioral change and creating and monitoring your personal change plan throughout the semester.

Internet Connections

www.acefitness.org

This website features information for the general public as well as for certified fitness trainers. The comprehensive site includes health and fitness news headlines, Fit Facts information sheets, a question and answer site, whole-body exercise workouts, daily fitness tips, discussion boards, newsletters, and information on ACE certification.

www.aahperd.org

This organization provides legislative advocacy for healthy lifestyles through high quality programs in health and physical education. The website features consumer news, career links, listing of graduate programs, research, and a link for the International Electronic Journal of Health Education.

www.shapeup.org/fitness/index.php

At this site, you can perform a battery of physical fitness assessments, including activity level, strength, flexibility, and an aerobic fitness test. You get started by entering your weight, height, age, and gender and then take a quick screen test to assess your physical readiness for physical activity. Your final results in each area will be based on your personal data.

www.heart.org/presenter.jhtml?identifier=3041198

At this website sponsored by the American Heart Association, after a free registration you can access an interactive exercise diary where you can keep track of your own exercise progress. An information resource called MyStart! provides health and fitness resources.

Key Terms

The terms listed are used on the page indicated. Definitions of the terms are in the Glossary at the end of the book.

active stretching 147
acute injuries 159
aerobic exercise 133
anaerobic exercise 133
ballistic stretching 147
body composition 123
body mass index (BMI) 149
cardiorespiratory fitness 123
dynamic flexibility 145
endorphins 129
FITT 133
flexibility 123
functional fitness 123
hypothermia 159
isokinetic 140
isometric 140
isotonic 140
muscular endurance 123
muscular strength 123
obesity 149
osteoporosis 129
overload principle 133
overloading 140
overtrain 159
overuse injuries 159
overweight 149
passive stretching 147
physical fitness 123
progressive overloading 133
range of motion 145
Rating of Perceived Exertion (RPE) 135
rep (or repetition) 140
resting heart rate 133
reversibility principle 133
set 140
specificity principle 133
static flexibility 145
static stretching 147
target heart rate 135
waist-to-hip ratio 149

Chapter 6 - Personal Nutrition

1. **An example of a macronutrient is: (Pg. 166)**
   A. vitamins
   B. minerals
   C. carbohydrates
   D. all of the above

2. **Grains would be considered to be which type of nutrient? (Pg. 169)**
   A. minerals
   B. complex carbohydrates
   C. protein
   D. fat

3. **Americans typically get most of their calories from eating what kinds of foods? (Pg. 171)**
   A. protein
   B. fat
   C. simple sugars
   D. complex carbohydrates

4. **It is recommended that no greater than 30% of our diet come from which nutrient? (Pg. 184)**
   A. protein
   B. starches
   C. sugars
   D. fats

5. **Which nutrient has the greatest number of calories? (Pg. 171)**
   A. protein
   B. fat
   C. carbohydrate
   D. vitamins

6. **Which nutrient does not contribute to any calories in our diet? (Pg. 174)**
   A. carbohydrates
   B. minerals
   C. fats
   D. proteins

7. **Kyle is trying to improve by eating more complex carbohydrates in his diet. Foods that he should stay away from would be: (Pg. 169)**
   A. whole grain breads
   B. pasta
   C. white bread
   D. nuts

8. **Dietary and functional fiber in the diet are both important except for which of the following benefits: (Pg. 170)**
   A. fastens the emptying of the stomach of food
   B. absorbs cholesterol so the arteries don't become plugged up
   C. helps to reduce heart disease
   D. may help to reduce colon cancer

9. **An example of an unhealthy saturated fat oil would be: (Pg. 172)**
   A. corn oil
   B. olive oil
   C. coconut oil
   D. canola oil

10. **A type of antioxidant food to include in the diet to prevent harmful effects caused by oxidation in the body is: (Pg. 174)**
    A. vitamin B-3
    B. vitamin C
    C. iron
    D. amino acids

11. **Which nutrient aids in fluid and electrolyte balance, maintains pH balance and transports molecules and cells throughout the body? (Pg. 168)**
    A. minerals
    B. water
    C. vitamins
    D. fats

12. **A key theme in the new MyPyramid food guidance system is: (Pg. 181)**
    A. proportionality
    B. moderation
    C. personalization
    D. all of the above

13. **'Proportionality' in the MyPyramid Food Guidance System refers to: (Pg. 181)**
    A. the portions and size of food servings one should be consuming
    B. the proportion of eating one category of food over another category of foods
    C. the ratio of eating more red meats and refined sugars compared to fruits and vegetables
    D. the proportion of calories one is consuming on a daily basis

14. **MyPyramid food guide suggests that we increase our daily servings of fruits and vegetables. What is one creative way to ensure that we do increase our number of portions? (Pg. 181)**
    A. force feed ourselves the five servings of fruits or vegetables each day
    B. toss fruit into a salad to add more crunchiness and varied flavor
    C. have extra fruit out on the kitchen counter to remind us to eat them
    D. buy one fruit or vegetable of each rainbow color to eat

15. **Sarah eats dairy products, cheese, eggs, grains, fruits and vegetables, but no meat of any kind. She is considered to be what type of vegetarian? (Pg. 192-193)**
    A. vegan
    B. lacto-ovo vegetarian
    C. pesco vegetarian
    D. lacto vegetarian

16. **An essential nutrient that can sometimes be difficult to provide for in the vegetarian diet is: (Pg. 192)**
    A. fiber
    B. carbohydrates
    C. minerals
    D. protein

17. **In order for a food item to be labeled "high fiber" on its food label, the product must have at least how many grams of fiber in it? (Pg. 195)**
    A. 2.5 grams
    B. 3.5 grams
    C. 5.0 grams
    D. 8.0 grams

18. **Which of the following examples would be considered the only correct nutritional information on its advertising? (Pg. 196)**
    A. 'one product does it all for your health problems'
    B. 'personal testimonies point to the success of this product'
    C. 'instant results guaranteed with using this product'
    D. 'consult with your doctor before attempting to use this product'

19. **Foodborne illnesses can be prevented through the use of: (Pg. 198)**
    A. proper handwashing
    B. adequate cooking of food to the right temperatures
    C. protection of food from unnecessary contamination
    D. all of the above

20. **A common pitfall in college student eating habits which needs to be avoided or changed is: (Pg. 201- 202)**
    A. eating too much sodium such as high salted snack foods
    B. eating too much high fat deep fried foods
    C. not eating at least 3-5 servings a day of fruits and vegetables
    D. all of the above should be looked at and changed in the diet

The freshmen on the fifth floor of a university dormitory decided to test a dubious premise: that man—and woman—can live on pizza alone. For a month, they vowed to eat nothing but pizza in all its savory varieties—mushroom, pepperoni, sausage, anchovies, extra cheese, thin crust, double crust. "In less than a week," said one coed, "most of us cringed at the very sight of a cardboard delivery box. It wasn't just the boredom of having the same meal that got to them. Some felt bloated. Others had stomachaches. A few complained of headaches and fatigue. One was

Personal Nutrition

convinced she had scurvy, a vitamin deficiency disease caused by a lack of fruit and vegetables. None of them managed to stick with pizza for an entire month.

As these students discovered, we are indeed what we eat—and it shows in everything from our stamina and strength to the sheen in our hair and the glow in our cheeks. Eating well helps us live and feel well.

As demonstrated by the science of **nutrition**, the field that explores the connections between our bodies and the foods we eat, our daily diet affects how long and how well we live. Sensible eating can provide energy for our daily tasks, protect us from many chronic illnesses, and may even extend longevity. A high-quality diet also enhances day-to-day vitality, energy, and sense of well-being. (See Making Change Happen, p. 167, and "Mind over Platter" in the *Labs for IPC* to develop greater awareness and appreciation of the food you eat.)

This chapter can help you make healthy food choices. It translates the latest scientific research into specific advice designed both to promote health and to prevent chronic disease. By learning more about nutrients, food groups, eating patterns, nutrition labels, and safety practices, you can nourish your body with foods that not only taste good but also are good for you.

> After studying the material in this chapter, you should be able to

- **List** the basic nutrients necessary for a healthy body and **describe** their functions.
- **Describe** the key themes of the USDA MyPyramid Food Guidance System.
- **List** five specific nutrition guidelines of the MyPyramid system.
- **Explain** how to interpret the nutritional information provided on food labels.
- **List** the food safety hazards and **describe** prevention measures.
- **List** your nutrition pitfalls and **define** a strategy to avoid them.

nutrition The science devoted to the study of dietary needs for food and the effects of food on organisms.

What You Need to Know about Nutrients

Every day your body needs certain **essential nutrients** that it cannot manufacture for itself. They provide energy, build and repair body tissues, and regulate body functions. The six classes of essential nutrients, which are discussed in this section, are water, protein, carbohydrates, fats, vitamins, and minerals (Table 6.1).

Water makes up about 60 percent of the body and is essential for health and survival. Besides water, we also need energy to live, and we receive our energy from the carbohydrates, proteins, and fats in the foods we eat. The digestive system (Figure 6.1, p. 168) breaks down food into these **macronutrients.** They are the nutrients required by the human body in the greatest amounts. The amount of energy that can be derived from the macronutrients is measured in **calories.** There are 9 calories in every gram of fat and 4 calories in every gram of protein or carbohydrate. The other two essential nutrients—the vitamins and minerals—are called **micronutrients** because our bodies need them in only very small amounts.

Your need for macronutrients depends on how much energy you expend. Because fats, carbohydrates, and protein can all serve as sources of energy, they can, to some extent, substitute for one another in providing calories. Adults, according to federal standards, should get 45 to 65 percent of calories from carbohydrates, 20 to 35 percent from fat, and 10 to 35 percent from protein. Children's fat intake should be slightly higher: 25 to 40 percent of their caloric intake.

To eat well without overeating, choose foods that are "nutrient-dense," that is, foods that provide the most nutritional value. For example, both a cup of nonfat milk and an

	TABLE 6.1

The Essential Nutrients

	Sources	Functions
Water	Liquids, fruits, and vegetables	Carries nutrients and removes waste; dissolves amino acids, glucose, and minerals; cleans body by removing toxins; regulates body temperature
Proteins	Meat, poultry, fish, eggs, beans, nuts, cheese, tofu, vegetables, some fruits, pastas, breads, cereal, and rice	Help build new tissue to keep hair, skin, and eyesight healthy; build antibodies, enzymes, hormones, and other compounds; provide fuel for body
Carbohydrates	Grains, cereal, pasta, fruits and vegetables, nuts, milk, and sugars	Provide energy
Fats		
Unsaturated Fats	Red meat, dairy products, egg yolks, coconut and palm oils, shortening, stick margarine, baked goods	Provide energy; trigger production of cholesterol
Saturated Fats	Some fish; avocados; olive, canola, and peanut oils	Also provide energy, but trigger more "good" cholesterol production and less "bad" cholesterol production
Vitamins	Fruits, vegetables, grains, some meat and dairy products	Facilitate use of other nutrients; involved in regulating growth, maintaining tissue, and manufacturing blood cells, hormones, and other body components
Minerals	Many foods	Help build bones and teeth; aid in muscle function and nervous system activity; assist in various body functions including growth and energy production

© Gregg Adams/Stone/Getty Images

Mind over Platter

If you want to transform your three daily meals from mundane chores to life-enhancing experiences, you have to learn to eat with your mind as well as your mouth. When you bring your mind to the table, you are practicing basic principles of personal change: You are making conscious choices. You are doing what's best for you. You are taking control of your care and feeding. And you are adding another dimension of pleasure to your life.

Whatever your eating circumstances, you always have choices. Maybe you eat in the dining hall every day. Maybe you commute home for meals with your family. Maybe you're rushing to and from a job and wolfing down the fastest food you can find. (See Reality Check, p. 169.) Even when you feel you can't completely control what you eat, you can control how you eat. By working through "Mind over Platter" in *Labs for IPC*, you can learn to bring to your meals a sense of awareness and appreciation that can transform even an ordinary doughnut into something worth savoring. Here's a preview.

Get Real

Among other activities in this stage, you will monitor what you put in your mouth for three days (including one weekend day) and record what you eat as well as when, where, and how (standing by a vending machine, sitting at the kitchen table with your husband, lying on your bed and watching a game, etc.). Include coffee, soda, the nibbles you took from your friend's dessert. You will analyze your food diary by answering several questions, including:

- If we are what we eat, what does you food log say about you?
- Are you a junk food junkie? A nonstop grazer? A breakfast skipper? A speed eater? A nocturnal nosher?

Get Ready

In this preparatory stage, you will plan and purchase specific foods and find time and a place to eat them. If your idea of a meal is inhaling some ramen noodles at your desk or munching on a pita on the way to class, you will need to make meals more of a time priority . . .

Get Going

The action stage of this lab includes activities on building bite awareness, mastering the mindful bite, and taste testing, as well as the exercises we call "The Mindful Doughnut" and "The Mindful Meal." However, our favorite is "Mindful Indulgence." Rather than banishing a particular food from your plate, you limit the amount you eat to four bites, which can deliver the maximum taste sensation.

If you're a chocoholic, for instance, mindful eating can take you to a new level of appreciation. Here's how:

- Go for quality. Buy a piece or two of handmade or gourmet chocolate rather than the biggest chocolate bar the supermarket sells.
- Set aside time to savor the chocolate. Enjoy the anticipation . . . Don't multitask or even watch television while you're eating it.
- Don't chew the chocolate. Put a piece in your mouth, and let it melt. Make each piece last at least 90 seconds . . .

Lock it In

In this stage, you will learn how to maintain mindfulness by exercises such as trying one new taste every week. The reason: When people try a new food, they generally "sample" the food by taking a very small piece and chewing it slowly but shallowly. This natural taste testing engages all the senses because . . .

---

ounce and a half of cheddar cheese provide about 300 mg of calcium, but the milk offers the same amount of calcium for half the calories. Foods that are extremely low in nutrient density—such as potato chips, candy, and soft drinks—deliver only calories. Fruits and vegetables are nutrient-dense foods that provide many health benefits. (The Self Survey on page 201 can help you evaluate how healthy your diet is.)

Calories

Calories are the measure of the amount of energy that can be derived from food. How many calories you need depends on your gender, age, body-frame size, weight, percentage of body fat, and your **basal metabolic rate** (BMR)—the number of calories needed to sustain your body at rest. Your activity level also affects your calorie requirements. Regardless of whether you consume fat, protein, or carbohydrates, if you take in more calories than required to maintain your size and don't work them off in some sort of physical activity, your body will convert the excess to fat (see Chapter 7). On average, daily calorie needs are:

- Most women, some older adults, children ages two to six: 1,600
- Average adult: 2,000
- Most men, active women, teenage girls, older children: 2,200
- Active men, teenage boys: 2,800

essential nutrients Nutrients that the body cannot manufacture for itself and must obtain from food.

macronutrients Nutrients required by the human body in the greatest amounts, including water, carbohydrates, proteins, and fats.

calorie The amount of energy required to raise the temperature of 1 gram of water by 1 degree Celsius. In everyday usage related to the energy content of foods and the energy expended in activities, a calorie is actually the equivalent of a thousand such calories, or a kilocalorie.

micronutrients Vitamins and minerals needed by the body in very small amounts.

basal metabolic rate (BMR) The number of calories required to sustain your body at rest.

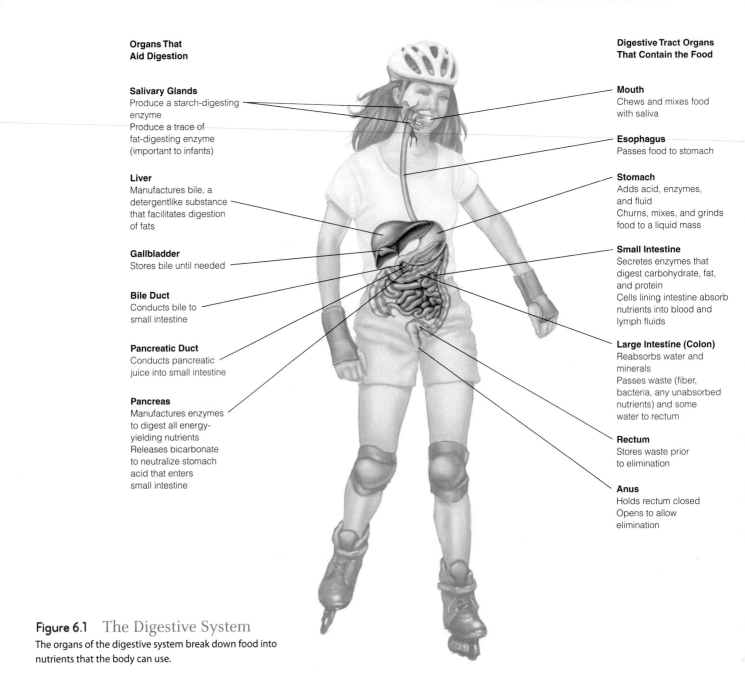

Organs That Aid Digestion

Salivary Glands
Produce a starch-digesting enzyme
Produce a trace of fat-digesting enzyme (important to infants)

Liver
Manufactures bile, a detergentlike substance that facilitates digestion of fats

Gallbladder
Stores bile until needed

Bile Duct
Conducts bile to small intestine

Pancreatic Duct
Conducts pancreatic juice into small intestine

Pancreas
Manufactures enzymes to digest all energy-yielding nutrients
Releases bicarbonate to neutralize stomach acid that enters small intestine

Digestive Tract Organs That Contain the Food

Mouth
Chews and mixes food with saliva

Esophagus
Passes food to stomach

Stomach
Adds acid, enzymes, and fluid
Churns, mixes, and grinds food to a liquid mass

Small Intestine
Secretes enzymes that digest carbohydrate, fat, and protein
Cells lining intestine absorb nutrients into blood and lymph fluids

Large Intestine (Colon)
Reabsorbs water and minerals
Passes waste (fiber, bacteria, any unabsorbed nutrients) and some water to rectum

Rectum
Stores waste prior to elimination

Anus
Holds rectum closed
Opens to allow elimination

Figure 6.1 The Digestive System
The organs of the digestive system break down food into nutrients that the body can use.

Water

Water, which makes up 85 percent of blood, 70 percent of muscles, and about 75 percent of the brain, performs many essential functions: It carries nutrients, maintains temperature, lubricates joints, helps with digestion, rids the body of waste through urine, and contributes to the production of sweat, which evaporates from the skin to cool the body. Research has correlated high fluid intake with a lower risk of kidney stones, colon cancer, and bladder cancer.

However, while water may indeed produce many benefits, researchers have found little scientific evidence to support the recommendation of eight glasses a day for healthy people.[1] (See Chapter 19 for a discussion of bottled water.)

You lose about 64 to 80 ounces of water a day—the equivalent of eight to ten 8-ounce glasses—through perspiration, urination, bowel movements, and normal exhalation. You lose water more rapidly if you exercise, live in a dry climate or at a high altitude, drink a lot of caffeine or alcohol (which increase urination), skip a meal, or become ill. To assure adequate water intake, nutritionists advise drinking enough so that your urine is not dark in color. Healthy individuals can get adequate hydration from beverages other than plain water, including juice.

Protein

Critical for growth and repair, **proteins** form the basic framework for our muscles, bones, blood, hair, and fingernails. Supplying 4 calories per gram, they are made of combinations of 20 **amino acids,** 9 of which we must get from our diet because the human body cannot produce them. These are called *essential amino acids.*

Animal proteins—meat, fish, poultry, and dairy products—are **complete proteins** that provide the nine essential amino acids. Not all protein sources are equally healthful. Diets high in red or processed meat may increase the risk of cancer, heart disease, Alzheimer's, and other conditions and shorten the lifespan.[2] Grains, dry beans, and nuts are **incomplete proteins** that may have relatively low levels of one or two essential amino acids but fairly high levels of others. Combining incomplete proteins, such as beans and rice, ensures that the body gets sufficient protein. The recommended level of daily protein intake is 0.8 gram per kilogram of body weight for adults.

Carbohydrates

Carbohydrates are organic compounds that provide our brains and bodies with *glucose,* their basic fuel. The major sources of carbohydrates are plants—including grains, vegetables, fruits, and beans—and milk. There are two types: *simple carbohydrates* (sugars) and *complex carbohydrates* (starches and fiber). All provide 4 calories per gram. Both adults and children should consume at least 130 grams of carbohydrates each day, the minimum needed to produce enough glucose for the brain to function.

Forms of Carbohydrates Simple carbohydrates include *natural sugars,* such as the lactose in milk and the fructose in fruit, and *added sugars* that are found in candy, soft drinks, fruit drinks, pastries, and other sweets. Those whose diets are higher in added sugars typically have lower intakes of other essential nutrients.

On average Americans consume more than 20 teaspoons of sweet calories a day. Some come from the teaspoons of sucrose (simple sugar) you add to coffee or tea. But many come from high-fructose corn syrup, a common sweetener and preservative made by changing the sugar glucose in cornstarch

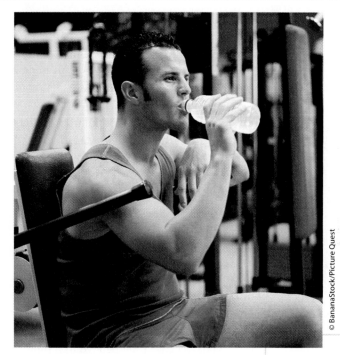

© BananaStock/Picture Quest

Be sure to get an adequate supply of water whenever and wherever you exercise.

to fructose. Because it extends the shelf life of processed foods and is cheaper than sugar, high-fructose corn syrup has become a popular ingredient in many sodas, fruit-flavored drinks, and other processed foods.[3]

High-fructose corn syrup isn't intrinsically less healthy than other sweeteners. However, it makes beverages very sweet, which may increase consumption and contribute to obesity and other health problems. With some people, this syrup accounts for 10 percent of daily calorie intake.[4]

Complex carbohydrates include grains, cereals, vegetables, beans, and nuts. Americans get most of their complex carbohydrates from refined grains, which have been stripped of fiber and many nutrients, in breads and desserts.[5]

Far more nutritious are whole grains, which are made up of all components of the grain: the *bran* (or fiber-rich outer layer), the *endosperm* (middle layer), and the *germ* (the nutrient-packed inner layer). Whole grains have proven effective in lowering the risk of diabetes and heart disease. Yet only 8 percent

proteins Organic compounds composed of amino acids; one of the essential nutrients.

amino acids Organic compounds containing nitrogen, carbon, hydrogen, and oxygen; the essential building blocks of proteins.

complete proteins Proteins that contain all the amino acids needed by the body for growth and maintenance.

incomplete proteins Proteins that lack one or more of the amino acids essential for protein synthesis.

carbohydrates Organic compounds, such as starches, sugars, and glycogen, that are composed of carbon, hydrogen, and oxygen, and are sources of bodily energy.

simple carbohydrates Sugars; like all carbohydrates, they provide the body with glucose.

complex carbohydrates Starches, including cereals, fruits, and vegetables.

PART 2: *Just the Facts*
• **35** *percent of college men and* **42** *percent of women feel they don't have time for a "social" meal.*
• **50** *percent of men and* **59** *percent of women tend to eat on the run.*

Source: Larson, N.I., et al. "Making Time for Meals: Meal Structure and Associations with Dietary Intake in Young Adults." *Journal of the American Dietetics Association*, Vol. 109, No. 1, January 2009, pp. 72–79.

of American adults consume three or more servings of whole grains; 42 percent eat no whole grains on a given day. One excellent source: popcorn. Popcorn eaters have higher intakes of fiber and other nutrients.[6]

Low-Carb Foods The popularity of diets that restrict carbohydrate intake, discussed in Chapter 7, prompted an explosion in products touted as "low-carb." You can get low-carb versions of everything from beer to bread. However, the Food and Drug Administration (FDA), which regulates health claims on food labels in the United States, hasn't defined what "low-carb" means. Words like "low-carb," "carb-wise," or "carb-free" are marketing terms created by manufacturers to sell their products.

Although many people may buy low-carb foods because they believe that they're healthier, that isn't necessarily the case. A low-carb nutrition bar, for instance, may be high in saturated fat and calories. Some low-carb food products cause digestive symptoms because food companies often replace the carbohydrates in a cookie or cracker with substances such as the sweetener sorbitol, which can cause diarrhea or stomach cramps.

Dieters often buy low-carb products in order to lose weight. According to proponents of low-carb diets, if carbohydrates raise blood sugar and insulin levels and cause weight gain, a decrease in carbs should result in lower blood sugar and insulin levels—and weight loss. With limited carbohydrates in the diet, the body would break down fat to provide needed energy.

Some people do lose weight when they switch to low-carb foods, but the reasons are probably that they consume fewer calories, lose water weight, and have decreased appetite because of a buildup of ketones (a by-product of fat metabolism) in the blood. As discussed in Chapter 7, a low-carb diet can lead to fairly rapid weight loss but is no easier to maintain over the long run

than any other diet. A 20-year study found that diets low in carbohydrates but high in animal fat and protein do not increase the risk of type 2 diabetes in women.[7]

Fiber **Dietary fiber** is the nondigestible form of complex carbohydrates occurring naturally in plant foods, such as leaves, stems, skins, seeds, and hulls. **Functional fiber** consists of isolated, nondigestible carbohydrates that may be added to foods and that provide beneficial effects in humans. Total fiber is the sum of both.

The various forms of fiber enhance health in different ways: They slow the emptying of the stomach, which creates a feeling of fullness and aids weight control. They interfere with absorption of dietary fat and cholesterol, which lowers the risk of heart disease and stroke in both middle-aged and elderly individuals. In addition, fiber helps prevent constipation, diverticulosis (a painful inflammation of the bowel), and diabetes. The link between fiber and colon cancer is complex. Some studies have indicated that increased fiber intake reduces risk; others found no such correlation.

The Institute of Medicine has set recommendations for daily intake levels of total fiber (dietary plus functional fiber): 38 grams of total fiber for men and 25 grams for women. For men and women over 50 years of age, who consume less food, the recommendations are, respectively, 30 and 21 grams. The American Dietetic Association recommends 25 to 35 grams of dietary fiber a day, much more than the amount Americans typically consume.

Good fiber sources include wheat and corn bran (the outer layer); leafy greens; the skins of fruits and root vegetables; oats, beans, and barley; and the pulp, skin, and seeds of many vegetables and fruits, such as apples and strawberries (see Table 6.2). Because sudden increases in fiber can cause symptoms like bloating and gas, experts recommend gradually adding more fiber to your diet with an additional serving or two of vegetables, fruit, or whole-wheat bread.

Glycemic Index and Glycemic Load The glycemic index is a ranking of carbohydrates, gram for gram, based on their immediate effect on blood glucose (sugar) levels.

TABLE 6.2

High-Fiber Foods

Grains
Whole-grain products provide about 1 to 2 grams (or more) of fiber per serving:
• 1 slice whole-wheat, pumpernickel, rye bread
• 1 oz ready-to-eat cereal (100% bran cereals contain 10 grams or more)
• 1/2 cup cooked barley, bulgar, grits, oatmeal

Vegetables
Most vegetables contain about 2 to 3 grams of fiber per serving:
• 1 cup raw bean sprouts
• 1/2 cup cooked broccoli, Brussels sprouts, cabbage, carrots, cauliflower, collards, corn, eggplant, green beans, green peas, kale, mushrooms, okra, parsnips, potatoes, pumpkin, spinach, sweet potatoes, swiss chard, winter squash
• 1/2 cup chopped raw carrots, peppers

Fruits
Fresh, frozen, and dried fruits have about 2 grams of fiber per serving:
• 1 medium apple, banana, kiwi, nectarine, orange, pear
• 1/2 cup applesauce, blackberries, blueberries, raspberries, strawberries
Fruit juices contain very little fiber.

Legumes
Many legumes provide about 6 to 8 grams of fiber per serving:
• 1/2 cup cooked baked beans, black beans, black-eyes peas, kidney beans, navy beans, pinto beans
Some legumes provide about 5 grams of fiber per serving:
• 1/2 cup cooked garbanzo beans, great northern beans, lentils, lima beans, split peas

Carbohydrates that break down quickly during digestion and trigger a fast, high glucose response have the highest glycemic index rating. Those that break down slowly, releasing glucose gradually into the bloodstream, have low glycemic index ratings. Potatoes, which raise blood sugar higher and faster than apples, for instance, earn a higher glycemic index rating than apples. Glycemic index does not account for the amount of food you typically eat in a serving.

Glycemic load is a measure of how much a typical serving size of a particular food raises blood glucose. For example, the glycemic index of table sugar is high, but you use so little to sweeten your coffee or tea that its glycemic load is low.

Some diets are based on the theory that high glycemic index foods raise blood sugar and insulin levels and cause weight gain, while low glycemic index foods lower your blood sugar and insulin levels so you'll lose weight. (See Chapter 7.)

Fats

Fats carry the fat-soluble vitamins A, D, E, and K; aid in their absorption in the intestine;

protect organs from injury; regulate body temperature; and play an important role in growth and development. They provide 9 calories per gram—more than twice the amount in carbohydrates or proteins.

Both high- and low-fat diets can be unhealthy. When people eat very low levels of fat and very high levels of carbohydrates, their levels of high-density lipoprotein, the so-called *good cholesterol*, decline. On the other hand, high-fat diets can lead to obesity and its related health dangers, discussed in Chapter 7.

Forms of Fat Saturated fats and unsaturated fats are distinguished by the type of fatty acids in their chemical structures. Unsaturated fats can be divided into monounsaturated or polyunsaturated, again depending on their chemical structure. All dietary fats are a mix of saturated and unsaturated fats but are predominantly one or the other. Unsaturated fats, like oils, are likely to be liquid at room temperature and saturated fats, like butter, are likely to be solid. In general, vegetable and fish oils are unsaturated,

dietary fiber The nondigestible form of carbohydrates found in plant foods, such as leaves, stems, skins, seeds, and hulls.

functional fiber Isolated, nondigestible carbohydrates with beneficial effects in humans.

saturated fats A chemical term indicating that a fat molecule contains as many hydrogen atoms as its carbon skeleton can hold. These fats are normally solid at room temperature.

unsaturated fats A chemical term indicating that a fat molecule contains fewer hydrogen atoms than its carbon skeleton can hold. These fats are normally liquid at room temperature.

TABLE 6.3

Major Sources of Various Fatty Acids

Healthful Fatty Acids

Monounsaturated	Polyunsaturated	Omega-3 Polyunsaturated
Avocado	Margarine (nonhydrogenated)	Fatty fish (herring, mackerel, salmon, tuna)
Oils (canola, olive, peanut, sesame)	Oils (corn, cottonseed, safflower, soybean)	Flaxseed
Nuts (almonds, cashews, filberts, hazelnuts, macadamia nuts, peanuts, pecans, pistachios)	Nuts (pine nuts, walnuts)	Nuts (walnuts)
Olives	Mayonnaise	
Peanut butter	Salad dressing	
Seeds (sesame)	Seeds (pumpkin, sunflower)	

Unhealthful Fatty Acids

Saturated	Trans
Bacon	Fried foods (hydrogenated shortening)
Butter	Margarine (hydrogenated or partially hydrogenated)
Chocolate	
Coconut	Nondairy creamers
Cream cheese	Many fast foods
Cream, half-and-half	Shortening
Lard	Commercial baked goods (including doughnuts, cakes, cookies)
Meat	
Milk and milk products (whole)	Many snack foods (including microwave popcorn, chips, crackers)
Oils (coconut, palm, palm kernel)	
Shortening	
Sour cream	

©Tim Hill/Alamy

and animal fats are saturated. Table 6.3 lists the major sources of healthful monounsaturated and polyunsaturated fats.

Olive, soybean, canola, cottonseed, corn, and other vegetable oils are unsaturated fats. Olive oil is considered a good fat and one of the best vegetable oils for salads and cooking. Used for thousands of years, this staple of the Mediterranean diet (discussed later in this chapter) has been correlated with a lower incidence of heart disease, including strokes and heart attacks.

Omega-3 and omega-6 are polyunsaturated fatty acids with slightly different chemical compositions. Regular consumption of omega-3 fatty acids, found in fatty fish such as salmon and sardines, flaxseed, walnuts, and canola oil, helps to prevent blood clots, protect against irregular heartbeats, and lower blood pressure, especially among people with high blood pressure or atherosclerosis. Omega-6 fatty acids are found in vegetable oils, nuts, seeds, meat, poultry, and eggs. The recommended ratio for consumption of omega-6 and omega-3 fatty acids is 6 to 1.

Some fish, such as mackerel, shark, tilefish, tuna, and swordfish, contain potentially harmful levels of mercury. To balance the benefits and risks of eating fish, the American Heart Association recommends two servings of fish a week, although even a single fish meal a month may be beneficial. Nutritionists do not advise fish oil supplements as a source of omega-3 fatty acids because high intake may increase bleeding time, interfere with wound healing, and suppress immune function.

Saturated fats can increase the risk of heart disease and should be avoided as much as possible. In response to consumer and health professionals' demand for less saturated fat in the food supply, many manufacturers switched to partially hydrogenated oils.

The process of hydrogenation creates unsaturated fatty acids called **trans fat.** They are found in some margarine products and most foods made with partially hydrogenated oils, such as baked goods and fried foods. Even though trans fats are unsaturated, they have an even more harmful effect on cholesterol than saturated fats because they

Butter

Nutrition Facts
Serving Size 1 Tbsp (14g)
Servings per container about 32

Amount per serving

Calories 100 Calories from Fat 100

%Daily Value*

Total Fat 11g	17%
Saturated Fat 7g	37%
Trans Fat 0g	
Cholesterol 30mg	10%
Sodium 95mg	4%
Total Carbohydrate 0g	0%
Protein 0g	

Vitamin A 8%

Not a significant source of dietary fiber, sugars, vitamin C, calcium, and iron.

*Percent Daily Values are based on a 2,000 calorie diet.

INGREDIENTS: Cream, salt.

Margarine (stick)

Nutrition Facts
Serving Size 1 Tbsp (14g)
Servings per container about 32

Amount per serving

Calories 100 Calories from Fat 100

%Daily Value*

Total Fat 11g	17%
Saturated Fat 2g	11%
Trans Fat 2.5g	
Polyunsaturated Fat 3.5g	
Monounsaturated Fat 2.5g	
Cholesterol 0mg	0%
Sodium 105mg	4%
Total Carbohydrate 0g	0%
Protein 0g	

Vitamin A 10%

Not a significant source of dietary fiber, sugars, vitamin C, calcium, and iron.

*Percent Daily Values are based on a 2,000 calorie diet.

INGREDIENTS: Liquid soybean oil, partially hydrogenated soybean oil, water, buttermilk, salt, soy lecithin, sodium benzoate (as a preservative), vegetable mono and diglycerides, artificial flavor, vitamin A palmitate, colored with beta carotene (provitamin A).

Margarine (tub)

Nutrition Facts
Serving size 1 Tbsp (14g)
Servings per container about 32

Amount per serving

Calories 100 Calories from Fat 100

%Daily Value*

Total Fat 11g	17%
Saturated Fat 2.5g	13%
Trans Fat 2g	
Polyunsaturated Fat 4g	
Monounsaturated Fat 2.5g	
Cholesterol 0mg	0%
Sodium 80mg	3%
Total Carbohydrate 0g	0%
Protein 0g	

Vitamin A 10%

Not a significant source of dietary fiber, sugars, vitamin C, calcium, and iron.

*Percent Daily Values are based on a 2,000 calorie diet.

INGREDIENTS: Liquid soybean oil, partially hydrogenated soybean oil, buttermilk, water, butter (cream, salt), salt, soy lecithin, vegetable mono and diglycerides, sodium benzoate added as a preservative, artificial flavor, vitamin A palmitate, colored with beta carotene.

Margarine (liquid)

Nutrition Facts
Serving size 1 Tbsp (14g)
Servings per container about 24

Amount per serving

Calories 70   Calories from Fat 70

%Daily Value*

Total Fat 8g	13%
Saturated Fat 1.5g	7%
Trans Fat 0g	
Polyunsaturated Fat 4.5g	
Monounsaturated Fat 2g	
Cholesterol 0mg	0%
Sodium 110mg	8%
Total Carbohydrate 0g	0%
Protein 0g	

Vitamin A 10%

Not a significant source of dietary fiber, sugars, vitamin C, calcium, and iron.

*Percent Daily Values are based on a 2,000 calorie diet.

INGREDIENTS: Liquid soybean oil, water, salt, hydrogenated cottonseed oil, vegetable monoglycerides and soy lecithin (emulsifiers), potassium sorbate and sodium benzoate (to preserve freshness), artificial flavor, phosphoric acid (acidulant), colored with beta carotene (source of vitamin A), vitamin A palmitate.

Figure 6.2   Butter or Margarine?
Most of the fat in butter is saturated fat. Most of the fat in margarine is unsaturated, but the trans fats are twice as damaging as saturated fat. (If the list of ingredients includes hydrogenated oils, you know the food contains trans fat. The closer "partially hydrogenated oils" is to the beginning of the ingredients list, the more trans fats the product contains.)

increase harmful LDL and, in large amounts, decrease helpful HDL. Epidemiological studies have suggested a possible link between cardiovascular disease risk and high intakes of trans fats, and researchers have concluded that they are, gram for gram, twice as damaging as saturated fats. There is no safe level for trans fats, which occur naturally in meats as well as in foods prepared with partially hydrogenated vegetable oils.

Some food manufacturers have reduced or eliminated trans fats in snacks and other products. Cities and communities across the country have banned trans fats in restaurants. Some campuses also have stopped using trans fats in their dining halls and food outlets.

To cut down on both saturated and trans fats, choose soybean, canola, corn, olive, safflower, and sunflower oils, which are naturally free of trans fats and lower in saturated fats—see Table 6.3. Look for reduced-fat, low-fat, fat-free, and trans-fat-free versions of baked goods, snacks, and other processed foods. Some choices—such as butter versus margarine—are more difficult to make (see Figure 6.2).

trans fat   Fat formed when liquid vegetable oils are processed to make table spreads or cooking fats; also found in dairy and beef products; considered to be especially dangerous dietary fats.

Vegetables and fruits are rich in antioxidants. By eating an orange at breakfast and half a carrot for lunch, you will get all the antioxidants you need for the day.

Vitamins and Minerals

Vitamins, which help put proteins, fats, and carbohydrates to use, are essential to regulating growth, maintaining tissue, and releasing energy from foods. Together with the enzymes in the body, they help produce the right chemical reactions at the right times. They're also involved in the manufacture of blood cells, hormones, and other compounds.

The body produces some vitamins, such as vitamin D, which is manufactured in the skin after exposure to sunlight. Other vitamins must be ingested.

Vitamins A, D, E, and K are fat-soluble; they are absorbed through the intestinal membranes and stored in the body.

© FoodPix/Jupiterimages

Vitamin D Vitamin D, which we get from sunlight as well as from fortified milk, eggs, liver, and sardines, aids in the absorption of calcium and helps to form and maintain strong bones. According to recent research, Vitamin D might help protect against osteoporosis, high blood pressure, colon cancer, diabetes, and several autoimmune diseases.[8] However, in the large-scale Women's Health Initiative, calcium and vitamin D supplements did not reduce postmenopausal women's risk of breast cancer[9] or high blood pressure.[10]

Many Americans of all ages, including those living in sunny places like southern California, are not getting enough of this important vitamin. Vitamin D deficiency, epidemiologists say, has reached epidemic proportions. A vitamin D deficit may contribute to low bone mineral density and increased risk of fractures and cognitive impairment in the elderly.[11] Low vitamin D levels also have been linked with Parkinson disease, stroke risk, and exacerbation of multiple sclerosis.[12]

Vitamin D may play a role in regulating weight and muscle strength. In one study of college-age young women (average age 19), those with too little vitamin D were heavier, weighing about 16 pounds more than those with adequate vitamin D intake. The researchers theorize that low vitamin D intake may be an independent predictor of obesity.[13] In another study of adolescent girls' muscle power and force, those lacking in vitamin D scored lower than others.[14]

The B vitamins and vitamin C are water-soluble; they are absorbed directly into the blood and then used up or washed out of the body in urine and sweat. They must be replaced daily. Table 6.4 summarizes key information about the vitamins.

Antioxidants **Antioxidants** prevent the harmful effects caused by oxidation within the body. They include vitamins C, E, and beta-carotene (a form of vitamin A), as well as compounds like carotenoids and flavonoids. All share a common enemy: renegade oxygen cells called free radicals released by normal metabolism as well as by pollution, smoking, radiation, and stress.

Diets high in antioxidant-rich fruits and vegetables have been linked with lower rates of esophageal, lung, colon, and stomach cancer. Nevertheless, scientific studies have not proved conclusively that any specific antioxidant, particularly in supplement form, can prevent cancer.

Minerals Carbon, oxygen, hydrogen, and nitrogen make up 96 percent of our body weight. The other 4 percent consists of **minerals** that help build bones and teeth, aid in muscle function, and help our nervous systems transmit messages. Every day we need about a tenth of a gram (100 milligrams) or more of the major minerals: sodium, potassium chloride, calcium, phosphorus, magnesium, and sulfur. We also need about a hundredth of a gram (10 milligrams) or less of each of the trace minerals: iron (although premenopausal women need more), zinc, selenium, molybdenum, iodine, copper, manganese, fluoride, and chromium. (See Table 6.5 for key information on minerals.)

Calcium Calcium, the most abundant mineral in the body, builds strong bone tissue throughout life and plays a vital role in blood clotting and muscle and nerve functioning. Pregnant or nursing women need more calcium to meet the additional needs of their babies' bodies. Calcium may also help control

vitamins Organic substances that are needed in very small amounts by the body and carry out a variety of functions in metabolism and nutrition.

antioxidants Substances that prevent the damaging effects of oxidation in cells.

minerals Naturally occurring inorganic substances, small amounts of some being essential in metabolism and nutrition.

TABLE 6.4

Key Information about Vitamins

Fat-Soluble Vitamins

Vitamin/Recommended Intake per Day	Significant Sources	Chief Functions	Signs of Severe, Prolonged Deficiency	Signs of Extreme Excess
Vitamin A Males 19–50: 900 µg RAE Females 19–50: 700 µg RAE	Fortified milk, cheese, cream, butter, fortified margarine, eggs, liver, spinach and other dark leafy greens, broccoli, deep orange fruits (apricots, cantaloupes), and vegetables (carrots, sweet potatoes, pumpkins)	Antioxidant; needed for vision, health of cornea, epithelial cells, mucous membranes, skin health, bone and tooth growth, reproduction, immunity, regulation of gene expression	Cracks in teeth, tendency toward tooth decay, night blindness, keratinization, corneal degeneration	Overstimulated cell division, skin rashes, hair loss, hemorrhage, bone abnormalities, birth defects, fractures, liver failure, death
Vitamin D Adults 19–50: 5 µg 51–70 years: 10 µg >70 years: 15 µg	Exposure to sunlight; fortified milk or margarine, eggs, liver, sardines	Mineralization of bones and teeth (promotes calcium and phosphorus absorption)	Abnormal growth, misshapen bones (bowing of legs), soft bones, joint pain, malformed teeth, muscle spasms	Raised blood calcium, excessive thirst, headaches, irritability, weakness, nausea, kidney stones, deposits in arteries
Vitamin E Males 19–50: 15 mg Females 19–50: 15 mg	Polyunsaturated plant oils (margarine, salad dressings, shortenings), green and leafy vegetables, wheat germ, whole-grain products, nuts, seeds	Antioxidant; needed for stabilization of cell membranes, regulation of oxidation reactions	Red blood cell breakage, anemia, muscle degeneration, difficulty walking, leg cramps, nerve damage	Augments the effects of anticlotting medication; general discomfort; blurred vision
Vitamin K Males 19–50: 120 µg Females 19–50: 90 µg	Green leafy vegetables, cabbage-type vegetables, soybeans, vegetable oils	Synthesis of blood-clotting proteins and proteins important in bone mineralization	Hemorrhage, abnormal bone formation	Interference with anticlotting medication

Water-Soluble Vitamins

Vitamin/Recommended Intake per Day	Significant Sources	Chief Functions	Signs of Severe, Prolonged Deficiency	Signs of Extreme Excess
Vitamin B$_6$ Males 19–50: 1.3 mg Females 19–50: 1.3 mg	Meats, fish, poultry, liver, legumes, fruits, whole grains, potatoes, soy products	Part of a coenzyme used in amino acid and fatty acid metabolism, helps make red blood cells	Anemia, depression, abnormal brain wave pattern, convulsions, skin rashes	Impaired memory, depression, irritability, headaches, numbness, damage to nerves, difficulty walking, loss of reflexes
Vitamin B$_{12}$ Males 19–50: 2.4 µg Females 19–50: 2.4 µg	Animal products (meat, fish, poultry, milk, cheese, eggs), fortified cereals	Part of a coenzyme used in new cell synthesis, helps maintain nerve cells	Anemia, nervous system degeneration progressing to paralysis, fatigue, memory loss, disorientation	None reported
Vitamin C Males 19–50: 90 mg Females 19–50: 75 mg Smokers: +35 mg	Citrus fruits, cabbage-type vegetables, dark green vegetables, cantaloupe, strawberries, peppers, lettuce, tomatoes, potatoes, papayas, mangoes	Antioxidant, collagen synthesis (strengthens blood vessel walls, forms scar tissue, matrix for bone growth), amino aid metabolism, strengthens resistance to infection, aids iron absorption, restores vitamin E to active form	Anemia, pinpoint hemorrhages, frequent infections, bleeding gums, loosened teeth, bone fragility, joint pain, blotchy bruises, failure of wounds to heal	Nausea, abdominal cramps, diarrhea, headache, fatigue, rashes, interference with drug therapies and medical tests
Thiamin Males 19–50: 1.2 mg Females 19–50: 1.1 mg	Pork, ham, bacon, liver, whole grains, legumes, nuts; occurs in all nutritious foods in moderate amounts	Part of a coenzyme used in energy metabolism, supports normal appetite and nervous system function	Beriberi, edema, enlarged heart, nervous/muscular system degeneration, difficulty walking, loss of reflexes, mental confusion	None reported

) TABLE 6.4

Key Information about Vitamins, continued

Vitamin/Recommended Intake per Day	Significant Sources	Chief Functions	Signs of Severe, Prolonged Deficiency	Signs of Extreme Excess
Riboflavin Males 19–50: 1.3 mg Females 19–50: 1.1 mg	Milk, yogurt, cottage cheese, meat, leafy green vegetables, whole-grain or enriched breads and cereals	Part of a coenzyme used in energy metabolism, supports normal vision and skin health	Cracks at corner of mouth, magenta tongue, hypersensitivity to light, reddening of cornea, skin rash, sore throat	None reported
Niacin Males 19–50: 16 mg NE Females 19–50: 14 mg NE	Meat, poultry, fish, whole-grain and enriched breads and cereals, nuts, and all protein-containing foods	Part of a coenzyme used in energy metabolism	Diarrhea, black smooth tongue, irritability, loss of appetite, weakness, dizziness, mental confusion, flaky skin rash on areas exposed to sun	Nausea, vomiting, painful flush and rash, sweating, liver damage, blurred vision, impaired glucose tolerance
Folate Males 19–50: 400 μg Females 19–50: 400 μg	Leafy green vegetables, legumes, seeds, liver, enriched breads, cereal, pasta, and grains	Part of a coenzyme needed for new cell synthesis	Anemia, heartburn, frequent infections, smooth red tongue, depression, mental confusion	Masks vitamin B_{12} deficiency
Pantothenic acid Males 19–50: 5 mg Females 19–50: 5 mg	Widespread in foods	Part of a coenzyme used in energy metabolism	Vomiting, intestinal distress, insomnia, fatigue, increased sensitivity to insulin	None reported
Biotin Males 19–50: 30 μg Females 19–50: 30 μg	Widespread in foods	Used in energy metabolism, fat synthesis, amino acid metabolism, and glycogen synthesis	Abnormal heart action, loss of appetite, nausea, depression, muscle pain, drying of facial skin	None reported

Source: Adapted from Sizer, Frances, and Ellie Whitney, *Nutrition: Concepts and Controversies,* 10th ed. Belmont, CA: Wadsworth, 2006.

) TABLE 6.5

Key Information about Minerals

Mineral	Significant Sources	Chief Functions	Signs of Severe, Prolonged Deficiency	Signs of Extreme Excess
Sodium	Salt, soy sauce, processed foods	Needed to maintain fluid balance and acid-base balance in body cells; critical to nerve impulse transmission	Mental apathy, poor appetite, muscle cramps	High blood pressure, edema
Potassium	All whole foods: meats, milk, fruits, vegetables, grains, legumes	Needed to maintain fluid balance and acid-base balance in body cells; needed for muscle and nerve activity	Muscle weakness, mental confusion, paralysis	Muscle weakness, irregular heartbeat, heart attacks, vomiting
Chloride	Salt, soy sauce, processed foods	Aids in digestion; needed to maintain fluid balance and acid-base balance in body cells	Does not occur under normal circumstances	Vomiting
Calcium	Milk and milk products, oysters, small fish (with bones), tofu, greens, legumes	Component of bones and teeth, needed for muscle and nerve activity, blood clotting	Stunted growth and weak bones in children, adult bone loss (osteoporosis)	Constipation; calcium deposits in kidneys, liver; decreased absorption of other minerals

TABLE 6.5

Key Information about Minerals, continued

Mineral	Significant Sources	Chief Functions	Signs of Severe, Prolonged Deficiency	Signs of Extreme Excess
Phosphorus	All animal tissues, milk and milk products, legumes	Component of bones and teeth, energy metabolism, needed to maintain cell membranes	Muscle weakness, impaired growth, bone pain	Calcification of soft tissue, particularly the kidneys
Magnesium	Nuts, legumes, whole grains, dark green vegetables, seafoods, chocolate, cocoa	Component of bones and teeth, nerve activity, energy and protein formation, immune function	Stunted growth in children, weakness, muscle spasms, personality changes, hallucinations	From nonfood sources: diarrhea, dehydration, pH imbalance
Sulfate	All protein-containing foods	Component of certain amino acids; stabilizes protein shape	None known; protein deficiency would occur first	None reported
Trace Minerals				
Iron	Red meats, fish, poultry, shellfish, eggs, legumes, dried fruits	Aids in transport of oxygen, component of myoglobin, energy metabolism	Anemia, weakness, fatigue, pale appearance, reduced attention span, developmental delays in children	Vomiting, abdominal pain, blue coloration of skin, shock, organ damage
Zinc	Protein-containing foods: fish, shellfish, poultry, grains, vegetables	Protein reproduction, component of insulin, activates many enzymes, transport of vitamin A	Growth failure, delayed sexual maturation, slow wound healing	Loss of appetite, impaired immunity, reduced copper and iron absorption, fatigue, metallic taste in mouth
Selenium	Meats and seafood, eggs, grains	Acts as an antioxidant in conjunction with vitamin E, regulates thyroid hormone	Anemia, heart failure	Hair and fingernail loss, weakness, skin rash, garlic or metallic breath
Molybdenum	Dried beans, grains, dark green vegetables, liver, milk and milk products	Aids in oxygen transfer from one molecule to another	Unknown	None reported
Iodine	Iodized salt, seaweed, seafood, bread	Component of thyroid hormones that helps regulate energy production and growth	Goiter, cretinism in newborns (mental retardation, hearing loss, growth failure)	Pimples, goiter, decreased thyroid function
Copper	Organ meats, whole grains, nuts and seeds, seafood, drinking water	Helps to form hemoglobin and collagen, component of enzymes involved in the body's utilization of iron and oxygen	Anemia, nerve and bone abnormalities in children, growth retardation	From nonfood sources: vomiting, diarrhea, liver disease
Manganese	Whole grains, coffee, tea, dried beans, nuts	Formation of body fat and bone	Rare	Infertility in men, disruptions in the nervous system, muscle spasms
Fluoride	Fluoridated water, foods, and beverages; tea; shrimp; crab	Component of bones and teeth (enamel), confers decay resistance on teeth	Tooth decay and other dental diseases	Fluorosis, brittle bones, mottled teeth, vomiting, diarrhea, chest pain
Chromium	Whole grains, liver, meat, beer, wine	Glucose utilization	Poor blood glucose control, weight loss	None reported

Source: Adapted from Brown, Judith E. *Nutrition Now,* 4th ed. Belmont, CA: Wadsworth, 2002; Sizer, Frances, and Ellie Whitney. *Nutrition: Concepts and Controversies,* 10th ed. Belmont, CA: Wadsworth, 2006.

high blood pressure, prevent colon cancer in adults, and promote weight loss. Adequate calcium and vitamin D intake during childhood, adolescence, and young adulthood is crucial to prevent osteoporosis, the bone-weakening disease that strikes one of every four women over the age of 60.

 National health organizations are promoting greater calcium consumption among college students, particularly women, to increase bone density and safeguard against osteoporosis. In both men and women, bone mass peaks between the ages of 25 and 35. Over the next 10 to 15 years, bone mass remains fairly stable. At about age 40, bone loss equivalent to 0.3 to 0.5 percent per year begins in both men and women. Women may experience greater bone loss, at a rate of 3 to 5 percent, at the time of menopause. This decline continues for approximately five to seven years and is the primary factor leading to post-menopausal osteoporosis.

The higher an individual's peak bone mass, the longer it takes for age- and menopause-related bone loss to increase the risk of fractures. Osteoporosis is less common in groups with higher peak bone mass—men versus women, blacks versus whites.

Calcium is a special concern for African Americans who, as a group, have a higher risk for high blood pressure and obesity than the rest of the population but, on average, consume less than one serving of dairy foods a day. In fact, more than 80 percent of African Americans fail to get their daily recommended amount of calcium.

Calcium and vitamin D supplements in healthy postmenopausal women provide a modest benefit in preserving bone mass and preventing hip fractures, but do not prevent other types of fractures or colorectal cancer, according to the results of a major clinical trial, part of the Women's Health Initiative, which studied more than 36,000 women over age 50.[15] Others have questioned the value of calcium supplementation in younger adults and children as well. The benefits for teenage girls who took supplements were short-lived, with no lasting differences in bone density.[16] A combination of regular exercise, dietary calcium, and vitamin D may be the best prescription for building and preserving strong bones.

Sodium Sodium helps maintain proper fluid balance, regulates blood pressure, transmits muscle impulses, and relaxes muscles. Excess sodium isn't a problem for most healthy people, but for those who are sodium-sensitive—as many as 30 percent of the population—too much sodium contributes to high blood pressure.

The National Heart, Lung, and Blood Institute recommends less than 2.4 grams (2,400 milligrams) of sodium a day, the equivalent of about one teaspoon of table salt a day. For someone with high blood pressure, a daily intake of less than 1,500 mg of sodium is better for lowering blood pressure.

 African Americans, who have higher rates of high blood pressure and diseases related to hypertension, such as stroke and kidney failure, tend to be more sensitive to salt. African Americans also have lower intakes of calcium and potassium—both of which can protect against heart disease.

Phytochemicals **Phytochemicals,** compounds that exist naturally in plants, serve many functions, including helping a plant protect itself from bacteria and disease. Some phytochemicals such as solanine, an insect-repelling chemical found in the leaves and stalks of potato plants, are natural toxins, but many are beneficial to humans.

Phytochemicals give tomatoes their red color and hot peppers their "fire." In the body, they act as antioxidants, mimic hormones, and reduce the risk of various illnesses, including cancer and heart disease (see Table 6.6). Broccoli may contain as many as 10,000 different phytochemicals, each capable of influencing some action or organ in the body. Tomatoes provide lycopene, a powerful antioxidant that seems to offer protection against cancers of the esophagus, lungs, prostate, and stomach. Soybeans, a rich source of an array of phytochemicals, appear to slow the growth of breast and prostate cancer.

The flavonoids, a large group of health-promoting phytochemicals found in whole grains, legumes, vegetables, fruits, herbs, spices, teas, chocolate, nuts, olive oil, and red wine, may lower the risk of chronic disease and improve cardiovascular health. Dark chocolate is the richest source of these substances, which lower harmful cholesterol, boost healthful cholesterol, improve the function of the arteries, modestly reduce blood pressure, and help prevent blood clots.[17] Flavonoids also may benefit the brain. In a study of flavonoid-rich wine, tea, and chocolate in the elderly, wine had the greatest impact on improving cognitive test performance, while chocolate had a more modest effect.[18]

Americans get adequate amounts of most nutrients. However, the 2005 Advisory Committee for Dietary Guidelines reported that intakes of several nutrients are low enough to be of concern.

- **For adults:** vitamins A, C, and E, calcium, magnesium, potassium, and fiber.
- **For children:** vitamin E, calcium, magnesium, potassium, and fiber.

Are you getting enough of these nutrients?

Among the groups at highest risk of nutritional deficiencies are:

- **Teenage girls.**
- **Women of child-bearing age** (iron and folic acid).

phytochemicals Chemicals such as indoles, coumarins, and capsaicin, which exist naturally in plants and have disease-fighting properties.

> ### TABLE 6.6

An Array of Phytochemicals in a Variety of Fruits and Vegetables

Broccoli and broccoli sprouts contain an abundance of the cancer-fighting phytochemical sulforaphane.

An apple a day—rich in flavonoids—may protect against lung cancer.

The phytoestrogens of soybeans seem to starve cancer cells and inhibit tumor growth; the phytosterols may lower blood cholesterol and protect cardiac arteries.

Garlic, with its abundant organosulfur compounds, may lower blood cholesterol and protect against stomach cancer.

The phytochemical resveratrol found in grapes (and nuts) protects against cancer by inhibiting cell growth and against heart disease by limiting clot formation and inflammation.

The ellagic acid of strawberries may inhibit certain types of cancer.

Tomatoes, with their abundant lycopene, may defend against cancer by protecting DNA from oxidative damage.

The monoterpenes of citrus fruits (and cherries) may inhibit cancer growth.

The flavonoids in black tea may protect against heart disease, whereas those in green tea may defend against cancer.

The flavonoids in cocoa and chocolate defend against oxidation and reduce the tendency of blood to clot.

Spinach and other colorful vegetables contain the carotenoids lutein and zeaxanthin, which help protect the eyes against macular degeneration.

Flaxseed, the richest source of lignans, may prevent the spread of cancer.

Blueberries, a rich source of flavonoids, improve memory in animals.

- **Persons over age 50** (vitamin B_{12}).
- **The elderly, persons with dark skin**, and those who do not get adequate exposure to sunshine (vitamin D).[19]

Dietary Supplements

About two out of five Americans take a vitamin or mineral supplement regularly. Should you be among them? Or are you getting enough of the vitamins and minerals you need from your food? Despite intensive marketing of a host of supplements, large-scale studies have cast doubts on the benefits of many, especially antioxidants.

Multivitamin supplements, long believed to be beneficial, did not prevent cancer or heart disease in a recent eight-year study of more than 160,000 postmenopausal women. After controlling for age, physical activity, family history of cancer, and many other factors, supplements had no effect on the risk of breast cancer, colorectal cancer, endometrial cancer, lung cancer, ovarian cancer, heart attack, stroke, blood clots, or mortality. Individuals who are less well nourished than the study participants may benefit from supplements, but there is no convincing scientific evidence to justify routine use of dietary supplements by the general population.[20] The bottom-line recommendation: Buying more fruits and vegetables might be a better choice than spending money on multivitamins.[21]

In another study, supplements of vitamins C and E and beta-carotene had no impact on the cancer risk of middle-aged women.[22]

Selenium and vitamin E also failed to protect men from prostate cancer.[23]

Yet certain supplements may have an impact on the risk for certain conditions. Women over age 40 who took folic acid, vitamin B_6 and vitamin B_{12} were less likely than a control group to develop a severe visual disorder called age-related macular degeneration.[24]

High doses of vitamins carry potential risks. Certain antioxidants can interfere with the efficacy of cholesterol-lowering medications. High doses of vitamin E may increase the chances of earlier death. In cancer patients, those taking large doses had an increased risk of a new cancer.

In particular, the fat-soluble vitamins, primarily A and D, can build up in our bodies and cause serious complications, such as damage to the kidneys, liver, or bones. Large doses of water-soluble vitamins, including the B vitamins, may also be harmful. Excessive intake of vitamin B_6 (pyridoxine), often used to relieve premenstrual bloating, can cause neurological damage, such as numbness in the mouth and tingling in the hands. (An excessive amount in this case is 250 to 300 times the recommended dose.) High doses of vitamin C can produce stomachaches and diarrhea. Niacin, often taken in high doses to lower cholesterol, can cause jaundice, liver damage, and irregular heartbeats as well as severe, uncomfortable flushing of the skin.

If you do feel a need for vitamins, be sure not to exceed the recommended doses listed in Tables 6.4 and 6.5.

Eating Guidelines for Americans

Over the years various governmental and health agencies have made recommendations for what Americans should eat. The three most influential are the U.S. Department of Agriculture's MyPyramid, the National Heart, Lung, and Blood Institute's Dietary Approaches to Stop Hypertension (DASH) Eating Plan, and Harvard University's Healthy Eating Plan. According to a recent comparative analysis, the three guides,

derived from the same scientific research, are more similar than different and convey the same key messages: Eat more fruits, vegetables, legumes, and whole grains. Eat less added sugar and saturated fat. Choose plant oils over animal fats. However, the Harvard plan (discussed on page 185) recommends only a small amount of milk because of the calories and fat in most of the milk and milk products that Americans consume.

Using the MyPyramid Food Guidance System

Making healthy choices about what and how to eat isn't easy. However, the federal government is trying to help. In its most recent edition of *Nutrition and Your Health: Dietary Guidelines for Americans,* the U.S. Departments of Health and Human Services and of Agriculture provide science-based advice both to promote wellness and to reduce the risk of major chronic diseases. The MyPyramid Food Guidance System (Figure 6.3) translates the guidelines into a personalized, balanced, total diet.

The key themes of MyPyramid are:

- **Variety.** Eating foods from all food groups and subgroups.

- **Proportionality.** Eating more of some foods (fruits, vegetables, whole grains, fat-free or low-fat milk products) and less of others (foods high in saturated or trans fats, added sugars, cholesterol, salt, and alcohol). Critics of the new pyramid point out that the guidelines still do not take a hard enough line on the amount of refined starches or red meat in the American diet.

- **Moderation.** Choosing forms of foods that limit intake of saturated or trans fats, added sugars, cholesterol, salt, and alcohol.

- **Activity.** Being physically active every day.

- **Personalization.** To make the most of the new MyPyramid system, you need to go online to www.mypyramid.gov. By filling in your age, gender, and typical level of activity, you will be linked to one of 12 versions of the pyramid, ranging from 1,000 to 3,200 daily calories. You can print out your customized pyramid and use it as a dietary guide. Track what you eat for a week to see how it compares with the recommendations, and go back to the website for specific suggestions.

Critics of the new MyPyramid charge that it does not go far enough in urging Americans to cut back on harmful fats and simple carbohydrates and also lumps together various protein sources (red meat, poultry, fish, and beans) as equally healthy. However, national surveys show that a large majority of Americans have heard of the revised guidelines and had a generally positive reaction. About a third said they would change their habits, another third said they might change, and a third said they wouldn't alter their lifestyles.

The following guidelines are based on the MyPyramid system.

You receive about the same amount and kinds of sugars from an orange as from a tablespoon of honey, but the packaging makes a big nutrition difference.

Consume a Variety of Foods
The six colors on the MyPyramid graphic represent the five food groups—grains, vegetables, fruits, milk, and meat and beans—and oils. The greater the variety of colors and of foods you choose, the more likely you are to obtain the nutrients you need. In general, the USDA recommends a diet that is high in fruits and vegetables, whole grains, and nonfat or low-fat milk products and low in saturated fat, cholesterol, added sugars, trans fat, and sodium.

Manage Your Weight
As discussed in Chapter 7, you must expend as much energy (calories) as you take in to stay at the same weight. Among the best ways to balance this energy equation are limiting portion sizes (discussed later in this chapter), substituting nutrient-dense foods (such as raw vegetables or low-fat soups) for nutrient-poor foods (such as candy and cake), and limiting added sugars, solid fats, and alcoholic beverages.

Get Physical Every Day
As discussed in Chapter 5, regular physical activity helps maintain a healthy weight and reduces risk for several chronic diseases. While 30 minutes of moderate physical activity (such as walking at a pace of three or four miles an hour) on most days provides important benefits, exercising more often and more intensely yields additional health dividends. Many adults need up to 60 minutes of moderate to vigorous physical activity—the equivalent of 150 to 200 calories, depending on body size—daily to prevent unhealthy weight gain. Men and women who have lost weight may need 60 to 90 minutes to keep off excess pounds.

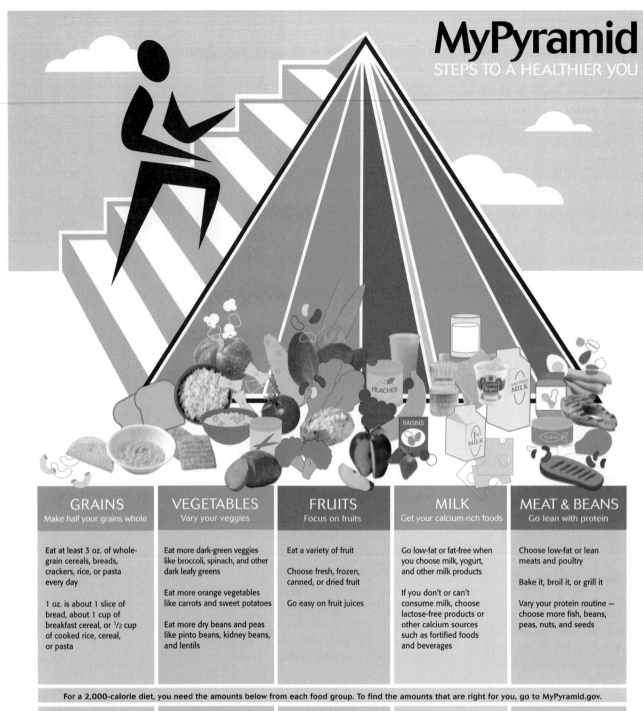

MyPyramid
STEPS TO A HEALTHIER YOU

GRAINS	VEGETABLES	FRUITS	MILK	MEAT & BEANS
Make half your grains whole	Vary your veggies	Focus on fruits	Get your calcium-rich foods	Go lean with protein
Eat at least 3 oz. of whole-grain cereals, breads, crackers, rice, or pasta every day 1 oz. is about 1 slice of bread, about 1 cup of breakfast cereal, or ½ cup of cooked rice, cereal, or pasta	Eat more dark-green veggies like broccoli, spinach, and other dark leafy greens Eat more orange vegetables like carrots and sweet potatoes Eat more dry beans and peas like pinto beans, kidney beans, and lentils	Eat a variety of fruit Choose fresh, frozen, canned, or dried fruit Go easy on fruit juices	Go low-fat or fat-free when you choose milk, yogurt, and other milk products If you don't or can't consume milk, choose lactose-free products or other calcium sources such as fortified foods and beverages	Choose low-fat or lean meats and poultry Bake it, broil it, or grill it Vary your protein routine — choose more fish, beans, peas, nuts, and seeds

For a 2,000-calorie diet, you need the amounts below from each food group. To find the amounts that are right for you, go to MyPyramid.gov.

Eat 6 oz. every day	Eat 2½ cups every day	Eat 2 cups every day	Get 3 cups every day; for kids aged 2 to 8, it's 2	Eat 5½ oz. every day

Find your balance between food and physical activity
- Be sure to stay within your daily calorie needs.
- Be physically active for at least 30 minutes most days of the week.
- About 60 minutes a day of physical activity may be needed to prevent weight gain.
- For sustaining weight loss, at least 60 to 90 minutes a day of physical activity may be required.
- Children and teenagers should be physically active for 60 minutes every day, or most days.

Know the limits on fats, sugars, and salt (sodium)
- Make most of your fat sources from fish, nuts, and vegetable oils.
- Limit solid fats like butter, stick margarine, shortening, and lard, as well as foods that contain these.
- Check the Nutrition Facts label to keep saturated fats, *trans* fats, and sodium low.
- Choose food and beverages low in added sugars. Added sugars contribute calories with few, if any, nutrients.

MyPyramid.gov
STEPS TO A HEALTHIER YOU

Figure 6.3   The MyPyramid Food Guidance System

Children and teenagers require at least 60 minutes of moderate physical activity every day.

Increase Foods from Certain Food Groups

Fewer than a third of American adults eat the recommended amounts of fruits and vegetables. College-age young adults between ages 18 and 24 eat the fewest vegetables. Nearly four-fifths of this group don't put vegetables on their plates—or scrape them to the side if they do.

Greater consumption of fruits and vegetables (5 to 13 servings or 2 1/2 to 6 1/2 cups per day, depending on how many calories you burn) may reduce the risk of stroke, certain cancers, and type 2 diabetes (vegetables more so than fruit) as well as helping reach and maintain a healthy weight. The more fruits and vegetables men and women consume, the lower their levels of harmful low-density lipoprotein (LDL) cholesterol. Plant-based foods also reduce the risk of rectal cancer in both men and women. To increase the fruits and vegetables in your diet, fill half of your plate with them (see Figure 6.4).

Among the ways to increase your fruit and vegetable intake:

- **Toss fruit into a green salad** for extra flavor, variety, color, and crunch.
- **Start the day with a daily double:** a glass of juice and a banana or other fruit on cereal.
- **Buy pre-cut vegetables** for snacking or dipping (instead of chips).
- **Make or order sandwiches** with extra tomatoes or other vegetable toppings.

Consuming at least three servings (the equivalent of 3 ounces) of whole grains per day can reduce the risk of diabetes and coronary heart disease and maintain a healthy weight. To increase your intake of grains:

- **Check labels of rolls and bread,** and choose those with at least 2 to 3 grams of fiber per slice.
- **Add brown rice or barley** to soups.
- **Choose whole-grain,** ready-to-eat cereals.

To get more dairy products with less fat, try the following:

- **Substitute fat-free sour cream** or non-fat, plain yogurt for sour cream.

Figure 6.4 Fruit and Vegetable Balance
Fill half your plate with fruits and vegetables.

- **Add nonfat milk** instead of water to oatmeal and hot cereals.
- **Eat cereals with added calcium** and with milk.
- **Top salads or soups with low-fat shredded cheese.**

Choose Carbohydrates Wisely Eating more fruits, vegetables, whole grains, and nonfat or low-fat milk and dairy products is a healthful way to get the carbohydrates you need. Fiber-rich choices—an apple rather than apple juice, for example—have the added benefits of promoting digestive health and reducing the risk of type 2 diabetes and heart disease.

The new guidelines do not include a specific message about sugar but caution against "added" sugars, those added to foods during processing or preparation or at the table. Carbohydrates (including sucrose, glucose, fructose, lactose, and starch) also can increase the risk of dental cavities. Drinking fluoridated water and/or using fluoride-containing dental hygiene products can protect your teeth.

To make sure your grains are whole, choose foods that name one of the following whole-grain ingredients first on the label's ingredient list: brown rice, bulgur, graham flour, oatmeal, whole-grain corn, whole oats, whole rye, whole wheat, wild rice. Foods labeled multigrain, stone-ground, 100% wheat, cracked wheat, seven-grain, or bran are usually not whole-grain products.

Be Finicky about Fats Reducing saturated fat, trans fat, and cholesterol can lower harmful LDL cholesterol and your risk of heart disease. You should keep saturated fat below 10 percent of total calories, trans fat as low as possible, and cholesterol intake below 300 mg per day. Your total fat intake should make up no more than 20 to 35 percent of calories. For children ages 2 and 3, recommended minimum fat intake is 30 percent of calories; for those between ages 4 and 18, it is 25 percent.

To keep within these limits:

- **Restrict animal fats** (such as those in cheese, milk, butter, ice cream, and other full-fat dairy products, fatty meat, bacon, sausage, poultry skin and fat).
- **Cut back** on foods made with partially hydrogenated vegetable oils.
- **Limit your intake** of eggs and organ meats.
- When preparing or ordering fish, choose grilled, baked, broiled, or poached fish, not fried. Fried fish at fast food restaurants is often low in omega-3 fatty acids and high in trans and saturated fats.

Limit Salt If Americans cut just one gram of salt from their daily diet, there would be 250,000 fewer new cases of heart disease and 200,000 fewer deaths over a decade.[25] Reducing salt in your diet can lower your blood pressure and reduce your risk of stroke, heart disease, and kidney disease. Another effective strategy is to eat more foods rich in potassium, which blunts the effects of salt on blood pressure, may decrease bone loss, and reduces the risk of kidney stones.

The USDA guidelines recommend less than 2,300 mg of sodium per day. Many people, including those with hypertension, African Americans, and older adults, should reduce their salt intake even more and increase potassium to at least 4,700 mg.

To reduce sodium intake:

- **Look for labels that say "low sodium."** They contain 140 mg or less of sodium per serving.
- **Learn to use spices and herbs** rather than salt to enhance the flavor of food.
- **Go easy on condiments** such as soy sauce, pickles, olives, ketchup, and mustard, which can add a lot of salt to your food.
- **Always check the amount of sodium** in processed foods, such as frozen dinners, packaged mixes, cereals, salad dressings, and sauces. The amount in different types and brands can vary widely.

If You Drink Alcoholic Beverages, Do So in Moderation As discussed in Chapter 12, alcohol has different effects on health for different age groups. In middle-aged and older adults, one to two drinks a day seem to lower the risk of dying, primarily because moderate alcohol consumption may protect against heart disease. Compared with non-drinkers, however, women who consume one alcoholic beverage per day appear to have a slightly higher risk of breast cancer. For younger people, alcohol provides little, if any, health benefits and increases the risk of traumatic injury and death. At any age, heavy drinking contributes to automotive accidents and deaths, assaults, liver disease, and other health problems.

MyPyramid includes a category for "discretionary calories," which can be used on fats, added sugar, alcohol, or more food from any food group. However, most people, especially those who are not physically active, "earn" very small discretionary calorie allowances, usually no more than 100 to 300 calories a day.

Keep Food Safe to Eat See page 198 for an in-depth discussion on food safety. The key steps you can take to ensure food safety and prevent a problem with foodborne illnesses are:

- **Thoroughly wash hands,** contact surfaces, and fruits and vegetables (but not meat and poultry).
- **Separate raw, cooked, and ready-to-eat foods** while shopping, preparing, or storing.
- **Cook foods to a safe temperature.**
- **Chill (refrigerate) perishable foods promptly.**

Alternative Guidelines

Critics of the Dietary Guidelines and the MyPyramid program challenge several key components. The guidelines, for instance, suggest that half of daily grain consumption can come from refined starches, such as white bread and rice, which critics say add empty calories and increase the risk of diabetes and obesity. The federal guidelines also lump together all forms of protein—red meat, poultry, fish, beans, and so on—and do not distinguish between the healthful fats found in fish and the harmful ones in red meat. Also controversial is the recommendation to consume three glasses of low-fat milk or the equivalent in other dairy products to prevent osteoporosis.[26]

Nutritionists at the Harvard School of Public Health have created the Healthy Eating Pyramid, revised in 2008, that they contend provides better guidance on healthy eating. (See Figure 6.5.) Its key components are:

- **Daily exercise and weight control,** with an emphasis on burning as many calories as you take in by means of regular physical activity.
- **Whole grains,** such as oatmeal, whole wheat bread, and brown rice.
- **Healthy fats and oil,** such as olive, canola, soy, corn, sunflower, peanut, and other vegetable oils, trans-fat-free margarines, nuts, seeds, avocadoes, and fatty fish such as salmon.
- **Vegetables and fruits.**
- **Nuts, seeds, beans, and tofu,** including black beans, navy beans, garbanzos, lentils, almonds, walnuts, pecans, peanuts, hazelnuts, and pistachios.
- **Fish, poultry, and eggs**
- **Dairy** (one or two servings a day) or a vitamin D/calcium supplement.
- **Red meat and butter** (only sparingly)

The basic guideline for using the Healthy Eating Pyramid is to eat more foods from the base of the pyramid than from the higher levels. A vegetarian can follow this approach by emphasizing nuts, beans, and other plant sources of protein and choosing nondairy sources of calcium and vitamin D.[27]

The Way We Eat

Just as there is no one perfect food, there is no one eating pattern that suits all people of all ages and backgrounds at all times. Your ethnic background and family makeup influenced the way you ate as a child. In college, you probably will find yourself eating in different—and not necessarily better—ways. Because the United States is so diverse, you also will have the opportunity to sample the cuisines of many cultures. However, in this country and others, many do not have enough to eat. (See Community Focus, p. 187.)

His Plate, Her Plate: Gender and Nutrition

Men and women do not need to eat different foods, but their nutritional needs are different. Because most men are bigger and taller than most women, they consume more calories. On average, a moderately active 125-pound woman needs 2,000 calories a day; a 175-pound man with a similar exercise pattern needs 2,800 calories. Eating more means it's easier for men to get the nutrients they need, even though many don't make the wisest food choices.

Women, particularly those who restrict their caloric intake or are chronically dieting, are more likely to develop specific deficiencies. Calcium is one example. Many teenage girls and young women under age 30 do not consume the recommended 800 to 1,200 milligrams of calcium daily and may be at increased risk of bone-weakening osteoporosis.

Many women also get too little iron. Even in adolescence, girls are more prone to iron deficiency than boys; some suffer memory and learning impairments as a result. In adult women, menstrual blood loss and poor eating habits can lead to low iron stores, which puts them at risk for anemia. According to U.S. Department of Agriculture research, most women consume only 60

USE SPARINGLY:
RED MEAT & BUTTER
REFINED GRAINS: WHITE RICE, BREAD & PASTA
POTATOES
SUGARY DRINKS & SWEETS
SALT

OPTIONAL: ALCOHOL IN MODERATION
(Not for everyone)

DAILY MULTIVITAMIN
PLUS EXTRA VITAMIN D
(For most people)

DAIRY (1–2 servings a day) OR
VITAMIN D/CALCIUM SUPPLEMENTS

NUTS, SEEDS, BEANS & TOFU

FISH, POULTRY & EGGS

HEALTHY FATS/OILS:
OLIVE, CANOLA, SOY, CORN,
SUNFLOWER, PEANUT
& OTHER VEGETABLE OILS;
TRANS-FREE MARGARINE

WHOLE GRAINS:
BROWN RICE,
WHOLE WHEAT PASTA,
OATS, ETC.

VEGETABLES & FRUITS

HEALTHY FATS/OILS

WHOLE GRAINS

DAILY EXERCISE & WEIGHT CONTROL

Figure 6.5   The Healthy Eating Pyramid

From Walter C. Willett, M.D. and Patrick J. Skerrett, *Eat, Drink, and Be Healthy*, ©2005 Harvard University Press.

percent of the recommended 18 milligrams of iron per day. (The recommendation for men is 8 milligrams.) Regular blood tests can monitor a woman's iron status.

Both genders should increase their fruit and vegetable intake to ensure that they are getting adequate amounts of vitamins and fiber in their daily diet.

Here are some gender-specific strategies for better nutrition:

- **Men should cut back on fat** and meat in their diets, two things they eat too much.

- **Women should increase their iron intake** by eating meat (iron from animal sources is absorbed better than that from vegetable sources) or a combination of meat and vegetable iron sources together (for example, a meat and bean burrito). Those with iron deficiencies should consult a physician. Because large doses of iron can be toxic, iron supplements should be taken only with medical supervision.

- **Women should consume more calcium-rich foods,** including low-fat and nonfat dairy products, leafy greens, and tofu. Women who cannot get adequate amounts of calcium from their daily diet should take calcium supplements. This is not advised for all men because of a possible connection between calcium and prostate cancer.

- **Women who could become pregnant should take a multivitamin** with 400 micrograms of **folic acid,** which helps prevent neural tube defects such as spina bifida. Folic acid is also useful to men because it may cut the risk of heart disease, stroke, and colon cancer.

Campus Cuisine: How College Students Eat

 Often on their own for the first time, college students typically change their usual eating patterns. In one recent survey, 59 percent of freshmen said their diet had changed since they began college. When they are making meal choices, the top two influences on students are price and convenience, with nutrition coming in third. However, eating right doesn't have to cost more. (See Health on a Budget, p. 188.)

According to various national samples, many students do not consume adequate amounts of fruits and vegetables and consume too many fried and fast foods. In one study that followed students through their freshman and sophomore years, more than half remained in the precontemplation stage for adopting healthier eating behaviors throughout this time. Only 30 percent of the students consumed at least five fruits and vegetables daily; more than half reported eating high-fat fried or fast foods at least three times during the previous week.

 The proportion of 18- to 24-year-olds who eat the recommended amounts of fruit and vegetables is generally lower than in the population as a whole. College men eat fewer fruits and vegetables than women do; Caucasian and Asian students eat more than African American undergraduates. Both African American and Hispanic students consume less than multiracial or other racial/ethnic groups. Students living in residence halls report greater fruit and vegetable intake than those living in other campus housing, off campus, or with their parents. Those in fraternity and sorority houses also report greater consumption than others living off campus.[28]

Student fruit-and-veggie eaters differ in other ways. According to an analysis of data from the ACHA-NCHA survey, they are more likely to exercise, use sunscreen, wear seatbelts and helmets, get more sleep, examine their breasts or testicles, report better health—and get better grades. They also are less likely to smoke, drink (and drink and drive), and feel hopeless. Researchers have found an association between higher fruit and vegetable consumption and lower BMI, as well as lower anorexia in both men and women and bulimia in women, possibly the result of "the preoccupation with food associated with both disorders."[29]

Time pressures often affect students' food choices. More than half say they tend to eat on the run, and they consume more soft drinks, fast food, total fat, and saturated fat. A significant number of undergraduates—35

percent of men and 42 percent of women—feel they don't have time to sit down and share a meal with friends or family. Yet students who take time for a social meal make better food choices, including eating more fruit and vegetables.[30]

Some colleges are doing their part to improve student nutrition. Many post nutritional information in dining halls; some have

PROBLEM One of every eight people on the planet is chronically hungry. Some 850 million are "undernourished," or lacking in adequate nutrition. The number of poor, hungry people is rising as the prices of basic foods such as rice, soy, and wheat have soared. You may be feeling the pinch in your wallet when you buy groceries or eat out, but for hundreds of millions around the world the impact is far more severe. Food riots have broken out in several developing countries.

Resolving the problem of world hunger may seem beyond any one individual's influence. Can recycling a bottle or volunteering in a food recovery program make a difference? The answer is yes. Your action may influence many others over time, and a repeated action becomes a habit, which compounds the benefits. Making choices with an awareness of their consequences also gives you a sense of personal control and efficacy. The daily actions of many members of a community can help provide adequate nutrition to their neighborhood or to a country on the other side of the globe.

BECOME INFORMED

- To learn more about the problem, check out websites such as **http://www.worldhunger.org**, an online magazine about world hunger and poverty, and **http://www.whyhunger.org**, the home page of World Hunger Year, a leading advocacy group for innovative, community-based solutions to hunger and poverty.

- To learn more about solutions, go to the websites of hunger-relief organizations, such as Bread for the World (**www.bread.org**), OxfamAmerica (**www.oxfamamerica.org**), and Feeding America (**http://feedingamerica.org**).

- Educate yourself about sustainability—using resources at such a rate that the earth can keep replacing them and producing pollutants at a rate with which cleanup efforts can keep pace so there is no net accumulation. More than 100 nations have agreed to a set of principles of sustainable development, that is, development that would meet the economic and environmental needs of both current and future generations.

- Find out about hunger in your community. Are there programs to provide free meals or to collect and distribute food for needy individuals and families? What is the local government doing? What about churches and charities? Identify campus groups that may work with them.

BECOME INVOLVED

- Learn more about what your school's food service is doing for the sake of sustainability. For instance, does it buy locally whenever possible? Are recycling bins available at all cafeterias and snack bars? Can students influence these policies?

- Identify at least one campus or community activity to reduce local hunger that you will participate in this month, and block out time to do so on your schedule.

- Eat "green." Choose more foods that are low on the food chain, that is, more plants and fewer animals. You can use the Center for Science in the Public Interest's "Eating Green Calculator" at **www.cspinet.org/EatingGreen/calculator.html** to assess the impact of your diet on the environment.

- Whenever possible, select foods with no or minimal and recyclable packages. Carry reusable cloth or string shopping bags. Buy from local suppliers. Use "real" plates and glasses rather than disposable ones.

folic acid A form of folate used in vitamin supplements and fortified foods.

Frugal Food Choices

Many people feeling a budget squeeze opt for the cheapest foods they can find, even if they're high in fat and calories and low in nutrients. Such short-term choices can lead to long-term health problems. Here are some ways to eat healthfully for less.

- **Drink tap water.** It's cheaper than bottled and just as safe. Don't waste money on fortified drinks, which offer no proven additional nutritional value. Sugar-sweetened drinks add extra calories as well as extra costs.
- **Consider the cost of convenience.** Prepackaged grab-and-go items such as individual packets of baby carrots or crackers and cheese may be handy but cost more. Buy larger bags or boxes and create your own easy-carry single servings with small reusable containers.
- **Avoid fad fruits.** Pomegranates and other exotic fruits are indeed rich in antioxidants but so are much cheaper oranges and seasonal berries.
- **Freeze.** If you have access to a freezer, take advantage of grocery store sales and stock up on frozen fruits and vegetables, which—thanks to advances in preservation and freezing methods—provide plenty of nutrients.
- **Bulk up.** Join with your roommates or friends and check for low prices on large quantities at the local co-op as well as national mega-stores.
- **Eat seasonally.** Take advantage of the low prices on watermelon in summer or apples in autumn.
- **Look for an Asian grocery store,** if you're a vegan and eat a lot of ramen dishes. Ramen usually costs much less at such stores, but be sure you're getting a vegetarian ramen package.

YOUR STRATEGIES FOR PREVENTION

A Guide to Fast Foods

- For breakfast, avoid croissants or muffins stuffed with eggs or meat; they pack as many as 700 calories. Better options include plain scrambled eggs (150–180 calories), pancakes without butter or syrup (400 calories), and English muffins (185 calories each).
- For lunch or dinner, if you want meat, go for plain hamburgers (no cheese), which average 275 to 350 calories. An even better choice is roast beef, which is lower in fat and calories.
- Be wary of fast-food fish. With frying oil trapped in the breading and creamy tartar sauce on top, fried-fish sandwiches supply more calories (425–500) and fat than do hamburgers.
- Avoid fried chicken; the coatings tend to retain grease. If you want bite-size chicken, select bites made of chicken breast, not processed chicken (which contains fatty, ground-up skin).
- Ask for unsalted items; they are available. (Many chains also have reduced the amount of sodium used in cooking.)
- If you sample the salad bar, steer clear of mayonnaise, bacon bits, oily vegetable salads, and rich dressings.
- See Table 6.7 for some specific choices.

expanded their offerings to include more salads, fewer fried foods, and more ethnic dishes. On some campuses, students are taking the lead in demanding more healthful, fresher, and more varied dishes in their dining halls. (See Point/Counterpoint, p. 189.)

Fast Food: Nutrition on the Run

On any given day, about 25 percent of adults in the United States go to a fast-food restaurant. The typical American consumes three hamburgers and four orders of french fries every week. Not all fast foods are junk foods—that is, high in calories, sugar, salt, and fat and low in beneficial nutrients (Table 6.7, p. 190). But while it's not all bad, fast food has definite disadvantages. A meal in a fast-food restaurant may cost twice as much as the same meal prepared at home and may provide half the daily calorie needs. The fat content of many items is extremely high. A Burger King Whopper with cheese contains

760 calories and 47 grams of fat, 16 grams from saturated fat. A McDonald's Sausage McMuffin with egg has 450 calories and 27 grams of fat, 10 grams from saturated fat. Many fast-food chains have switched from beef tallow or lard to unsaturated vegetable oils for frying, but the total fat content of the foods remains the same.

When provided with nutrition information on fast food choices, college women chose meals significantly lower in calories than women who did not get such information. However, information on calories and nutrition had no effect on men's choices. In one study, college men tended to choose higher-calorie foods when supplied with nutrition information.[31]

You Are What You Drink

About 20 percent of the calories Americans over age two consume come from sweetened beverages, predominantly soft drinks and fruit drinks. The consumption of sweetened beverages has surged in recent decades. Calories from these drinks, which some call "liquid candy," account for half the rise in caloric intake by Americans since the 1970s

Water—tap or bottled, sparkling or still, chilled or room temperature—is the medical experts' beverage of choice. But don't think that "fortified" or "enriched" water is better. There is no evidence that nutrients added to water confer any health benefits. Consumers who assume they're getting vitamins in their drinks may think they don't need to eat healthful foods and could end up short-changing themselves of vital nutrients.

Soft Drinks According to a national survey, two-thirds of adults drink sugar-sweetened beverages, averaging 28 ounces per drink and almost 300 calories daily (15 percent of recommended total calories). Young adults, particularly those with lower incomes and education, consume the most soda.[32]

These beverages can add five pounds every year. Cutting 300 liquid calories from your daily intake by cutting out sweetened beverages would translate into a 2.5 pound loss every month.[33] In a recent review of 88 studies, researchers linked soft drinks with increased calorie intake, higher body weight, lower consumption of calcium and other nutrients, and greater risk of other medical problems, such as diabetes. Women who consume two or more cans of soda daily are almost twice as likely as other women to show early evidence of kidney disease. No one knows if the culprit is the amount of sugar they consume or the type. Some samples of the high-fructose syrup used to make and preserve soda have contained mercury, which is toxic to the kidneys.[34]

Researchers also have found a strong association between soft drink consumption and greater risk of heart disease.[35] A single daily soft drink, either diet or regular, also increases the likelihood of metabolic syndrome. Sweetened iced tea and many carbonated beverages can damage tooth enamel, especially when not consumed with food. Drinking regular and diet cola has been linked with the thinning of hip bones in women.

POINT COUNTERPOINT

POINT

At some college campuses students are demanding more healthful foods in their dining halls, including organically grown fruits and vegetables, more culturally diverse dishes, and alternatives to trans fats. Universities, they argue, should practice the lessons of good nutrition taught in their classrooms.

COUNTERPOINT

Cost can be a limiting factor in choosing food suppliers and products for campus food vendors. Organic food can be more expensive and, in some locations, difficult to obtain. Not all students care about good nutrition, and many are content with a steady diet of burgers, fries, and pizza.

YOUR VIEW

What do you think of the food options available on your campus? Does your school encourage healthful food choices? What would you like to see on the menu? Would you eat differently if more healthful choices were available? Would you be willing to pay more for these items?

© AP Images

Many dining halls are providing nutritional information and more healthful food options for students.

People who consume a lot of soft drinks generally take in more calories than others—and not just from the beverages. Instead of satisfying a sweet tooth, soft drinks seem to do the opposite. Although researchers cannot explain exactly why, soft drinks may increase hunger or decrease feelings of satiety or fullness. Even diet drinks made with artificial sweeteners may "condition" people to eat more sweets.

TABLE 6.7

Some Fast-Food Choices

	Calories	Fat (g)	% Calories from Fat	Protein (g)	Carb (g)	Fiber (g)
Arby's						
Martha's Vineyard Salad	276	8	25	26	24	4
Santa Fe Salad w/ Grilled Chicken	283	9	27	29	20	5
Burger King						
Tendergrill Chicken Sandwich w/o mayo	450	10	20	37	53	4
Big Fish Sandwich w/o tartar sauce	470	13	25	23	65	3
Veggie Burger w/o mayo	40	8	21	23	46	7
Tendergrill Chicken Garden Salad	240	9	34	33	8	4
Domino's						
1 slice 12" Classic Hand-Tossed:						
with any veggies	220	7	28	9	32	1
with grilled chicke.	235	8	30	11	32	1
Jack in the Box						
Chicken Fajita Pita	290	9	28	21	31	2
Asian Grilled Chicken Salad	160	2	10	22	18	5
Southwest Grilled Chicken Salad	320	12	34	31	27	7
KFC						
Original Recipe Chicken Breast w/o skin or breading	140	2	14	29	1	0
Honey BBQ Sandwich	280	3.5	11	22	40	3
Tender Roast Sandwich w/o sauce	300	4.5	13	37	28	2
KFC Snacker, Buffalo	260	8	27	15	31	1
Long John Silver's						
Baked Cod—1 piece	120	4.5	33	22	1	0
Buttered Lobster Bites—snack box	250	9	32	14	27	2
1 Corn Cobbette	90	3	28	3	14	3
McDonald's						
Hamburger	250	9	32	12	31	2
Premium Grilled Chicken Classic Sandwich	420	10	21	33	51	3
Ranch Snack Wrap w/ Grilled Chicken	270	10	33	18	26	1
Subway						
6" Ham	290	5	16	18	47	4
6" Roast Beef	290	5	156	19	45	4
6" Sweet Onion Teriyaki	370	5	12	26	59	5
Subway Club Wrap	310	8	23	22	40	3
Taco Bell						
Bean Burrito	340	9	23	13	54	8
Fiesta Burrito—Chicken	350	10	26	18	47	3
Fiesta Burrito—Steak	340	11	29	15	47	3
Spicy Chicken Soft Taco	170	6	30	10	20	2
(Order "Fresco Style" to substitute cheese and sauce with Fiesta Salsa)						
Wendy's						
Jr. Hamburger	280	9	29	15	34	1
Ultimate Chicken Grill Sandwich	320	7	20	28	36	2
Large Chili	330	9	24	25	35	8

© Spencer Grant/PhotoEdit

College students say they consume sugar-sweetened beverages—including soft drinks, energy drinks, and fruit-based drinks—on social occasions, sometimes mixed with alcohol. Some think of these drinks as part of the enjoyment of going to a movie or hanging out with friends; others drink more caffeinated beverages at exam times. Even when aware of negative health consequences, most do not feel these consequences pertain to them.[36]

Energy Drinks Coffee and tea, which both contain caffeine, are the classic "pick-me-up" beverages. As discussed in Chapter 11, regular coffee consumption may reduce the risk of several serious illnesses—including type 2 diabetes, colon cancer, and Parkinson's disease—and may protect against age-related memory and thinking defects. Studies of tea's benefits have produced mixed results, although some research suggests that tea may improve blood flow to the heart and help prevent kidney stones.

Consumption of energy drinks such as Red Bull and Rockstar has more than doubled in the last three years, particularly among young people. The main ingredient in these drinks, including diet brands, is caffeine, sometimes in doses that can cause physical and psychological complications, including disrupted sleep, exaggerated stress response, heart palpitations, and increased risk of high blood pressure.

Red Bull, for instance, contains nearly 80 mg of caffeine per can, about the same amount of caffeine as a cup of brewed coffee and twice the caffeine of a cup of tea. Other energy drinks contain several times this amount—see Table 6.8.

The drink formulations vary widely, and manufacturers make many different claims about their effects. Some brands contain fruit juices, teas, and dietary supplements such as ginseng and glucuronolactone. One can of Red Bull contains 1,000 mg of taurine, a substance that plays an important role in muscle contraction (especially in the heart) and the nervous system. Some energy drinks contain guarana, a South American herbal caffeine source that could pose additional risks. We know very little about the effects of such combinations of ingredients, which may work synergistically with caffeine to boost its stimulant power.

Millions of college students consume energy drinks for the jolt provided or because they believe the drinks enhance sports performance or sexual function. Yet health experts warn that these sugar- and caffeine-laden drinks pose serious health risks, including dehydration, accidents, and alcohol poisoning.

Dietary Diversity

Whatever your cultural heritage, you have probably sampled Chinese, Mexican, Indian, Italian, and Japanese foods. If you belong to any of these ethnic groups, you may eat these cuisines regularly. Each type of ethnic cooking has its own nutritional benefits and potential drawbacks.

 Mediterranean Diet Several years ago epidemiologists noticed something unexpected in the residents of regions along the Mediterranean Sea: a lower incidence of deaths from heart disease. Scientists have identified antioxidants in red wine and olive oil that may account for the beneficial effects on the heart of the Mediterranean diet, which features lots of fruits and vegetables, legumes, nuts, and grains (see Figure 6.6). The Mediterranean diet also has beneficial effects on the lungs, reducing the risk of asthma and progressive lung disease as well as cardiovascular disease.[37]

Meat is used mainly as a condiment rather than as a main course, and fish, yogurt, and low-fat feta cheese are the predominant animal foods. The diet is relatively high in fat, but the main source is olive oil, an unsaturated fat.

With its emphasis on low-glycemic foods such as fruits, vegetables, and nuts, this has proven superior to cereal-based diets in lowering blood sugar and other risk factors for heart disease in people with diabetes.[38] The more closely individuals adhere to the diet, the greater the benefits to their hearts' health.[39]

 Ethnic Cuisines The cuisine served in Mexico features rice, corn, and beans, which are low in fat and high in nutrients. However, the dishes Americans think of as Mexican are far less healthful. Burritos, especially when topped

TABLE 6.8	
Energy drinks: Caffeine in Cans and Cups	
Type or Drink	**Amount of Caffeine**
Regular Cola (12-oz can)	40 mg
Red Bull (8.3-oz ca)	75 mg
Coffee (standard 8-oz cup)	95 g
Monster (16-oz container)	140 mg
Rockstar (16-oz container)	240 mg

Figure 6.6 The Traditional Healthy Mediterranean Diet Pyramid

©2009 Oldways Preservation and Exchange Trust. Reprinted by permission.

with cheese and sour cream, are very high in fat. Although guacamole has a high fat content, it contains mostly monounsaturated fatty acids, a better form of fat.

African American cuisine traces some of its roots to food preferences from west Africa (for example, peanuts, okra, and black-eyed peas), as well as to traditional American foods, such as fish, game, greens, and sweet potatoes. It uses many nutritious vegetables, such as collard greens and sweet potatoes, as well as legumes. However, some dishes include high-fat food products such as peanuts and pecans or involve frying, sometimes in saturated fat.

The mainland Chinese diet, which is plant-based, high in carbohydrates, and low in fats and animal protein, is considered one of the healthiest in the world. However, Chinese restaurants in the United States serve more meat and sauces than are generally eaten in China. According to laboratory tests of typical take-out dishes from Chinese restaurants, many have more fats and cholesterol than hamburger or egg dishes from fast-food outlets.

Traditional French cuisine, which includes rich, high-fat sauces and dishes, has never been considered healthful. Yet, nutritionists have been stumped to explain the so-called French paradox. Despite a diet high in saturated fats, the French have had one of the lowest rates of coronary artery disease in the world. The French diet increasingly resembles the American diet, but French portions tend to be one-third to one-half the size of American portions.

Many Indian dishes highlight healthful ingredients such as vegetables and legumes (beans and peas). However, many also use *ghee* (a form of butter) or coconut oil; both are rich in harmful saturated fats. The best advice in an Indian restaurant is to ask how each dish is prepared. Good choices include *daal* or *dal* (lentils), *karbi* or *karni* (chickpea soup), and *chapati* (tortilla-like bread).

The traditional Japanese diet is very low in fat, which may account for the low incidence of heart disease in Japan. Dietary staples include soybean products, fish, vegetables, noodles, and rice. A variety of fruits and vegetables are also included in many dishes. However, Japanese cuisine is high in salted, smoked, and pickled foods. Watch out for deep-fried dishes such as tempura and salty soups and sauces.

Table 6.9 summarizes some of the ethnic food choices by food group.

Vegetarian Diets Not all vegetarians avoid all meats. Some, who call themselves *lacto-ovo-pesco-vegetarians*, eat dairy products, eggs, and fish but not red meat. **Lacto-vegetarians** eat dairy products as well as grains, fruits, and vegetables; **ovo-lacto-vegetarians** also eat eggs. Pure vegetarians, called **vegans**, eat only plant foods; often they take vitamin B_{12} supplements because that vitamin is normally found only in animal products. If they select their food with care, vegetarians can get sufficient amounts of protein, vitamin B_{12}, iron, and calcium without supplements.

The key to getting sufficient protein from a vegetarian diet is understanding the concept of **complementary proteins.** Recall that meat, poultry, fish, eggs, and dairy products are complete proteins that provide the nine essential amino acids—substances that the human body cannot produce itself. Incomplete proteins, such as legumes or nuts, may have relatively low levels of one or two essential amino acids but fairly high levels of others. By combining complementary protein sources, vegetarians can make sure

lacto-vegetarians People who eat dairy products as well as fruits and vegetables (but not meat, poultry, or fish).

ovo-lacto-vegetarians People who eat eggs, dairy products, and fruits and vegetables (but not meat, poultry, or fish).

vegans People who eat only plant foods.

complementary proteins Incomplete proteins that, when combined, provide all the amino acids essential for protein synthesis.

TABLE 6.9

Ethnic Food Choices

	Grains	Vegetables	Fruits	Meats and Legumes	Milk
Asian	Rice, noodles, millet	Amaranth, baby corn, bamboo shoots, chayote, bok choy, mung bean sprouts, sugar peas, straw mushrooms, water chestnuts, kelp	Carambola, guava, kumquat, lychee, persimmon, melons, mandarin orange	Soybeans and soy products such as soy milk and tofu, squid, duck eggs, pork, poultry, fish and other seafood peanuts, cashews	Usually excluded
Mediterranean	Pita pocket bread, pastas, rice, couscous, polenta, bulgur, focaccia, Italian bread	Eggplant, tomatoes, peppers, cucumbers, grape leaves	Olives, grapes, figs	Fish and other seafood, gyros, lamb, chicken, beef, port, sausage, lentils, fava beans	Ricotta, provolone, parmesan, feta, mozzarella, and goat cheeses; yogurt
Mexican	Tortillas (corn or flour), taco shells, rice	Chayote, corn, jicama, tomato salsa, cactus, cassava, tomatoes, yams, chilies	Guava, mango, papaya, avocado, plantain, bananas, oranges	Refried beans, fish, chicken, chorizo, beef, eggs	Cheese, custard

their bodies make the most of the nonanimal proteins they eat. Many cultures rely heavily on complementary foods for protein. In Middle Eastern cooking, sesame seeds and chickpeas are a popular combination; in Latin American dishes, beans and rice, or beans and tortillas; in Chinese cuisine, soy and rice.

According to the Dietary Guidelines, vegetarians can best meet their nutrient needs by paying special attention to protein, iron, vitamin B_{12}, calcium, and vitamin D. Instead of a 6-ounce serving of meat, they can substitute one egg, 1.5 ounces of nuts, or two-thirds cup of legumes. Those who avoid milk because of its lactose content may obtain all the nutrients of milk by using lactose-reduced milk or eating other calcium-rich foods, such as broccoli, calcium-fortified orange juice, and fortified soy milk. Figure 6.7 shows a vegetarian food pyramid.

Vegetarian diets have proven health benefits. Studies show that vegetarians' cholesterol levels are low, and vegetarians are seldom overweight. As a result, they're less apt to be candidates for heart disease than those who consume large quantities of meat. Vegetarians also have lower incidences of breast, colon, and prostate cancer; high blood pressure; and osteoporosis.

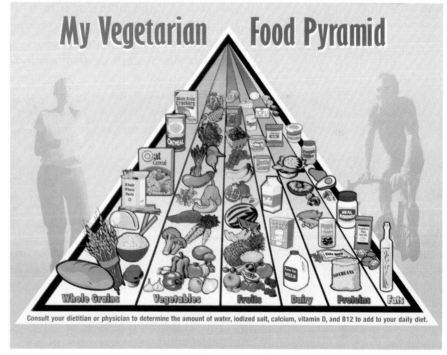

Figure 6.7 A Vegetarian Food Pyramid

Tips for planning a vegetarian diet can be found at MyPyramid.gov.

Source: © GC Nutrition Council, 2006, adapted from USDA 2005 Dietary Guidelines and www.MyPyramid.gov. Copies can be ordered from 301-680-6717.

Portions and Servings

Consumers often are confused by what a *serving* actually is, especially since many American restaurants have super-sized the amount of food they put on their customers'

Figure 6.8
Understanding Nutrition Labels
Quick and easy estimates of portion sizes

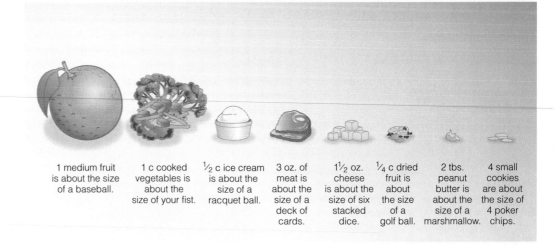

1 medium fruit is about the size of a baseball.

1 c cooked vegetables is about the size of your fist.

½ c ice cream is about the size of a racquet ball.

3 oz. of meat is about the size of a deck of cards.

1½ oz. cheese is about the size of six stacked dice.

¼ c dried fruit is about the size of a golf ball.

2 tbs. peanut butter is about the size of a marshmallow.

4 small cookies are about the size of 4 poker chips.

plates. The average bagel has doubled in size in the last ten to fifteen years. A standard fast-food serving of french fries is larger in the United States than in the United Kingdom.

A food-label *serving* is a specific amount of food that contains the quantity of nutrients described on the Nutrition Facts label. A *portion* is the amount of a specific food that an individual eats at one time. Portions can be bigger or smaller than the servings on food labels. According to nutritionists, "marketplace portions"—the actual amounts served to customers—are two to eight times larger than the standard serving sizes defined by the USDA. In fast-food chains, today's portions are two to five times larger than the original sizes. As studies have shown, people presented with larger portions eat 30 to 50 percent more than they otherwise would.

If you are trying to balance your diet or control your weight, it's important to keep track of the size of your portions so that you do not exceed recommended servings. For instance, a 3-ounce serving of meat is about the size of a pack of playing cards—see Figure 6.8. If you eat a larger amount, count it as more than one serving. (See Making Change Happen, p. 167, and "Mind over Platter" in the *Labs for IPC* for more on developing greater awareness of what and how you eat.)

Taking Charge of What You Eat

You can't control what you don't know. Because of the Nutrition Labeling and Education Act, food manufacturers must provide information about fat, calories, and ingredients in large type on packaged food labels, and they must show how a food item fits into a daily diet of 2,000 calories. The law also restricts nutritional claims for terms such as *healthy, low-fat,* and *high-fiber.*

At one university, almost two-thirds of the freshmen reported that they were aware of the nutrition labels posted in the dining commons. One-third used them to help make food choices. Female students were significantly more likely to base their food choices on the labels than were the men. Students primarily checked overall good/balanced nutrition content of foods, calories, fat, saturated fat, and protein. Their top reason for checking labels: to be healthy now.

In evaluating food labels and product claims, keep in mind that while individual foods vary in their nutritional value, what matters is your total diet. If you eat too much of any one food—regardless of what its label states—you may not be getting the variety and balance of nutrients that you need.

How to Read Nutrition Labels

As Figure 6.9 shows, the Nutrition Facts on food labels present a wealth of information—if you know what to look for. The label focuses on those nutrients most clearly associated with disease risk and health: total fat, saturated fat, cholesterol, sodium, total carbohydrate, dietary fiber, sugar, and protein.

- **Calories.** Calories are the measure of the amount of energy that can be derived from food. Scientists define a calorie as the amount of energy required to raise the temperature of 1 gram of water by 1 degree Celsius. In the laboratory, the caloric content of food is measured in 1,000-calorie units called kilocalories.

Figure 6.9   Understanding Nutrition Labels
The Nutrition Facts label lists the essential nutrient content of packaged food as well as the amount of potentially harmful substances such as fat and sodium.

The calorie referred to in everyday usage is actually the equivalent of the laboratory kilocalorie.

The Nutrition Facts label lists two numbers for calories: calories per serving and calories from fat per serving. This allows consumers to calculate how many calories they'll consume and to determine the percentage of fat in an item.

- **Serving size.** Rather than the tiny portions manufacturers sometimes used in the past to keep down the number of calories per serving, the new labels reflect more realistic portions. Serving sizes, which have been defined for approximately 150 food categories, must be the same for similar products (for example, different brands of potato chips) and for similar products within a category (for example, snack foods such as pretzels, potato chips, and popcorn). This makes it easier to compare the nutritional content of foods.

- **Daily Values (DVs).** DVs refer to the total amount of a nutrient that the average adult should aim to get or not exceed on a daily basis. The DVs for cholesterol, sodium, vitamins, and minerals are the same for all adults. The DVs for total fat, saturated fat, carbohydrate, fiber, and protein are based on a 2,000-calorie daily diet—the amount of food ingested by many American men and active women.

- **Percent Daily Values (%DVs).** The goal for a full day's diet is to select foods that together add up to 100 percent of the DVs. The %DVs show how a particular food's nutrient content fits into a 2,000-calorie diet. Individuals who consume (or should consume) fewer than 2,000 total calories a day have to lower their DVs for total fat, saturated fat, and carbohydrates. For example, if their caloric intake is 10 percent less than 2,000 calories, they would lower the DV by 10 percent. Similarly, those who consume more than 2,000 calories should adjust the DVs upward.

- **Calories per gram.** The bottom of the food label lists the number of calories per gram for fat, carbohydrates, and protein.

People zero in on different figures on the food label—for example, calories if they're watching their weight, specific ingredients if they have food allergies. Among the useful items to check are the following:

- **Calories from fat.** Get into the habit of calculating the percentage of fat calories in a food before buying or eating it.

- **Total fat.** Since the average person munches on 15 to 20 food items a day, it's easy to overload on fat. Saturated fat and trans fat numbers deserve special attention because of their link to several diseases.

- **Cholesterol.** Cholesterol is made by and contained in products of animal origin only. Many high-fat products, such as potato chips, contain 0 percent cholesterol because they're made from plants and are cooked in vegetable fats. However, if the vegetable fats are hydrogenated, the resulting trans fat is more harmful to the heart than cholesterol.

- **Sugars.** There is no Daily Value for sugars because health experts have yet to agree on a daily limit. The figure on the label includes naturally present sugars, such as lactose in milk and fructose in fruit, as well as those added to the food, such as table sugar, corn syrup, or dextrose.

- **Fiber.** A "high-fiber" food has 5 or more grams of fiber per serving. A "good" source of fiber provides at least 2.5 grams. "More" or "added" fiber means at least 2.5 grams more per serving than similar foods—10 percent more of the DV for fiber.

- **Calcium.** "High" equals 200 mg or more per serving. "Good" means at least 100 mg, while "more" indicates that the food contains at least 100 mg more calcium—10 percent more of the DV—than the item usually would have.

- **Sodium.** Most of us routinely get more sodium than we need. Read labels carefully to avoid excess sodium, which can be a health threat.

- **Vitamins.** A Daily Value of 10 percent of any vitamin makes a food a "good" source; 20 percent qualifies it as "high" in a certain vitamin.

What Is Organic?

Foods certified as **organic** by the USDA must meet strict criteria, including:

- Processing or preservation only with substances approved by the USDA for organic foods.
- Processing without genetic modification or ionizing radiation.
- No use of most synthetic chemicals, such as pesticides, herbicides, or fertilizers.
- Fertilization without sewage sludge.
- Food-producing animals grown without medication such as antibiotics or hormones, provided with living conditions similar to their natural habitat, and fed organic feed.

Are organic foods better for you? There has been limited research as to whether organic foods are nutritionally superior to conventional foods. Some studies have shown higher levels of specific nutrients, such as flavonoids, in organic produce, but no one knows if this translates into specific health benefits. However, you can avoid exposure to pesticides and other chemicals by opting for organic foods.

Functional Foods

As the American Dietetic Association has noted, all foods are functional at some physiological level. However, the term *functional* generally applies to a food specifically created to have health-promoting benefits. The International Food Information Council defines functional foods as those "that provide health benefits beyond basic nutrition."

Some manufacturers are adding biologically active components such as beta-carotene to food products and promoting them as functional foods. However, the amounts added are often too low to have any effect, and many such foods are high-sugared drinks and snack foods. More research is needed to evaluate their claims of health benefits.

Choosing Healthful Snacks

Snacking has become more widespread on campuses, as in other places. College students snack primarily "to satisfy hunger"; the second-most common reason is "no time for meals." Other reasons for munching between meals: "for energy," "to be sociable," and "to relieve stress." One-third snack at 9:00 p.m. or later.

Snacking has increased dramatically across all age groups, and more people are getting more of their total calories and nutrients from "grazing," a term coined for eating throughout the day rather than mainly at mealtimes. In a study of teenagers, snacks contributed to their daily intake of fruit and vitamin C (primarily from orange juice). The more the teens snacked, the higher their sugar intake and total daily calorie consumption.[40]

In response to consumer demands for smart snack choices, food manufacturers are offering "better-for-you" options that are lower in salt and sugar or free of trans fat and artificial colors. Some new snack items promoted as healthful options, such as sugar-free chocolate or organic potato chips, offer little nutritional value. Meat-based snacks, increasingly popular among young men, also can be high in fat and sodium. Read labels carefully, and be sure to check total calories and fat.

A best-for-you option is fruit such as bananas, apples, or berries—rich in vitamins, low in calories, and packed with fiber. Other nutritious snacks include nuts, trail mix, granola bars, yogurt, sunflower seeds, soy nuts, and dried fruit (such as cranberries). If you enjoy fruit juice, buy 100 percent fruit juice without added sugar. Limit yourself to one serving of these calorie-rich beverages a day.

If you rely on snacks to keep you energized throughout the day, take time to plan in advance so you have choices other than the nearest vending machine. Try to prepare snacks from different food groups: low- or no-fat milk and a few graham crackers, for instance, or celery sticks with peanut butter and raisins. Save part of one meal—half of your breakfast bagel or lunch sandwich—to eat a few hours later. If you're trying to add fiber to your diet, eat high-fiber snacks, such as prunes, popcorn, or sunflower seeds.

organic Term designating food produced with, or production based on the use of, fertilizers originating from plants or animals, without the use of pesticides or chemically formulated fertilizers.

Food Safety

Foodborne infections cause an estimated 76 million illnesses, 325,000 hospitalizations, and 5,000 deaths in the United States every year. Three organisms—*Salmonella, Listeria, and Toxoplasma*—are responsible for more than 75 percent of these deaths. Although most foodborne infections cause mild illness, severe infections and serious complications—including death—do occur.

Scares about tainted food have led to massive recalls of such popular foods as peanut butter, jalapenos, lettuce, spinach, and tomatoes.[41] As a result, consumer advocates, as well as manufacturers and trade associations, are calling for stricter regulations.[42]

What can you do to protect yourself? Pay attention when you hear that a food or product is under suspicion. Make note of the brands, the production dates, and the manufacturer(s) involved. Check the labels of the foods in your pantry and refrigerator, and throw out any that may be contaminated.

Fight BAC!

To improve food safety awareness and practices, government and private agencies have developed the Fight BAC! campaign, which identifies four key culprits in foodborne illness:

- **Improper cooling.**
- **Improper hand washing.**
- **Inadequate cooking.**
- **Failure to avoid cross-contamination.**

Avoiding *E. coli* Infection

Eating unwashed produce, such as spinach or lettuce, or undercooked beef, especially hamburger, can increase your risk of infection with *Escherichia coli (E. coli)* bacteria. These bacteria, which live in the intestinal tract of healthy people and animals, are usually harmless. However, infection with the strain *E. coli* O157:H7 produces symptoms that can range from mild to life-threatening. This strain has made its way into hamburger in fast-food chains and into packaged spinach. *E. coli* can cause severe bloody diarrhea, kidney failure, and even death. Symptoms usually develop within two to ten days and can include severe stomach cramps, vomiting, mild fever, and bloody diarrhea. Most people recover within seven to ten days. Others—especially older adults, children under the age of five, and those with weakened immune systems—may develop complications that lead to kidney failure.

Proper handling and cooking of food can practically eliminate infection from meat. Especially if grilled, meat is likely to brown before it's completely cooked, so a meat thermometer should be used to ensure that meat is heated to at least 160°F at its thickest point. If a thermometer is not available, ground meat should be cooked until no pink shows in the center.

Food Poisoning

Salmonella is a bacterium that contaminates many foods, particularly undercooked chicken, eggs, and sometimes processed meat. Eating contaminated food can result in salmonella poisoning, which causes diarrhea and vomiting. The Centers for Disease Control and Prevention (CDC) estimates 40,000 reported cases of salmonella poisoning a year; the actual number of cases could be anywhere from 400,000 to 4 million. The FDA has warned consumers about the dangers of unpasteurized orange juice because of the risk of salmonella contamination.

Another bacterium, *Campylobacter jejuni*, may cause even more stomach infections than salmonella. Found in water, milk, and some foods, campylobacter poisoning causes severe diarrhea and has been implicated in the growth of stomach ulcers.

Bacteria can also cause illness by producing toxins in food. *Staphylococcus aureus* is the most common culprit. When cooked foods are cross-contaminated with the bacteria from raw foods and not stored properly, staph infections can result, causing nausea and abdominal pain anywhere from 30 minutes to 8 hours after ingestion.

Even many healthful foods can pose dangers. The FDA has urged consumers to avoid eating raw sprouts because of the risk of getting sick. Sprouts, particularly alfalfa and clover, can be contaminated by salmonella or *E. coli* bacteria. The FDA advises people to either cook sprouts before eating them or request that they be left off sandwiches and other food ordered in restaurants. Home-grown sprouts can also present a risk if they come from contaminated seeds.

An uncommon but sometimes fatal form of food poisoning is botulism, caused by the *Clostridium botulinum* organism. Improper home-canning procedures are the most common cause of this potentially fatal problem.

There have been several outbreaks of listeriosis, caused by the bacterium *Listeria,* commonly found in deli meats, hot dogs, soft cheeses, raw meat, and unpasteurized milk. Although rare, listeriosis can be life-threatening. At greatest risk are pregnant women, infants, and those with weakened immune systems. You can reduce your risk by cooking meats and leftovers thoroughly and by washing everything that may come into contact with raw meat.

Pesticides

Plants and animals naturally produce compounds that act as pesticides to aid in their survival. The vast majority of the pesticides we consume are therefore natural, not added by farmers or food processors. *Commercial pesticides* save billions of dollars of valuable crops from pests, but they also may endanger human health and life. Fearful of potential risks in pesticides, many consumers are purchasing organic foods.

Food Allergies

Food allergies are more common in children than adults, and there is controversy over whether they have been overdiagnosed.

Physicians disagree as to which foods are the most common triggers of food allergies. Cow's milk, eggs, seafood, wheat, soybeans, nuts, seeds, and chocolate have all been identified as culprits. The symptoms they provoke vary. One person might sneeze if exposed to an irritating food; another might vomit or develop diarrhea; others might suffer headaches, dizziness, hives, or a rapid heartbeat. Symptoms may not develop for up to 72 hours, making it hard to pinpoint which food was responsible.

If you suspect that you have a food allergy, see a physician with specialized training in allergy diagnosis. Medical opinion about the merits of many treatments for food allergies is divided. Once you've identified the culprit, the wisest and sometimes simplest course is to avoid it.

Nutritional Quackery

The American Dietetic Association describes nutritional quackery as a growing problem for unsuspecting consumers. Because so much nutritional nonsense is garbed in scientific-sounding terms, it can be hard to recognize bad advice when you get it. One basic rule: If the promises of a nutritional claim sound too good to be true, they probably are (see Consumer Alert, p. 200).

If you seek the advice of a nutrition consultant, carefully check his or her credentials and professional associations. Because licensing isn't required in all states, almost anyone can use the label "nutritionist," regardless of qualifications. Be wary of diplomas from obscure schools and organizations that allow anyone who pays dues to join. (One physician obtained a membership for his dog!) A registered dietitian (R.D.), who has a bachelor's degree and specialized training (including an internship) and who passed a certification examination, is usually a member of the American Dietetic Association (ADA), which sets the standard for quality in diets. A nutrition expert with an M.D. or Ph.D. generally belongs to the ADA, the American Institute of Nutrition, or the American Society of Clinical Nutrition; all have stringent membership requirements.

Spot the Hype!

Facts to Know

Nutritional supplements sold in health stores or through health and body-building magazines may contain ingredients that have not been tested and proven safe.

- Be wary of anyone who recommends megadoses of vitamins or nutritional supplements, which can be dangerous. High doses of vitamin A, which some people take to clear up acne, can be toxic.
- A quick way to spot a bad nutrition self-help book is to look in the index for a diet to prevent or treat rheumatoid arthritis (none exists). If you find one, don't buy the book.

Steps to Take

- Before you try any new nutritional approach, check with your doctor or a registered dietitian or call the American Dietetic Association's consumer hotline, (800) 366–1655.
- Don't believe ads or advisers basing their nutritional recommendations on hair analysis, which is not accurate in detecting nutritional deficiencies.
- Question personal testimonies about the powers of some magical pill or powder, and be wary of "scientific articles" in journals that aren't reviewed by health professionals.

Satisfaction guaranteed
Marketers may make generous promises, but consumers won't be able to collect on them.

One product does it all
No one product can possibly treat such a diverse array of conditions.

Time tested
Such findings would be widely publicized and accepted by health professionals.

Paranoid accusations
And this product's company doesn't want money? At least the drug company has scientific research proving the safety and effectiveness of its products.

Quick and easy fixes
Even proven treatments take time to be effective.

Natural
Natural is not necessarily better or safer; any product that is strong enough to be effective is strong enough to cause side effects.

Personal testimonials
Hearsay is the weakest form of evidence.

Meaningless medical jargon
Phony terms hide the lack of scientific proof.

Guaranteed! OR your money back!

Instant recovery, back to your everyday schedule

"Best pills around"

"Cures gout, ulcers, diabetes and cancer"

Wonder Pills

W

The natural way to becoming a better you

Revolutionary product, based on ancient medicine

Money grabbing drug companies further corporate means

Super Trim

S

"My friends feel good as new!"

Beats the hunger stimulation point (HSP)

As nutritional knowledge expands and evolves, it's easy to be confused by changing advice on which foods to avoid and which to eat. But even though research may challenge or change thinking on a specific food, some basic principles always apply.

- **Eat breakfast.** Easy-to-prepare breakfasts include cold cereal with fruit and low-fat milk, whole-wheat toast with peanut butter, yogurt with fruit, or whole-grain waffles.
- **Don't eat too much of one thing.** Your body needs protein, carbohydrates, fat, and many different vitamins and minerals, such as vitamins C and A, iron, and calcium, from a variety of foods.
- **Eat more grains, fruits, and vegetables.** These foods give you carbohydrates for energy, plus vitamins, minerals, and fiber. Try breads such as whole-wheat, bagels, and pita. Spaghetti and oatmeal are also in the grain group.
- **Don't ban any food.** Fit in a higher-fat food, like pepperoni pizza, at dinner by choosing lower-fat foods at other meals. And don't forget about moderation. If two pieces of pizza fill you up, don't eat a third.
- **Make every calorie count.** Load up on nutrients, not on big portions. Choosing foods that are nutrient dense will help protect against disease and keep you healthy.

SELF SURVEY   How Healthful Is Your Diet?

Step 1
Keep a food diary for a week, writing down everything you eat and drink for meals and snacks. Include the approximate amount eaten (for example, 1/2 cup, 1 large, 12-oz can, and so on).

	Mon	Tues	Wed	Thurs	Fri	Sat	Sun
Grains							
Vegetables							
Fruits							
Milk, yogurt, cheese							
Meat, poultry, dry beans, eggs, nuts							
Fats, oil, sweets							

STEP 2: Are You Getting Enough Vegetables, Fruits, and Grains?

How often do you eat:	Seldom/Never	1–2 times a week	3–5 times a week	Almost daily
At least three servings of vegetables a day?				
Starchy vegetables like potatoes, corn, or peas?				
Foods made with dry beans, lentils, or peas?				
Dark green or deep yellow vegetables (broccoli, spinach, collards, carrots, sweet potatoes, squash)?				
At least two servings of fruit a day?				
Citrus fruits and 100% fruit juices (oranges, grapefruit, tangerines)?				
Whole fruit with skin or seeds (berries, apples, pears)?				
At least six servings of breads, cereals, pasta, or rice a day?				

The best answer for each is "almost daily." Use your food diary to see which foods you should be eating more often.

STEP 3: Are You Getting Too Much Fat?

How often do you eat:	Seldom/Never	1–2 times a week	3–5 times a week	Almost daily
Fried, deep-fat fried, or breaded food?				
Fatty meats, such as sausages, luncheon meat, fatty steaks or roasts?				
Whole milk, high-fat cheeses, ice cream?				
Pies, pastries, rich cakes?				
Rich cream sauces and gravies?				
Oily salad dressings or mayonnaise?				
Butter or margarine on vegetables, rolls, bread, or toast?				

Ideally, you should be eating these foods no more than one or two times a week. If your food diary indicates that you're eating them more frequently, your fat intake may well be too high.

STEP 4: Are You Getting Too Much Sodium?

How often do you eat:	Seldom/Never	1–2 times a week	3–5 times a week	Almost daily
Cured or processed meats, such as ham, sausage, frankfurters, or luncheon meats?				
Canned vegetables or frozen vegetables with sauce?				
Frozen TV dinners, entrees, or canned or dehydrated soups?				
Salted nuts, popcorn, pretzels, corn chips, or potato chips?				
Seasoning mixes or sauces containing salt?				
Processed cheese?				
Salt added to table foods before you taste them?				

Ideally, you should be eating these high-sodium items no more than one or two times a week. If your food diary indicates that you're eating them more frequently, your sodium intake may well be too high.

Your Health Action Plan for Better Nutrition

- **Eat five servings of fruits and vegetables per day.** For breakfast, have 100% fruit juice or add raisins, berries, or sliced fruit to cereal, pancakes, or waffles. For lunch, have vegetable soup or salad with your meal or pile vegetables on your sandwich. For dinner, choose vegetables that are green, orange (such as carrots or squash), and red (such as tomatoes or bell peppers).

- **Include three servings of whole-grain foods every day.** To identify whole-grain products, check the ingredient list. The first ingredient should be a whole grain, such as "whole-grain oats," "whole-grain wheat," or "whole wheat."

- **Consume a calcium-rich food at each meal.** Good options include low-fat and nonfat milk; cheese; or yogurt; tofu; broccoli; dried beans; spinach; and fortified soy milk.

- **Eat less meat.** Rather than making meat the heart of a meal, think of it as a flavoring ingredient.

- **Avoid high-fat fast foods.** Hot dogs, fried foods, packaged snack foods, and pastries are most likely to be laden with fat.

- **Check the numbers.** When buying prepared foods, choose items that contain no more than 3 grams of fat per 100 calories.

- **Think small.** A dinner-size serving of meat should be about the size of a deck of cards; half a cup is the size of a woman's fist; a pancake is the diameter of a CD.

- **Read labels carefully.** Remember that "cholesterol-free" doesn't necessarily mean fat-free. Avoid products that contain saturated coconut oil, palm oil, lard, or hydrogenated fats.

- **Switch to low-fat and nonfat dairy products.** Rather than buying whole-fat dairy products, choose skim milk, fat-free sour cream, and low- or nonfat yogurt.

- **The brighter the better.** When selecting fruits and vegetables, choose the most intense color. A bright orange carrot has more beta-carotene than a pale one. Dark green lettuce leaves have more vitamins than lighter ones. Orange sweet potatoes pack more vitamin A than yellow ones.

CENGAGENOW™ If you want to write your own goals for more nutritious choices, go to the Wellness Journal at CengageNow for Health: **www.cengage.com/sso.**

MAKING THIS CHAPTER WORK FOR YOU

Review Questions

1. An example of an unhealthy saturated fat would be:
   a. olive oil
   b. canola oil
   c. corn oil
   d. coconut oil

2. The 2005 Dietary Guidelines for Americans include:
   a. Maintain intake of added sugars.
   b. Decrease consumption of olive oil.
   c. Control calorie intake to manage body weight.
   d. Eat dessert no more than three days a week.

3. Common causes of foodborne infections include which of the following?
   a. the influenza virus
   b. *Salmonella* and *E. coli* bacteria
   c. avian flu virus
   d. pesticides

4. The classes of essential nutrients include which of the following?
   a. amino acids, antioxidants, fiber, and cholesterol
   b. proteins, calcium, calories, and folic acid
   c. carbohydrates, minerals, fat, and water
   d. iron, whole grains, fruits, and vegetables

5. Some vegetarians may
   a. include fish in their diets.
   b. avoid vitamin B_{12} supplements if they eat only plant foods.
   c. eat only legumes or nuts because these provide complete proteins.
   d. have high cholesterol levels because of the saturated fats in fruits and vegetables.

6. Which nutrient has the greatest number of calories?
   a. protein
   b. carbohydrate
   c. vitamins
   d. fats

7. Since Sam plays poker, it's been easy for him to remember that a recommended serving of 3 ounces of meat means a piece of meat about the size of
   a. one deck of cards.
   b. eight poker chips.
   c. two decks of cards.
   d. a roll of quarters.

8. It is recommended that no greater than 30% of a healthy diet come from
   a. fats.
   b. sugars.
   c. starches.
   d. protein.

9. Food labels on packaged foods include all of the following *except*
   a. total weight of the package.
   b. total amount of nutrients contained in the food.
   c. the percent of nutrient Daily Values provided in the food.
   d. serving size.

10. Antioxidants
    a. are nutrients important in the production of hemoglobin.
    b. are substances added to foods to make them more flavorful or physically appealing.
    c. are suspected triggers of food allergies.
    d. are substances that prevent the harmful effects of free radicals.

Answers to these questions can be found on page 650.

Critical Thinking

1. Which alternative or ethnic diet do you think has the best tasting food? Which is the most healthy? Why?

2. Is it possible to meet nutritional requirements on a limited budget? Have you ever been in this situation? What would you recommend to someone who wanted to eat healthfully on $30 a week?

3. Consider the number of times a week you eat fast food. How much money would you have saved if you had eaten home-prepared meals? Which fast foods could you have selected that would have provided more nutritional value?

Media Menu

CENGAGENOW™ Go to the CengageNOW for Health website at **www .cengage.com/sso** that will:
- Help you evaluate your knowledge of the material.
- Allow you to take an exam-prep quiz.
- Provide a personalized Learning Plan targeting resources that address areas you should study.
- Coach you through identifying target goals for behavioral change and creating and monitoring your personal change plan throughout the semester.

Internet Connections

www.nal.usda.gov/fnic/
This comprehensive governmental website features reports and scientific studies on a variety of nutrition information, including the 2005 USDA Dietary Guidelines, MyPyramid, dietary supplements, dietary assessment, food composition searchable databases, educational brochures, historical food guides, and a topics "A-Z" section.

www.MyPyramid.gov
This interactive site features MyPyramid Plan, which gives you a personal eating plan, and MyPyramid Tracker, which offers a detailed assessment of your food intake and physical activity level.

http://nat.crgq.com
This site, provided as a public service by the Food Science and Human Nutrition Department at the University of Illinois, features a free nutrient analysis interactive program that calculates the amount of calories, carbohydrates, protein, fat, vitamins, minerals, and fiber in the foods that make up your daily diet.

www.nhlbisupport.com/chd1/Tipsheets/cyberkit.htm
This interactive site helps you discover how much you are really eating with an activity on comparing standard serving sizes versus real serving sizes. You also can provide personal information regarding your age, gender, height, weight, and activity level, and the Cyberkitchen will provide you with a healthy diet plan to meet your weight management goals. It's fun and educational.

Key Terms

The terms listed are used on the page indicated. Definitions of the terms are in the Glossary at the end of the book.

amino acids 169
antioxidants 174
basal metabolic rate (BMR) 167
calorie 167
carbohydrates 169
complementary proteins 192
complete proteins 169
complex carbohydrates 169
dietary fiber 171
essential nutrients 167
folic acid 187
functional fiber 171
incomplete proteins 169
lacto-vegetarians 192

macronutrients 167
micronutrients 167
minerals 174
nutrition 165
organic 197
ovo-lacto-vegetarians 192
phytochemicals 179
proteins 169
saturated fats 171
simple carbohydrates 169
trans fat 173
unsaturated fats 171
vegans 192
vitamins 174

Chapter 7 - Managing Your Weight

1. It is estimated that Americans are exercising much less than 25 years ago which leads to more overweight issues. Americans are now burning how many less calories than in the past? (Pg. 208)
   - A. less than 50 calories
   - B. 100- 150 calories
   - C. 200- 300 calories
   - D. more than 400 calories

2. Which of the following is not a factor associated with the global increase in obesity? (Pg. 207- 208)
   - A. our fast food menus have increased serving size and portions
   - B. technology has allowed people to be more sedentary in their behaviors
   - C. babies are being born fatter and also starting the overweight trend at birth
   - D. physical activity is taking a set back to passive television viewing

3. An accumulation of fat beyond what is considered to be normal for a person's sex, age, and body type is called: (Pg. 212)
   - A. overweight
   - B. obesity
   - C. body fat
   - D. body composition

4. What is the basal metabolism rate and why is this so important for weight control? (Pg. 211)
   - A. it is another way to define body mass index
   - B. it is the metabolic breathing rate
   - C. it is the number of calories needed to sustain the body at rest
   - D. it is the number of calories to maintain the body after physical activity

5. A body mass index (BMI) of 30 would indicate: (Pg. 212)
   - A. underweight
   - B. average weight for height and weight
   - C. borderline overweight
   - D. obese

6. One is considered to be overweight when their BMI is at what range: (Pg. 212)
   - A. BMI 15- 19
   - B. BMI 19- 24
   - C. BMI 25- 29
   - D. BMI 30- 35

7. What percent of overweight people in this country suffer from Type 2 diabetes? (Pg. 213)
   - A. 20%
   - B. 33%
   - C. 50%
   - D. 80%

8. Being grossly overweight or obese can lead to all of the following health conditions except: (Pg. 212)
   - A. developing gallstones
   - B. hardening of the arteries
   - C. impotence in males
   - D. colon cancer

9. Obesity surgery should not be attempted unless a person has a BMI of 40 or greater and also meets which qualification?:
   (Pg. 223)
   - A. has made many unsuccessful attempts to diet and lose weight
   - B. has trouble fitting into smaller size clothing
   - C. is not able to exercise or walk very well
   - D. none of the above

10. Which of the following would not be a sensible plan for losing weight in a weight loss program Lynn is trying to accomplish?
    (Pg. 230)
    - A. start slowly with the weight loss program
    - B. set a goal to lose ten pounds in the first week of your loss weight plan
    - C. adopt the 90% rule of good eating habits 90% of the time
    - D. make a graph and keep track of what you are losing each week

11. **Explain what the physiological desire to consume food is know as:** (Pg. 215)
   - A. caloric need
   - B. appetite
   - C. satiety
   - D. hunger

12. **All of the following behaviors may signal compulsive overeating except:** (Pg. 225)
   - A. eating only at set meal times
   - B. history of failed diets
   - C. refusing to talk about food
   - D. turning to food as a reward

13. **All of the following can increase the risk of developing an eating disorder except:** (Pg. 226)
   - A. social pressure
   - B. preoccupation with a thin body
   - C. perfectionism
   - D. having no siblings

14. **All of the following are characteristic of anorexia except:** (Pg. 227)
   - A. fear of gaining weight
   - B. severe menstrual cramps
   - C. distorted body image
   - D. refusal to maintain normal body weight

15. **Megan binge eats and then secretly vomits her food. What eating disorder is she likely suffering from?** (Pg. 228)
   - A. pica
   - B. anorexia
   - C. bulimia
   - D. binge eating disorder

16. **All of the following may play a role in the development of bulimia except:** (Pg. 229)
   - A. depression
   - B. family conflicts
   - C. being accepted to college
   - D. transitioning to adulthood

17. **Which would not be used by those who binge eat and purge afterwards?** (Pg. 228)
   - A. laxative use
   - B. vomiting
   - C. using diuretics
   - D. fasting

18. **For many people who suffer from eating disorders, a helpful solution is for the person to:** (Pg. 226)
   - A. focus on the feelings and not use food to stuff their emotions
   - B. put your body in charge of what you eat
   - C. know what your triggers are that get you going to over eat
   - D. all of the above

19. **Carrie suffers from an acute form of self starvation motivated by a fear of gaining weight and how she perceives her body image. She is likely suffering from:** (Pg. 227)
   - A. anorexia
   - B. bulimia
   - C. binge eating disorder
   - D. compulsive eating disorder

20. **All of the following but one are important considerations to starting a personal weight management program to lose or maintain your weight.** (Pg. 230)
   - A. being realistic with small weigh loss goals
   - B. practicing good eating habits at least 90% of the time
   - C. mentally beating yourself up when your weight loss plan is not going well
   - D. plotting or graphing your weekly weigh losses to see the progress

ina's mother called it "baby fat." "You'll outgrow it soon enough," she said. Yet Lina's cheeks grew chubbier and her waist wider every year. "Wait for your growth spurt," her mother reassured her. But Lina remained one of the shortest girls in her class—and, she was convinced, the roundest.

Lina went on her first diet in high school. For three days she ate nothing but carrot sticks, cottage cheese, and apples. Then she scarfed down two double cheese-

Managing Your Weight

burgers with fries and a chocolate shake. Her other attempts at dieting didn't last much longer. By graduation Lina was grateful to hide under the flowing black robe as she walked on stage to get her diploma.

When Lina heard about the "freshman 15," the extra pounds many students acquire during their first year at college, she groaned at the prospect of putting on more weight. In her Personal Health class, Lina set one primary goal: not to gain another pound. Rather than going on—and inevitably falling off—one diet after another, she developed a weight management plan that included healthful food choices and regular exercise. Armed with the information and tools provided in this chapter, Lina, for the first time in her life, took charge of her weight.

You can do the same.

This chapter explains how we grew so big, tells what obesity is and why excess pounds are dangerous, describes current approaches to weight loss, discusses diets that work (and some that don't), offers practical guidelines for exercise and behavioral approaches to losing weight, and examines unhealthy eating patterns and eating disorders. Using the Making Change Happen on p. 221 and in *Labs for IPC*, you can practice "Thinking Thinner." If you're already at a healthy weight, this chapter can ensure that you remain so in the future. If, like two-thirds of Americans, you are overweight, you will find help in these pages. Remember: You *can* choose to lose.

After studying the material in this chapter, you should be able to

- **List** the factors besides genetics that have contributed to the global increase in overweight and obesity.
- **Define** overweight and obesity.
- **Identify** the main health risks of excess weight.
- **Assess** various approaches to weight loss.
- **Identify** and **describe** the symptoms and dangers associated with eating disorders.
- **Design** a personal plan for sensible weight management.

Log on to CengageNOW for Health at **www.cengage.com/sso** to find your Behavior Change Planner and to explore self-assessments, interactive tutorials, and practice quizzes.

The Global Epidemic

 An estimated 1.1 billion people around the world—seven in ten of the Dutch and Spanish, two in three Americans and Canadians, and one in two Britons, Germans, and Italians—are overweight or obese. In Europe, excess weight ranks as the most common childhood disorder. Since 1980, obesity rates have tripled in parts of Eastern Europe, the Middle East, China, and the Pacific Islands. In many poor countries, obesity is common among city dwellers, while people in rural areas remain underweight and malnourished.

The World Health Organization, in its first global diet, exercise, and health program to combat obesity, recommends that governments promote public knowledge about diet, exercise, and health; offer information that makes healthy choices easier for consumers to make; and require accurate, comprehensible food labels.[1] Although ultimately each individual decides what and how much to eat, policy makers agree that governments also must act to reverse the obesity epidemic.

Exposure to a Western lifestyle seems to bring out susceptibility to excess weight. Obesity is much more common among the Pima Indians of Arizona compared to Pimas living in Mexico, who have maintained a more traditional lifestyle, with more physical activity and a diet lower in fat and richer in complex carbohydrates. Native Hawaiians who follow a more traditional diet and lifestyle also have lower rates of obesity and cardiovascular disease.

Millions of men and women in the United States weigh more—often two times more— than their recommended ideal weights.

© iStockphoto.com/Joanna Pecha

Supersized Nation

 Obesity rates among young adults have tripled in the last three decades, rising from 8 percent to 24 percent.[2] The prevalence of obesity among men has increased significantly since 1999, rising to 31 percent. The rate of obesity among women has remained the same: 33 percent. About 3 percent of men and 7 percent of women are extremely obese. By some estimates, Americans are collectively more than 5 billion pounds overweight. Some 200 million men and women weigh more—often much more—than their recommended target weights.

Obesity rates vary by ethnic groups as well as by gender and age. About 30 percent of white Americans are obese, compared with 45 percent of African Americans and 37 percent of Mexican Americans. In some Native American communities, up to 70 percent of all adults are dangerously overweight. Differences in metabolic rates may be one factor.

Not all Americans are equally likely to be overweight or obese. As Figure 7.1 shows, the southern states have the highest concentration of obese residents. Mississippi is home to the county with the highest percentage of people with a body mass index (BMI) between 30 and 40. (BMI, as discussed in Chapter 5, is defined as the ratio between weight and height that correlates with percentage of body fat.)

Weight problems are starting earlier than ever. About one in four children between ages 2 and 5 is overweight or at risk of becoming overweight. Among those between ages 6 and 11, the percentage rises to 37 percent. About one in three teenagers falls into this category. The earlier the weight gain, the greater the danger posed. Obesity at age 20 can cut 20 years off a person's life.

How Did We Get So Fat?

A variety of factors, ranging from behavior to environment to genetics, played a role in the increase in overweight and obesity. They include:

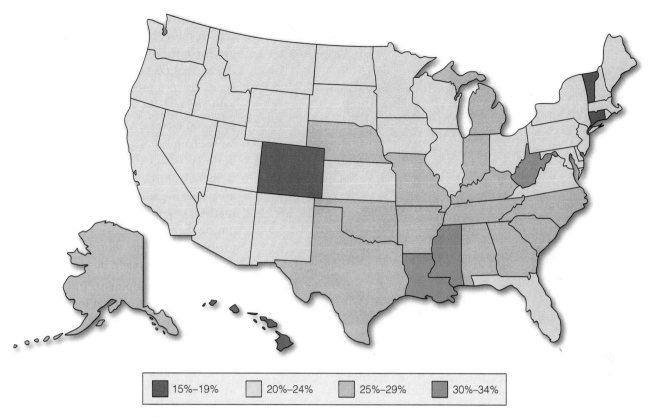

	15%–19%		20%–24%		25%–29%		30%–34%

Figure 7.1 Obesity in the United States

This map shows the percentage of people in each state who are obese—they have a body mass index between 30 and 40.

Source: Data from National Center for Chronic Disease Prevention and Health Promotion, "At a Glance 2007," www.cdc.gov.nccdphp/publications/aag/dnpa.htm.

- **More calories.** Bombarded by nonstop commercials for taste treats, tempted by foods in every form to munch and crunch, in the last 30 years the average man has added 168 calories and the average woman 335 calories to their daily diets. Many of these extra calories come from refined carbohydrates, which can raise levels of heart-damaging blood fats called triglycerides and increase the risk of diabetes as well as obesity. As discussed in Chapter 6, soft drinks account for half of the increase in caloric intake.

- **Bigger portions.** As Table 7.1 shows, the size of many popular restaurant and packaged foods has increased two to five times during the past 20 years. Some foods, like chocolate bars, have grown more than ten times since they were first introduced. Popular 64-ounce sodas can pack a whopping 800 calories. According to studies of appetite and satiety, people presented with larger portions eat up to 30 percent more than they otherwise would.

TABLE 7.1

Supersized Portions

Food/Beverage	Original Size (year introduced)	Today (largest available)
Soda (Coca-Cola)	6.5 oz (1916)	34 oz
French fries (Burger King)	2.6 oz (1954)	6.9 oz
Hamburger (McDonald's); (beef only)	1.6 oz (1965)	8 oz
Nestlés Crunch	1.6 oz (1938)	5 oz
Budweiser (bottle)	7 oz (1976)	40 oz

Matthew Farruggio (both)

Source: Are Growing Portion Sizes Leading to Expanding Waistlines?" American Dietetic Association, www.eatright.org.

- **Fast food.** Young adults who eat frequently at fast-food restaurants gain more weight and develop metabolic abnormalities that increase their risk of diabetes in early middle age. In a recent

Round-the-clock snacking, fast-food restaurants on every corner, and hours in front of the TV have all contributed to the increase in overweight and obesity.

study, those who ate fast food at least twice a week gained an extra ten pounds and had a twofold greater increase in insulin resistance, a risk factor for diabetes. The men in the study visited fast-food restaurants more often than the women; African Americans did so more frequently than whites.

- **Physical inactivity.** As Americans eat more, they exercise less. Experts estimate that most adults expend 200 to 300 fewer calories than people did 25 years ago. The most dramatic drop in physical activity often occurs during the college years.

- **Passive entertainment.** Television is a culprit in an estimated 30 percent of new cases of obesity. TV viewing may increase weight in several ways: It takes up time that otherwise might be spent in physical activities. It increases food intake since people tend to eat more while watching TV. And compared with sewing, reading, driving, or other relatively sedentary pursuits, watching television lowers metabolic rate so viewers burn fewer calories. The combination of watching television (at least two and one-half hours a day) and eating fast food more than twice a week can triple the risk of obesity.

- **Genetics.** Scientists have identified a specific gene, found in one-sixth of people of European descent, that

increases the risk of obesity by 30 percent or more. It also may be that various genes contribute a small increase in risk or that rare abnormalities in many genes create a predisposition to weight gain and obesity.

- **Prenatal factors.** A woman's weight before conception and weight gain during pregnancy influence her child's weight. A substantial number of children are prone to gaining weight because their mothers developed gestational diabetes during their pregnancies. Children born to obese women are more than twice as likely to be overweight by age four.

- **Childhood development.** Today's children don't necessarily eat more food than in the past, but they eat more high-fat, high-calorie foods and they exercise much, much less. On days when they eat fast food, youngsters consume an average of 187 more calories per day. Fewer than half of grade schoolers participate in daily physical education classes. Many spend five hours or more a day in front of a computer or television screen.

- **Emotional influences.** Obese people are neither more nor less psychologically troubled than others. Psychological problems, such as irritability, depression, and anxiety, are more likely to be the result of obesity than the cause. As discussed later in this chapter, emotions do play a role in weight problems. Just as some people reach for a drink or a drug when they're upset, others cope by overeating, bingeing, or purging.

- **Social networks.** Friends may have a significant effect on a person's risk of obesity. A 32-year detailed analysis of a large social network of 12,067 people found that when one close friend became obese, the others' chances of doing the same increased by 171 percent. Among pairs of adult siblings, if one became obese, the chance that the other would become obese increased by 40 percent. Researchers cannot fully explain why this happens. Perhaps one explanation is that friends alter each others' perception of fatness: When a close friend is obese, obesity seems normal and acceptable.

The Social Context

Is obesity an individual problem or a societal one? Some experts argue that obesity may be a problem that cannot be solved by individual persons but that requires community action. Two small towns in France illustrate this point. Starting in 2000 everyone from the mayor to shop owners, schoolteachers, doctors, restaurant owners, the media, and various government officials joined in an effort to encourage children to eat better and move around more. The towns built more playgrounds, trails, and sports facilities and hired sports instructors. By 2005 the prevalence of overweight children had fallen to 8.8 percent while it had risen to 17.8 percent in a neighboring town. This preventive community approach is being extended to 200 towns in Europe under the name EPODE (for the French equivalent of "Together, let's prevent obesity in children").[3]

Whatever your age, wherever you live, the less money you make, the more likely you are to be overweight. One in four adults below the poverty level is obese, compared with one in six in households earning $67,000 or more. Minorities are at even greater risk. One in three poor African Americans is obese.

 Location is important because where you live influences the availability of healthful food choices and the quality of your diet. In studies of diverse neighborhoods in Baltimore, Maryland, researchers found a much lower availability of healthful foods in predominately black, low-income areas, compared with more affluent white ones.[4] Lower-income and minority neighborhoods generally have greater access to fast-food restaurants and high-calorie foods.[5] Obesity rates are consistently higher in neighborhoods with more small grocery stores and fast-food restaurants and fewer supermarkets.[6] However, suburban sprawl also directly contributes to obesity, according to research. People who live in neighborhoods where they must drive to get anywhere are significantly more likely to be obese than those who can easily walk to their destinations.

Body Image

Throughout most of history, bigger was better. The great beauties of centuries past, as painted by such artistic masters as Rubens and Renoir, were soft and fleshy, with rounded bellies and dimpled thighs. Culture often shapes views of beauty and health.

 Many developing countries still regard a full figure, rather than a thin one, as the ideal. Fattening huts, in which brides-to-be eat extra food to plump up before marriage, still exist in some African cultures. Among certain Native American tribes of the Southwest, if a girl is thin at puberty, a fat woman places her foot on the girl's back so she will magically gain weight and become more attractive.

Influenced by the media, many Americans are paying more attention to their body images than ever before. The "perfect body" ideal popularized by television, magazines, and movies can undermine a positive body image and cause girls and women to go to extreme measures to control their weight.[7]

The more time that women spend reading fashion magazines, the more "antifat" their attitudes are and the greater dissatisfaction with their bodies.[8] Boys' body images also are influenced by media images depicting superstrong, highly muscular males.

Being overweight for a long period of time has a cumulative negative impact on body image. In a study of 266 college women, those who described themselves as "always overweight" ranked much lower in current body self-esteem than those with more recent weight problems.

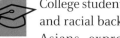 College students of different ethnic and racial backgrounds, including Asians, express as much—and sometimes more—concern about their body shape and weight as whites. In a study of university students, African American and Caucasian men were similar in their ideals for body size and in their perceptions of their own shapes. Both African American and white women perceive themselves as

Some people have a distorted view of their weight. How do you decide what your ideal body size is?

© Rubberball/Jupiterimages

smaller than they actually were and desire an even smaller body size. However, African American women are more accepting of larger size.

Male and Female Body Image

 Although women generally report a more negative body image, many men are dissatisfied with their bodies but for different reasons. Often they want either to lose or gain weight or to add muscle and bulk. Women compare their appearance to others more frequently than

men and worry more that others will think negatively about their looks. Yet appearance matters just as much to men, who are as likely as women to engage in efforts to improve their bodies.

Women have long been bombarded by idealized images in the media of female bodies that bear little resemblance to the way most women look. Increasingly, more advertisements and men's magazines are featuring idealized male bodies. Sleek, strong, and sculpted, they do not resemble the bodies most men inhabit. The gap between reality and ideal is getting bigger for both genders.

When college men and women step on a scale or look in a mirror, they react in different ways. In a study of 525 undergraduates, the women failed to see themselves as underweight, even when they were, and perceived themselves as overweight, even when they were not. Many of the women who considered themselves normal weight nonetheless desired to be thinner. Men in the study generally saw themselves as underweight, even when they were not. Most desired to be heavier, though not obese.

The higher their body fat percentage, the more dissatisfied college women tend to be with their shape. Women at all-female schools are just as prone to distorted perceptions of body size and body dissatisfaction as those at coed institutions.

The greater the discrepancy between a woman's current view of her body shape and the ideal she considers most attractive to men, the more likely she is to worry about how others will view her and to doubt her ability to make a desirable impression. Such "social physique anxiety" occurs often in women who feel they do not measure up to what they or others consider most desirable in terms of weight or appearance. Women with high BMIs and greater body-related anxiety may exercise to become thinner or more attractive. Those reporting the greatest distress because of body image are at highest risk of disordered eating or actual eating disorders (discussed later in this chapter).

Health educators are tackling the thorny issue of body image in various ways, including discussions of the media's role in influencing how people perceive their bodies. "Health educators should demand that airbrushed, touched up, and computer-enhanced images be replaced with those of real, beautiful women complete with freckles, stretch marks, scars, and, on occasion, cellulite," argues Catherine Rasberry of Texas A&M University.[9] Do you think more realistic media images would affect how you feel about your body?

Understanding Weight Problems

Weight problems don't develop overnight. Fat accumulates meal by meal, day by day, pound by pound. Ultimately, all weight problems are the result of a prolonged energy imbalance—of consuming too many calories and burning too few in daily activities.

How many calories you need depends on your gender, age, body-frame size, weight, percentage of body fat, and your *basal metabolic rate* (BMR)—the number of calories needed to sustain your body at rest. Your activity level also affects your calorie requirements. Regardless of whether you consume fat, protein, or carbohydrates, if you take in more calories than required to maintain your size and don't work them off in some sort of physical activity, your body will convert the excess to fat.

The average American consumes about 1 million calories a year. Given that number, what difference does an extra 100-calorie soda or 300-calorie brownie make? A lot, because the extra calories that you don't burn every day accumulate, adding an average of two to four pounds to your weight every year.

Weight and the College Student

 Obesity rates have increased most rapidly among 18- to 29-year-olds, including college students.[10] (See "Reality Check", p. 213.) One in five college students has an unhealthy weight as well as at least one risk factor for metabolic disorder, an important cause of cardiovascular disease (discussed in Chapter 14).

As many students discover, it's easy to gain weight on campuses, which are typically crammed with vending machines, fast-food counters, and cafeterias serving up hearty meals. As discussed in Chapter 6, students who eat on the run often opt for fast food and consume more fatty foods and soft drinks, which increase their risk of obesity

and other health problems.[11] However. it is possible to hold the line on calories—and costs. (See Health on a Budget.)

The infamous *freshman 15,* the extra pounds acquired in the first year at college, seems to be a myth. Several studies have documented much lower weight gains, ranging from 2.45 to 7 pounds—still much more than the average yearly weight gain of .8 pounds by other Americans. In one recent study, more than half of freshmen at a southern university gained weight by the end of their first year. The mean number of pounds was seven. About a quarter of freshmen lost weight; the others showed no difference. Freshmen who were already overweight gained more weight than those whose weights, as determined by body mass index, were in the desirable range. Male freshmen were almost twice as likely to be classified as overweight as women.[12]

HEALTH ON A BUDGET

Hold the Line!

You can leave college a whole lot smarter but no heavier than when you entered—without spending extra money. Here are some suggestions:

- **Plan meals.** Most campus cafeterias post the week's menus in advance. Plan which items you will eat before you see or smell high-fat dishes.
- **Don't linger.** If you use the cafeteria as a social gathering place, you may end up eating with two or three different groups of people. Set a time limit to eat—then leave.
- **Develop alternative behavior.** People who eat when they are stressed or bored need substitute activities ready when they need them. Make a list of things you can do—shower, phone a friend, take a hike—when stress strikes.
- **Eat at "home."** If the dormitory has a small kitchen, cook some healthful dishes and invite friends to join you.
- **Take advantage of physical activity programs.** Many college students become less active during their years in college. Aim to maintain or increase the amount of exercise you did in high school. Join a biking club, take a salsa class, learn yoga, try tennis or raquetball.

Researchers have found other gender differences in first-year weight gain. In men, increased alcohol consumption and peer pressure to drink account for extra pounds. In women, the strongest correlation of weight gain was with an increased workload, which may lead to more stress-related eating, greater snacking, or less exercise.[13]

Although students do put on the most weight in their first term of college, many continue to gain weight as sophomores. Among the suspected culprits in college weight gain are alcohol, socializing that involves eating, high-fat foods in dorm cafeterias, and less physical activity.

What Is a Healthy Weight?

Rather than relying on a range of ideal weights for various heights, as they did in the past, medical experts use various methods to assess body composition and weight. The best indicators of weight-related health risks are body mass index (BMI); waist circumference (WC); and waist-to-hip ratio (WHR). (All are discussed in depth in Chapter 5.)

If you have a BMI higher than 25, you are **overweight** and at greater risk of health problems. If your BMI is between 30 and 34.9, you have class 1 **obesity.** If it is between 35 and 39.9, you have class 2 obesity. Both indicate increased risk of dying of weight-related problems. A BMI over 40 signifies class 3 or severe obesity and poses the greatest threat to health and longevity.

If you're a young adult, even mild to moderate overweight poses a threat to your health because it puts you at risk for gaining even more weight—and for facing greater health risks. Obesity has been implicated as a culprit in rising rates of disability among younger Americans as well as a factor in chronic health problems. If you are older than a traditional-aged student, the risks to your health are more immediate.

Health Dangers of Excess Weight

The federal government has recognized obesity as a serious, potentially fatal disease. This designation cleared the way for insurance coverage for obesity treatments, rather than just for the medical problems it can cause. The effects of obesity on health are the equivalent of 20 years of aging. They include increased risk of cardiovascular disease, diabetes, and cancer, as well as rheumatoid arthritis, sleep apnea, gout, and liver disease (Figure 7.2). Being overweight or obese at age 25 increases your likelihood of difficulties in walking, balance, and rising from a chair. Total medical costs, both direct and indirect, amount to more than $117 billion a year.

The Impact on the Body

The incidence of diabetes, gallstones, hypertension, heart disease, and colon cancer increases with the degree of overweight in both sexes. Those with BMIs of 35 or more are approximately 20 times more likely to develop diabetes. Overweight men and women are at least three times more likely to suffer knee injuries that require surgery to repair.

Health risks may vary in different races, ethnic groups, and at-risk populations. Even relatively small amounts of excess fat—as little as five pounds—can add to the dangers in those already at risk for hypertension and diabetes. Obesity also causes alterations in various measures of immune function and increases the risk of kidney stones and disease. It may also affect the brain and contribute to cognitive problems and dementia.

Overweight young adults have a 70 percent chance of becoming overweight or obese adults. They are two to three times more likely to have high total cholesterol levels and more than 43 times more likely to have cardiovascular disease risk factors such as elevated blood pressure. They also have a higher prevalence of type 2 diabetes.

Excess pounds affect people around the clock. Overweight and obese individuals sleep less than those with normal weights.

(See Chapter 2 for a discussion of sleep.) The lost sleep could add to the risk of medical problems.

Major diseases linked to obesity include:

- **Type 2 diabetes.** More than 80 percent of people with type 2 diabetes are overweight. Although the reasons are not known, being overweight may make cells less efficient at using sugar from the blood. This then puts stress on the cells that produce insulin (a hormone that carries sugar from the blood to cells) and makes them gradually fail. You can lower your risk for developing type 2 diabetes by losing weight and increasing the amount of physical activity you do. If you have type 2 diabetes, losing weight and becoming more physically active can help you control your blood sugar levels and may allow you to reduce the amount of diabetes medication you take.

- **Heart disease and stroke.** People who are overweight are more likely to suffer from high blood pressure, high levels of triglycerides (blood fats) and harmful LDL cholesterol, and low levels of beneficial HDL cholesterol. In addition, people with more body fat have higher blood levels of substances that cause inflammation, which may raise heart disease risk. Losing 5 to 15 percent of your weight can lower your chances for developing heart disease or having a stroke.

People who both smoke and are obese are at especially high risk of cardiovascular disease. Although some smokers have felt that they couldn't lose weight until they stopped smoking,

Cancer:

Breast, ovary, cervix, endometrium (women)

esophagus

kidney

gallbladder

non-Hodgkin's disease

stomach

colorectal

prostate (men)

Type 2 diabetes

High blood cholesterol

High blood pressure

Stroke

Daytime sleepiness/Sleep apnea

Impaired breathing

Heart disease

Pancreatitis

Kidney disease

Liver disease

Gallbladder disease

Carpal tunnel syndrome

Low back pain

Pain

Urinary stress incontinence

Surgical complications

Infections following wounds

Infertility

Impaired immunity

Osteoarthritis

Gout

Figure 7.2 Health Dangers of Excess Weight

overweight A condition of having a BMI between 25.0 and 29.9.

obesity The excessive accumulation of fat in the body; class 1 obesity is defined by a BMI between 30.0 and 34.9; class 2 obesity by a BMI between 35.0 and 39.9; class 3, or severe obesity, by a BMI of 40 or higher.

PART 2: *Just the Facts*
• **22** *percent of college students are overweight.*
• *Almost* **10** *percent are obese.*

Source: Pedersen, P. J., and P. L. Ketcham. "Exploring the Climate for Overweight and Obese Students in a Student Health Setting." *Journal of American College Health*, Vol. 57, No. 4, January–February 2009, 465–480.

researchers have found that weight loss among smokers is possible and beneficial, leading to a reduction in other risk factors, such as lower blood pressure and lower cholesterol.

- **Cancer.** Excess weight may account for 14 percent of all cancer deaths in men and 20 percent of those in women. Losing weight, researchers estimate, could prevent as many as one of every six cancer deaths. Excess weight has been linked to cancers of the colon and rectum, kidney, esophagus, and gallbladder; non-Hodgkin's lymphoma; multiple myeloma; and cancers of the pancreas and liver, the breast, uterus, cervix, and ovary (in women), and the stomach and prostate (in men).

  Body size and higher BMI are linked with increased risk of breast cancer in premenopausal women and in post-menopausal women not using hormone replacement therapy. Women who are overweight or obese tend to have more aggressive cancers and lower survival rates.[14]

The Impact on Life Expectancy

Obesity kills. Researchers attribute 112,000 to 280,000 deaths every year to excess weight. Your weight in early adulthood and middle age can have an impact on how long and how well you live. Life expectancy at age 20 is five years less for someone who is obese.

The Emotional Toll

In our calorie-conscious and thinness-obsessed society, obesity also affects quality of life, including sense of vitality and physical pain. Many see it as a psychological burden, a sign of failure, laziness, or inadequate willpower. Overweight men and women often blame themselves for becoming heavy and feel guilty and depressed as a result. In fact, the psychological problems once considered the cause of obesity may be its consequence. (See Point/Counterpoint, p. 216.)

 Weight may affect risky sexual behaviors among college students. In a study of almost 1,000 undergraduates, sexually active women with the highest BMIs were more likely to have sex with a casual partner, to have multiple same-sex partners, and to recall being intoxicated at the time of their most recent sexual intercourse. There was no correlation between men's weight and their sexual behavior.

If You're Too Thin: How to Gain Weight

Being underweight is not an uncommon problem, particularly among adolescent and young adult men as well as among those who diet excessively or suffer from an eating disorder (discussed later in this chapter). If you lose weight suddenly and don't know the reason, talk to a doctor. Rapid weight loss can be an early symptom of a health problem.

If you're trying to put on pounds, you need to do the opposite of dieters: Consume more calories than you burn. But as with losing weight, you should try to gain weight in healthy ways. Here are some suggestions:

- **Eat more of a variety of foods** rather than more high-fat, high-calorie foods. Get no more than 30 percent of your daily calories from fat. A higher percentage poses a threat to your heart and your health.

- **If your appetite is small, eat more frequently.** Try for five or six smaller meals rather than a big lunch and dinner.

- **Choose some calorie-rich foods,** such as dried fruits rather than fresh ones.

Add nuts and cheese to salads and main dishes.

- **Drink juice** rather than regular or diet soda.

- **Try adding a commercial liquid meal** replacement as a snack.

- **Exercise regularly** to build up both appetite and muscle.

A Practical Guide to Weight Loss

More than half of college women and about a third of college men intend to lose weight. Readiness to change is the key to successful weight loss. However, individuals vary in their readiness to change their diets, increase their physical activity, and seek professional counseling. Take the Self Survey on page 230 to determine your readiness to lose weight.

Why We Overeat

The answer lies not just in the belly but in the brain. Both **hunger,** the physiological drive to consume food, and **appetite,** the psychological desire to eat, influence and control our desire for food. Scientists have discovered appetite receptors within the brain that specifically respond to hunger messages carried by hormones produced in the digestive tract (Figure 7.3).

Appetite usually begins with the fear of the unpleasant sensation of hunger. We learn to avoid hunger by eating a certain amount of food at certain times of the day, just as dogs in the laboratory learn to avoid electric shocks by jumping at the sound of a warning bell. But appetite is easily led into temptation. In one famous experiment, psychologists bought high-calorie goodies—peanut butter, marshmallows, chocolate-chip cookies, and salami—for their test rats. The animals ate so much on this "supermarket diet" that they gained more weight than any laboratory rats ever had before. The snack-food diet that fattened up these rats was particularly high in fats. Biologists speculate that creamy, buttery, or greasy foods may cause internal changes that increase appetite and, consequently, weight.

A hormone called leptin, produced by fat cells, sends signals to the brain that affect appetite. When leptin levels are normal, people eat just enough to maintain weight.

When leptin is low, the brain responds as if fat stores had been depleted and slows down metabolism. This may be one reason why it is so difficult to lose weight by dieting alone. However, as discussed in Chapter 5, vigorous exercise can lower appetite control hormones, including ghrelin.[15]

Ghrelin, a natural appetite stimulant, is one of the hormones made in the stomach that influence how hungry we feel. When given shots of ghrelin, people become very hungry and eat 30 percent more than they normally would. Ghrelin typically rises before meals and falls afterward. Dieters tend to have high levels of ghrelin, as if their bodies were trying to stimulate appetite so they regain lost fat.

We stop eating when we feel satisfied; this is called **satiety,** a feeling of fullness and relief from hunger. The neurotransmitter serotonin has been shown to produce

hunger The physiological drive to consume food.

appetite A desire for food, stimulated by anticipated hunger, physiological changes within the brain and body, the availability of food, and other environmental and psychological factors.

satiety A feeling of fullness after eating.

Appetite receptors in hypothalamus respond to hormonal messages

Ghrelin stimulates appetite before meals

Leptin regulates appetite to maintain weight

© Bestie Van der Meer/Stone/Getty Images

Figure 7.3 Hormones Help Regulate Our Appetites

POINT

Many people assume that obesity occurs because of a failure of willpower. If they chose more healthful foods, didn't overeat, and exercised more, the 200 million overweight and obese Americans could take control of their weight. If they don't, they deserve to suffer the consequences, which include health problems, social prejudice, and discrimination on the job.

COUNTERPOINT

Society sets people up to get fat. The food industry spends $30 billion a year urging us to eat. Fast-food outlets peddle high-calorie treats on practically every street corner and in every shopping mall. Changes in the social environment to make it easier to eat healthfully and exercise more are essential to solving America's weight problems.

YOUR VIEW

Who do you think is responsible for the widening of our waistlines? Do you see weight as a personal responsibility? Should society do more to prevent obesity and help the overweight lose excess pounds? What could your school do to prevent weight problems or help heavy students slim down?

feelings of satiety. In addition, several peptides, released from the digestive tract as we ingest food, may signal the brain to stop or restrict eating. However, it takes 20 minutes for the brain to register fullness.

Weight Loss Diets

The diet debates over low-fat versus low-carbohydrate versus high-protein have raged for years. Which is best? Several studies over recent years found little difference in the ultimate results. In 2009 the largest-ever controlled study of dietary methods reached a clear conclusion: It doesn't matter whether you count carbohydrates, protein, or fat—as long as you eat less.

In the study, more than 800 overweight men and women were assigned to one of four diets, each loosely based on popular weight loss programs, such as the Atkins high-protein diet and Dean Ornish's low-fat approach. Here is how they compared in terms of macronutrients:

- **High fat, high protein:** 40 percent fat, 25 percent protein, 35 percent carbohydrates.
- **High fat, modified protein:** 40 percent fat, 15 percent protein, 45 percent carbohydrates.
- **Low fat, high protein:** 20 percent fat, 25 percent protein, 55 percent carbohydrates.
- **Low fat, average protein:** 20 percent fat, 15 percent protein, 65 percent carbohydrates.

Each participant consumed about 750 calories less than normal, but all ate at least 1,200 calories a day. After six months every diet group had lost about the same amount of weight, regardless of the weight loss plan, for an average of 13 pounds per person. About 15 percent lost more than ten percent of their body weight by the end of the two-year study. Those who lost the most attended more counseling sessions and followed the diets more closely than the others.[16]

Most of the dieters regained some of the weight they shed, although on average the volunteers were nine pounds lighter and their waistlines two inches smaller at the end of two years. They also reduced their risk factors for cardiovascular disease and diabetes.

Although people lose weight on any diet that helps them eat less, most dieters only lose about 5 percent of their initial weight. However, even a modest weight loss can lower cardiovascular risk factors, such as blood pressure, total cholesterol, and elevated blood glucose.

Following is a brief overview of some of the current approaches to dieting.

High-Carbohydrate, Low-Fat (Ornish)

The basic principle of Dr. Dean Ornish's approach is that by strictly limiting fat (whether animal or vegetable) by eating high-fiber, low-fat foods, you eat fewer calories without eating less food.

Promise

- Weight loss plus significant health benefits, including lower blood pressure and cholesterol.

Pitfalls

- Many people find low-fat diets so unsatisfying that they cannot stay on them.
- The diet limits the healthy fats in fish, nuts, and olive oil.
- With so little fat, some people may not get adequate essential fatty acids.

Low-Carbohydrate, High-Protein (Atkins)

The late Dr. Robert Atkins theorized that eating too many carbohydrates could create a metabolic imbalance that leads to overweight or obesity. Restricting carbohydrates corrects these imbalances so people can lose weight without having to eat fewer calories.

Promise
- Quick, short-term weight loss without hunger.

Pitfalls
- Severe restriction of carbohydrates can induce ketosis, which is caused by an incomplete breakdown of fats that can lead to nausea, fatigue, and light-headedness and can worsen kidney disease and other medical problems.
- Low-carb diets may impair memory and cognition.[17]
- A high-fat diet may increase the long-term risk of heart disease and some cancers.

Low-Carbohydrate (Zone)
The premise of this approach is that eating the correct proportions of carbohydrates, fat, and protein leads to hormonal balance, weight loss, greater vitality, and less risk of disease.

Promise
- Quick weight loss because of low calorie intake.

Pitfalls
- The plan is so rigid, restrictive, and complicated that many find it hard to follow.
- There is no sound scientific basis for the diet's health claims.

Carbohydrate-Modified (South Beach)
This diet encourages eating "good carbohydrates," such as vegetables, whole-wheat pasta, and brown rice, in order to feel full and resist cravings for "bad carbs," such as potatoes and white rice.

Promise
- Enhanced health due to emphasis on nutritious foods such as fish, lean meats, vegetables, and unsaturated oils and restriction on fatty meats, cheeses, and sweets.

Pitfalls
- The complete exclusion of starchy carbohydrates and all fruits during the first two weeks is difficult for many people.

Low-Calorie (Weight Watchers)
Nothing is forbidden on this diet. Instead, a point system assigns a value to portions of all sorts of foods, and dieters track the number of points taken in every day.

Promise
- Steady weight loss with portion control and moderation.

Pitfalls
- Hunger makes the diet hard to maintain.

Avoiding Diet Traps
Whatever your eating style, there are only two effective strategies for losing weight: eating less and exercising more. Unfortunately, most people search for easier alternatives that almost invariably turn into dietary dead ends or unexpected dangers (see Consumer Alert, p. 218.) Common traps to avoid are very-low-calorie diets, diet pills, diet foods, and the yo-yo syndrome.

Very-Low-Calorie Diets
Very-low-calorie diets, which provide fewer than 800 calories a day, lead to rapid weight loss but pose serious, potentially deadly health risks. Whenever people cut back drastically on calories, they immediately lose several pounds because of a loss of fluid. As soon as they return to a more normal way of eating, they regain this weight.

Very low-calorie diets, which provide fewer than 800 calories a day, lead to rapid weight loss but pose serious, potentially deadly health risks. Whenever people cut back drastically on calories, they immediately lose several pounds because of a loss of fluid. As soon as they return to a more normal way of eating, they regain this weight.

On a very low-calorie diet, as much as 50 percent of the weight you lose may be muscle (so you'll actually look flabbier). Because your heart is a muscle, it may become so weak that it can no longer pump blood through your body. In addition, your blood pressure may plummet, causing dizziness, light-headedness, and fatigue. You may develop nausea and abdominal pain. You may lose hair. If you're a woman, your menstrual cycle may become irregular, or you may stop menstruating altogether. As you lose more water, you also lose essential vitamins, and your metabolism slows down. Even reaction time slows, and crash dieters may not be able to respond as quickly as usual.

YOUR STRATEGIES FOR CHANGE
How to Design a Diet

There is no one perfect diet that will work for everyone who needs to lose weight. "Experiment with various methods for weight control," suggests Dr. Walter Willett of the Harvard School of Public Health. "Patients should focus on finding ways to eat that they can maintain indefinitely rather than seeking diets that promote rapid weight loss." In other words, design an eating plan that you can stick with for the rest of your life.

Whether you decide to focus on carbohydrates, fat, or calories, the following strategies can help you get to and maintain a healthy weight:

- Avoid "bad" fats, including trans-fatty acids and partially hydrogenated fats.
- Consume "good" fats, such as omega-3 fatty acids, every day.
- Eat fewer "bad" carbohydrates, such as sugar and white flour.
- Eat more "good" carbs, including fruits, vegetables, legumes, and unrefined grains like whole-wheat flour and brown rice.
- Opt for quality over quantity. Eating a smaller amount of something delicious and nutritious can be far more satisfying than larger portions of junk foods.
- Exercise more. The key to balancing the equation between calories consumed and calories used is physical activity.
- Eliminate sweetened soft drinks and drink water instead.

Dubious Diets

Facts to Know

The National Council Against Health Fraud cautions dieters to watch for these warnings of dangerous or fraudulent programs.

- Promises of very rapid weight loss.
- Claims that the diet can eliminate "cellulite" (a term used to describe dimply fatty tissue on the arms and legs).
- "Counselors" who are really salespersons pushing a product or program.
- No mention of any risks associated with the diet.
- Unproven gimmicks, such as body wraps, starch blockers, hormones, diuretics, or "unique" pills or potions.
- No maintenance program.

Steps to Take

If you hear about a new diet that promises to melt away fat, don't try it until you get answers to the following questions:

- Does it include a wide variety of nutritious foods?
- Does it provide at least 1,200 calories a day?
- Is it designed to reduce your weight by one-half to two pounds per week?
- Does it emphasize moderate portions?
- Does it use foods that are easy to find and prepare?
- Can you follow it wherever you eat—at home, work, restaurants, or parties?
- Is its cost reasonable?

If the answer to any of these questions is no, don't try the diet; then ask yourself one more question: Is losing weight worth losing your well-being?

Once you go off an extreme diet—as you inevitably must—your metabolism remains slow, even though you're no longer restricting your food intake. The human body appears to alter its energy use to compensate for weight loss. These metabolic changes may make it harder for people to maintain a reduced body weight after dieting.

Over-the-Counter Diet Pills An estimated 15 percent of adults—21 percent of women and 10 percent of men—have used weight loss supplements. Women between ages 18 and 34 are the highest users. In the 1920s, some women swallowed patented weight loss capsules that turned out to be tapeworm eggs. In the 1960s and 1970s, addictive amphetamines were common diet aids. In the 1990s, appetite suppressants known as fen-phen became popular but were taken off the market after being linked to heart valve problems.

In the last decade dieters tried ephedra products for weight loss, but a major study reported more than 16,000 adverse events associated with the use of ephedra-containing dietary supplements, including heart palpitations, tremors, and insomnia. The study also found little evidence that ephedra is effective in boosting physical activities and weight loss. The Food and Drug Administration has prohibited the sale of dietary supplements containing ephedra, because they present an unreasonable risk of illness or injury.

The weight loss prescription drug Orlistat is available as an over-the-counter weight loss pill called Alli. The drug, which blocks about a quarter of the fat consumed, works best with a low-fat diet. If dieters eat a meal made up of more than 15 fat grams, they can suffer nasty side effects, including flatulence, an urgent need to defecate, oily stools, and diarrhea.

Dozens of weight loss products contain undeclared ingredients that could pose serious health risks, according to the FDA. Sold online and in some stores, the products claim only "natural" or "herbal" ingredients but also contain substances such as an antiseizure medication and a suspected carcinogen. The risks from these unlabeled ingredients include high blood pressure, seizures, palpitations, heart attacks, and stroke. If you have purchased or taken any herbal weight loss products, check the FDA website to see if they are included in the consumer alert.[18]

Diet Foods According to the Calorie Control Council, 90 percent of Americans choose some foods labeled "light." But even though these foods keep growing in popularity, Americans' weight keeps rising. There are several reasons: Many people think choosing a food that's lower in calories, fat-free, or light gives them a license to eat as much as they want. What they don't realize is that many foods that are low in fat are still high in sugar and calories. Refined carbohydrates, rapidly absorbed into the bloodstream, raise blood glucose levels. As those levels fall, appetite increases.

Diet products, including diet sodas and low-fat foods, are a very big business. Many people rely on meal replacements, usually shakes or snack bars, to lose or keep off weight. If used appropriately—as actual replacements rather than supplements to regular meals and snacks—they can be a useful strategy for weight loss. Yet people who use these products often gain weight because they think that they can afford to add high-calorie treats to their diets.

What about the artificial sweeteners and fake fats that appear in many diet products? Nutritionists caution to use them in moderation and not to substitute them for basic foods, such as grains, fruits, and vegetables. Foods made with fat substitutes may have fewer grams of fat, but they don't necessarily have significantly fewer calories. Many people who consume reduced-fat, fat-free, or sugar-free sodas, cookies, chips, and other snacks often cut back on more nutritious foods, such as fruits and vegetables. They also tend to eat more of the low- or no-fat foods so that their daily calorie intake either stays the same or actually increases.

The Yo-Yo Syndrome

On-and-off-again dieting, especially by means of very-low-calorie diets (under 800 calories a day), can be self-defeating and dangerous. Some studies have shown that weight cycling may make it more difficult to lose weight or keep it off (Figure 7.5). Repeated cycles of rapid weight loss followed by weight gain may even change food preferences. Chronic crash dieters often come to prefer foods that combine sugar and fat, such as cake frosting.

To avoid the yo-yo syndrome and overcome its negative effects: Exercise. Researchers at the University of Pennsylvania found that when overweight women who also exercised went off a very-low-calorie diet, their metabolism did not stay slow but bounced back to the appropriate level for their new, lower body weight. The reason may be exercise's ability to preserve muscle tissue. The more muscle tissue you have, the higher your metabolic rate.

If you've been losing (and regaining) the same five or ten pounds for years, try the following suggestions for long-term success:

- **Set a danger zone.** Once you've reached your desired weight, don't let your weight climb more than three or four pounds higher. Take into account normal fluctuations, but watch out for an upward trend. Once you hit your upper weight limit, take action immediately rather than waiting until you gain ten pounds.

- **Be patient.** Think of weight loss as a road trip. If you're going across town, you expect to get there in 20 minutes. If your destination is 400 miles away, you know it'll take longer. Give yourself the time you need to lose weight safely and steadily.

- **Try, try again.** Dieters don't usually keep weight off on their first attempt. The people who eventually succeed don't give up. Through trial and error, they find a plan that works for them.

However, in the long run, dieting usually doesn't keep off excess pounds. Regardless of the diets they follow, people lose only about 5 percent of their initial weight after one year. Even in programs that provide intensive counseling by doctors, nurses, or dietitians, participants regain about half the weight they lost within three years. Five years after a successful diet, they typically have put on all the weight they lost. What can keep off extra pounds for good? A minimum of 200-300 minutes of exercise a week.[19]

Physical Activity

Unplanned daily activity, such as fidgeting or pacing, can make a difference in preventing weight gain. Scientists use the acronym **NEAT**—for **nonexercise activity thermogenesis**—to describe such "nonvolitional" movement and have verified that it can be an effective way of burning calories. In a study of ten lean and ten mildly obese people—all self-confessed couch potatoes—the thinner ones sat an average of two hours less and moved and stood more often than the heavier individuals. Small steps such as taking the stairs for a flight or two or parking farther away can make a difference.

Although physical activity and exercise can prevent weight gain and improve health,

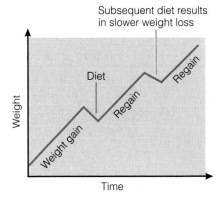

Figure 7.4 Weight-Cycling Effect of Repeated Dieting
Each round of dieting is typically followed by a rebound leading to a greater weight gain.

NEAT (nonexercise activity thermogenesis) Nonvolitional movement that can be an effective way of burning calories.

usually it does not lead to significant weight loss. However, when combined with diet, exercise ensures that you lose fat rather than muscle and helps keep off excess pounds. Moderate exercise, such as 30 to 60 minutes of daily physical activity, has proved effective in reducing the risk of heart disease and other health threats. But more exercise—a minimum of 200 to 300 minutes weekly of moderately intense activity—is necessary to maintain weight loss.[20] Recommending such higher levels of activity to overweight men and women does indeed lead to more exercise—and more lasting weight loss.

Exercise has other benefits: It increases energy expenditure, builds up muscle tissue, burns off fat stores, and stimulates the immune system. Exercise also may reprogram metabolism so that more calories are burned during and after a workout.

An exercise program designed for both health benefits and weight loss should include both aerobic activity and resistance training. (See Chapter 5.) People who start and stick with an exercise program during or after a weight loss program are consistently more successful in keeping off most of the pounds they've shed.

Can a Person Be Fat and Fit?   Most people assume that fitness comes in only one size: small. That's not necessarily so. There is considerable controversy over how to define a healthy weight. But individuals of every size can improve their physical fitness.

Physical fitness can buffer some, but not all of the ill effects of obesity. Individuals who are both overweight and sedentary face the greatest risk of disease and premature death. Those who are obese but physically active can be healthier, in many ways, than sedentary individuals whose weight is considered healthy. But working out cannot overcome all the dangers of weighing too much. The current recommendation from medical researchers is to increase physical activity so you can both lower your weight and enhance your fitness.[21]

The Psychology of Losing Weight

Diets change what you eat. Exercise changes body composition, stamina, and strength. But changing your food-related thoughts and behaviors can be the key to lasting weight loss. If you think that you can shed pounds, if you think that you can control what you put in your mouth, if you think that there is a form of exercise that you could enjoy, then you are on your way to reaching your weight loss goals. (See Making Change Happen, p. 221, and *Labs for IPC.)*

Get a Grip on Emotional Eating

Occasionally all of us seek comfort at the tip of a spoon. However, many people use food as a way of coping with anger, frustration, stress, boredom, or fatigue. Whatever its motivation, emotional eating always involves eating for reasons other than physiological hunger. If you're not sure whether you do this, ask yourself the following questions:

- Do you eat when you're not hungry?
- Do you eat or continue eating even if the food doesn't taste good?
- Do you eat when you can't think of anything else to do?
- Do you eat when you're emotionally vulnerable—tired, frustrated, or worried?
- Do you eat after an argument or stressful situation to calm down?
- Do you eat as one of your favorite ways of enjoying yourself?
- Do you eat to reward yourself?
- Do you keep eating even after you're full?

If you answer yes to more than three of these, you're eating in response to what you feel, not what you need. Diets may work for you, but the extra weight will inevitably creep back unless you confront your hidden motives for overeating. Since neither emotions nor food ever go away, you have to learn to deal with both for as long as you live.

Thinking Thinner

Good news: The "freshman 15" is a myth. Bad news: Even though most students put on less than 15 pounds their first year, they continue gaining weight throughout college. Have you gained weight at school? Are you trying to lose it?

If you eat less and exercise more, you will lose weight—at least for a while. Unfortunately, most people regain the pounds they lose. The reason is that diets aim for the wrong target: the belly. "Thinking Thinner" in *Labs for IPC* targets the brain. If you want to lose weight, the lab can help change the way you think about food and your body. Don't go on a diet; that's always something you do only for a while. Instead, permanently change the way you eat and exercise.

Get Real

In this stage, you will realistically assess whether you need to lose weight by answering questions about what you weigh, whether your weight is healthy, and what you see when you look in the mirror. You'll also find out who's in control of your weight by rating your weight-related sense of self-efficacy and locus of control (discussed in Chapter 1). Among the ten statements that you will respond to with True or False are these three:

- I am overweight because I eat too much.
- Diet pills are my best hope for losing weight.
- I could make time for exercise if I really wanted to.

Get Ready

As you prepare your weight loss plan, you will redefine your target weight by defining your "if-only," "happy," "acceptable," "disappointed," and "never-again" weights, identifying your resources, and systematically analyzing barriers by planning for situations that could throw you off track, such as:

- For each snack that is all too easy to reach and munch, what obstacles can you put in your way?
- What if the break room at work overflows with goodies?
- What if you can't resist nibbling on your kids' french fries when you take them out to eat?

Get Going

In the action stage of this lab, you will utilize some of the most effective tools for weight loss, including affirmations, prior planning, keeping a food log, journaling about your feelings, and eliminating environmental cues that trigger eating. Among the steps you'll take are:

- Declare "food-free zones," such as your bedroom (or at least your bed and desk). Rid your shelves of snacks and sweets.
- At mealtime, position yourself so you aren't looking at food and have to think twice before taking seconds . . .

Lock it In

Weight management is a lifelong commitment, so this lab will equip you with tools to stay on top of your weight loss. For instance, you will do a quarter-day review, a weekly weigh-in, and a monthly report card. But you don't have to wait until you lose weight to complete one of the maintenance tasks: to love the body you're in. Among the questions that can remind you of why your body deserves appreciation are these two:

- Do your eyes allow you to see the people you love?
- Do your ears allow you to hear laughter and music?

To get a grip on your emotional eating, try this three-step plan:

Step 1: Know Your Triggers Whatever its specific motivation, emotional eating always involves eating for reasons other than physiological hunger. The key to getting it under control is awareness.

Did any of these possibilities hit home? If so, train yourself to take a step back and ask yourself a series of questions before you take a bite: Are you hungry? If not, what are you feeling? Stressed, tired, bored, anxious, sad, happy? Once you identify your true feeling, push deeper and ask why you feel this way. Try writing down your answers in a notebook. This is an even more effective way to help make sure that every bite you take is a conscious one.

Step 2: Put Your Body, Not Your Emotions, in Charge of What You Eat To keep mind and body on an even keel, avoid getting so hungry and feeling so deprived that you become desperate and panicky. If you're facing an emotionally intense period—exam week or a visit from an ornery relative—plan your meals and snacks in advance and try, as much as you can, to stick with your program.

Step 3: Focus on Your Feelings Let yourself feel how you're feeling without eating. Breathe deeply for a minute or two. Focus on the places in your body that feel tense. Rate the intensity of the emotion on a scale from ten (life or death) to one (truly trivial). Ask yourself: What's the worst-case scenario of feeling this way? Is food going to make it better in any way? Will it make it worse?

Maintaining Weight Loss

Vigilance helps keep weight off. If the number on the scale creeps upward, take action.

©iStockphoto.com/Ernesto Solla Domínguez

Surveys of people who lost significant amounts of weight and kept it off for several years show that most did so on their own—without medication, meal substitutes, or membership in an organized weight loss group. When a National Institutes of Health panel reviewed 48 separate weight loss trials, they found that participants lost about 8 percent of their body weight on average and kept it off.

Rather than focusing on why dieters fail, the creators of the National Weight Control Registry study the habits and lifestyles of those who've maintained a weight loss of at least 30 pounds for at least a year. The nearly 6,000 people in the registry have maintained their weight loss for almost six years.

No one diet or commercial weight loss program helped all these formerly overweight individuals. Many, through years of trial and error, eventually came up with a permanent exercise and eating program that worked for them. Despite the immense variety, their customized approaches share certain characteristics:

- **Personal responsibility for change.** Weight loss winners develop an internal locus of control. Rather than blaming others for their weight problem or relying on a doctor or trainer to fix it, they believe that the keys to a healthy weight lie within themselves.

- **Exercise.** Registry members report an hour of moderate physical activity almost every day. Their favorite exercise? Three in four say walking, followed by cycling, weight lifting, aerobics, running, and stair climbing. On average, they burn about 2,545 calories per week through physical activity.

- **Monitoring.** About 44 percent of registry members count calories, and almost all keep track of their food intake in some way, written or not.

- **Vigilance.** Rather than avoiding the scale or telling themselves their jeans shrank in the wash, successful losers keep tabs on their weight and size. About a third check the scale every week. If the scale notches upward or their waistbands start to pinch, they take action.

- **Breakfast.** Your mother probably told you that breakfast is the most important meal of the day, and 40 years of breakfast-related studies, as well as the experience of registry members, have proved her right. A morning meal improves concentration and problem-solving ability, boosts energy levels, and helps control weight in children, adolescents, and adults.[22]

Treating Severe Obesity

The biggest Americans are getting bigger. The prevalence of severe or "morbid" obesity is increasing faster than obesity itself. The number of extremely obese adults—those at least 100 pounds overweight with BMIs over 40—has quadrupled in the last two decades from 1 in 200 to about 1 in every 50 men and women. The number with BMIs greater than 50 has jumped from 1 in 2,000 in the 1980s to 1 in 400.

Extreme obesity poses extreme danger to health and survival and undermines quality of life. White women report more impairment than men or African American women, even when they have lower BMIs. Severe obesity also has a profound effect on every aspect of an adolescent's life.

Drug Therapy

Obesity medications are recommended only for patients with BMIs equal to or greater than 30 or those with a BMI equal to or greater than 27 with risk factors (like high blood pressure) that increase their risk of disease. Researchers are experimenting with other medications, such as rimonabant and the epilepsy drug zonisamide, to enhance weight loss. Currently, only two weight loss drugs are FDA approved.

Xenical (orlistat) (also available in a lower dose as the over-the-counter drug Alli) blocks fat absorption by the gut but also inhibits absorption of water and vitamins in some patients and may cause cramping and diarrhea. It produces a weight loss of 2 to 3 percent of initial weight beyond the weight lost by dieting over the course of a year.

Meridia (sibutramine) is in the same chemical class as amphetamines and works by suppressing appetite. It also may increase blood pressure, heart rate, or both. Other side effects include headache, insomnia, dry mouth, and constipation. Patients taking these drugs generally lose less than 10 percent of their body weight, and many regain weight after they stop treatment.

Obesity Surgery

Obesity, or bariatric, surgery is becoming the most popular weight loss approach for the estimated 15 million men and women who qualify as "morbidly obese" (100 or more pounds overweight) because of their increased health risks. This year as many as 200,000 Americans will undergo obesity surgery—four times the number who did so in 2000. Eight in ten are women. A growing number are teenagers, although adolescents make up less than 1 percent of patients having such procedures. According to the Agency for Healthcare Research and Quality, three in four bariatric patients lose 50 to 75 percent of their excess weight within two years and keep it off.

As recent research has shown, bariatric surgery eliminates or improves diabetes, hypertension, sleep apnea, and

© Alex Segre/Alamy

high cholesterol in most patients.[23] However, these operations—particularly in the hands of poorly trained or inexperienced surgeons—pose serious risks, including potentially fatal leaks, infection, bleeding, hernias, and pneumonia. According to federal estimates, four in ten patients suffer complications within six months. The mortality rate averages about two deaths in 1,000 operations. Long-term dangers—both physical and psychological—are unknown, particularly for adolescents. Even with excellent medical results, extreme weight loss creates drapes of excess skin that sag over the belly, buttocks, thighs, breasts, or upper arms.

Gastric bypass surgery has proven effective in helping patients lose weight, extending their lives, and improving, even eliminating, type 2 diabetes. Following gastric bypass surgery, obese teenagers lose weight and no longer suffer from diabetes, according to recent research.[24] The benefits extend beyond the physical, with many reporting better psychological health and social ease.[25]

The two most common types of procedures are:

- **Gastric bypass.** Surgeons create an egg-sized pouch with staples and reroute food around part of the upper intestine to block absorption of calories and nutrients. About 75 percent of bypass patients lose 50 to 75 percent of their excess weight within two years. For the "super obese," a more extensive procedure that bypasses most of the small intestine can lead to a loss of 80 percent

The long-term health benefits of obesity or bariatric surgery may outweigh the risks for individuals who are "morbidly obese" (100 or more pounds overweight).

of excess weight. However, the latter procedure carries the highest risks of complications, including serious vitamin and mineral deficiencies. Too little thiamine, for instance, can lead to a serious neurological condition called Wernicke encephalopathy.

- **Banding.** In this newer, less risky procedure, surgeons slip an inflatable silicon band around the stomach; it can be tightened or loosened at a doctor's office without the need for further surgery. Patients lose about 40 to 55 percent of excess weight but may be more likely to regain lost pounds. The band also may slip or erode.

The individuals most likely to benefit from obesity surgery generally:

- Have a body mass index over 40.
- Have a BMI over 35 and a serious obesity-related problem, such as type 2 diabetes or severe sleep apnea (when breathing stops for brief periods during sleep).
- Have made repeated unsuccessful attempts to lose weight.
- Do not have any significant or untreated psychological problems.
- Are well-informed about the risks of the surgery.
- Recognize the need for lifestyle changes and daily vitamin and mineral supplements.

Unhealthy Eating Behaviors

Unhealthy eating behavior takes many forms, ranging from not eating enough to eating too much too quickly. Its roots are complex. In addition to media and external pressures, family history can play a role. Researchers have linked specific genes to some cases of anorexia nervosa and binge eating, but most believe that a variety of factors, including stress and culture, combine to cause disordered eating.

Sooner or later many people don't eat the way they should. They may skip meals, thereby increasing the likelihood that they'll end up with more body fat, a higher weight, and a higher blood cholesterol level. They may live on diet foods, but consume so much of them that they gain weight anyway. Some even engage in more extreme eating behavior: Dissatisfied with almost all aspects of their appearance, they continuously go on and off diets, eat compulsively, or binge on high-fat treats. Such behaviors can be warning signs of potentially serious eating disorders that should not be ignored.

Unhealthy Eating in College Students

College students—particularly women, including varsity athletes—are at risk for

 unhealthy eating behaviors. Researchers estimate that only about a third of college women maintain healthy eating patterns.[26] Some college women have full-blown eating disorders; others develop "partial syndromes" and experience symptoms that are not severe or numerous enough for a diagnosis of anorexia nervosa or bulimia nervosa. Distress over body image increases the risk of all forms of disordered eating in college women.

 In a survey at a large, public, rural university in the mid-Atlantic states, 17 percent of the women were struggling with disordered eating. Younger women (ages 18 to 21) were more likely than older students to have an eating disorder. In this study, eating disorders did not discriminate, equally affecting women of different races (white, Asian, African American, Native American, and Hispanic), religions, athletic involvement, and living arrangements (on or off campus; with roommates, boyfriends, or family). Although the students viewed eating disorders as both mental and physical problems and felt that individual therapy would be most helpful, all said that they would first turn to a friend for help. Women in sororities are at slightly increased risk of an eating disorder compared with those in dormitories. Loneliness also has emerged as a risk factor for eating disorders in college women.[27]

Extreme Dieting

Extreme dieters go beyond cutting back on calories or increasing physical activity. They become preoccupied with what they eat and weigh. Although their weight never falls below 85 percent of normal, their weight loss is severe enough to cause uncomfortable physical consequences, such as weakness and sensitivity to cold. Technically, these dieters do not have anorexia nervosa (discussed later in this chapter), but they are at increased risk for it.

Extreme dieters may think they know a great deal about nutrition, yet many of their beliefs about food and weight are misconceptions or myths. For instance, they may eat only protein because they believe complex carbohydrates, including fruits and whole-grain breads, are fattening.

Sometimes nutritional education alone can help change these eating patterns. However, many avid dieters who deny that they have a problem with food may need counseling (which they usually agree to only at their family's insistence) to correct dangerous eating behavior and prevent further complications.

Compulsive Overeating

People who eat compulsively cannot stop putting food in their mouths. They eat fast and they eat a lot. They eat even when they're full. They may eat around the clock rather than at set mealtimes, often in private because of embarrassment over how much they consume.

Some mental health professionals describe compulsive eating as a food addiction that is much more likely to develop in women. According to Overeaters Anonymous (OA), an international 12-step program, many women who eat compulsively view food as a source of comfort against feelings of inner emptiness, low self-esteem, and fear of abandonment.

The following behaviors may signal a potential problem with compulsive overeating:

- **Turning to food** when depressed or lonely, when feeling rejected, or as a reward.

- **A history of failed diets** and anxiety when dieting.
- **Thinking about food** throughout the day.
- **Eating quickly** and without pleasure.
- **Continuing to eat** even when no longer hungry.
- **Frequently talking about food** or refusing to talk about food.
- **Fear of not being able to stop** eating after starting.

Recovery from compulsive eating can be challenging because people with this problem cannot give up entirely the substance they abuse. Like everyone else, they must eat. However, they can learn new eating habits and ways of dealing with underlying emotional problems. An OA survey found that most of its members joined to lose weight but later felt the most important effect was their improved emotional, mental, and physical health. As one woman put it, "I came for vanity but stayed for sanity."

Binge Eating

Binge eating—the rapid consumption of an abnormally large amount of food in a relatively short time—often occurs in compulsive eaters. The 25 million Americans with a binge-eating disorder typically eat a larger than ordinary amount of food during a relatively brief period, feel a lack of control over eating, and binge at least twice a week for at least a six-month period. During most of these episodes, binge eaters experience at least three of the following:

- **Eating much more rapidly** than usual.
- **Eating until they feel uncomfortably full.**
- **Eating large amounts of food** when not feeling physically hungry.
- **Eating large amounts of food** throughout the day with no planned mealtimes.
- **Eating alone** because they are embarrassed by how much they eat and by their eating habits.

Binge eaters may spend up to several hours eating, and consume 2,000 or more calories worth of food in a single binge—more than many people eat in a day. After

binge eating The rapid consumption of an abnormally large amount of food in a relatively short time.

binge—more than many people eat in a day. After such binges, they usually do not do anything to control weight, but simply get fatter. As their weight climbs, they become depressed, anxious, or troubled by other psychological symptoms to a much greater extent than others of comparable weight.

Binge eating is probably the most common eating disorder. An estimated 8 to 19 percent of obese patients in weight loss programs are binge eaters.

If you occasionally go on eating binges, use the behavioral technique called *habit reversal*, and replace your bingeing with a competing behavior. For example, every time you're tempted to binge, immediately do something—text-message a friend, play solitaire, check your e-mail—that keeps food out of your mouth.

If you binge twice a week or more for at least a six-month period, you may have binge-eating disorder, which can require professional help. Treatment usually consists of cognitive-behavioral therapy, either individually or in a group setting. As chronic binge eaters recognize their unhealthy behavior and confront the underlying issues, they usually are able to stop binge-ing and resume normal eating patterns.

Eating Disorders

According to the American Psychiatric Association, patients with **eating disorders** display a broad range of symptoms that occur along a continuum between those of anorexia nervosa and those of bulimia nervosa.

As many as 10 percent of teenage girls develop symptoms of or full-blown eating disorders. Among the factors that increase the risk are preoccupation with a thin body; social pressure; and childhood traits such as perfectionism and excessive cautiousness, which can reflect an obsessive-compulsive personality. Teenage girls who diet and have four specific risk factors—a high BMI, menarche (first menstruation) before sixth grade, extreme concern with weight or shape, and teasing by peers—are most likely to have an eating disorder.

The best known eating disorders are anorexia nervosa, which affects fewer than 1 percent of adolescent women, and bulimia nervosa, which strikes 2 to 3 percent. The American Psychiatric Association has developed practice guidelines for the treatment of patients with eating disorders, which include medical, psychological, and behavioral approaches. One of the most scientifically supported is cognitive-behavioral therapy.

Who Develops Eating Disorders?

Eating disorders affect an estimated 5 to 10 million women and 1 million men. Despite evidence that 5 to 10 percent of those with eating disorders are male, many college students believe mainly young white women develop eating disorders.[28]

 In the few studies of eating disorders in minority college students that have been completed, African American female undergraduates had a slightly lower prevalence of eating disorders than did whites. Asian Americans reported fewer symptoms of eating disorders but more body dissatisfaction, concerns about shape, and more intense efforts to lose weight.

In a survey of health-care professionals at the country's largest colleges and universities, 69 percent have professionals on staff who specialize in diagnosing and treating eating disorders. Of all the hurdles to helping students with eating disorders, 39 percent said denial is the biggest, while 24 percent felt it was unwillingness to seek treatment, and 20 percent blamed pressure from peers and the media to stay thin.

Eating disorders affect every aspect of college students' lives, including dating. Both men and women tend to avoid dating individuals with eating disorders, but men are far less accepting of obesity than women.

Male and female athletes are vulnerable to eating disorders, because of the pressure either to maintain ideal body weight or to achieve a weight that might enhance their performance. Many female athletes, particularly those participating in sports or activities that emphasize leanness (such as gymnastics, distance running, diving, figure skating, and classical ballet) have subclinical eating disorders that could undermine their nutritional status and energy levels. Male wrestlers, cyclists, triathletes, and Nordic skiers are also developing unhealthy eating behaviors.[29] However, there is often little awareness or recognition of their disordered eating. On the other hand, a recent study found that many female athletes rely on exercise rather than vomiting or diet pills to control their weight.[30]

If someone you know has an eating disorder, let your friend know you're concerned and that you care. Don't criticize or make fun of his or her eating habits. Encourage your friend to talk about other problems and feelings, and suggest that he or she talk to the school counselor or someone at the mental health center, the family doctor, or another trusted person. Offer to go along if you think that will make a difference.

Anorexia Nervosa

Although *anorexia* means "loss of appetite," most individuals with **anorexia nervosa** are, in fact, hungry all the time. For them, food is an enemy—a threat to their sense of self, identity, and autonomy. In the distorted mirror of their mind's eye, they see themselves as fat or flabby even at a normal or below-normal body weight. Some simply feel fat; others think that they are thin in some places and too fat in others, such as the abdomen, buttocks, or thighs.

The characteristics of anorexia nervosa include:

- A refusal to maintain normal body weight (weight loss leading to body weight of less than 85 percent of that expected for age and height).

- An intense fear of gaining weight or becoming fat, even though underweight.

- A distorted body image so that the person feels fat even when emaciated.

- In women, the absence of at least three menstrual cycles.

The incidence of anorexia nervosa has increased in the last three decades in most developed countries. The peak ages for its onset are 14 1/2 to 18 years. According to the American Psychiatric Association's Work Group on Eating Disorders, cases are increasing among males, minorities, women of all ages, and possibly preteens. About 1 percent of American women develop anorexia.

In the *restricting type* of anorexia, individuals lose weight by avoiding any fatty foods and by dieting, fasting, and exercising. Some start smoking as a way of controlling their weight. In the *binge-eating/purging* type, they engage in binge eating, purging (through self-induced vomiting, laxatives, diuretics, or enemas), or both. Obsessed with an intense fear of fatness, they may weigh themselves several times a day, measure various parts of their body, check mirrors to see if they look fat, and try on different items of clothing to see if they feel tight.

What Causes Anorexia Nervosa? Many complex factors interact and contribute to this disorder, including biological, psychological, and social ones. Anorexia is more common among close relatives, particularly sisters, than it is in the general population. The relatives of anorexics also have a higher than expected frequency of depressive disorders.

Anorexia is associated with changes within the brain, including abnormalities in the stress hormone cortisol and the neurotransmitters dopamine, serotonin, and norepinephrine—all of which influence appetite and satiety. Brain chemistry returns to normal after treatment and recovery.

Anorexia also may be a response to a personal loss or a sign of a driven, perfectionist personality. Often young anorexics have above-average grades and an unwarranted fear of failure. Girls who develop anorexia often have little insight into or awareness of their feelings, needs, and wants.

 In one study that followed 21 college women with eating disorders for six years, 11 got better during their postcollege years, while 10 continued to struggle with disordered eating. The major difference between the two groups revolved around issues of autonomy and relation. Those who could better negotiate the tension between being independent and relating to others had higher self-esteem, a more positive self-concept, and a healthier relationship with food.

eating disorders Bizarre, often dangerous patterns of food consumption, including anorexia nervosa and bulimia nervosa.

anorexia nervosa A psychological disorder in which refusal to eat and/or an extreme loss of appetite leads to malnutrition, severe weight loss, and possibly death.

Loss of fat and muscle mass, including heart muscle

Increased sensitivity to cold

Irregular heartbeats

Bloating, constipation, abdominal pain

Amenorrhea (absence of menstruation)

Growth of fine, babylike hair over body

Abnormal taste sensations

Osteoporosis

Depression

Sudden death

Figure 7.5 Medical Complications of Weight Loss from Anorexia Nervosa

About one-third of those with those anorexia initially were mildly overweight and cut back on food just to lose a few pounds. Others had normal weights but began to diet to look more attractive or, in the case of male and female athletes and dancers, to gain a performance advantage. Sometimes illness, stress, or surgery triggers weight loss. Often the initial response to their weight loss—from parents, coaches, or friends—is positive. However, starvation seems to take on a life of its own, and anorexics cannot return to a healthy eating pattern. In time, they may place so much value on thinness that they cannot recognize the dangers to their health.

 Health Dangers and Treatment
The medical consequences of anorexia nervosa are serious (Figure 7.5). Menstrual periods stop in women; testosterone levels decline in men. Adolescents with this disorder do not undergo normal sexual maturation, such as breast development, and may not reach their anticipated height. Even individuals who look and feel reasonably healthy may have subtle or hidden abnormalities, including heart irregularities and arrhythmias that can increase their risk of sudden death. Women who do not menstruate for six months or more may develop osteoporosis and suffer irreversible weakening and thinning of their bones as a result.

Even when they realize that they are jeopardizing their health, people with anorexia tend to fear that treatment will make them worse—that is, fatter. They need repeated reassurance that they will not become overweight and that they can and will find healthier ways of coping with life.

According to current practice guidelines, treatment of anorexia nervosa includes medical therapy (such as "refeeding" to overcome malnutrition) and behavioral, cognitive, psychodynamic, and family therapy. Antidepressant medication sometimes can help, particularly when there is a personal or family history of depression. Most people who get help do return to normal weight, but it can take a long time for their eating behaviors to become normal and for them to deal with troubling body image issues. Nutritional therapy is critical for a return to regular menstrual periods and an improvement in bone density.

Bulimia Nervosa

Individuals with **bulimia nervosa** go on repeated eating binges and rapidly consume large amounts of food, usually sweets, stopping only because of severe abdominal pain or sleep, or because they are interrupted. Those with *purging bulimia* induce vomiting or take large doses of laxatives to relieve guilt and control their weight. In *nonpurging* bulimia, individuals use other means, such as fasting or excessive exercise, to compensate for binges.

The characteristics of bulimia nervosa include:

- Repeated binge eating.
- A feeling of lack of control over eating behavior.
- Regular reliance on self-induced vomiting, laxatives, or diuretics.
- Strict dieting or fasting, or vigorous exercise, to prevent weight gain.
- A minimum average of two bingeing episodes a week for at least three months.
- A preoccupation with body shape and weight.

An estimated 1 to 3 percent of adolescent and young American women develop bulimia. Some experiment with bingeing and purging for a few months and then stop when they change their social or living situation. Others develop longer-term bulimia. Among males, this disorder is about one-tenth as common. The average age for developing bulimia is 18.

What Causes Bulimia Nervosa? Bulimia usually begins after a rigid diet that lasted from several weeks to a year or more. Strict dieting may affect brain chemistry in such a way as to disrupt the normal mechanisms for appetite and satiety. Semi-starvation eventually sets off a binge; bingeing leads to purging. Once dieters realize that vomiting reduces the anxiety triggered by gorging, they no longer fear overeating. When this happens, bingeing may become more frequent and severe until, in time, it becomes an all-purpose way of coping with stress. However, the driving force in this disorder may not be the overeating but the vomiting or laxative use. If individuals felt they couldn't get rid of food, they might not overeat.

Obesity in adolescence may increase the likelihood of bulimia in adulthood. Extremely obese individuals may lose weight by vomiting and not want to stop because they fear regaining it. Sometimes bulimia develops after recovery from anorexia. Purging becomes an alternative way of staying thin. People with bulimia may spend thousands of dollars—a third of their food budget—on foods for binge episodes and for laxatives and diet pills.[31]

As with anorexia, bulimia is associated with changes in brain chemistry, particularly low levels of the peptide cholescystokinin, which produces feelings of satiety. The cycle of bingeing and purging seems to wreak havoc on the biological controls that keep weight at a certain level. Neuroimaging scans show differences in areas of the brain responsible for regulating behavior in individuals with bulimia.[32]

Family conflicts, life stresses such as going away to school, and struggles with the transition to independent adulthood also may play a role. Bulimia also may be a symptom of depression. About 20 to 30 percent of those with this problem are chronically depressed; others have a history of depressive episodes. Bulimic individuals also are more likely to experience other problems, including anxiety disorders, substance abuse, and impulse disorders, such as shoplifting (kleptomania) and cutting themselves. A significant percentage of bulimics—from a quarter to a half, by some estimates—may have been victims of incest, sexual molestation, or rape, but this correlation is controversial.

Bulimia may continue for many years, with binges alternating with periods of normal eating. Physiological consequences are cumulative. Often dentists are the first to detect bulimia because they notice damage to teeth and gums, including erosion of the enamel from the stomach acids in vomit. Repeated vomiting can lead to other complications as it robs the body of essential nutrients and fluids, causes dehydration and electrolyte imbalances, and impairs the ability of the heart and other muscles to function. Bulimia can trigger cardiac arrhythmias and, occasionally, sudden death.

Cognitive-behavioral therapy has proved more effective than other psychological approaches. Antidepressant medications that increase levels of the neurotransmitter serotonin can also help.

Group therapy has proven effective in allowing university students with bulimia the opportunity to experience, express, and understand the emotions related to their disorder. About 70 percent of those who complete treatment programs reduce their bingeing and purging, although flareups are common in times of stress.

One of the health complications of purging is erosion and decay of dental enamel from the acid in vomit.

bulimia nervosa Episodic binge eating, often followed by forced vomiting or laxative abuse, and accompanied by a persistent preoccupation with body shape and weight.

No diet—high-protein, low-fat, or high-carbohydrate—can produce permanent weight loss. Successful weight management, the American Dietetic Association has concluded, "requires a lifelong commitment to healthful lifestyle behaviors emphasizing sustainable and enjoyable eating practices and daily physical activity." Studies have shown that successful dieters are highly motivated, monitor their food intake, increase their activity, set realistic goals, and receive social support from others. Another key to long-term success is tailoring any weight loss program to an individual's gender, lifestyle, and cultural, racial, and ethnic values.

Here are some practical guidelines.

- **Be realistic.** Trying to shrink to an impossibly low weight dooms you to defeat. Start off slowly and make steady progress. If your weight creeps up five pounds, go back to the basics of your program. Take into account normal fluctuations, but watch out for an upward trend. If you let your weight continue to creep up, it may not stop until you have a serious weight problem—again.

- **Recognize that there are no quick fixes.** Ultimately, quick-loss diets are very damaging physically and psy-chologically because when you stop dieting and put the pounds back on, you feel like a failure.

- **Note your progress.** Make a graph, with your initial weight as the base, to indicate your progress. View plateaus or occasional gains as temporary setbacks rather than disasters.

- **Adopt the 90 percent rule.** If you practice good eating habits 90 percent of the time, a few indiscretions won't make a difference. In effect, you should allow for occasional cheating, so that you don't have to feel guilty about it.

- **Look for joy and meaning beyond your food life.** Make your personal goals and your relationships your priorities, and treat food as the fuel that allows you to bring your best to both.

- **Try, try again.** Remember, dieters usually don't keep weight off on their first attempt. The people who eventually succeed try various methods until they find the plan that works for them.

SELF SURVEY | Are You Ready to Lose Weight?

As discussed in Chapter 1, people change the way they behave stage by stage and step by step. The same is true for changing behaviors related to weight. If you need to lose excess pounds, knowing your stage of readiness for change is a crucial first step. Here is a guide to identifying where you are right now.

If you are still in the *precontemplation* stage, you don't think of yourself as having a weight problem, even though others may. If you can't fit into some of your clothes, you blame the dry cleaners. Or you look around and think, "I'm no bigger than anyone else in this class." Unconsciously, you may feel helpless to do anything about your weight. So you deny or dismiss its importance.

In the *contemplation* stage, you would prefer not to have to change, but you can't avoid reality. Your coach or doctor may comment on your weight. You wince at the vacation photos of you in a swimsuit. You look in the mirror, try to suck in your stomach, and say, "I've got to do something about my weight."

In the *preparation* stage, you're gearing up by taking small but necessary steps. You may buy athletic shoes or check out several diet books from the library. Maybe you experiment with some minor changes, such as having fruit instead of cookies for an afternoon snack. Internally, you are getting accustomed to the idea of change.

In the *action* stage of change, you are deliberately working to lose weight. You no longer snack all evening long. You stick to a specific diet and track calories, carbs, or points. You hop on a treadmill or stationary bike for 30 minutes a day. Your resolve is strong, and you know you're on your way to a thinner, healthier you.

In the *maintenance* stage, you strengthen, enhance, and extend the changes you've made. Whether or not you have lost all the weight you want, you've made significant progress. As you continue to watch what you eat and to be physically active, you lock-in healthy new habits.

Where are you right now? Read each of the following statements and decide which best applies to you.

1. I never think about my weight.　　　　　　　　　　　　　　　　　　　Precontemplation Stage
2. I'm trying to zip up a pair of jeans and wondering when was the last time they fit.　　Contemplation Stage
3. I'm downloading a food diary to keep track of what I eat.　　　　　　　Preparation Stage
4. I have been following a diet for three weeks and have started working out.　　Action Stage
5. I have been sticking to a diet and engaging in regular physical activity for at least six months.　　Maintenance Stage

Here is a guide to strategies most likely to help you at your particular stage of readiness to change.

Your Health Action Plan for Losing Weight

Precontemplation (not active and not thinking about becoming active)

- **Set a small, reasonable goal** that does not involve working up a sweat, such as standing rather than sitting when blow-drying your hair or doing squats while brushing your teeth.
- **Start paying attention** to what, when, where, and why you eat. Take note of the times you eat or continue eating even though you're not hungry.
- **List what you see** as the cons of physical activity. For example, do you fear it will take up too much time? Write down three activities you could do if you woke up half an hour earlier.

Contemplation (not active but thinking about becoming active)

- **Think back to activities** you found enjoyable in the past. Did you ever try inline skating? Play softball? Row? Ask friends if they can put you in touch with others with the same interest.
- **Start drinking more water.** Get used to the idea of ending every meal with water to wash away the taste of what you've eaten and signal that you've stopped putting food in your mouth.
- **Determine the types of activity** you can realistically fit into your daily schedule. If you have classes and work most of the day, sign up for an evening body-sculpting or spinning class.
- **Find an image of a slimmer body** you'd like to have—from a magazine advertisement, for example—and post it where you can see it often.

Preparation (active but not at recommended levels)

- **Record everything you put in your mouth.** List calories and carbs next to each entry. Also describe how you feel as you eat.
- **Set specific daily and weekly action-oriented goals.** Your daily goal might begin with 10 or 15 minutes of activity and increase by 5 minutes every week or two. Your weekly goal might be to try a new activity, such as kick-boxing or a dance class.

- **Document your progress.** You could use a monthly calendar to keep track of the number of days you've exercised as well as the length of each workout. Or you can keep a more detailed record, noting the types of exercise you do every day, the intensity you work at, the duration of each workout, and so forth

Action and Maintenance (active at recommended levels for less than six months)

- **Find new comfort foods.** Good options include air-popped popcorn, chocolate fruit sundaes (fresh fruit with a spoonful of rich syrup), hot chocolate (with skim milk), and fudgsicles (creamy but low in calories).
- **Avoid boredom.** Think through ways to vary your exercise routine. Take different routes on your walks. Invite different friends to join you. Alternate working with free weights with resistance machines at the gym.
- **Try new athletic and sports skills.** Try snowshoeing, kayaking, rock climbing, dancing. Don't expect instant expertise. It usually takes four to six weeks to feel competent and get in the swing of a new activity.

Don't expect to progress through these stages just once. Most people "recycle" several times before a change becomes permanent. Whether you're moving forward or have temporarily fallen back, remember that change is a journey that happens step by step, meal by meal, day by day, stage by stage.

CENGAGENOW™ If you want to write your own goals for losing weight, go to the Wellness Journal at CengageNow for Health: **www.cengage .com/sso.**

MAKING THIS CHAPTER WORK FOR YOU

Review Questions

1. If you have gone online to check out weight reduction support groups in your area, which stage of readiness for weight behavior change are you in?
   a. precontemplation stage
   b. contemplation stage
   c. preparation stage
   d. action stage

2. Successful weight management strategies include which of the following?
   a. Learn to distinguish between actual and emotional hunger.
   b. Ask friends for recommendations for methods that helped them to lose weight quickly.
   c. Practice good eating habits 50 percent of the time so that you can balance your cravings with healthy food.
   d. Look at celebrity photos and pick one for a model.

3. Jacob is an average build 26-year-old college student who is much thinner than his friends. What should he focus on to gain more weight?
   a. Consume more calories than he burns on an average day.

   b. Eat a large lunch and dinner each day.
   c. Eat foods that will provide at least 50% of caloric intake from fats.
   d. Bench press more weights to build up muscle mass.

4. Individuals with anorexia nervosa
   a. believe they are overweight even if they are extremely thin.
   b. typically feel full all the time, which limits their food intake.
   c. usually look overweight, even though their body mass index is normal.
   d. have a reduced risk for heart-related abnormalities.

5. What is basal metabolic rate?
   a. Another way to define body mass index.
   b. The number of calories needed to maintain the body after physical activity.
   c. Another term for breathing rate.
   d. The number of calories needed to sustain the body at rest.

6. People gain weight when
   a. their basal metabolic rate increases.
   b. they consume more calories than they use up in daily activity.

    c. they eat fast food more than two times a week.

    d. they watch two hours of television a day.

7. Bulimia nervosa

    a. is characterized by excessive sleeping followed by periods of insomnia.

    b. is found primarily in older women who are concerned with the aging process.

    c. is associated with the use of laxatives or excessive exercise to control weight.

    d. does not have serious health consequences.

8. Which of the following statements is *incorrect?*

    a. I can lose weight successfully on a low-carbohydrate diet.

    b. I can lose weight successfully on a low-fat diet.

    c. I can lose weight successfully on a low-calorie diet.

    d. I can lose weight successfully by working out once a week.

9. Which of the following statements is true?

    a. Very-low-calorie diets increase metabolism, which helps burn calories more quickly.

    b. An individual eating low-calorie or fat-free foods can increase the serving sizes.

    c. Low-carbohydrate diets have been shown safe over the short term but long-term studies have not been completed.

    d. Yo-yo dieting works best for long-term weight loss.

10. Satiety occurs when

    a. one's caloric needs have been met.

    b. one feels full.

    c. one has had dessert.

    d. one has no appetite.

Answers to these questions can be found on page 650.

Critical Thinking

1. Do you think you have a weight problem? If so, what makes you think so? Is your perception based on your actual BMI measurement or on how you believe you look? If you found out that your BMI was within the ideal range, would that change your opinion about your body? Why or why not?

2. Suppose a good friend appears to have symptoms of an eating disorder. You have told him or her of your concerns, but your friend has denied having a problem and brushed off your fears. What can you do to help this individual? Should you contact his or her parent or spouse? Why or why not?

Media Menu

CENGAGENOW Go to the CengageNOW for Health website at **www.cengage.com/sso** that will:

- Help you evaluate your knowledge of the material.
- Allow you to take an exam-prep quiz.
- Provide a personalized Learning Plan targeting resources that address areas you should study.
- Coach you through identifying target goals for behavioral change and creating and monitoring your personal change plan throughout the semester.

Internet Connections

www.obesity.org

The American Obesity Association is the leading organization for advocacy and education on the nation's obesity epidemic. This comprehensive website features statistics on overweight and obesity in the United States, research articles, consumer protection links, prevention topics, library resources, fact sheets on a variety of weight management topics, and more.

http://win.niddk.nih.gov

This government-sponsored website features a variety of publications in English and Spanish on nutrition, physical activity, and weight control for the general public and for health-care professionals. In addition, there are links for research, a newsletter, statistical data, and a bibliographic collection of journal articles on various aspects of weight management and obesity.

www.something-fishy.org

This very comprehensive and popular site features the latest news on eating disorders, as well as links regarding signs to watch for, "Recovery: Reach Out," treatment finders, doctors and patients, cultural issues, and a support chat.

Key Terms

The terms listed are used on the page indicated. Definitions of the terms are in the Glossary at the end of the book.

anorexia nervosa 227

appetite 215

binge eating 225

bulimia nervosa 229

eating disorders 227

hunger 215

NEAT (nonexercise activity thermogenesis) 219

obesity 213

overweight 213

satiety 215

SECTION 3

Responsible Sexuality

Our most special relationships are those that bring us closer to others—our friends, partners, spouses, parents, and children. Such intimacy is the most rewarding and the most demanding of human involvements. The giving of ourselves to another—sharing thoughts, feelings, experiences, and sexual pleasure—touches the essence of what it means to be human. This section provides a comprehensive philosophical and practical view of relating to others. Each of the chapters focuses on the unique form of personal responsibility involved in every close relationship: a responsibility that looks beyond the self to those we care for and love.

Chapter 8 - Communicating and Relating

1. **Hooking up refers to:** (Pg. 242- 243)
   - A. hanging out with a friend
   - B. dating another person
   - C. sexual encounter with a non-serious acquaintance
   - D. becoming romantically involved with a partner

2. **It is estimated that ____ of communications we do with others is non-verbal in nature.** (Pg. 238)
   - A. 20%
   - B. 50%
   - C. 75%
   - D. 90%

3. **All of the following are true statements concerning gender differences in communication except:** (Pg. 240)
   - A. men tend to be better listeners than women
   - B. men interrupt more during a conversation
   - C. women speak more in private conversations
   - D. women use more words related to emotions

4. **In order to sustain a close friendship and allow it to deepen even more, the two people in the friendship must:** (Pg. 241)
   - A. see each other's perspective on issues
   - B. anticipate each other's needs
   - C. be supportive and be there in the other's need
   - D. all of the above

5. **The term intimacy means:** (Pg. 244)
   - A. desire
   - B. commitment
   - C. within
   - D. love

6. **Intimate relationships are characterized by all of the following except:** (Pg. 244)
   - A. emotional attachment
   - B. financial commitment
   - C. behavioral independence
   - D. need fulfillment

7. **Smart suggestions for online dating include all the following except for:** (Pg. 242)
   - A. don't give out your phone number or address
   - B. tell your roommate or a friend when you first meet this person live where you will be going and what time you expect to return
   - C. schedule your first live encounter late at night so no one will see who the person is
   - D. don't 'date' on the office or university computer

8. **Healthy relationships should be built on:** (Pg. 244)
   - A. mutual respect
   - B. being listened and responded to in a courteous manner
   - C. the right to express your own view or opinion without harassment
   - D. all of the above

9. **The difference between intimacy and infatuation is:** (Pg. 245)
   - A. infatuation is falling in love that doesn't last or materialize into anything more deeply
   - B. intimacy is the heavy amount of sexual activity that goes on between two people
   - C. infatuation is the deep emotional bonds of companionship
   - D. intimacy and infatuation mean the same thing

10. **Breakdowns in relationships usually begin with:** (Pg. 247- 248)
    - A. spending time apart
    - B. sexual difficulties
    - C. change in communications
    - D. unresolved conflicts over money

11. **Relationships that do not promote healthy communications, honesty, and intimacy are called:** (Pg. 247)
   A. blended
   B. dysfunctional
   C. disruptive
   D. codependent

12. **Which example would describe Calvin's self-disclosure to his girlfriend Laura?** (Pg. 243)
   A. Calvin discusses a dream trip he wants to take to Australia
   B. Calvin tells about his mom's bout with breast cancer
   C. Calvin shares that he is bisexual
   D. Calvin talks about his younger brother who is good in sports

13. **When your partner enables you to continue your self-destructive behavior because they worry or care for you too much, this is known as:** (Pg. 249)
   A. controlling
   B. shielding
   C. codependent
   D. rescuing

14. **When a wife covers up her husband's alcoholic hangover by lying to his supervisor that he is sick and can't come to work today, this is an example of:** (Pg. 249)
   A. rescuing
   B. enabling
   C. shielding
   D. loving

15. **The term cohabitation means to:** (Pg. 250)
   A. live together
   B. get married
   C. date another person of the same sex
   D. be codependent on each other

16. **The difference between a couple co-habitating together versus having a domestic partnership living arrangement is that:** (Pg. 250)
   A. it is cheaper to live together as a partnership
   B. domestic partners can register their relationship which may entitle them to certain benefits
   C. domestic partnership is only for homosexual couples
   D. co-habitation always precedes marriage for the couple

17. **When ending a relationship, one of the most important things to remember is:** (Pg. 250)
   A. make sure there is a third party around to help mediate
   B. break up by sending an email or text message so as not to face the other person
   C. lie to your ex-partner so you don't hurt their feelings
   D. treat your ex-partner the way you will would want to be treated during this breakup

18. **Although couples have conflicts in their relationships where arguing and fighting may result, it is said that couples will likely not fight over:** (Pg. 253)
   A. money matters
   B. sexual difficulties
   C. poor communications
   D. child discipline issues

19. **Which of the following ways to improve a relationship in which there is both intimacy and autonomy is suggested to keep the relationship healthy and sustaining?** (Pg. 255)
   A. physical affection
   B. togetherness
   C. expressiveness
   D. staying power

20. **To create a better relationship with a partner, both individuals must agree to:** (Pg. 257)
   A. confide and trust in each other
   B. respect each other's boundaries
   C. have humor and laugh a lot
   D. all of the above are important for a healthy relationship

riana compares the people in her life to threads in a magnificent tapestry. Each brings different tones and textures that complement and contrast with others. Her earliest childhood memories are of loving circles of family and friends that she once thought revolved around only her. Now she sees that she is part of these concentric rings and that the friendship and support she offers others enrich all of their lives.

When she left for a college thousands of miles from her home, Briana worried about the people she was leaving behind and the strangers she would be living among.

Communicating and Relating

"I wondered if I'd be welcomed or shunned, judged by my looks or my race, invited to join social groups or excluded from them." Briana admitted, "What I discovered was that the choice was largely mine." She could reach out to others, smile, and hope that others would smile in return, communicate clearly and honestly, strive to forge connections. Within months of her arrival, Briana was sure she had made friends she would keep forever.

Whether we are shy or outgoing, reserved or exuberant, we all crave human connection. As individuals and as part of society, we need to care about others and to know that others care about us, to feel for others and have others feel for us, to share what we know and to learn from what others know.

Learning to listen (see "Listen Up" in Making Change Happen and *Labs for IPC*) and to send clear messages is the essence of good communication. The more effectively we communicate, the more likely we are to create good relationships built on honesty, understanding, and mutual trust. Such relationships can infuse our lives with a richness no solitary pleasure can match.

This chapter discusses the social needs we all share, the ways some of us respond to those needs, healthy and unhealthy relationships, and the possibilities that exist for coming together from our solitude to warm ourselves in each other's glow.

After studying the material in this chapter, you should be able to

- **Define** social networking and
- **Describe** some of the ways social networks have affected ways people communicate.
- Describe the role verbal and nonverbal communication plays in forming and maintaining relationships and **discuss** gender differences in communication.
- **Define** friendship and **explain** how friendship grows.
- **Discuss** the behavior and emotional expectations for friendship, dating, and intimate relationships.
- **Identify** the behaviors that may result in dysfunctional relationships.
- **List** and **describe** the various living arrangements today's adults might choose.
- **Identify** the problems likely to affect long-term relationships and **explain** how they can be prevented.
- **Describe** at least two ways to improve one of your relationships.

Log on to CengageNOW for Health at **www.cengage.com/sso** to find your Behavior Change Planner and to explore self-assessments, interactive tutorials, and practice quizzes.

235

Your Social Health

Your relationships with your family, friends, coworkers, and loved ones may amaze, irritate, exhilarate, frustrate, and delight you. They also may affect your health. As noted in Chapter 1, your ability to communicate, to develop satisfying relationships, and to live in harmony with others is an important dimension of health and wellness.

Social networks also have a direct impact on health. As discussed in previous chapters, friends and acquaintances can affect both mind and body. Happy individuals transmit their sunny outlook, while individuals whose friends are overweight tend to put on excess pounds as well.[1]

Specific qualities in a relationship affect physical health, particularly *social support.* This term refers to the ways in which we provide information or assistance, show affection, comfort, and confide in others. As mounting evidence shows, people of all ages function best in socially supportive environments.

This is particularly true of college students, who report more stress and more physical symptoms when they feel a lack of family support. More than any other component of social support, a sense of belonging may have the greatest impact on college students' health. In a study of undergraduates, belonging to a social network enhanced women's perceptions of their health and lowered the number of symptoms that men reported. Because college is a transition time, forming new attachments may be especially important—and beneficial to overall health.

Social Networking

Modern technology has revolutionized the way people connect and communicate. Today you can call almost anyone from almost anywhere with a cell phone, send a text message, e-mail, check in with Facebook, MySpace, Twitter, or other networking services, blog, drop in on a chat room or forum, write on a message board, or upload your photos and videos to share with the world.

"Computer-mediated communication refers to the conveying of written text via the Internet, whether by e-mail, texting, or posting on Facebook, MySpace, Twitter, or

Some young people spend more time texting than talking to others face to face.

blogs." More than 90 percent of adolescents and young adults in the United States have access to the Internet; about half of them use social working sites. Facebook and MySpace, the two largest, have hundreds of millions of members and keep growing.[2]

What draws people, particularly young ones, to social networking sites? According to researchers, the appeal comes from the opportunity they offer to:

- Explore their identities.
- Make new friends.
- Continue to develop long-standing relationships.
- Explore their sexuality.
- Voice their opinions.
- Be creative.[3]

 More than three-quarters of college students have created a social networking profile. (See Reality Check.) They score higher on tests of risk-taking attitudes than those who have not. Women express more privacy concerns than men and are less likely to provide their cell phone numbers online. They also are less likely to accept strangers as "friends," perhaps because of fear of stalking or sexual approaches.[4]

In many ways computer-mediated communication has made the world a smaller, friendlier place. The majority of college students communicate in cyberspace on a daily basis. Online they can keep up with friends from high school, see a picture of little brother's new puppy, and celebrate birthdays from afar. Despite all these benefits, communication in cyberspace also poses risks—some of which could affect your health. Already stressed by time and money pressures, students may find it hard to stay in touch with their closest friends

and family—let alone the hundreds of friends they make online. As discussed in Chapter 1, many students look for and share health information online, which can be misleading or inaccurate.[5] Others are looking for love the same place they look for everything else: online. Some may reveal personal information they later regret disclosing.

In a recent study, more than half of 18-year-olds on MySpace had posted information about sexual behavior (24 percent), substance abuse (41 percent), or violence (14 percent).[6] Comments about sexual behavior or explicit language and images increase the risk of sexual harassment and solicitation online. References to drugs and alcohol can lead to trouble at home, on campus, and with authorities and might jeopardize future applications for jobs or graduate schools.

Simply being made aware of such risks has an impact on student behavior. As part of a research study, a physician sent a message to 18- to 20-year-olds who had revealed risky behavior online. "Are you sure that's a good idea?" she asked. "If I could see it, nearly anybody could. That probably includes some people you do not want seeing your profile or who would take things the wrong way." After getting this message, 14 percent of the young adults deleted references to sexual behavior. However, the warning had no effect on disclosure of drinking or drug use.[7]

Personal Communications

Getting to know someone is one of life's greatest challenges and pleasures. When you find another person intriguing—as a friend, as a teacher, as a colleague, as a possible partner—you want to find out as much as you can about him or her and to share more and more information about yourself. Roommates may talk for endless hours. Friends may spend years getting to know each other. Partners in committed relationships may delight in learning new things about each other.

Communication stems from a desire to know and a decision to tell. The first step is learning how to listen. (See Making Change Happen, p. 239, and "Listen Up" in *Labs for IPC.*) Then you mostly choose what information about yourself to disclose and what to keep private. But in opening up to others, you increase your own self-knowledge and understanding.

A great deal of daily communication focuses on facts: on the who, what, where, when, and how. Information is easy to convey and comprehend. Emotions are not. Some people have great difficulty saying "I appreciate you" or "I care about you," even though they are genuinely appreciative and caring. Others find it hard to know what to say in response and how to accept such expressions of affection. Men and women vary in their communication styles.

Some people feel that relationships shouldn't require any effort, that there's no need to talk of responsibility between people who care about each other. Yet responsibility is implicit in our dealings with anyone or anything we value—and what can be more valuable than those with whom we share our lives? Friendships and other intimate relationships always demand an emotional investment, but the rewards they yield are great.

Sometimes people convey strong emotions with a kiss or a hug, a pat or a punch, but such actions aren't precise enough to communicate exact thoughts. Stalking out of a room and slamming the door may be clear signs of anger, but they don't explain what caused the anger or suggest what to do about it. You must learn how to communicate all feelings clearly and appropriately if you hope to become truly close to another person.

As two people build a relationship, they must sharpen their communication skills so that they can discuss all the issues they may confront. They must learn how to communicate anger as well as affection, hurt as well as joy—and they must listen as carefully as they speak.

Listening involves more than waiting for the other person to stop talking. Listening is an active process of trying to understand the other person's feelings and motivation. Effective listeners ask questions when they're not sure they understand the other person and prompt the other person to continue.

Nonverbal Communication

More than 90 percent of communication may be nonverbal. While we speak with our vocal cords, we communicate with our facial expressions, tone of voice, hands, shoulders, legs, torsos, posture. Body language is the building block upon which more advanced verbal forms of communication rest.

Learning to interpret what people *don't* say can reveal more than what they *do* say. "Understanding nonverbal communication is probably the best tool there is for a good life of communicating, be it personally or professionally," says Marilyn Maple, an educator at the University of Florida. "It's one of the most practical skills you can develop. When you can consciously read what others are saying unconsciously, you can deal with issues before they become problems."[8]

In a survey of undergraduates at a large southeastern university, those who saw themselves as "involved" daters were more concerned about nonverbal communication than "casual" daters. These individuals were

Listen Up

The essence of good listening is to seek to understand another person before you seek to be understood. In the process you not only will get an earful but also will learn more than you might imagine. If you would like to take a relationship to another level, see what happens when you listen up. And if you're shy or feel self-conscious in social settings, expect an added return on your investment. Knowing how to listen can help you—and the people around you—feel at ease. "Listen Up" in *Labs for IPC* shows you how to "be all ears." Here's a preview.

Get Real

In this stage, you will replay three conversations you've had in the last 24 hours with three different people and answer eleven questions about them, including the following:

- What was the purpose of the conversation? Killing time? Flirting? Trying to get information you needed for a class or assignment?
- What questions did you ask, if any?
- What do you remember?

On the basis of your answers, rate your listening skills on a scale of 1 (you talkin' to me?) to 10 (competition for Oprah).

Get Ready

In this stage, you will check your schedule and make time for listening opportunities.

Get Going

In this stage you will embark on a comprehensive program that includes four steps:

- **Enhance basic skills** by engaging in at least one conversation each day in which you focus on specifics such as making eye contact and reading body language.
- **Observe listening styles** in yourself and others as you converse in varied settings.
- **Master interviewing skills.** You will set up situations in which you might pretend you're a reporter doing a "person-on-the-street" interview or talk with an instructor about some class material that you're struggling to comprehend.
- **Apply listening skills.** You will seek out real-life encounters, for instance, with a friend seeking advice or with someone you don't like talking with and usually avoid.

Lock it In

To keep your listening muscles in shape, you will consciously practice intensive listening on a daily basis. You might ask a sales clerk how the day is going, and then listen—really listen—to the answer, or ask a classmate about . . .

---

more likely to "work hard" to ensure that their nonverbal behavior backed up the words they said—and to say their partners did the same. Regardless of their dating status, the female students valued nonverbal behavior more than men. They also engaged in more forms of nonverbal communication, such as looking their partners straight in the eye and nodding their heads as their partners spoke.

Culture has a great deal of influence over body language. In some cultures, for example, establishing eye contact is considered hostile or challenging; in others, it conveys friendliness. A person's sense of personal space—the distance he or she feels most comfortable in keeping from others—also varies in different societies.

How Men and Women Communicate

Gender differences in communication start early. By age one, boys make less eye contact than girls and pay more attention to moving objects like cars than to human faces. Both mothers and fathers talk less about feelings (except anger) to sons than daughters, and boys' vocabularies include fewer "feeling" words. In the playground, if not at home, boys learn to choke back tears and show no fear. Their faces—once as openly emotional as girls—become less expressive as they move through the elementary years.

As adults, men use fewer words and talk, at least in public, as a means of putting themselves in a one-up situation—unlike women, who talk to draw others closer. Even with friends, men mainly swap information as they talk shop, sports, cars, computers. "Women talk to clear their heads, but men think before they talk," says psychiatrist Mark Goulston, author of *The 6 Secrets of a Lasting Relationship.* "If they didn't, they'd risk saying something stupid and being humiliated or offending another man and getting beaten up. They're safer not saying anything."[9]

In studies of language, Deborah Tannen and other linguists have identified the following gender differences, which may be based on sex or gender roles:

Men:

- Speak more often and for longer periods in public.

- Interrupt more, breaking in on another's monologue if they aren't getting the information they need.

- Look into a woman's eyes more often when talking than they would if talking with another man.

- When writing, use more numbers, more prepositions, and more articles such as "an" and "the."

- Write briefer, more utilitarian e-mails.

- Write blogs for the sake of a personal expectation or motive.[10]

- In blogs or chat rooms, are more likely to make strong assertions, disagree wit others, and use profanity and sarcasm.

Women:

- Speak more in private, usually to build better connections with others.

- Are generally better listeners, facilitating conversation by nodding, asking questions, and signaling interest by saying "uh-huh," or "yes."

- Are more likely to wait for a speaker to finish rather than interrupting.

- Look into another woman's eyes more often than they would if talking with a man.

- When writing, use more words overall, more words related to emotion (positive and negative), more idea words, more hearing, feeling, and sensing words, more causal words (such as *because),* and more modal words *(would, should, could).*

- Write e-mails in much the same way they talk, using words to build a connection with people.

- Write blogs for the sake of self-expression.[11]

- In blogs or chat rooms, are more prone to posing questions, making suggestions, and including polite expressions. Communication researchers studying the differences between "he-mails" and "she-mails" have also found that people who are not generally verbally expressive—mainly but not exclusively men—often convey more feelings in e-mails than they do in face-to-face conversations.

Forming Relationships

We first learn how to relate in our families as children. Our relationships with parents and siblings change dramatically as we grow toward independence. Relationships between friends also change as they move or develop different interests; between lovers, as they come to know more about each other; between spouses, as they pass through life together; and between parents and children, as youngsters develop and mature. But throughout life, close relationships, tested and strengthened by time, allow us to explore the depths of our souls and the heights of our emotions. (See Self Survey, "How Strong Are the Communication and Affection in Your Relationship?" on p. 258.)

I, Myself, and Me

The way each of us perceives himself or herself affects all the ways we reach out and relate to others. If we feel unworthy of love, others may share that opinion. Self-esteem (discussed in Chapter 2) provides a positive foundation for our relationships with others. Self-esteem doesn't mean vanity or preoccupation with our own needs; rather, it is a genuine concern and respect for ourselves so that we remain true to our own feelings and beliefs. We can't know or love or accept others until we know and love and accept ourselves, however imperfect we may be.

Partners with low self-esteem may feel responsible for a partner's unhappiness. In studies of college students, those who scored low on measures of self-esteem were far more likely to feel rejected or hostile if their partners seemed distraught. Regardless of the reason for the distress, insecure, self-doubting individuals may read nonexistent meaning into their partners' ambiguous cues. As a result, they may unwittingly sabotage their relationships. This misreading of cues occurs not just in dating couples, but among long-married partners who still fear that their spouses love them less than they actually do.

Friendship

Friendship has been described as "the most holy bond of society." Every culture has prized the ties of respect, tolerance, and loyalty that friendship builds and nurtures. An anonymous writer put it well:

> A friend is one who knows you as you are,
> Understands where you've been,
> Accepts who you've become,
> And still gently invites you to grow.

Friends can be a basic source of happiness, a connection to a larger world, a source of solace in times of trouble. Although we have different friends throughout life, often the friendships of adolescence and young adulthood are the closest we ever form. They ease the normal break from parents and the transition from childhood to independence.

In the past, many people believed that men and women couldn't become close friends without getting romantically involved. But as the genders have worked together and come to share more interests, this belief has changed. Yet unique obstacles arise in male-female friendships, such as distinguishing between friendship and romantic attraction and dealing with sexual tension. However, men and women who overcome such barriers and become friends benefit from their relationship—but in different ways. For men, a friendship with a woman offers support and nurturance. What they report liking most is talking and relating to women, something they don't do with their male buddies. Women view their friendships with men as more lighthearted and casual, with more joking and less fear of hurt feelings. They especially like getting insight into what guys really think.

Women and men view friendships on the job somewhat differently. Women are significantly more likely than men to describe the benefits of workplace friendship in terms of social and emotional support in times of stress, while men focus mainly on the practical benefits of having friends help them get a job done or succeed in their careers.[12]

Dating on Campus

Dating isn't what it used to be. Many young people socialize in groups until a couple pairs off into a romantic relationship. Rather than the conventional dinner and a movie, college students may just get together to hang out. Is one person interested in something more? Is the other? Often it can take a while for couples to figure out if they are in fact dating. With more people remaining single longer, the search for a good date has become more complex. Singles bars have become less popular; cafés, laundromats, health clubs, and bookstores have become more acceptable as places to meet new people.

Many young people meet or maintain contact online. Text-messaging, Facebook, and e-mail may be convenient and fun, but virtual encounters can be tricky. Because you can't observe body language or detect the tone in a voice, it can be hard to tell if a person is being sincere or sarcastic, informal or inappropriate. Flirting in the digital world tends to be bolder and racier than in real life, in part because two people are looking at a screen rather than into each other's eyes. Caught up in the "conversation," they

Online Flirting and Dating

E-mail flirtations can be fun, but they also entail some risks, particularly if you decide to go off-line and meet in person. Here are some guidelines:

Facts to Know

- Remember that you have no way of verifying if a correspondent is telling the truth about anything—sex, age, occupation, marital status. If your online partner seems insincere or strange in any way, stop corresponding.

- Be careful of what you type. Anything you put on the Internet can end up almost anywhere, including with potential employers. To avoid embarrassment, don't say anything you wouldn't want to see in newspaper print.

Steps to Take

- Don't give out your address, telephone number, or any other identifying information. The people you meet online are strangers, and you should keep your guard up.

- Don't "date" on an office or university computer. You could end up supplying your professors, classmates, or coworkers with unintentional entertainment. Also, many organizations and institutions consider e-mail messages company property.

- Don't rely on the Internet as your only method of meeting people. Continue to get out in the real world and meet potential dates the old-fashioned way: live and in person.

- If you do decide to meet, make your first face-to-face encounter a double or group date and make it somewhere public, like a café or museum. Don't plan a full-day outing. Coffee or a drink in a crowded place makes the best transition from e-mail.

- Don't let your expectations run wild. Finding Mr. or Ms. Right is no easier in cyberspace than anywhere else, so be realistic about where your relationship might lead.

---

may not reflect on the message they're sending—or whether they should be sending it at all. (See Consumer Alert.)

Dating can do more than help you meet people. By dating, you can learn how to make conversation, get to know more about others as well as yourself, and share feelings, opinions, and interests. In adolescence and young adulthood, dating also provides an opportunity for exploring your sexual identity. Some people date for months and never share more than a good-night kiss. Others may fall into bed together before they fall in love or even "like."

Separating your emotional feelings about someone you're dating from your sexual desire is often difficult. The first step to making responsible sexual decisions is respecting your sexual values and those of your partner. If you care about the other person—not just his or her body—and the relationship you're creating, sex will be an important, but not the all-important, factor while you're dating.

Should You Keep Seeing Each Other?

You've met someone, gone out a few times, and enjoyed yourself. Is it infatuation, "like," or love? Here are some positive indications of a relationship worth continuing:

- You feel at ease with your new partner.

- You feel good about your new partner when you're together and when you're not.

- Your partner is open with you about his or her life—past, present, and future.

- You can say no to each other without feeling guilty.

- You feel cared for, appreciated, and accepted as you are.

- Your partner really listens to what you have to say.

Following are some reasons to rethink your relationship:

- You don't feel comfortable together.

- You feel angry or let down when you're together or apart.

- Your partner is very secretive about his or her life.

- You feel your partner isn't attentive to you.

- You don't feel cared for and appreciated.

Hooking Up

Hooking up refers to a sexual encounter between two people who usually are not seriously dating and who may or may not know each other well. College students use the term to describe a variety of sexual interactions, including kissing, fondling, oral sex, and sexual intercourse. What makes hooking up unique is that the couple agrees there will be no commitment, no exclusivity, no feelings.

 Why do people hook up? According to a recent book on the subject, college students, focused on academic and career success, don't have time for a real relationship. But social commentators speculate that by not seeking a connection beyond the physical, young people may be shortchanging themselves of the richness of a caring, committed relationship. They also face a higher risk of sexually transmitted infections and of date rape (discussed in Chapters 16 and 18).

In an informal survey of college hookups, a sexuality instructor found that over 85 percent of students had engaged in a hookup. Ninety percent reported having had a "really good" hookup for reasons that included good sex, no interruptions, or a resulting relationship. However, 78 percent reported a bad hookup experience because of bad sex, interruptions, or a partner wanting more out of the hookup than they did.[13]

Alcohol often plays a role in hooking up. Under its influence, individuals may engage in sexual activities, including unsafe sex, that they normally would avoid or with someone they usually would not choose. Most students surveyed believe that hooking up is more common than it may in fact be and that their peers—particularly men—are more comfortable with hooking up than they are.

Some young people also engage in sexual activities with friends with whom they are not romantically involved. Many "friends with benefits" may have had a sexual relationship in the past. Others have no expectation of any serious involvement.

Self-Disclosure in Relationships

A key element of relationships—whether friendships or romantic ones—is **self-disclosure,** that is, how much we reveal about ourselves to another person. What you share about yourself is a critical building block that affects the nature and quality of the

bonds you establish with others. But both cultural and individual factors can influence self-disclosure.

Talking about your feelings and listening intently move a relationship to a deeper and more meaningful level.

 In a study of American and Japanese college students, the Japanese undergraduates reported significantly less self-disclosure, whether in passionate love relationships, companionate love relationships, cross-sex friendships, or same-sex friendships. As previous studies have shown, Japanese people talk less about themselves than Americans do and may think that talking about their personal issues would hurt the feelings of people around them. On the other hand, Americans generally strive to express themselves.

Yet both American and Japanese students disclosed more in romantic relationships than in friendships and more in same-sex than in cross-sex friendships. This might be because we talk about more topics with a romantic partner than with a friend. We also may have more in common with people of the same sex so we discuss more with them than with a friend of the other sex.

Single Life

 Perhaps because there are so many singles, more and more Americans are living alone. The number of women living alone has doubled since 1970 and has nearly tripled for men. Approximately one-quarter of the households in the nation are one-person homes.

Among Americans between 25 and 34 years old, about 35 percent (14 million) have never been married. Of African Americans in this age group, 53 percent have never been married. Being single no longer marks a transition phase between living with parents and living with a spouse, but is an accepted, appealing lifestyle for millions of men and women.

self-disclosure Sharing personal information and experiences with another that he or she would not otherwise discover; self-disclosure involves risk and vulnerability.

Healthy Relationships

- Fill your life with meaningful work, experiences, and people.
- Build a network of supportive friends who care for and about you.
- Be open to new experiences that can expand your feelings about yourself and your world.
- Don't miss out on a special event because you don't have someone to accompany you: Go alone.
- Enjoy your own company. Allow yourself to be amazed by your own witty or off-the-wall observations.
- Volunteer to help others less fortunate, or become involved in church and social organizations.

A healthy relationship requires empathy, the ability to appreciate what another person is experiencing. You may not agree with your roommate's political opinions or your sibling's wardrobe choices, yet you respect their rights to think and dress as the individuals they are.

The term **intimacy**—the open, trusting sharing of close, confidential thoughts and feelings—comes from the Latin word for *within.* Intimacy doesn't happen at first sight, or in a day or a week or a number of weeks. Intimacy requires time and nurturing; it is a process of revealing rather than hiding, of wanting to know another and to be known by that other. Although intimacy doesn't require sex, an intimate relationship often includes a sexual relationship, heterosexual or homosexual.

In an intimate relationship, empathy becomes even more important. You can develop your capacity for empathy by pulling back periodically, particularly in moments of stress or conflict, and asking yourself: "What is my partner or spouse feeling right now? What does he or she need?" (See "Your Intimacy Quotient" in *Labs for IPC.*)

We tend to be attracted to people who are similar to ourselves in age, race, ethnicity, socioeconomic class, and education.

What Attracts Two People to Each Other?

What draws two people to each other and keeps them together: chemistry or fate, survival instincts or sexual longings? "Probably it's a host of different things," reports sociologist Edward Laumann, coauthor of *Sex in America,* a landmark survey conducted by the National Opinion Research Center at the University of Chicago.[14] "But what's remarkable is that most of us end up with partners much like ourselves—in age, race, ethnicity, socioeconomic class, education."

Why? "You've got to get close for sexual chemistry to occur," says Laumann. "Sparks may fly when you see someone across a crowded room, but you only see a preselected group of people—people enough like you to be in the same room in the first place. This makes sense because initiating a sexual relationship is very uncertain."

Scientists have tried to analyze the combination of factors that attracts two people to each other. In several studies of college students, four predictors ranked as the most important reasons for attraction: warmth and kindness, desirable personality, something specific about the person, and reciprocal liking. Economic factors, including money or lack thereof, didn't make the list. (See Health on a Budget, p. 247.)

Do opposites attract, or do people find greater happiness with partners who are similar to them? One of the most comprehensive studies ever undertaken on these questions found no evidence that opposites attract. Most people, the researchers found, tend to marry those who are similar in attitudes, religion, and values. However, these similarities have little to do with having a happy marriage. What does matter are similarities in personality, such as being extroverted or conscientious. These take more time to recognize but have a greater impact on how a couple gets along over the long term.

In his cross-cultural research, psychologist David Buss, author of *The Evolution of Desire,* found that men in 37 sample groups

© Comstock/Jupiterimages

drawn from Africa, Asia, Europe, North and South America, Australia, and New Zealand rated youth and attractiveness as more important in a possible mate than did women. Women placed greater value on potential mates who were somewhat older, had good financial prospects, and were dependable and hardworking.[15]

Attractive women in different cultures, including the United States, use different mating strategies than less attractive ones, including more "attractiveness enhancement tactics" (such as wearing makeup), flirting with other men to make a date jealous, and acting possessively. Attractive women also may have more opportunities for "trial liaisons" in selecting long-term partners and for replacing a mate who fails to live up to expectations.

Infatuation

It is tempting to think of love as scenes from a movie script: blazing sunsets and misty nights, fiery glances and passionate embraces, consuming desire and happily-ever-after endings. However, movies only last for 2 hours; ideally, love lasts a lifetime. Infatuation falls somewhere in between.

Certainly, falling in love is an intense, dizzying experience. A person not only enters our life, but also takes possession. We are intrigued, flattered, captivated, delighted—but is this love or a love of loving?

At the time you're experiencing it, there is no difference between infatuation and lasting love. You feel the same giddy, wonderful way. However, if it's infatuation, it won't last. Infatuation refers only to falling in love. People genuinely in love with each other do more than fall: They start building a relationship together.

Infatuation also can be a disguise for something quite different: a strong sex drive, a fear of loneliness, loneliness itself, or a hunger for approval. Sometimes lovers in love with love may become infatuated with someone who doesn't even exist: the projection of their unmet needs for unconditional love.

intimacy A state of closeness between two people, characterized by the desire and ability to share one's innermost thoughts and feelings with eachother either verbally or nonverbally.

The Science of Romantic Love

We like to think of this powerful force, this source of both danger and delight, as something that defies analysis. However, scientists have provided new perspectives on its true nature.

A Psychological View

According to psychologist Robert Sternberg, love can be viewed as a triangle with three faces: passion, intimacy, and commitment (Figure 8.1). Each person brings his or her own triangle to a relationship. If they match well, their relationship is likely to be satisfying.

Sternberg also identified six types of love:

- **Liking,** the intimacy friends share.
- **Infatuation,** the passion that stems from physical and emotional attraction.
- **Romantic love,** a combination of intimacy and passion.

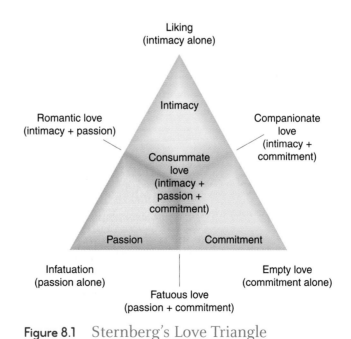

Figure 8.1 Sternberg's Love Triangle
The three components of love are intimacy, passion, and commitment. The various kinds of love are composed of different combinations of the three components.

- **Companionate love,** a deep emotional bond in a relationship that may have had romantic components.
- **Fatuous love,** a combination of passion and commitment in two people who lack a deep emotional intimacy.
- **Consummate love,** which combines passion, intimacy, and commitment over time.

An Anthropological View

When you first fall in love, you may be sure that no one else has ever known the same dizzying, wonderful feelings. Yet, while every romance may be unique, romantic love is anything but. Anthropologists have found evidence of romantic love between individuals in most of the cultures they have studied—it seems to be a human universal or, at the least, a near-universal.

Anthropologist Helen Fisher, author of *Anatomy of Love: The Natural History of Monogamy, Adultery and Divorce,* describes romantic love "as a very primitive, basic human emotion, as basic as fear, anger or joy." As she explains, it pulled men and women of prehistoric times into the sort of partnerships that were essential to child rearing. But after about four years—just "long enough to rear one child through infancy," says Fisher—romantic love seemed to wane, and primitive couples tended to break up and find new partners. This "four-year itch" may well have endured through the centuries, contends Fisher, who notes that divorce statistics from most of the 62 cultures she has studied still show a pattern of restlessness four years into a marriage.[16]

A Biochemical View

The heart is the organ we associate with love, but the brain may be where the action really is. According to research on neurotransmitters (the messenger chemicals within the brain), love sets off a chemical chain reaction that causes our skin to flush, our palms to sweat, and our lungs to breathe more deeply and rapidly. The "love chemicals" within the brain—dopamine, norepinephrine, and phenylethylamine (PEA)—have effects similar to those of amphetamines, stimulant drugs that intensify physiological reactions (see Chapter 11).

Infatuation may indeed be a natural high, but like other highs, this rush doesn't last—possibly because the body develops tolerance for love-induced chemicals, just as it does with amphetamines. However, as the initial lovers' high fades, other brain chemicals may come into play: the endorphins, morphine-like chemicals that can help produce feelings of well-being, security, and tranquility. These feel-good molecules may increase in partners who develop a deep attachment.

The hormone *oxytocin,* best known for its role in inducing labor during childbirth, seems particularly important in our ability to bond with others. By measuring blood levels of women as they recalled positive and negative relationships, researchers have found that women whose oxytocin levels rose when remembering a positive relationship reported having little difficulty setting appropriate boundaries, being alone, or trying too hard to please others. Women whose oxytocin levels fell in response to remembering a negative emotional relationship reported greater anxiety in close relationships.

Assessing a Relationship

How do you know if you're in a healthy relationship? Ask yourself the following questions:

- **Do you have a clear sense of who you are,** what you believe and value, the goals you want? Such self-knowledge is critical for forming any mature relationship.

- **Do you feel that you can be yourself** when you're with this person? Do you feel good about yourself? Do you get—and give—compliments, support, and praise?

- **Do you share interests and values?** When you have things in common, you have a foundation to expand and build your relationship.

- **Do you respect the other person** and feel respected in return?
- **Do you have differences in values,** politics, religion, age, or race? Can you accept them?
- **Do you still feel like a unique, strong individual within this relationship?**

Mature Love

Social scientists have distinguished between *passionate love* (characterized by intense feelings of elation, sexual desire, and ecstasy) and *companionate love* (characterized by friendly affection and deep attachment). Often relationships begin with passionate love and evolve into a more companionate love. Sometimes the opposite happens and two people who know each other well discover that their friendship has "caught fire" and the sparks have flamed an unexpected passion.

Mature love is a complex combination of sexual excitement, tenderness, commitment, and—most of all—an overriding passion that sets it apart from all other love relationships in one's life. This passion isn't simply a matter of orgasm but also entails a crossing of the psychological boundaries between oneself and one's lover. You feel as if you're becoming one with your partner while simultaneously retaining a sense of yourself.

Dysfunctional Relationships

Although they enrich and fulfill us in many ways, our relationships with friends, siblings, parents, or colleagues can also sabotage our health. Mental health professionals define a "toxic" relationship as one in which either person is made to feel worthless or incompetent. In the most recent ACHA-NCHA survey, one in ten college students reported being in an emotionally abusive intimate relationship.[17] (See the accompanying table.)

Relationships that don't promote healthy communication, honesty, and intimacy are sometimes called **dysfunctional.** Individuals with addictive behaviors or dependence on drugs or alcohol (see Chapters 11 and 12),

Within the last 12 months, college students reported experiencing:	M	F	Total
An emotionally abusive intimate relationship	7.3	11.5	10.3
A physically abusive intimate relationship	2.1	2.4	2.4
A sexually abusive intimate relationship	0.6	1.8	1.5

American College Health Association. *American College Health Association-National College Health Assessment II: Reference Group Executive Summary Fall 2008.* Baltimore: American College Health Association, 2009.

dysfunctional Characterized by negative and destructive patterns of behavior between partners or between parents and children.

- **Start a dialogue.** Focus on communication, not confrontation. Start with a positive statement, for instance, saying what you really value in the relationship. Volunteer what you might do to make it better, and state what you need from the other person.
- **Distance yourself.** Take a vacation from a toxic friendship. Skip the family reunion or Thanksgiving dinner. When forced into proximity, be polite. If you refuse to engage—not arguing, not getting angry, not trying to make things better—toxic people give up trying to get under your skin.
- **Consult a professional.** A therapist or minister can help people recognize and change toxic behavior patterns. Changes you make in how you act and react may trigger changes in others.
- **Save yourself.** If you can never get what you need in a relationship, you may need to let it go. Nothing is worth compromising your mental or physical health.

and the children or partners of such people, are especially likely to find themselves in such relationships, although they occur in all economic and social groups.

Often partners have magical, unrealistic expectations (e.g., they expect that a relationship with the right person will make their life okay), and one person uses the other almost as if he or she were a mood-altering drug. The partners may compulsively try to get the other to act the way they want. Both persons may distrust or may deceive each other. Often they isolate themselves from others, thus trapping themselves in a recurring cycle of pain.

"Physical symptoms, such as headaches, digestive troubles, tics, and inability to sleep well, can be signs of a destructive relationship," says sociologist Robert Billingham, professor of human development and family studies at Indiana University.[18] Yet, although one person may repeatedly attack, abandon, betray, badger, bully, criticize, deceive, dominate, or demean the other, the responsibility for changing the unhealthy dynamic belongs to both.

"The big question is, 'Do I want or have to keep this relationship going?'" says sociologist Jan Yager, author of *When Friendship Hurts.* "If yes, are you willing to invest time and energy to turn it around?"[19]

Emotional Abuse

Abuse consists of any behavior that uses fear, humiliation, or verbal or physical assaults to control and subjugate another human being. Rather than being physical, emotional abuse often takes the form of constant berating, belittling, and criticism. Aggressive verbal abuse includes calling names, blaming, threatening, accusing, demeaning, and judging. Trivializing, minimizing, or denying what a person says or feels is a more subtle but equally destructive type of abuse. Even if done for the sake of "teaching" or "helping," emotional abuse wears away at self-confidence, sense of self-worth, and trust and belief in one's self. Because it is more than skin deep, emotional abuse can leave deeper, longer-lasting scars.

 In a survey of more than 1,500 never-married undergraduates, 25 percent reported that they had experienced at least two acts of physical abuse in a dating relationship. Far fewer (12 percent) believed that they had ever physically abused their current or most recent dating partner. The majority of students who abuse or are physically abused by a dating partner, the researchers concluded, may not identify themselves as being in an abusive relationship. This may be because of denial, ignorance, or acceptance of physical violence as a norm in a dating relationship.

No one wants to get into an abusive relationship, but often people who were emotionally abused in childhood find themselves in similar circumstances as adults. Dealing with an emotional abuser, regardless of how painful, may feel familiar or even comfortable. Individuals who think very little of themselves also may pick partners who treat them as badly as they believe they deserve.

Abusers also may have grown up with emotional abuse and view it as a way of coping with feelings of fear, hurt, powerlessness, or anger. They may seek partners who see themselves as helpless and who make them feel more powerful.

Among the signs of emotional abuse are:

- **Attempting to control various aspects of your life,** such as what you say or wear.
- **Frequently humiliating you** or making you feel bad about yourself.
- **Making you feel as if you are to blame** for what your partner does.
- **Wanting to know where you are** and whom you're with at all times.
- **Becoming jealous or angry** when you spend time with friends.
- **Threatening to harm you** if you break up.
- **Trying to coerce you** into unwanted sexual activity with statements such as, "If you loved me, you would . . ."

If you can never get what you need or if you're afraid, you need to get out of the relationship. Take whatever steps necessary to ensure your safety. Find a trusted friend who can help. Don't isolate yourself from family and friends. This is the time when you need their support and often the support of a counselor, minister, or doctor as well.

Codependency

Codependency has expanded its definition to include any maladaptive behaviors learned by family members in order to survive great emotional pain and stress, such as addiction, chronic mental or physical illness, and abuse. Some therapists refer to codependency as a "relationship addiction" because codependent people often form or maintain relationships that are one-sided, emotionally destructive, or abusive. First identified in studies of the relationships in families of alcoholics, codependent behavior can occur in any dysfunctional family.

Among the characteristics of codependency are:

- **An exaggerated sense of responsibility** for the actions of others.
- **An attraction to people who need rescuing.**
- **Always trying to do more than one's share.**
- **Doing anything to cling to a relationship** and avoid feeling abandoned.
- **An extreme need for approval and recognition.**
- **A sense of guilt** about asserting needs and desires.
- **A compelling need to control others.**
- **Lack of trust in self and/or others.**
- **Fear of being alone.**
- **Difficulty identifying feelings.**
- **Rigidity/difficulty** adjusting to change.
- **Chronic anger.**
- **Lying/dishonesty.**
- **Poor communications.**
- **Difficulty making decisions.**

Because the roots of codependency run so deep, people don't just "outgrow" this problem or magically find themselves in a healthy relationship. Treatment to resolve childhood hurts and deal with emotional issues may take the form of individual or group therapy, education, or programs such as Codependents Anonymous (www.codependents.org). The goal is to help individuals get in touch with long-buried feelings and build healthier family and relationship dynamics.

Enabling Experts on the subject of addiction first identified traits of codependency in spouses of alcoholics, who followed a predictable pattern of behavior: While intensely trying to control the drinkers, the codependent mates would act in ways that allowed the drinkers to keep drinking. For example, if an alcoholic found it hard to get up in the morning, his wife would wake him up, pull him out of bed and into the shower, and drop him off at work. If he was late, she made excuses to his boss. The husband was the one with the substance-abuse problem, but without realizing it, his wife was **enabling** him to continue drinking. In fact, he might not have been able to keep up his habit without her unintentional cooperation.

Codependency progresses just as an addiction does, and codependents excuse their own behavior with many of the same defense mechanisms used by addicts, such as rationalization ("I cut class so I could catch up on my reading, not to keep an eye on my partner") and denial ("He likes to gamble, but he never loses more than he can afford"). In time, codependents lose sight of everything but their loved one. They feel that if they can only "fix" this person, everything will be fine.

When Love Ends

As the old song says, breaking up is indeed hard to do. Sometimes two people grow apart gradually, and both of them realize that they must go their separate ways. More often, one person falls out of love first. It hurts to be rejected; it also hurts to inflict pain on someone who once meant a great deal to you.

 In surveys, college students say it's more difficult to initiate a breakup than to be rejected. Those who decided to end a relationship report greater feelings of guilt, uncertainty, discomfort, and awkwardness than their girlfriends or boyfriends. However, students with high levels of jealousy are likely to feel a desire for vengeance that can lead to aggressive behavior.

Research suggests that people do not end their relationships because of the disappearance of love. Rather a sense of dissatisfaction or unhappiness develops, which may then cause love to stop growing. The

YOUR STRATEGIES FOR CHANGE
How to Deal with Rejection

- Remind yourself of your own worth. You are no less attractive, intelligent, interesting, or lovable because someone ends a relationship with you.
- Accept the rejection as a statement of the other person's preference rather than trying to debate or defend yourself.
- Think of other people who value or have valued you, who accept and even see as appealing the same characteristics the rejecting person viewed as undesirable.
- Don't withdraw from others. Although you may not want to risk further rejection, it's worth the gamble to get involved again. The only individuals who've never been rejected are those who've never reached out to connect with another.

codependency An emotional and psychological behavioral pattern in which the spouses, partners, parents, children, and friends of individuals with addictive behaviors allow or enable their loved ones to continue their self-destructive habits.

enabling Unwittingly contributing to a person's addictive or abusive behavior. Components of enabling include shielding or covering up for an abuser/addict; controlling him or her; taking over responsibilities; rationalizing addictive behavior; or cooperating with him or her.

fact that love does not dissipate completely may be why breakups are so painful. While the pain does ease over time, it can help both parties if they end their relationship in a way that shows kindness and respect. Your basic guideline should be to think of how you would like to be treated if someone were breaking up with you. Would it hurt more to find out from someone else? Would it be more painful if the person you cared for lied to you or deceived you, rather than admitted the truth? Saying "I don't feel the way I once did about you; I don't want to continue our relationship" is hard, but it's also honest and direct.

Committed Relationships

Even though men and women today may have more sexual partners than in the past, most still yearn for an intense, supportive, exclusive relationship, based on mutual commitment and enduring over time. In our society, most such relationships take the form of heterosexual marriages, but partners of the same sex or heterosexual partners who never marry also may sustain long-lasting, deeply committed relationships. These couples are much like married people: They make a home, handle daily chores, cope with problems, celebrate special occasions, plan for the future—all the while knowing that they are not alone, that they are part of a pair that adds up to far more than just the sum of two individual souls.

Cohabitation

Although couples have always shared homes in informal relationships without any official ties, "living together," or **cohabitation,** has become more common (see Figure 8.2). Some 5 million couples are cohabiting in the United States; the vast majority are heterosexual; 40 percent have children.

About a quarter of unmarried women age 25 to 39 are currently living with a partner; an additional quarter lived with a partner in the past. Couples live together before more than half of all marriages, a practice that was practically unknown 50 years ago. In addition, the proportion of cohabiting women between the ages of 20 and 50 has tripled in the last 50 years.

Cohabitation can be a prelude to marriage, an alternative to living alone, or an alternative to marriage. Couples choose to cohabit for different reasons. In one study, spending more time together and convenience were the most common motivations. Couples who move in together to "test" their relationship report more problems—including more negative communication, physical aggression, and symptoms of depression and anxiety—than others.[20]

The timing of a decision to move in together also matters. Couples who cohabited before getting engaged later reported less marital satisfaction, dedication, and confidence as well as more negative communication and greater potential for divorce than those who lived together after engagement or after getting married.[21]

 Asians and non-Hispanic white couples are the least likely to cohabit. A higher percentage of Native American, black, and Hispanic couples are unmarried. "Cohabiters" tend to have lower income and education levels. They also are younger—on average, some 12 years younger than married men and women.

According to the U.S. Census Bureau, unmarried couples tend to cluster in several zones in the United States, including the western states and the Northeast. In these regions, married couples flock to the suburbs, while unmarried couples, especially same-sex ones, are most likely to live in central cities. As more states and nations are increasing the legal obligations of all intimate partners, the lines between cohabitation and conventional marriage are blurring.

Domestic Partners

Committed couples, both heterosexual and homosexual, can register as domestic partners in certain areas. This may enable them to qualify for benefits such as health insurance.

Employers may require that the couple has lived together for a specified period (generally, at least six months) and are responsible for each other's financial welfare. Recent court rulings have placed domestic partners on the same legal footing as married couples in dealings with businesses.

Long-Term Same-Sex Relationships

Contrary to the stereotype that same-sex relationships tend to be brief, researchers have studied couples who have been together for more than 20 years. Like heterosexual ("straight") couples, same-sex relationships progress through various stages. The first, blending, is a time of intense passion and romantic love. Gradually the couples move through nesting (starting a home together), to building trust and dependability, to merging assets, to establishing a strong sense of partnership.

Because there are no social norms for same-sex unions, researchers describe these relationships as more egalitarian. Each partner tends to be more self-reliant, and homosexual men and women tend to be more willing to communicate and experiment in terms of sexual behaviors.

Gay and lesbian relationships are comparable to straight relationships in many ways. But same-sex couples have to deal with everyday ups-and-downs in a social context of isolation from family, workplace prejudice, and other social barriers. However, gay and lesbian couples are more upbeat in the face of conflict. Compared to straight couples, they use more affection and humor when they bring up a disagreement and remain more positive after a disagreement. They also display less belligerence, domineering, and fear with each other than straight couples do. When they argue, they are better able to soothe each other so they show fewer signs of physiological arousal, such as an elevated heart rate or sweaty palms, than heterosexual couples.

Marriage

Like everything which is not the involuntary result of fleeting emotion but the creation of time and will, any marriage, happy or unhappy, is infinitely more interesting and significant than any romance, however passionate.

W. H. Auden

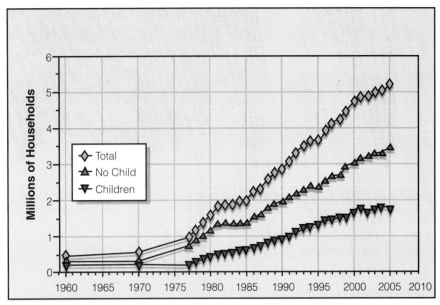

Figure 8.2 Unmarried Couple Households
The number of unmarried couples living together, both with and without children, has risen dramatically in the last 50 years.
Source: U.S. Census Bureau

Contemporary marriage has been described as an institution that everyone on the outside wants to enter and everyone on the inside wants to leave. According to the U.S. Census Bureau, nine in ten people marry, but about half of first marriages end in divorce after an average of seven or eight years.

The proportion of married people, especially among younger age groups, has been declining for decades. Across North America and many European countries, the age of first marriage has risen, with both men and women waiting an extra three years before saying "I do," and the rate of first marriages among men has been cut in half.

Not too long ago, marriage was often a business deal, a contract made by parents for economic or political reasons when the spouses-to-be were still very young. Today, in some countries, it is still culturally acceptable to arrange marriages in this manner. Even in America, certain ethnic groups, such as Asians who have recently immigrated to the United States, plan marriages for their children. In such arrangements, the marriage partners are likely to have similar values and expectations. However, the newlyweds also start out as strangers who may not even know whether they like—let alone love—each other. Sometimes arranged marriages do lead to loving unions; sometimes

cohabitation Two people living together as a couple, without official ties such as marriage.

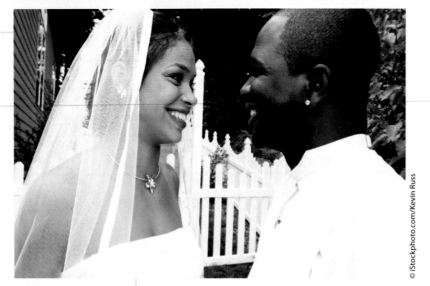

Couples are more likely to live happily long after their wedding day if they share the same values and religious beliefs, tolerate flaws, and communicate effectively.

they trap both partners in loneliness and longing.

Preparing for Marriage

Most people say they marry for one far-from-simple reason: love. However, with more than half of all marriages ending in divorce, there's little doubt that modern marriages aren't made in heaven. Are some couples doomed to divorce even before they swap vows? Could counseling before a marriage increase its odds of success? According to recent research findings, the answer to both questions is yes.

There have been government attempts to set requirements for couples who want to marry. Some states, such as Arizona and Louisiana, have established "covenant" marriages in which engaged couples are required to get premarital counseling. Utah allows counties to require counseling before issuing marriage licenses to minors and people who have been divorced. Florida requires high school students to take marriage education classes.

Finding Mr. or Ms. Right

Generally, men and women marry people from the geographical area they grew up in and from the same social background. Differences in religion and race can add to the pressures of marriage, but they also can enrich the relationship if they aren't viewed as obstacles. In our culturally diverse society, interracial and cross-cultural marriages are becoming more common and widely accepted, although the odds are much greater for partners of the same race to live together or marry.

Some of the traits that appeal to us in a date become less important when we select a mate; others become key ingredients in the emotional cement holding two people together. According to psychologist Robert Sternberg of Yale University, the crucial ingredients for commitment are the following:

- Shared values.
- A willingness to change in response to each other.
- A willingness to tolerate flaws.
- A match in religious beliefs.
- The ability to communicate effectively.

The single best predictor of how satisfied one will be in a relationship, according to Sternberg, is not how one feels toward a lover, but rather the difference between how one would like the lover to feel and how the lover actually feels. Feeling that the partner you've chosen loves too little or too much is, as he puts it, "the best predictor of failure."[22] For other predictors, see Your Strategies for Prevention: "Think Twice about Getting Married If . . ."

Premarital Assessments

There are scientific ways of predicting marital happiness. Some premarital assessment inventories identify strengths and weaknesses in many aspects of a relationship: realistic expectations, personality issues, communication, conflict resolution, financial management, leisure activities, sex, children, family and friends, egalitarian roles, and religious orientation. Couples who become aware of potential conflicts by means of such inventories may be able to resolve them through professional counseling. In some cases, they may want to reconsider or postpone their wedding.

Other common predictors of marital discord, unhappiness, and separation are:

- **A high level of arousal during a discussion.**
- **Defensive behaviors** such as making excuses and denying responsibility for disagreements.
- **A wife's expressions of contempt.**
- **A husband's stonewalling** (showing no response when a wife expresses her concerns).

By looking for such behaviors, researchers have been able to predict with better than 90 percent accuracy whether a couple will separate within the first few years of marriage.

The Benefits of Marriage Despite its problems, marriage endures because it is a fulfilling way for two people to live. As researchers have proved, saying "I do" can do wonders for your health. According to a DCD study of more than 127,000 adults, married people are healthier than those who are divorced, widowed, never-married, or live with a partner. The connection between marriage and health was strongest in the youngest group, aged 18 to 44.[23]

Married people are less likely to suffer from health conditions like back pain, headaches, and serious psychological distress. That is true for all ages, ethnicities, and levels of income and education. Married people are less likely to smoke, drink heavily, and be physically inactive.

Marriage does pose one health hazard: weight gain. Married men are more likely to be overweight or obese. Three in four married men aged 45 to 64 are overweight or obese. The slimmest groups are men and women who have never married.

Married men and women also have lower rates of most mental disorders than single or divorced individuals. Both husbands and wives live longer than single or divorced individuals. In one national survey, about 90 percent of husbands and wives survived until at least age 65, compared with only about 60 to 70 percent of divorced and never-married men and women. Although there has not been much research on same-sex committed relationships, most experts believe that gay couples are likely to enjoy similar benefits, as long as they remain together and receive social support for doing so.

For years researchers thought that marriage was especially beneficial to men. Married men have lower rates of alcohol and drug abuse, depression, and risk-taking behavior than divorced men. They also earn more money—possibly because they have more incentive to do so. However, more recent research indicates that a happy marriage boosts mental health and well-being in both spouses.

 Same-Sex Marriage **Same-sex marriage,** also called gay or single-sex or gender-neutral marriage, refers to a governmentally, socially, or religiously recognized marriage in which two people of the same sex live together as a family. Several countries, including Canada, the Netherlands, Belgium, and Spain, have legitimized same-sex marriages. Several states now recognize same-sex marriages. Several other states recognize domestic partnerships and civil unions that grant some of the legal and economic benefits of marriage.

Same-sex marriages have triggered intense controversy. (See Point/Counterpoint, p. 254.) Some oppose gay unions on religious and moral grounds. Others argue that marriage is a right based on procreation and designed to protect the children of a man and a woman. Advocates of gay marriage contend that the ban on same-gender unions discriminates against homosexuals and denies them the civil rights and legal protection that heterosexual couples have.

Is marriage as beneficial to the health of same-sex partners as it is for male-female couples? In terms of physical well-being, researchers found no difference between heterosexual and homosexual spouses.[24] In a Danish study, mortality rates were higher among gay men and lesbian women in same-sex marriages than they are in the general population, particularly in the first years of marriage. However, the primary reason, according to the researchers, is an illness that existed at the time of marriage.[25]

Issues Couples Confront No two people can live together in perfect harmony all the time. Some of the issues that crop up in any long-term relationship include expectations, money, sex, and careers.

Money Money may make the business world go around, but it has the opposite effect on relationships: It knocks them off their tracks, brings them to a halt, twists them upside down. However, even though almost all couples quarrel about money, they rarely fight over how much they have. What matters more—whether they make $10,000 or $100,000 a year—is what money means to both partners. How does each person use money to meet emotional needs? Who decides how the

same-sex marriage
Governmentally, socially, or religiously recognized marriage in which two people of the same sex live together as a family.

POINT

Marriage "by definition" can only unite a man and a woman. Any attempt to extend it beyond heterosexuals would threaten and devalue the institution of marriage. Homosexual unions are abnormal, immoral, and unworthy of the law's protection.

COUNTERPOINT

All human being should have the same fundamental rights. The fact that they were denied equality in the past does not justify continuing to treat lesbians and gays unfairly. Same-sex couples should have the same economic and civil rights guaranteed in a legally recognized marriage as heterosexual couples have.

YOUR VIEW

Should marriage be restricted to heterosexual couples? Should homosexual couples have the same recognition? Are committed relationships between gay or lesbians different or less deserving of legal protection than those between heterosexuals?

© John Riley/Stone/Getty Images

Understanding that your partner may have different money values can help avoid arguments.

money is spent? Who keeps track? Until they resolve these issues, couples may quarrel over money as long as they're together.

To avoid fighting over money, understand that having different money values or expectations doesn't make one of you right and the other wrong. Recognize the value of unpaid work. A partner who's finishing school or taking care of the children is making an important contribution to the family and its future. It also helps to go over your finances together so that you have a firm basis in reality for what you can and can't afford. Talk about the financial goals you hope to attain five years from now. Set priorities to meet them. Also, set aside money for each of you to spend without asking or answering to the other. Even a small amount can make each partner feel more independent.

Sex   Like every other aspect of a relationship, sex evolves and changes over the course of marriage. The redhot sexual chemistry of

the early stages of intimacy invariably cools down. Even so, the happiest couples have sex more often than unhappily married pairs do.

What matters most isn't quantity alone, but the quality of sexual activity and intimacy. Are both partners satisfied with their sexual relationship? Does one partner always initiate sex? Do the partners talk about their preferences and pleasures? Sexuality, like personality, is dynamic and changes throughout life. Do the partners acknowledge and adapt to these changes? Do they feel sufficiently at ease with each other to discuss anxieties about sex? The answers to these questions can determine how sexually gratifying a marriage is for both spouses.

Extramarital Affairs   How faithful are American mates? The answer depends on the questions researchers ask and who they ask. In face-to-face interviews, University of Chicago researchers found that 25 percent of men and 15 percent of women had had affairs and that 94 percent of the married subjects had been monogamous in the last year. Another survey of Americans found that one out of six Americans had had an extramarital relationship—19 percent of the men and 15 percent of the women.[26]

High or low, numbers are little comfort when affairs do occur. A husband or wife who learns about a spouse's affair typically feels a devastating sense of betrayal as well as deep feelings of shame, fear of abandonment, depression, and anger. Two crucial questions determine whether a marriage can survive: Do the spouses still feel a serious commitment to each other? And do they love each other and want to remain together?

Two-Career Couples   More than 75 percent of women with children work—a dramatic increase from the 1960s, when only 30 percent of mothers worked outside the home. Two careers can bring pressure to a relationship: Both individuals may come home tired and irritable; both may have to spend a great deal of time on their jobs; both may have to travel or work on weekends. Two-career couples must be able to discuss their problems openly to resolve these pressures.

Couples pursuing individual careers sometimes face difficult choices. What happens, for example, if one of them is offered a promising job in another city? Does the spouse quit his or her job, pack up, and move? Some couples resolve such dilemmas by working in different cities and spending weekends together. Others try to alternate career and home priorities. However imperfect these arrangements may be, they work for some couples.

Conflict in Marriage

While all couples may wish to live happily and peacefully ever after, sooner or later, they argue. In a five-year study of newly married couples, about a third (36 percent) sought some form of help for their relationship, most often from books on relationships and marital therapy.[27] Years of research have shown that while conflict is inevitable, the key difference between happy and unhappy couples is the way they fight.

Happier couples interject positive interactions, like a joke or a smile, into their arguments. As long as the ratio of positive to negative interactions remains at least five to one, the relationship remains intact. By comparison, unhappy couples unfurl a barrage of negative words, gestures, criticisms, and hostility at their mates with hardly any positive interactions. Based on observations of couples in conflict, researchers have been able to predict which would divorce with 94 percent accuracy. Both men and women feel the strain of arguing and being angry because of marital difficulties, but wives are more likely to develop high blood pressure, high cholesterol, high blood sugar, and other markers of metabolic syndrome (discussed in Chapter 14). The reason may be that many women take negativity to heart and become depressed.[28]

Among the other suggestions therapists offer couples are:

- **Focus on friendship.** If a marriage is not built on a strong friendship, it may be difficult to stay connected over time.

- **Remember what you loved and admired in your partner in the first place.** Focusing on these qualities can foster a much more positive attitude toward him or her.

- **Show respect.** Your spouse deserves the same courtesy and civility that your colleagues do. Without respect, love cannot survive.

- **Compliment what your partner does right.** Noticing the positive can change how both of you feel about each other.

- **Forgive one another.** When your partner hurts your feelings but then reaches out, don't reject his or her attempts to make things better.

Saving Marriages Fewer than two-thirds of couples—65 percent of husbands and 60 percent of wives—say they are "very happy" in their marriages. Each year, hundreds of thousands of couples go into counseling in an effort to make their unions happier. Among the approaches currently in use are marriage education and various forms of couples therapy.

Marriage education consists of workshops that teach couples practical skills so they get along better. Some studies indicate that graduates of these programs have a lower divorce rate than unhappy couples who do not enroll in them.

Couples therapy, also called marriage counseling or marriage therapy, uses a variety of psychological techniques to help couples understand and overcome their conflicts. These include:

- **Behavioral marital therapy,** which teaches partners to communicate better and to improve their conflict resolution skills.

- **Emotionally focused therapy,** which helps couples identify and break free of destructive emotional cycles.

- **Insight-oriented marital therapy,** which combines behavioral therapy with techniques for understanding negative behaviors, such as power struggles, within the relationship.

Divorce

According to the most recent U.S. Census Bureau data, 2,230,000 marriages occur every year. The marriage rate now stands at 7.5 per 1,000 Americans.[29] The divorce rate is almost 50 percent: 3.6 per 1,000 Americans. Your risk of divorce depends on many factors. Simply having some college education improves your odds of a happy marriage. Other factors that do the same are an income higher than $50,000, marrying at age 25 or older, not having a baby during the first seven months after the wedding, coming from an intact family, and having some religious affiliation.

Race also influences marriage and divorce rates. African American couples are more likely to break up than white couples, and black divorcées are less likely to marry again. Researchers have found that African Americans place an equally high value on marriage. However, there is a smaller "marriageable pool" of black men for a variety of reasons, including a higher mortality rate.

Children whose parents divorced are less likely to marry and to stay married. However, their adult relationships aren't doomed to fail. "Divorce isn't in the genes," says child psychologist Judith Wallerstein, who has studied divorced families for thirty years. "Divorce is an avoidable human error."

Family Ties

Children have become the exception rather than the rule in American households. A century ago most households contained children under age 18. In 1960, slightly fewer than half did. In 2000, fewer than a third of households included children, and this figure is expected to drop to 28 percent by 2010.

Attitudes also have changed. While many traditionally viewed having children as the primary purpose for getting married, nearly 70 percent of Americans now cite another reason. When young adults—ages 18 to 34—react to the statement, "Those who want children should get married," only about half of men and even fewer women agree.

Fertility has declined in the United States since 1960. At that time, the average woman had about three and one-half children over the course of her life. Today's woman has an average of about two children, which is lower than the "replacement level" of 2.1 children per woman. This is the level at which the population would be replaced by births alone. In most European and several Asian countries, fertility has dropped even lower.

Diversity Within Families

 Families have become as diverse as the American population and reflect different traditions, beliefs, and values. Within African American families, for instance, traditional gender roles are often reversed, with women serving as head of the household, a kinship bond uniting several households, and a strong religious commitment or orientation. In Chinese American families, both spouses may work and see themselves as breadwinners, but the wife may not have an equal role in decision making. In Hispanic families, wives and mothers are acknowledged and respected as healers and dispensers of wisdom. At the same time, they are expected to defer to their husbands, who see themselves as the strong, protective, dominant head of the family. As time passes and families from different cultures become more integrated into American life, traditional gender roles and decision-making patterns often change, particularly among the youngest family members.

American families are diverse in other ways. *Multigenerational families*, with children, parents, and grandparents, make up 3.7 percent of households. They occur most often in areas where new immigrants live with relatives, where housing shortages or high costs force families to double up their living arrangements, or where high rates of out-of-wedlock childbearing force unwed mothers to live with their children in their parents' home.

Three of every ten households consist of **blended families,** formed when one or both of the partners bring children from a previous union. In the future, social scientists predict, American families will become even more diverse, or pluralistic. But as norms or expectations about the configurations of families have changed, values or ideas about the intents and purposes of families have not. American families of every type still support each other and strive toward values such as commitment and caring.

Working Parents

The traditional family with a breadwinner and a homemaker has been replaced by what some call "the juggler family." Two working parents or an unmarried working parent head 70 percent of American families with children. As a result, American parents have fewer hours to spend with their children. Women, balancing multiple roles as parents, spouses, caregivers, and employees often give their own personal needs the lowest priority.

The Family and Work Institute of New York calculates that American husbands put in 75 percent as much time as wives on workday chores—a dramatic rise from 30 percent in 1977. In actual clocktime, the gender difference in domestic "scutwork" amounts to just 45 minutes a day.

Single Parents

About 35 percent of births—up from 5 percent a half-century ago—occur outside of marriage. About 28 percent of all children under age 18 live with just one parent, the majority with their mothers. The number of families headed by single mothers has increased 25 percent since 1990, to more than 7.5 million households.

The new breed of single mother doesn't fit the old stereotype of an unwed, minority teenager. The median age for unmarried mothers is the late 20s; the fastest growing group is white women. She may be divorced or unmarried. Forty percent live with men

© Image Source Pink/Jupiterimages

Whether married or single, fathers play an important role in their children's lives.

who may be the fathers of one or more of their children.

Single fathers head over two million households. The typical single father is 38 years old. One in 9 is under age 25; and 1 in 70 is 60 or older. About 5 of every 6 (83 percent) of the nation's single fathers are white. African Americans and Hispanics together constitute about 13 percent.

Median family income for one-parent families is significantly lower than the median for two-parent families. Twenty percent are poor, compared with 9 percent of two-parent families. Half live in rental housing, compared with one-quarter of two-parent families.

family A group of people united by marriage, blood, or adoption; residing in the same household; maintaining a common culture; and interacting with one another on the basis of their roles within the group.
blended family A family formed when one or both of the partners bring children from a previous union to the new marriage.

LEARN IT LIVE IT Creating Better Relationships

We are born social. From our first days of life, we reach out to others, struggle to express ourselves, strive to forge connections. The fabric of our lives becomes richer as family and friends weave through it the threads of their experiences. No solitary pleasure can match the gifts that we gain by reaching out and connecting with others.

As with other significant endeavors, good relationships require work—through hard times, despite conflicts, over months and years and decades. As you strive to improve the ties that bind you to others, keep in mind the characteristics of a good relationship. They can serve as the goals you strive to attain:

- **Trust.** Partners are able to confide in each other openly, knowing their confidences will be respected.

- **Togetherness.** In a healthy relationship, two people create a sense of both intimacy and autonomy. They enjoy each other's company but also pursue solitary interests.

- **Expressiveness.** Partners in healthy relationships say what they feel, need, and desire.

- **Staying power.** People in committed relationships keep their bond strong through tough times by proving that they will be there for each other.

- **Security.** Because a good relationship is strong enough to absorb conflict and anger, partners know they can express their feelings honestly. They also are willing to risk vulnerability for the sake of becoming closer.

- **Laughter.** Humor keeps things in perspective—always crucial in any sort of ongoing relationship or enterprise.

- **Support.** Partners in good relationships continually offer each other encouragement, comfort, and acceptance.

- **Physical affection.** Sexual desire may fluctuate or diminish over the years, but partners in loving, long-term relationships usually retain some physical connection.

- **Personal growth.** In the best relationships, partners are committed to bringing out the best in each other and have the other's best interests at heart.

- **Respect.** Caring partners are aware of each other's boundaries, need for personal space, and vulnerabilities. They do not take each other or their relationship for granted.

How Strong Are the Communication and Affection in Your Relationship?

Effective, caring communication and loving affection markedly enhance a couple's relationship. The following self-test may help you to assess the degree of good communication, love, and respect in your intimate relationship. If you agree or mostly agree with a statement, answer yes. If you disagree or mostly disagree, answer no. You may wish to have your partner respond to this assessment as well. If so, mark your answers on a separate sheet.

1.	My partner seeks out my opinion.	Yes	No	11.	There's lots of love in our relationship.	Yes	No
2.	My partner cares about my feelings.	Yes	No	12.	We are genuinely interested in one another.	Yes	No
3.	I don't feel ignored very often.	Yes	No	13.	I love spending time with my partner.	Yes	No
4.	We touch each other a lot.	Yes	No	14.	We are very good friends.	Yes	No
5.	We listen to each other.	Yes	No	15.	Even during rough times, we can be empathetic.	Yes	No
6.	We respect each other's ideas.	Yes	No	16.	My partner is considerate of my viewpoint.	Yes	No
7.	We are affectionate toward one another.	Yes	No	17.	My partner finds me physically attractive.	Yes	No
8.	I feel my partner takes good care of me.	Yes	No	18.	My partner expresses warmth toward me.	Yes	No
9.	What I say counts.	Yes	No	19.	I feel included in my partner's life.	Yes	No
10.	I am important in our decisions.	Yes	No	20.	My partner admires me.	Yes	No

Scoring:

A preponderance of yes answers indicates that you enjoy a strong relationship characterized by good communication and loving affection. If you answered yes to fewer than seven items, it is likely that you are not feeling loved and respected and that the communication in your relationship is decidedly lacking.

Source: John Gottman, *Why Marriages Succeed or Fail.* New York: Simon & Schuster, 1994.

Your Health Action Plan for Improving Your Relationships

Being in a relationship should be an opportunity for fun, personal growth, and mutual support, never an excuse for hurting or controlling someone else. The following guidelines can help keep a relationship healthy:

- **Recognize that both people in the relationship have the right to be accepted** as they are, to be treated with respect, to feel safe, to ask for what they want, to say no without feeling guilty, to express themselves, to give and receive affection, and to make some mistakes and be forgiven.

- **Remember that no one in a relationship has the right to force the other to do anything,** to tell the other where or when to speak up or go out, to humiliate the other in public or private, to isolate the other from friends and family, to read personal material without permission, to pressure the other to give up goals or interests, or to abuse the other person verbally or physically.

- **Be willing to open up.** The more you share, the deeper the bond between you and your friend will become.

- **Be sensitive to your friend's or partner's feelings.** Keep in mind that, like you, he or she has unique needs, desires, and dreams.

- **Express appreciation.** Be generous with your compliments. Let your friends and family know you recognize their kindnesses.

- **Know that people will disappoint you from time to time.** We are only human. Accept your loved ones as they are. Admitting their faults need not reduce your respect for them.

- **Talk about your relationship.** If you have any gripes or frustrations, air them.

CENGAGENOW If you want to write your own goals for enhanced relationships, go to the Wellness Journal at CengageNow for Health: **www.cengage.com/sso.**

MAKING THIS CHAPTER WORK FOR YOU

Review Questions

1. Romantic love
   a. is associated with the depletion of the hormone oxytocin.
   b. is an emotional phenomenon between humans that has its roots in prehistoric times and occurs in almost all cultures.
   c. can only occur between people who share interests and goals.
   d. always results in a committed long-term relationship.

2. Which of the following is most likely a sign of a dysfunctional relationship?
   a. The partners have frequent disagreements about money.
   b. One partner makes all the decisions for the couple and the other partner.
   c. Each partner has a demanding career.
   d. One partner is much older than the other partner.

3. Smart suggestions for online dating include:
   a. Use your office or school computer so that contacts can't access your personal computer.
   b. Give out only your cell phone number, not your address.
   c. Plan a full-day outing so that you will have plenty of time to get to know each other.
   d. Plan to meet in a busy place, like the local coffee house.

4. In friendships and other intimate relationships, which of the following is *not* true?
   a. Friends can communicate feelings as well as facts.

b. Listening is just as important as talking.

c. Emotional investment is required but the rewards are great.

d. There is no need to pay attention to nonverbal communication.

5. Which of these is an example of self-disclosure?

a. Steve tells his friend Twana that he would really like to change jobs sometime in the next year.

b. Mike and Nicole talk about which cars they prefer.

c. Maria mentions to Carrie that she and her brother don't get along so he won't be at the picnic.

d. Angela lets her boyfriend Paul know that she used to be bulimic.

6. Married people

a. have sex less frequently than unmarried partners.

b. are more likely to become alcoholics and drug users.

c. typically have at least one extramarital affair during their marriage.

d. live longer than single or divorced individuals.

7. Which of the following scenarios demonstrates what might be considered gender differences in verbal and nonverbal communication styles?

a. While Alyssa and Peter are discussing their vacation plans, Alyssa is gazing at the television and Peter is looking at Alyssa.

b. Good friends Eva and Julia see each other for the first time after Christmas break and greet each other with a nod and a quick "Hi."

c. New bank manager Alejandro tells the staff that they should consider him "the team coach and the keeper of the playbook."

d. During an argument, Tony complains to Nicki, "I don't appreciate your crude jokes and constant swearing."

8. Which of the following statements is *false?*

a. College education increases your chances of a happy marriage.

b. African American couples are more likely to divorce than white couples.

c. Children whose parents divorced are more likely to stay married.

d. The divorce rate is lower now than it was in 1980.

9. Partners in successful marital relationships

a. are generally from the same social and ethnic background.

b. usually lived together before marrying.

c. were usually very young at the time of their marriage.

d. have premarital agreements.

10. The characteristics of a good relationship include which of the following?

a. trust   c. identical interests

b. financial stability   d. physical attractiveness

Answers to these questions can be found on page 650.

Critical Thinking

1. While our society has become more tolerant, marriages between people of different religious and racial groups still face special pressures. What issues might arise if a Christian marries a Jew or Muslim? What about the issues facing partners of different races? How could these issues be resolved? What are your own feelings about mixed marriages? Would you date someone of a different religion or race? Why or why not?

2. What are your personal criteria for a successful relationship? Develop a brief list of factors you consider important, and support your choices with examples or experiences from your own life.

Media Menu

CENGAGENOW™ Go to the CengageNOW for Health website at **www .cengage.com/sso** that will:

• Help you evaluate your knowledge of the material.

• Allow you to take an exam-prep quiz.

• Provide a personalized Learning Plan targeting resources that address areas you should study.

• Coach you through identifying target goals for behavioral change and creating and monitoring your personal change plan throughout the semester.

Internet Connections

www.goaskalice.columbia.edu
Sponsored by the health education and wellness program of the Columbia University Health Service, this site features educators' answers to questions on a wide variety of topics, including those related to relationships and marriage and family.

www.apahelpcenter.org/articles/topic.php?id=2
The American Psychological Association provides a wealth of articles and information on sustaining healthy relationships.

www.cyfc.umn.edu/family/index.html
This site offers research, programs, publications, and information on all types of parenting, relationships, and family issues.

Key Terms

The terms listed are used on the page indicated. Definitions of the terms are in the Glossary at the end of the book.

blended families 257
codependency 249
cohabitation 251
dysfunctional 247
enabling 249
family 257
intimacy 245
same-sex marriages 253
self-disclosure 243

Chapter 9 - Personal Sexuality

1. **Males and females have the same endocrine hormone system except for which organ in the body?** (Pg. 264)
    A. respiratory system organs
    B. sex organs
    C. brain
    D. alimentary organs

2. **The primary sex hormone in men is:** (Pg. 264)
    A. estrogen
    B. progesterone
    C. adrenaline
    D. testosterone

3. **The physical, psychological, and social aspects of one's male or female core make up are known as their:** (Pg. 262)
    A. sexual orientation
    B. sexual identity
    C. gender
    D. sexual preference

4. **The most sensitive female organ for sexual arousal is the:** (Pg. 266)
    A. vagina
    B. cervix
    C. clitoris
    D. labia minora

5. **The female organ that produces the egg cells needed for fertilization is the:** (Pg. 266)
    A. labia majora
    B. ovaries
    C. endometrium
    D. fallopian tubes

6. **When a girl begins to have her first menstrual cycle at puberty, this is known as:** (Pg. 267)
    A. amenorrhea
    B. menarche
    C. dyspareunia
    D. nocturnal emissions

7. **Approximately half of all women during their menstrual cycle phase of life suffer from:** (Pg. 267)
    A. amenorrhea
    B. dysphoric disorder
    C. toxic shock syndrome
    D. dysmenorrheal

8. **Teenage boys often experience non-sexual erections and ejaculation while they are sleeping at night, which is known as:** (Pg. 273)
    A. nocturnal malfunction
    B. sex nightmares
    C. wet dreams
    D. sexual dysfunction

9. **The number one reason that both men and women say why they want to have sex with their partner is:** (Pg. 276)
    A. because it feels good
    B. to express their love for each other
    C. they are attracted to their partner
    D. because it is fun

10. **Which of the following is not considered to be a characteristic of a sexually healthy relationship?** (Pg. 271- 272)
    A. it is consensual and agreeable to both partners
    B. it is permissible for the man to exploit the female partner in sexual ways
    C. it is protected against unwanted pregnancy or sexually transmitted infections
    D. it is mutually satisfying to both partners

11. **Androgyny is another term for:** (Pg. 265)
    A. homosexuals
    B. female gender with male characteristics
    C. transgenderism
    D. individuals who possess both male and female characteristics

12. **When one is sexually attracted exclusively to the opposite sex, they are considered to be:** (Pg. 278)
    A. monogamous
    B. homosexual
    C. heterosexual
    D. polyamorous

13. **When a partner performs fellatio, this means that a:** (Pg. 283)
    A. man's genitals are being orally stimulated
    B. woman's genitals are being stimulated by her partner's mouth
    C. man is having anal sex with his partner
    D. mutual masturbation is occurring

14. **A type of safer sex which employs pleasure, yet is non-penetrative to the partner is called:** (Pg. 282)
    A. intercourse
    B. outercourse
    C. cunnilingus
    D. coitus

15. **A person who obtains sexual pleasure or finds eroticism from inanimate objects is known to be into:** (Pg. 291)
    A. voyeurism
    B. sadism
    C. fetishism
    D. masochism

16. **The most powerful sex organ is the:** (Pg. 281)
    A. penis
    B. clitoris
    C. mind
    D. lips

17. **In what stage of sexual intercourse does the penis continue to engorge wider and longer and the vagina also becomes wider to absorb the penis during sex?** (Pg. 284)
    A. excitement phase
    B. plateau phase
    C. orgasm phase
    D. resolution phase

18. **Men who are heavier smokers and alcoholic drinkers will tend to have greater sexual dysfunction known as:** (Pg. 287)
    A. premature ejaculation
    B. impotence
    C. dyspareunia
    D. anxiety performance

19. **Which ethnic group tends to be more nonverbal and intuitive (private) when dealing with sexual matters in the relationship?** (Pg. 283)
    A. African Americans
    B. Hispanic Americans
    C. Whites
    D. Asian Americans

20. **To communicate about sex to your partner also means being sexually responsible. Which of the following would not be acceptable in communicating or being responsible about sexual matters?** (Pg. 272 & 292)
    A. if you cannot talk comfortably about sexual matters, you should not be having sex with your partner
    B. sexual harassment is okay as it is a prelude to good sex with your partner
    C. both partners should share in the responsibility of protecting one's self from unwanted pregnancy, HIV or other STIs
    D. both partners should respect sexual privacy of each other's prior sexual activities

Charles, several years older than the typical college freshman, usually doesn't think much about the age difference—until the conversation turns to sex. He understands his younger classmates' seemingly endless fascination with sex, but his perspective is different. As a teenager, he had plunged recklessly into dangerous territory of every type. Sex—casual and sometimes unprotected—was one of them. "Looking back," Charles muses, "I feel lucky that I didn't end up a statistic. But he still regrets the irresponsible ways he acted.

Personal Sexuality

At 28 Charles is a veteran of military service, a married man, and an expectant father. His enjoyment of sex hasn't faded—in many ways, it's deepened and become more gratifying. He now realizes that there is no such thing as casual sex, that sexual choices have consequences and effects on one's own life and on other people. These are the lessons he hopes someday to pass on to his own children.

As Charles learned with time and experience, you are ultimately responsible for your sexual health and behavior. You make decisions that affect how you express your sexuality, how you respond sexually, and how you give and get sexual pleasure. Yet most sexual activity involves another person. Therefore, your decisions about sex—more so than those you make about nutrition, drugs, or exercise—have important effects on other people. Recognizing this fact is the key to responsible sexuality. (See Making Change Happen, p. 263, and "What's Your Intimacy Quotient?" in *Labs for IPC*.)

Sexual responsibility means learning about your body, your partner's body, your sexual development and preferences, and the health risks associated with sexual activity. This chapter is an introduction to your sexual self and an exploration of sexual issues in today's world. It provides the information and insight you can use in making decisions and choosing behaviors that are responsible for all concerned.

After studying the material in this chapter, you should be able to

- **Explain** the roles of hormones in sexual development.
- **Describe** the male and female reproductive systems and the functions of the individual structures of each system.
- **Describe** conditions or issues unique to women's and men's sexual health.
- **Define** sexual health and list behaviors that can contribute to sexually healthy relationships.
- **Define** sexual orientation and **give examples** of sexual diversity.
- **List** the range of sexual behaviors practiced by adults.
- **Describe** the phases of sexual response.
- **List** the common sexual concerns of men and women.
- **Evaluate** your ability to communicate about sex with a potential partner.

Log on to CengageNOW for Health at **www.cengage.com/sso** to find your Behavior Change Planner and to explore self-assessments, interactive tutorials, and practice quizzes.

Human Sexuality

Human **sexuality**—the quality of being sexual—is as rich, varied, and complex as life itself. Along with our **sex,** or biological maleness or femaleness, it is an integral part of who we are, how we see ourselves, and how we relate to others. Of all of our involvements with others, sexual **intimacy,** or physical closeness, can be the most rewarding. But while sexual expression and experience can provide intense joy, they also can involve great emotional turmoil.

Sexuality and the Dimensions of Health

sexuality The behaviors, instincts, and attitudes associated with being sexual.

sex Maleness or femaleness, resulting from genetic, structural, and functional factors.

intimacy A state of closeness between two people, characterized by the desire and ability to share one's innermost thoughts and feelings with each other either verbally or nonverbally.

sexual health The integration of the physical, emotional, intellectual, social, and spiritual aspects of sexual being in ways that are positively enriching and that enhance personality, communication, and love.

gender Maleness or femaleness, as determined by a combination of anatomical and physiological factors, psychological factors, and learned behaviors.

Our sexuality both affects and is affected by the various dimensions of health. Responsible sexuality and high-level **sexual health** contribute to the fullest possible functioning of body, mind, spirit, and social relationships. In turn, other aspects of health enhance our sexuality. Here are some examples:

- **Physical.** As described in Chapter 16, safer sex practices reduce the risk of sexually transmitted infections that can threaten sexual health, physical health, and even survival. When our bodies are healthy and well, we feel better about how we look and move—which enhances both self-esteem and healthy sexuality.

- **Emotional.** By acknowledging and respecting the intimacy of a sexual relationship, responsible sexuality builds trust and commitment. When our emotional health is high, we can better understand and cope with the complex feelings related to being sexual.

- **Social.** From dating to mating, we express and fulfill our sexual identities in the context of families, friends, and society as a whole. Having strong friendships, intimate relationships, and caring partnerships enables us to explore our sexuality in safe and healthy ways.

- **Intellectual.** Our most fulfilling relationships involve a meeting of minds as well as bodies. High-level intellectual health enables us to acquire and understand sexual information, analyze it critically, and make healthy sexual decisions.

- **Spiritual.** At its deepest, most fulfilling level, sexuality uplifts the soul by allowing us to connect to something greater than oneself. Individuals who have developed their spirituality bring to their most intimate relationships an awareness and appreciation that lifts them beyond the physical.

- **Environmental.** Responsible sexuality makes people more aware of the impact of their decisions on others. Protecting yourself from sexual threats and creating a supportive environment in which to study and work are crucial to high-level health and to healthy sexuality.

Becoming Male or Female

 Physiological maleness or femaleness, or biological sex, is indicated by the sex chromosomes, hormonal balance, and genital anatomy. **Gender** refers to the psychological and sociological, as well as the physical, aspects of being male or

What's Your Intimacy Quotient?

Intimacy doesn't happen at first sight—or in a day or a week or a string of weeks. Intimacy needs time and nurturing. It is a process of self-revelation, of exposing rather than hiding, or expressing rather than suppressing, or wanting someone to know us as fully as possible, and of wanting to know that someone as fully as possible. Although intimacy isn't the same as sex, it often includes a sexual relationship.

Like every other worthwhile endeavor in life, quality relationships require attention and effort—but of the most delightful and rewarding type. "What's Your Intimacy Quotient?" in *Labs for IPC* assesses and strengthens the skills you need to enrich your life with warm, close, supportive intimate relationships. Here's a preview.

Get Real

To create and maintain intimate relationships, you need to assess nine essential skills, including the following three:

- **Receptivity.**
  If you are text-messaging or checking e-mail while talking to your partner, friend, or child, the message you're sending them is, "Don't bother me. I've got something better to do" . . .
  Do you spend some time every day simply sitting and reconnecting with your partner? Do you spend some time every day simply sitting and reconnecting with you?

- **Expressing your self.**
  Don't expect your partner to read your mind. Avoid the "If-you-loved-me-you'd-know" trap. Avoid fuzzy expressions like "sort of" and "kind of maybe."
  Do you spend time every day communicating your thoughts, needs, and wishes to your self and your partner?

- **Trust.**
  . . . In an intimate relationship, trust creates a safe harbor where you can be who you are without being attacked, rejected, or abandoned—and without attacking, rejecting, or abandoning.
  Do you honor the trust between you every day by following a basic rule: no secrets, no lies, no deceptions, no excuses, no illusions.
  On a scale of 0 (clueless) to 10 (masterful), how did you rate yourself?

Get Ready

For the sake of your future, you and your partner need to coordinate your schedules and, if necessary, make appointments for quality time together. You also have to ask whether you spend more time on intimacy substitutes like blogging, gaming, gambling, shopping, or working out than you do enjoying your relationship.

Get Going

This section consists of seven exercises, each with daily, weekly, and monthly components and designed to create more intimacy in your most personal relationship. Here are three examples:

- **Receptivity.**
  Every day: Clear the decks for some real one-on-one time. But beware . . .
  Every week: Make a date to go out for a meal, walk together, or curl up on the couch and just talk . . .

- **Expressing yourself.**
  Every day: Let your partner in on things you know would be of interest . . .
  Every week: Share your perspective on the issues that came up during your week . . .
  Every month: If you journal, review the themes that have been on your mind. Are you rethinking your major? Concerned about expenses?

- **Trust.**
  Every day: Honor your partner's trust by not discussing private matters with friends.
  Every week or so: Confide in your partner to demonstrate your trust.
  Every month or so: Let your partner know how much you value the trust you have in each other. Be consistently trustworthy.

Lock It In

In this stage you set a goal for which intimacy skills to focus on in the coming week. Continue working to deepen and enrich your relationships throughout your life.

---

female. You are born with a certain *sexual identity* based on your sexual anatomy and appearance; you, your parents, and society mold your gender identity.

Are You an X or a Y?

Biologically, few absolute differences separate the sexes: Males alone can make sperm and contribute the chromosome that causes embryos to develop as males; females alone are born with sex cells (eggs, or ova), menstruate, give birth, and breast-feed babies.

But the process of becoming male or female is a long and complex one.

In the beginning, all human embryos have undifferentiated sex organs. Only after several weeks do the sex organs differentiate, becoming either male or female *gonads* (testes or ovaries), the structures that produce the future reproductive cells of an individual. This initial differentiation process depends on genetic instructions in the form of the sex chromosomes, referred to as X and Y. If a Y (or male) chromosome is present in the embryo, about seven weeks after conception, it signals the sex organs to develop into testes. If a Y chromosome isn't present, an embryo begins developing ovaries in the eighth week. From this point on, the sex hormones produced by the gonads, not the chromosomes, play the crucial role in making a male or female.

How Hormones Work

In Greek, *hormone* means "set into motion"—and that's exactly what our **hormones** do. These chemical messengers, produced by various organs in the body, including the sex organs, and carried to target structures by the bloodstream, arouse cells and organs to specific activities and influence the way we look, feel, develop, and behave.

The group of organs that produce hormones is referred to as the **endocrine system**. Except for the sex organs, males and females have identical endocrine systems. Directing the endocrine system is the hypothalamus, a pea-sized section of the brain. The pituitary gland, directly beneath the hypothalamus, turns the various glands on and off in response to messages from it.

The ovaries produce the sex hormones most crucial to women, **estrogen** and **progesterone**. The primary sex hormone in men is **testosterone**, which is produced by the testes and the adrenal glands. However, both men and women have small amounts of the hormones of the opposite sex. Estrogen, in fact, is crucial to male fertility and gives sperm what researchers describe as their "reproductive punch."

The sex hormones begin their work early in an embryo's development. As soon as the testes are formed, they start releasing testosterone, which stimulates the development of other structures, such as the penis. The absence of testosterone in an embryo causes female genitals to form. (If the testes of a genetic male don't produce testosterone, the fetus will develop female genitals. Similarly, if a genetic female is exposed to excessive testosterone, the fetus will have ovaries but will also develop male genitals.)

As puberty begins, the pituitary gland initiates the changes that transform boys into men and girls into women (Figure 9.1). When a boy is about 14 years old and a girl about 12, their brains stimulate the hypothalamus to secrete a hormone called gonadotropin-releasing hormone (GnRH). This substance causes the pituitary gland to release hormones called **gonadotropins**.

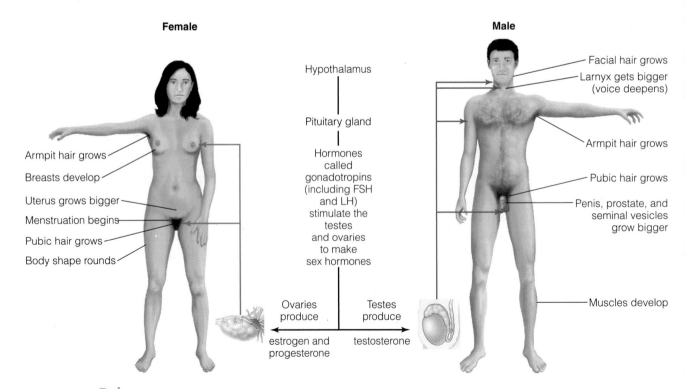

Female

Armpit hair grows
Breasts develop
Uterus grows bigger
Menstruation begins
Pubic hair grows
Body shape rounds

Hypothalamus

Pituitary gland

Hormones called gonadotropins (including FSH and LH) stimulate the testes and ovaries to make sex hormones

Ovaries produce estrogen and progesterone

Testes produce testosterone

Male

Facial hair grows
Larnyx gets bigger (voice deepens)
Armpit hair grows
Pubic hair grows
Penis, prostate, and seminal vesicles grow bigger
Muscles develop

Figure 9.1 Puberty

The body's endocrine system produces hormones that trigger body changes, including growth spurts, in boys and girls.

These, in turn, stimulate the gonads to make sex hormones.

The gonadotropins are *follicle-stimulating hormone (FSH)* and *luteinizing hormone (LH)*. In girls, these hormones travel to the ovary and stimulate the production of estrogen. As estrogen increases, a girl's **secondary sex characteristics** develop. Her breasts become fuller, her external genitals enlarge, and fat is deposited on her hips and buttocks. Estrogen keeps her hair thick and skin smooth. She begins menstruating because she has begun ovulating, the process that prepares her body to conceive and carry a baby.

This process seems to be beginning earlier than in the past. "By eight, 15 percent of white girls and 48 percent of African American girls show signs of sexual development," says Marcia Herman-Giddens, Ph.D., of the University of North Carolina at Chapel Hill, who analyzed 17,077 growth charts from pediatricians around the country. In her study, the mean ages for breast development were 8.87 years for African American girls and 9.96 years for white girls. African American girls reach **menarche**—the term for first menstruation—at a mean age of 12.16 years; white girls, at 12.88 years. By comparison, a hundred years ago girls didn't reach menarche until the relatively ripe age of fifteen.[1]

Improved nutrition and good health seem to be the primary factors. Girls today are bigger, taller, better fed, more sedentary, and have a higher percentage of body fat (one of the triggers of sexual maturation). They also grow up amid a host of environmental influences that may further speed development.

Cultural influences affect a girl's response to menarche. In a cross-cultural study of college students, the most common emotions expressed by American women at menarche were embarrassment, pride, and anxiety. Malaysian women cited fear, embarrassment, and worry. Lithuanian women described themselves as happy or scared, while Sudanese women cited fear, anxiety, embarrassment, and anger. On the positive side, the Lithuanian women reported feeling more valuable and believing they had entered the world of women. American girls worried about whether they could still play sports but felt superior to friends who had not reached menarche and became eager to learn about sex. Malaysians described feeling wise, respected, and mature. Sudanese women felt more beautiful and aware that they could now have children.

In boys, the gonadotropins stimulate the testes to produce testosterone, which triggers the development of male secondary sex characteristics. Their voices deepen, hair grows on their faces and bodies, their penises become thicker and longer, and their muscles become stronger.

The sex hormones released during puberty change the growth pattern of childhood, so that a boy or girl may now spurt up 4 to 6 inches in a single year. The skeleton matures very rapidly until, at the end of puberty (usually around age 18), the growth centers at the ends of the bones close off. Estrogen causes girls' bones to stop growing at an earlier age than boys' bones.

Sexual and Gender Identity

It's a boy! It's a girl! These statements confer an instant identity on a newborn. However, in recent years, researchers have challenged such either/or distinctions as male or female, masculine or feminine, heterosexual or homosexual. Although most people have the biological characteristics of a male or a female, some possess some degree of both male and female reproductive structures. They are referred to as intersexual.

The continuum for gender identity ranges from extreme stereotypical masculine notions to extreme stereotypical feminine behaviors. Different cultures vary in defining what is masculine or feminine. Individuals who consider themselves androgynous choose not to conform to sexual stereotypes. **Androgyny** includes those who are "positively androgynous," combining positive attributes linked with both sexes, for example, feminine compassion and masculine independence, and individuals who are "negatively androgynous" and might show less desirable characteristics of each gender, such as feminine dependency and masculine assertiveness. (Transgenderism is discussed on page 279.)

hormone Substance released in the blood that regulates specific bodily functions.

endocrine system The group of ductless glands that produce hormones and secrete them directly into the blood for transport to target organs.

estrogen The female sex hormone that stimulates female secondary sex characteristics.

progesterone The female sex hormone that stimulates the uterus, preparing it for the arrival of a fertilized egg.

testosterone The male sex hormone that stimulates male secondary sex characteristics.

gonadotropins Gonad-stimulating hormones produced by the pituitary gland.

secondary sex characteristics Physical changes associated with maleness or femaleness, induced by the sex hormones.

menarche The onset of menstruation at puberty.

androgyny The expression of both masculine and feminine traits.

Women's Sexual Health

mons pubis The rounded, fleshy area over the junction of the female pubic bones.

labia majora The fleshy outer folds that border the female genital area.

labia minora The fleshy inner folds that border the female genital area.

clitoris A small erectile structure on the female, corresponding to the penis on the male.

urethral opening The outer opening of the thin tube that carries urine from the bladder.

vagina The canal leading from the exterior opening in the female genital area to the uterus.

perineum The area between the anus and vagina in the female and between the anus and scrotum in the male.

cervix The narrow, lower end of the uterus that opens into the vagina.

uterus The female organ that houses the developing fetus until birth.

endometrium The mucous membrane lining the uterus.

ovary The female sex organ that produces egg cells, estrogen, and progesterone.

ovum (plural, **ova**) The female gamete (egg cell).

fallopian tubes The pair of channels that transport ova from the ovaries to the uterus; the usual site of fertilization.

ovulation The release of a mature ovum from an ovary approximately 14 days prior to the onset of menstruation.

corpus luteum A yellowish mass of tissue that is formed, immediately after ovulation, from the remaining cells of the follicle; it secretes estrogen and progesterone for the remainder of the menstrual cycle.

menstruation Discharge of blood from the vagina as a result of the shedding of the uterine lining at the end of the menstrual cycle.

Only recently has medical research devoted major scientific investigations to issues in women's health. Until about a decade ago, the National Institutes of Health routinely excluded women from experimental studies because of concerns about menstrual cycles and pregnancy. In clinical settings, women are more likely to have their symptoms dismissed as psychological and not to be referred to a specialist than are men with identical complaints. Some physicians are suggesting the creation of a new medical specialty (distinct from obstetrics and gynecology) that would be devoted to women's health.

Female Sexual Anatomy

As illustrated in Figure 9.2a, the **mons pubis** is the rounded, fleshy area over the junction of the pubic bones. The folds of skin that form the outer lips of a woman's genital area are called the **labia majora.** They cover soft flaps of skin (inner lips) called the **labia minora.** The inner lips join at the top to form a hood over the **clitoris,** a small elongated erectile organ, and the most sensitive spot in the entire female genital area. Below the clitoris is the **urethral opening,** the outer opening of the thin tube that carries urine from the bladder. Below that is a larger opening, the mouth of the **vagina,** the canal that leads to the primary internal organs of reproduction. The **perineum** is the area between the vagina and the anus (the opening to the rectum and large intestine).

At the back of the vagina is the **cervix,** the opening to the womb, or **uterus** (see Figure 9.2b). The uterine walls are lined by a layer of tissue called the **endometrium.** The **ovaries,** about the size and shape of almonds, are located on either side of the uterus and contain egg cells called **ova** (singular, **ovum**). Extending outward and back from the upper uterus are the **fallopian tubes,** the canals that transport ova from the ovaries to the uterus. When an egg is released from an ovary, the fingerlike ends of the adjacent fallopian tube "catch" the egg and direct it into the tube.

Discharge and changes in odor normally occur in a healthy vagina. They typically fluctuate through the menstrual cycle, depending on hormone level. In the past, many women practiced douching, the introduction of a liquid into the vagina, to cleanse the vagina. However, particularly if done frequently, douching may increase the risk of pelvic inflammatory disease (discussed in Chapter 16) and ectopic or out-of-uterus pregnancy. Despite the potential dangers, according to data from a southern university, four in ten female students had douched in the past; half currently douche.

African American women were encouraged to douche by their mothers; white women were more influenced by television advertisements. When advised to stop douching by a doctor or nurse, most students do so.

The Menstrual Cycle

Scientists have discovered that the menstrual cycle actually begins in the brain with the production of gonadotropin-releasing hormone (GnRH). Each month a surge of GnRH sets into motion the sequence of steps that lead to ovulation, the potential for conception, and if conception doesn't occur, menstruation. The hypothalamus monitors hormone levels in the blood and sends messages to the pituitary gland to release follicle-stimulating hormone (FSH) and luteinizing hormone (LH).

As shown in Figure 9.3 on p. 268, in the ovaries, these hormones stimulate the growth of a few of the immature eggs, or ova, stored in follicles in every woman's body. Usually, only one ovum matures completely during each monthly cycle. As it does, it increases its production of the female sex hormone estrogen, which in turn triggers the release of a larger surge of LH.

At midcycle, the increased LH hormone levels trigger **ovulation,** the release of the egg cell, or ovum, from the follicle. Estrogen levels drop, and the remaining cells of the follicle then enlarge, change character, and form the **corpus luteum,** or yellow body. In the second half of the menstrual cycle, the corpus luteum secretes estrogen and larger amounts of progesterone. The endometrium (uterine lining) is stimulated by progesterone to thicken and become more engorged with blood in preparation for nourishing an implanted, fertilized ovum.

If the ovum is not fertilized, the corpus luteum disintegrates. As the level of progesterone drops, **menstruation** occurs; the uterine lining is shed during the course of a menstrual period. If the egg is fertilized and pregnancy occurs, the cells that eventually develop into the placenta secrete *human chorionic gonadotropin (HCG),* a messenger hormone that signals the pituitary not to start a new cycle. The corpus luteum then steps up its production of progesterone.

Many women experience physical or psychological changes, or both, during their monthly cycles. Usually the changes are minor, but more serious problems can occur. One recently recognized culprit is work stress. Women who are overcommitted or in jobs in which they put in a great deal of effort are more likely to report painful periods, possibly because of the effect of stress on the hormones that regulate menstruation.[2]

Premenstrual Syndrome
Women with **premenstrual syndrome (PMS)** experience bodily discomfort and emotional distress for up to two weeks, from ovulation until the onset of menstruation. Up to 75 percent of menstruating women report one or more premenstrual symptoms; 3 to 9 percent experience disabling, incapacitating symptoms.

Once dismissed as a psychological problem, PMS has been recognized as a very real physiological disorder that may be caused by a hormonal deficiency; abnormal levels of thyroid hormone; an imbalance of estrogen and progesterone; or social and environmental factors, particularly stress. Recent studies indicate that PMS may originate in the brain. Changes in brain receptors during the ovarian cycle may be responsible.

The most common symptoms of PMS are mood changes, anxiety, irritability, difficulty concentrating, forgetfulness, impaired judgment, tearfulness, digestive symptoms (diarrhea, bloating, constipation), hot flashes, palpitations, dizziness, headache, fatigue, changes in appetite, cravings (usually for sweets or salt), water retention,

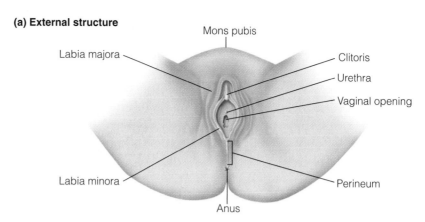

(a) External structure

Mons pubis · Labia majora · Clitoris · Urethra · Vaginal opening · Labia minora · Perineum · Anus

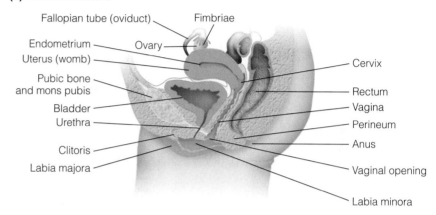

(b) Internal structure

Fallopian tube (oviduct) · Fimbriae · Endometrium · Ovary · Uterus (womb) · Pubic bone and mons pubis · Bladder · Urethra · Clitoris · Labia majora · Cervix · Rectum · Vagina · Perineum · Anus · Vaginal opening · Labia minora

Figure 9.2   The Female Sex Organs and Reproductive Structures

breast tenderness, and insomnia. For a diagnosis to be made, women—using a self-rating symptom scale or calendar—must report troubling premenstrual symptoms in the period before menstruation in at least two successive menstrual cycles.

Treatments   Treatments for PMS depend on specific symptoms. Diuretics (drugs that speed up fluid elimination) can relieve water retention and bloating. Relaxation techniques have led to a 60 percent reduction in anxiety symptoms. Sleep deprivation, or the use of bright light to adjust a woman's circadian or daily rhythm, also has proven beneficial. Behavioral approaches, such as exercise or charting cycles, help by letting women know when they're vulnerable.

Low doses of medications known as *selective serotonin-reuptake inhibitor (SSRIs)* (discussed in Chapter 4), such as fluoxetine (marketed as Prozac, Sarafem, and in generic forms) provide relief for

premenstrual syndrome (PMS)
A disorder that causes physical discomfort and psychological distress prior to a woman's menstrual period.

Figure 9.3 Menstrual Cycle

(a) In response to the hypothalamus, the pituitary gland releases the gonadotropins FSH and LH. Levels of FSH and LH stimulate the cycle (and in turn are affected by production of estrogen and progesterone).

(b) FSH does what its name says—it stimulates follicle development in the ovary. The follicle matures and ruptures, releasing an ovum (egg) into the fallopian tube.

(c) The follicle produces estrogen, and the corpus luteum produces estrogen and progesterone. The high level of estrogen at the middle of the cycle produces a surge of LH, which triggers ovulation.

(d) Estrogen and progesterone stimulate the endometrium, which becomes thicker and prepares to receive an implanted, fertilized egg. If a fertilized egg is deposited in the uterus, pregnancy begins. If the egg is not fertilized, progesterone production decreases, and the endometrium is shed (menstruation). At this point, both estrogen and progesterone levels have dropped, so the pituitary responds by producing FSH, and the cycle begins again.

symptoms such as tension, depression, irritability, and mood swings, even when taken only during the premenstrual phase rather than daily throughout the month. SSRIs are not effective in all women with PMS, and other factors, including a genetic susceptibility, may play a role. YAZ, a low-dose combination birth control pill made up of the hormones drospirenone and ethinyl estradiol, is the only oral contraceptive approved by the FDA to treat emotional and physical premenstrual symptoms. (See Chapter 10 on birth control.)[3]

A diet rich in calcium and vitamin D reduces the risk of PMS; supplements of the two decrease the severity of symptoms.[4] Cognitive-behavioral therapy, discussed in Chapter 4, may be the most effective psychological approach; simply educating women about PMS has not proven useful.[5] Other treatments with some reported success include exercise; less caffeine, alcohol, salt, and sugar; acupuncture; and stress management techniques such as meditation or relaxation training. Chinese herbal medicine is popular in several nations, but a recent study concluded that there is insufficient evidence to support its use.[6]

 In a study of women in five countries—the United States, Canada, United Kingdom, France, and Germany—a very small percentage of women (less than 0.1 percent) sought medical help for PMS. Women in the United States and Germany were most likely to consult gynecologists, while those in Canada and the United Kingdom turned to family physicians. No matter which type of doctor they saw, women were prescribed medication. American and British physicians generally recommended SSRIs. French physicians favored hormonal treatments and painkillers, while German physicians recommended the plant extract *Vitex agnuscastus*, which is considered an unproven alternative therapy in the United States.[7]

Premenstrual Dysphoric Disorder

Premenstrual dysphoric disorder (PMDD), which is not related to PMS, occurs in an estimated 3 to 5 percent of all menstruating women. It is characterized by regular symptoms of depression (depressed mood, anxiety, mood swings, diminished interest or pleasure) during the last week of the menstrual cycle. Women with PMDD cannot function as usual at work, school, or home. They feel better a few days after menstruation begins. SSRIs, which are often used to treat PMS, also are effective in relieving symptoms of PMDD.

Menstrual Cramps **Dysmenorrhea** is the medical name for the discomforts—abdominal cramps and pain, back and leg pain, diarrhea, tension, water retention, fatigue, and depression—that can occur during menstruation. About half of all menstruating women suffer from dysmenorrhea. The cause seems to be an overproduction of bodily substances called prostaglandins, which typically rise during menstruation. Medications that inhibit prostaglandins can reduce menstrual pain, and exercise can also relieve cramps.

Amenorrhea Women may stop menstruating—a condition called **amenorrhea**—for a variety of reasons, including a hormonal disorder, drastic weight loss, strenuous exercise, or change in the environment. "Boarding-school amenorrhea" is common among young women who leave home for school. Distance running and strenuous exercise also can lead to amenorrhea. The reason may be a drop in body fat from the normal range of 18 to 22 percent to a range of 9 to 12 percent. To be considered amenorrheic, a woman's menstrual cycle is typically absent for three or more consecutive months. Prolonged amenorrhea can have serious health consequences, including a loss of bone density that may lead to stress fractures or osteoporosis.

Scientists have developed chemical mimics, or analogues, of GnRH—usually administered by nasal spray—that trigger ovulation in women who don't ovulate or menstruate normally.

Toxic Shock Syndrome This rare, potentially deadly bacterial infection primarily strikes menstruating women under the age of 30 who use tampons. Both *Staphylococcus aureus* and group A *Streptococcus pyogenes* can produce **toxic shock syndrome (TSS)**. Symptoms include a high fever; a rash that leads to peeling of the skin on the fingers, toes, palms, and soles; dizziness; dangerously

premenstrual dysphoric disorder (PMDD) A disorder that causes symptoms of psychological depression during the last week of the menstrual cycle.

dysmenorrhea Painful menstruation.

amenorrhea The absence or suppression of menstruation.

toxic shock syndrome (TSS) A disease characterized by fever, vomiting, diarrhea, and often shock, caused by a bacterium that releases toxic waste products into the bloodstream.

low blood pressure; and abnormalities in several organ systems (the digestive tract and the kidneys) and in the muscles and blood. Treatment usually consists of antibiotics and intense supportive care; intravenous administration of immunoglobulins that attack the toxins produced by these bacteria also may be beneficial.

Men's Sexual Health

Because the male reproductive system is simpler in many ways than the female, it's often ignored—especially by healthy young men. However, men should make regular self-exams (including checking the penis and testes, as described in Chapter 16) part of their routine.

Male Sexual Anatomy

The visible parts of the male sexual anatomy are the **penis** and the **scrotum,** the pouch that contains the **testes** (Figure 9.4). The testes manufacture testosterone, the hormone that stimulates the development of a male's secondary sex characteristics, and **sperm,** the male reproductive cells. Immature sperm are stored in the **epididymis,** a collection of coiled tubes adjacent to each testis.

The penis contains three hollow cylinders loosely covered with skin. The two major cylinders, the *corpora cavernosa,* extend side by side through the length of the penis. The third cylinder, the *corpus spongiosum,* surrounds the **urethra,** the channel for both seminal fluid and urine; see Figure 9.4.

When hanging down loosely, the average penis is about $3^3/_4$ inches long. During erection, its internal cylinders fill with so much blood that they become rigid, and the penis stretches to an average length of $6^1/_4$ inches. About 90 percent of all men have erect penises measuring between 5 and 7 inches in length. There is no relation, however, between penis size and female sexual satisfaction: A woman's vagina naturally adjusts during intercourse to the size of her partner's penis.

Inside the body are several structures involved in the production of seminal fluid, or **semen,** the liquid in which sperm cells are carried out of the body during ejaculation.

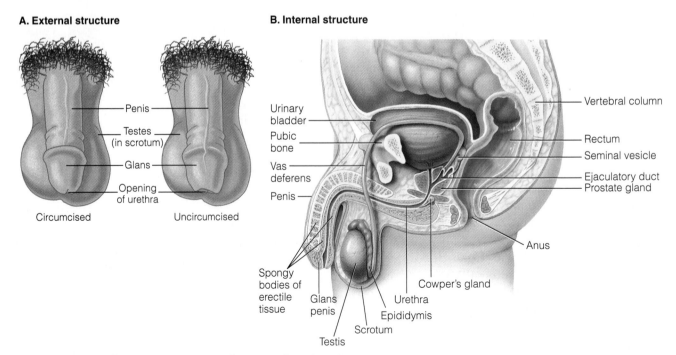

A. External structure

Penis
Testes (in scrotum)
Glans
Opening of urethra

Circumcised

Uncircumcised

B. Internal structure

Urinary bladder
Pubic bone
Vas deferens
Penis

Vertebral column
Rectum
Seminal vesicle
Ejaculatory duct
Prostate gland
Anus

Spongy bodies of erectile tissue
Glans penis
Cowper's gland
Urethra
Epididymis
Scrotum
Testis

Figure 9.4 Male Sex Organs and Reproductive Structures

The **vas deferens** are two tubes that carry sperm from the epididymis into the urethra. The **seminal vesicles,** which make some of the seminal fluid, join with the vas deferens to form the **ejaculatory ducts.** The **prostate gland** produces some of the seminal fluid, which it secretes into the urethra during ejaculation. The **Cowper's glands** are two pea-sized structures on either side of the urethra (just below where it emerges from the prostate gland) and connected to it via tiny ducts. When a man is sexually aroused, the Cowper's glands often secrete a fluid that appears as a droplet at the tip of the penis. This fluid is not semen, although it occasionally contains sperm.

Circumcision

In its natural state, the tip of the penis is covered by a fold of skin called the *foreskin.* About 60 percent of baby boys in the United States undergo **circumcision,** the surgical removal of the foreskin.

An estimated 1.2 million newborn males are circumcised in the United States annually for reasons that vary from religious traditions to preventive health measures. Circumcision rates are highest in the Midwest and Northeast and lowest in the West. They are significantly higher in states that provide Medicaid coverage for routine circumcision.[8] Until the last half century, scientific evidence to support or repudiate routine circumcision was limited. Large, carefully controlled studies in sub-Saharan Africa have shown that circumcision significantly reduces a man's risk of acquiring HIV through heterosexual intercourse. It is still not known whether circumcision also lowers the risk in men who have sex with men. Male circumcision may help to prevent the spread of HIV in part because the cells on the foreskin of the penis are more susceptible to HIV infection. Circumcision does not protect against herpes, syphilis, or gonorrhea, suggesting a biological rather than a behavioral explanation for the protective effect of circumcision against HIV.

Boys who are not circumcised are four times as likely to develop urinary tract infections in their first year; however, such infections develop in only 1 percent of circumcised boys. Uncircumcised men are three times as likely to develop penile cancer, but the absolute risk is low. (Only about nine in every million American men ever gets cancer of the penis.)

The drawbacks of circumcision include the risk of complications (which tend to be uncommon and minor) and pain. The AAP recommends that when circumcision is performed, analgesic creams or anesthetic shots be used to minimize discomfort. There is little consensus on what impact the presence or absence of a foreskin has on sexual functioning or satisfaction.

Responsible Sexuality

The World Health Organization defines sexual health as "the integration of the physical, emotional, intellectual, and social aspects of sexual being in ways that are positively enriching, and that enhance personality, communication, and love. . . . Every person has a right to receive sexual information and to consider sexual relationships for pleasure as well as for procreation."

Sexuality education is a lifelong process. Your own knowledge about sex may not be as extensive as you might assume. Most people grow up with a lot of myths and misconceptions about sex. (See this chapter's Self Survey: "How Much Do You Know About Sex?"). Rather than relying on what peers say or what you've always thought was true, find out the facts. This textbook is a good place to start. The student health center and the library can provide additional materials on sexual identity, orientation, behavior, and health, as well as on options for reducing your risk of acquiring sexually transmitted infections (discussed in Chapter 16) or becoming pregnant.

Creating a Sexually Healthy Relationship

A sexually healthy relationship, as defined by the Sexuality Information and Education

penis The male organ of sex and urination.

scrotum The external sac or pouch that holds the testes.

testes (singular, **testis**) The male sex organs that produce sperm and testosterone.

sperm The male gamete produced by the testes and transported outside the body through ejaculation.

epididymis That portion of the male duct system in which sperm mature.

urethra The canal through which urine from the bladder leaves the body; in the male, also serves as the channel for seminal fluid.

semen The viscous whitish fluid that is the complete male ejaculate; a combination of sperm and secretions from the prostate gland, seminal vesicles, and other glands.

vas deferens Two tubes that carry sperm from the epididymis into the urethra.

seminal vesicles Glands in the male reproductive system that produce the major portion of the fluid of semen.

ejaculatory duct The canal connecting the seminal vesicles and vas deferens.

prostate gland A structure surrounding the male urethra that produces a secretion that helps liquefy the semen from the testes.

Cowper's glands Two small glands that discharge into the male urethra; also called bulbourethral glands.

circumcision The surgical removal of the foreskin of the penis.

Council of the United States (SIECUS), is based on shared values and has five characteristics: It is

- Consensual.
- Nonexploitative.
- Honest.
- Mutually pleasurable.
- Protected against unintended pregnancy and sexually transmitted infections.

All individuals also have sexual rights, which include the right to the information, education, skills, support, and services they need to make responsible decisions about their sexuality consistent with their own values, as well as the right to express their sexual orientation without violence or discrimination.

Communication is vital in a sexually healthy relationship, even though these discussions can be awkward. Yet if you have a need or a problem that relates to your partner, it is your responsibility to bring it up. (See Health on a Budget, p. 274.)

Making Sexual Decisions

Sexual decision making should always take place within the context of an individual's values and perceptions of right and wrong behavior. Making responsible sexual decisions means considering all the possible consequences—including emotional consequences—of sexual behavior for both yourself and your partner.

Prior to any sexual activity that involves a risk of sexually transmitted infection or pregnancy, both partners should talk about their prior sexual histories (including number of partners and exposure to STIs) and other high-risk behavior, such as the use of injection drugs. They should also discuss the issue of birth control and which methods might be best for them to use. If you know someone well enough to consider having sex with that person, you should be

The key to a healthy, happy sexual relationship is open, honest communication—even when you and your partner have different points of view.

©T. Ozonas/Masterfile

able to talk about such sensitive subjects. If a potential partner is unwilling to talk or hedges on crucial questions, you shouldn't be engaging in sex.

Here are some questions to consider as you think and talk about the significance of becoming sexually intimate with a partner:

- **What role do we want relationships and sex to have in our life at this time?**
- **What are my values and my potential partner's values as they pertain to sexual relationships?** Does each of us believe that intercourse should be reserved for a permanent partnership or committed relationship?
- **Will a decision to engage in sex enhance my positive feelings about myself or my partner?** Does either of us have questions about sexual orientation or the kinds of people we are attracted to?
- **Do I and my partner both want to have sex?** Is my partner pressuring me in any way? Am I pressuring my partner? Am I making this decision for myself or for my partner?
- **Have my partner and I discussed our sexual histories and risk factors?** Have I spoken honestly about any STIs I've had in the past? Am I sure that neither my partner nor I have a sexually transmitted infection?
- **Have we taken precautions against unwanted pregnancy and STIs?**

Saying No to Sex

Whether couples are on a first date or have been married for years, each partner always has the right not to have sex. Unfortunately, "no" sometimes seems to mean different things to men and women.

The following strategies can help you assert yourself when saying no to sex:

- **First of all, recognize** your own values and feelings. If you believe that sex is something to be shared only by people who've already become close in other ways, be true to that belief.
- **Be direct.** Look the person in the eyes, keep your head up, and speak clearly and firmly.

- **Just say no.** Make it clear you're rejecting the offer, not the person. You don't owe anyone an explanation for what you want, but if you want to expand on your reasons, you might say, "I enjoy your company, and I'd like to do something together, but no," or "Thank you. I appreciate your interest, but no."

- **If you're still at a loss for words,** try these responses: "I like you a lot, but I'm not ready to have sex." "You're a great person, but sex isn't something I do to prove I like someone." "I'd like to wait until I'm married to have sex."

- **If you're feeling pressured,** let your date know that you're uncomfortable. Be simple and direct. Watch out for emotional blackmail. If your date says, "If you really like me, you'd want to make love," point out that if he or she really likes you, he or she wouldn't try to force you to do something you don't want to do.

☑ **REALITY CHECK**
- *How many college students report at least one hookup (casual sexual experience)?* _____
- *Who is more likely to feel more distress after a hookup?* Men _____ Women _____
- *What is the most common regret expressed by men after a hookup?* ____
- *What is the most common regret expressed by women?* _____
Answers on next page.

- **If you're a woman, monitor your sexual signals.** Men impute more sexual meaning to gestures (such as casual touching) that women perceive as friendly and innocent.

- **Communicate your feelings** to your date sooner rather than later. It's far easier to say, "I don't want to go to your apartment" than to fight off unwelcome advances once you're there.

- **Remember that if saying no to sex** puts an end to a relationship, it wasn't much of a relationship in the first place.

Sexual Behavior

From birth to death, we are sexual beings. Our sexual identities, needs, likes, and dislikes emerge in adolescence and become clearer as we enter adulthood, but we continue to change and evolve throughout our lives. In men, sexual interest is most intense at age 18; in women, it reaches a peak in the 30s. Although age brings changes in sexual responsiveness, we never outgrow our sexuality.

Adolescent Sexuality

Early in adolescence, sexual curiosity explodes, and sexual exploration—both alone and with a partner—takes on new meaning and intensity. Sexual education programs can make a difference by helping young people become sexually responsible, enabling them to form satisfying relationships, helping them assess their own attitudes toward sex, and giving them information on sexuality. Good programs can clarify values and enhance communication.

It's not unusual for teenage boys to experience frequent erections during the day and night, including **nocturnal emissions,** or wet dreams, during which ejaculation occurs. **Masturbation** (discussed later in this chapter) is the primary form of sexual expression for many teenagers, especially boys. Self-stimulation helps teens learn about their bodies and their sexual potential and serves as an outlet for sexual tension. By the end of adolescence, the majority of teens have masturbated to orgasm.

Other common sexual activities during adolescence include kissing and petting—erotic physical contact that may include holding, touching, manual stimulation of the genitals, and oral sex. As many as 25 percent of teens experience some same-sex attractions. Although many experiment with heterosexual and homosexual sexual experiences, adolescent sexual behavior does not always foretell sexual orientation. Young people, who often feel confused about their sexual identity, may engage in sexual activity with members of the same or the other sex as a way of testing how they really feel.

nocturnal emissions
Ejaculations while dreaming; wet dreams.

masturbation Manual (or non-manual) self-stimulation of the genitals, often resulting in orgasm.

PART 2: *Just the Facts*
- *The percentage of students engaging in hookups ranges from* **70 to 85 percent** *in different studies.*
- **Women** *are significantly more likely to experience psychological distress than men after a hookup.*
- *The regret men express most often is hooking up with* **an unattractive partner**.
- *The regret women express most often is* **feeling used**.

Source: Fielder, R. L., and M. P. Carey. "Predictors and Consequences of Sexual 'Hookups' among College Students: A Short-term Prospective Study." *Archives of Sex Behavior,* January 9, 2009, epub.

HEALTH ON A BUDGET ⑤

The Secret to a Good Sexual Relationship

The secret to a healthy, happy sexual relationship isn't a hot car or sexy outfit. It's the ability to communicate openly, honestly, and respectfully with your partner. Here are some specific suggestions:

- **Choose an appropriate time and place** for an intimate discussion. In a new relationship, talking in a public place, such as a park bench or a quiet table at a coffee house, can seem safer. If you're in an established relationship, choose a time when you can give each other complete attention and a setting in which you can both relax.
- **Ask open-ended questions** that encourage a dialogue, for instance, "How do you feel about . . . ?" or "What are your thoughts about . . . ?"
- **Listen actively** rather than passively when your partner speaks. Show that you're paying attention by nodding, smiling, and leaning forward. Paraphrase what he or she says to show you understand it fully. (See "Listen Up" in *Labs for IPC*)
- **Use "I" statements,** such as "I really enjoy making love, but I'm so tired right now that I won't be a responsive partner. Why don't we get the kids to bed early tomorrow so we can enjoy ourselves a little earlier?"
- **If you would like to try something different, say so.** Practice saying the words first if they embarrass you. If your partner feels uncomfortable, don't force the issue, but do try talking it through.
- **If you want to request changes** or tackle a touchy topic, start with positive statements. Let your partner know how much you enjoy having sex, and then express your desire to enjoy lovemaking more often or in different ways.
- **Encourage small changes.** If you want your partner to be less inhibited, start slowly, perhaps by suggesting sex in a different room or place.

Teen Sexual Behaviors

For the first time since the federal government started keeping statistics in the early 1970s, fewer American teenagers are becoming sexually active. According to the National Youth Risk Behavior, fewer than half of all high school students have had sex, down from 54 percent in 1991. Teenagers also are waiting longer to have sex than in the past. The percentage of 15- to 17-year-old girls who had experienced sex has fallen from 38 percent in 1995 to 30 percent; the percentage of boys, from 43 percent to 31 percent. About 16 percent of teens say they have had oral sex but haven't yet had intercourse.[9]

Teenagers report that they get information about sex from many sources. Those who learn about sex from parents, grandparents, and religious leaders express more beliefs indicating they are likely to delay sex. Those who get sex information from friends, cousins, and media express beliefs that increase their likelihood of having sexual intercourse.[10]

Are students who take a "virginity pledge," a key component of many sexual abstinence programs, less likely to become sexually active? The answer is no, according to a study that followed a nationally representative sample of young teens for five years. "Pledgers" were just as likely as "nonpledgers" to engage in premarital sex and did not differ in age of first sex, number of sexual partners, sexually transmitted infections, and rates of oral and anal sex. About eight in ten denied ever having taken a virginity pledge. Many were less likely to protect themselves from pregnancy and disease.[11]

After dropping steadily for years, teen pregnancy rates have risen (see discussion in Chapter 10). There may be more teen pregnancies, researchers theorize, not because more teens are having sex but because fewer teens are using contraception.[12]

Sex on Campus

Sexual behavior on campus has changed dramatically in the last 25 years. Surveys conducted in the United States and in Canada since 1980 reveal a steady increase in the number of students who have had intercourse and an increase in safer sex practices among sexually active students. Today's undergraduates are more likely to question potential partners about their past, use condoms with a new partner, and maintain fairly long-term monogamous relationships.

College students see sexual activity as normal behavior for their peer group. When researchers at Pennsylvania State University conducted focus groups with undergraduates, most agreed that the majority of college students (80 to 90 percent, in their estimate) are sexually active and that alcohol and drug use make sexual activity more likely.

College students tend to overestimate how much sex their peers are having. According to the American College Health Association National College Health Assessment, about a third of undergraduates reported having no sexual partners within the last 12 months. Among sexually active students, the mean number of partners was one.[13]

College students who binge drink or participate in drinking games, which often involve physical skills (such as bouncing a coin into a glass) or word play, increase their odds of sexually risky behavior. Both men and women report being taken advantage of sexually, including someone having sex with them when they were too drunk to give consent, after such games.

Annual spring breaks provide what researchers describe as "ideal conditions for the potentially lethal interaction between alcohol, drugs, and sexual risk-taking." Students typically engage in binge drinking, illicit drug use, and unsafe sexual practices. The likelihood of casual sex depends on several factors, including peer influences, prior experiences with casual sex, alcohol consumption prior to sex, and impulsivity.

 As with other aspects of health, cultural, religious, and personal values affect students' sexual behaviors. Researchers raised concern about young Latina women, who have the highest teen birth rate in the United States (twice the national rate) and are at greater risk of sexually transmitted infections. Although Latinas represent about 10 percent of women over age 21, they account for 20 percent of female AIDS cases. Among college students and other populations, Latinas are more likely to engage in unprotected intercourse than women from other ethnic groups.

Acculturation—the process of adaptation that occurs when immigrants enter a new country—also affects sexual behavior. As Latina immigrants become more acculturated in the United States, some aspects of their sexual behavior become more Americanized; for instance, they become more likely to engage in nonmarital sexual activity and to have multiple partners. In a study of Cuban American college women, older, less

During adolescence, teens explore different social and intimate relationships as they begin to develop a sexual identity.

religious, and U.S.-born Latinas were more likely to be sexually active and to engage in risky sexual behavior than other Latinas.

The Sex Life of American Adults

The scientific study of Americans' sexual behavior began in 1938, when Alfred Kinsey, Ph.D., a professor of biology at the University of Indiana, and his colleagues asked 5,300 white men and 5,940 white women about their sexual practices. In his landmark studies—*Sexual Behavior in the Human Male,* published in 1948, and *Sexual Behavior in the Human Female,* published in 1953—Kinsey reported that 73 percent of men and 20 percent of women had premarital intercourse by age 20, and 37 percent of men and 17 percent of women had some homosexual experience in their lifetime.

The Janus Report on Sexual Behavior, published in 1993, was based on a survey of 2,765 individuals across the United States. A larger survey, conducted by researchers at the University of Chicago, was based on face-to-face interviews with 3,432 Americans, age 18 to 59. It became the basis for two books published in 1994: *Sex in America,* aimed at a lay audience, and *The Social Organization of Sexuality,* a more scholarly work. Since then, the researchers' General Social Survey (GSS) database on sexual activity has grown to nearly 10,000 respondents.

© Stephen Mallon/Photonica/Getty Images

In a loving, committed relationship, every form of physical contact can serve as an intimate form of expressing deep emotion.

© iStockphoto.com/Adam Kazmierski

the frequency reports of husbands and wives (not in the same couples) are within one episode per year—58.6 for married men and 57.9 for married women. If other differences between men and women are statistically controlled (such as sexual preference, age, and educational attainment), married women actually report a slightly higher frequency than men.

Sexual frequency peaks among those with some college education, then decreases among four-year college graduates, and declines even further among those with professional degrees. Americans who have attended graduate school are the least sexually active educational group in the population. These respondents may be more honest than others in reporting sexual activity, or they may be more precise in their definition of what counts as sex.

Does sex make people happier or healthier? Researchers have concluded that the more sex a person has, the more likely he or she is to report having a happy life and a happy marriage. This connection is stronger among women than among men. A second and more important predictor of sexual frequency is the feeling that one's life is exciting rather than routine or dull. "Being excited by life is most strongly associated with being happier," the researchers noted. "It seems that increased sexual activity is one of the many benefits of having a positive attitude."

Why People Have Sex

The reasons people engage in sex long seemed so obvious that scientists didn't bother to investigate them. They assumed that heterosexuals had sex primarily to reproduce, experience sexual pleasure, and relieve sexual tension.

In the most extensive study of why humans have sex, researchers identified 237 motivations. The study sample included 1,549 undergraduates ranging in age from 16 to 42. The reasons people gave fell into nine categories:

- Pure attraction to the other person in general.
- Experiencing physical pleasure.
- Expressing love.
- Feeling desired by the other.

In a recent national survey of about 1,500 men and women between the ages of 40 and 80, 79 percent of the men and 69 percent of the women had engaged in sexual intercourse in the previous year.[14]

The average American adult reports having sex about once a week. However, 1 in 5 Americans has been celibate for at least a year, and 1 in 20 engages in sex at least every other day. Men report more sexual frequency than women—not because men are more boastful about their prowess, the researchers contend, but because the sample of women includes many widows and older women without partners. Among married people,

TABLE 9.1

Top 10 Reasons Why Men and Women Have Sex

Women	Men
1. I was attracted to the person.	I was attracted to the person.
2. I wanted to experience the physical pleasure.	It feels good.
3. It feels good.	I wanted to experience the physical pleasure.
4. I wanted to show my affection to the person.	It's fun.
5. I wanted to express my love for the person.	I wanted to show my affection to the person.
6. I was sexually aroused and wanted the release.	I was sexually aroused and wanted the release.
7. I was "horny."	I was "horny."
8. It's fun.	I wanted to express my love for the person.
9. I realized I was in love.	I wanted to achieve an orgasm.
10. I was "in the heat of the moment."	I wanted to please my partner.

Source: Meston, Cindy, and David Buss, "Why Humans Have Sex." *Archives of Sexual Behavior*, Vol. 36, August 2007, pp. 477–507.

© Marili Forastieri/Digital Vision/Getty Images

- Escalating the depth of a relationship.
- Curiosity or seeking new adventures.
- Marking a special occasion for celebration.
- Mere opportunity.
- Sex "just happening" due to seemingly uncontrollable circumstances.

The responses of men and women were generally similar (see Table 9.1). However, men were significantly more likely to report having sex for reasons of opportunity and experience—for instance, because a person "was available" or wanting "to increase the number of partners I experienced." Women were more likely to endorse certain emotional motivations, such as, "I wanted to express my love for the person," or "I realized I was in love." Men also endorsed more reasons related to pure physical pleasure, such as wanting to have sex because it felt good or because they were "horny."

Sexual Diversity

Human beings are diverse in all ways—including sexual preferences and practices. Physiological, psychological, and social factors determine whether we are attracted to members of the same sex or the other sex. This attraction is our **sexual orientation.** Sigmund Freud argued that we all start off **bisexual,** or attracted to both sexes. But by the time we reach adulthood, most males prefer female sexual partners, and most females prefer male partners. **Heterosexual** is the term used for individuals whose primary orientation is toward members of the other sex. In virtually all cultures, some men and women are **homosexuals,** preferring partners of their own sex.

In our society, we tend to view heterosexuality and homosexuality as very different. In reality, these orientations are opposite ends of a spectrum. Sex researcher Alfred Kinsey devised a seven-point continuum representing sexual orientation in American

sexual orientation The direction of an individual's sexual interest, either to members of the opposite sex or to members of the same sex.

bisexual Sexually oriented toward both sexes.

heterosexual Primary sexual orientation toward members of the other sex.

homosexual Primary sexual orientation toward members of the same sex.

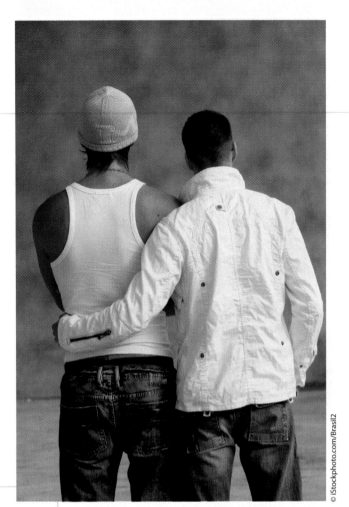

© iStockphoto.com/Brasil2

Close-couple homosexual relationships are similar to stable heterosexual relationships.

with a man (at the median age of 18) and that sex with a woman followed a few years later (at median age 21).

Heterosexuality

Heterosexuality, the most common sexual orientation, refers to sexual or romantic attraction between opposite sexes. The adjective *heterosexual* describes intimate relationships and/or sexual relations between a man and a woman. The term *straight* is used predominantly for self-identified heterosexuals of either sex. In his landmark research in the 1940s, Alfred Kinsey reported that while many men and women were exclusively heterosexual, a significant number (37 percent of men and 13 percent of women) had at least one adult sexual experience with a member of the same sex.

Bisexuality

Bisexuality—sexual attraction to both males and females—can develop at any point in one's life. In some cultures, bisexual activity is considered part of normal sexual experimentation. Among the Sabmia Highlanders in Papua New Guinea, for instance, boys perform oral sex on one another as part of the rites of passage into manhood.

Some people identify themselves as bisexual even if they don't behave bisexually. Some are *serial bisexuals*—that is, they are sexually involved with same-sex partners for a while and then with partners of the other sex, or vice versa. An estimated 7 to 9 million men, about twice the number thought to be exclusively homosexual, could be described as bisexual during some extended period of their lives. The largest group are married, rarely have sexual relations with women other than their wives, and have secret sexual involvements with men.

Fear of HIV infection has sparked great concern about bisexuality, particularly among heterosexual women who worry about becoming involved with a bisexual man. About 20 to 30 percent of women with AIDS were infected by bisexual partners, and health officials fear that bisexual men who hide their homosexual affairs could transmit HIV to many more women.

society. At one end of the continuum are those exclusively attracted to members of the other sex; at the opposite end are people exclusively attracted to members of the same sex. In between are varying degrees of homosexual, bisexual, and heterosexual orientation.

According to Kinsey's original data, 4 percent of men and 2 percent of women are exclusively homosexual. More recent studies have found lower numbers. For instance, in the University of Chicago's national survey, 2.8 percent of men and 1.4 percent of women defined themselves as homosexual. However, when asked if they'd had sex with a person of the same gender since age 18, about 5 percent of men and 4 percent of women said yes. When asked if they found members of the same gender sexually attractive, 6 percent of men and 5.5 percent of women said yes.

Most lesbian and bisexual women report that their first sexual experience occurred

Homosexuality

Homosexuality—social, emotional, and sexual attraction to members of the same sex—exists in almost all cultures. Men and women homosexuals are commonly referred to as *gays;* women homosexuals are also called *lesbians.*

Homosexuality threatens and upsets many people, perhaps because homosexuals are viewed as different, or perhaps because no one understands why some people are heterosexual and others homosexual. *Homophobia* has led to an increase in *gay bashing* (attacking homosexuals) in many communities, including college campuses. Some blame the emergence of AIDS as a societal danger. However, researchers have found that fear of AIDS has not created new hostility but has simply given bigots an excuse to act out their hatred.

 Different ethnic groups respond to homosexuality in different ways. To a greater extent than white homosexuals, gays and lesbians from ethnic groups tend to stay in the closet longer rather than risk alienation from their families and communities. Often they feel forced to choose between their gay and their ethnic identities.

In general, the African American community has stronger negative views of homosexuals than whites, possibly because of the influence of strong fundamentalist Christian beliefs. Stigma may contribute to a phenomenon called "the Down Low" or DL, which refers to African American men who publicly present themselves as heterosexuals while secretly having sex with other men. This practice, which is neither new nor limited to African American men, can increase the risk of HIV infection in unsuspecting female partners. Hispanic culture, with its emphasis on machismo, also has a very negative view of male homosexuality. Asian cultures, which tend to view an individual as a representative of his or her family, tend to view open declarations of sexual orientation as shaming the family and challenging their reputation and future.

Roots of Homosexuality Most mental health experts agree that nobody knows what causes a person's sexual orientation. Research has discredited theories tracing homosexuality to troubled childhoods or abnormal psychological development. Sexual orientation probably emerges from a complex interaction that includes biological and environmental factors.

 Homosexuality on Campus In a study of almost 700 heterosexual students at six small liberal arts colleges, attitudes toward homosexuals and homosexuality varied, depending on students' membership in fraternities or sororities, sex-role attitudes, religion and religiosity, and contact with and knowledge of gays, lesbians, and bisexuals. The students most likely to be accepting were those who were women, had less traditional sex-role attitudes, were less religious, attended colleges that did not have Greek social clubs, and had gay, lesbian, and/or bisexual friends.

 In a study of heterosexual African American college students, women expressed positive attitudes toward homosexuality, whereas men's attitudes were slightly negative. Church attendance influenced students' attitudes: Those who did not attend regularly expressed more positive opinions.[15]

A survey of colleges and universities found great variation in the resources available to gay, lesbian, and bisexual students. Most (71 percent) have a student organization; 32 percent provide a paid staff member to deal with the students' needs and issues; 40 percent provide a support identification program; 36 percent offered at least one course on gay, lesbian, and bisexual issues.

Transgenderism and Transsexuality

The term **transgender** is used as an umbrella term to describe people who have gender identities, expressions, or behaviors not traditionally associated with their birth sex. Male-to-female transgenders have been assigned a male gender at birth, but identify their gender as female. Female-to-male people were assigned a female gender at birth, but identify their gender as male.

Transgender individuals may be happy with the biological sex in which they are born but enjoy dressing up and behaving like the other sex. Most do so for psychological and social pleasure rather than sexual gratification.

transgender Having a gender identity opposite one's biological sex.

Transsexuals feel trapped in the body of the wrong gender—a condition called *gender dysphoria.* In general, more men than women have this experience. Transsexualism is now viewed as a disorder that can be treated with sexual reassignment surgery. However, this intervention, which requires long psychological counseling, hormonal treatments, and complicated operations, remains controversial. Some studies report healthy postoperative functioning, while others note that many male and female transsexuals do not escape their psychological misery.[16]

Transgender individuals face varied health risks, including unprotected sex, sexually transmitted diseases, and HIV infection. Violence, including rape, sexual abuse, physical abuse, and suicide, is a major public health issue.

Sexual Activity

Part of learning about your own sexuality is having a clear understanding of human sexual behaviors. Understanding frees us from fear and anxiety so that we can accept ourselves and others as the natural sexual beings we all are.

Celibacy

A celibate person does not engage in sexual activity. Complete **celibacy** means that the person doesn't masturbate (stimulate himself or herself sexually) or engage in sexual activity with a partner. In partial celibacy, the person masturbates but doesn't have sexual contact with others. Many people decide to be celibate at certain times of their lives. Some don't have sex because of concerns about pregnancy or STIs; others haven't found a partner for a permanent, monogamous relationship. Many simply have other priorities, such as finishing school or starting a career, and realize that sex outside of a committed relationship is a threat to their physical and psychological well-being.

Abstinence

The CDC defines **abstinence** as "refraining from sexual activities which involve vaginal, anal, and oral intercourse." The definition of abstinence remains a subject of debate and controversy, with some emphasizing positive choices and others avoidance of specific behaviors. In reality, abstinence means different things to different people, cultures, and religious groups.

Increasing numbers of adolescents and young adults are choosing to remain virgins and abstain from sexual intercourse until they enter a permanent, committed, monogamous relationship. About 2.5 million teens have taken pledges to abstain from sex. (See Point/Counterpoint, p. 282.)

Many people who were sexually active in the past also are choosing abstinence because the risk of medical complications associated with STIs increases with the number of sexual partners a person has. Practicing abstinence is the safest, healthiest option for many. However, there is confusion about what it means to abstain, and individuals who think they are abstaining may still be engaging in behaviors that put them at risk for HIV and STIs. (See Chapter 10 for more on abstinence as a form of birth control.)

Why abstain? Among the reasons students give are:

- Remaining a virgin until you meet someone you love and see as a life partner.
- Being true to your religious and moral values.
- Getting to know a partner better.
- If you're heterosexual, to avoid pregnancy.
- To be sure you're safe from sexually transmitted infections.

Abstinence education programs, which received federal support and became widespread in American schools, have had little, if any, impact on teen sexual behavior. In a five-year study of adolescents, the same percentage—49 percent—of teens did not have

Sex in Cyberspace

Sex is the number-one word searched for online. About 15 percent of Americans logging onto the Internet visit sexually oriented sites. Most people who check out sex sites on the Internet do not suffer any negative impact, but be aware of some potential risks.

Facts to Know
- Men are the largest consumers of sexually explicit material and outnumber women by a ratio of six to one. However, while men look for visual erotica, women are more likely to visit chat rooms, which offer more interactions.
- While most individuals use their home computers when surfing the Internet for sex-related sites, one in ten has used a school computer. Some universities have strict policies barring such practices and may take punitive actions against students or employees who violate the rules.

Steps to Take
- **Limit time online.** Individuals who spend 11 hours or more a week online in sexual pursuits show signs of psychological distress and admit that their behavior interferes with some areas of their lives.
- **Be skeptical.** Most Internet surfers admit that they occasionally "pretend" about their age on the Internet. Most keep secret how much time they spend on sexual pursuits in cyberspace.
- **Monitor yourself for signs of compulsivity.** A small but significant number of users are at risk of a serious problem as a result of their heavy Internet use.
- **Don't do anything "virtually" that you wouldn't do in real life.** For instance, "sexting" a photo of yourself nude or partially nude to your boyfriend or girlfriend might seem funny and flirty at the time. But would you flash your body on the quad or at a mall? Remember that nothing remains totally private once it makes its way into cyberspace.

---

sex, regardless of whether or not they'd had abstinence education. Scientists have found no difference in age of first intercourse for students who had graduated from abstinence programs and those who had not.[17]

Fantasy

The mind is the most powerful sex organ in the body, and erotic mental images can be sexually stimulating. Sexual fantasies can accompany sexual activity or be pleasurable in themselves.

Fantasies generally enhance sexual arousal, reduce anxiety, and boost sexual desire. They're also a way to anticipate and rehearse new sexual experiences, as well as to bolster a person's self-image and feelings of desirability. Part of what makes fantasies exciting is that they provide an opportunity for expressing forbidden desires, such as sex with a different partner or with a past lover.

 Men and women have different types of sexy thoughts, with men's fantasies containing more explicit genital images and culminating in sexual acts more quickly than women's. In women's fantasies, emotional feelings play a greater role, and there is more kissing and caressing rather than genital contact. For many women, fantasy helps in reaching orgasm during intercourse; a loss of fantasy often is a sign of low sexual desire.

Fantasies lived out via the Internet are becoming more common but may also be harmful to psychological health. (See Consumer Alert.)

Masturbation

Not everybody masturbates, but most people do. Kinsey estimated that 7 out of 10 women and 19 out of 20 men masturbate (and admit they do). Their reason is simple: It feels good. Masturbation produces the same physical responses as sexual activity with a partner and can be an enjoyable form of sexual release.

Masturbation has been described as immature; unsocial; tiring; frustrating; and a cause of hairy palms, warts, blemishes, and blindness. None of these myths is true. Sex educators recommend masturbation to adolescents as a means of releasing tension and becoming familiar with their sexual organs. Throughout adulthood, masturbation often is the primary sexual activity of individuals not involved in a sexual relationship and can be particularly useful when illness, absence, divorce, or death deprives a person of a partner. In the University of Chicago survey, about 25 percent of men and 9 percent of women said they masturbate at least once a week.

 White men and women have a higher incidence of masturbation than African American men

celibacy Abstention from sexual activity; can be partial or complete, permanent or temporary.

abstinence Voluntary refrainment from sexual intercourse.

POINT

Campus abstinence clubs are gaining in popularity at Ivy League schools and other colleges around the country. They sponsor parties, lectures, and discussion panels that encourage abstinence. By publicly committing themselves to a chaste lifestyle, their members are presenting an alternative to casual hookups between two people who make no commitment to each other.

COUNTERPOINT

Sexual choices are private and personal. If students organized clubs to promote hookups and casual sex, there would be immediate protests. Rightly so, but neither should campus abstinence clubs be allowed. Consenting adults have the right to choose not to have sex, but not the right to impose their moral values and judgments on others.

YOUR VIEW

Do students have the right to proclaim and defend their personal values in a club setting? Do you think abstinence clubs are a reaction to the anything-goes sexual culture on many campuses? Are these clubs trying to impose a certain standard of behavior on others? What do you think of the students who join such groups? Are you or would you become a member?

© Arlene Collins/The Image Works

Touch—thrilling, soothing, stimulating—is a powerful way to communicate affection and sexual pleasure.

and women. Latina women have the lowest rate of masturbation, compared with Latino men, white men and women, and African American men and women. Individuals with a higher level of education are more likely to masturbate than those with less schooling, and people living with sexual partners masturbate more than those who live alone.

Nonpenetrative Sexual Activity (Outercourse)

Various pleasurable behaviors can lead to orgasm with little risk of pregnancy or sexually transmitted infection. The options for "outercourse" include kissing, hugging, and touching but do not involve genital-to-genital, mouth-to-genital, or insertive anal sexual contact.

A kiss is a universal sign of affection. A kiss can be just a kiss—a quick press of the lips—or it can lead to much more. Usually kissing is the first sexual activity that couples engage in, and even after years of sexual experimentation and sharing, it remains an enduring pleasure for partners.

Touching is a silent form of communication between friends and lovers. Although a touch to any part of the body can be thrilling, some areas, such as the breasts and genitals, are especially sensitive. Stimulating these **erogenous** regions can lead to orgasm in both men and women. Though such forms of stimulation often accompany intercourse, more couples are gaining an appreciation of these activities as primary sources of sexual fulfillment—and as safer alternatives to intercourse.

Intercourse

Vaginal **intercourse,** or coitus, refers to the penetration of the vagina by the penis (Figure 9.5). This is the preferred form of sexual intimacy for most heterosexual couples, who may use a wide variety of positions. The most familiar position for intercourse in our society is the so-called missionary position, with the man on top, facing the woman. An alternative is the woman on top, either lying down or sitting upright. Other positions include lying side by side (either face-to-face or with the man behind the woman, his penis entering her vagina from the rear); lying with the man on top of the woman in a rear-entry position; and kneeling or standing (again, in either a face-to-face or rear-entry position). Many couples move into several different positions for intercourse during a single episode of lovemaking; others may have a personal favorite or may choose different positions at different times.

Sexual activity, including intercourse, is possible throughout a woman's menstrual cycle. However, some women prefer to avoid sex while menstruating because of uncomfortable physical symptoms, such as cramps, or concern about bleeding or messiness. Others use a diaphragm or cervical cap (see Chapter 10) to hold back menstrual flow. Since different cultures have different views on intercourse during a woman's period, partners should discuss their own feelings and try to respect each other's views. If they choose not to have intercourse, there are other gratifying forms of sexual activity.

Vaginal intercourse, like other forms of sexual activity involving an exchange of body fluids, carries a risk of sexually transmitted infections, including HIV infection. In many other parts of the world, in fact, heterosexual intercourse is the most common means of HIV transmission (see Chapter 16).

Oral Sex

Our mouths and genitals give us some of our most intense pleasures. Though it might seem logical to combine the two, some people are very uncomfortable with it. Some people consider oral–genital sex a perversion; it is against the law in some states and a sin in some religions. However, others find it normal and acceptable. (The same comments apply to anal sex as well—see the next section.)

The formal terms for oral sex are **cunnilingus,** which refers to oral stimulation of the woman's genitals, and **fellatio,** oral stimulation of the man's genitals. For many couples, oral sex is a regular part of their lovemaking. For others, it's an occasional experiment. Oral sex with a partner carrying a sexually transmitted infection, such as herpes or HIV infection, can lead to infection, so a condom should be used (with cunnilingus, a condom cut in half to lay flat can be used).

Anal Stimulation and Intercourse

Because the anus has many nerve endings, it can produce intense erotic responses. Stimulation of the anus by the fingers or mouth can be a source of sexual arousal; anal intercourse involves penile penetration of the anus. An estimated 25 percent of adults have experienced anal intercourse at least once. However, anal sex involves important health risks, such as damage to sensitive rectal tissues and the transmission of various intestinal infections, hepatitis, and STIs, including HIV.

Cultural Variations

 While the biological mechanisms underlying human sexual arousal

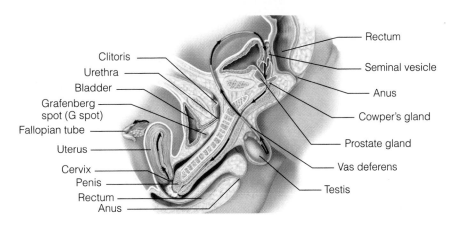

Figure 9.5 A Cross-Sectional View of Sexual Intercourse

Sperm are formed in each of the testes and stored in the epididymis. When a man ejaculates, sperm carried in semen travel up the vas deferens. (The prostate gland and seminal vesicles contribute components of the semen.) The semen is expelled from the penis through the urethra and deposited in the vagina, near the cervix. During sexual excitement and orgasm in a woman, the upper end of the vagina enlarges and the uterus elevates. After orgasm, these organs return to their normal states, and the cervix descends into the pool of semen.

and response are essentially universal, the particular sexual stimuli or behaviors that people find arousing are greatly influenced by cultural conditioning. For example, in Western societies, where the emphasis during sexual activity tends to be heavily weighted toward achieving orgasm, genitally focused activities are frequently defined as optimally arousing. In contrast, devotees to Eastern Tantric traditions (where spirituality is interwoven with sexuality) often achieve optimal pleasure by emphasizing the sensual and spiritual aspects of shared intimacy rather than orgasmic release.

Kissing on the mouth, a universal source of sexual arousal in Western society, may be rare or absent in many other parts of the world. Certain North American Eskimo people and inhabitants of the Trobriand Islands would rather rub noses than lips, and among the Thonga of South Africa, kissing is viewed as odious behavior. The Hindu people of India are also disinclined to kiss because they believe such contact symbolically contaminates the act of sexual intercourse. One survey of 190 societies found that mouth kissing was acknowledged in only 21 societies and practiced as a prelude or accompaniment to coitus in only 13.

Oral sex (both cunnilingus and fellatio) is a common source of sexual arousal among island societies of the South Pacific, in

erogenous Sexually sensitive.

intercourse Sexual stimulation by means of entry of the penis into the vagina; coitus.

cunnilingus Sexual stimulation of a woman's genitals by means of oral manipulation.

fellatio Sexual stimulation of a man's genitals by means of oral manipulation.

industrialized nations of Asia, and in much of the Western world. In contrast, in Africa (with the exception of northern regions), such practices are likely to be viewed as unnatural or disgusting behavior.

Foreplay in general, whether it be oral sex, sensual touching, or passionate kissing, is subject to wide cultural variation. In some societies, most notably those with Eastern traditions, couples may strive to prolong intense states of sexual arousal for several hours. While varied patterns of foreplay are common in Western cultures, these activities often are of short duration as lovers move rapidly toward the "main event" of coitus. In still other societies, foreplay is either sharply curtailed or absent altogether. For example, the Lepcha farmers of the southeastern Himalayas limit foreplay to men briefly caressing their partners' breasts, and among the Irish inhabitants of Inis Beag, precoital sexual activity is reported to be limited to mouth kissing and rough fondling of the woman's lower body by her partner.

Sexual Response

Sexuality involves every part of you: mind and body, muscles and skin, glands and genitals. The pioneers in finding out exactly how human beings respond to sex were William Masters and Virginia Johnson, who first studied more than 800 individuals in their laboratory in the 1950s. They discovered that sexual response is a well-ordered sequence of events, so predictable it could be divided into four phases: excitement, plateau, orgasm, and resolution (Figure 9.6). In real life, individuals don't necessarily follow this well-ordered pattern. But the responses for both sexes are remarkably similar. And sexual response always follows the same sequence, whatever the means of stimulation.

Excitement

Stimulation is the first step: a touch, a look, a fantasy. In men, sexual stimuli set off a rush of blood to the genitals, filling the blood vessels in the penis. Because these vessels are wrapped in a thick sheath of tissue, the penis becomes erect. The testes lift.

Women respond to stimulation with vaginal lubrication within 10 to 20 seconds of exposure to sexual stimuli. The clitoris becomes larger, as do the vaginal lips (the labia), the nipples, and later the breasts. The vagina lengthens, and its inner two-thirds increase in size. The uterus lifts, further increasing the free space in the vagina.

Plateau

During this stage, the changes begun in the excitement stage continue and intensify. The penis further increases in both length and diameter. The outer one-third of the vagina swells. During intercourse, the vaginal muscles grasp the penis to increase stimulation for both partners. The upper two-thirds of the vagina become wider as the uterus moves up; eventually its diameter is $2\frac{1}{2}$ to 3 inches.

Orgasm

Men and women have remarkably similar **orgasm** experiences. Both men and women typically have 3 to 12 pelvic muscle contractions approximately four-fifths of a second apart and lasting up to 60 seconds. Both undergo contractions and spasms of other muscles, as well as increases in breathing and pulse rates, and blood pressure. Both can sometimes have orgasms simply from kisses, stimulation of the breasts or other parts of the body, or fantasy alone.

The process of **ejaculation** (the discharge of semen by a male) requires two separate events. First, the vas deferens, the seminal vesicles, the prostate, and the upper portion of the urethra contract. The man perceives these subtle contractions deep in his pelvis just before the point of no return—which therapists refer to as the point of "ejaculatory inevitability." Then, seconds later, muscle contractions force semen out of the penis via the urethra.

Key Terms

The terms listed are used on the page indicated. Definitions of the terms are in the Glossary at the end of the book.

Chapter 10 - Reproductive Choices

1. **Ovulation occurs in a woman when:** (Pg. 298)
   - A. sperm are created
   - B. an egg is released
   - C. the sperm and ovum merge
   - D. the egg implants

2. **The term contraception means:** (Pg. 298)
   - A. the release of an ovum
   - B. implantation
   - C. methods of preventing pregnancy
   - D. methods to stop spermatogenesis

3. **Kimberly wants to start using birth control. Which consideration would be least important to her decision-making?** (Pg. 303)
   - A. failure rate
   - B. effectiveness
   - C. adverse reactions
   - D. which methods her girlfriends use

4. **An example of a barrier form of birth control is the:** (Pg. 305)
   - A. pill
   - B. ortho patch
   - C. IUD
   - D. diaphragm

5. **Among college-aged students using contraceptive methods, the most popular choice is the:** (Pg. 311)
   - A. condom
   - B. coitus interruptus
   - C. pill
   - D. inter uterine device

6. **Which form of contraceptive provides protection against sexually transmitted infections (STIs)?** (Pg. 306)
   - A. cervical cap
   - B. IUD
   - C. condom
   - D. diaphragm

7. **To be most effective, what needs to also be used when a woman uses a diaphragm?** (Pg. 309)
   - A. her male partner needs to use a condom
   - B. she needs to be on the oral pill
   - C. spermicide needs to be placed inside the diaphragm
   - D. an IUD should also be in place

8. **Which of the female barrier contraceptives does not require a physician's prescription for use?** (Pg. 308)
   - A. FemCap
   - B. diaphragm
   - C. female condom
   - D. cervical cap

9. **A disadvantage for women taking the progestin-only mini-pill is:** (Pg. 312)
   - A. it may relieve painful menstruation
   - B. the pill must be taken the same time every day
   - C. it is reversible within three months of stopping the pill
   - D. risk of heart disease is lower

10. **Which birth control method administers the drug transdermally?** (Pg. 314)
    - A. contraceptive injections
    - B. Ortho Evra patch
    - C. intrauterine device
    - D. NuvaRing

11. **Abortifacients are:** (Pg. 322)
  A. artifacts found from the caveman era
  B. facts and information to learn about abortions
  C. drugs used to terminate a pregnancy
  D. a type of sterilization technique

12. **In an ectopic pregnancy, the fertilized embryo is located in the:** (Pg. 327)
  A. uterus
  B. cervix
  C. anus
  D. fallopian tubes

13. **At what stage is the embryo now called a fetus (the unborn child in the womb)?** (Pg. 326)
  A. 2 weeks
  B. 9 weeks
  C. 12 weeks
  D. 30 weeks

14. **In which trimester of a woman's pregnancy is it most likely for her to experience nausea and vomiting?** (Pg. 326)
  A. preconception
  B. first trimester
  C. second trimester
  D. third trimester

15. **One of the most important aspects of prenatal care for a woman should be:** (Pg. 325)
  A. not engaging in sexual activity while pregnant
  B. not dieting during pregnancy, but rather consume about 300 calories more each day
  C. doing back exercises everyday on the floor to strengthen the abdominal muscles
  D. restrict salt intake to lower the blood pressure

16. **In which stage of labor and delivery is the woman's cervix (birth canal) completely open and ready for the baby's arrival?** (Pg. 329)
  A. prelabor contractions
  B. first stage
  C. second stage
  D. third stage

17. **Women who are not able to become pregnant can opt to have a procedure done where upon male sperm is artificially inseminated into the woman's vagina. This procedure is known as:** (Pg. 331)
  A. in vitro fertilization
  B. assisted reproductive technology
  C. artificial insemination
  D. tubal ligation

18. **In the natural family planning method of birth control, the main premise for controlling the woman's chances of getting pregnant are based on:** (Pg. 318)
  A. the woman's rhythm of safe or unsafe days to get pregnant
  B. the woman's basal temperature which rises after ovulation
  C. observing changes in the woman's cervical mucus
  D. all of the above

19. **When a woman decides to undergo sterilization to prevent further pregnancies, this is known as:** (Pg. 320)
  A. vasectomy
  B. tubal ligation
  C. abortion
  D. coitus interruptus

20. **When a man undergoes a vasectomy, what part of the genitals is surgically treated to prevent further sperm travel to impregnate the female?** (Pg. 320)
  A. urethra
  B. penis
  C. testicles
  D. vas deferens

Justin and Sara, sophomores at the same community college, can't remember a time when abortion was illegal, when AIDS wasn't a deadly threat, and when safe sex wasn't a concern of every sexually active individual. Yet even though they were aware of the risks and the realities involved, neither used contraception during every single sexual encounter. Then one of Justin's partners had a pregnancy scare. He decided never again to engage in unprotected sex. Sara had a different reality check: At her regular physical, she learned that she had contracted chlamydia, the most common sexually transmitted infection in the United States.

Reproductive Choices

"When we started dating," Sara recalls, "both of us felt that something was special about our relationship." Despite their mutual attraction, they decided to take every step toward intimacy slowly. Both considered and talked about their personal priorities and concerns. Even though it was awkward, they also discussed their own sexual histories and underwent tests for STIs. Looking toward a continuing committed relationship, they decided on not one but two forms of contraception: the birth control pill and a condom. In the future, they realized that they might switch to other forms of birth control—and might well consider different options, including both marriage and parenthood.

As human beings, we have a unique power: the ability to choose to conceive or not to conceive. No other species on earth can separate sexual activity and pleasure from reproduction. However, simply not wanting to get pregnant is never enough to prevent conception, nor is wanting to have a child always enough to get pregnant. Both desires require individual decisions and actions. (See Making Change Happen, p. 300, and "To Have or Have Not" in *Labs for IPC*.)

This chapter provides information on conception, birth control, abortion, infertility, adoption, and the processes by which a new human life develops and enters the world.

After studying the material in this chapter, you should be able to

- **Describe** the process of human conception.
- **List** the major options available for contraception, and **identify** the advantages and disadvantages of each.
- **Describe** the commonly used abortion methods.
- **Discuss** the physiological effects of pregnancy on a woman and **describe** fetal development.
- **Describe** the three stages of labor and the birth process.
- **Identify** the options available to infertile couples wanting children.
- If contraception is one of your reproductive choices for the next three years, **name** the methods you will likely use and why.

Log on to CengageNOW for Health at **www.cengage.com/sso** to find your Behavior Change Planner and to explore self-assessments, interactive tutorials, and practice quizzes.

297

Reproductive Responsibility

Anyone who engages in vaginal intercourse must be willing to accept the consequences of that activity—the possibility of pregnancy and responsibility for the child who might be conceived—or take action to avoid those consequences. Although many people are concerned about the risks associated with contraception, using birth control is safer and healthier than not using it. According to the Population Reference Bureau, the use of contraceptives, including oral contraceptives, saves millions of lives each year.

The typical American woman who wants two children spends about five years pregnant or trying to become pregnant and three decades—more than three-quarters of her reproductive life—trying to avoid pregnancy. About half of all pregnancies in the United States each year—more than three million—are unintended. By age 45, more than half of all American women will have experienced an unintended pregnancy, and about one-third will have had an abortion.[1]

Conception

The equation for making a baby is quite simple: One sperm plus one egg equals one fertilized egg, which can develop into an infant. But the processes that affect or permit **conception** are quite complicated. The creation of sperm, or **spermatogenesis,** starts in the male at puberty, and the production of sperm is regulated by hormones. Sperm cells form in the seminiferous tubules of the testes and are passed into the epididymis, where they are stored until ejaculation; a single male ejaculation may contain 500 million sperm. Each sperm released into the vagina during intercourse moves on its own, propelling itself toward its target, an ovum.

To reach its goal, the sperm must move through the acidic secretions of the vagina, enter the uterus, travel up the fallopian tube containing the ovum, then fuse with the nucleus of the egg (**fertilization**). Just about every sperm produced by a man in his lifetime fails to accomplish its mission.

There are far fewer human egg cells than there are sperm cells. Each woman is born with her lifetime supply of ova, and between 300 and 500 eggs eventually mature and leave her ovaries during ovulation. As discussed in Chapter 9, every month, one or the other of the woman's ovaries releases an ovum to the nearby fallopian tube. It travels through the fallopian tube until it reaches the uterus, a journey that takes three to four days. An unfertilized egg lives for about 24 to 36 hours, disintegrates, and during menstruation is expelled along with the uterine lining.

Even if a sperm, which can survive in the female reproductive tract for two to five days, meets a ripe egg in a fallopian tube, its success is not ensured. A mature ovum releases the chemical allurin, which attracts the sperm. A sperm is able to penetrate the ovum's outer membrane because of a protein called fertilin. The egg then pulls the sperm inside toward its nucleus (Figure 10.1). The fertilized egg, called the **zygote,** travels down the fallopian tube, dividing to form a tiny clump of cells called a **blastocyst.** When it reaches the uterus, about a week after fertilization, it burrows into the endometrial, the lining of the uterus. This process is called **implantation.**

Conception can be prevented by **contraception.** Some contraceptive methods prevent ovulation or implantation, and others block the sperm from reaching the egg. Some methods are temporary; others permanently alter one's fertility.

conception The merging of a sperm and an ovum.

spermatogenesis The process by which sperm cells are produced.

fertilization The fusion of sperm and egg nucleus.

zygote A fertilized egg.

blastocyst In embryonic development, a ball of cells with a surface layer and an inner cell mass.

implantation The embedding of the fertilized ovum in the uterine lining.

contraception The prevention of conception; birth control.

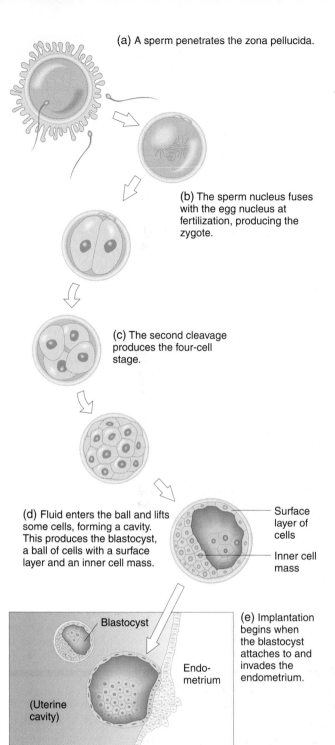

(a) A sperm penetrates the zona pellucida.

(b) The sperm nucleus fuses with the egg nucleus at fertilization, producing the zygote.

(c) The second cleavage produces the four-cell stage.

(d) Fluid enters the ball and lifts some cells, forming a cavity. This produces the blastocyst, a ball of cells with a surface layer and an inner cell mass.

Surface layer of cells

Inner cell mass

Blastocyst

Endo-metrium

(Uterine cavity)

(e) Implantation begins when the blastocyst attaches to and invades the endometrium.

Figure 10.1 Fertilization

(a) The efforts of hundreds of sperm may allow one to penetrate the ovum's corona radiate, an outer layer of cells, and then the zone pel-lucid, a thick inner membrane. (b) The nuclei of the sperm and the egg cells merge, and the male and female chromosomes in the nuclei come together, forming a zygote. (c) The zygote divides into two cells, then four cells, and so on. (d) As fluid enters the ball, cells form a ball of cells called a blastocyst. (e) The blastocyst implants itself in the endometrium.

Birth Control Basics

Most sexually active women use some form of birth control. According to the Centers for Disease Control and Prevention, more than 98 percent of women between the ages of 15 and 44 who have ever had intercourse have used at least one contraceptive method. Most of the women not using any form of contraception are pregnant, trying to get pregnant, unable to conceive, or not having intercourse.

The use of contraception has declined in recent years, particularly among poor women. As a result, they are more likely to get pregnant unintentionally and to have abortions. An estimated 11 percent of sexually active women, including white, Hispanic, and African American women, who are not trying to get pregnant do not use birth control, up from 7 percent in 1994. Half of unintended pregnancies are carried to term. About 14,000 women who continue their pregnancies put the children up for adoption; 1.2 million women have abortions.[2]

If you are engaging in sexual activity that could lead to conception, you have to be realistic about your situation. This means assuming full responsibility for your reproductive ability, whether you're a man or a woman. The more you know about contraception, the more likely you are to use birth control. Contraceptives cost money; not using contraception can cost much more. (See Health on a Budget, p. 302.)

You also have to recognize the risks associated with various methods of contraception. If you're a woman, the risks are chiefly yours. Various methods of birth control have side effects, but

Maybe you can't imagine not having a child. Maybe you feel that you're still a kid yourself but maybe someday you'll want a baby. Or maybe you're married and are seriously thinking about starting a family. Regardless of whether your answer to the question of wanting a child is yes, no, maybe, not yet, or it depends, "To Have or Have Not" in *Labs for IPC* can help you sort through your feelings so you can make a conscious, responsible decision. Here's a preview.

In this stage, you test your parental readiness by answering 17 questions including the following three:

Get Real

- How much experience have you had in caring for children in the past? As an older sibling, babysitter, camp counselor? What did you enjoy about it? What didn't you enjoy?
- What did you enjoy about being a child? What didn't you enjoy?
- What did you get from your parents that you would like to pass on to your children? What wouldn't you want to pass on?

You also complete several exercises, including this one: Imagine that you or your partner (or a woman you slept with a few weeks ago) will take a pregnancy test tomorrow. Spend the next 24 hours thinking about how you might feel if it turns out positive and how you might feel if it's negative . . .

Get Ready

In this stage you complete several preparatory exercises, including the following:

- **Make a wish list.** In your *IPC Journal,* write down everything you want for any child you bring into the world. This list might include:
- A loving home.
- Two committed parents.
- Financial security.
- An excellent education.

Put a check mark next to every one that you are confident you and your partner could give to a child at this point in your life. Write a second set of check marks for what you could give to this child if for some reason you become solely responsible for this child . . .

- **Budget for a baby.** Make a list of all the supplies, equipment, and furniture new parents have to get for their baby's first year. "Shop" for these items online, and calculate how much they would cost . . .

Get Going

Over an eight-week period, you will engage in five exercises, such as:

- **"Shadowing" a new parent.** Ask a friend with a baby, or a friend of a friend, or a cousin or neighbor, if you can follow her or him during a typical day. Take notes of when the baby wakes, cries, frets, and sleeps. You get extra credit if you volunteer to change a diaper . . .
- **Having a virtual baby.** Based on your research, come up with a typical day in the life of a three-month-old baby. Name your baby boy or girl. Record when your baby wakes up. Calculate how much time you would need to drop the baby off at day care on your way to class . . . Throw in some unexpecteds, such as the baby fussing all afternoon so you don't have time to study . . .

Lock It In

Keep talking—with your partner, your friends, parents you know. Also seek out and talk to people who have decided not to have children. Imagine that you have decided not to have children, and live with this decision for a week. Then imagine you've decided to have a child. Think of all the ways your life would change. How does that make you feel?

---

pregnancy and childbirth account for much higher rates of medical complications and deaths than any contraceptive. Although most women never experience any serious complications, it's important to be aware of the potential for long-term risks. Risks that are acceptable to others may not be acceptable to you. (See Reality Check, p. 301.)

Abstinence and Nonpenetrative Sexual Activity

The contraceptive methods discussed in this chapter are designed to prevent pregnancy as a consequence of vaginal intercourse.

Couples who choose abstinence make a very different decision—to abstain from vaginal intercourse and forms of nonpenetrative sexual activity that could result in conception (any in which ejaculation occurs near the vaginal opening).

For many individuals, abstinence represents a deliberate choice regarding their bodies, minds, spirits, and sexuality. People choose abstinence for various reasons, including waiting until they are ready for a sexual relationship or until they find the "right" partner, respecting religious or moral values, enjoying friendships without sexual involvement, recovering from a breakup, or preventing pregnancy and sexually transmitted infection.

Practicing abstinence is the only form of birth control that is 100 percent effective and risk-free. It is also an important, increasingly valued lifestyle choice. A growing number of individuals, including some who have been sexually active in the past, are choosing abstinence until they establish a relationship with a long-term partner.

Abstinence offers special health benefits for women. Those who abstain until their twenties and engage in sex with fewer partners during their lifetime are less likely to get sexually transmitted infections, to suffer infertility, or to develop cervical cancer. However, some people find it difficult to abstain for long periods of time. There also is a risk that people will abruptly end their abstinence without being prepared to protect themselves against pregnancy or infection.

Individuals who choose abstinence from vaginal intercourse often engage in activities sometimes called *outercourse,* such as kissing, hugging, sensual touching, and mutual masturbation. Outercourse is nearly 100 percent effective as a contraceptive measure, but pregnancy is possible if there is genital contact. If the man ejaculates near the vaginal opening, sperm can swim up into the vagina and fallopian tubes to fertilize an egg. Outercourse also may lower the risk of contracting

• *What percent of college students engaging in vaginal intercourse rely on condoms to prevent pregnancy?* _____
• *What percent rely on birth control pills?* _____
• *What percent reported using (or their partner using) emergency contraception within the last 12 months?* _____
• *What percent of students who had vaginal intercourse within the last 12 months reported experiencing an unintended pregnancy or getting someone pregnant?* _____

Answers on next page.

Some couples refrain from intercourse by engage in "outercourse," or intimacy that includes kissing and hugging.

sexually transmitted infections. It is an effective form of safe sex as long as no body fluids are exchanged.

Some couples routinely restrict themselves to outercourse; others temporarily choose such sexual activities when it is inadvisable for them to have vaginal intercourse, for example, after childbirth. Other benefits: Outercourse has no medical or hormonal side effects; it may prolong sex play and enhance orgasm; it can be used when no other birth control methods are available.

A Cross-Cultural Perspective

Culture, religion, gender roles, and folklore can affect birth control options and decisions. In countries that are predominantly Catholic, such as Ireland, Italy, and the

Philippines, the Church promotes fertility awareness and the rhythm method and condemns other contraceptive methods. Because Jewish law teaches men not to "spill

PART 2: *Just the Facts*
- *64 percent of college students engaging in vaginal intercourse use condoms to prevent pregnancy.*
- *61 percent use birth control pills.*
- *14 percent of sexually active college students used emergency contraception within the last 12 months.*
- *3 percent of those who had vaginal intercourse within the last 12 months reported an unintentional pregnancy.*

Source: American College Health Association. American College Health Association-National College Health Assessment II: Reference Group Executive Summary Fall 2008. Baltimore: American College Health Association, 2009.

their seed," methods that can cause damage to sperm, such as vasectomy, condoms, or spermicides, are less acceptable in Israel than oral contraceptives are. In Japan, which has one of the lowest birth rates in the world (see Figure 10.2), men are primarily responsible for birth control decisions. In Kenya, married couples view the use of a condom as an indicator of a husband's infidelity. In Scandinavian countries, where birth control is free and easily accessible, many women

HEALTH ON A BUDGET $

The Cost of Contraception

The only free forms of birth control are abstinence and the rhythm method. But even the most expensive methods cost less (much, much less) than having and caring for a child. If you're on a tight budget, you might want to consider the relative cost of a year's prescription of oral contraceptives compared to the annual cost of condoms or spermicidal foam or jelly.

Here are some cost estimates from the FDA that can help you make sense of the dollars-and-cents of contraception:

Spermicide	Less than a dollar per time
Contraceptive sponge	$2.50 to $3 per sponge
Cervical cap	$65 or more for cap; $50 to $200 for fitting
Diaphragm	$30 to $50 plus fitting
Female condom	$2 to $4 each
Male condom	$.50 to $2 each
Progestin-only pill	$15 to $60 a month
Injection	$30 to $70 per shot plus exam
Combination pill	$15 to $60 per cycle
Contraceptive patch	$35 to $70 a month
NuvaRing	$25 to $35 a month
Seasonale	$90 to $100 for three-month supply
Copper-coated IUD	$150 to $300
Mirena	$150 to $300 every five years
Female sterilization	$2,000 to $4,000
Male sterilization	$300 to $1,000
Emergency contraception	$8 to $25 for Plan B

The cost of each method depends on where you purchase it. Contraceptives are generally less expensive at health care clinics than in pharmacies or private medical practices.

Source of cost estimates: Carroll, Janell. *Sexuality Now,* 3rd ed. Belmont, CA: Wadsworth-Cengage, 2010.

begin taking oral contraceptives before becoming sexually active.[3]

Worldwide, sterilization is used by more people than any other birth control method. The intrauterine device (IUD) is the most commonly used reversible form of contraception. Among the countries with the highest usage rates are Turkey, China (where an IUD is often inserted immediately after a woman gives birth to her first child), Nigeria, England, Russia, and Korea. About two percent of women in the United States rely on IUDs for birth control.[4]

In developing countries, conception and contraception are life-and-death issues. One in three women give birth before age 20. Some 20 million women have unsafe abortions, which claim the lives of about 70,000 women between the ages of 15 and 19. Effective contraception could prevent about 90 percent of these deaths.[5]

The reasons why young women in developing countries do not use effective birth control are complex. In a recent analysis of studies in four African countries and Vietnam, the key factors were:

- Lack of education and information about sex and reproduction.
- Limited access to modern birth control methods.
- Limited understanding of how they work (for example, the belief that a woman only needs to take a birth control pill before or after sex).
- Fears that hormonal contraceptives would endanger future fertility.
- Association of condoms with disease and promiscuity.
- Partners' refusal to use condoms.

Even when premarital sex is widespread, many of these young women view birth control as appropriate only for married couples and feel ashamed to visit a family planning center. These women rely on traditional methods, such as herbs or withdrawal, and seek abortions if they become pregnant.[6]

Costs and insurance coverage also influence contraceptive choices (see Health on a Budget). Young women between ages 18 and 24 who lack insurance coverage are less likely to use prescription contraceptives, which are generally more effective, than women with private insurance.[7]

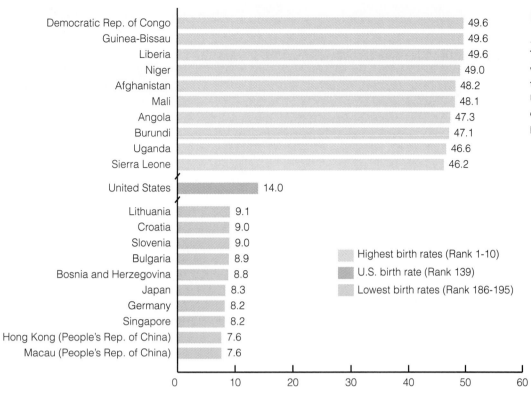

Figure 10.2 Birth Rates Around the World
The average birth rate for the entire world is 20.3 births per 1,000 population. These figures come from the United Nations Population Division's estimates for births in the five-year period from 2005 to 2010.

Birth rate (births per 1,000 persons)

Choosing a Birth Control Method

When it comes to deciding which form of birth control to use, there's no one "right" decision. Good decisions are based on sound information. You should consult a physician or family-planning counselor if you have questions or want to know how certain methods might affect existing or familial medical conditions, such as high blood pressure or diabetes.

Table 10.1 presents your contraceptive choices. As the table indicates, contraception doesn't always work. When you evaluate any contraceptive, always consider its effectiveness (the likelihood that it will indeed prevent pregnancy). The **failure rate** refers to the number of pregnancies that occur per year for every 100 women using a particular method of birth control.

The reliability of contraceptives in actual, real-life use is much lower than that reported in national surveys or clinical trials. In general, failure rates are highest among cohabiting and other unmarried women, very poor families, African American and Hispanic women, adolescents, and women in their twenties.

Some couples use withdrawal or **coitus interruptus** (removal of the penis from the vagina before ejaculation), to prevent pregnancy, even though this is not a reliable form of birth control. About half the men who have tried coitus interruptus find it unsatisfactory, either because they don't know when they're going to ejaculate or because they can't withdraw quickly enough. Also, the Cowper's glands, two pea-size structures located on each side of the urethra, often produce a fluid that appears as drops at the tip of the penis any time from arousal and erection to orgasm. This fluid can contain active sperm and, in infected men, human immunodeficiency virus (HIV).

Many unintentional pregnancies are the result of contraceptive failure, either from problems with the drug or device itself or from improper use. Partners can lower the risk of unwanted pregnancy by using backup methods—that is, more than one form of contraception simultaneously. Emergency or after-intercourse contraception (discussed later in this chapter) could

failure rate The number of pregnancies that occur per year for every 100 women using a particular method of birth control.

coitus interruptus The removal of the penis from the vagina before ejaculation.

TABLE 10.1

Birth Control Guide

Methods	Number of pregnancies expected per 100 women	MD Visit	How to use it	Some Risks	Noncontraceptive Benefits
Sterilization Surgery for Women	1	yes	One-time procedure; nothing to do or remember	• Pain • Bleeding • Infection or other complications after surgery • Ectopic (tubal) pregnancy	Reduces rist of ovarian cancer
Surgical Sterilization Implant for Women	1	yes	One-time procedure; nothing to do or remember	• Mild to moderate pain after insertion • Ectopic (tubal) pregnancy	Reduces rist of ovarian cancer
Sterilization Surgery for Men	1	yes	One-time procedure; nothing to do or remember	• Pain • Bleeding • Infection	Possible reduction in risk for prostate cancer
Implantable Rod	1	yes	One-time procedure; nothing to do or remember	• Acne • Hair loss • Weight gain • Headache • Cysts of the ovaries • Upset stomach • Mood changes • Dizziness • Depression • Sore breasts	Can use while breast-feeding; reduced menstrual flow and cramping
IUD	1	yes	One-time procedure; nothing to do or remember	• Cramps • Lower interest in sexual activity • Bleeding • Changes in your periods • Pelvic inflammatory disease • Infertility • Tear or hole in the uterus	Decreased menstrual flow and cramping; can use while breast-feeding; reduced risk of endometrial cancer
Shot/Injection	1	yes	Need a shot every 3 months	• Bone loss • Bleeding between periods • Weight gain • Breast tenderness • Headaches	
Oral Contraceptives (Combined Pill) "The Pill"	5	yes	Must swallow a pill every day	• Dizziness • High blood pressure • Nausea • Blood clots • Changes in your cycle (period) • Heart attack • Changes in your mood • Strokes • Weight gain	Decreases menstrual flow and cramping, PMS, acne, ovarian and endometrial cancers, and the development of ovarian cysts
Oral Contraceptives (Progestin-only) "The Pill"	5	yes	Must swallow a pill every day	• Irregular bleeding • Weight gain • Breast tenderness	May have similar noncontraceptive benefits as combined pills; reduction of uterine and ovarian cancers
Oral Contraceptives Extended/ Continued Use "The Pill"	5	yes	Must swallow a pill every day	• Risks are similar to other oral contraceptives • Bleeding • Spotting between periods	Four periods per year and fewer menstrual-related problems; may reduce uterine fibroids and endometriosis symptoms
Patch	5	yes	Must wear a patch every day	• Exposure to higher average levels of estrogen than most oral contraceptives	Decreases menstrual flow and cramping, PMS, acne, ovarian and endometrial cancers, and the development of ovarian cysts
Vaginal Contraceptive Ring	5	yes	Must leave the ring in every day for 3 weeks	• Vaginal discharge • Swelling of the vagina • Irritation • Similar to oral contraceptives	Decreases menstrual flow and cramping, PMS, acne, ovarian and endometrial cancers, and the development of ovarian cysts
Male Condom	11–16	no	Must use every time you have sex; requires partners cooperation Except for abstinence, latex condoms are the best protection against HIV/AIDS and other STIs	• Allergic reactions	Protects against STIs; delays premature ejaculation
Diaphram with Spermicide	15	yes	Must use every time you have sex	• Irritation • Urinary tract infection • Allergic reactions • Toxic shock	Possible STI protection; may reduce cervical dysplasia
Sponge with Spermicide	16–32	no	Must use every time you have sex	• Irritation • Allergic reactions • Hard time removing • Toxic shock	Possible STI protection
Cervial Cap with Spermicide	17–23	yes	Must use every time you have sex	• Irritation • Allergic reactions • Abnormal Pap test • Toxic shock	Possible STI protection
Female Condom	20	no	Must use every time you have sex May give some protection against STIs	• Irritation • Allergic reactions	Possible STI protection
Spermicide	30	no	Must use every time you have sex	• Irritation • Allergic reactions • Urinary tract infection	Possible STI protection
Emergency Contraception—If your primary method of birth control fails					
Emergency Contraceptives "The Morning After Pill"	15	no, if over 18	Must be used within 72 hours of unprotected sex It should not be used as a regular form of birth control	• Nausea • Vomiting • Abdominal pain • Fatigue • Headache	

> TABLE 10.2

Contraceptive Choices on Campus

Contraceptive use reported by students or their partner the last time they had vaginal intercourse:

Percent (%)	Male	Female	Total
Yes, used a method of contraception	49.5	53.7	52.4
Not applicable/Didn't use a method/Don't know	50.5	46.3	47.6

If YES to contraceptive use the last time student had vaginal intercourse, reported means of birth control used among college students or their partner to prevent pregnancy:

Percent (%)	Male	Female	Total
Birth control pills (monthly or extended cycle)	6.27	60.1	60.9
Birth control shots	2.6	2.4	25.
Birth control implants	1.2	0.3	0.6
Birth control patch	1.5	1.0	1.2
Vaginal ring	4.6	5.8	5.4
Intrauterine device	3.1	3.4	3.3
Male condom	69.4	61.2	63.6
Female condom	0.8	0.6	0.7
Diaphragm or cervical cap	0.8	0.4	0.5
Contraceptive sponge	0.6	0.2	0.4
Spermicide (foam, jelly, cream)	9.4	5.5	6.6
Fertility awareness (calendar, mucous, basal body temperature)	4.7	5.9	5.6
Withdrawal	24.5	28.5	27.4
Sterilization (hysterectomy, tubes tied, vasectomy)	1.8	2.7	2.5
Other method	2.2	2.1	2.1
Male condom use plus another method	51.1	45.7	47.2
Any two or more methods (excluding male condoms)	26.6	26.6	26.6

American College Health Association, *American College Health Association-National College Health Assessment II: Reference Group Executive Summary Fall 2008*. Baltimore: American College Health Association, 2009.

© Peter Ardito/Index Stock Imagery/Photolibrary

prevent as many as 1.7 million unwanted pregnancies each year.

Even college students aware of the risks associated with unprotected sexual intercourse often do not practice safe-sex behaviors (see Table 10.2). There are many reasons, ranging from the influence of drugs and alcohol to embarrassment about buying condoms. Generally, the ability to talk about a desire to use condoms has been found to be associated with a greater use of condoms.

The bottom line is that it takes two people to conceive a baby, and two people should be involved in deciding not to conceive a baby. In the process, they can also enhance their skills in communication, critical thinking, and negotiating.

barrier contraceptives Birth control devices that block the meeting of egg and sperm, either by physical barriers, such as condoms, diaphragms, or cervical caps, or by chemical barriers, such as spermicide, or both.

Barrier Contraceptives

As their name implies, **barrier contraceptives** block the meeting of egg and sperm by means of a physical barrier (condom, sponge, diaphragm, cervical cap, or FemCap) or a chemical one (vaginal spermicide in jellies, foams, creams, suppositories, or film).

Nonprescription Barriers

The nonprescription barrier contraceptives include the male and female condom, the contraceptive sponge, and vaginal spermicides. Condoms provide some protection against HIV infection and other STIs; spermicides, sponges, and films do not.

Male Condom   The male **condom** covers the erect penis and catches the ejaculate, thus preventing sperm from entering the woman's reproductive tract (Figure 10.3). Most are made of thin surgical latex or sheep membrane; a new type is made of polyurethane, which is thinner, stronger, more heat sensitive, and more comfortable than latex. In a study of 901 couples over six months, the polyurethane condom was not as effective as the latex condom for pregnancy prevention. Experts now advise against use of condoms with nonoxynol-9, which may increase rather than lower the risk of sexual infections (see discussion in Chapter 16).

Although the theoretical effectiveness rate for condoms is 97 percent, the actual rate is only 80 to 85 percent. The condom can be torn during the manufacturing process or during its use; testing by the manufacturer may not be as strenuous as it could or should be. Careless removal can also decrease the effectiveness of condoms. However, the major reason that condoms have such a low actual effectiveness rate is that couples don't use them each and every time they have sex. Users who have little experience with condoms—who are young, single, or childless, or who engage in risky behaviors—are more likely to have condoms break.

Condoms are second only to the pill in popularity among college-age adults. Half of sexually active students report using condoms the last time they had vaginal intercourse.[8] Nearly one-third of students in one survey reported discomfort, such as a too-tight fit or loss of pleasurable sensation. These students were less likely to use condoms correctly and more likely to report condom breakage. Larger-size condoms and/or vaginal lubricants can eliminate many complaints of discomfort.

College men also may try to avoid condom use because of concern about erectile dysfunction (ED), the inability to maintain a penile erection sufficient for sexual relations. In an anonymous survey of 234 sexually active males between the ages of 18 and 25 on three university campuses, 25 percent reported ED with condom use. These men were much more inconsistent in their use of condoms than other students. Six percent of all the students surveyed had taken ED medications, such as Viagra. Almost two-thirds mixed these medications with alcohol and drugs, such as ecstasy or methamphetamine.

Female Condom   The female condom, made of polyurethane, consists of two rings and a polyurethane sheath, and is inserted into the vagina with a tamponlike applicator (Figure 10.4). Once in place, the device loosely lines the walls of the vagina. Internally, a thickened rubber ring keeps it anchored near

Pinch or twist the tip of the condom, leaving one-half inch at the tip to catch the semen.

Holding the tip, unroll the condom.

Unroll the condom until it reaches the pubic hairs.

Figure 10.3 'Male Condom

Condoms effectively reduce the risk of pregnancy as well as STIs if used consistently and correctly.

the cervix. Externally, another rubber ring, two inches in diameter, rests on the labia and resists slippage.

Although not widely used in the West, female condoms have been distributed in 142 countries.[9] Properly used, it is believed to be as good as or better than the male condom for preventing infections, including HIV, because it is stronger and covers a slightly larger area. Female condoms may be more prone to slipping and other mechanical problems but are as effective as male condoms in blocking semen.[10] The efficacy of female condoms does increase with a woman's experience in using them.

How They Work

Male Condoms Most physicians recommend prelubricated, spermicide-treated, American-made latex or polyurethane condoms, not membrane condoms ("natural" or "sheepskin"). Before using a condom, check the expiration date and make sure it's soft and pliable. If it's yellow or sticky, throw it out. Don't check for leaks by blowing up a condom before using it; you may weaken or tear it.

The condom should be put on at the beginning of sexual activity, before genital contact occurs. There should be a little space left at the top of the condom to catch the semen (Figure 10.3). Any vaginal lubricant should be water-based. Petroleum-based creams or jellies (such as Vaseline, baby oil, massage oil, vegetable oils, or oil-based hand lotions) can deteriorate the latex. After ejaculation, the condom should be held firmly against the penis so that it doesn't slip off or leak during withdrawal. Couples engaging in anal intercourse should use a water-based lubricant as well as a condom, but should never assume the condom will provide 100 percent protection from HIV infection or other STIs.

Female Condom As illustrated in Figure 10.4, a woman removes the condom and applicator from the wrapper and inserts the condom slowly by gently pushing the applicator toward the small of the back. When properly inserted, the outer ring should rest on the folds of skin around the vaginal opening, and the inner ring (the closed end) should fit against the cervix.

Advantages

- Effective when used correctly.

- Lowers a woman's risk of pelvic inflammatory disease (PID) and may protect against some urinary tract and genital infections.

- No side effects, unless the woman is allergic to latex.

- No prescription required.

- Inexpensive.

- The female condom gives women more control in reducing their risk of pregnancy and STIs and does not require a prescription or medical appointment.

Disadvantages

- Requires consistent and diligent use.

- Not 100 percent effective in preventing pregnancy or STIs.

- Risk of manufacturing defects, such as pin-size holes, and breaking or slipping off during intercourse.

- May inhibit sexual spontaneity.

- Users or partners may complain about odor, lubrication (too much or too little), feel, taste, difficulty opening the packages, and disposal.

- Some men dislike reduced penile sensitivity or cannot sustain an erection while putting on a condom.

- Some women complain that the female condom is difficult to use, squeaks, and looks odd.

© Joel Gordon Photography

Figure 10.4
Female Condom
No spermicide is used with the female condom. Like the male condom, this method does not require a prescription.

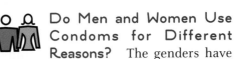 **Do Men and Women Use Condoms for Different Reasons?** The genders have very different motives both for engaging in sex and for using condoms. In focus groups, young women say they engage in sexual relations because of a desire for physical intimacy and a committed relationship. They generally report having sex only with men they care for

condom A latex sheath worn over the penis during sexual acts to prevent conception and/or the transmission of disease; the female condom lines the walls of the vagina.

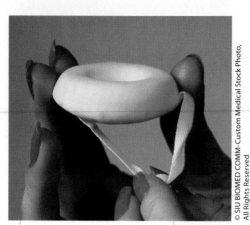

The contraceptive sponge prevents sperm from entering the uterus and is available without a prescription.

and deeply trust and expect that these men would be honest and forthright about their sexual history. This trust plays a significant role in their decision whether to insist on condom use.

In contrast, few young men say relationships are an important dimension of their sexual involvements. Their primary motivation is a desire for physical and sexual satisfaction. Most say they are not interested in commitment and view emotional expectations as a complication of becoming sexually involved with a woman. Young men also admit to making judgments about types of girls. To them, young women they didn't care about were "sluts" with whom they used a condom for their own protection.

Which partner determines whether a couple uses a condom? The answer is often the women—if they choose to do so. Regardless of race or ethnicity, many young women are adamant in demanding that their partners use condoms—and many young men say they would not challenge such a demand out of fear of losing the opportunity for sex. Men often expect potential partners to want to use condoms and describe themselves as "suspicious" of women who do not.

Both sexes name two primary reasons for using condoms: preventing pregnancy and protecting against sexually transmitted infections. Young women see an unwanted pregnancy as an occurrence that would be disruptive and expensive and that could "ruin" their lives and their parents' lives. Young men see condom use as a way of protecting themselves against emotional entanglements and paternity issues. But young adults of both sexes tend to overestimate how consistently they use condoms.[11]

Contraceptive Sponge The Today Sponge, which is made of soft polyurethane foam laced with spermicide, was sold as an over-the-counter contraceptive in the United States from 1983 to 1995, when it was withdrawn because of contamination problems at the manufacturing plant. It has returned to stores several times.

How It Works The contraceptive sponge acts as a barrier by blocking the entrance to the uterus and absorbing and deactivating sperm. Prior to inserting it in the vagina, moisten the sponge with water to activate the spermicide. Then fold it in half and insert deep into the vagina. Check to make sure it is covering the cervix. Intercourse can occur immediately or at any time during the next 24 hours. However, the sponge must remain in place for six hours after intercourse. To remove, gently pull the cloth loop or the tabs on the outside.

Advantages

- Easy to carry and use.
- Can be inserted up to 24 hours before intercourse.
- Effective immediately if used correctly.
- No effect on fertility.
- Generally cannot be felt by a woman or her partner.
- Can be used by women who are breastfeeding.

Contraceptive Sponge

- May be difficult to remove.
- May be less effective in women who have had children.
- No reliable protection against STIs.
- Requires advance planning to place the sponge.
- Side effects include vaginal irritation and allergic reactions.
- Should not be used during menstruation.
- Slightly increased risk of toxic shock syndrome (see Chapter 9).

Vaginal Spermicides The various forms of **vaginal spermicide** include chemical foams, creams, jellies, vaginal suppositories, gels, and film. Some creams and jellies are made for use with a diaphragm; others can be used alone. Several vaginal suppositories claim high effectiveness, but no American studies have confirmed these claims. In general, failure rates for vaginal suppositories are as high as 10 to 25 percent.

One widely used spermicide, nonoxynol-9, has proven to be less effective than once believed. It does not protect against many STIs, including chlamydia and gonorrhea. Nonoxynol-9 also may increase the risk of infection with human papillomavirus (HPV). The CDC has concluded that it is ineffective against HIV, and the World Health Organization describes it as only "moderately effective" for pregnancy prevention.

Vaginal contraceptive film (VCF), a thin two-inch square film laced with spermicide, is folded and inserted into the vagina, where it dissolves into a stay-in-place gel (see Figure 10.5). VCF, which can be used by people allergic to foams and jellies, is as effective as most spermicides and almost 100 percent effective when paired with a condom.

Although more effective methods of birth control now provide good alternatives to spermicides, they remain popular as a means of lowering the risk of STIs.

How They Work Spermicides consist of a chemical that kills sperm and potential pathogens and an inert base, such as jelly, cream, foam, or film, that holds the spermicide close to the cervix. The jelly, cream, or foam spermicide is inserted into the vagina with an applicator or finger. Vaginal suppositories take about 20 minutes to dissolve and cover the vaginal walls. Follow package directions precisely.

You must apply additional spermicide or insert another VCF film before each additional intercourse. After sex, women should shower rather than bathe to prevent the spermicide from being rinsed out of the vagina, and they should not douche for at least six hours.

Advantages

- Easy to use.
- Effective if used with another form of contraception, such as condoms.
- Reduces the risk of some vaginal infections, PID, and STIs.
- No effect on fertility.

Disadvantages

- Insertion interrupts sexual spontaneity.
- May cause irritation.

- Some people cannot use foams or jellies because of an allergic reaction.
- Some users complain that spermicides are messy or interfere with oral-genital contact.
- Spermicidal suppositories that do not dissolve completely can feel gritty.

Prescription Barriers

The prescription barrier contraceptives are used by women: the diaphragm, cervical cap, and FemCap. They are placed in the vagina with a spermicide. They do not protect against HIV infection and most STIs.

Diaphragm The **diaphragm** is a bowl-like rubber cup with a flexible rim that is inserted into the vagina to cover the cervix and prevent the passage of sperm into the uterus during sexual intercourse (Figure 10.6). When used with a spermicide, the diaphragm is both a physical and a chemical barrier to sperm. The effectiveness of the diaphragm in preventing pregnancy depends on strong motivation (to use it faithfully) and a precise understanding of its use. If diaphragms with spermicide are used consistently and carefully, they can be 95 to 98 percent effective. Without a spermicide, the diaphragm is not effective.

Cervical Cap Like the diaphragm, the **cervical cap** combined with spermicide serves as both a chemical and physical barrier blocking the path of the sperm to the uterus. The rubber or plastic cap is smaller and thicker than a diaphragm. It resembles a large thimble that fits snugly around the cervix and may work better for some women. It is about as effective as a diaphragm (95 to 98 percent).

© Joel Gordon Photography

FemCap The FemCap is a nonhormonal, latex-free barrier contraceptive that works with a spermicide (Figure 10.7). The FemCap,

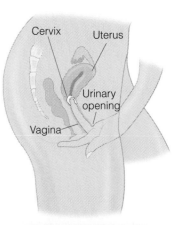

Cervix
Uterus
Urinary opening
Vagina

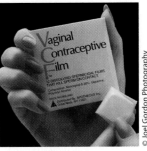
© Joel Gordon Photography

Figure 10.5 Vaginal Contraceptive Film
The effectiveness of this thin film, laced with spermicide, is similar to other spermicides and greatest when used with a condom.

vaginal spermicide A substance that kills or neutralizes sperm, inserted into the vagina in the form of a foam, cream, jelly, suppository, or film.

vaginal contraceptive film (VCF) A small dissolvable sheet saturated with spermicide that can be inserted into the vagina and placed over the cervix.

diaphragm A bowl-like rubber cup with a flexible rim that is inserted into the vagina to cover the cervix and prevent the passage of sperm into the uterus during sexual intercourse; used with a spermicidal foam or jelly, it serves as both a chemical and a physical barrier to sperm.

cervical cap A thimble-size rubber or plastic cap that is inserted into the vagina to fit over the cervix and prevent the passage of sperm into the uterus during sexual intercourse; used with a spermicidal foam or jelly, it serves as both a chemical and a physical barrier to sperm.

Spermicidal cream or jelly

Diaphragm

Squeeze spermicide into dome of diaphragm and around the rim.

Squeeze rim together; insert jelly-side up.   Check placement to make certain cervix is covered.

Figure 10.6 Diaphragm

When used correctly and consistently with a spermicide, the diaphragm is effective in preventing pregnancy. It must be fitted by a health-care professional.

Courtesy of FemCap, Inc., and Alfred Shihata, MD

Figure 10.7 FemCap

The FemCap must be used with spermicide and correctly positioned to cover the cervix completely.

Source: Reproduced with permission from FemCap, Inc., and Alfred Shihata, M.D.

designed to conform to the anatomy of the cervix and vagina, comes in three sizes. The smallest usually best suits women who have never been pregnant; the medium size, for women who have been pregnant but have not had a vaginal delivery; the largest, for those who have delivered a full-term baby vaginally.

How They Work

Diaphragm   Diaphragms are fitted and prescribed by a qualified health-care professional in diameter sizes ranging from two to four inches (50 to 105 millimeters). The diaphragm's main function is to serve as a container for a spermicidal (sperm-killing) foam or jelly, which is available at pharmacies without a prescription. A diaphragm should remain in the vagina for at least six hours after intercourse to ensure that all sperm are killed. If intercourse occurs again during this period, additional spermicide must be inserted with an applicator tube.

The key to proper use of the diaphragm is having it available. A sexually active woman should keep it in the most accessible place— her purse, bedroom, bathroom. Before every use, a diaphragm should be checked for tiny leaks (hold up to the light or place water in the dome). A health-care provider should check its fit and condition every year when the woman has her annual Pap smear. Oil-based lubricants will deteriorate the latex of the diaphragm and should not be used.

Cervical Cap   Like the diaphragm, the cervical cap is fitted by a qualified health-care professional. For use, the woman fills it one-third to two-thirds full with spermicide and inserts it by holding its edges together and sliding it into the vagina. The cup is then pressed onto the cervix. (Most women find it easiest to do so while squatting or in an upright sitting position.) The cap can be inserted up to six hours prior to intercourse and should not be removed for at least six hours afterward. It can be left in place up to 24 hours. Pulling on one side of the rim breaks the suction and allows easy removal. Oil-based lubricants should not be used with the cap because they can deteriorate the latex.

FemCap   A prescription is required to purchase FemCap, and the woman selects the appropriate size. Apply spermicide to the bowl of the FemCap (which goes over the cervix), to the outer brim, and to the groove that will face into the vagina. Insert the squeezed, flattened cap into the vagina with the bowl facing upward. The FemCap must be pushed all the way in to cover the cervix completely and left in place at least six hours after intercourse.

Advantages

- Relatively inexpensive.
- Doesn't interrupt sexual activity; can be inserted hours ahead of time.
- Usually not felt by either partner.
- Can easily be carried in pocket or purse.
- No hormones or side effects.
- Cervical caps are an alternative for women who cannot use diaphragms or find them too messy.

Disadvantages

- Less effective than hormonal contraceptives.
- Available by prescription only.
- Requires advance planning or interruption of sexual activity to position the device before intercourse.
- May slip out of place during intercourse.
- May be uncomfortable for some women and their partners.
- Spermicidal foams, creams, and jellies may be messy, cause irritation, and detract from oral–genital sex.
- Some diaphragm users report bladder discomfort, urethral irritation, or recurrent cystitis.
- Some cap users find it difficult to insert and remove and uncomfortable to wear.
- Slightly increased risk of toxic shock syndrome.

Hormonal Contraceptives

In recent years, birth control methods made with synthetic hormones have become available in a variety of forms. Oral contraceptives have been available for decades, and the birth control pill is one of the most well-researched medications. Other options for hormonal birth control include a skin patch, a vaginal ring, a three-month injection, and a three-year implant. All are extremely effective when used consistently and conscientiously.

Hormonal contraceptives do not protect against HIV infection and other STIs, so condoms and spermicides should also be used to get protection against infections.

Oral Contraceptives

The *pill*—the popular term for **oral contraceptives**—is the method of birth control preferred by unmarried women and by those under age 30, including college students. About one in five American women of childbearing age uses the pill.[12] Women 18 to 24 years old are most likely to choose oral contraceptives. In use for 40 years, the pill is one of the most researched, tested, and carefully followed medications in medical history—and one of the most controversial.

Although many women incorrectly think that the risks of the pill are greater than those of pregnancy and childbirth, long-term studies show that oral contraceptive use does not increase mortality rates. Combination oral contraceptives significantly reduce the risk of ovarian and endometrial cancer and produce no increase in diabetes, multiple sclerosis, rheumatoid arthritis, and liver disease. However, there is evidence of increased risk of breast cancer in women who have taken the pill within the last ten years for more than a year.[13]

Common antibiotics, including many prescribed for dental procedures or skin conditions, may lower the effectiveness of oral contraceptives, particularly low-dose birth control pills. Always ask a dentist or doctor who prescribes an antibiotic about its potential effect on your oral contraceptive, and check with your gynecologist or primary physician about using an additional nonhormonal means of contraception (such as a condom) to ensure protection against an unwanted pregnancy. Other medicines and supplements that may make hormonal contraceptives less effective include St. John's wort, certain pills prescribed for yeast infections, certain HIV medications, and certain antiseizure medication.

Combination Pills These pills consist of two hormones, synthetic estrogen and progestin, which play important roles in

oral contraceptives Preparations of synthetic hormones that inhibit ovulation; also referred to as birth control pills or simply the pill.

Various types of birth control pills contain different hormones and combinations of hormones.

controlling ovulation and the menstrual cycle. The doses in today's oral contraceptives are much lower—less than one-fourth the amount of estrogen and one-twentieth the progestin in the original pill. This means fewer side effects and lower risk of heart disease and stroke.[14] Stroke risk among women taking newer, low-dose formulations of oral contraceptive pills may be extremely low. However, these pills appear to be less effective than those approved decades ago, with twice the failure rate of previous products. The reason seems to be lower doses of hormones that stop ovulation. Women on low-dose oral contraceptives should take their pills at the same time every day and follow their doctor's advice if they miss a dose.[15]

Monophasic pills release a constant dose of estrogen and progestin throughout a woman's menstrual cycle. **Multiphasic pills** mimic normal hormonal fluctuations of the natural menstrual cycle by providing different levels of estrogen and progesterone at different times of the month. Multiphasic pills reduce total hormonal dose and side effects. Both monophasic and multiphasic pills block the release of hormones that would stimulate the process leading to ovulation. They also thicken and alter the cervical mucus, making it more hostile to sperm, and they make implantation of a fertilized egg in the uterine lining more difficult.

One combination pill, Yasmin, contains a unique progestin that works like a mild diuretic and prevents fluid retention. YAZ, a lower-dose 24-day version, can ease the emotional and physical symptoms of premenstrual dysphoric disorder (discussed in Chapter 9).[16] Women who are taking

potassium supplements, daily anti-inflammatory drugs, or heparin (a blood-thinner) should talk with their doctor because of potentially dangerous drug interactions. Other pills offer different benefits, such as clearer skin and reduced facial hair, and less spotting.

Progestin–Only Pills Progestin-only "minipills" contain only a small amount of progestin and no estrogen. They work somewhat differently than combination pills. Women taking **progestin-only pills** probably ovulate, at least occasionally. In those cycles, the pills prevent pregnancy by thickening cervical mucus, making it hard for sperm to penetrate, and by interfering with implantation of a fertilized egg.

The risk of heart disease and stroke is lower with progestin-only pills than with any combination pill. For this reason, they are a good choice for women over age 35 and others who cannot take estrogen-containing pills because of high blood pressure, diabetes, or clotting disorders. Because they do not affect the quality or quantity of breast milk, progestin-only pills often are recommended for nursing mothers, and they are recommended for smokers. Because progestin can affect mood and worsen the symptoms of depression, progestin-only pills are not recommended for women with a history of depression. Antiseizure medications, such as Dilantin, which accelerate liver metabolism, may make the minipill less effective.

Users of progestin-only pills have to be conscientious about taking these pills, not just every day, but at the same time every day. If you take a progestin-only pill three or more hours later than usual, use a backup method of contraception, such as a condom, for two days after you resume taking the pill.

How They Work The pill usually comes in 28-day packets: 21 of the pills contain the hormones, and 7 are "blanks," included so that the woman can take a pill every day, even during her menstrual period. If a woman forgets to take one pill, she should take it as soon as she remembers. However, if she forgets during the first week of her cycle or misses more than one pill, she should rely on another form of birth control until her next menstrual period.

Even if you experience no discomfort or side effects while on the pill, see a physician at least once a year for an examination, which should include a blood pressure test, a pelvic exam, and a breast exam. Notify your doctor at once if you develop severe abdominal pain, chest pain, coughing, shortness of breath, pain or tenderness in the calf or thigh, severe headaches, dizziness, faintness, muscle weakness or numbness, speech disturbance, blurred vision, a sensation of flashing lights, a breast lump, severe depression, or yellowing of your skin.

Generally, when a woman stops taking the pill, her menstrual cycle resumes the next month, but it may be irregular for the next couple of months. However, 2 to 4 percent of pill users experience prolonged delays. Women who become pregnant during the first or second cycle after discontinuing use of the pill may be at greater risk of miscarriage; they also are more likely to conceive twins.

Advantages

- Extremely effective when taken consistently.
- Convenient.
- Moderately priced.
- Does not interrupt sexual activity.
- Reversible within three months of stopping the pill.
- Reduces the risk of benign breast lumps, ovarian cysts, iron-deficiency anemia, pelvic inflammatory disease, endometrial and ovarian cancer.
- May relieve painful menstruation.

Disadvantages

- Requires a prescription.
- Increases risk of cardiovascular problems, primarily for women over age 35 who smoke and those with high blood pressure or other health problems.
- Side effects vary with different brands but include spotting between periods, weight gain or loss, nausea and vomiting, breast tenderness, and decreased sex drive.
- Must be taken at the same time every day (especially critical with low-dose estrogen and progestin-only pills).

- No protection against STIs.
- Must use a secondary form of birth control for the initial seven days of use.

Before Using Oral Contraceptives Before starting on the pill, you should undergo a thorough physical examination that includes the following tests:

- Routine blood pressure test.
- Pelvic exam, including a Pap smear.
- Breast exam.
- Blood test.
- Urine sample.

Let your doctor know about any personal or family incidence of high blood pressure or heart disease; diabetes; liver dysfunction; hepatitis; unusual menstrual history; severe depression; sickle-cell anemia; cancer of the breast, ovaries, or uterus; high cholesterol levels; or migraine headaches. (See Consumer Alert, p. 314.)

Extended-Use Pills

For years physicians have prescribed prolonged use of birth control pills to lessen the number of menstrual cycles for women with asthma, migraines, rashes, or other conditions that flare up during their periods. Eliminating periods eliminates symptoms, and having fewer cycles also may lower a woman's long-term risk of ovarian cancer. However, some women are wary of long-term hormone use or consider a lack of menstrual cycles unnatural.

Seasonale and Seasonique Seasonale and Seasonique are prescription forms of oral contraception that prevent pregnancy as effectively as other birth control pills but produce only four menstrual periods a year.

How They Work Unlike traditional birth control pills, women take "active" pills continuously for three months or 84 days. During this time, Seasonale prevents the uterine lining from thickening enough to produce a full menstrual period. Every three months, a woman takes one week of inactive pills to produce a "pill period," which may be lighter than a regular period. With Seasonique, women take a very low dose of estrogen for

monophasic pill An oral contraceptive that releases synthetic estrogen and progestin at constant levels throughout the menstrual cycle.

multiphasic pill An oral contraceptive that releases different levels of estrogen and progestin to mimic the hormonal fluctuations of the natural menstrual cycle.

minipill, progestin-only pill An oral contraceptive containing a small amount of progestin and no estrogen, which prevents contraception by making the mucus in the cervix so thick that sperm cannot enter the uterus.

The Risks of Contraceptives

For individuals with certain medical conditions, specific types of birth control can pose a health risk.

Facts to Know

If you have one of the following conditions, you should talk with your doctor about which types of contraceptive may increase your health risks:

- High blood pressure.
- Episodes of depression.
- Seizure disorder.
- Ectopic pregnancy.
- Hepatitis.

Steps to Take

- **High blood pressure** (180/110 mmHg or higher): Avoid birth control pills or injections containing estrogen, which may increase your risk of a heart attack or stroke.
- **Episodes of depression:** Avoid products that contain progestin, such as Depo-Provera, the contraceptive implant and the minipill. In some women with depression, progestin may worsen depressive symptoms. Also, check with your doctor if you are taking an antidepressant medication; it may affect or be affected by oral contraceptives and you may require a different dose.
- **Seizure disorder:** Avoid low-dose birth control pills. Some antiseizure medications, such as Dilantin, accelerate liver metabolism of all substances, including oral contraceptives, and make them less effective.
- **Ectopic pregnancy:** Avoid IUDs. Although IUDs do not cause ectopic pregnancies, if your fallopian tubes have been scarred by a previous ectopic gestation, you're more likely to have another ectopic if you use an IUD.
- **Hepatitis:** Avoid birth control pills or injections containing estrogen, which is metabolized in the liver—an organ damaged by hepatitis.

seven days to eliminate any symptoms of complete hormone withdrawal.

The chance of getting pregnant ranges from 5 percent with typical use to 1 percent with perfect use. For maximum effectiveness, each pill should be taken at the same time of day.

Advantages

- Fewer periods.
- Tri-monthly periods are usually lighter, with less blood flow.

Disadvantages

- Similar to those of other oral contraceptives in terms of health risks, costs, and side effects. Cigarette smoking increases these risks.
- No protection from STIs.

- More spotting and breakthrough bleeding than with a 28-day pill.
- Determining pregnancy is difficult without a monthly period.

Lybrel, the "No-Period" Pill Lybrel, described as a continuous contraceptive, works the same way as other combination hormonal birth control pills. However, women take the "365-day" pill every single day without interruption.

How It Works Like other oral contraceptives, Lybrel stops the body's monthly preparation for pregnancy by lowering the production of hormones that make pregnancy possible. However, it does not include the "week-off" of placebo pills that leads to vaginal bleeding. Most women resume menstruation within 90 days of stopping Lybrel.

Medical experts see no long-term risk in doing away with regular monthly periods, but the long-term safety of menstrual suppression is unknown.

Advantages

- No menstrual periods, cramps, or other symptoms.
- No need to stop taking pills or to switch to dummy pills for a week.
- Relief from menstruation-linked conditions such as endometriosis and menstrual migraine.

Disadvantages

- Spotting, which generally tapers off over the first year of use.
- Health risks similar to those of other combination pills.
- Determining pregnancy is difficult without a monthly period.
- Some women feel that eliminating periods is unnatural.

The Patch (Ortho Evra)

The Ortho Evra birth control patch, the first transdermal (through the skin) contraceptive, works like a combination pill but looks like a Band-Aid. Embedded in its adhesive layer are two hormones, a low-dose estrogen and a progestin. It prevents pregnancy by delivering continuous levels of estrogen and progestin through the skin directly into the bloodstream so women are exposed to higher overall levels of estrogen, which may increase their risk of blood clots. The patch is waterproof and stays on in the shower, swimming pool, or hot tub.

© Ortho McNeil Pharmaceutical

How It Works   A woman applies the 1 3/4-inch square to her back, upper arm, lower abdomen, or buttocks and changes it every seven days for three weeks. During the patch-free week, she experiences menstrual bleeding. A user should check every day to make sure the patch is still in place. If you don't replace a detached patch within 24 hours, use a backup method of contraception until your next period.

Advantages

- Good alternative for women who can't remember, don't like, or have problems swallowing daily pills.
- Highly effective when used correctly.
- Does not interrupt sexual activity.
- Fewer side effects, such as nausea, breakthrough bleeding, and mood swings, than pills.
- Fertility returns quickly after you stop using it.

Disadvantages

- Must apply a new patch every week.
- Requires a prescription.
- No protection against STIs.
- Increases risk of blood clots, heart attack, and stroke, particularly for women who smoke or have certain health conditions. The risk of dying or suffering a survivable blood clot while using the patch is estimated to be about three times higher than while using birth control pills.

- Less effective in women who weigh more than 198 pounds.
- Some women report breast tenderness, headaches, bleeding between periods, upper respiratory infections, or self-consciousness wearing the patch.
- Contact lens wearers may experience vision changes.
- Five percent of women report that at least one patch slipped off; 2 percent report skin irritation.
- Must use another form of birth control for the initial seven days of use.

The NuvaRing

The silver-dollar-size NuvaRing, a two-inch ring made of flexible, transparent plastic, slowly emits the same hormones as oral contraceptives through the vaginal tissues (Figure 10.8). Smaller than the smallest diaphragm, it contains less estrogen than any pill. As effective as the pill, it provides a steady dose of hormones and causes fewer side effects.

How It Works   Unlike a diaphragm, the NuvaRing does not have to be exactly positioned within the vagina or used with a spermicide. The flexible, plastic two-inch ring compresses so a woman can easily insert it. Each ring stays in place for three weeks, then is removed for the fourth week of the menstrual cycle.

   If a NuvaRing pops out (uncommon but possible), it should be washed, dried, and replaced within three hours. If a longer time passes, users should rely on a backup form of birth control until the ring has been reinserted for a week and the medications have risen to protective levels again.

Advantages

- Under medical supervision, may be safer than birth control pills for women with mild hypertension or diabetes.
- Less likelihood of pill-related side effects, such as nausea, mood swings, spotting, and cramping.
- No need to remember a daily pill or weekly patch.
- Fertility returns quickly when ring is removed.

ORGANON Communications

Figure 10.8   NuvaRing
The NuvaRing releases estrogen and progestin, preventing ovulation. The exact position of the NuvaRing in the vagina is not critical.

Disadvantages

- Some women do not feel comfortable placing and removing something inside their vagina.
- Possible side effects include vaginal discharge, irritation, and infection.
- Cannot use oil-based vaginal medications for yeast infections while ring is in place.
- No protection against STIs.

Contraceptive Injections

A progestin-only contraceptive is available in the form of a birth control "shot" or injection. Depo-Provera or its newer form, Depo-subQ Provera, must be given every 12 weeks. Contraceptive injections provide no protection against HIV and other STIs.

Because of the risk of significant bone mineral loss, the FDA has recommended that women not use Depo-Provera for longer than two years. Although mineral loss is common and greater in the first year of use, most individuals regain bone density after discontinuing its use.[17]

How It Works   One injection of this synthetic version of the natural hormone progesterone provides three months of contraceptive protection. This long-acting hormonal contraceptive raises levels of progesterone, thereby simulating pregnancy. The pituitary gland doesn't produce FSH and LH, which normally cause egg ripening and release. The endometrial lining of the uterus thins, preventing implantation of a fertilized egg.

Advantages

- Because it contains only progestin, it is safe for women who cannot take combination birth control pills.
- No risk of user error.
- No worry about buying, storing, or using contraceptives.
- No need to think about contraception for three months at a time.
- Possible protection against endometrial and ovarian cancer.

- Can be used by women who are breast-feeding.

Disadvantages

- Must visit a doctor or clinic every three months for injection.
- Menstrual cycles become irregular. After a year, 50 percent of women stop having periods.
- Potential side effects include decreased sex drive, depression, headaches, dizziness, frequent urination, allergic reactions, hair loss or increased hair growth.
- Increased weight gain, especially for obese women and teenage girls.
- No protection against STIs.
- According to a recent NIH study, appears to triple risk of acquiring chlamydia and gonorrhea compared with women not using a hormonal contraceptive. Scientists do not know the reason for this increased risk.
- Delayed return of fertility.
- Long-term use may significantly reduce bone density.

Contraceptive Implant (Implanon)

This thin, flexible, plastic implant—about the size of a matchstick—is inserted under the skin of the upper arm to provide birth control that is 99 percent effective for up to three years. Easier to insert and remove than earlier implants, Implanon is not yet widely available in the United States, but has been used in other countries for years.

How It Works   Implanon works primarily by releasing progestin and suppressing ovulation. It also thickens cervical mucus, which inhibits sperm movement, inhibits the development and growth of the uterine lining, and limits secretion of progesterone during the second half of the menstrual cycle.

Advantages

- Can be used while breast-feeding.
- Can be used by women who cannot take estrogen.
- Provides continuous long-lasting birth control without sterilization.
- No medicine to take every day.

of contraception. An X-ray called a hystero-salpingogram must confirm that the inserts are correctly placed and the fallopian tubes are completely blocked.

Like traditional forms of tubal ligation, Essure cannot be reversed. It is recommended only for women who definitely do not want more children and especially for those with medical and health problems (such as diabetes, heart disease, or obesity) that make surgery and anesthesia more dangerous. There is a risk that the micro-inserts may not be placed correctly at the first attempt (this occurred in 14 percent of women in one study). Long-term data on the effectiveness of Essure are not yet available.

Advantages of Sterilization

- Offers permanent protection against unwanted pregnancy.
- No effect on sex drive in men or women. Many couples report greater sexual activity and pleasure because they no longer have to worry about pregnancy or deal with contraceptives.
- Vasectomy and tubal ligation are performed as outpatient procedures, with a quick recovery time.
- Use of Essure requires no incision, so there's less discomfort and very rapid recovery. Essure may be an option for women with chronic health conditions,

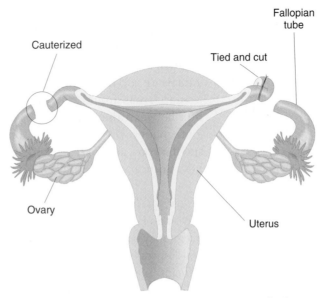

Figure 10.11 Female Sterilization, or Tubal Ligation

such as obesity, diabetes, or heart disease.

Disadvantages of Sterilization

- All procedures should be considered permanent and used only if both partners are certain they want no more children.
- No protection against STIs.
- Must use another form of birth control for first three months.
- Many long-term risks remain unknown, but there is no evidence of any link between vasectomy and prostate cancer.

sterilization A surgical procedure to end a person's reproductive capability.

vasectomy A surgical sterilization procedure in which each vas deferens is cut and tied shut to stop the passage of sperm to the urethra for ejaculation.

tubal ligation The suturing or tying shut of the fallopian tubes to prevent pregnancy.

tubal occlusion The blocking of the fallopian tubes to prevent pregnancy.

laparoscopy A surgical sterilization procedure in which the fallopian tubes are observed, with a laparoscope inserted through a small incision, and then cut or blocked.

Abortion

No woman in any country ever chooses to be in a situation where she has to consider abortion. But if faced with an unwanted pregnancy, many women consider *elective abortion* as an option.

 The U.S. abortion rate, which has declined in the last two decades, still remains higher than that of many Western countries, including Canada, Great Britain, the Netherlands, and Sweden. Although there is no one single or simple explanation for this difference, researchers focus on America's high rate of unintended

pregnancies. In many nations with fewer unwanted pregnancies and lower abortion rates, contraceptives are generally easier and cheaper to obtain, and early sex education strongly emphasizes their importance.

After rising steadily through the 1970s, the number of legal abortions leveled off in the 1980s and has declined since.[26] Although women of all backgrounds have abortions, abortion in the United States is most likely to occur among single women, racial or ethnic minorities, low-income women, and women who have had at least one child.

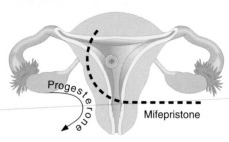

Step 1. Taken early in pregnancy, mifepristone blocks the action of progesterone and makes the body react as if it weren't pregnant.

Step 2. Prostaglandins, taken two days later, cause the uterus to contract and the cervix to soften and dilate. As a result, the fertilized egg is expelled in 97 percent of cases.

Figure 10.12
Medical Abortion

Mifepristone works by blocking the action of progesterone, a hormone produced by the ovaries that is necessary for the implantation and development of a fertilized egg.

medical abortion Method of ending a pregnancy within nine weeks of conception using hormonal medications that cause expulsion of the fertilized egg.

Claims that abortion increases the risk of breast cancer, based on retrospective studies that are less accurate because they rely on individuals' recall, have proved false. Research has found no correlation between the termination of a pregnancy, whether induced or spontaneous, and increased risk of breast cancer.

Thinking Through the Options

A woman faced with an unwanted pregnancy—often alone, unwed, and desperate—can find it extremely difficult to decide what to do. The political debate over the right to life almost always is secondary to practical and emotional matters, such as the quality of her relationship with the baby's father, their capacity to provide for the child, the impact on any children she already has, and other important life issues.

Giving up her child for adoption is an option for women who do not feel abortion is right for them. Because the number of would-be adoptive parents greatly exceeds the number of available newborns, some women considering adoption may feel pressured by offers of money from couples eager to adopt. Others, particularly minority women, may feel cultural pressures to keep a child—regardless of their age, economic situation, or ability to care for an infant. Advocates of adoption reform are pressing for mandatory counseling for all pregnant women considering adoption (available now in agency-arranged, but not private, adoptions) and for extending the period of time during which a new mother can change her mind about giving up her child for adoption.

Medical Abortion

The term **medical abortion** describes the use of drugs, also called *abortifacients*, to terminate a pregnancy. In 2000, the abortion pill mifepristone *(Mifeprex)*, formerly known as RU-486, became available for use in the United States. Mifepristone, which is 97 percent effective in inducing abortion, blocks progesterone, the hormone that prepares the uterine lining for pregnancy. Two

days after taking this compound, a woman takes a prostaglandin to increase uterine contractions. The uterine lining is expelled along with the fertilized egg (Figure 10.12).

Women have compared the discomfort of this experience to severe menstrual cramps. Common side effects include excessive bleeding, nausea, fatigue, abdominal pain, and dizziness. About 1 woman in 100 requires a blood transfusion. The FDA has warned doctors about rare but deadly bloodstream infections in women using mifepristone. The rate of infection is about 1 in 100,000 uses, comparable to infection risks with surgical abortions and childbirth.

Although condemned by right-to-life advocates, abortion medications may in time lower the public profile of pregnancy termination. They are not painless, cheap, or equally available to all, but they do offer women a chance to carry through on their personal choice in greater privacy and safety.

Medical abortion does not require anesthesia and can be performed very early in pregnancy. However, women experience more cramping and bleeding during medical abortion than during surgical abortion, and bleeding lasts for a longer period.

Other Abortion Methods

About half of all abortions (54 percent) are performed within the first 8 weeks of pregnancy. Only about 1 percent of abortions occur after 20 weeks. Medically, first-trimester abortion is less risky than childbirth. However, the likelihood of complications increases when abortions are performed in the second trimester (the second three-month period) of pregnancy.

The majority of abortions performed in the United States today are surgical. **Suction curettage,** usually done from 7 to 13 weeks after the last menstrual period, involves the gradual dilation (opening) of the cervix, often by inserting into the cervix one or more sticks of *laminaria* (a sterilized seaweed that absorbs moisture and expands, thus gradually stretching the cervix). Some women feel pressure or cramping with the laminaria in place. Occasionally, the laminaria itself starts to bring on a miscarriage.

At the time of abortion, the laminaria is removed, and dilators are used to further enlarge the cervical opening, if needed. The physician inserts a suction tip into the cervix, and the uterine contents are drawn out via a vacuum system (Figure 10.13). A *curette* (a spoon-shaped surgical instrument used for scraping) is used to check for complete removal of the contents of the uterus. With suction curettage, the risks of complication are low. Major complications, such as perforation of the uterus, occur in fewer than 1 in 100 cases.

For early second-trimester abortions, physicians generally use a technique called **dilation and evacuation (D and E),** in which they open the cervix and use medical instruments to remove the fetus from the uterus. D and E procedures are performed under local or general anesthesia.

To induce abortion from week 16 to week 20, prostaglandins (natural substances found in most body tissues) are administered as vaginal suppositories or injected into the amniotic sac by inserting a needle through the abdominal wall. They induce uterine contractions, and the fetus and placenta are expelled within 24 hours. Injecting saline or urea solutions into the amniotic sac also can terminate the pregnancy by triggering contractions that expel the fetus and placenta. Sometimes vaginal suppositories or drugs that help the uterus contract are used. Complications from abortion techniques that induce labor include nausea, vomiting, diarrhea, tearing of the cervix, excessive bleeding, and possible shock and death.

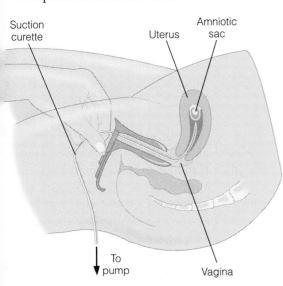

Suction curette

Uterus

Amniotic sac

To pump

Vagina

Figure 10.13 Suction Curettage
The contents of the uterus are extracted through the cervix with a vacuum apparatus.

The Psychological Impact of Abortion

Abortion can have various psychological effects. As decades of research have shown, the primary emotion of women who have just had an abortion is relief. Although many women also express feelings of guilt or sadness, usually their anxiety levels drop to lower levels than immediately before the abortion. Women who experienced violence, including rape, or high anxiety levels prior to becoming pregnant have more anxiety symptoms following an abortion.[27] A Scandinavian study recently found a higher prevalence of depression among young adult women who have had an abortion.[28]

A woman's responses to abortion often change with passing days, weeks, months, or years. Anniversaries—of conception, of the date a woman found out she was pregnant, of the abortion, of the delivery date—can trigger memories and a sense of loss, but most women deal with these and move on with their lives.

The best predictor of psychological well-being after abortion is a woman's emotional well-being prior to pregnancy. At highest risk are women who have had a psychiatric illness, such as an anxiety disorder or clinical depression, prior to an abortion, and those whose abortions occurred among complicated circumstances (such as a rape, or coercion by parents or a partner). The vast majority of women manage to put the abortion into perspective as one of many life events.

The Politics of Abortion

Abortion is one of the most controversial political, religious, and ethical issues of our time. The issues of when life begins, a woman's right to choose, and an unborn child's right to survival are among the most divisive Americans face. Abortions were legal in the United States until the 1860s. For decades after that, women who decided to terminate unwanted pregnancies did so by attempting to abort on their own or by obtaining illegal abortions—often performed by untrained individuals using unsanitary and unsafe procedures. In the late 1960s, some states changed their laws to make abortions legal. In 1973, the U.S. Supreme Court, following a 1970 ruling on the case of *Roe v. Wade* by the

suction curettage A procedure in which the contents of the uterus are removed by means of suction and scraping.

dilation and evacuation (D and E) A medical procedure in which the contents of the uterus are removed through the use of instruments.

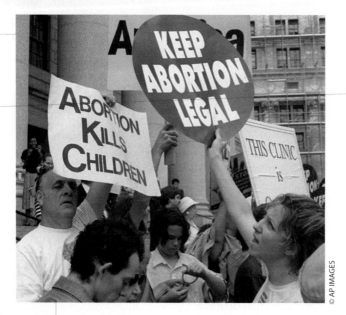

The controversy over abortion has resulted in countless demonstrations and encounters between pro-choice and pro-life supports.

patients and staff members. Although the majority of Americans continue to support abortion, many feel that it should be more restricted and difficult to obtain.

The Supreme Court has upheld a federal law banning "partial-birth" abortions, a late-term procedure involving the removal of a fetus from the uterus and the collapsing of its skull. Pro-life groups hailed this ruling as a step toward the overthrow of *Roe v. Wade.*[29] More than 40 years after this landmark ruling, the controversy over abortion and the conflict between pro-lifers and pro-choicers remains intense. (See Point/Counterpoint, p. 325.)

A Cross-Cultural Perspective

More than one in four pregnancies worldwide ends in abortion. Of the estimated 46 million global abortions, an estimated 20 million are illegal and lead to the death of about 70,000 women.

More than 50 countries now allow abortion up to at least the twelfth week of pregnancy. Some, such as Great Britain, permit it up to 24 weeks; others have no time limit. In recent years abortion has become more restrictive in terms of limits on timing, grounds, or methods in the United States, Russia, Hungary, and Poland. Nicaragua and El Salvador have banned the practice outright. Romania has the world's highest abortion rate; three in four pregnancies are terminated. In the United States, Australia, Canada, Great Britain, and most of Western Europe, around 15 to 25 percent of pregnancies end in abortion.

New York Supreme Court, said that an abortion in the first trimester of pregnancy was a decision between a woman and her physician and was protected by privacy laws. The Court further ruled that abortion during the second trimester could be performed on the basis of health risks and that abortion during the final trimester could be performed only for the sake of the mother's health.

The debate over abortion continues to stir passionate emotions, with pro-life supporters arguing that life begins at conception and that abortion is therefore immoral, and pro-choice advocates countering that an individual woman should have the right to make decisions about her body and health. The controversy over abortion has at times become violent: Physicians who perform abortions have been shot and killed; abortion clinics have been bombed, wounding and killing

Childfree by Choice

More women and men are deliberately choosing to remain "childfree." According to the limited data available, single childfree women tend to be better educated, more cosmopolitan, less religious, and more professional than those in the general population. In general, childfree women are high achievers, often in demanding careers, who describe their work as exciting and satisfying. Childfree couples are predominantly urban,

well-educated, and upper middle class, with egalitarian and long-running marriages.

Their reasons for not having children are diverse: a desire to maintain their freedom and have more time with their partners, career ambitions, concern about overpopulation and the fate of the earth. Some women cite the hostile work environment for mothers and the inadequacy of day care. Others say they're disillusioned with the have-it-all hopes of baby boomers and believe in a have-most-of-it philosophy.

POINT

Life, from the moment of conception, is sacred, and no one has the right to end it. The laws permitting abortion in this country should be overturned. Because abortion is morally wrong, women should be counseled toward other options, such as adoption.

COUNTERPOINT

A woman's body is her own, and she alone has the right to choose whether to carry a pregnancy to term. Rather than forcing women to jeopardize their own lives by resorting to illegal abortions, the government should guarantee safe, legal abortions to women who choose to terminate a pregnancy.

YOUR VIEW

Where do you stand on one of the most heated controversies of our time? Do you see abortion as a moral or a political issue? How do you feel about those with opposing views? Why do you think that the issue of abortion ignites such intense and emotional debate?

Pregnancy

Birth rates rose to the highest ever recorded in the U.S. in 2007. Births rose among all racial and age groups, including teenagers and unmarried women.[30] The average age of mothers in the United States has risen, but about 70 percent of babies are still born to women in their twenties. Mothers are now averaging about two children each.

The number of never-married, college-educated, career women who are becoming single parents has risen dramatically. They want children—with or without an ongoing relationship with a man—and may feel that, because of their age, they can't delay getting pregnant any longer.

Preconception Care

The time *before* a child is conceived can be crucial in ensuring that an infant is born healthy, full-size, and full-term. Women who smoke, drink alcohol, take drugs, eat poorly, are too thin or too heavy, suffer from unrecognized infections or illnesses, or are exposed to toxins at work or home may start pregnancy with one or more strikes against them and their unborn babies. The best chance for lowering the infant mortality rate and preventing birth defects is before pregnancy. **Preconception care**—the enhancement of a woman's health and well-being prior to conception in order to ensure a healthy pregnancy and baby—includes risk assessment (evaluation of medical, genetic, and lifestyle risks), health promotion (such as teaching good nutrition), and

interventions to reduce risk (such as treatment of infections and other diseases, and assistance in quitting smoking or drug use).

Home Pregnancy Tests

The sooner a woman realizes she is pregnant, the more she can do to take care of herself and her child. Home pregnancy tests detect the presence of human chorionic gonadotropin (hCG), which is secreted as the fertilized egg implants in the uterus. If the concentration of hCG is high enough, a woman will test positive for pregnancy. If the test is done too early, the result will be a false negative. A follow-up test a week later can usually confirm a pregnancy. Although home pregnancy tests are 85 to 95 percent accurate, medical laboratory tests provide definitive confirmation of a pregnancy.

How a Woman's Body Changes During Pregnancy

The 40 weeks of pregnancy transform a woman's body. At the beginning of pregnancy, the woman's uterus becomes slightly larger, and the cervix becomes softer and bluish due to increased blood flow. Progesterone and estrogen trigger changes in the milk glands and ducts in the breasts, which increase in size and feel somewhat tender. The pressure of the growing uterus against the bladder causes a more frequent need to urinate. As the pregnancy progresses, the woman's skin

preconception care Health care to prepare for pregnancy.

stretches as her body shape changes, her center of gravity changes as her abdomen protrudes, and her internal organs shift as the baby grows (Figure 10.14). Pregnancy is typically divided into three-month periods called trimesters.

How a Baby Grows

Silently and invisibly, over a nine-month period, a fertilized egg develops into a human being. When the zygote reaches the uterus, it's still smaller than the head of a pin. Once nestled into the spongy uterine lining, it becomes an **embryo.** The embryo takes on an elongated shape, rounded at one end. A sac called the **amnion** envelops it (see photo in Fig. 10.15). As water and other small molecules cross the amniotic membrane, the embryo floats freely in the absorbed fluid, cushioned from shocks and bumps. At nine weeks the embryo is called a **fetus.**

A special organ, the **placenta,** forms. Attached to the embryo by the umbilical cord, it supplies the growing baby with fluid and nutrients from the maternal bloodstream and carries waste back to the mother's body for disposal (Figure 10.15).

Complications of Pregnancy

In about 10 to 15 percent of all pregnancies, there is increased risk of some problem, such as a baby's failure to grow normally. *Perinatology*, or maternal-fetal medicine, focuses on the special needs of high-risk mothers and their unborn babies. Perinatal centers, with state-of-the-art equipment and 24-hour staffs of specialists in this field, have been set up around the country. Several of the most frequent potential complications of pregnancy are discussed next.

Ectopic Pregnancy Any woman who is of childbearing age, has had intercourse, and feels abdominal pain with no reasonable

First Trimester

Increased urination because of hormonal changes and the pressure of the enlarging uterus on the bladder.
Enlarged breasts as milk glands develop.
Darkening of the nipples and the area around them.
Nausea or vomiting, particularly in the morning, may occur.
Fatigue.
Increased vaginal secretions.
Pinching of the sciatic nerve, which runs from the buttocks down through the back of the legs, may occur as the pelvic bones widen and begin to separate.

Second Trimester

Thickening of the waist as the uterus grows.
Weight gain.
Increase in total blood volume.
Slight increase in size and change in position of the heart.
Darkening of the pigment around the nipple and from the navel to the pubic region.
Darkening of the face.
Increased salivation and perspiration.
Secretion of colostrum from the breasts.

Third Trimester

Increased urination because of pressure from the uterus.
Tightening of the uterine muscles (called Braxton-Hicks contractions).
Shortness of breath because of increased pressure by the uterus on the lungs and diaphragm.
Interrupted sleep because of the baby's movements or the need to urinate.
Descending ("dropping") of the baby's head into the pelvis about two to four weeks before birth.
Navel pushed out.

Figure 10.14 Physiological Changes of Pregnancy

cause may have an **ectopic pregnancy.** In this type of pregnancy, the fertilized egg remains in the fallopian tube instead of traveling to the uterus. Ectopic, or tubal, pregnancies have increased dramatically in recent years, now accounting for 2 percent of all reported pregnancies. STIs, particularly chlamydia infections (discussed in Chapter 16), have become a major cause of ectopic pregnancy. Other risk factors include previous pelvic surgery, particularly involving the fallopian tubes; pelvic inflammatory disease; infertility; and use of an IUD.

Miscarriage About 10 to 20 percent of pregnancies end in **miscarriage,** or spontaneous abortion, before the twentieth week of gestation. Major genetic disorders may be responsible for 33 to 50 percent of pregnancy losses. The most common cause is an abnormal number of chromosomes. About 0.5 to 1 percent of women suffer three or more miscarriages, possibly because of genetic, anatomic, hormonal, infectious, or autoimmune factors. An estimated 70 to 90 percent of women who miscarry eventually become pregnant again.

Infections The infectious disease most clearly linked to birth defects is **rubella** (German measles). All women should be vaccinated against this disease at least three months prior to conception, to protect themselves and any children they may bear. (See Chapter 15 for more on immunization.) The most common prenatal infection today is *cytomegalovirus.* This infection produces mild flulike symptoms in adults but can cause brain damage, retardation, liver disease, cerebral palsy, hearing problems, and other malformations in unborn babies.

STIs, such as syphilis, gonorrhea, and genital herpes, can be particularly dangerous during pregnancy if not recognized and treated. If a woman has a herpes outbreak around the date her baby is due, her physician will deliver the baby by caesarean section to prevent infecting the baby. HIV infection endangers both a pregnant woman and her unborn baby, and all pregnant women and new mothers should be aware of the HIV epidemic, the risks to them and their babies, and the availability of anonymous testing.

© Petit/Format/Nestle/Science Source/Photo Researchers, Inc.

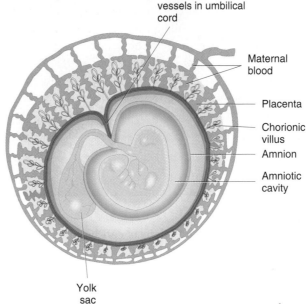

Figure 10.15 The Placenta

The placenta supplies the growing embryo with fluid and nutrients from the maternal bloodstream and carries waste back for disposal.

© Petit/Format/Nestle/Science Source/Photo Researchers, Inc.

Genetic Disorders In some sense, each of us is a carrier of a genetic problem. Every individual has an estimated four to six defective genes, but the chances of passing them on to a child are slim. Almost all are recessive, which means they are "masked" by a more influential dominant gene. The likelihood of a child inheriting the same faulty recessive gene from both parents is remote—unless the parents are so closely related that they have very similar genetic makeup.

The child of a parent with an abnormal dominant gene has a 50 percent likelihood of inheriting it. The most common of such defects are minor, such as the growth of an extra finger or toe. However, some

embryo An organism in its early stage of development; in humans, the embryonic period lasts from the second to the eighth week of pregnancy.

amnion The innermost membrane of the sac enclosing the embryo or fetus.

fetus The human organism developing in the uterus from the ninth week until birth.

placenta An organ that develops after implantation and to which the embryo attaches, via the umbilical cord, for nourishment and waste removal.

ectopic pregnancy A pregnancy in which the fertilized egg has implanted itself outside the uterine cavity, usually in the fallopian tube.

miscarriage A pregnancy that terminates before the twentieth week of gestation; also called spontaneous abortion.

rubella An infectious disease that may cause birth defects if contracted by a pregnant woman; also called German measles.

genetic disorder among African Americans), beta-thalassemia (found in families of Mediterranean origin), and Tay-Sachs (found in Jews of Eastern European origin). Two carriers of the same abnormal recessive genes can pass such problems on to their children.

The American College of Obstetricians and Gynecologists recommends a blood test for biochemical markers and ultrasound to screen for chromosomal abnormalities for all women in their first trimester. More invasive techniques, such as chorionic villus sampling (CVS) and second-trimester amniocentesis, can provide a precise diagnosis but carry a small risk for pregnancy loss.

Premature Labor Approximately 10 percent of all babies are born too soon (before the thirty-seventh week of pregnancy). According to researchers, prematurity is the main underlying cause of stillbirth and infant deaths within the first few weeks after birth. Bed rest, close monitoring, and, if necessary, medications for at-risk women can buy more time in the womb for their babies. But women must recognize the warning signs of **premature labor**—dull, low backache; a feeling of tightness or pressure on the lower abdomen; and intestinal cramps, sometimes with diarrhea. Low–birth weight premature babies face the highest risks, but comprehensive, enriched programs can reduce developmental and health problems.

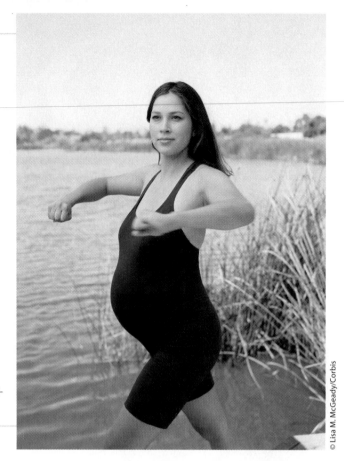

Most pregnant women benefit from regular moderate exercise.

© Lisa M. McGeady/Corbis

single-gene defects can be fatal. Huntington's chorea, for example, is a degenerative disease that in the past was usually not diagnosed until midlife.

Genetic tests can identify "carriers" of abnormal recessive genes for diseases such as sickle-cell anemia (the most common

Childbirth

A generation ago, delivering a baby was something a doctor did in a hospital. Today parents can choose from many birthing options, including a birth attendant, who can be a physician or a nurse-midwife, and a birthing center, hospital, or home birth.

Preparing for Childbirth

The most widespread method of childbirth preparation is the **Lamaze method** (*psychoprophylaxis*). Fernand Lamaze, a French doctor, instructed women to respond to labor contractions with prelearned, controlled breathing techniques. As the intensity of each contraction increases, the

laboring woman concentrates on increasing her breathing rate in a prescribed way. Her partner coaches her during each contraction and helps her cope with discomfort.

Women who attend prenatal classes are less likely to undergo caesarean deliveries and more likely to breast-feed. They also tend to have fewer complications and require fewer medications. However, painkillers or anesthesia are always an option if labor is longer or more painful than expected. The lower body can be numbed with an *epidural block*, which involves injecting an anesthetic into the membrane around the spinal cord, or a spinal block, in which the injection goes directly into the spinal canal. General anesthesia is usually used only for emergency caesarean births.

Labor and Delivery

There are three stages of **labor.** The first starts with *effacement* (thinning) and *dilation* (opening up) of the cervix. Effacement is measured in percentages, and dilation in centimeters or finger-widths. Around this time, the amniotic sac of fluids usually breaks, a sign that the woman should call her doctor or midwife.

The first contractions of the early, or *latent*, phase of labor are usually not uncomfortable; they last 15 to 30 seconds, occur every 15 to 30 minutes, and gradually increase in intensity and frequency. The most difficult contractions come after the cervix is dilated to about 8 centimeters, as the woman feels greater pressure from the fetus. The first stage ends when the cervix is completely dilated to a diameter of 10 centimeters (or five finger-widths) and the baby is ready to come down the birth canal (Figure 10.16). For women having their first baby, this first stage of labor averages 12 to 13 hours. Women having another child often experience shorter first-stage labor.

When the cervix is completely dilated, the second stage of labor occurs, during which the baby moves into the vagina, or birth canal, and out of the mother's body. As this stage begins, women who have gone through childbirth preparation training often feel a sense of relief from the acute pain of the transition phase and at the prospect of giving birth.

This second stage can take up to an hour or more. Strong contractions may last 60 to 90 seconds and occur every two to three minutes. As the baby's head descends, the mother feels an urge to push. By bearing down, she helps the baby complete its passage to the outside.

As the baby's head appears, or *crowns*, the doctor may perform an *episiotomy*—an incision from the lower end of the vagina toward the anus to enlarge the vaginal opening. The purpose of the episiotomy is to prevent the baby's head from causing an irregular tear in the vagina, but routine episiotomies have been criticized as unnecessary. Women may be able to avoid this procedure by trying different birthing positions or having an attendant massage the perineal tissue.

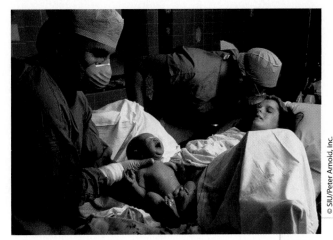

© SIU/Peter Arnold, Inc.

Today's fathers are active participants at the birth of their children.

Usually the baby's head emerges first, then its shoulders, then its body. With each contraction, a new part is born. However, the baby can be in a more difficult position, facing up rather than down, or with the feet or buttocks first (a *breech birth)*, and a caesarean birth may then be necessary.

In the third stage of labor, the uterus contracts firmly after the birth of the baby and, usually within five minutes, the placenta separates from the uterine wall. The woman may bear down to help expel the placenta, or the doctor may exert gentle external pressure. If an episiotomy has been performed, the doctor sews up the incision. To help the uterus contract and return to its normal size, it may be massaged manually, or the baby may be put to the mother's breast to stimulate contraction of the uterus.

Caesarean Birth

In a **caesarean delivery** (also referred to as a *caesarean section,* or *C-section*), the doctor lifts the baby out of the woman's body through an incision made in the lower abdomen and uterus. The most common reason for caesarean birth is *failure to progress*, a vague term indicating that labor has gone on too long and may put the baby or mother at risk. Other reasons include the baby's position (if feet or buttocks are first) and signs that the fetus is in danger.

Thirty years ago, only 5 percent of babies born in America were delivered by caesarean birth. Nearly one in three babies is delivered by this method, many in women who had a previous C-section. A recent analysis of data on more than half a million caesarean births found that more than 95 percent are performed because of risk factors complicating labor or delivery.[31]

premature labor Labor that occurs after the twentieth week but before the thirty-seventh week of pregnancy.

Lamaze method A method of childbirth preparation taught to expectant parents to help the woman cope with the discomfort of labor; combines breathing and psychological techniques.

labor The process leading up to birth: effacement and dilation of the cervix; the movement of the baby into and through the birth canal, accompanied by strong contractions; and contraction of the uterus and expulsion of the placenta after the birth.

caesarean delivery The surgical procedure in which an infant is delivered through an incision made in the abdominal wall and uterus.

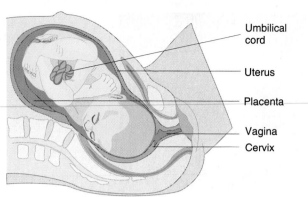

Umbilical cord

Uterus

Placenta

Vagina

Cervix

(a) The cervix is partially dilated, and the baby's head enters the birth canal.

Sacrum

(b) The cervix is nearly completely dilated. The baby's head rotates so that it can move through the birth canal.

Perineum

(c) The baby's head extends as it reaches the vaginal opening, and the head and the rest of the body pass through the birth canal.

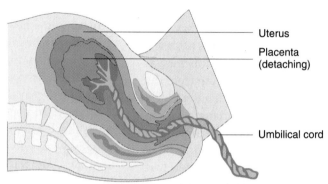

Uterus

Placenta (detaching)

Umbilical cord

(d) After the baby is born, the placenta detaches from the uterus and is expelled from the woman's body.

Figure 10.16   Birth

Infertility

The World Health Organization defines **infertility** as the failure to conceive after one year of unprotected intercourse. Infertility affects one in seven couples. Women between age 35 and 44 are about twice as likely to have fertility problems as women age 30 to 34.

Infertility is a problem of the couple, not of the individual man or woman. In 40 percent of cases, infertility is caused by female problems, in 40 percent by male problems, in 10 percent by a combination of male and female problems, and in 10 percent by unexplained causes. A thorough diagnostic workup can reveal a cause for infertility in 90 percent of cases.

In women, the most common causes of subfertility or infertility are age, abnormal menstrual patterns, suppression of ovulation, and blocked fallopian tubes. A woman's fertility peaks between age 20 and 30 and then drops quickly: by 20 percent after 30, by 50 percent after 35, and by 95 percent after 40.

Male subfertility or infertility is usually linked to either the quantity or the quality of sperm, which may be inactive, misshapen, or insufficient (less than 20 million sperm per milliliter of semen in an ejaculation of 3 to 5 milliliters). Sometimes the problem is hormonal or a blockage of a sperm duct. Some men suffer from the inability to ejaculate normally, or from retrograde ejaculation, in which some of the semen travels in the wrong direction, back into the body of the male.

Infertility can have an enormous emotional impact. Many women long to experience pregnancy and childbirth and feel great loss if they cannot conceive. Women in their thirties and forties fear that their biological clock is running out of time. Men may be confused and surprised by the intensity of their partner's emotions.

Options for Infertile Couples

The treatment of infertility has become a $2 billion a year enterprise in the United States. The odds of successful pregnancy range from 30 to 70 percent, depending on the specific cause of infertility. One result of successful infertility treatments has been a boom in multiple births, including quintuplets and sextuplets. Multiple births are associated with greater risk, both to the babies—including prematurity, low birth weight, neonatal death, and lifelong disability—and to the mothers, including caesarean section and hemorrhage.

Artificial Insemination
Artificial insemination—the introduction of viable sperm into the vagina by artificial means—is used primarily by couples in which the husband is infertile. Some states do not recognize such children as legitimate; others do, but only if the woman's husband gives consent for the insemination.

Assisted Reproductive Technology
An estimated 500,000 babies have been born in the United States through assisted reproductive technology (ART) since 1985.[32] The most common ART procedure is *in vitro fertilization (IVF)*, which removes the ova from a woman's ovary and places the woman's egg and her mate's sperm in a laboratory dish for fertilization. If the fertilized egg cell shows signs of development, within several days it is returned to the woman's uterus, the egg cell implants itself in the lining of the uterus, and the pregnancy continues as normal.

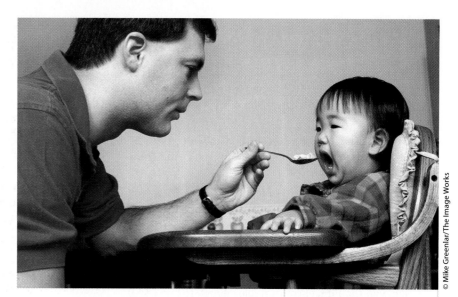

© Mike Greenlar/The Image Works

Adoption matches would-be parents yearning for youngsters to love with infants or children who need loving homes.

One of the most common complications of ART is the birth of as many as eight babies. More than half of ART-conceived twins and more than 95 percent of ART triplets are born prematurely or have low birth weights. Born too soon or too small, they face greater risks of short- and long-term complications.

Adoption

Men and women who cannot conceive children biologically can still become parents. **Adoption** matches would-be parents yearning for youngsters to love with infants or children who need loving. Couples interested in adoption can work with either public agencies or private counselors who contact obstetricians directly. Or they can contact organizations that arrange adoptions of children in need from other countries.

There are no reliable statistics on the annual number of adoptions in the United States, but census records indicate there are currently 1.6 million adopted children in the United States. Each year some 50,000 U.S. children become available for adoption—far fewer than the number of would-be parents looking for youngsters to adopt. An estimated 13 percent of adopted children are foreign-born.

infertility The inability to conceive a child.

artificial insemination The introduction of viable sperm into the vagina by artificial means for the purpose of inducing conception.

adoption The legal process for becoming the parent to a child of other biological parents.

The decisions you make about birth control can affect your reproductive health—and your partner's. Here are guidelines that can help prevent pregnancy and protect your reproductive well-being.

- **Abstain.** The only 100 percent safe and effective way to avoid unwanted pregnancy is not to engage in heterosexual intercourse.

- **Limit sexual activity to outercourse or oral sex.** You can engage in many sexual activities—kissing, hugging, touching, massage, oral–genital sex—without risking pregnancy.

- **Talk about birth control with any potential sex partner.** If you are considering sexual intimacy with a person, you should feel comfortable enough to talk about contraception.

- **Know what doesn't work—and don't rely on it.** There are many misconceptions about ways to avoid getting pregnant, such as having sex in a standing position or during menstruation. Only the methods described in this chapter are reliable forms of birth control.

- **Talk with a health-care professional.** A great deal of information and advice is available—in writing, from family planning counselors, from physicians on the Internet. Check it out.

- **Choose a contraceptive method that matches your personal habits and preferences.** If you can't remember to take a pill every day, oral contraceptives aren't for you. If you're constantly forgetting where you put things, a diaphragm might not be a good choice.

- **Consider long-term implications.** Since you may well wish to have children in the future, find out about the reversibility of various methods and possible effects on future fertility.

- **Resist having sex without contraceptive protection "just this once."** It only takes once—even the very first time—to get pregnant. Be wary of drugs and alcohol. They can impair your judgment and make you less conscientious about using birth control—or using it properly.

- **Use backup methods.** If there's a possibility that a contraceptive method might not offer adequate protection (for instance, if it's been almost three months since your last injection of Depo-Provera), use an additional form of birth control.

- **Inform yourself about emergency contraception.** Just in case a condom breaks or a diaphragm slips, find out about the availability of forms of after-intercourse contraception.

> **SELF SURVEY**   Which Contraceptive Method is Best for You?

Answer Yes or No to each statement as it applies to you and, if appropriate, your partner.

1. You have high blood pressure or cardiovascular disease.
2. You smoke cigarettes.
3. You have a new sexual partner.
4. An unwanted pregnancy would be devastating to you.
5. You have a good memory.
6. You or your partner have multiple sexual partners.
7. You prefer a method with little or no bother.
8. You have heavy, crampy periods.
9. You need protection against STIs.
10. You are concerned about endometrial and ovarian cancer.
11. You are forgetful.
12. You need a method right away.
13. You're comfortable touching your own and your partner's genitals.
14. You have a cooperative partner.
15. You like a little extra vaginal lubrication.
16. You have sex at unpredictable times and places.
17. You are in a monogamous relationship and have at least one child.

Scoring:

Recommendations are based on Yes answers to the following numbered statements:

> The combination pill: 4, 5, 6, 8, 10, 16
> The progestin-only pill: 1, 2, 5, 7, 16
> The patch: 4, 7, 8, 11, 16
> The NuvaRing: 4, 7, 8, 11, 13, 16
> Condoms: 1, 2, 3, 6, 9, 12, 13, 14
> Depo-Provera: 1, 2, 4, 7, 11, 16
> Diaphragm, cervical cap, or FemCap: 1, 2, 13, 14
> Mirena IUD: 1, 2, 7, 8, 11, 13, 16, 17
> Spermicides: 1, 2, 12, 13, 14, 15
> Sponge: 1, 2, 12, 13

Your Health Action Plan for Choosing a Contraceptive

Your responses may indicate that there's more than one appropriate method of birth control for you. Remember that you may choose different types of birth control at different stages of your life, or switch contraceptives for various reasons. You and your partner should always consider and discuss these factors:

- **Effectiveness.** Keep in mind that your own conscientiousness will play an important role. If you forget to take your daily pill, or if you decide not to use a condom "just this once," you'll increase the odds of pregnancy by interfering with effective birth control.
- **Suitability.** If you don't have sex very often, a contraceptive with many risks and side effects, such as the pill, may be wrong for you. If you have many sexual partners and are at risk of contracting a sexually transmitted infection, a condom may provide protection against pregnancy and infection, especially if used with a diaphragm or cervical cap.
- **Side effects.** Some complications related to contraceptives are serious health threats. Be sure to ask questions and gather as much information as possible about what side effects to expect.
- **Safety.** The risks of certain contraceptives, such as the pill, may be too great to allow their use if, for example, you have high blood pressure. Be honest in describing your medical history to your physician.
- **Future fertility.** Some women don't return to regular menstrual cycles for six months to a year after discontinuing oral contraceptives. This possibility may or may not be important to you now, but you should try to look ahead.
- **Reduced risk of sexually transmitted infections.** Some forms of contraception, in particular barrier contraceptives and spermicides, help reduce the risk of transmission of some STIs. However, none provides complete protection.

CENGAGENOW™ If you want to write your own goals for for safe and effective contraception, go to the Wellness Journal at CengageNOW for Health: **www.cengage.com/sso**

MAKING THIS CHAPTER WORK FOR YOU

Review Questions

1. Which statement about prescription contraceptives is *not* true?
   a. Prescription contraceptives do not offer protection against STIs.
   b. Some prescription contraceptives contain estrogen and progestin, and some contain only progestin.
   c. The contraceptive ring must be changed every week.
   d. IUDs prevent pregnancy by preventing or interfering with implantation.

2. Which of the following statements is true about infertility?
   a. Infertility is most often caused by female problems.
   b. In men, infertility is usually caused by a combination of excess sperm production and an ejaculation problem.
   c. In vitro fertilization involves introducing sperm into the vagina with a long needle.
   d. In some cases of infertility, no cause can be demonstrated.

3. Conception occurs
   a. when a fertilized egg implants in the lining of the uterus.
   b. when sperm is blocked from reaching the egg.
   c. when a sperm fertilizes the egg.
   d. after the uterine lining is discharged during the menstrual cycle.

4. Which of the following statements is true about sterilization?
   a. In women, the most frequently performed sterilization technique is Essure.
   b. Many couples experience an increase in sexual encounters after sterilization.
   c. Vasectomies are easily reversed with surgery.
   d. Sterilization is recommended for single men and women who are unsure about whether they want children.

5. Factors to consider when choosing a contraceptive method include all of the following *except*
   a. cost.
   b. failure rate.
   c. effectiveness in preventing sexually transmitted infections.
   d. preferred sexual position.

6. During childbirth,
   a. breech birth can be prevented by practicing the Lamaze method.
   b. the cervix thins and dilates so that the baby can exit the uterus.
   c. the intensity of contractions decreases during the second stage of labor.
   d. the placenta is expelled immediately before the baby's head appears.

7. When used correctly, which is the most effective non-hormonal contraceptive method?
   a. male condom
   b. female condom
   c. spermicide
   d. diaphragm

8. Which statement about abortion is *false?*
   a. The abortion rate in the United States started declining in the 1990s.
   b. The U.S. abortion rate is higher than the rate in Canada and England.
   c. Most women are traumatized by an abortion.
   d. Mifepristone is 97 percent effective in inducing abortion.

9. Which of the following contraceptive choices offers the best protection against STIs?
    a. condom alone
    b. condom plus spermicide
    c. abstinence
    d. withdrawal plus spermicide

10. In the third trimester of pregnancy,
    a. the woman experiences shortness of breath as the enlarged uterus presses on the lungs and diaphragm.
    b. the embryo is now called a fetus.
    c. the woman should begin regular prenatal checkups.
    d. the woman should increase her activity level to ensure that she is fit for childbirth.

    Answers to these questions can be found on page 650.

Critical Thinking

1. After reading about the various methods of contraception, which do you think would be most effective for you? What factors enter into your decision (convenience, risks, effectiveness, etc.)?

2. If you are sexually active, how do you start the conversation about contraception with a potential partner? What do you say and do if your partner is not ready for sex? What would you do if you do not have condoms with you to prevent sexually transmitted infection and do not have another form of birth control, such as a diaphragm?

3. Suppose that you and your partner were told that your only chance of having a child is by using fertility drugs. After taking the drugs, you and your partner are informed that there are seven fetuses. Would you carry them all to term? What if you knew that the chances of them all surviving were very slim and that eliminating some of them would improve the odds for the others? What ethical issues do cases like this raise?

Media Menu

CENGAGENOW™ Go to the CengageNOW for Health website at **www .cengage.com/sso** that will:
- Help you evaluate your knowledge of the material.
- Allow you to take an exam-prep quiz.
- Provide a Personalized Learning Plan targeting resources that address areas you should study.
- Coach you through identifying target goals for behavioral change and creating and monitoring your personal change plan throughout the semester.

Internet Connections

www.guttmacher.org
This site offers excellent resources on teen pregnancy rates and sexual health for teens and young adults, including discussions on contraceptives versus abstinence.

www.arhp.org
ARHP calls their website "the ultimate resource offering comprehensive information and education on all reproductive health topics to healthcare professionals, policymakers, the media, and the public."

www.naral.org
The website of this national organization provides information on the politics of the pro-choice movement.

www.nrlc.org
The website of this national organization provides information on the politics of the pro-life movement.

www.plannedparenthood.org
The website for the Planned Parenthood Federation of America offers a wealth of information on sexual and reproductive health, reproductive choices, methods of contraception, and reproductive policy.

Key Terms

The terms listed are used on the page indicated. Definitions of the terms are in the Glossary at the end of the book.

adoption 331
amnion 327
artificial insemination 331
barrier contraceptives 305
blastocyst 298
caesarean delivery 329
cervical cap 309
coitus interruptus 303
conception 298
condom 307
contraception 298
diaphragm 309
dilation and evacuation (D and E) 323
ectopic pregnancy 327
embryo 327
emergency contraception (EC) 319
failure rate 303
fertilization 298
fetus 327
implantation 298
infertility 331
intrauterine device (IUD) 317
labor 329

Lamaze method 329
laparoscopy 321
medical abortion 322
minipill, progestin-only pill 313
miscarriage 327
monophasic pills 313
multiphasic pills 313
oral contraceptives 311
placenta 327
preconception care 325
premature labor 329
rhythm method 319
rubella 327
spermatogenesis 298
sterilization 321
suction curettage 323
tubal ligation 321
tubal occlusion 321
vaginal contraceptive film (VCF) 309
vaginal spermicide 309
vasectomy 321
zygote 298

Avoiding Health Risks

People may encourage you to take risks with your health—to try drugs, to have another drink, to smoke cigarettes. But remember: You have nothing to gain and everything to lose when you let an addiction run your life. You also live with the consequences of others' drug abuse, alcoholism, and smoking. That's why it's important to know about potentially harmful habits—even if you never rely on drugs to pick you up or bring you down, never drink to excess, and never smoke. This section provides information you can use to avoid or overcome habits that jeopardize or destroy health, happiness, and life.

Chapter 11 - Avoiding Addictions

1. **Problem gambling refers to those who have: (Pg. 339)**
   A. lied to friends or family about their gambling use
   B. gotten into arguments with family or friends about their gambling
   C. experience the gambling to be a rush (high) but wanting it over and over again
   to continue to gamble
   D. all of the above are indications of problem or addictive gambling

2. **The following behaviors indicate an increased risk for problem gambling except for one: (Pg. 341)**
   A. feeling excited before going to gamble
   B. betting more money to recoup losses
   C. skipping classes to go gambling
   D. feeling aroused while gambling

3. **The biggest reason why college students say they use illicit or prescription drugs is: (Pg. 343)**
   A. to experiment with drugs
   B. to get high
   C. to reduce stress
   D. to lose their sexual inhibitions

4. **One of the biggest reasons why college students choose not to use drugs or alcohol is because: (Pg. 342)**
   A. they are too busy working outside of school
   B. their heavy involvement with religiosity and church activities keeps them busy
   C. involvement with athletics keeps them away from drugs and alcohol
   D. none of the above

5. **When sleeping pills are taken with alcohol, the interaction between these two drugs can cause a situation known as a(n): (Pg. 346)**
   A. additive reaction
   B. synergistic interaction
   C. potentiating mixing effect
   D. antagonistic neutralizing effect

6. **One of the mostly widely abused prescription medicines by college males is: (Pg. 352)**
   A. marijuana
   B. narcotic pain medicines
   C. stimulants such as Ritalin used for attention deficient disorders
   D. alcohol

7. **An example of drug misuse would be: (Pg. 344)**
   A. shooting up on heroin 5 times a day
   B. taking your roommate's penicillin prescription to fight a strep throat infection
   C. taking more than the recommended dosages of aspirin
   D. illegally smoking marijuana in your dorm room

8. **Drug abuse means: (Pg. 344)**
   A. the same as drug misuse
   B. taking your girlfriend's pain narcotic medicine to help with a painful shoulder
   injury
   C. taking much more of a prescription medicine even though you don't need it
   any longer
   D. using illegal drugs

9. **Which characteristic best describes Tyler becoming addicted to alcohol: (Pg. 353)**
   A. he is drinking his roommate's brand of alcohol
   B. he is mixing different types of alcohol together
   C. he is becoming dependent on drinking alcohol much more than he can handle
   D. he is a social drinker only at parties

10. Jack has become dependent on his alcohol use but is also abusing marijuana, stimulants, and tobacco. He is suffering from a condition known as: (Pg. 353)
    A. intoxication
    B. psychoactive substance abuse disorder
    C. dual diagnosis
    D. polyabuse

11. **Which of the following is not a factor that would determine the effects of a drug on an individual? (Pg. 344)**
    A.   how the drug enters the body
    B.   the amount of the drug being taken
    C.   the brand of the medicine being taken
    D.   the presence of other drugs in the body

12. **One of the strongest negative effects of marijuana use that can be damaging to college-aged students is: (Pg. 359)**
    A. throat damage from marijuana inhalation which will lead to throat cancer
    B. difficulty in concentration, attention to details, and learning new complex materials
    C. decreases the heart rate
    D. the possibility of reproduction capability

13. **The toxicity of a drug refers to: (Pg. 345)**
    A. the amount of inert ingredients it has
    B. the strength of its poison to the body
    C. how strong the medicine is to take effect
    D. the breakdown capability of the drug in the liver

14. **Drugs that have a greater effect on one specific organ are said to be acting: (Pg. 346)**
    A. locally
    B. generally
    C. selectively
    D. cumulatively

15. **A drug abuser who becomes dependent or addicted to several drugs at once is known as: (Pg. 353)**
    A. multiple addicted personality
    B. polyabuse
    C. physical tolerance
    D. maladaptive intoxication

16. **An intense risk related to overdosing on amphetamines is that of: (Pg. 362)**
    A. crashing
    B. roboing
    C. hallucinating
    D. chipping

17. **Jack was in total denial about his cocaine addiction and his family had to confront Jack and force him into a rehab program to get clean. This type of dependency treatment is known as: (Pg. 370)**
    A. relapse prevention
    B. 12 step recovery programming
    C. intervention
    D. motivational interviewing by the family

18. **A brief intervention whereas a counselor shows empathy in supporting personal change of the student who has violated a drug or alcohol policy at the school is known as: (Pg. 370)**
    A. relapse prevention
    B. minor intervention
    C. 12-step therapy
    D. motivational interviewing

T anner had too many papers to write and too little time to finish them. One of the guys in his fraternity suggested a prescription stimulant a friend took for an attention deficit disorder. The jolt felt like just what Tanner needed. During midterms Tanner bought another prescription stimulant from a classmate. As finals approached, he started hoarding stimulants from several people. He popped the final ones to rev up for the last bash of the school year parties. Without realizing it, Tanner put himself at risk for drug-related problems—physical, psychological, and legal.

Avoiding Addictions

People who try drugs or engage in addictive behaviors don't think they'll ever lose control. Even regular users believe they are smart enough, strong enough, lucky enough not to get caught or hooked. However, over time addictions produce changes in an individual's body, brain, and behavior. In time they can outweigh everything else a person values and holds dearest.

The impact of addictions in college ranges from short-term consequences, such as academic difficulties, to long-term physical and psychological problems. The toll of drug abuse, for instance, includes more than 1,700 deaths, 700,000 assaults, and almost 100,000 sexual attacks and rapes. But knowing the risks isn't enough to keep many students from heading down the dead-end road of addiction. (See "Don't Go There" in Making Change Happen and *Labs for IPC.*)

Going beyond warnings, this chapter provides information and insights into how addictions start, why students use and abuse drugs, the nature and effect of drugs, and the most commonly used, misused, and abused drugs. It also offers practical strategies for preventing, recognizing the signs of, and seeking help for addiction.

> After studying the material in this chapter, you should be able to

- **Name** some of the risk factors for problem gambling.
- **Discuss** reasons why people choose to use or not to use drugs.
- **Give examples** of appropriate and inappropriate use of over-the-counter and prescription medications.
- **Identify** the types of drug dependence, and discuss the factors affecting drug dependence.
- **Describe** the effects and health risks of common drugs of abuse.
- **Describe** the treatment methods available for individuals seeking help for drug dependence.
- **Review** your drug history (legal and illegal) and **assess** the health risks you chose to take.

Log on to CengageNOW for Health at **www.cengage.com/sso** to find your Behavior Change Planner and to explore self-assessments, interactive tutorials, and practice quizzes.

337

Risky Behaviors

College is a time when students want to experiment, enjoy, stretch—and take some risks. But there is a difference between the risks of smoking marijuana and the risks of forming a band or trying out for a team. One is an illegal activity that can get you in serious trouble in the short term and cause adverse health consequences in the long run The others impart the thrill that comes with trying something new and mastering a challenge. Are you taking risks that don't make sense and that don't add pleasure or passion to your life? Or are you taking risks that empower and inspire you? (See Chapter 3 in *IPC* for a discussion of good risks, bad risks, and knowing the difference between them.)

The vast majority of college students do not engage in addictive behaviors. However, some do, and the reasons why are complex. According to recent research, risk-takers—individuals who engage in impulsive, rule-breaking behaviors that may involve food, money, sex, alcohol, or drugs—may lack the ability to limit the release of dopamine, a "feel good" chemical in the brain. Because they have fewer dopamine "autoreceptors," exciting or dangerous activities may trigger higher levels of dopamine than normal, which encourages thrill-seeking behavior.[1] However, biology is not destiny. Although there are promising treatments for addictions (discussed later in this chapter), prevention is the smarter, safer—and far less costly—choice (see Health on a Budget).

Addictive Behaviors and the Dimensions of Health

Young adults have the highest rates of illicit drug use (see Figure 11.1). Many do not realize that substance abuse and other self-destructive behaviors, such as gambling or compulsive eating, can affect every dimension of health. Some of the harmful effects are:

- **Physical health.** As shown in this and the following chapters, the abuse of alcohol, tobacco, and drugs takes a toll on every organ system in the body, increasing the likelihood of disease, disability, and premature death.

- **Psychological health.** Sometimes people begin abusing substances or engaging in addictive behavior as a way of "self-medicating" symptoms of anxiety or depression. However, alcohol or drugs provide only temporary relief. As abuse continues, shame and guilt increase, and coping with daily stressors becomes more difficult. Depression and anxiety are as likely to be the consequences as the causes of substance abuse.

- **Spiritual health.** Addictive behavior blocks the pursuit of meaning and inner fulfillment. As they rely more and more

---

HEALTH ON A BUDGET $

Develop a Positive Addiction

When you're anxious, bored, restless, or confused, when drugs seem all too appealing as a "quick fix," there are real solutions, "positive addictions" that can help you solve your problems without creating new and bigger ones. A positive addiction—whether it is exercising, mountain climbing, or listening to music—can produce very real "highs," often for very little money. There's a crucial difference between this sort of stimulation and drug dependency: one is real, the other is chemical. With one, you're in control; with the other, drugs are.

Here are some examples:

- **If you feel a need for physical relaxation,** if you want more energy or distraction from physical discomforts, you can turn to athletics, exercise (including walking and hiking), dance, or outdoor hobbies.

- **If you want to stimulate your senses,** enhance sexual stimulation, or magnify the sensations of sight, sound, and touch, train yourself to be more sensitive to nature and beauty. Take time to appreciate the sensations you experience when you're walking in the woods or embracing a person you love. Through activities like sailing or sky-diving, you can literally fill up your senses without relying on chemicals.

- **If you want to escape mental boredom,** gain new understanding of the world around you, study better, experiment with your levels of awareness, or indulge your intellectual curiosity, you can challenge your mind through reading, classes, creative games, discussion groups, memory training, or travel.

- **If you're looking for kicks,** adventure, danger, and excitement, sign up for a wilderness survival course. Take up an adventurous sport, like hang gliding or rock climbing. Set a challenging professional or personal goal and direct your energies to meeting it.

---

on a chemical or behavioral escape, individuals lose their sense of self and of connection with others and with a higher power.

- **Social health.** Addictive behavior strains and, in time, severs the ties that bind an individual to family, friends, colleagues, and classmates. The primary relationship in the life of alcoholics or addicts is with a behavior or a drug. They withdraw from others and become increasingly isolated.

- **Intellectual health.** The brain is one of the targets of alcohol and drugs. Under their influence, logic and reasoning break down. Impulses become more difficult to control. Judgment falters. Certain substances, such as ecstasy, can lead to permanent changes in brain chemistry.

- **Environmental health.** The use of some substances, such as tobacco, directly harms the environment. Abusers of alcohol and drugs also pose indirect threats to others because their behavior can lead to injury and damage.

See Making Change Happen, p. 340, and "Don't Go There" in *Labs for IPC*.

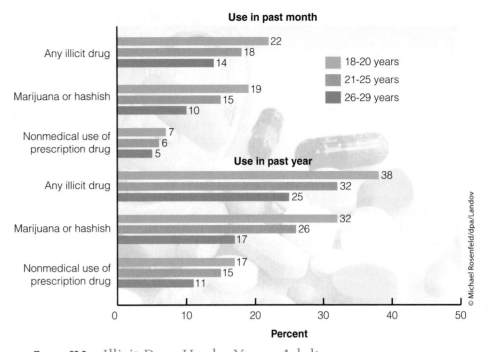

Figure 11.1 Illicit Drug Use by Young Adults

Sources: CDC/NCHS, *Health, United States, 2008*, Figure 32. Data from the National Survey on Drug Use and Health.

Gambling on Campus

Gambling can take many forms, from slot machines to online poker, to March Madness or Superbowl pools. The National Council on Problem Gambling defines "problem gambling" as gambling that causes disruptions in any major area of life: psychological, physical, social, or vocational. It is a progressive addiction characterized by increasing preoccupation with betting, a need to gamble more money more frequently, restlessness or irritability when attempting to stop, "chasing" losses, and inability to stop gambling despite mounting serious negative consequences.

Roughly 1 percent of American adults—some 2.3 million people—are addicted to the risk and excitement of betting. Another 2 to 3 percent have serious gambling problems, while 5 to 6 percent are considered

at risk, including a growing number of college students.[2] Although gambling is illegal for anyone under 18 to 21 years of age, depending on individual state law, underage gambling is a significant and growing problem across the country. Many college students buy lottery or scratch tickets, bet on sporting events, or go to casinos. About half of those who gamble at least once a month experience significant problems related to their gambling, including poor academic performance, heavy alcohol consumption, illicit drug use, unprotected sex, and other risky behaviors.[3] An estimated 3 to 6 percent of college students engage in "pathological gambling," which is characterized by "persistent and recurrent maladaptive gambling behavior."[4]

MAKING CHANGE HAPPEN

Don't Go There

The use of illegal drugs can lead to terrible, life-changing consequences for you and your family. Legal drugs, when used for reasons other than those for which they were prescribed, can be even stronger and more deadly. Drugs interfere with learning and education by making it more difficult to pay attention, concentrate, and remember. They create problems for and with people who love you. Drugs produce short- and long-term side effects that can range from mood changes to potentially fatal abnormalities in your breathing and heart rate. Most important, drugs can steal control of your life and your future—or can steal life itself.

But there are other, perhaps less obvious, reasons not to go down the path of drug use or other compulsive behaviors. For one thing, there is no need to. As you'll learn in "Don't Go There" in *Labs for IPC,* you can experience the sensations drugs can offer in other ways yet remain in charge and in control. Here's a preview.

Get Real
In this stage you complete an inventory of your drug-related behaviors by means of a checklist with 26 items, including the following three:

_____ • Used marijuana.
_____ • Felt that you could not control or stop using a particular drug.
_____ • Took any medicine, including painkillers and stimulants, for a reason other than that for which it was prescribed.

The more checks you see, the greater your risk of losing control of your life to a compulsive behavior or a substance of abuse . . .

In another exercise, you answer the question "What if?" by writing brief essays that begin with three different phrases, including:

• "As long as I stuck to prescription meds, I was sure I'd be able to stop whenever I wanted. But . . ."

Get Ready
In this stage you list all the advantages and benefits that your compulsive substance use has brought you. You might mention things such as:

• It made me feel that I fit in with a certain group.
• It was a way to blow off steam and relax . . .

You then list the disadvantages and negative consequences you've experienced as a result of your compulsive substance use, such as:

• Being unable to afford other things because of money spent on drugs or gambling.
• Side effects from drugs, which can include elevated blood pressure, heart rate, and breathing problems . . .

You also start tracking compulsive behavior or substance use by recording every time you engage in the behavior (such as gambling), when, how long, how much you gamble . . .

Get Going
This stage consists of five steps, including the following three:

• Consciously choosing an alternative behavior rather than your drug or escape of choice the next time you're stressed out or feeling lonely, down, or anxious . . .
• Quitting for 90 days. If you claim you can stop any time, prove it . . . Just stop. Yes, stop. And don't go back to your drug use or compulsive behavior for three consecutive months.
• Creating positive diversions, noncompulsive, nonchemical ways of achieving physical relaxation, sensory stimulation, greater creativity . . .

Lock It In
You continue self-monitoring to prove to yourself that you really are in the driver's seat regarding your use of drugs, alcohol, and other addictive substances and behaviors. You also keep expanding your repertoire of positive activities and coping skills . . .

Researchers identified key indicators associated with "pathological" gambling: gambling more than once a month, gambling more than two hours a month, and wagering more than 10 percent of monthly income. A combination of parental gambling problems, gambling frequency, and psychological distress also is associated with college gambling.[5]

College students who gamble say they do so for fun or excitement, to socialize, to win money, or to "just have something to do"—reasons similar to those for adults who gamble. Simply having access to casino machines, ongoing card games, or Internet gambling sites increases the likelihood that students will gamble.

Although most people who gamble limit the time and money they spend, some cross the line and lose control of their gambling "habit." The term *problem gambling* refers to all individuals with gambling-related problems, including mild or occasional ones.

Researchers now view problem or pathological gambling as an addiction that runs in families. Individuals predisposed to gambling because of their family history are more likely to develop a problem if they are regularly exposed to gambling. Alcoholism and drug abuse often occur along with gambling, leading to chaotic lives and greater health risks.

Risk Factors for Problem Gambling

Among young people (age 16 to 25) the following behaviors indicate increased risk of problem gambling:

- Being male.
- Gambling at an early age (as young as age 8).
- Having a big win earlier in one's gambling career.
- Consistently chasing losses (betting more to recover money already lost).
- Gambling alone.
- Feeling depressed before gambling.
- Feeling excited and aroused during gambling.
- Behaving irrationally during gambling.
- Having poor grades at school.
- Engaging in other addictive behaviors (smoking, drinking alcohol, illegal drug use).
- Being in a lower socioeconomic class.
- Having parents with a gambling or other addiction problem.
- Having a history of delinquency or stealing money to fund gambling.
- Skipping class to go gambling.

Pathological Gamblers

Adult pathological gamblers are more likely to be male, single, nonwhite, and less educated. Women start gambling later than men, but they progress more rapidly to pathological gambling. Genetics and exposure to gambling in childhood are significant influences. More than half of pathological gamblers report at least one first-degree relative with symptoms consistent with gambling problems.

Gamblers typically progress through various stages. In the winning phase, they feel empowered by their winnings and success. Next comes the losing phase, during which gamblers try to win back their losses. This is followed by the desperation phase, during which a gambler may resort to illegal activity, including stealing, to continue gambling. Some gamblers experience a fourth phase, the giving-up phase, where they desperately try to stay afloat in a game even though they realize they can't win.

As many as three-fourths of adult pathological gamblers suffer from depression. They also are at higher risk of other mood or anxiety disorders, such as panic disorder, phobias, obsessive-compulsive disorder, generalized anxiety, or post-traumatic stress disorder. An estimated 20 percent suffer from attention-deficit/hyperactivity disorder (ADHD). Even more—30 to 50 percent of pathological gamblers—abuse drugs or alcohol.

No standard or proven treatment exists for pathological gambling, but inpatient treatment centers, self-help groups, cognitive-behavioral psychotherapy, and addiction-based psychotherapy can help.

An evening of playing poker with friends can be a great way to relax. But for some college students, gambling can become addictive.

© Comstock Images/Jupiterimages

Drug Use on Campus

The percentage o undergraduates who abuse drugs has grown in recent years. Almost half of students (49 percent) report that they've smoked marijuana at least once in their lifetime; 27 percent have used another illegal drug.[6]

The nature of drug users as well as drug use has changed on campus. Marijuana remains the most widely used drug of abuse, but the nonmedical use of prescription drugs now outranks other forms of substance abuse.[7] Students who engage only in nonmedical use of prescription pills (dubbed "pill-poppers" in one study) and those who use only illicit drugs ("dopers" in the same study) are similar in some ways and different in others.

Characteristics of illicit drug users:

- Most in late teens and early twenties.
- More likely to be male.
- More likely to be white.
- Lower GPAs.
- More likely to be sexually active.
- Less likely to report strong religious values.
- More likely not to be or have never been married.
- Less likely to report good physical or mental health.
- More likely than nonusers to misuse prescription drugs.

Characteristics of users of prescription drugs for nonmedical reasons:

- Unclear if women or men have higher rates.
- More likely to be white.
- Lower GPA.
- Less likely to report good physical or mental health.
- More likely to report knowing a member of the faculty administration (possibly because of their concern about grades and academic performance).[8]

Why Students Don't Use Drugs

The majority of undergraduates do not use illegal drugs or abuse prescription drugs. What keeps them drug-free? Here are some important factors:

- **Spirituality and religion.** The greater a student's religiosity—a term that encompasses hours spent in prayer, attendance at religious services, and reading spiritual materials—the less likely the student is to use alcohol, illegal drugs, or tobacco. Unfortunately, researchers have noted a drop in students' religiosity during college, along with an increase in their alcohol and marijuana use.

- **Academic engagement.** Illicit drug use is much less common among students who actively participate in classes and feel connected with the subject matter. However, many students report never working closely with a faculty member, never being inspired by an educational experience, or never having an educational or extracurricular experience that motivates them to make an active contribution to a greater goal.[9]

- **Perceived harmfulness.** Although nonmedical use of prescription drugs has increased on college campuses, students—about one in four in a recent survey—who perceived a great risk of harm from repeated or occasional use were the least likely to misuse medications.

- **Athletics.** Although male and female college athletes drink at higher rates than nonathletes, they are less likely to use illegal drugs. One exception is the use of anabolic steroids (discussed in Chapter 5), which college athletes use more than other students.[10]

Why Students Use Drugs

Various factors influence which students use drugs, including the following:

- **Genetics and family history.** Some college students inherit a genetic or biological predisposition to substance abuse. Researchers have identified specific genes tied to all types of addictions. Some of the genes associated with alcohol dependence are closely linked with addictions to nicotine, cocaine, heroin, and other substances.[11] Also, the risk for problem drinking and alcohol abuse is higher among children of substance abusers.

- **Parental attitudes and behavior.** Parents' concerns or expectations influence whether or how much most students drink, smoke, or use drugs. Those who perceive that their parents approve of their drinking, for instance, are more likely to report a drinking-related problem, such as memory loss or missing class. More than one in five underage students report acquiring alcohol from their parents or relatives.[12]

- **Substance use in high school.** Many students start abusing drugs or alcohol well before getting to college. Only 8 percent of undergraduate marijuana users and even fewer cocaine users began their use in college. Misusing prescription drugs before age 16 increases the risk of a substance abuse disorder later in life.[13]

- **Social norms.** College students tend to overestimate drug use on campus. In the American College Health Association National College Health Assessment survey, students reported believing that 20 percent of undergraduates had never used marijuana. In fact, 69 percent never had. Students believed that 58 percent of their peers had used marijuana one or more times in the last 30 days and that 22 percent used it daily. The true incidence was much lower: 11 percent had used marijuana at least once in the previous month and 1 percent smoked it daily.[14] (see Reality Check, p. 345.)

- **Positive expectations.** Many students expect a drug to make them feel less stressed or anxious, more relaxed or confident, less shy or inhibited. Among students who use illicit drugs, many say they do so to relieve stress. Others self-medicate, taking drugs to relieve

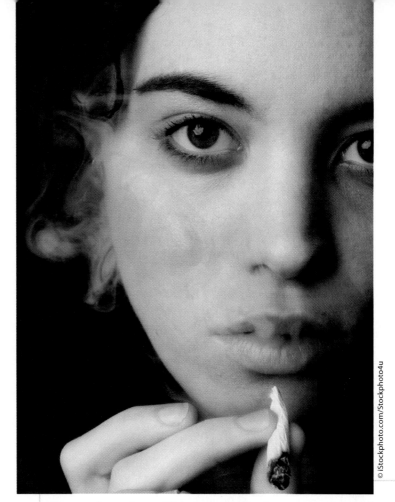

Many students who use illicit drugs say they do so to relieve stress, depression, or anxiety.

© iStockphoto.com/Stockphoto4u

depression or anxiety. Some abuse prescription medications, such as Adderall and Ritalin, because they think these drugs will energize them to study longer or perform better. Even when drugs don't live up to students' expectations, they may continue taking them for some short-term relief or because they have become addicted and cannot stop.

- **Mental health problems.** Students with feelings of hopelessness, sadness, depression, and anxiety as well as those with clinical mental disorders have higher rates of prescription drug abuse and illegal drug use. Students diagnosed with depression in the past school year have higher rates of marijuana, cocaine, alcohol, and tobacco use. The combination of mental illness and substance use is a strong predictor of violent behavior.[15]

- **Social influences.** More than nine in ten students who use illegal drugs were introduced to the habit through friends;

most use drugs with friends. Sorority and fraternity members, who tend to socialize more often, are likelier to abuse prescription stimulants, but students who live off campus have higher rates of marijuana and cocaine use.

- **Alcohol use.** Often individuals engage in more than one risky behavior. Researchers have found that those students who report binge drinking are much more likely than other students to report current or past use of marijuana, cocaine, or other illegal drugs.

- **Race/ethnicity.** In general, white students have higher levels of alcohol and drug use than do African American students. In a comparison of African American students at predominantly white and predominantly black colleges, those at historically black colleges had lower rates of alcohol and drug use than did either white or African American students at white schools. The reason, according to the researchers, may be that these colleges provide a greater sense of self-esteem, which helps prevent alcohol and drug use.

- **Sexual identity.** Gay, lesbian, and bisexual teens may rely on alcohol and marijuana to lessen social anxiety and boost self-confidence when they first come out. However, once they become more involved in the gay community, many are less likely to do so. Nonetheless, lesbians are significantly more likely than heterosexual women to use marijuana, Ecstasy, and other drugs. Gay and bisexual men are significantly less likely than heterosexual men to drink heavily but more likely to use drugs.

Understanding Drugs and Their Effects

A **drug** is a chemical substance that affects the way you feel and function. In some circumstances, taking a drug can help the body heal or relieve physical and mental distress. In other circumstances, taking a drug can distort reality, undermine well-being, and threaten survival. No drug is completely safe; all drugs have multiple effects that vary greatly in different people at different times. Knowing how drugs affect the brain, body, and behavior is crucial to understanding their impact and making responsible decisions about their use.

Drug abuse is the widely used term for the improper use of drugs, but some researchers have broken down the behavior into several categories:

- **Drug abuse** is a pattern of substance use resulting in negative consequences or impairment.

- **Drug dependence** is a pattern of continuing substance use despite cognitive, behavioral, and physical symptoms.

- **Drug misuse** is taking a drug for a purpose or by a person other than that for which it was intended or not taking the recommended doses.

- **Drug diversion** is the transfer of a medication from the individual to whom it was prescribed to another person.[16]

Risks are involved with all forms of drug use. Even medications that help cure illnesses or soothe symptoms have side effects and can be misused. Some substances that millions of people use every day, such as caffeine, pose some health risks. Others— like the most commonly used drugs in our society, alcohol and tobacco—can lead to potentially life-threatening problems. With some illicit drugs, any form of use can be dangerous.

Many factors determine the effects a drug has on an individual. These include how the drug enters the body, the dosage, the drug action, and the presence of other drugs in the body—as well as the physical and psychological makeup of the person taking the drug and the setting in which the drug is used.

Routes of Administration

Drugs can enter the body in a number of ways (Figure 11.2). The most common way of taking a drug is by swallowing a tablet, capsule, or liquid. However, drugs taken orally don't reach the bloodstream as quickly as drugs introduced into the body by other means. A drug taken orally may not have any effect for 30 minutes or more.

Drugs can enter the body through the lungs either by inhaling smoke, for example, from marijuana, or by inhaling gases, aerosol sprays, or fumes from solvents or other compounds that evaporate quickly. Young users of such inhalants, discussed later in this chapter, often soak a rag with fluid and press it over their nose. Or they may place inhalants in a plastic bag, put the bag over their nose and mouth, and take deep breaths—a practice called *huffing* and one that can produce serious, even fatal consequences.

Drugs can also be injected with a syringe subcutaneously (beneath the skin), intramuscularly (into muscle tissue, which is richly supplied with blood vessels), or intravenously (directly into a vein). **Intravenous** (IV) injection gets the drug into the bloodstream immediately (within seconds in most cases); **intramuscular** injection, moderately fast (within a few minutes); and **subcutaneous** injection, more slowly (within ten minutes).

Injecting drugs is extremely dangerous because many diseases, including hepatitis and infection with human immunodeficiency virus (HIV), can be transmitted by sharing contaminated needles. Injection-drug users who are HIV-positive are a major source of transmission of HIV among heterosexuals (see Chapter 16).

Dosage and Toxicity

The effects of any drug depend on the amount an individual takes. Increasing the dose usually intensifies the effects produced by smaller doses. Also, the kind of effect may change at different dose levels. For example, low doses of barbiturates may relieve anxiety, while higher doses can induce sleep, loss of sensation, even coma and death.

✓ REALITYCHECK

- *What percent of college students have never used marijuana?* _____
- *What percent do other students think have never used marijuana?* _____
- *What percent of students use marijuana daily?* _____
- *What percent do other students think use marijuana daily?* _____

Answers on next page.

Figure 11.2 Routes of Administration of Drugs

The dosage level at which a drug becomes poisonous to the body, causing either temporary or permanent damage, is called its **toxicity.** In most cases, drugs are eventually broken down in the liver by special body chemicals called *detoxification enzymes.*

Individual Differences

Each person responds differently to different drugs, depending on circumstances or setting. The enzymes in the body reduce the levels of drugs in the bloodstream; because there can be 80 variants of each enzyme, every person's body may react differently.

Often drugs intensify the emotional state a person is in. If you're feeling depressed, a drug may make you feel more depressed. A generalized physical problem, such as having the flu, may make your body more vulnerable to the effects of a drug. Genetic differences among individuals also may account for varying reactions.

Personality and psychological attitude also play a role in drug effects. Each user's *mind-set*—his or her expectations

drug Any substance, other than food, that affects bodily functions and structures when taken into the body.

drug abuse The excessive use of a drug in a manner inconsistent with accepted medical practice.

drug dependence Continued substance use even when its use causes cognitive, behavioral, and physical symptoms.

drug misuse The use of a drug for a purpose (or person) other than that for which it was medically intended.

drug diversion The transfer of a drug from the person for whom it was prescribed to another individual.

intravenous Into a vein.

intramuscular Into or within a muscle.

subcutaneous Under the skin.

toxicity Poisonousness; the dosage level at which a drug becomes poisonous to the body, causing either temporary or permanent damage.

or preconceptions about using the drug—affects the experience. Someone who takes a "club drug" (discussed further later in this chapter) to feel more "connected" may feel more sociable simply because that's what he or she expects.

Setting

The setting for drug use also influences its effects. Passing around a marijuana joint at a friend's is not a healthy or safe behavior, but the experience of going to a crack house is very different—and entails greater dangers.

Types of Action

A drug can act *locally,* as novocaine does to deaden pain in a tooth; *generally,* throughout a body system, as barbiturates do on the central nervous system; or *selectively,* as a drug does when it has a greater effect on one specific organ or system than on others, such as a spinal anesthetic. A drug that accumulates in the body because it's taken in faster than it can be metabolized and excreted is called *cumulative;* alcohol is such a drug.

Interaction with Other Drugs or Alcohol

A drug can interact with other drugs in four different ways:

- An **additive** interaction is one in which the resulting effect is equal to the sum of the effects of the different drugs used.

- A **synergistic** interaction is one in which the total effect of the two drugs taken together is greater than the sum of the effects the two drugs would have had if taken by themselves on separate occasions. Mixing barbiturates and alcohol, for example, has up to four times the depressant effect that either drug has alone.

- A drug can be **potentiating**—that is, one drug can increase the effect of another. Alcohol, for instance, can increase the drowsiness caused by antihistamines (antiallergy medications).

- Drugs can interact in an **antagonistic** fashion—that is, one drug can neutralize or block another drug with opposite effects. Tranquilizers, for example, may counter some of the nervousness and anxiety produced by cocaine.

The danger of mixing alcohol with other drugs cannot be emphasized too strongly. Alcohol and marijuana intensify each other's effects, making driving and many other activities extremely dangerous. Some people who have mixed sedatives or tranquilizers with alcohol never regained consciousness.

Men, Women, and Drugs

Beginning at a very early age, males and females show different patterns in drug use. Men generally encounter more opportunities to use drugs than women, but given an opportunity to use drugs for the first time, both genders are equally likely to do so and to progress from initial use to dependence. Vulnerability to some drugs varies with gender. Both are equally likely to become addicted to or dependent on cocaine, heroin, hallucinogens, tobacco, and inhalants. Women are more likely than men to become addicted to or dependent on sedatives and drugs designed to treat anxiety or sleeplessness and less likely than men to abuse alcohol and marijuana.

Males and females may differ in their biological responses to drugs. In studies of animals given the opportunity to self-administer intravenous doses of cocaine or heroin, females began self-administration sooner than males and administered larger amounts of the drugs. Male and female long-term cocaine users showed similar impairment in tests of concentration, memory, and academic achievement following sustained abstinence, even though women in the study had substantially greater exposure to cocaine. Female cocaine users also were less likely than men to exhibit abnormalities of blood flow in the brain's frontal lobes. These findings suggest a gender-related mechanism that may protect women from some of the damage cocaine inflicts on the brain. However, women are more vulnerable to poor nutrition and below-average weight, depression, physical abuse, and if pregnant, preterm labor or early delivery.

Caffeine and Its Effects

Caffeine, which has been drunk, chewed, and swallowed since the Stone Age, is the most widely used **psychoactive** (mind-affecting) drug in the world. Eighty percent of Americans drink coffee, our principal caffeine source—an average of 3.5 cups a day. Coffee contains 100 to 150 milligrams of caffeine per cup; tea, 40 to 100 milligrams; cola, about 45 milligrams. Most medications that contain caffeine are one-third to one-half the strength of a cup of coffee. However, some, such as Excedrin, are very high in caffeine (Table 11.1).

As a stimulant, caffeine relieves drowsiness, helps in the performance of repetitive tasks, and improves the capacity for work. Caffeine improves performance and endurance during prolonged, exhaustive exercise and, to a lesser degree, enhances short-term, high-intensity athletic performance. Additional benefits include improved concentration, reduced fatigue, and sharpened alertness.

You'll stay more alert, particularly if you are fighting sleep deprivation, if you spread your coffee consumption over the course of the day. For instance, rather than drinking two 8-ounce cups in the morning, try consuming smaller servings of an ounce or two during the course of the day.

In recent decades, some 19,000 studies have examined caffeine's impact on health. Their conclusion: For most people, caffeine poses few serious health risks—and may convey a surprising range of benefits. Drinking up to six cups a day of caffeinated or decaffeinated coffee won't shorten your lifespan and may convey some health benefits, including a lower risk of type 2 diabetes and cardiovascular disease.[17] Caffeine may also protect against Alzheimer's

TABLE 11.1

Caffeine Counts

Substance (Typical Serving)	Caffeine (milligrams)
No Doz, one pill	200
Coffee (drip), one 5-ounce cup	130
Excedrin, two pills	130
Espresso, one 2-ounce cup	100
Energy drink (Red Bull), one can	80
Instant coffee, one 5-ounce cup	74
Coca-Cola, 12 ounces	46
Tea, one 5-ounce cup	40
Dark chocolate, 1 ounce	20
Milk chocolate, 1 ounce	6
Cocoa, 5 ounces	4
Decaffeinated coffee, one 5-ounce cup	3

disease,[18] Parkinson's disease, colon cancer, liver cirrhosis, and gallstones. There is some evidence that coffee may relieve migraines, boost mood, and even prevent cavities. Researchers have found no significant relationship between coffee and tea consumption and the risk of breast cancer.[19]

Despite these positive findings, doctors still advise pregnant women, heart patients, and those at risk for osteoporosis to limit or avoid coffee. High doses of daily caffeine—whether from coffee, tea, caffeinated soda, or hot chocolate—increase the risk of miscarriage.[20] Too much caffeine, particularly in high-powered energy drinks (discussed in Chapter 5), can be dangerous for everyone.

You can overdose on caffeine and develop symptoms such as restlessness, nervousness, excitement, insomnia, flushed face,

additive Characterized by a combined effect that is equal to the sum of the individual effects.

synergistic Characterized by a combined effect that is greater than the sum of the individual effects.

potentiating Making more effective or powerful.

antagonistic Opposing or counteracting.

psychoative Mind-affecting.

increased urination, digestive complaints, muscle twitching, rambling thoughts and speech, rapid heart rate or arrhythmias, periods of inexhaustibility, and physical restlessness. Some people develop these symptoms after as little as 250 milligrams of caffeine a day; others, only with much larger doses. Higher doses may produce ringing in the ears or flashes of light, grand mal seizures, and potentially fatal respiratory failure.

Caffeine withdrawal for those dependent on this substance can cause headaches and other neurological symptoms. Those who must cut back should taper off gradually. One approach is to mix regular and decaffeinated coffee, gradually decreasing the quantity of the former.

Medications

As many as half of all patients take the wrong medications, in the wrong doses, at the wrong times, or in the wrong ways. Every year these inadvertent errors lead to an estimated 125,000 deaths and more than $8.5 billion in hospital costs. Mistakes occur among people of all ages, both genders, and every race, occupation, level of education, and personality type. Their number one cause: not understanding directions (see Consumer Alert, p. 349).

Doctors occasionally make errors when it comes to prescription drugs. The most frequent are over- or underdosing, omitting information from prescriptions, ordering the wrong dosage form (a pill instead of a liquid, for example), and not recognizing a patient's allergy to a drug.

Always read the consumer-information label before using an over-the-counter drug.

© Geri Engberg Photography

Over-the-Counter Drugs

More than half a million health products— remedies for everything from bad breath to bunions—are readily available without a doctor's prescription. This doesn't mean that they're necessarily safe or effective. Indeed, many widely used **over-the-counter (OTC) drugs** pose unsuspected hazards.

Federal regulators have issued warnings for many popular painkillers, including over-the-counter pills like Advil (ibuprofen) and Aleve (naproxin). Their labels cite risks to the heart, stomach, and skin. Tylenol (acetaminophen) and aspirin are generally considered safe for people with temporary pain like headaches and muscle aches. However, aspirin can cause stomach irritation and bleeding. Tylenol and other products containing acetaminophen account for 40 to 50 percent of all acute cases of liver failure, many the result of unintentional overdose. Doctors caution against taking more than eight Tylenol Extra Strength pills (which contain 500 mg per tablet) in a 24-hour period.

Like other drugs, OTC medications can be used improperly, often simply because of a lack of education about proper use. Among those most often misused are the following:

- **Nasal sprays.** Nasal sprays relieve congestion by shrinking blood vessels in the nose. If they are used too often or for too many days in a row, the blood vessels widen instead of contracting, and the surrounding tissues become swollen, causing more congestion. To make the vessels shrink again, many people use

Avoid Medication Mistakes

Whenever you get a prescription, be sure to find out from your doctor and pharmacist the name of the drug, what it's supposed to do, and how and when to take it and for how long. Are there foods, drinks, other medications, or activities you should avoid while taking the medication? Ask if the drug causes any side effects and what you should do if any occur.

Facts to Know

- Popular herbal supplements like gingko biloba and common over-the-counter drugs like aspirin can interact with many prescription drugs to cause serious problems, such as excessive bleeding. Inform your doctor if you take any.
- Don't use a kitchen spoon to dispense liquid medications. Household teaspoons can hold between 3 and 7 milliliters; a prescription "teaspoon" means 5 milliliters. Either measure the dose in the cup or dropper that came with the medicine or ask the pharmacist for a measuring device.
- Don't crush or chew a medicine without checking with your doctor or pharmacist first. Some medications are designed for gradual release rather than all at once and could be harmful if absorbed too quickly.

Steps to Take

- Keep a record of all your medicines, listing both their brand and generic (chemical) names and the reason you are taking them, and update it regularly. Give a copy of this list to every physician and every pharmacy providing health-care services.
- Always turn on the lights when you take your medication. Familiarize yourself with the imprint on each tablet or capsule so you can recognize each pill. If a refill looks different, check with your pharmacist or doctor before taking it.
- Never take someone else's medications. They could interact with your medications or the dose may be different.
- Always check labels for warnings on interactions with alcohol and instructions on whether or not to take before, with, or after meals.
- Don't take medicine with grapefruit juice, which can interact with more than 200 medications, including cholesterol-lowering statins, sleeping pills, and antianxiety agents.
- Don't leave medicines in a car for prolonged periods. Temperature extremes, along with moisture, light, and oxygen, can affect the potency of many medications.

---

more spray more often. The result can be permanent damage to nasal membranes, bleeding, infection, and partial or complete loss of smell.

- **Laxatives.** Believing that they must have one bowel movement a day (a common misconception), many people rely on laxatives. Brands that contain phenolphthalein irritate the lining of the intestines and cause muscles to contract or tighten, often making constipation worse rather than better. Bulk laxatives are less dangerous, but regular use is not advised. A high-fiber diet and more exercise are safer and more effective remedies for constipation.

- **Eye drops.** Eye drops make the blood vessels of the eye contract. However, as in the case of nasal sprays, with overuse (several times a day for several weeks), the blood vessels expand, making the eye look redder than before.

- **Sleep aids.** Although OTC sleeping pills are widely used, there has been little research on their use and possible risks. A national consensus panel on insomnia concluded that they are not effective and cause side effects such as morning-after grogginess. Medications like

Tylenol PM and Excedrin PM combine a pain reliever with a sleep-inducing antihistamine, the same ingredient that people take for hay fever or cold symptoms. Although they make people drowsy, they can leave a groggy feeling the next day, and they dry out the nose and mouth.

- **Cough syrup.** Many of the "active" ingredients in over-the-counter cough preparations may be ineffective. Young people may chug cough syrup (called *roboing,* after the OTC medication Robitussin) because they think of dextromethorphan (DXM), a common ingredient in cough medicine, as a "poor man's version" of the popular drug Ecstasy.

Prescription Drugs

 Most undergraduates have used prescription drugs for medical reasons at some point in their lives. The most widely used ones are pain medications, sedative or anxiety medications, sleeping medications, and stimulant medications. College women use more pain, anxiety, and sleeping pills; college men, more medically prescribed stimulants.

over-the-counter (OTC) drugs Medications that can be obtained legally without a prescription from a medical professional.

Nonadherence Many prescribed medications aren't taken the way they should be; millions simply aren't taken at all. As many as 70 percent of adults have trouble understanding dosage information and 30 percent can't read standard labels, according to the FDA, which has called for larger, clearer drug labeling. The dangers of nonadherence (not properly taking prescription drugs) include recurrent infections, serious medical complications, and emergency hospital treatment. The drugs most likely to be taken incorrectly are those that treat problems with no obvious symptoms (such as high blood pressure), require complex dosage schedules, treat psychiatric disorders, or have unpleasant side effects.

The most common reason that college students fail to take medicines as directed is forgetting. Others are concerned about cost, or they stop when they feel better.

Physical Side Effects Most medications, taken correctly, cause only minor complications. However, no drug is entirely without side effects for all individuals taking it. Serious complications that may occur include heart failure, heart attack, seizures, kidney and liver failure, severe blood disorders, birth defects, blindness, memory problems, and allergic reactions.

Allergic reactions to drugs are common. The drugs that most often provoke allergic responses are penicillin and other antibiotics (drugs used to treat infection). Aspirin, sulfa drugs, barbiturates, anticonvulsants, insulin, and local anesthetics can also provoke allergic responses.

Psychological Side Effects Dozens of drugs—both over-the-counter and prescription—can cause changes in the way people think, feel, and behave. Unfortunately, neither patients nor their physicians usually connect such symptoms with medications. Doctors may not even mention potential mental and emotional problems because they don't want to scare patients away from what otherwise may be a very effective treatment. What you don't know about a drug's effects on your mind *can* hurt you.

Among the medications most likely to cause psychiatric side effects are drugs for high blood pressure, heart disease, asthma,

epilepsy, arthritis, Parkinson's disease, anxiety, insomnia, and depression. Some drugs—such as the powerful hormones called *corticosteroids*, used for asthma, autoimmune diseases, and cancer—can cause different psychiatric symptoms, depending on dosage and other factors. The older you are, the sicker you are, and the more medications you're taking, the greater your risk of developing some psychiatric side effects.

Drug Interactions OTC and prescription drugs can interact in a variety of ways. For example, mixing some cold medications with tranquilizers can cause drowsiness and coordination problems, thus making driving dangerous. Moreover, what you eat or drink can impair or completely wipe out the effectiveness of drugs or lead to unexpected effects on the body. For instance, aspirin takes five to ten times as long to be absorbed when taken with food or shortly after a meal than when taken on an empty stomach. If tetracyclines encounter calcium in the stomach, they bind together and cancel each other out.

To avoid potentially dangerous interactions, check the label(s) for any instructions on how or when to take a medication, such as "with a meal." If the directions say that you should take a drug on an empty stomach, take it at least one hour before eating or two or three hours after eating. Don't drink a hot beverage with a medication; the temperature may interfere with the effectiveness of the drug.

Whenever you take a drug, be especially careful of your intake of alcohol, which can change the rate of metabolism and the effects of many different drugs. Because it dilates the blood vessels, alcohol can add to the dizziness sometimes caused by drugs for high blood pressure, angina, or depression. Also, its irritating effects on the stomach can worsen stomach upset from aspirin, ibuprofen, and other anti-inflammatory drugs.

Generic Drugs The **generic** name is the chemical name for a drug. A specific drug may appear on the pharmacist's shelf under a variety of brand names, which may cost more than twice the generic equivalent. About 75 percent of all prescriptions specify a brand name, but pharmacists may—and in some states must—switch to a generic drug

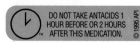

Check the labels on prescription medications.

unless the doctor specifically tells them not to. Prescriptions filled with generic drugs cost 20 to 85 percent less than their brand-name counterparts.

Generic drugs have the same active ingredients as brand-name prescriptions, but their fillers and binders, which can affect the absorption of a drug, may be different. For some serious illnesses, the generics may not be as effective; some experts recommend sticking with brand names for heart medications, psychiatric drugs, and anti-convulsant drugs (for epilepsy and other seizure disorders).

To determine whether you should buy the generic version of a drug, ask your physician whether it matters if you get a brand-name or generic drug. If it does, ask which brand name is best. Also, find out if switching to a generic or from one generic to another might harm your condition in any way.

Buying Drugs Online Millions of people in the United States purchase prescription medications online. Although some websites fill only faxed prescriptions from medical doctors, others ignore or sidestep traditional regulations and safeguards. Cyberspace distributors often ship pills across state lines without requiring a physical examination by a medical doctor. Instead, a "cyberdoc," who may or may not be qualified or up-to-date in a given specialty, reviews information submitted by a "patient." International pharmacies sometimes sell drugs that are not available or approved in the United States. And patients themselves use bulletin boards and other online resources to sell unused or unwanted medications to each other.

Many individuals turn to the Internet for "lifestyle" drugs such as pills for erectile dysfunction, weight control, and smoking cessation. Customers like the convenience and anonymity of buying drugs online. Although many assume drugs cost less on the Internet, shipping costs tend to drive prices up to the same amount or more than the price at a pharmacy.

The dangers of unregulated distribution of medications have alarmed government agencies and medical groups. The American Medical Association has declared it unethical for physicians to write prescriptions for people they've never met. The National Association of Boards of Pharmacy has developed a seal of approval to help customers determine which sites are legitimate. The FDA and other federal agencies, such as the Federal Trade Commission, which regulates advertising, are trying to find ways to impose some controls.

Consumers have to be wary. Ordering a drug like Accutane, an acne treatment, online may seem harmless. However, without close monitoring by a physician, you could develop complications, such as a bad reaction that aggravates hepatitis or inflames the pancreas. Quality control is another concern. Counterfeit drugs, increasingly sold online, may do little, if any, good and could be harmful. Cyberspace pharmacies provide no information on how the drug was stored or whether its expiration date has passed. In addition, since importing medications without a prescription is against the law, you could find yourself in legal trouble.

Prescription Drug Abuse on Campus

 The abuse of prescription medications on college campuses has increased in the last 15 years. As many as one in five college students misuses or abuses a prescription medication every year. Young adults (between ages 18 and 24) have the highest rates of prescription painkiller abuse of any age group in the country.[21] Only marijuana use is more widespread on campus.

 College men have higher rates of prescription drug abuse than women. White and Hispanic undergraduates are significantly more likely to abuse medications than are African American and Asian students. Many students taking prescription drugs for medical purposes report being approached by classmates seeking drugs. Undergraduates who misuse or

generic A consumer product with no brand name or registered trademark.

> **TABLE 11.2**

Why College Students Abuse Prescription Medications

- Boost concentration and alertness
- Improve academic performance
- Pain relief
- Sleep
- Get high
- Experimentation
- Weight control

Source: Judson, Rachel, and Susan W. Langdon. "Illicit Use of Prescription Stimulants among College Students: Prescription Status, Motives, Theory of Planned Behaviour, Knowledge and Self-Diagnostic Tendencies." *Psychology, Health & Medicine,* Vol. 14, No. 1, 2009, pp. 97–104.

abuse prescription medications are much more likely to report heavy binge drinking and use of illicit drugs.

Students who abuse prescription drugs may use both stimulants and painkillers. However, most students choose these agents for different reasons. Students who abuse stimulants say they do so to help improve performance at school, to increase alertness, or to enjoy partying more. A much smaller number take stimulants to lose weight or prevent weight gain. Students who abuse prescription painkillers say they do so to relax or get high, although some report taking the drugs to help with depression and anxiety or for chronic pain. (See Table 11.2.)

Prescription Stimulants

The most widely abused prescription drugs are stimulant medications such as Ritalin. Students think that stimulants can help them focus, concentrate, and study longer. Yet users of these drugs actually have lower GPAs than nonusers, and there is little evidence that stimulants provide any boost. One study found that the lowest dose might provide some benefit, but that increased doses actually impair performance.[22]

Here are some other reasons behind non-medical use of prescription drugs:

- **Legitimate goal.** Students may feel that since they are using stimulants to achieve a positive goal—getting good grades—their use is more acceptable than simply taking drugs to get high.[23]
- **Acceptability.** Prescription drugs are easier to obtain, pose less risk of arrest, and are more socially acceptable than street drugs.[24]
- **Self-diagnosed ADHD.** In one study, about 40 percent of those using stimulants without a prescription reported that they believe they have an attention disorder or were thought to have one in the past.[25]
- **Academic strain.** Researchers have found an indirect connection between students who feel stressed by academic demands and stimulant use. Academic strain leads to higher levels of depression, and students with higher levels of depression are more likely to report nonmedical use of stimulants.[26]

- **Perceived harmlessness.** Almost half of adolescents in one survey believe that prescription drugs are much safer to use than illegal drugs.[27] College students who abuse prescription stimulants also consider these drugs safer because they are manufactured legally and used for legitimate medical reasons.

In various studies, 5 to 35 percent of college-age individuals have reported non-prescribed use of stimulants, and 16 to 29 percent of students prescribed stimulants for ADHD reported being asked to give, sell, or trade their medications. Students who are white, are traditional college age (under 24), belong to fraternities or sororities, have lower grade-point averages, and report some symptoms of ADHD are most likely to misuse or pass on stimulants to others.[28] Most illicit users obtain the drugs from friends or peers for free or at a cost of $1 to $5. In a study of 1,550 undergraduates at a large southern university, about four in ten reported illicit stimulant use. These users, along with students with ADHD, reported significantly greater drug use than others.[29]

Although proper medical use of this agent appears safe, misuse or abuse of any stimulant medication can be dangerous, even deadly. When taken in high doses, either orally or nasally, the risk of addiction increases. Physical side effects include cardiorespiratory complications, increased blood pressure, and headache. High doses can trigger panic attacks, aggressive behavior, and suicidal or homicidal impulses. Overdoses can kill.

Prescription Painkillers

Abuse of prescription painkillers, such as OxyContin and Vicodin, is also widespread on campuses. Students who are members of fraternities and sororities, enrolled at more competitive schools, earning lower grade-point averages, and engaging in substance use and other risky behaviors are more likely to abuse these drugs.

Like other addictions, a prescription painkiller "habit" is a treatable brain disease. Recovery usually requires carefully supervised detoxification, appropriate medications (similar to those used for opioid dependence), behavioral therapy, and ongoing support.

Substance Use Disorders

People have been using psychoactive chemicals for centuries. Citizens of ancient Mesopotamia and Egypt used opium. More than 3,000 years ago, Hindus included cannabis products in religious ceremonies. For centuries the Inca in South America have chewed the leaves of the coca bush. Yet while drugs existed in most societies, their use was usually limited to small groups. Today millions of people regularly turn to drugs to pick them up, bring them down, alter perceptions, or ease psychological pain.

The word **addiction,** as used by the general population, refers to the compulsive use of a substance, loss of control, negative consequences, and denial. Mental health professionals describe drug-related problems in terms of *dependence* and *abuse*.

Dependence

Individuals may develop **psychological dependence** and feel a strong craving for a drug because it produces pleasurable feelings or relieves stress and anxiety. **Physical dependence** occurs when a person develops *tolerance* to the effects of a drug and needs larger and larger doses to achieve intoxication or another desired effect. Individuals who are physically dependent and have a high tolerance to a drug may take amounts many times those that would produce intoxication or an overdose in someone who was not a regular user.

Men and women with a substance dependence disorder may use a drug to avoid or relieve withdrawal symptoms, or they may consume larger amounts of a drug or use it over a longer period than they'd originally intended. They may repeatedly try to cut down or control drug use without success; spend a great deal of time obtaining or using drugs or recovering from their effects; give up or reduce important social, occupational, or recreational activities because of their drug use; or continue to use a drug despite knowledge that the drug is likely to cause or worsen a persistent or recurring physical or psychological problem.

Specific symptoms of dependence vary with particular drugs. Some drugs, such as marijuana, hallucinogens, and phencyclidine, do not cause withdrawal symptoms. The degree of dependence also varies. In mild cases, a person may function normally most of the time. In severe cases, the person's entire life may revolve around obtaining, using, and recuperating from the effects of a drug.

Individuals with drug dependence become intoxicated or high on a regular basis—whether every day, every weekend, or several binges a year. They may try repeatedly to stop using a drug and yet fail, even though they realize their drug use is interfering with their health, family life, relationships, and work.

Abuse

Some drug users do not develop the symptoms of tolerance and withdrawal that characterize dependence, yet they use drugs in ways that clearly have a harmful effect on them. These individuals are diagnosed as having a *psychoactive substance abuse disorder*. They continue to use drugs despite their awareness of persistent or repeated social, occupational, psychological, or physical problems related to drug use, or they use drugs in dangerous ways or situations (before driving, for instance).

Intoxication and Withdrawal

Intoxication refers to maladaptive behavioral, psychological, and physiologic changes that occur as a result of substance use. **Withdrawal** is the development of symptoms that cause significant psychological and physical distress when an individual reduces or stops drug use. (Intoxication and withdrawal from specific drugs are discussed later in this chapter.)

Polyabuse

Most users prefer a certain type of drug but also use several others; this behavior is called **polyabuse.** The average user who enters treatment is on five different drugs. The more drugs anyone uses, the greater the chance of side effects, complications, and possibly life-threatening interactions.

addiction A behavioral pattern characterized by compulsion, loss of control, and continued repetition of a behavior or activity in spite of adverse consequences.

psychological dependence The emotional or mental attachment to the use of a drug.

physical dependence The physiological attachment to, and need for, a drug.

intoxication Maladaptive behavioral, psychological, and physiologic changes that occur as a result of substance abuse.

withdrawal Development of symptoms that cause significant psychological and physical distress when an individual reduces or stops drug use.

polyabuse The misuse or abuse of more than one drug.

Coexisting Conditions

Mental disorders and substance abuse disorders have a great deal of overlap.[30] Many individuals with substance abuse disorders also have another psychiatric disorder, such as depression. Individuals with such *dual diagnoses* require careful evaluation and appropriate treatment for the complete range of complex and chronic difficulties they face. However, they can benefit from participation in 12-step groups, like Double Trouble in Recovery, that provide treatment for both.

Causes of Drug Dependence and Abuse

No one fully understands why some people develop drug dependence or abuse disorders, whereas others, who may experiment briefly with drugs, do not. Inherited body chemistry, genetic factors, and sensitivity to drugs may make some individuals more susceptible. These disorders may stem from many complex causes.

The Biology of Dependence   Scientists now view drug dependence as a brain disease triggered by frequent use of drugs that change the biochemistry and anatomy of neurons and alter the way they work. A major breakthrough in understanding dependence has been the discovery that certain mood-altering substances and experiences—a puff of marijuana, a slug of whiskey, a snort of cocaine, a big win at blackjack—trigger a rise in a brain chemical called **dopamine,** which is associated with feelings of satisfaction and euphoria. This brain chemical or neurotransmitter is one of the crucial messengers that links nerve cells in the brain and its level rises during any pleasurable experience, whether it be a loving hug or a taste of chocolate.

The mechanism governing the rise in dopamine levels is not the same for all drugs. Figure 11.3 shows the one for cocaine. Normally, after dopamine is released from the axon terminal of a neuron and activates dopamine receptors on the adjacent neuron, the dopamine is then transported back to its original neuron by "uptake pumps." Cocaine binds to the uptake pumps and prevents them from transporting dopamine back into the neuron terminal. So more dopamine builds up in the synapse and is free to activate more dopamine receptors.

Addictive drugs have such a powerful impact on dopamine and its receptors that they change the pathways within the brain's pleasure centers. Various psychoactive chemicals create a craving for more of the same. According to this hypothesis, addicts do not specifically yearn for heroin, cocaine, or nicotine but for the rush of dopamine that these drugs produce. Some individuals, born with low levels of dopamine, may be particularly susceptible to this craving and thus to addiction.

The Psychology of Vulnerability

Although scientists do not believe there is an addictive personality, certain individuals are at greater risk of drug dependence because of psychological factors, including difficulty controlling impulses, a lack of values that might constrain drug use (whether based in religion, family, or society), low self-esteem, feelings of powerlessness, and depression. The one psychological trait most often linked with drug use is denial. Young people in particular are absolutely convinced that they will never lose control or suffer in any way as a result of drug use.

Many diagnosed drug users have at least one mental disorder, particularly depression or anxiety. Disorders that emerge in adolescence, such as bipolar disorder, may increase the risk of substance abuse. Many

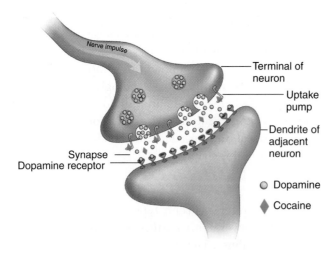

Figure 11.3   Dopamine Levels for Cocaine

Within the synapses between adjacent neurons, cocaine binds to the dopamine uptake pumps and thus allows the neurotransmitter dopamine to build up in the synapse and bind to more dopamine receptors.

people with psychiatric disorders abuse drugs. Individuals may self-administer drugs to treat psychiatric symptoms; for example, they may take sedating drugs to suppress a panic attack.

Early Influences

Teen drug abuse has declined in the last decade, but some teens remain more vulnerable. Young people from lower socioeconomic backgrounds are more likely to use drugs than their more affluent peers, possibly because of economic disadvantage; family instability; a lack of realistic, rewarding alternatives and role models; and increased hopelessness.

Those whose companions are substance abusers are far more likely to use drugs. Peer pressure to use drugs can be a powerful factor for adolescents, although having a drug-using roommate does not increase the odds that a college student will use drugs. The likelihood of drug abuse is also related to family instability, parental rejection, and divorce.

Parents' own attitudes and drug-use history affect their children's likelihood of using marijuana, according to the Substance Abuse and Mental Health Services Administration. Parents who perceive little risk associated with marijuana use have children with similar attitudes, and the children of parents who used marijuana are more likely to try the drug than children whose parents never used the drug.

Drugs and Driving

About one in three adult drivers ages 21 to 25 has driven under the influence of alcohol or drugs during the past year, according to the Substance Abuse and Mental Health Services Administration. Older drivers are less likely than younger drivers to drive while under the influence of alcohol or illicit drugs. Among those ages 26 to 34, 24 percent drove while under the influence of alcohol or illicit drugs in the past year, as did 19 percent of those ages 35 to 49.

Different drugs affect driving ability in different ways. Here are the facts from the National Institute on Drug Abuse:

- **Alcohol** affects perception, coordination, and judgment, and increases the sedative effects of tranquilizers and barbiturates.
- **Marijuana** affects a wide range of driving skills—including the ability to track (stay in the lane) through curves, brake quickly, and maintain speed and a safe distance between cars—and slows thinking and reflexes. Normal driving skills remain impaired for four to six hours after smoking a single joint.
- **Sedatives, sedative-hypnotics, and anti-anxiety agents** slow reaction time and interfere with hand–eye coordination and judgment; the greatest impairment is in the first hour after taking the drug. The effects depend on the particular drug: some build up in the body and can impair driving skills the morning after use; others make drivers very sleepy and therefore incapable of driving safely.
- **Amphetamines,** after repeated use, impair coordination. They can also make a driver more edgy and less coordinated and thus more likely to be involved in an accident.
- **Hallucinogens** distort judgment and reality and cause confusion and panic, thus making driving extremely dangerous.

dopamine A brain chemical associated with feelings of satisfaction and euphoria.

marijuana The drug derived from the cannabis plant, containing the psychoactive ingredient THC, which causes a mild sense of euphoria when inhaled or eaten.

hashish A concentrated form of a drug, derived from the cannabis plant, containing the psychoactive ingredient THC, which causes a sense of euphoria when inhaled or eaten.

Common Drugs of Abuse

Table 11.3 describes the common drugs of abuse within these categories: cannabis, "club drugs," stimulants, depressants, hallucinogens, and inhalants.

Cannabis

Marijuana (pot) and **hashish** (hash)—the most widely used illegal drugs—are derived from the cannabis plant. The major psychoactive ingredient in both is *THC*

> **TABLE 11.3**

Commonly Abused Drugs

Drug	Street Names	How It's Used	Intoxication Effects/Potential Health Consequences
Cannabis			
Marijuana **Hashish**	Pot, grass, reefer, weed, blunt, dope, ganja, herb, joints, Mary Jane, sinsemilla, skunk	Smoked, swallowed	Euphoria, slowed thinking and reaction time, confusion, impaired balance and coordination/Cough, frequent respiratory infections; impaired memory and learning; increased heart rate, anxiety; panic attacks; tolerance, addiction
Club Drugs			
MDMA	Ecstasy, E, Eve, X, XTC, clarity, lover's speed, peace, STP, hug, beans, love drug	Swallowed	Mild hallucinogenic effects, increased tactile sensitivity, empathic feelings/Impaired memory and learning, hyperthermia, cardiac toxicity, renal failure, liver toxicity
GHB	G, Georgia home boy, grievous bodily harm, liquid ecstasy	Swallowed	Reduced anxiety, feeling of well-being, lowered inhibitions, slowed pulse and breathing, lowered blood pressure, poor concentration/Fatigue; confusion; impaired coordination, memory, judgment; addiction; drowsiness; nausea/vomiting; headache; loss of consciousness; loss of reflexes; seizures; coma; death
Ketamine	Cat valium, K, Special-K, vitamin K	Injected, snorted, smoked	Increased heart rate and blood pressure, impaired motor function/ Memory loss; numbness; nausea/vomiting; at high doses, delirium, depression, respiratory depression and arrest
Nitrites	Poppers	Inhaled	Stimulation, loss of inhibition; headache; nausea/vomiting; slurred speech; loss of motor coordination; wheezing/ Unconsciousness, cramps, weight loss, muscle weakness, depression, memory impairment, damage to cardiovascular and nervous systems, sudden death
Stimulants			
			Increased heart rate, blood pressure, metabolism; feelings of exhilaration, energy, increased mental alertness/Rapid or irregular heart beat; reduced appetite; weight loss; heart failure; nervousness; insomnia
Amphetamine	Bennies, black beauties, crosses, hearts, LA turnaround, speed, truck drivers, uppers	Injected, swallowed, smoked, snorted	In addition to preceding: Rapid breathing/Tremor, loss of coordination; irritability; anxiousness; restlessness; delirium; panic; paranoia; impulsive behavior; aggressiveness; tolerance; addiction; psychosis
Methamphetamine	Chalk, crank, crystal, fire, glass, go fast, ice, meth, speed	Injected, swallowed, smoked, snorted	In addition to preceding: Aggression, violence, psychotic behavior/Memory loss; cardiac and neurological damage; impaired memory and learning; tolerance; addiction
Cocaine	Blow, bump, C, candy, Charlie, coke, crack, flake, rock, snow, toot, white girl, lady	Injected, smoked, snorted	In addition to preceding: Increased temperature/Chest pain, respiratory failure, nausea, abdominal pain, strokes, seizures, headaches, malnutrition, panic attacks
Depressants			
			Reduced anxiety, feeling of well-being, lowered inhibitions; slowed pulse and breathing, lowered blood pressure, poor concentration/Fatigue; confusion; impaired coordination, memory, judgment; addiction; respiratory depression and arrest; death
Benzodiazepines	Candy, downers, sleeping pills, tranks	Swallowed, injected	In addition to preceding: Sedation, drowsiness/Dizziness
Rohypnol	Forget-me pill, Mexican Valium, R2, Roche, roofies, roofinol, rope, rophies	Swallowed, snorted	Visual and gastrointestinal disturbances, urinary retention, memory loss for the time under the drug's effects

continued

TABLE 11.3

Commonly Abused Drugs, *continued*

Drug	Street Names	How It's Used	Intoxication Effects/Potential Health Consequences
Barbiturates	Barbs, reds, red birds, phennies, tooies, yellows, yellow jackets	Injected, swallowed	In addition to preceding: Sedation, drowsiness/Depression, unusual excitement, fever, irritability, poor judgment, slurred speech, dizziness, life-threatening withdrawal
Opioids			
			Pain relief, euphoria, drowsiness/Nausea, constipation, confusion, sedation, respiratory depression and arrest, tolerance, addiction, unconsciousness, coma, death
Heroin	Brown sugar, dope, H, horse, junk, skag, skunk, smack, white horse	injected, smoked, snorted	
Morphine	Miss Emma, monkey, white stuff	Injected, swallowed, smoked	
Codeine	Captain Cody, Cody, schoolboy	Injected, swallowed	
OxyContin	Oxy, OC, Killer	Swallowed, snorted, injected	
Vicodin	Vike, Watson-387	Swallowed	
Hallucinogens			
			Altered states of perception and feeling/Nausea, persisting perception disorder (flashbacks)
LSD	Acid, blotter, boomers, cubes, microdot, yellow sunshines	Swallowed, absorbed through mouth tissues	In addition to preceding: Increased body temperature, heart rate, blood pressure; loss of appetite; sleeplessness; numbness; weakness; tremors; persistent mental disorders
PCP	Angel dust, boat, hog, love boat, peace pill	Injected, swallowed, smoked	Impaired motor function, possible decrease in blood pressure and heart rate, panic, aggression, violence/Memory loss, numbness, nausea/vomiting, loss of appetite, depression
Inhalants			
			Stimulation, loss of inhibition; headache; nausea/vomiting; slurred speech, loss of motor coordination; wheezing/Unconsciousness, cramps, weight loss, muscle weakness, depression, memory impairment, damage to cardiovascular and nervous systems, sudden death
Solvents (paint thinners, gasoline, glues)		Inhaled through nose or mouth	
Gases (butane, propane, aerosol propellants, nitrous oxide)		Inhaled through nose or mouth	

Source: National Institute on Drug Abuse, www.nida.nih.gov/DrugPages/DrugsofAbuse.html

(delta-9-tetrahydrocannabinol). Marijuana is the most widely abused substance, with more than 150 million people reporting they've used it at least once in the last year. Some 12 million Americans use cannabis; more than 1 million cannot control this use.

Teens and young adults who use marijuana are more likely to develop serious mental health problems. Researchers have documented an association between frequent marijuana use and increased anxiety and depression in young adults, regardless of whether they use other illicit drugs.

Some people, particularly advocates for its legalization, argue that marijuana is relatively harmless. However, scientific research has confirmed that long-term use causes many adverse health consequences, including significant brain injury. When used

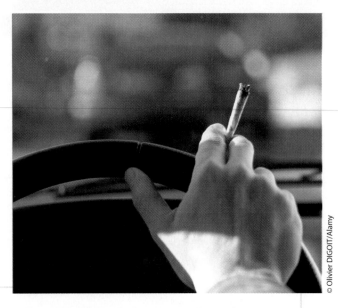

All psychoactive drugs affect driving ability. For instance, marijuana decreases the ability to stay in the lane through curves and to brake quickly, and it slows thinking and reflexes.

© Olivier DIGOIT/Alamy

Marijuana has shown some medical benefits, including boosting appetite in patients who are HIV-positive or undergoing chemotherapy, alleviating cancer and neck pain, reducing pressure on the eyeball in glaucoma patients, and helping people with spasticity (extreme muscle tension) due to multiple sclerosis or injuries.

A growing number of states have passed voter referenda (or legislative actions) making marijuana available to smoke for a variety of medical conditions upon a doctor's recommendation. However, the FDA, after a comprehensive investigation, concluded that "no sound scientific studies supported medical use of marijuana for treatment in the United States, and no animal or human data supported the safety or efficacy of marijuana for general medical use."[33] FDA-approved medications are available as treatment alternatives for many of the proposed uses of smoked marijuana, such as relief of nausea and vomiting induced by chemotherapy. Synthetic versions of the active ingredient in marijuana, developed for medical use, act on the brain like the THC in smoked marijuana but eliminate the need to inhale harmful smoke.

chronically, cannabis can produce dependence, respiratory disease and psychotic symptoms, especially in vulnerable young adults. It also may interfere with normal brain development in adolescents and young adults.[31] Another recently recognized danger is increased risk of a particularly aggressive form of testicular cancer, the most common cancer in men between ages 15 and 34.[32]

 Marijuana use is generally less pervasive than binge drinking (see Chapter 12) on most campuses, although at some schools as many as a third of students report smoking pot. Students who used marijuana in high school are more likely to do so in college. Roommates have very little impact on drug use. Men who have not used marijuana before college seem, if anything, turned off rather than turned on by roommates who have smoked pot. Peers have no clear impact on women's marijuana use.

Different types of marijuana have different percentages of THC. Because of careful cultivation, the strength of today's marijuana is much greater than that used in the 1970s. Today a marijuana joint contains 150 mg of THC, compared to 10 mg in the 1960s. Usually, marijuana is smoked in a joint (hand-rolled cigarette) or pipe; it may also be eaten as an ingredient in other foods (as when baked in brownies), though with a less predictable effect.

How Users Feel   The circumstances in which marijuana is smoked, the communal aspects of its use, and the user's experience all can affect the way a marijuana-induced high feels.

In low to moderate doses, marijuana typically creates a mild sense of euphoria, a sense of slowed time (five minutes may feel like an hour), a dreamy sort of self-absorption, and some impairment in thinking and communicating. Users report heightened sensations of color, sound, and other stimuli, relaxation, and increased confidence. The sense of being stoned peaks within half an hour and usually lasts about three hours. Even when alterations in perception seem slight, it is not safe to drive a car for as long as four to six hours after smoking a single joint.

Some users—particularly those smoking marijuana for the first time or taking a high dose in an unpleasant or unfamiliar setting—experience acute anxiety, which may be accompanied by a panicky fear of losing control. They may believe that their companions are ridiculing or threatening them and experience a panic attack, a state of intense terror.

The immediate physical effects of marijuana include increased pulse rate, bloodshot eyes, dry mouth and throat, slowed reaction times, impaired motor skills, increased appetite, and diminished short-term memory (Figure 11.4). High doses reduce the ability to perceive and to react; all the reactions experienced with low doses are intensified, leading to sensory distortion and, in the case of hashish, vivid hallucinations and LSD-like, psychedelic reactions. The drug remains in the body's fat cells 50 hours or more after use, so people may experience psychoactive effects for several days after use. Drug tests may produce positive results for days or weeks after last use.

Risks Marijuana produces a range of effects in different body systems, such as depression, diminished immune responses, and impaired fertility in men. Other risks include damage to the brain, lungs, and heart and to babies born to mothers who use marijuana during pregnancy or while nursing (see Figure 11.4).

Brain As brain scans have documented, long-term marijuana use causes significant brain abnormalities, including shrinkage of key structures involved in memory, learning, and emotion, that can lead to memory loss, difficulty learning new information, and psychotic symptoms.[34] Short-term effects include problems with memory and learning; distorted perceptions; difficulty thinking and problem solving; loss of coordination; increased anxiety; and panic attacks. Long-term heavy users of marijuana perform significantly worse on tests of verbal fluency, memory, and coordination than short-term users or nonusers, even after abstaining from pot for more than 24 hours.

Over time, continued heavy marijuana use can disrupt sleep[35] and interfere with students' ability to learn and perform well in school and in challenging careers. Marijuana contributes significantly to accidental death and injury among adolescents, especially through motor vehicle crashes.

Lungs Smoking cannabis may cause effects similar to those of smoking tobacco, with many of them appearing at a younger age. They include chronic bronchitis, emphysema, and other lung disorders and increased risk of heart attacks and sudden death. The amount of tar inhaled by marijuana smokers and the level of carbon monoxide absorbed are three to five times greater than among tobacco smokers. The reasons may be that marijuana users inhale more deeply, hold the smoke in the lungs longer, and do not use filters. Smoking a single joint can be as damaging to the lungs as smoking five tobacco cigarettes. Someone who smokes five joints a week may take in as many cancer-causing chemicals as a person who smokes a pack of cigarettes a day.

Heart Otherwise healthy people have suffered heart attacks shortly after smoking marijuana. Experiments have also linked marijuana use to elevated blood pressure and decreased oxygen supply to the heart muscle. The risk of heart attack triples within an hour of smoking pot. Smoking marijuana while

Negative Long-Term Effects

Brain and central nervous system
- Causes brain abnormalities
- Dulls sensory and cognitive skills
- Impairs short-term memory
- Alters motor coordination
- Causes changes in brain chemistry
- Leads to difficulty in concentration, attention to detail, and learning new complex information
- Increases risk of stroke
- Increases risk of psychotic symptoms
- Causes disturbed sleep

Cardiovascular system
- Increases heart rate
- Increases blood pressure
- Decreases blood flow to the limbs

Respiratory system
- Damages the lungs (50% more tar than tobacco)
- May cause lung cancer
- May damage throat from inhalation

Reproductive system
- In women, may impair ovulation and cause fetal abnormalities if used during pregnancy
- In men, may suppress sexual functioning and may reduce the number, quality, and motility of sperm, possibly affecting fertility

Figure 11.4 Impact of Marijuana

Marijuana has negative long-term effects on many systems of the body.

shooting cocaine can potentially cause deadly increases in heart rate and blood pressure.

Pregnancy   Babies born to mothers who used marijuana during pregnancy are smaller than those born to mothers who did not use the drug, and the babies are more likely to develop health problems. A nursing mother who uses marijuana passes some of the THC to the baby in her breast milk. This may impair the infant's motor development (control of muscle movement).

Withdrawal   Marijuana users can develop a compulsive, often uncontrollable craving for the drug. More than 120,000 people enter treatment every year for marijuana addiction. Marijuana withdrawal has proven as difficult as quitting smoking.[36] Stopping after long-term marijuana use can produce *marijuana withdrawal syndrome*, which is characterized by insomnia, restlessness, loss of appetite, and irritability. People who smoke marijuana daily for many years may become aggressive after they stop using it and may relapse to prevent aggression and other symptoms.

Club Drugs (Designer Drugs)

The National Institute on Drug Abuse identifies a variety of drugs—alcohol, LSD (acid), MDMA (Ecstasy), GHB, GBL, ketamine (Special-K), fentanyl, Rohypnol, and nitrites—as **"club drugs."** They first became popular among teens and young adults at nightclubs, bars, or night-long dances often held in warehouses or other unusual settings. Their use by teenagers has been dropping in recent years.

Young people may take club drugs to relax, energize, and enhance their social interactions, but a large number also experience negative consequences. As many as three in four report side effects such as profuse sweating, hot and cold flashes, tingling or numbness, blurred vision, trouble sleeping, hallucinations, depression, confusion, anxiety, irritability, paranoia, and loss of libido (sex drive). Some also experience difficulty with their usual daily activities and financial and work troubles.

Ecstasy   Ecstasy (E, XTC, X, hug, beans, love drug) is the most common street name

for methylenedioxymethamphetamine (MDMA), a synthetic compound with both stimulant and mildly hallucinogenic properties.

According to various studies, students who take Ecstasy were more likely to use marijuana, binge-drink, smoke cigarettes, have multiple sexual partners, spend more time socializing with friends and less time studying, and consider parties important and religion less important. However, researchers who compared students who used Ecstasy and other illicit drugs with those who used only marijuana have concluded that undergraduates who use Ecstasy may be a subgroup of marijuana users who tend to engage in many risk-taking behaviors. Ecstasy users also think that their peers smoke more marijuana and use more Ecstasy than they actually do.

How Users Feel   Although it can be smoked, inhaled (snorted), or injected, Ecstasy is almost always taken as a pill or tablet. Its effects begin in 45 minutes and last for three to six hours.

MDMA belongs to a family of drugs called *enactogens*, which literally means "touching within." As a mood elevator, it produces a relaxed, euphoric state but does not produce hallucinations. Users of Ecstasy often say they feel at peace with themselves and a sense of connectedness with others. In some settings, they reveal intimate details of their lives (which they may later regret); in other settings, they join in collective rejoicing. Like hallucinogenic drugs, MDMA can enhance sensory experience, but it rarely causes visual distortions, sudden mood changes, or psychotic reactions. Regular users may experience depression and anxiety the week after taking MDMA.

Risks   Ecstasy poses risks similar to those of cocaine and amphetamines. These include psychological difficulties (confusion, depression, sleep problems, drug craving, severe anxiety, and paranoia) and physical symptoms (muscle tension, involuntary teeth clenching, nausea, blurred vision, rapid eye movement, faintness, chills, sweating, and increases in heart rate and blood pressure that pose a special risk for people with circulatory or heart disease).

Ecstasy can produce nausea, vomiting, and dizziness. When combined with extended physical exertion like dancing, club drugs can lead to hyperthermia (severe overheating), severe dehydration, serious increases in blood pressure, stroke, and heart attack. Without sufficient water, dancers at raves may suffer dehydration and heat stroke, which can be fatal. Individuals with high blood pressure, heart trouble, or liver or kidney disease are in the greatest danger. Several deaths have occurred in teens who suffered brain damage by drinking large amounts of water to counteract the raised body temperature induced by the drug.

MDMA has been implicated in some cases of acute hepatitis, which can lead to liver failure. Even after liver transplantation, the mortality rate for individuals with this condition is 50 percent. Another danger comes from the practice of taking SSRIs (see Chapter 4), which modulate the mood-altering brain chemical serotonin, before Ecstasy. This can cause jaw clenching, nausea, tremors, and, in extreme cases, potentially fatal elevations in body temperature.

Although not a sexual stimulant (if anything, MDMA has the opposite effect), Ecstasy fosters strong feelings of intimacy that may lead to risky sexual behavior. The psychological effects of Ecstasy become less intriguing with repeated use, and the physical side effects become more uncomfortable. Ecstasy poses risks to a developing fetus, including a greater likelihood of heart and skeletal abnormalities and long-term learning and memory impairments in children born to women who used MDMA during pregnancy.

GHB and GBL Once sold in health-food stores for its muscle-building and alleged fat-burning properties, **gamma hydroxybutyrate** (GHB, G, Georgia home boy, grievous bodily harm, liquid ecstasy) was banned because of its effects on the brain and nervous system. The main ingredient is **GBL (gamma butyrolactone)**, an industrial solvent often used to strip floors, which converts into GHB once ingested. GHB acts as a sedative while producing feelings of euphoria and heightened sexuality. Because of its amnesic properties, GHB has been used as a "date rape" drug, similar to Rohypnol.

Alcohol intensifies its effects, which typically last up to four hours.

Large doses can cause someone to pass out in 15 minutes and fall into a coma within half an hour. Death can occur. Other side effects include nausea, amnesia, hallucinations, decreased heart rate, convulsions, and sometimes blackouts. Long-term use at high doses can lead to a withdrawal reaction: rapid heartbeat, tremor, insomnia, anxiety, and occasionally hallucinations that last a few days to a week.

GHB is addictive. Users who attempt to quit may experience significant withdrawal symptoms, including anxiety, tremors, and insomnia. Most symptoms decrease within one to two weeks of cessation, but severe psychological effects can last for weeks to months.

Ketamine Ketamine—called K, Special-K, and vitamin K—is an anesthetic used by veterinarians. When cooked, dried, and ground into powder for snorting, ketamine blocks chemical messengers in the brain that carry sensory input. As a result, the brain fills the void with hallucinations. Users may report an "out-of-body" experience with distorted perceptions of time and space. The effects typically begin within 30 minutes and last for approximately two hours.

Ketamine has become common in club scenes and has been used as a date rape drug. Low doses can cause impaired attention and memory, anxiety, agitation, paranoia, and vomiting. Higher doses can cause delirium, amnesia, impaired motor function, high blood pressure, depression, and potentially deadly breathing problems. Repeated ketamine use can be addictive and even a single use can occasionally produce audiovisual "flashbacks," similar to those described by phencyclidine (PCP) users, and long-term memory loss.

Nitrites Nitrites (amyl, butyl, and isobutyl nitrite) are clear, amber-colored liquids that have had a history of abuse for more than three decades, especially in gay and bisexual men. Popular in dance clubs, they are used recreationally for a high feeling, a slowed sense of time, a carefree sense of well-being, and intensified sexual experiences.

club drugs Illegally manufactured psychoactive drugs that have dangerous physical and psychological effects.

Ecstasy (MDMA) A synthetic compound, also known as methylenedioxymethamphetamine, that is similar in structure to methamphetamine and has both stimulant and hallucinogenic effects.

GHB (gamma hydroxybutyrate) A brain messenger chemical that stimulates the release of human growth hormone; commonly abused for its high and its alleged ability to trim fat and build muscles. Also known as "blue nitro" or the "date rape drug."

GBL (gamma butyrolactone) The main ingredient in gamma hydroxybutyrate (GHB); once ingested, GBL converts to GHB and can cause the ingestor to lose consciousness.

Sold in small glass ampules containing individual doses, nitrites are usually inhaled and rapidly absorbed into the bloodstream. Users feel their physiological and psychological impact in seconds. Acute adverse effects include headache, dizziness, a drop in blood pressure, changes in heart rate, increased pressure within the eye, and skin flushing. Some individuals develop respiratory irritation and cough, sneezing, or difficulty breathing. Chronic use can lead to crusty skin lesions and chemical burns around the nose, mouth, and lips.

Herbal Ecstasy Herbal ecstasy, also known as herbal bliss, cloud 9, and herbal X, is a mixture of stimulants such as ephedrine, pseudoephedrine, and caffeine. Sold in tablet or capsule form as a "natural" and safe alternative to Ecstasy, its ingredients vary greatly. Herbal ecstasy can have dangerous and unpleasant side effects, including stroke, heart attack, and a disfiguring skin condition.

Stimulants

Central nervous system **stimulants** are drugs that increase activity in some portion of the brain or spinal cord. Some stimulants increase motor activity and enhance mental alertness, and some combat mental fatigue. Amphetamine, methamphetamine, caffeine, cocaine, and khat are stimulants. Stimulant medications are used to treat conditions such as ADHD.

Amphetamine Amphetamines trigger the release of epinephrine (adrenaline), which stimulates the central nervous system. They were once widely prescribed for weight control because they suppress appetite, but they have emerged as a global danger. Amphetamines are sold under a variety of names: amphetamine (brand name Benzedrine, street name bennies), dextroamphetamine (Dexedrine, dex), methamphetamine (Methedrine, meth, speed, crank), and Desoxyn (copilots). Related *uppers* include the prescription drugs methylphenidate (Ritalin), pemoline (Cylert), and phenmetrazine (Preludin). Amphetamines are available in tablet or capsule form.

How Users Feel Amphetamines produce a state of hyper-alertness and energy. Users feel confident in their ability to think clearly and to perform any task exceptionally well—although amphetamines do not, in fact, significantly boost performance or thinking. Higher doses make users feel *wired:* talkative, excited, restless, irritable, anxious, moody.

If taken intravenously, amphetamines produce a characteristic rush of elation and confidence, as well as adverse effects, including confusion, rambling or incoherent speech, anxiety, headache, and palpitations. Individuals may become paranoid; be convinced they are having profound thoughts; feel increased sexual interest; and experience unusual perceptions, such as ringing in the ears, a sensation of insects crawling on their skin, or hearing their name called. Methamphetamine users may feel high and sleepy or may hallucinate and lose contact with reality.

Risks Dependence on amphetamines can develop with episodic or daily use. Bingeing—taking high doses over a period of several days—can lead to an extremely intense and unpleasant *crash,* characterized by a craving for the drug, shakiness, irritability, anxiety, and depression. Two or more days are required for recuperation.

Amphetamine intoxication may cause the following symptoms:

- Feelings of grandiosity, anxiety, tension, hypervigilance, anger, social hypersensitivity, fighting, jitteriness or agitation, paranoia, and impaired judgment in social or occupational functioning.

- Increased heart rate, dilated pupils, elevated blood pressure, perspiration or chills, and nausea or vomiting.

- Less frequent effects such as speeding up or slowing down of physical movement; muscular weakness; impaired breathing, chest pain, heart arrhythmia; confusion, seizures, impaired movements or muscle tone; or even coma.

- In high doses, a rapid or irregular heartbeat, tremors, loss of coordination, and collapse.

The long-term effects of amphetamine abuse include malnutrition, skin disorders, ulcers, insomnia, depression, vitamin deficiencies, and, in some cases, brain damage that results in speech and thought disturbances. Sexual dysfunction and impaired concentration or memory also may occur.

Withdrawal   When the immediate effects of amphetamines wear off, users experience a *crash* and become shaky, irritable, anxious, and depressed. Amphetamine withdrawal usually persists for more than 24 hours after cessation of prolonged, heavy use. Its characteristic features include fatigue, disturbing dreams, much more or less than usual sleep, increased appetite, and speeding up or slowing down of physical movements. Those who are unable to sleep despite their exhaustion often take sedative-hypnotics (discussed later in this chapter) to help them rest and may then become dependent on them in addition to amphetamines. Symptoms usually reach a peak in two to four days, although depression and irritability may persist for months. Suicide is a major risk.

Methamphetamine   Methamphetamine, an addictive stimulant that is less expensive and possibly more addictive than cocaine or heroin, has become America's leading drug problem. More than 12 million Americans have tried methamphetamine, and 1.5 million are regular users, according to federal estimates. Its estimated annual economic cost is $23.4 billion.[37]

Methamphetamine is chemically related to amphetamine, but its effects on the central nervous system are greater. Made in illegal laboratories, street methamphetamine is referred to by many names, such as speed, crystal, fire, glass, meth, and chalk. Methamphetamine hydrochloride, clear chunky crystals resembling ice that can be inhaled by smoking, is called ice, crystal, glass, and tina. Methamphetamine can be snorted, smoked, injected, or ingested orally.

How Users Feel   Methamphetamine causes the release of large amounts of dopamine, which creates a sensation of euphoria, increased self-esteem, and alertness. Users also report a marked increase in sexual appetite, which often leads to risky sexual behaviors while under the drug's influence.

Smoking or intravenous injection leads to an intense, pleasurable sensation, called a rush or flash, that lasts only a few minutes.

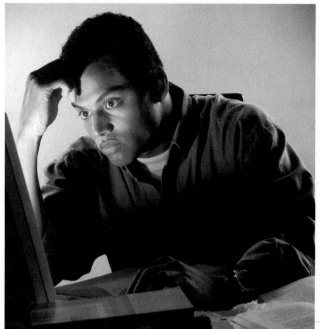

Some college students try stimulants to stay alert while cramming for exams, but these medications do not improve academic performance and can cause harmful side effects.

Oral or intranasal use produces a high but not a rush. Users may become addicted quickly, using more methamphetamine more and more frequently. Despair and suicidal thinking can develop when the stimulant effect wears off.

Risks   Even small amounts of methamphetamine can increase wakefulness and physical activity, depress appetite, and raise body temperature. Other effects on the central nervous system include irritability, insomnia, confusion, tremors, convulsions, anxiety, paranoia, and aggressiveness.

Methamphetamine increases heart rate and blood pressure and can cause irreversible damage to blood vessels in the brain, producing strokes. Other effects of methamphetamine include respiratory problems, irregular heartbeat, and extreme loss of appetite and weight. During intoxication, the body (and probably brain) temperature rises, sometimes resulting in convulsions. High fevers or collapse of the circulatory system can cause death.

Common psychiatric symptoms are insomnia, irritability, and aggressive behavior. The drug causes intellectual impairment, anxiety, and depression. Chronic users become disorganized and unable to cope

stimulant   An agent, such as a drug, that temporarily relieves drowsiness, helps in the performance of repetitive tasks, and improves capacity for work.

amphetamine   Any of a class of stimulants that trigger the release of epinephrine, which stimulates the central nervous system; users experience a state of hyper-alertness and energy, followed by a crash as the drug wears off.

© Esbin-Anderson/The Image Works

Ya-ba/Thai Tabs are a powerful form of methamphetamine that tastes sweet like candy.

with everyday problems. The risk of developing psychotic symptoms—hallucinations and delusions—is very high. They may persist for months or years after use stops.

Another side effect is called meth mouth. In short periods of time, sometimes just months, teeth can turn a grayish-brown, twist, begin to fall out, and take on a peculiar texture. This may be the result of methamphetamine's effects on the metabolic system, plus the huge quantities of sugary soft drinks that users consume for the dry mouth caused by the drug.

Meth users engage in more sex, more carelessly. Meth has become popular among gay and bisexual men, and it has been linked to an increase in unsafe sex practices. Methamphetamine use and needle sharing have been linked to a spike in HIV and hepatitis C infections in gay communities.

Methamphetamine causes abnormalities in brain regions associated with selective attention and in those associated with memory. The brain may recover somewhat after months of abstinence, but problems often remain. Long-term use causes changes in brain chemistry that may lead to compulsive drug-seeking and make addiction especially hard to overcome.[38] Former methamphetamine addicts may suffer from chronic apathy and anhedonia (inability to experience pleasure) for years.

The Toll on Society   Law enforcement officials consider methamphetamine their biggest drug problem. Meth-related arrests have soared. Meth addicts are pouring into prisons and recovery centers at an ever-increasing rate. "Meth babies" are crowding

the foster-care system. Meth-making operations have been uncovered in all 50 states, with the greatest number in Missouri. Production releases poisonous gases and results in toxic waste that is often dumped down household drains, in a backyard, or at a roadside. The cost of cleaning up the environment is a growing problem for many communities.

Over-the-counter cold medicines (ephedrine and pseudoephedrine) are commonly used in meth production, which is one reason for federal and state restrictions on their sale. As drugstores and retailers have placed nonprescription cold pills behind the pharmacy counter, meth manufacturing has moved into Mexico, where labs produce hundreds of pounds of meth a year and smuggle it into the United States.

Withdrawal   Methamphetamine addiction is difficult to treat. As with cocaine, coming off methamphetamine causes intense distress, so users often seek out the drug to relieve their pain. Treatment usually requires the intervention of the patient's family as well as a substance abuse specialist team experienced in treating methamphetamine addiction. Standard substance abuse treatment methods such as education, behavior therapy, individual and family counseling, and support groups may be effective for some. Methamphetamine abusers often use other illicit drugs as well, a problem that can be addressed as part of a comprehensive program.

Cocaine   Cocaine (coke, snow, lady) is a white crystalline powder extracted from the leaves of the South American coca plant. Usually mixed with various sugars and local anesthetics like lidocaine and procaine, cocaine powder is generally inhaled. When sniffed or snorted, cocaine anesthetizes the nerve endings in the nose and relaxes the lung's bronchial muscles.

Cocaine can be dissolved in water and injected intravenously. The drug is rapidly metabolized by the liver, so the high is relatively brief, typically lasting only about 20 minutes. This means that users will commonly inject the drug repeatedly, increasing the risk of infection and damage to their veins.

In addition to respiratory problems, brain damage, and mental impairment, methamphetamine damages teeth. This is how "meth mouth" looks.

Cocaine alkaloid, or *freebase*, is obtained by removing the hydrochloride salt from cocaine powder. *Freebasing* is smoking the fumes of the alkaloid form of cocaine. *Crack,* pharmacologically identical to freebase, is a cheap, easy-to-use, widely available, smokeable, and potent form of cocaine named for the popping sound it makes when burned. Because it is absorbed rapidly into the bloodstream and large doses reach the brain very quickly, it is particularly dangerous. However, its low price and easy availability have made it a common drug of abuse in poor urban areas.

How Users Feel A powerful stimulant to the central nervous system, cocaine targets several chemical sites in the brain, producing feelings of soaring well-being and boundless energy. Users feel they have enormous physical and mental ability, yet are also restless and anxious. After a brief period of euphoria, users slump into a depression. They often go on cocaine binges, lasting from a few hours to several days, and consume large quantities of cocaine.

With crack, dependence develops quickly. As soon as crack users come down from one high, they want more crack. Whereas heroin addicts may shoot up several times a day, crack addicts need another hit within minutes. Thus, a crack habit can quickly become more expensive than heroin addiction.

Risks Cocaine dependence is an easy habit to acquire. With repeated use, the brain becomes tolerant of the drug's stimulant effects, and users must take more of it to get high. Those who smoke or inject cocaine can develop dependence within weeks. Those who sniff cocaine may not become dependent on the drug for months or years. It is thought that 5 to 20 percent of all coke users—a group as large as the estimated total number of heroin addicts—are dependent on the drug.

The physical effects of acute cocaine intoxication include dilated pupils, elevated or lowered blood pressure, perspiration or chills, nausea or vomiting, speeding up or slowing down of physical activity, muscular weakness, impaired breathing, chest pain, and impaired movements or muscle tone. Prolonged cocaine snorting can result in ulceration of the mucous membrane of the nose and damage to the nasal septum (the membrane between the nostrils) severe enough to cause it to collapse.

Although some users initially try cocaine as a sexual stimulant, it does not enhance sexual performance. At low doses, it may delay orgasm and cause heightened sensory awareness, but men who use cocaine regularly have problems maintaining erections and ejaculating. They also tend to have low sperm counts, less active sperm, and more abnormal sperm than nonusers. Both male and female chronic cocaine users tend to lose interest in sex and have difficulty reaching orgasm.

Cocaine use can cause blood vessels in the brain to clamp shut and can trigger a stroke, bleeding in the brain, and potentially fatal brain seizures. Cocaine users can also develop psychiatric or neurological complications (Figure 11.5). Repeated or high doses of cocaine can lead to impaired judgment, hyperactivity, nonstop babbling, feelings of suspicion and paranoia, and violent behavior. The brain never learns to tolerate cocaine's negative effects; users may become incoherent and paranoid and may experience unusual sensations, such as ringing in their ears, feeling insects crawling on the skin, or hearing their name called.

Cocaine can damage the liver and cause lung damage in freebasers. Smoking crack causes bronchitis as well as lung damage and may promote the transmission of HIV through burned and bleeding lips. Some smokers have died of respiratory complications, such as pulmonary edema (the buildup of fluid in the lungs).

Cocaine can trigger the symptoms of a heart attack in young people; the wrong therapeutic responses can be fatal.[39] Cocaine causes the heart rate to speed up and blood pressure to rise suddenly. Its use is associated with many cardiac complications, including arrhythmia (disruption of heart rhythm), angina (chest pain), and acute myocardial infarction (heart attack).

The combination of alcohol and cocaine is particularly lethal. The liver combines the two agents and manufactures cocaethylene, which intensifies cocaine's euphoric effects, while possibly increasing the risk of sudden death. Cocaine users who inject the drug and share

cocaine A white crystalline powder extracted from the leaves of the coca plant that stimulates the central nervous system and produces a brief period of euphoria followed by a depression.

Central nervous system
- Repeated use or high dosages may cause severe psychological problems
- Suppresses desire for food, sex, and sleep
- Can cause strokes, seizures, and neurological damage

Nose
- Damages mucous membrane

Cardiovascular system
- Increases blood pressure by constricting blood vessels
- Causes irregular heartbeat
- Damages heart tissue

Respiratory system
- Freebasing causes lung damage
- Overdose can lead to respiratory arrest

Reproductive system
- In men, affects ability to maintain erections and ejaculate; also causes sperm abnormalities
- In women, may affect ability to carry pregnancy to term

Figure 11.5 Some Effects of Cocaine on the Body

needles put themselves at risk for another potentially lethal problem: HIV infection.

Cocaine is dangerous for pregnant women and their babies, causing miscarriages, developmental disorders, and life-threatening complications during birth. Cocaine can reduce the fetal oxygen supply, possibly interfering with the development of the fetus's nervous system.

Withdrawal When addicted individuals stop using cocaine, they often become depressed. This may lead to further cocaine use to alleviate depression. Other symptoms of cocaine withdrawal include fatigue, vivid and disturbing dreams, excessive or too little sleep, irritability, increased appetite, and physical slowing down or speeding up. This initial crash may last one to three days after cutting down or stopping the heavy use of cocaine. Some individuals become violent, paranoid, and suicidal.

Symptoms usually reach a peak in two to four days, although depression, anxiety, irritability, lack of pleasure in usual activities, and low-level cravings may continue for weeks. As memories of the crash fade, the desire for cocaine intensifies. For many

weeks after stopping, individuals may feel an intense craving for the drug.

Treatment Overcoming an addiction to cocaine or other stimulant drug can be challenging. Among the behavioral approaches that have shown the greatest success are:

- Cognitive-behavioral therapy (CBT), which helps patients recognize and avoid drug triggers and learn new ways of coping with them.
- Contingency management, which uses tangible rewards such as vouchers for movies, to encourage abstinence.
- The Matrix Model, which combines a 12-step program, behavioral therapy, family education, and individual counseling.

The FDA has not approved any medications for these addictions, but several drugs have shown promise. These include Antabuse, widely used for alcohol dependence; the muscle relaxant baclofen (Lioresal); the anticonvulsant topiramate (Topamax); and the stimulant modafinil (Provigil), used to treat narcolepsy.[40]

Khat (Kat, Catha, Chat, Abyssinian Tea)

For centuries people in East Africa and the Arabian peninsula consumed the fresh young leaves of the *Catha edulis shrub* in ways similar to our drinking coffee. Its active ingredients are two controlled substances, cathinone and cathine. Chewing alleviates fatigue and reduces appetite. Compulsive use may result in manic behavior, grandiose illusions, paranoia, and hallucinations.

Depressants

Depressants depress the central nervous system, reduce activity, and induce relaxation, drowsiness, or sleep. They include the benzodiazepines and the barbiturates, the opioids, and alcohol.

Benzodiazepines and Barbiturates These depressants are the sedative-hypnotics, also known as anxiolytic or antianxiety drugs. The **benzodiazepines**—the most widely used drugs in this category—are commonly prescribed for tension, muscular strain, sleep problems, anxiety, panic attacks, anesthesia, and in the treatment of alcohol withdrawal. They include such drugs as *chlordiazepoxide*

(Librium), *diazepam* (Valium), *oxazepam* (Serax), *lorazepam* (Ativan), *flurazepam* (Dalmane), and *alprazolam* (Xanax). They differ widely in their mechanism of action, absorption rate, and metabolism, but all produce similar intoxication and withdrawal symptoms.

Rohypnol, a trade name for flunitrazepam—called roofies, rophie, roche, or the forget-me pill—is one of the benzodiazepines that has been of particular concern for the last few years because of its abuse in date rape. When mixed with alcohol, Rohypnol, which is tasteless and odorless, can incapacitate victims and prevent them from resisting sexual assault. It produces "anterograde amnesia," which means individuals may not remember events they experienced while under the effects of the drug. Other adverse effects include decreased blood pressure, drowsiness, visual disturbances, dizziness, confusion, urinary retention, and digestive problems. Rohypnol may be lethal when mixed with alcohol or other depressants.

Benzodiazepine sleeping pills have largely replaced the **barbiturates,** which were used medically in the past for inducing relaxation and sleep, relieving tension, and treating epileptic seizures. These drugs are usually taken by mouth in tablet, capsule, or liquid form. When used as a general anesthetic, they are administered intravenously.

How Users Feel Low doses of these drugs may reduce or relieve tension, but increasing doses can cause a loosening of sexual or aggressive inhibitions. Individuals using this class of drugs may experience rapid mood changes, impaired judgment, and impaired social or occupational functioning.

Risks All sedative-hypnotic drugs can produce physical and psychological dependence within two to four weeks. A complication specific to sedatives is *cross-tolerance* (cross-addiction), which occurs when users develop tolerance for one sedative or become dependent on it and develop tolerance for other sedatives as well.

Intoxication with these drugs can produce changes in mood or behavior, such as inappropriate sexual or aggressive acts,

mood swings, and impaired judgment. Physical signs include slurred speech, poor coordination, unsteady gait, involuntary eye movements, impaired attention or memory, and stupor or coma.

Taken in combination with alcohol, these drugs have a synergistic effect that can be dangerous or even lethal. For example, an individual's driving ability, already impaired by alcohol, will be made even worse, increasing the risk of an accident. Alcohol in combination with sedative-hypnotics leads to respiratory depression and may result in respiratory arrest and death. Regular users of any of these drugs who become physically dependent should not try to cut down or quit on their own. If they try to quit suddenly, they run the risk of seizures, coma, and death.

Withdrawal Withdrawal from sedative-hypnotic drugs may range from relatively mild discomfort to a severe syndrome with grand mal seizures, depending on the degree of dependence. Withdrawal symptoms include malaise or weakness, sweating, rapid pulse, coarse tremors (of the hands, tongue, or eyelids), insomnia, nausea or vomiting, temporary hallucinations or illusions, physical restlessness, anxiety or irritability, and grand mal seizures. Withdrawal may begin within two to three days after stopping drug use, and symptoms may persist for many weeks.

Opioids The **opioids** include *opium* and its derivatives *(morphine, codeine,* and *heroin)* and synthetic drugs that have similar sleep-inducing and pain-relieving properties. The opioids come from a resin taken from the seedpod of the Asian poppy. Synthetic opioids, such as *meperidine* (Demerol), *methadone,* and *propoxyphene* (Darvon), are synthesized in a chemical laboratory. Whether natural or synthetic, these drugs are powerful *narcotics,* or painkillers.

Heroin (also known as horse, junk, smack, or downtown), the most widely abused opioid, is illegal in this country. In other nations it is used as a potent painkiller for conditions such as terminal cancer. There are an estimated 600,000 heroin addicts in the United States, with men outnumbering women addicts by three to one. Among

Because Rohypnol is colorless, tasteless, and odorless, it can be added to beverages without your knowledge.

benzodiazepines Antianxiety drugs that depress the central nervous system, reduce activity, and induce relaxation, drowsiness, or sleep; often prescribed to relieve tension, muscular strain, sleep problems, anxiety, and panic attacks; also used as an anesthetic and in the treatment of alcohol withdrawal.

barbiturates Antianxiety drugs that depress the central nervous system, reduce activity, and induce relaxation, drowsiness, or sleep; often prescribed to relieve tension and treat epileptic seizures or as a general anesthetic.

opioids Drugs that have sleep-inducing and pain-relieving properties, including opium and its derivatives and nonopioid, synthetic drugs.

© Roy Morsch

Opioid drugs, made from the Asian poppy, come in both legal and illegal forms. All are highly addictive.

people age 18 to 25, the percentage of heroin users who inject the drug has doubled in the last decade. While the number of young heroin users in major cities has dropped by 50 percent, their numbers have almost tripled in suburban and rural areas.

Heroin users typically inject the drug into their veins. However, individuals who experiment with recreational drugs often prefer *skin-popping* (subcutaneous injection) rather than *mainlining* (intravenous injection); they also may snort heroin as a powder or dissolve it and inhale the vapors. To try to avoid addiction, some users begin by *chipping*, taking small or intermittent doses. Regardless of the method of administration, tolerance can develop rapidly.

Morphine, used as a painkiller and anesthetic, acts primarily on the central nervous system, eyes, and digestive tract. By producing mental clouding, drowsiness, and euphoria, it does not decrease the physical sensation of pain as much as it alters a person's awareness of the pain; in effect, he or she no longer cares about it.

How Users Feel All opioids relax the user. When injected, they can produce an immediate rush (high) that lasts 10 to 30 minutes. For two to six hours thereafter, users may feel indifferent, lethargic, and drowsy; they may slur their words and have problems paying attention, remembering, and going about their normal routine. The primary attractions of heroin are the euphoria and pain relief it produces. However, some people experience very unpleasant feelings, such as anxiety and fear. Other effects include a sensation of warmth or heaviness, dry mouth, facial

flushing, and nausea and vomiting (particularly in first-time users).

Risks Addiction is common. Almost all regular users of opioids rapidly develop drug dependence, which can lead to lethargy, weight loss, loss of sex drive, and the continual effort to avoid withdrawal symptoms through repeated drug administration. In addition, they experience anxiety, insomnia, restlessness, and craving for the drug. Users continue taking opioids as much to avoid the discomfort of withdrawal, a classic sign of opioid addiction, as to experience pleasure.

Physical symptoms include constricted pupils (although pupils may dilate from a severe overdose), drowsiness, slurred speech, and impaired attention or memory. Morphine affects blood pressure, heart rate, and blood circulation in the brain. Both morphine and heroin slow down the respiratory system; overdoses can cause fatal respiratory arrest.

Over time, users who inject opioids may develop infections of the heart lining and valves, skin abscesses, and lung congestion. Infections from unsterile solutions, syringes, and shared needles can lead to hepatitis, tetanus, liver disease, and HIV. Depression is common and may be both an antecedent and a risk factor for needle sharing.

Opioid abuse during pregnancy can cause miscarriage, stillbirth, or low birth weight. Babies born to addicted mothers experience withdrawal symptoms after birth.

Withdrawal If a regular user stops taking an opioid, withdrawal begins within 6 to 12 hours. The intensity of the symptoms depends on the degree of the addiction; they may grow stronger for 24 to 72 hours and gradually subside over a period of 7 to 14 days, though some symptoms, such as insomnia, may persist for several months. Individuals may develop craving for an opioid, irritability, nausea or vomiting, muscle aches, runny nose or eyes, dilated pupils, sweating, diarrhea, yawning, fever, and insomnia. Opioid withdrawal usually is not life-threatening.

Hallucinogens

The drugs known as **hallucinogens** produce vivid and unusual changes in thought, feeling, and perception. Hallucinogens do not produce dependence in the same way as cocaine or heroin. Individuals who have an unpleasant experience after trying a hallucinogen may stop using the drug completely without suffering withdrawal symptoms. Others continue regular or occasional use because they enjoy the effects.

LSD (lysergic acid diethylamide, acid) was initially developed as a tool to explore mental illness. It became popular in the 1960s and resurfaced among teenagers in the 1990s. LSD is taken orally, either blotted onto pieces of paper that are held in the mouth or chewed along with another substance, such as a sugar cube. Peyote (whose active ingredient is *mescaline*) is another hallucinogen, but it is much less commonly used in this country.

PCP (phencyclidine, brand name Sernyl; street names angel dust, peace pill, lovely, and green) is an illicit drug manufactured as a tablet, capsule, liquid, flake, spray, or crystal-like white powder that can be swallowed, smoked, sniffed, or injected. Sometimes it is sprinkled on crack, marijuana, tobacco, or parsley, and smoked. A fine-powdered form of PCP can be snorted or injected.

PCP use peaked in the 1970s, but it remains a popular drug of abuse in both inner-city ghettos and suburban high schools. Users often think that the PCP they take together with another illegal psychoactive substance, such as amphetamines, coke, or hallucinogens, is responsible for the highs they feel, so they seek it out specifically.

The effects of PCP are utterly unpredictable. It may trigger violent behavior or irreversible psychosis the first time it is used, or the twentieth time, or never. In low doses, PCP produces changes—from hallucinations or euphoria to feelings of emptiness or numbness—similar to those produced by other psychoactive drugs. Higher doses may produce a stupor that lasts several days, increased heart rate and blood pressure, skin flushing, sweating, dizziness, and numbness.

Some people experience repetitive motor movements (such as facial grimacing), hallucinations, and paranoia. Suicide is a definite risk. Intoxication typically lasts four to six hours, but some effects can linger for several days. Delirium may occur within 24 hours of taking PCP or after recovery from an overdose and can last as much as a week.

Inhalants

Inhalants or *deleriants* are chemicals that produce vapors with psychoactive effects. The most commonly abused inhalants are solvents, aerosols, model-airplane glue, cleaning fluids, and petroleum products like kerosene and butane. Some anesthetics and nitrous oxide (laughing gas) are also abused.

Young people who have been treated for mental health problems, have a history of foster care, or already abuse other drugs have an increased risk of abusing or becoming dependent on inhalants. In addition, adolescents who first begin using inhalants at an early age are more likely to become dependent on them. Approximately 11 percent of adolescents nationwide report having used inhalants in their lifetime. Teens with inhalant use disorders report coexisting multiple drug abuse and dependence, mental health treatment, and delinquent behaviors.

Inhalants very rapidly reach the lungs, bloodstream, and other parts of the body. At low doses, users may feel slightly stimulated; at higher doses, they may feel less inhibited. Intoxication often occurs within five minutes and can last more than an hour. Inhalant users do not report the intense rush associated with other drugs; nor do they experience the perceptual changes associated with LSD. However, inhalants interfere with thinking and impulse control, so users may act in dangerous or destructive ways.

Often there are visible external signs of use: a rash around the nose and mouth; breath odors; residue on face, hands, and clothing; redness, swelling, and tearing of the eyes; and irritation of throat, lungs, and nose that leads to coughing and gagging. Nausea and headache also may occur.

Regular use of inhalants leads to tolerance, so the sniffer needs more and more to attain the desired effects. Younger children who use inhalants several times a week may develop dependence. Older users who become dependent may use the drugs many times a day.

Although some young people believe inhalants are safe, this is far from true.

hallucinogen A drug that causes hallucinations.

LSD (lysergic acid) A synthetic psychoactive substance originally developed to explore mental illness.

PCP (phencyclidine) A synthetic psychoactive substance that produces effects similar to other psychoactive drugs when swallowed, smoked, sniffed, or injected, but also may trigger unpredictable behavioral changes.

inhalants Substances that produce vapors having psychoactive effects when sniffed.

Inhalation of butane from cigarette lighters displaces oxygen in the lungs, causing suffocation. Users also can suffocate while covering their heads with a plastic bag to inhale the substance or from inhaling vomit into their lungs while high. The effects of inhalants are unpredictable, and even a single episode can trigger asphyxiation or cardiac arrhythmia, leading to disability or death. Abusers also can develop difficulties with memory and abstract reasoning, problems with coordination, and uncontrollable movements of the extremities.

Treating Substance Dependence and Abuse

An estimated 6.1 million Americans are in need of drug treatment, but the majority—some 5 million—never get treatment. (See Point/Counterpoint, p. 371, for different perspectives on treatment vs. criminal prosecution.) The most difficult step for a drug user is to admit that he or she *is* in fact an addict. If drug abusers are not forced to deal with their problem through some unexpected trauma, such as being fired or going bankrupt, those who care—family, friends, coworkers, doctors—may have to confront them and insist that they do something about their addiction. Often this *intervention* can be the turning point for addicts and their families. Treatment has proved equally successful for young people and for older adults.

Some universities offer interventions for students who violate college substance abuse policies. *Motivational interviewing*, a brief intervention in which counselors express empathy to support personal change, has proved effective in reducing alcohol and drug consumption.

Treatment may take place in an outpatient setting, a residential facility, or a hospital. Increasingly, treatment thereafter is tailored to address coexisting or dual diagnoses. A personal treatment plan may consist of individual psychotherapy, marital and family therapy, medication, and behavior therapy. Once an individual has made the decision to seek help for substance abuse, the first step usually is detoxification, which involves clearing the drug from the body.

Controlled and supervised withdrawal within a medical or psychiatric hospital may be recommended if an individual has not been able to stop using drugs as an outpatient or in a residential treatment program. Detoxification is most likely to be complicated in a polysubstance abuser, who may require close monitoring and treatment of potentially fatal withdrawal symptoms. Other reasons for inpatient treatment include lack of psychosocial support for maintaining abstinence and the absence of a drug-free living environment. Restrictions on insurance coverage may limit the number of days of inpatient care. Increasingly, once individuals complete detoxification, they continue treatment in residential programs or as outpatients.

Anti-addiction medications that target neurotransmitters in the brain are becoming safer and more effective. With treatment, substance abusers are less prone to relapse. If they do return to drug use, their relapses tend to be shorter and less frequent.

The aim of chemical dependence treatment is to help individuals establish and maintain their recovery from alcohol and drugs of abuse. Recovery is a dynamic process of personal growth and healing in which the drug user makes the transition from a lifestyle of active substance use to a drug-free lifestyle.

Whatever their setting, chemical dependence treatment programs initially involve some period of intensive treatment followed by one or two years of continuing aftercare. Most freestanding programs

Chapter 12 - Alcohol Use, Misuse, and Abuse

1. Kristy has joined a sorority on campus and when she goes to a mixer with a fraternity she usually ends up having five or six drinks in a row. This type of high risk drinking is called: (Pg. 382- 383)
   A. drinking over abuse
   B. alcoholic addiction
   C. binge drinking
   D. alcohol over consumption

2. What is the most common consequence college students feel after a heavy drinking episode? (Pg. 386)
   A. had unprotected sex
   B. physically injured themselves
   C. got involved in a fight
   D. did something they later regretted

3. The absorption rate of alcohol through the body will be faster if the alcohol is mixed with: (Pg. 392)
   A. juice
   B. water
   C. milk
   D. soda pop

4. When students on campus announce they are going to be "pre-loading", they are referring to a phenomena known as: (Pg. 384)
   A. social drinking
   B. predrinking
   C. binge drinking
   D. confirmatory drinking

5. Which of the following is not considered to be a 'standard drink' measurement? (Pg. 389)
   A. a 12 oz bottle or can of beer
   B. a 16 oz bottle of malt beer
   C. a 4-5oz glass of wine
   D. a 1-1.5 shot of 100 proof vodka

6. A bottle of gin that is 40% by volume of alcohol is what proof? (Pg. 390)
   A. 20 proof
   B. 40 proof
   C. 80 proof
   D. 100 proof

7. What is a smart thing for a person who is planning to go out to a drinking party but does not want to get drunk at the party? (Pg. 386)
   A. alternate an alcoholic drink with a non alcoholic drink
   B. have had some food in their stomach to slow absorption of the alcohol
   C. sip and enjoy your drink and don't guzzle it down
   D. all of the above

8. If you suspect a friend at a drinking party has suffered from acute alcohol poisoning, what is one thing you should not do: (Pg. 393)
   A. call for medical assistance
   B. let him sleep it off
   C. have person lie down and tilt head to the side in case of vomiting
   D. keep the person covered if their skin is cold or clammy

9. Alcohol is metabolized or broken down in which organ of the body? (Pg: 394)
   A. stomach
   B. small intestines
   C. liver
   D. pancreas

10. Blood alcohol concentration (BAC) is the: (Pg. 390)
    A. concentration of sugars in the bloodstream
    B. percentage of alcohol in a beverage
    C. ratio of alcohol to the total blood volume
    D. level of alcohol in the blood before getting drunk

11. What is one reason why women tend to get drunk faster than men even having the same amount of alcohol that the man is having? (Pg. 397)
    A. women have very little or no enzyme that is needed to break down alcohol
    B. men have more muscle mass and water weight to dilute their alcohol than women do
    C. women tend to be more slender than men and don't have as much body fat
    D. all of the above

12. At a party, Alan has been downing many shots of tequila over a short period of time. He has become unconscious, his skin is turning bluish, his breathing is shallow, and he cannot be aroused. If Alan does not get medical help soon, he can die from: (Pg. 393)
    A. alcohol abuse
    B. inflamed cirrhosis of the liver
    C. acute alcohol poisoning
    D. delirium tremors

13. Because alcohol slows down the brain, it is classified as a(n): (Pg. 396)
    A. stimulant
    B. hallucinogen
    C. depressant
    D. opioid

14. All of the following can be health effects of alcohol abuse to the body except: (Pg. 394)
    A. malnutrition
    B. stronger heart muscle
    C. cancer of the stomach
    D. suppressed immune system

15. The difference between alcohol abuse and alcohol dependence is that alcohol dependence involves: (Pg. 400)
    A. continued use of alcohol even when it is known to cause personal problems
    B. stronger cravings and without the alcohol, the body goes into withdrawal
    C. chronic drinking that leads to cirrhosis of the liver
    D. binge drinking excessively in the previous two week period

16. Medical complications of chronic alcohol abuse can include: (Pg. 401)
    A. liver disease
    B. vitamin deficiencies
    C. brain and memory loss
    D. all of the above

17. When a chronic alcoholic goes into detox to rid the body of alcohol, it is common for the body to respond to having no alcohol in its system by going into: (Pg. 402)
    A. seizures
    B. delirium tremors
    C. hallucinations
    D. shock

18. Which of the following is not a characteristic of a child with fetal alcohol syndrome who was born of an alcoholic drinking mother? (Pg. 397)
    A. enlarged head
    B. mental retardation
    C. hyperactivity
    D. abnormal facial features

Jake never thought he had an alcohol problem. He didn't crave a drink first thing in the morning or carry a flask like some guys in his frat house. But by the end of the week he was ready to let it rip. "If you're gonna party, party!" he'd say. And if you're going to drink, he might have added, you might as well get drunk.

Jake didn't pay much attention to exactly how much he drank. He was too busy doing keg headstands, playing beer pong, chugging tequila shooters, or posting photos of his wasted buddies on Facebook. He'd crash into bed near dawn and

Alcohol Use, Misuse, and Abuse

sleep till noon. The moment Jake woke up he'd reach for some ibuprofen for his throbbing head. He certainly wasn't in any shape for studying. No wonder he ended up on academic probation.

One Saturday night Jake passed out after six games of beer pong. At the emergency room the doctor asked how often he went on drinking binges. Jake tried to explain that he was just playing a popular game with his buddies, but his words came out slurred.

According to recent surveys, almost 80 percent of college students drink alcohol; about 40 percent, like Jake, engage in dangerous drinking.[1] More students today binge, drink to get drunk, participate in drinking games, or drink to excess at athletic rallies, celebrations, and Spring Breaks. As a result, more students are being injured, assaulted, arrested, or raped in alcohol-related crimes—and are dying as a result of alcohol poisoning or alcohol-related accidents. Yet like Jake, many deny that they have a problem with alcohol until the consequences of their drinking finally catch up with them.

After studying the material in this chapter, you should be able to

- **Describe** the impact of alcohol misuse among college students, and **define** binge drinking.
- **Define** a standard drink.
- **Describe** the symptoms of alcohol poisoning and **state** what you should do if someone exhibits any of the symptoms.
- **Define** alcohol abuse, dependence, and alcoholism, and **list** their symptoms.
- **List** the effects of alcohol on the body's systems.
- **Evaluate** your drinking habits and **list** any health risks you are taking.

Drinking in America

Alcohol is the most widely used drug in the United States. No medical conditions, other than heart disease, cause more disability and premature death than alcohol-related problems. No mental or medical disorders touch the lives of more families. No other form of disability costs individuals, employers, and the government more for treatment, injuries, reduced worker productivity, and property damage. The costs in emotional pain and in lost and shattered lives because of irresponsible drinking are beyond measure.

Many Americans drink alcohol; most do not misuse or abuse it. According to the most recent statistics available from the National Institute on Alcohol Abuse and Alcoholism, two-thirds of American adults use alcohol, although they vary in how much and how often they drink.

Whites are more likely to be daily or near-daily drinkers than nonwhites. Men tend to drink more and more often than women. In general the rates of women who drink have not changed much in the last 20 years. However, the drinking behavior of women in their twenties has changed in two seemingly contradictory ways: More young women don't drink at all, and more of the women who do consume alcohol drink to intoxication.[2]

The median age of first alcohol use is 15. Drinking typically increases in the late teens, peaks in the early 20s, and decreases as people age. The median age of onset for alcohol-use disorders is 19 to 20.

Why People Don't Drink

More Americans are choosing not to drink, and alcohol consumption is at its lowest level in decades. About a third of adults over age 21 report not using alcohol in the last year.[3]

With fewer people drinking alcohol, nonalcoholic beverages have grown in popularity. They appeal to drivers, boaters, individuals with health problems that could worsen with alcohol, those who are older and can't tolerate alcohol, anyone taking medicines that interact with alcohol (including antibiotics, antidepressants, and muscle relaxers), and everyone interested in limiting alcohol intake. Under federal law, these drinks can contain some alcohol but a much smaller amount than regular beer or wine. Nonalcoholic beers and wines on the market also are lower in calories than alcoholic varieties.

Certain people should not drink at all. These include:

- Anyone younger than age 21. Underage drinking (discussed later in this chapter) poses many medical, behavioral, and legal dangers.

- Anyone who plans to drive, operate motorized equipment, or engage in other activities that require alertness and skill (including sports and recreational activities).

- Women who are pregnant or trying to become pregnant.

- Individuals taking certain over-the-counter or prescription medications. (See Consumer Alert, p. 396.)

- People with medical conditions that can be made worse by alcohol.

- Recovering alcoholics.

Some people feel they can be more relaxed when they have a drink. However, alcohol lowers inhibitions and can lead to behavior that one or both people regret later.

© iStockphoto.com/Chris Schmidt

Why People Drink

 The most common reason people drink alcohol is to relax. Because it depresses the central nervous system, alcohol can make people feel less tense. Some psychologists theorize that men engage in *confirmatory drinking*; that is, they drink to reinforce the image of masculinity associated with alcohol consumption. Both genders may engage in *compensatory drinking,* consuming alcohol to heighten their sense of masculinity or femininity.

Here are some other reasons why men and women, drink:

- **Social ease.** When people use alcohol, they may seem bolder, wittier, sexier. At the same time, they become more relaxed and seem to enjoy each other's company more. Because alcohol lowers inhibitions, some people see it as a prelude to seduction.

- **Role models.** Athletes, some of the biggest celebrities in our country, have a long history of appearing in commercials for alcohol. Many advertisements feature glamorous men and women holding or sipping alcoholic beverages.

- **Advertising.** Brewers and beer distributors spend multimillions of dollars every year promoting the message: If you want to have fun, have a drink. Young people may be especially responsive to such sales pitches.

- **Relationship issues.** Single, separated, or divorced men and women drink more and more often than married ones.

Individuals with drinking problems often turn to alcohol for other reasons, including:

- **Psychological factors.** Both men and women may drink to compensate for feelings of inadequacy. Yet women who tend to ruminate or mull over bad feelings may find that alcohol increases this tendency and makes them feel more distressed.

- **Self-medication.** More so than men, some women feel it's permissible to use alcohol as if it were a medicine. As long as they're taking it for a reason, it seems acceptable to them.

- **Childhood traumas.** Female alcoholics often report that they were physically or sexually abused as children or suffered great distress because of poverty or a parent's death.

- **Depression.** Women are more likely than men to be depressed prior to drinking and to suffer from both depression and a drinking problem at the same time.

- **Inherited susceptibility.** In both women and men, genetics accounts for 50 to 60 percent of a person's vulnerability to a serious drinking problem.

Drinking on Campus

 Young adults are the most frequent users of alcohol in the United States, and college students consume more alcohol more often and more dangerously than nonstudents the same age. (See Table 12.1) Many health experts consider the use and abuse of alcohol as the primary health concern for college students.

In a National Center on Addiction and Substance Abuse survey conducted at Columbia University, about two-thirds of undergraduates reported having a drink within the last 30 days. About 60 percent drank one to five days in the month. On the days that they drank, 45 percent consumed fewer than three drinks. Compared to the amount of drinking they did in high school, 64 percent said they drink more in college.[4]

However, even though the percentage of students who drink hasn't changed much, drinking on campus has. At many schools, students' social lives revolve around parties, games, and bar crawls. More students drink simply to get drunk and drink more per drinking episode. "Blowouts" on big game

TABLE 12.1

Percent of Students Who Report They Used Alcohol (Beer, Wine, Liquor) in the Past 30 Days/Past Year

Student Groups	30 Days	Past Year
All college students	72%	84%
Under 21	69%	82%
Athletes	78%	88%
Greeks	86%	93%
Freshmen	67%	80%
Female college students	71%	85%

Source: Core Drug and Alcohol Survey, www.med.unc.edu/alcohol/prevention/coresurvey.html.

© Colin Young-Wolff/PhotoEdit

TABLE 12.2

The Toll of Campus Drinking

Deaths from alcohol-related injuries	**1,700**
Unintentional injuries due to drinking	**599,000**
Assaulted by another student who had been drinking	**696,000**
Victims of alcohol-related acquaintance rape and sexual assault	**97,000**

Source: http://www.collegedrinkingprevention.gov/.

weekends, twenty-first birthdays, or Spring Break have turned into nonstop booze fests—often displayed on Facebook or YouTube, described in real time on Twitter or in text messages, and discussed in blogs.

The misuse and abuse of alcohol affect every dimension of students' lives. When high or hungover, they cannot think clearly, focus, apply themselves, or nurture their creativity. Their academic grades may plummet, and they may fail courses or lose merit-based financial aid. Their social life consists of superficial drinking games and rowdy parties rather than meaningful relationships. Their physical health suffers, and their risk of serious, even fatal, injuries increases. An arrest for driving under the influence or disruptive behavior can haunt them years later when they apply for jobs or graduate school. (See Table 12.2.)

More college women drink, and they drink more than in the past. They face unique risks. As discussed later in this chapter, women have less water in their bodies to dilute alcohol and lack the stomach enzyme alcohol dehydrogenase to break it down, so they achieve higher levels of blood alcohol more quickly and with less alcohol than men. College women who drink are at much greater risk of unwanted sexual activity. In one study more than one in five reported some type of sexual assault.[5]

  College men drink more, more often, and more intensely than women. Caucasians drink more than African or Asian Americans. Fraternity and sorority members, athletes, and vigorous exercisers also use more alcohol more often than other students.[6] The students who drink the least are those attending two-year institutions, religious schools, commuter schools, and historically black colleges and universities. How does your drinking compare? (See "Making Change Happen, p. 381.)

Why Students Don't Drink

According to the National College Health Assessment, 23 percent of students report never using alcohol. Students who don't drink give various reasons for their choice, including not having access to alcohol, parental or peer pressure, being underage, costs, religious reasons, and not liking the taste.[7]

African American students are more likely than white undergraduates to abstain and to report never having had an alcoholic drink or not having a drink in the past 30 days. They also drink less frequently and consume fewer drinks per occasion than whites. Black undergraduates experience fewer negative consequences of drinking and more regularly use strategies to prevent problem drinking, such as eating before drinking and keeping track of how many drinks they consume.

Why Students Drink

Undergraduates have always turned to alcohol for the same reasons. Away from home, often for the first time, many are excited by and apprehensive about their newfound independence. When new pressures seem overwhelming, when they feel awkward or insecure, when they just want to let loose and have a good time, they reach for a drink.[8]

The following list summarizes the most common influences on student drinking.

- **Social Norms.** Compared with other factors, such as race, gender, year in school, and fraternity/sorority membership, social norms (discussed in Chapter 1) have the strongest association with how much college students drink. Students' perceptions of how much their peers, particularly those closest to them, drink have more influence on their own drinking than do parents or resident advisors.[9] Yet, students generally overestimate how much and how often their classmates drink. (See Reality Check, p. 383.)

Women, psychologists have theorized, may be more sensitive to social norms and other influences than men. But just as women tend to overestimate how much men value thin bodies (discussed in Chapter 7), they also have distorted ideas about how much alcohol men prefer their female

Your Alcohol Audit

We have no objection to drinking. What does concern us is drinking without thinking. When you drink without thinking, you give up control and turn your life over to alcohol. And when you lose control, you lose. You can end up a hapless spectator or a victim of consequences you never intended. A third of students report doing something they later regretted as a result of their drinking. "Your Alcohol Audit" in *Labs for IPC* can help you avoid this experience—ever or again. If just thinking about drinking makes you uneasy, definitely read the following and do this lab. The feeling is a red flag you shouldn't ignore.

Get Real

In this section, you analyze your drinking by answering twelve questions, including the following three:

- When did you last have a drink? How many drinks did you have? Why did you choose to drink?
- How often do you drink? When do you drink? Where?
- Have you ever failed to do what was expected of you because of drinking? How often?

On a scale of 1 (no reason for concern) to 10 (I have a drinking problem), you rate your concern about the role of alcohol in your life.

Get Ready

In this stage, you research alcoholism in your family, going back to your grandparents. If drinking problems run in your family, you need to think about drinking even more carefully than other students. You also list what you see as the advantages of drinking (such as feeling less socially anxious) and then its negative consequences (such as headaches, hangovers, or blowing a test because you were too wasted to study).

Get Going

In this stage you set a drinking quota and write in your *IPC Journal:*

"My limit is _____ drink(s) whenever I drink."

You keep to this limit through a variety of strategies, including the following:

- **When "No" Isn't Enough**

Being with people who are drinking doesn't mean you have to drink as much as they do. Here are some effective ways to get your message across. Rehearse the following two examples before you go out:

"Just have one beer."	"I have a bet with someone (no need to say it's you) to see how long I can go without drinking." OR "I can't stop at one, and I'm not going there tonight."
"Why aren't you drinking?"	"I've got practice/work/a job interview/whatever first thing tomorrow."

Lock It In

Responsible drinking requires attention. Among other steps, you continue your alcohol audit for the rest of the term by using this format:

Day of Week	Number of Drinks	Type of Drinks	Place Consumed
Monday			
Tuesday			
Wednesday			
Thursday			
Friday			
Saturday			
Sunday			

Check how the amounts recorded compare with the goal you set at the beginning of the "Get Going" section.

---

friends, dates, and partners to consume. In a recent study, 26 percent of women stated that men would most likely want to be friends with a woman who drinks five or more drinks; 17 percent thought men would be most attracted to that woman. Both estimates were nearly double what men actually said.[10]

- **Party schools.** Colleges and universities in the Northeast, those with a strong Greek system, and those where athletics predominate have higher drinking rates than others.

  Students who drank heavily before college are more likely to join a fraternity or sorority, and the environment in many Greek organizations fosters continued drinking. Students who never join or who drop out of a fraternity or sorority report less risky drinking behavior.[11]

- **Living arrangements.** Drinking rates are highest among students living in fraternity and sorority houses, followed by those in on-campus housing (dormitories, residence halls) and off-campus apartments or houses. Students living at home with their families drink the least. In a study at the University of Michigan, women living in same-sex residential learning communities had lower rates of alcohol use and binge drinking than those living in other types of housing.

- **Celebrations.** A twenty-first birthday poses a common and serious risk. In a study of some 2,500 college drinkers, four in five reported drinking to celebrate their twenty-first birthdays, 12 percent (men and women) reported having 21 drinks, and about half drank more than they ever had before.[12] Tailgating parties, big game rallies, Halloween bonfires, and other events fueled by "fun" also become occasions for drinking. Students have more drinks on the days of a semifinal or championship game—and on the Monday after a victory. The most notorious celebratory drinking occurs during Spring Break.

- **Participation in sports.** College athletes drink more often and more heavily than nonathletes. They may be at greater risk because many are younger than 21, belong to Greek organizations, have lower GPAs, or spend more time socializing than other students.[13] Individual sports also matter. Male hockey and female soccer players drink the most; male basketball players and cross-country or track athletes of both sexes, the least. Female athletes may drink more than other college women because they are following the male athletic model of taking the lead, not just on the field, but also at the party or bar.

- **Parental approval.** Students who believe that their parents approve of drinking are more likely to drink and to report a drinking-related problem. This relationship is even stronger in younger students and those who perceive that their mothers approve of drinking.

- **First-year transition.** Some students who drank less in high school than classmates who weren't headed for college start drinking, and drinking heavily, in college—often during their first six weeks on campus and peaking during school breaks. Students who engaged in binge drinking and other dangerous behaviors in high school also are at risk for heavy drinking in college.[14] Alcohol consumption declines over the course of an undergraduate education, but a substantial number of students continue to drink heavily through their third year.

- **Positive expectations.** College students drink because they believe alcohol will make them feel better—more at ease, less stressed, more sociable, less self-conscious. The behaviors most commonly reported by students when they drink reflect these expectations: flirting, dancing, telling jokes, and laughing harder or more frequently. The primary expectations of students who go to bars and nightclubs are intoxication, socializing with friends, romance/sex-seeking, and problem relief (feeling less depressed, stress, etc.).[15]

- **Coping.** Students turn to alcohol to cope with everyday problems and personal issues. Those with symptoms of depression who lack skills to cope with daily problems, particularly males, are more likely to drink than others. Students who feel angry, hostile, nervous, guilty, or ashamed are more likely to drink in their dorm rooms and apartments than those who report positive moods.[16]

Media Messages

Simply watching commercials for alcohol or wearing clothing emblazoned with alcohol brand names can increase the likelihood of drinking. In a study of young men between ages 18 and 29, those who watched a movie interspersed with alcohol commercials were more apt to drink beer or wine during it than those who didn't see such cues.[17] Other research found that young teenagers who have T-shirts, caps, jewelry, and key chains with brands of alcoholic beverages on them seem more prone to becoming binge drinkers.[18]

High-Risk Drinking on Campus

The most common types of student high-risk drinking are binge drinking, predrinking, and underage drinking.

Binge Drinking   According to the National Institute of Alcohol Abuse and Alcoholism, a **binge** is a pattern of drinking alcohol that brings blood alcohol concentration (BAC) (discussed later in this chapter) to 0.08 gram-percent or above. For a typical adult man, this pattern corresponds to consuming five or more drinks in about two hours; for a woman, four or more drinks.

Colleges vary widely in their binge-drinking rates—from 1 percent to more than 70 percent. The federal government set a goal of cutting the current binge-drinking rate of 40 percent among college students in half as a goal for *Healthy People 2010*. How do you think your campus compared?

One of the most common ways in which students binge is playing drinking games such as beer pong. In this paddle-less game, called "Beirut" in some regions, players try to toss a ping-pong ball into one of six to ten cups on the other end of a table. Although there are endless variations and no official rules, when one side gets a ball in a cup, the other must consume the beer inside it. When one side eliminates the other team's cups, the losers must drink all the remaining beer.

Beer pong is so widespread on college campuses that there are campus and regional tournaments and Facebook pages dedicated to the game. However, beer pong presents real dangers. The sharing and reusing of cups readily spreads infections. Players, who don't monitor or regulate how much they're drinking, are at risk of extreme intoxication. Beer pong has been implicated in alcohol-related injuries and deaths from alcohol poisoning.

  Who Binge-Drinks in College? An estimated four in ten college students drink at binge levels or greater. They consume 91 percent of all alcohol that undergraduates report drinking.[19] Hundreds of studies have created a portrait of who they are and how they differ from others. Here are some of their characteristics.

- More likely to be male than female, although one in three women—up from one in four—reports binge drinking.

- More likely to be white than any other ethnic or racial group (least likely to be African American women).

- More likely to be under age 24 than older.

- More likely to be enrolled in four-year colleges than two-year ones.

- More likely to live in states with fewer alcohol control policies.

✓ REALITYCHECK

• *What percentage of college students have never drunk alcohol?* _____
• *What percentage do students believe have never had an alcoholic drink?* _____
• *What percentage of students drink alcohol daily?* _____
• *What percentage do students believe do so?* _____

Answers on next page.

- More likely to be involved in athletics and socialize frequently.

- More likely to be in a fraternity or sorority.

- More likely to be dissatisfied with their bodies, not exercise, eat poorly, and go on unhealthy diets.[20]

- More likely to put themselves or others at risk by driving after drinking.

- Much more likely to miss classes or fall behind in schoolwork.

- More likely to abuse other substances, including nicotine, marijuana, cocaine, and LSD.

- Much more likely to engage in vandalism, be injured or hurt, engage in unplanned or unprotected sexual activity, or get in trouble with campus police.

Why Students Binge-Drink Young people who came from, socialized within, or were exposed to "wet" environments—settings in which alcohol is cheap and accessible and drinking is prevalent—are more likely to engage in binge drinking. Students who report drinking at least once a month during their final year of high school are over three times more likely to binge-drink in college than those who drank less frequently in high school.

The factors that most influence students to binge-drink are:

- **Low price for alcohol.** Beer, which is cheap and easy to obtain, is the beverage of choice among binge drinkers.

- **Easy access to alcohol.** In one study, the density of alcohol outlets (such as bars) near campus affected the drinking of students.

- **Attending a school** or living in a residence with many binge drinkers.

- **Belief** that close friends were likely to binge.

binge For a man, having five or more alcoholic drinks at a single sitting; for a woman, having four drinks or more at a single sitting.

PART 2: *Just the Facts*
- *23 percent of college students have never drunk alcohol.*
- *Students believe that 3 percent have never had an alcoholic drink.*
- *Less than 1 percent of students drink daily.*
- *Students believe that 14 percent do so.*

Source: American College Health Association. *American College Health Association National College Health Assessment II: Reference Group Executive Summary Fall 2008.* Baltimore: American College Health Association, 2009.

© Sean Murphy/Stone/Getty Images

Young people in "wet" environments where alcohol is cheap and accessible are more likely to engage in binge drinking.

- **Drinking games**—such as beer pong or drinking whenever a certain phrase is mentioned in a song or on a TV program—can result in high levels of intoxication in a short period of time.
- **Parents who drank** or did not disapprove of their children drinking.
- **Recreational drinking** before age 16.

Some educators view bingeing as a product of the college environment. More students binge-drink at the beginning of the school year and then cut back as the semester progresses and academic demands increase. Binge drinking also peaks following exam times, during home football weekends, and during Spring Break. Many new students engage in binge drinking for the first time very soon after they arrive on campus. Binges become less common in their subsequent years at school and almost always end with education. Real life, one educator notes, is "a strong disincentive" to this type of drinking.

Predrinking Drinking before going out has become increasing common on college campuses, where **predrinking** (also called "pre-gaming," "pre-loading," or "front-loading") is announced and celebrated in text messages, emails, blogs, YouTube videos, and Facebook entries. In one of the few studies of predrinking, 55 percent of college men and 60 percent of college women drank before going to a pub, bar, or nightclub. Predrinkers consistently reported much higher alcohol consumption during the evening and more negative consequences, such as getting into a fight or being referred to a university's mandatory alcohol intervention program.[21]

Why Is Predrinking Popular? College students predrink for a variety of reasons, including:

- **Economic.** Many say they want to avoid paying for expensive drinks at a bar, although most end up drinking just as much if not more than they do when they don't drink beforehand. (For better ways to save money on booze, see Health on a Budget.)
- **Intoxication.** A growing number of students seem to want to get drunk as quickly as possible.
- **Socializing.** Predrinking gives students a chance to chat with their friends, which often isn't possible in noisy, crowded clubs or bars.
- **Anxiety reduction.** By drinking before meeting strangers, students say they feel less shy or self-conscious.
- **Group bonding.** Young men may use predrinking as what one research calls "a collective ritual of confidence building to prepare themselves for subsequent interactions with the opposite sex."[22]

The Perils of Predrinking When students get together to drink before a game or a night out, they usually consume large quantities of alcohol quite rapidly. In part that's because they're drinking in places without restraints on how much they can drink. Various studies have shown that students drink more and have higher blood-alcohol concentrations on days when they predrink. They also are at greater risk of blackouts, passing out, hangovers, and alcohol poisoning (discussed on page 393).

In addition to drinking more alcohol, predrinkers are more likely to use other drugs, such as marijuana and cocaine. The combined effects of these substances (discussed on page 396) further increase the risk of injury, violence, or victimization. Because students tend to predrink in groups, college men are more likely to get into or provoke fights. Because their driving skills are often impaired before a game, party, or evening begins, predrinkers are at greater risk of driving under the influence, being arrested, and being injured or injuring others.[24]

Underage Drinking on Campus

Each year, approximately 5,000 young people under the age of 21 die as a result of underage drinking. This figure includes about 1,900 deaths from motor vehicle crashes, 1,600 as a result of homicides, 300 from suicide, as well as hundreds from other injuries such as falls, burns, and drownings. Students under age 21 drink less often than older students, but tend to drink more heavily and to experience more negative alcohol-related consequences. More underage students report drinking "to get drunk" and drinking at binge levels when they consumed alcohol.

Some college presidents have called for a lowering of the drinking age from 21 to 18 to prevent underage drinkers' dangerous habits. This has provoked controversy among health and safety advocates. (See Point/Counterpoint, p. 386.)

Underage college students are most likely to drink if they can easily obtain cheap alcohol, especially beer. They tend to drink in private settings, such as dorms and fraternity parties, and to experience such drinking-related consequences as doing something they regretted, forgetting where they were or what they did, causing property damage, getting into trouble with police, and being hurt or injured. (See Table 12.2.) The drinking behavior of underage students also depends on their living arrangements. Those in controlled settings, such as their parents' home or a substance-free dorm, are less likely to binge-drink. Students living in fraternities or sororities are most likely to binge-drink, regardless of age.

Why Students Stop Drinking

Only 1 percent of students ages 18 to 24 receive treatment for alcohol or drug abuse. Nonetheless, as many as 22 percent of alcohol-abusing college students "spontaneously" reduce their drinking as they progress through college. Unlike older adults, who often hit bottom before they change their drinking behaviors, many college students go through a gradual process of reduced drinking. Researchers refer to this behavioral change as early cessation, natural reduction, natural recovery, or spontaneous recovery.

Even though most are underage, freshmen drink more—and often more recklessly—than upperclassmen. The reason may be their fervent, even desperate desire to fit in and feel connected. Unsure of their social skills, anxious about being accepted, they rely on alcohol to make them feel more at ease. Because freshmen seem more susceptible to external influences, perceived drinking norms on campus may have a greater impact on them than on older students.

Why do students say they stop heavy drinking? One common response: "It was just getting old." Some describe more specific reasons why alcohol lost its appeal, including vomiting, urinating in hallways, being physically fondled, sexual assault, violence, accidents, injuries, unprotected intercourse, and emergency room visits. Alcohol-induced blackouts scare many students, especially women, into cutting back, at least temporarily. Vicarious experiences, such as a roommate's arrest for driving under the influence or a sorority sister's date rape, also have a powerful impact.

Students often change their lifestyles during college. They may move out of a dorm or Greek house. As they

HEALTH ON A BUDGET $

Drink Less, Save More

Yet another good reason to control how much you drink is economic. The less spending money that college students have, the less they drink—and the less likely they are to get drunk and to suffer alcohol-related negative consequences.[23] Here are some simple ways to spend less on alcohol:

- **Pace yourself.** Start with a soft drink and have a nonalcoholic drink every second or third drink.
- **Stay busy.** You will drink less if you play pool or dance rather than just sitting and drinking.
- **Try low-alcohol alternatives,** such as light beers and low- or no-alcohol wines.
- **Have alcohol-free days.** Don't drink at all at least two days a week.
- **Drink slowly.** Take sips and not gulps. Put your glass down between sips.
- **Avoid salty snacks.** Salty foods like chips or nuts make you thirsty so you drink more.
- **Have one drink at a time.** Don't let people top up your drinks. It makes it harder to keep track of how much alcohol you're consuming.

predrinking Consuming alcoholic beverages, usually with friends, before going out to bars or parties; also called pre-gaming, pre-loading, or front-loading.

YOUR STRATEGIES
FOR PREVENTION

*How to Manage
Predrinking and
Drinking Without
Getting Drunk*

Here are some strategies
students frequently use:
- Eat before and/or during drinking.
- Keep track of how many drinks you're having.
- Avoid drinking games.
- Decide in advance how many drinks to have.
- Alternate alcoholic and nonalcoholic beverages.
- Limit yourself to no more than one drink an hour.
- Have a friend let you know when you've had enough.
- Choose not to drink.[25]

POINT COUNTERPOINT *Should the Drinking Age Be Lowered?*

POINT
More than 100 college presidents are supporting an initiative to lower the drinking age from 21 to 18. Underage drinkers, they argue, engage in dangerous, hidden drinking practices, such as binges, break the law by using fake IDs, and hesitate to get help for alcohol-related injuries for fear of legal consequences.

COUNTERPOINT
Groups such as Mothers Against Drunk Driving and the National Transportation Safety Board counter that lowering the drinking age will increase traffic fatalities and alcohol-related injuries, along with drinking and drinking problems among high school students.

YOUR VIEW
Since 18-year-olds can vote and join the military, should they also have the right to buy and consume alcohol? Or would lowering the drinking age jeopardize thousands of lives on the road and encourage drinking at even younger ages?

choose majors, they may meet different friends and form relationships that don't revolve around drinking. Looking toward graduate school and finding a job, many focus more on grades. And as research has shown, students who believe that dedicated studying and high GPAs will enhance their future employment opportunities, economic rewards, and respect from other students are less likely to engage in excessive alcohol consumption. As they approach graduation, students also take on increasingly adult roles and responsibilities, such as an internship or job, marriage, or parenthood.

Alcohol-Related Problems on Campus
The consequences of excessive drinking by students are more significant, more destructive, and more costly than many students or parents realize. As many as 10 to 30 percent of college students experience some negative consequences of drinking. Those at highest risk are men, fraternity or sorority members, and college athletes, who are more likely than other students to drive under the influence, engage in unplanned or unprotected sex, or participate in illegal activities while drunk.

In the National College Health Assessment, 36 percent of students who drank did something they later regretted; 30 percent forgot who they were with or what they did. Men were more likely than women to injure themselves, have unprotected sex, get involved in

a fight, or physically injure another person. Women were more likely to have someone use force or threat of force to have sex with them. Students who drink heavily also are much more likely to abuse prescription drugs (see Chapter 11).

Consequences of Drinking Among the other problems linked to drinking are:

- **Atypical behavior.** Under the influence of alcohol, students behave in ways they normally wouldn't. Many become more outgoing and sociable. Others become more emotional and cry, tell secrets, or become verbally aggressive. Male heavy drinkers are more prone to behave in ways that are considered "antisocial," or contrary to the standards of our society, such as forcing or trying to force unwanted sexual contact, driving drunk, exposing themselves, or having sex with a stranger.

- **Academic problems.** The more that students drink, the more likely they are to fall behind in schoolwork, miss classes, have lower GPAs, and face suspensions. In general, students with an A average have three to four drinks per week, while students with D or F averages drink almost 10 drinks a week. About 30 percent of students who drink and 68 percent of binge drinkers say they have missed a class because of alcohol use.

- **Risky sexual behavior.** About one in five college students reports engaging in unplanned sexual activity, including having sex with someone they just met, while drunk. In one study, 15 percent reported having unprotected sex as a result of drinking.

• **Sexual assault.** In a recent survey, almost 20 percent of undergraduate women reported some type of completed sexual assault since entering college. Most occurred after women voluntarily consumed alcohol; a few after they were unknowingly given a drug in their drinks.[26]

• **Unintentional injury.** More than 30 percent of college drinkers have been hurt or injured as a result of drinking. They also are more likely to cause injury to others, to have a car accident, to suffer burns, and to suffer a fall serious enough to require medical attention. Alcohol-related injuries result in more than 1,700 deaths every year.

• **Consequences beyond college.** The majority of student drinkers do not develop alcohol abuse disorders. However, heavy drinkers are at greater risk for alcohol dependence. Alcohol-related convictions, including carrying a false I.D. or driving under the influence of alcohol, remain on an individual's criminal record and could affect a student's graduate school and professional opportunities.

• **Illness and death.** Many students suffer short-term health consequences of drinking, such as headaches and hangovers. Heavy alcohol use in college students is associated with immunological problems and digestive and upper respiratory disorders. Even moderate drinking can contribute to infertility in women. Longer term consequences of heavy drinking include liver disease, stroke, heart disease, and certain types of cancer. About 300,000 of today's college students will eventually die from alcohol-related causes, including drunk-driving accidents, cirrhosis of the liver, various cancers, and heart disease.

"Secondhand" Drinking Problems Heavy alcohol use can endanger both drinkers and others. Secondhand problems caused by other's alcohol use include loss of sleep, interruption of studies, assaults, vandalism, and unwanted sexual advances. Students living on campuses with high rates of binge drinking are two or more times as likely to experience these secondhand effects as those living on campuses with low rates. In one study, nearly three-quarters of campus rapes happened when the victims were so intoxicated that they were unable to consent or refuse.

You can share in the fun and toast a happy occasion with nonalcoholic or alcoholic beverages.

© Jeff Greenberg/Alamy

*How to Prevent Drunk-
Driving Disasters*

- When going out in a group, always designate one person who won't drink at all to serve as the driver.
- Never get behind the wheel if you've had more than two drinks within two hours, especially if you haven't eaten.
- Never let intoxicated friends drive home. Call a taxi, drive them yourself, or arrange for them to spend the night in a safe place.

Drinking and Driving Drunk driving is the most frequently committed crime in the United States. Alcohol impairs driving-related skills regardless of the age of the driver or the time of day it is consumed. However, younger drinkers and drivers are at greatest risk. Underage drinkers are more likely to drive after drinking, to ride with intoxicated drivers, and to be injured after drinking—at least in part because they believe that people can drive safely and legally after drinking.

Of the 5,000 alcohol-related deaths among 18- to 24-year-olds, 80 percent were caused by alcohol-related traffic accidents. A young person dies in an alcohol-related traffic crash an average of once every three hours.[27] Since states began setting the legal drinking age at 21, the National Highway Safety Board estimates that over 26,000 lives have been saved.[28]

Safety groups also attribute the decline in alcohol-related deaths to enforcement tools like sobriety checkpoints and to the states' adoption of a uniform drunken-driving standard of a BAC of 0.08 percent.

In the last two decades, families of the victims of drunk drivers have organized to change the way the nation treats its drunk drivers. Because of the efforts of MADD (Mothers Against Drunk Driving), SADD (Students Against Destructive Decisions), and other lobbying groups, cities, counties, and states are cracking down on drivers who drink. Since courts have held

establishments that serve alcohol liable for the consequences of allowing drunk customers to drive, many bars and restaurants have joined the campaign against drunk driving.

How Schools Are Sobering Up

The National Institute on Alcohol Abuse and Alcoholism has studied interventions that effectively deal with college drinking problems. Programs that address alcohol-related attitudes and behaviors, use survey data to counter students' misconceptions about their fellow students' drinking practices, and increase students' motivation to change their drinking habits have proved effective.[29]

- **Social norms.** This approach, which communicates actual facts about drinking behavior to dispel myths, is simple, cost-efficient, and effective. Its positive message is that most students on virtually every campus believe in and practice safety, responsibility, and moderation, rather than excess drinking.

- **Motivational enhancement.** This nonjudgmental, supportive approach to personal change also has proved beneficial. In brief interventions, specially trained counselors help build students' self-efficacy (discussed in Chapter 2), in this case, their belief in their ability to change their drinking behavior.

- **Freshman education.** Since first-year students are at particular risk for alcohol-related problems, some schools focus on incoming freshmen with interventions that include self-surveys, group discussions about normal drinking behavior, and practical strategies for high-risk situations.

- **"E-interventions."** Electronically based interventions including text messages, e-mails, and podcasts have become increasingly popular.[30] Sending a greeting card about the negative consequences of excess drinking just before a student's twenty-first birthday did lead to the consumption of fewer drinks and lower BACs, especially among women, in one recent study.[31]

- **Alcohol policies.** University alcohol policies include campus alcohol bans, no alcohol at university-sponsored events,

Alcohol impairs driving-related skills regardless of the time of day or the age of the driver.

© Martin Heitner/Stock Connection/Jupiterimages

prohibition of beer kegs, limits on the maximum number of drinks served per student, and dry sorority and fraternity initiation activities. Studies suggest that students who attend schools that ban alcohol are less likely to engage in heavy binge drinking, more likely to abstain from using alcohol, and less likely to experience the secondhand effects of drinking. (See Community Focus.)

Understanding Alcohol

Pure alcohol is a colorless liquid obtained through the fermentation of a liquid containing sugar. **Ethyl alcohol,** or *ethanol,* is the type of alcohol in alcoholic beverages. Another type—methyl, or wood, alcohol—is a poison that should never be drunk. Any liquid containing 0.5 to 80 percent ethyl alcohol by volume is an alcoholic beverage. However, different drinks contain different amounts of alcohol.

The types of alcohol consumed vary around the world. Beer accounts for most of the alcohol consumed in the United States. People in southern European countries such as France, Spain, Italy, and Portugal prefer wine. In Guatemala, Nicaragua, Costa Rica, and Peru, liquor ranks first, while beer is the most frequently consumed alcoholic beverage in most of Central and South America.[32]

Do you know what a "drink" is? Most students don't. In one experiment undergraduates defined a "drink" as one serving, regardless of how big it was or how much alcohol it contained. In fact, one standard drink can be any of the following:

- **One bottle or can** (12 ounces) of beer, which is 5 percent alcohol.
- **One glass** (4 or 5 ounces) of table wine, such as burgundy, which is 12 percent alcohol.
- **One small glass** (2 1/2 ounces) of fortified wine, which is 20 percent alcohol.
- **One shot** (1 ounce) of distilled spirits (such as whiskey, vodka, or rum), which is 50 percent alcohol.

All of these drinks contain close to the same amount of alcohol—that is, if the number of ounces in each drink is multiplied by the percentage of alcohol, each drink contains the equivalent of approximately 1/2 ounce of 100 percent ethyl alcohol.

Drinks at college parties vary greatly in their alcoholic content. It may be impossible for students to monitor their alcohol intake simply by counting the number of drinks they have. In one study, when asked to pour a liquid into cups of various sizes to reflect what they perceived to be one beer,

ethyl alcohol The intoxicating agent in alcoholic beverages; also called ethanol.

COMMUNITY FOCUS *Changing the Culture of Campus Drinking*

PROBLEM Regardless of how much you drink, you can play a role in changing drinking attitudes and habits on your campus.

BECOME INFORMED

- Learn about the consequences of college drinking, including 1,700 alcohol-related deaths, 599,000 injuries, more than 696,000 physical attacks, and more than 97,000 sexual assaults. Check out http://www.collegedrinkingprevention.gov/ for more statistics.
- Find alternative ways to soothe stress. Daily sessions of meditation have proven effective in helping high-risk student drinkers relax. Try some of the alternatives in "Rx Relax" in *Labs for IPC.*
- Develop a defensive drinking program. Make a list of simple strategies you can use to reduce your risk of alcohol-related problems, such as planning in advance not to exceed a set number of drinks and avoiding drinking games.

BECOME INVOLVED

- Do a reality check. Ask your friends and classmates how much and how often they think students at your school drink. Then play the role of a reporter or objective observer and get an accurate picture of how much they actually drink.
- Check out community resources. Are there chapters of AA and Al-Anon on campus? Find out more about the BACCHUS (Boost Alcohol Consciousness Concerning the Health of University Students) network, including programs in your area. Do these groups offer volunteer opportunities that interest you?
- Talk to your dorm, fraternity, sorority, or roommates about steps you could take collectively, such as restricting drinking in rooms or setting up a "Seize the Keys" policy to prevent drunk driving.
- Read your school's alcohol policy. Are beer kegs allowed at social events? Is drinking banned in stadiums? What are the consequences for violating these rules or for underage drinking and alcohol-related behaviors such as disrupting others' studies or vandalizing property? Share this information with your peers.

one shot, or the amount of liquor in one mixed drink, undergraduates overpoured beer by 25 percent, shots by 26 percent, and mixed drinks by 80 percent.[33]

The words *bottle* and *glass* also can be deceiving. Drinking a 16-ounce bottle of malt liquor, which is 6.4 percent alcohol, is not the same as drinking a 12-ounce glass of light beer (3.2 percent alcohol): The malt liquor contains 1 ounce of alcohol and is the equivalent of two drinks. Two bottles of high-alcohol wines (such as Cisco), packaged to resemble much less powerful wine coolers, can lead to alcohol poisoning, especially in those who weigh less than 150 pounds.

With distilled spirits (such as bourbon, scotch, vodka, gin, and rum), alcohol content is expressed in terms of **proof**, a number that is twice the percentage of alcohol: 100-proof bourbon is 50 percent alcohol; 80-proof gin is 40 percent alcohol. Many mixed drinks are equivalent to one and a half or two standard drinks; for instance, see the margarita in Figure 12.1.

Blood–Alcohol Concentration

The amount of alcohol in your blood at any given time is your **blood-alcohol concentration (BAC).** It is expressed in terms of the percentage of alcohol in the blood and is often measured from breath or urine samples.

Law enforcement officers use BAC to determine whether a driver is legally drunk. All the states have followed the recommendation of the federal Department of Transportation to set 0.08 percent—the BAC that a 150-pound man would have after consuming about three mixed drinks within an hour—as the threshold at which a person can be cited for drunk driving (Figure 12.2).

Using a formula for blood-alcohol concentration developed by highway transportation officials, researchers calculate that when college students drink, their typical BAC is 0.079, dangerously close to the legal limit.

A BAC of 0.05 percent indicates approximately 5 parts alcohol to 10,000 parts other blood components. Most people reach this level after consuming one or two drinks and experience all the positive sensations of drinking—relaxation, euphoria, and well-being—without feeling intoxicated. If they continue to drink past the 0.05 percent BAC level, they start feeling worse rather than better, gradually losing control of speech, balance, and emotions. At a BAC of 0.2 percent, they may pass out. At a BAC of 0.3 percent, they could lapse into a coma; at 0.4 percent, they could die.

Many factors affect an individual's BAC and response to alcohol, including the following:

- **How much and how quickly you drink.** The more alcohol you put into your body, the higher your BAC. If you chug drink after drink, your liver, which metabolizes about 1/2 ounce of alcohol an hour, won't be able to keep up—and your BAC will soar.

- **What you're drinking.** The stronger the drink, the faster and harder the alcohol hits. Straight shots of liquor and cocktails such as martinis will get alcohol into your bloodstream faster than beer or table wine. Beer and wine not only contain lower concentrations of alcohol, but they also contain nonalcoholic

Figure 12.1 How Many Standard Drinks Are You Drinking?

Margarita:

1¹/₂ oz. tequila (80 proof) = 1.5 oz. × 40 percent alcohol = 0.6 oz. alcohol

³/₄ oz. triple sec (60 proof) = 0.75 oz. × 30 percent alcohol = 0.23 oz. alcohol

Splash of sour mix

Dash of lime juice   0.83 oz. alcohol = 1¹/₂ drinks

Salt for the rim

Malt liquor:

16 oz. × 6.4 percent alcohol = 1 oz. alcohol = 2 drinks

Immune system
• Lowers resistance to diseases

Heart
• Weakens heart muscle
• May raise blood pressure
• Causes irregular heartbeat

Reproductive system
• In men, hormone levels may be altered; impotence may occur
• In women, menstrual cycles become irregular; pregnant women have an increased risk of bearing children with birth defects

Brain
• Damages and eventually destroys brain cells
• Impairs memory
• Dulls senses
• Impairs physical coordination

Breast cancer in women

Stomach and intestines
• Causes bleeding and inflammation
• May trigger cancer

Pancreas
• Increases risk of cancer

Liver
• Damages and eventually destroys liver cells
• Displaces important nutrients, which can cause malnutrition

Figure 12.3 The Effects of Alcohol Abuse on the Body

Alcohol has a major effect on the brain, damaging brain cells, impairing judgment and perceptions, and often leading to accidents and altercations. Alcohol also damages the digestive system, especially the liver.

Cancer

Long-term heavy drinking increases the risk of certain forms of cancer, especially cancer of the esophagus, mouth, throat, and larynx. Even a small amount of alcohol may increase a woman's cancer risk. In a British study of more than a million women over five years, women who had a drink a day had an increased risk of several common cancers, including breast, rectum, liver, esophagus, and throat. Alcohol, the researchers theorize, may contribute to 13 percent of these cancers.[37] In another study, neither red nor white wine provided any protection against breast cancer for women. Consumption of either increases their risk.[38]

Brain and Behavior

At first when you drink, you feel up. In low dosages, alcohol affects the regions of the brain that inhibit or control behavior, so you feel looser and act in ways you might not otherwise. However, you also experience losses of concentration, memory, judgment, and fine motor control; and you have mood swings and emotional outbursts.

Moderate amounts of alcohol can have disturbing effects on perception and judgment, including the following:

• **Impaired perceptions.** You're less able to adjust your eyes to bright lights because glare bothers you more. Although you can still hear sounds, you can't distinguish between them or judge their direction well.

• **Dulled smell and taste.** Alcohol itself may cause some vitamin deficiencies, and the poor eating habits of heavy drinkers result in further nutrition problems.

• **Diminished sensation.** On a freezing winter night, you may walk outside without a coat and not feel the cold.

• **Altered sense of space.** You may not realize, for instance, that you have been in one place for several hours.

• **Impaired motor skills.** Writing, typing, driving, and other abilities involving your muscles are impaired. This is why law enforcement officers sometimes ask suspected drunk drivers to touch their nose with a finger or to walk a straight line. Drinking large amounts of alcohol impairs reaction time, speed, accuracy, and consistency, as well as judgment.

- **Impaired sexual performance.** While drinking may increase your interest in sex, it may also impair sexual response, especially a man's ability to achieve or maintain an erection. As Shakespeare wrote, "It provokes the desire, but it takes away the performance."

Moderate and heavy drinkers show signs of impaired intelligence, slowed-down reflexes, and difficulty remembering. Because alcohol is a central nervous system depressant, it slows down the activity of the neurons in the brain, gradually dulling the responses of the brain and nervous system. One or two drinks act as a tranquilizer or relaxant. Additional drinks result in a progressive reduction in central nervous system activity, leading to sleep, general anesthesia, coma, and even death.

Heavy alcohol use may pose special dangers to the brains of drinkers at both ends of the age spectrum. Adolescents who drink regularly show impairments in their neurological and cognitive functioning. Elderly people who drink heavily appear to have more brain shrinkage, or atrophy, than those who drink lightly or not at all. In general, moderate drinkers have healthier brains and a lower risk of dementia than those who don't drink and those who drink to excess.

Interaction with Other Drugs

Alcohol can interact with other drugs—prescription and nonprescription, legal and illegal. Of the 100 most frequently prescribed drugs, more than half contain at least one ingredient that interacts adversely with alcohol. Because alcohol and other psychoactive drugs may work on the same areas of the brain, their combination can produce an effect much greater than that expected of either drug by itself. For example, the liver combines alcohol and cocaine to produce cocaethylene, which intensifies the drug's effects and may increase the risk of sudden death. Alcohol is particularly dangerous when combined with other depressants and antianxiety medications. (See Consumer Alert.)

CONSUMER**ALERT**

Alcohol and Drug Interactions

Drug	Possible Effects of Interaction
Allergy, cold, flu medicines (Allegra, Benadryl, Carlitin, Dimetapp, Sudafed, Tylenol Cold & Flu)	Drowsiness, dizziness, increased risk for overdose.

Analgesics (painkillers)
   Narcotic (Codeine, Demerol, Percodan, Vicodin)
   Nonnarcotic (aspirin, acetaminophen, ibuprofen)
	Increase in central nervous system depression, possibly leading to respiratory failure and death.
	Irritation of stomach resulting in bleeding and increased susceptibility to liver damage.

Antabuse (disulfiram: an aid to quit drinking)	Nausea, vomiting, headache, high blood pressure, and erratic heartbeat.
Antianxiety drugs (Valium, Librium, Ativan, Xanax)	Increase in central nervous system depression; decreased alertness and impaired judgment.
Antidepressants (Prozac, Zoloft, Celexa, Lexapro, Paxil, Wellbutrin, Luvox, and others)	Increase in central nervous system depression; certain antidepressants in combination with red wine could cause a sudden increase in blood pressure.
Antihistamines (Actifed, Dimetapp, and other cold medications)	Increase in drowsiness; decrease in ability to drive.
Antibiotics	Nausea, vomiting, headache; some medications rendered less effective.
Central nervous system stimulants (caffeine, Dexedrine, Ritalin)	Stimulant effects of these drugs may reverse depressant effect of alcohol but do not decrease its intoxicating effects.
Cocaine	Intensification of cocaine's effects; increased risk of sudden death.
Sedatives (Dalmane, Nembutal, Quaalude)	Increase in central nervous system depression, possibly leading to coma, respiratory failure, and death.

Immune System

Chronic alcohol use can inhibit the production of both white blood cells, which fight off infections, and red blood cells, which carry oxygen to all the organs and tissues of the body. Alcohol may increase the risk of infection with human immunodeficiency virus (HIV), by altering the judgment of users so that they more readily engage in activities such as unsafe sex that put them in danger. If you drink when you have a cold or the flu, alcohol interferes with the body's ability to recover. It also increases the chance of bacterial pneumonia in flu sufferers.

Increased Risk of Dying

Alcohol kills. Alcohol is responsible for 100,000 deaths each year and is the third leading cause of death after tobacco and improper diet and lack of exercise. The leading alcohol-related cause of death is injury. Alcohol plays a role in almost half of all traffic fatalities, half of all homicides, and a quarter of all suicides. The second leading cause of alcohol-related deaths is cirrhosis of the liver, a chronic disease that causes extensive scarring and irreversible damage. In addition, as many as half of patients admitted to hospitals and 15 percent of those making office visits seek or need medical care because of the direct or indirect effects of alcohol.

Young drinkers—teens and those in their early twenties—are at highest risk of dying from injuries, mostly car accidents. Older drinkers over age 50 face the greatest danger of premature death from cirrhosis of the liver, hepatitis, and other alcohol-linked illnesses.

Most studies of the relationship between alcohol consumption and death from all causes show that moderate drinkers—those who consume approximately seven drinks per week—have a lower risk of death than abstainers, while heavy drinkers have a higher risk than either group. In one ten-year study, never-drinkers showed no elevated risk of dying, while consistent heavier drinkers were at higher risk of dying of any cause than other men.

Alcohol, Gender, and Race

Experts in alcohol treatment are increasingly recognizing racial and ethnic differences in risk factors for drinking problems, patterns of drinking, and most effective types of treatment.

Gender

According to conventional gender stereotypes, drinking is a symbol of manliness. In the past, far more men than women drank. In the United States today, both genders are likely to consume alcohol. However, there are well-documented differences in how often and how much men and women drink. In general, men drink more frequently, consume a larger quantity of alcohol per drinking occasion, and report more problems related to drinking. More than half of women drink: They drink alone more often, binge less, have more regular drinking patterns, and drink smaller quantities than men.[39]

The bodies of men and women respond to alcohol in different ways. Because they have a far smaller quantity of a protective enzyme in the stomach to break down alcohol before it's absorbed into the bloodstream, women absorb about 30 percent more alcohol into their bloodstream than men—see Table 12.3. The alcohol travels through the blood to the brain, so women become intoxicated much more quickly. And because there's more alcohol in the bloodstream to break down, the liver may also be adversely affected. In alcoholic women, the stomach seems to completely stop digesting alcohol, which may explain why female alcoholics are more likely to suffer liver damage than men.

An estimated 15 percent of women drink alcohol while pregnant, most having one drink or less per day. Even light consumption of alcohol can lead to **fetal alcohol effects (FAE):** low birth weight, irritability as newborns, and permanent mental impairment. A few drinking binges of four or more drinks a day during pregnancy may significantly increase the risk of childhood mental health and learning problems.[40]

fetal alcohol effects (FAE)
Milder forms of FAS, including low birth weight, irritability as newborns, and permanent mental impairment as a result of the mother's alcohol consumption during pregnancy.

TABLE 12.3

How Alcohol Discriminates

	Women	Men
Ability to Dilute Alcohol	Average total body water: 52%	Average total body water: 61%
Ability to Metabolize Alcohol	Women have a smaller quantity of dehydrogenase, an enzyme that breaks down alcohol.	Men have a larger quantity of dehydrogenase, which allows them to break down the alcohol they take in more quickly.
Hormonal Factors, Part 1	Premenstrual hormonal changes cause intoxication to set in faster during the days right before a woman gets her period.	Their susceptibility to getting drunk does not fluctuate dramatically at certain times of the month.
Hormonal Factors, Part 2	Alcohol increases estrogen levels. Birth control pills or other medicine with estrogen increase intoxication.	Alcohol also increases estrogen levels in men. Chronic alcoholism has been associated with loss of body hair and muscle mass, development of swollen breasts and shrunken testicles, and impotence.

Source: www.factsontap.org/factsontap/risky/discrimination.htm.

The babies of women who consume three or more ounces of alcohol (the equivalent of six or seven cocktails) are at risk of more severe problems. One of every 750 newborns has a cluster of physical and mental defects called **fetal alcohol syndrome (FAS):** small head, abnormal facial features, jitters, poor muscle tone, sleep disorders, sluggish motor development, failure to thrive, short stature, delayed speech, mental retardation, and hyperactivity.

About a third of the symptoms of alcohol abuse are gender-specific, but men exhibit more obvious ones, such as violent behavior. Because women develop more subtle problems such as feelings of guilt about alcohol consumption, they are less likely to be diagnosed as early as men.

Both men and women experience blackouts after heavy drinking, but women black out after consuming half as much alcohol as men. Women also may be more susceptible to alcohol-induced memory problems when given comparable amounts of alcohol. In addition, they are at greater risk of engaging in risky behavior, including unprotected sex, than men.

Alcohol interferes with male sexual function and fertility through direct effects on testosterone and the testicles. In half of alcoholic men, increased levels of female hormones lead to breast enlargement and a feminine pubic hair pattern. Damage to the nerves in the penis by heavy drinking can lead to impotence. In women who drink heavily, a drop in female hormone production may cause menstrual irregularity and infertility.

As women age, their risk of osteoporosis, a condition characterized by calcium loss and bone thinning, increases. Alcohol can block the absorption of many nutrients, including calcium, and heavy drinking may worsen the deterioration of bone tissue.

Race

 African American Community Overall, African Americans consume less alcohol per person than whites, yet twice as many blacks die of cirrhosis of the liver each year. In some cities, the rate of cirrhosis is ten times higher among African American than white men. Alcohol also contributes to high rates of hypertension, esophageal cancer, and homicide among African American men.

Hispanic Community The various Hispanic cultures tend to discourage any drinking by women but encourage heavy drinking by men as part of machismo, or feelings of manhood. Hispanic men have higher rates of alcohol use and abuse than the general population and suffer a high rate of cirrhosis. Moreover, American-born Hispanic men drink more than those born in other countries.

Few Hispanics with severe alcohol problems enter treatment, partly because of a lack of information, language barriers, and poor community-based services. Hispanic families generally try to resolve problems themselves, and their cultural values discourage the sharing of intimate personal stories, which characterizes Alcoholics Anonymous and other support groups. Churches often provide the most effective forms of help.

Native American Community European settlers introduced alcohol to Native Americans. Because of the societal and physical problems resulting from excessive drinking, at the request of tribal leaders, the U.S. Congress in 1832 prohibited the use of alcohol by Native Americans. Many reservations still ban alcohol use, so Native Americans who want to drink may have to travel long distances to obtain alcohol, which may contribute to the high death rate from hypothermia and pedestrian and motor-vehicle accidents among Native Americans. (Injuries are the leading cause of death among this group.)

Certainly, not all Native Americans drink, and not all who drink do so to excess. However, they have three times the general population's rate of alcohol-related injury and illness. Cirrhosis of the liver is the fourth leading cause of death among this cultural group. While many Native American women don't drink, those who do have high rates of alcohol-related problems, which affect both them and their children.

Liquor advertisers use billboards like this to promote their products to Hispanic Americans.

Their rate of cirrhosis of the liver is 36 times that of white women. In some tribes, 10.5 out of every 1,000 newborns have fetal alcohol syndrome, compared with 1 to 3 out of 1,000 in the general population.

Asian American Community Asian Americans tend to drink very little or not at all, in part because of an inborn physiological reaction to alcohol that causes facial flushing, rapid heart rate, lowered blood pressure, nausea, vomiting, and other symptoms. A very high percentage of women of all Asian American nationalities abstain completely. Some sociologists have expressed concern, however, that as Asian Americans become more assimilated into American culture, they'll drink more—and possibly suffer very adverse effects from alcohol.

Alcohol Problems

By the simplest definition, problem drinking is the use of alcohol in any way that creates difficulties, potential difficulties, or health risks for an individual. Like alcoholics, problem drinkers are individuals whose lives are in some way impaired by their drinking. The only difference is one of degree. Alcohol becomes a problem, and a person becomes an alcoholic, when the drinker can't "take it or leave it." He or she spends more and more time anticipating the next drink, planning when and where to get it, buying and hiding alcohol, and covering up secret drinking. As many as one in six adults in the United States may have a problem with drinking.

Alcohol abuse involves continued use of alcohol despite awareness of social, occupational, psychological, or physical problems related to drinking, or drinking in dangerous ways or situations (before driving, for instance). A diagnosis of alcohol abuse is based on one or more of the following occurring at any time during a 12-month period:

- A failure to fulfill major role obligations at work, school, or home (such as missing work or school).

- The use of alcohol in situations in which it is physically hazardous (such as before driving).

fetal alcohol syndrome (FAS) A cluster of physical and mental defects in the newborn, including low birth weight, smaller-than-normal head circumference, intra-uterine growth retardation, and permanent mental impairment caused by the mother's alcohol consumption during pregnancy.

alcohol abuse Continued use of alcohol despite awareness of social, occupational, psychological, or physical problems related to its use, or use of alcohol in dangerous ways or situations, such as before driving.

A normal liver (top) compared to one with cirrhosis.

Mark Nielsen (both)

- Alcohol-related legal problems (such as drunk-driving arrests).
- Continued alcohol use despite persistent or recurring social or interpersonal problems caused or exacerbated by alcohol (such as fighting while drunk).

Alcohol dependence is a separate disorder in which individuals develop a strong craving for alcohol because it produces pleasurable feelings or relieves stress or anxiety. Over time they experience physiological changes that lead to *tolerance* of its effects; this means that they must consume larger and larger amounts to achieve intoxication. If they abruptly stop drinking, they suffer *withdrawal,* a state of acute physical and psychological discomfort. A diagnosis of alcohol dependence is based on three or more of the following symptoms occurring during any 12-month period:

- Tolerance, as defined by either a need for markedly increased amounts of alcohol to achieve intoxication or desired effect, or a markedly diminished effect with continued drinking of the same amount of alcohol as in the past.
- Withdrawal, including at least two of the following symptoms: sweating, rapid pulse, or other signs of autonomic hyperactivity; increased hand tremor; insomnia; nausea or vomiting;

alcohol dependence
Development of a strong craving for alcohol due to the pleasurable feelings or relief of stress or anxiety produced by drinking.

temporary hallucinations or illusions; physical agitation or restlessness; anxiety; or grand mal seizures.

- Drinking to avoid or relieve the symptoms of withdrawal.
- Consuming larger amounts of alcohol, or drinking over a longer period than was intended.
- Persistent desire or unsuccessful efforts to cut down or control drinking.
- A great deal of time spent in activities necessary to obtain alcohol, drink it, or recover from its effects.
- Important social, occupational, or recreational activities given up or reduced because of alcohol use.
- Continued alcohol use despite knowledge that alcohol is likely to cause or exacerbate a persistent or recurring physical or psychological problem.

According to a survey of more than 14,000 undergraduates at four-year colleges, 6 percent of college students met criteria for a diagnosis of alcohol dependence or alcoholism, 31 percent for alcohol abuse. More than two of every five students reported at least one symptom of these conditions and were at increased risk of developing a true alcohol disorder. Few reported seeking treatment since coming to college.

Alcoholism, as defined by the National Council on Alcoholism and Drug Dependence and the American Society of Addiction, is a primary, chronic disease in which genetic, psychosocial, and environmental factors influence its development and manifestations. The disease is often progressive and fatal. Its characteristics include an inability to control drinking; a preoccupation with alcohol; continued use of alcohol despite adverse consequences; and distorted thinking, most notably denial. Like other diseases, alcoholism is not simply a matter of insufficient willpower but a complex problem that causes many symptoms, can have serious consequences, yet can improve with treatment.

Causes of Alcohol Dependence and Abuse

Although the exact cause of alcohol dependence and abuse is not known, certain

Daytime drinking and drinking alone can be signs of a serious problem, even though the drinker may otherwise appear to be in control.

© Catherine Ursillo/Photo Researchers, Inc.

factors—including biochemical imbalances in the brain, heredity, cultural acceptability, and stress—all seem to play a role. They include the following:

- **Genetics.** Scientists have not yet identified conclusively a specific gene that puts people at risk for alcoholism. However, epidemiological studies have shown evidence of heredity's role. Studies of twins suggest that heredity accounts for two-thirds of the risk of becoming alcoholic in both men and women.

- **Stress and traumatic experiences.** Many people start drinking heavily as a way of coping with psychological problems.

- **Parental alcoholism.** According to researchers, alcoholism is four to five times more common among the children of alcoholics, who may be influenced by the behavior they see in their parents.

- **Drug abuse.** Alcoholism is also associated with the abuse of other psychoactive drugs, including marijuana, cocaine, heroin, amphetamines, and various anti-anxiety medications.

Medical Complications of Alcohol Abuse and Dependence

As previously discussed, excessive alcohol use adversely affects virtually every organ system in the body, including the brain, the digestive tract, the heart, muscles, blood, and hormones (look back at Figure 12.3, page 395). In addition, because alcohol interacts with many drugs, it can increase the risk of potentially lethal overdoses and harmful interactions. A summary of the major risks and complications follows:

- **Liver disease.** Chronic heavy drinking can lead to alcoholic hepatitis (inflammation and destruction of liver cells) and in the 15 percent of people who continue drinking beyond this stage, cirrhosis (irreversible scarring and destruction of liver cells). The liver eventually may fail completely, resulting in coma and death.

- **Cardiorespiratory disease.** Heavy drinking can weaken the heart muscle (causing cardiac myopathy), elevate blood pressure, and increase the risk of stroke.

- **Cancer.** Heavy alcohol use may contribute to cancer of the liver, stomach, and colon, as well as malignant melanoma, a deadly form of skin cancer.

- **Brain damage.** Long-term heavy drinkers may suffer memory loss and be unable to think abstractly, recall names of common objects, and follow simple instructions. Chronic brain damage resulting from alcohol consumption is second only to Alzheimer's disease as a cause of cognitive deterioration in adults.

- **Vitamin deficiencies.** Alcoholism is associated with vitamin deficiencies, especially of thiamin (B_1). Lack of thiamin may result in Wernicke-Korsakoff syndrome, which is characterized by disorientation, memory failure, hallucinations, and jerky eye movements, and can be disabling enough to require life-long custodial care.

- **Digestive problems.** Alcohol triggers the secretion of acids in the stomach that irritate the mucous lining and cause gastritis. Chronic drinking may result in peptic ulcers (breaks in the stomach lining) and bleeding from the stomach lining.

- **Accidents and injuries.** Alcohol may contribute to almost half of the deaths caused by car accidents, burns, falls, and choking. Nearly half of those convicted and jailed for criminal acts committed these crimes while under the influence of alcohol.

- **Higher mortality.** As discussed earlier, the mortality rate for alcoholics is two to three times higher than that for non-alcoholics of the same age. Injury is the leading alcohol-related cause of death, chiefly in auto accidents involving a drunk driver. Alcohol is a factor in about 30 percent of all suicides.

alcoholism A chronic, progressive, potentially fatal disease characterized by impaired control of drinking; a preoccupation with alcohol; continued use of alcohol despite adverse consequences; and distorted thinking, most notably denial.

Alcoholism Treatments

An estimated 8 million adults in the United States have alcohol dependence. Only a minority ever undergo treatment for alcohol-related problems. Until recent years, the

- Try to remain calm, unemotional, and factually honest in speaking about the drinker's behavior. Include the drinker in family life.
- Discuss the situation with someone you trust: a member of the clergy, social worker, friend, or someone who has experienced alcoholism directly.
- Never cover up or make excuses for the drinker, or shield him or her from the consequences of drinking. Assuming the drinker's responsibilities undermines his or her dignity and sense of importance.
- Refuse to ride with the drinker if he or she is driving while intoxicated.
- Encourage new interests and participate in leisure-time activities that the drinker enjoys.
- Try to accept setbacks and relapses calmly.

only options for professional alcohol treatment were, as one expert puts it, "intensive, extensive, and expensive," such as residential programs at hospitals or specialized treatment centers. Today individuals whose drinking could be hazardous to their health may choose from a variety of approaches, including medication, behavioral therapy, or both. Treatment that works well for one person may not work for another. As research into the outcomes of alcohol treatments has grown, more attempts have been made to match individuals to approaches tailored to their needs and more likely to help them overcome their alcohol problems.

Men and women who have seriously remained sober for more than a decade credit a variety of approaches, including Alcoholics Anonymous (AA), individual psychotherapy, and other groups, such as Women for Sobriety. There is no one sure path to sobriety—a wide variety of treatments may offer help and hope to those with alcohol-related problems.

Detoxification

The first phase of treatment for alcohol dependence focuses on **detoxification,** the gradual withdrawal of alcohol from the body. For 90 to 95 percent of alcoholics, withdrawal symptoms are mild to moderate. They include sweating; rapid pulse; elevated blood pressure; hand tremor; insomnia; nausea or vomiting; malaise or weakness; anxiety; depressed mood or irritability; headache; and temporary hallucinations or illusions. Withdrawal can be life-threatening when accompanied by medical problems, such as grand mal seizures, pneumonia, liver failure, or gastrointestinal bleeding. The standard treatment is a safer sedative, such as Valium or Ativan, with a gradual reduction in the dose.

Alcohol withdrawal delirium, commonly known as **delirium tremens,** or **DTs,** is most common in chronic heavy drinkers who also suffer from a physical illness, fatigue, depression, or malnutrition. Delirium tremens are characterized by agitated behavior, delusions, rapid heart rate, sweating, vivid hallucinations, trembling hands, and fever. The symptoms usually appear over several days after heavy drinking stops. Individuals

frequently report terrifying visual hallucinations, such as seeing insects all over their bodies. With treatment, most cases subside after several days, although delirium tremens has been known to last as long as four or five weeks. In some cases, complications such as infections or heart arrhythmias prove fatal.

Medical Treatments

Antianxiety and antidepressant drugs are sometimes used in early treatment for alcoholism, especially for those with underlying mental disorders. Three drugs—naltrexone, acamprosate, and topiramate—are approved to reduce the persistent craving for alcohol. Vitamin supplements, especially thiamin and folic acid, can help overcome some of the nutritional deficiencies linked with alcoholism.

The drug disulfiram (Antabuse), given to deter drinking, causes individuals to become nauseated and acutely ill when they consume alcohol. Antabuse interrupts the removal of acetaldehye by the liver, so this toxic substance accumulates and causes nausea or vomiting. If individuals taking Antabuse drink at all or consume foods with alcoholic content, they become extremely ill. They must avoid foods cooked or marinated in wine and cough syrup preparations containing alcohol. Some individuals have reactions to the alcohol in after-shave lotion. A large amount of alcohol can make them dangerously ill; fatalities have occurred. Side effects are usually mild and include drowsiness, bad breath, skin rash, and temporary impotence. Because Antabuse does not reduce cravings for alcohol, psychotherapy and support groups remain a necessary part of treatment.

Inpatient or Residential Treatment

In the past, 28-day treatment programs in a medical or psychiatric hospital or a residential facility were the cornerstone of early recovery treatment. According to outcome studies, inpatient treatment was effective, with as many as 70 percent of "graduates" remaining abstinent or stable, nonproblem drinkers for five years after. However, because of cost pressures from the insurance industry, the length of stay has been reduced, and there's been increasing emphasis on outpatient care.

Outpatient Treatment

Outpatient treatment may involve group therapy, individual supportive therapy, marital or family therapy, regular attendance at Alcoholics Anonymous (AA) or another support group, brief interventions, and relapse prevention. According to outcome studies, intensive outpatient treatment at a day hospital (with individuals returning home every evening) are as effective as inpatient care. Outpatient therapy continues for at least a year, but many individuals continue to participate in outpatient programs for the rest of their lives.

Brief Interventions These methods include individual counseling, group therapy, and training in specific skills—such as assertiveness—all packed into a six- to eight-week period. Offered at a growing number of centers, brief interventions may be most helpful for problem drinkers who are not physically dependent on alcohol. They have proved effective in reducing alcohol consumption up to one year compared with no intervention or standard care. However, at ten years, there is no difference in alcohol consumption among those who had a brief intervention and those who did not. This indicates the need for follow-up advice and counseling.

Moderation Training Highly controversial, this approach uses cognitive-behavioral techniques, such as keeping a diary to chart drinking patterns and learning "consumption management" techniques, such as never having more than one drink an hour.

Treatment programs in other countries, such as Great Britain and Canada, have long offered moderation training for problem drinkers who consume too much alcohol. However, most experts agree that the best—and perhaps only—hope for recovery for chronic alcoholics who are physically dependent on alcohol is complete abstinence.

12-Step Self-Help Programs The best-known and most commonly used self-help program for alcohol problems is Alcoholics Anonymous (AA), which was founded more than 60 years ago and which has grown into an international organization that includes 2 million members and 185,000 groups worldwide. Acknowledging the power of alcohol,

AA offers support from others struggling with the same illness, from a sponsor available at any time of the day or night, and from fellowship meetings that are held every day of the year. Because anonymity is a key part of AA, it has been difficult for researchers to study its success, but it is generally believed to be a highly effective means of overcoming alcoholism and maintaining abstinence. Its 12 steps, which emphasize honesty, sobriety, and acknowledgment of a "higher power," have become the model for self-help groups for other addictive behaviors, including drug abuse (discussed in Chapter 11) and compulsive eating.

The average age of entry into AA is 30; about 60 percent of the members are men. Members encompass a wide range of ages, occupations, nationalities, and socioeconomic classes. People generally attend 12-step meetings every day when they first begin recovery; most programs recommend 90 meetings in 90 days. Many people taper off to one or two meetings a week as their recovery progresses. No one knows exactly how 12-step programs help people break out of addictions. Some individuals stop their drinking, or other destructive behavior, simply on the basis of the information they get at meetings. Others bond to the group and use it as a social support and refuge while they explore and release their inner feelings—a process similar to what happens in psychotherapy.

Many individuals recovering from substance abuse—as many as 1 in 10 Americans, by some estimates—will attend a 12-step meeting in their lifetime. For many with alcohol-related problems, AA is the first and only treatment they receive. Does AA work? Some studies have found that fewer than 1 in 30 people remain in AA after one year, although this may be because many are coerced to make their initial visits. However, continued AA attendance is modestly associated with abstinence and improved social functioning.

Spirituality is a key and controversial component of AA, with 11 of its 12 steps explicitly referring to the importance of God or a higher power for recovery. Yet both spiritually oriented and atheistic individuals benefit equally from AA programs. In a 10-year study, individuals involved with

detoxification The supervised removal of a poisonous or harmful substance (such as a drug) from the body; a therapy for alcoholics in which they are denied alcohol in a controlled environment.

delirium tremens (DTs) The delusions, hallucinations, and agitated behavior following withdrawal from long-term chronic alcohol abuse.

AA reported significantly larger gains in religious practices, such as prayer, compared with those without such exposure. Individuals who maintain consistent AA membership reported the greatest increases in "God consciousness" and religious practices.

Harm Reduction Therapy   This controversial approach aims to help substance abusers reduce the negative impact of alcohol or drugs on their lives. Its fundamental principles include:

- While absolute abstinence may be preferable for many or most substance abusers, very few achieve it. Even these few will take time to reach this point and may relapse periodically.

- The field of medicine accepts and practices other types of treatments that preserve health and well-being even when people fail to comply with all recommended behaviors.

- Therapists cannot make judgments for clients, even though they should present accurate information and may even express their own beliefs.

- There are many shades of improvement in every kind of therapy. If a certain level of improvement is all a person is capable of reaching, that person should be encouraged.

Alternatives to AA   Secular Organizations for Sobriety (SOS) was founded in 1986 as an alternative for people who couldn't accept the spirituality of AA. Like AA, SOS holds confidential meetings, celebrates sobriety anniversaries, and views recovery as a one-day-at-a-time process.

Rational Recovery, which also emphasizes anonymity and total abstinence, focuses on the self rather than spirituality. Members use reason instead of prayer and learn to control the impulse to drink by learning how to control the emotions that lead them to drink.

Recovery

Recovery from alcoholism is a lifelong process of personal growth and healing. The first two years are the most difficult, and relapses are extremely common. By some estimates, more than 90 percent of those recovering from substance use will use alcohol or drugs in any one 12-month period after treatment. However, approximately 70 percent of those who get formal treatment stop drinking for prolonged periods. Even without treatment, 30 percent of alcoholics are able to stop drinking for long periods. Those most likely to remain sober after treatment have the most to lose by continuing to drink: they tend to be employed, married, and upper-middle class. Recovering alcoholics who help other alcoholics stay sober are better able to maintain their own sobriety.

Most recovering alcoholics experience urges to drink, especially during early recovery when they are likely to feel considerable stress. These urges are a natural consequence of years of drinking and diminish with time. Mood swings are common during recovery, and individuals typically describe themselves as alternately feeling relieved or elated and then discouraged or tearful. Such disconcerting ups and downs also decrease over time. Patience—learning to take "one day at a time"—is crucial.

Increasingly, treatment programs focus on **relapse prevention,** which includes the development of coping strategies and learning techniques that make it easier to live with alcohol cravings and rehearsal of various ways of saying "no" to offers of a drink. According to outcomes research, social skills training—a combination of stress management therapy, assertiveness and communication skills training, behavioral self-control training, and behavioral marital therapy—has proved effective in decreasing the duration and severity of relapses after one year in a group of alcoholics. A new approach to relapse behavior, "Mindfulness-Based-Relapse Prevention" teaches clients meditation techniques as a way of coping with cravings and high-risk relapse situations.

Alcoholism's Impact on Relationships

Alcoholism shatters families and creates unhealthy patterns of communicating and relating. Separation and divorce rates are high among alcoholics.

Growing Up with an Alcoholic Parent

An estimated 28 million children in the United States (or one of every four) are living in a household with an alcoholic adult. Parental alcoholism increases the likelihood of childhood ADHD, conduct disorder, and anxiety disorders. The experience often leads youngsters to play certain roles: The adjuster or "lost child" does whatever the parent says. The responsible child, or "family hero," typically takes over many household tasks and responsibilities. The acting-out child, or "scapegoat," shows his or her anger early in life by causing problems at home or in school and taking on the role of troublemaker. The "mascot" disrupts tense situations by focusing attention on himself or herself, often by clowning. Regardless of which roles they assume, the children of alcoholics are prone to learning disabilities, eating disorders, and addictive behavior.

Numerous studies have linked parental drinking to child abuse and neglect. Children of women who are problem drinkers have twice the risk of serious injury as children of mothers who don't drink. Children with two parents who are problem drinkers are at even higher risk. As teenagers, children of alcoholics are more likely to report early sexual intercourse and face a greater risk of adolescent pregnancy.

Adult Children of Alcoholics

Growing up with an alcoholic parent can have a long-lasting effect. Adult children of alcoholics are at risk for many problems. Some try to fill the emptiness inside with alcohol, drugs, or addictive habits. Others find themselves caught up in destructive relationships that repeat the patterns of their childhood. They are likely to have difficulty solving problems, identifying and expressing their feelings, trusting others, and being intimate. In addition to their own increased risk of addictive behavior, they are likely to marry individuals with some form of addiction and keep on playing out the roles of their childhood. They may feel inadequate, not know how to set limits or recognize normal behavior, be perfectionistic, and want to control all aspects of their lives. However, not all adult children are alike or necessarily suffer from psychological problems or face an increased risk of substance abuse themselves.

Because the impact of alcoholism can be so enduring, support groups—such as Adult Children of Alcoholics, Children of Alcoholics, and Adult Children of Dysfunctional Families—have spread throughout the country in the last decade. These organizations provide adult children of alcoholics a mutually supportive group setting to discuss their childhood experiences with alcoholic parents and the emotional consequences they carry into adult life. Through such groups or other forms of therapy, individuals may learn to move beyond anger and blame, see the part they themselves play in their current state of unhappiness, and create a future that is healthier and happier than their past.

relapse prevention An alcohol recovery treatment method that focuses on social skills training to develop ways of preventing or minimizing a relapse.

LEARN IT   LIVE IT   Responsible Drinking

Problems with drinking aren't just the serious ones such as drunk driving and alcoholism. They can start with minor problems, such as missing classes and term paper deadlines. Or they can start with the belief that a party is no fun unless there is a bottle or a six-pack.

As you decide about the role alcohol should play in your life, you might want to follow these guidelines, proposed by BACCHUS, a volunteer college student organization that promotes responsible alcohol-related behavior:

- Set a limit on how many drinks you're going to have ahead of time—and stick to it.
- When you're mixing a drink, measure the alcohol.
- Alternate nonalcoholic and alcoholic drinks.
- Drink slowly; don't guzzle.

- Eat before and while drinking.
- Develop alternatives to drinking so you don't turn to alcohol whenever you're depressed or upset. Exercise is a wonderful release for tension; meditation or relaxation techniques can also help you cope.
- Avoid performing tasks that require skilled reactions during or after drinking.
- Don't encourage or reinforce others' irresponsible behavior.

Above all, keep in mind that drinking should not be the primary focus of any activity. Responsible drinking is a matter of you controlling your drinking rather than the drinking controlling you.

SELF SURVEY   Do You Have a Drinking Problem?

This self-assessment, the Michigan Alcoholism Screening Test (MAST), is widely used to identify potential problems. This test screens for the major psychological, sociological, and physiological consequences of alcoholism.

Answer Yes or No to the following questions, and add up the points shown in the right column for your answers.

	Yes	No	Points
1. Do you enjoy a drink now and then?			(0 for either)
2. Do you think that you're a normal drinker? (By normal, we mean that you drink less than or as much as most other people.)			(2 for no)
3. Have you ever awakened the morning after some drinking the night before and found that you couldn't remember part of the evening?			(2 for yes)
4. Does your wife, husband, a parent, or other near relative ever worry or complain about your drinking?			(1 for yes)
5. Can you stop drinking without a struggle after one or two drinks?			(2 for no)
6. Do you ever feel guilty about your drinking?			(1 for yes)
7. Do friends or relatives think that you're a normal drinker?			(2 for no)
8. Do you ever try to limit your drinking to certain times of the day or to certain places?			(0 for either)
9. Have you ever attended a meeting of Alcoholics Anonymous?			(2 for yes)
10. Have you ever gotten into physical fights when drinking?			(1 for yes)
11. Has your drinking ever created problems for you and your wife, husband, a parent, or other relative?			(2 for yes)
12. Have your wife, husband, or other family members ever gone to anyone for help about your drinking?			(2 for yes)
13. Have you ever lost friends because of your drinking?			(2 for yes)
14. Have you ever gotten into trouble at work or school because of your drinking?			(2 for yes)
15. Have you ever lost a job because of your drinking?			(2 for yes)
16. Have you ever neglected your obligations, your family, or your work for two or more days in a row because of drinking?			(2 for yes)
17. Do you drink before noon fairly often?			(1 for yes)
18. Have you ever been told you have liver trouble? Cirrhosis?			(2 for yes)
19. After heavy drinking, have you ever had delirium tremens (DTs) or severe shaking, or heard voices or seen things that weren't actually there?			(2 for yes*)
20. Have you ever gone to anyone for help about your drinking?			(5 for yes)
21. Have you ever been in a hospital because of your drinking?			(5 for yes)
22. Have you ever been a patient in a psychiatric hospital or on a psychiatric ward of a general hospital where drinking was part of the problem that resulted in hospitalization?			(2 for yes)

23. Have you ever been seen at a psychiatric or mental health clinic or gone to any doctor, social worker, or clergyman for help with any emotional problem where drinking was part of the problem? _____ _____ (2 for yes)

24. Have you ever been arrested for drunk driving, driving while intoxicated, or driving under the influence of alcoholic beverages? _____ _____ (2 for yes)

25. Have you ever been arrested, or taken into custody, even for a few hours, because of drunken behavior _____ _____ (2 for yes)
(If Yes, how many times?) _____ **

*Five points for delirium tremens
**Two points for each arrest

Scoring

In general, five or more points places you in an alcoholic category; four points suggests alcoholism; while three or fewer points indicates that you're *not* an alcoholic.

Your Health Action Plan for Avoiding Destructive Decisions

Students Against Destructive Decisions (originally founded as Students Against Driving Drunk) developed the following statement and contract for college students to discuss and sign. Use it as your health action plan for making responsible decisions about alcohol, drugs, and other behaviors that could put your health at risk:

Despite increased public and legislative awareness, the abuse of legal and illegal alcohol and other drugs is rampant in our society. The consequences of alcohol abuse and drug addiction are devastating and pose a major threat to young people in our society. No age group is more vulnerable to the tragic consequences of this abuse and addiction than are college students and other young adults.

College students across the nation have begun to band together to fight the substance abuse problems affecting their campuses. Innovative SADD programs have highlighted the power of college students to effectively deal with critical problems. The SADD College Contract for Life is designed to facilitate communication between college friends about potentially destructive decisions related to alcohol, drug use, HIV/AIDS, sexuality, date rape, impaired driving, and many more challenges. The Contract provides a practical tool for opening discussion, raising awareness, and demonstrating the desire to help friends find any assistance they need.

Source: http://www.sadd.org/contract.htm#collegecfl

CENGAGENOW™ If you want to write your own goals for healthy drinking, go to the Wellness Journal at CengageNOW for Health: **www.cengage .com/sso**

COLLEGE CONTRACT FOR LIFE
Between Friends
STUDENTS AGAINST DESTRUCTIVE DECISIONS

As students at _____, we recognize that we will be faced with many difficult decisions. Throughout our college experience we may encounter issues such as alcohol and other drug use, HIV/AIDS, risky sexual behaviors, date rape, impaired driving, abusive relationships, and many more challenges.

By signing below, we have entered into a contract in which we agree that we will always attempt to choose the best option that considers our own well-being, health, and safety. In addition, we will help friends whom we see making destructive decisions find any assistance they need.

When I find myself in a situation that makes me uncomfortable or that I feel unequipped to handle, I will discuss it with someone I trust.

SIGNATURE OF 1ST PARTY _____ DATE _____

SIGNATURE OF 2ND PARTY _____ DATE _____

Students Against Destructive Decisions

©2005 SADD, Inc., a Massachusetts nonprofit corporation. All rights reserved. SADD and all SADD logos are registered trademarks of SADD, Inc. SADD chapters and their individual students have permission to reproduce this material in its entirety for use by the students. Copying of this material by other entities (publishers or other individuals), either in whole or in part, without written permission is strictly prohibited. SADD, Inc. sponsors Students Against Destructive Decisions and other health and safety programs.

SADD, Inc. | 255 Main Street | Marlborough, MA 01752
877-SADD-INC TOLL-FREE | 508-481-3568 | 508-481-5759 FAX
www.sadd.org

COLLEGE CONTRACT FOR LIFE
Between Friends
STUDENTS AGAINST DESTRUCTIVE DECISIONS

As students at _____, we recognize that we will be faced with many difficult decisions. Throughout our college experience we may encounter issues such as alcohol and other drug use, HIV/AIDS, risky sexual behaviors, date rape, impaired driving, abusive relationships, and many more challenges.

By signing below, we have entered into a contract in which we agree that we will always attempt to choose the best option that considers our own well-being, health, and safety. In addition, we will help friends whom we see making destructive decisions find any assistance they need.

When I find myself in a situation that makes me uncomfortable or that I feel unequipped to handle, I will discuss it with someone I trust.

SIGNATURE OF 1ST PARTY _____ DATE _____

SIGNATURE OF 2ND PARTY _____ DATE _____

Students Against Destructive Decisions

©2005 SADD, Inc., a Massachusetts nonprofit corporation. All rights reserved. SADD and all SADD logos are registered trademarks of SADD, Inc. SADD chapters and their individual students have permission to reproduce this material in its entirety for use by the students. Copying of this material by other entities (publishers or other individuals), either in whole or in part, without written permission is strictly prohibited. SADD, Inc. sponsors Students Against Destructive Decisions and other health and safety programs.

SADD, Inc. | 255 Main Street | Marlborough, MA 01752
877-SADD-INC TOLL-FREE | 508-481-3568 | 508-481-5759 FAX
www.sadd.org

MAKING THIS CHAPTER WORK FOR YOU

Review Questions

1. Which of the following statements about the effects of alcohol on the body systems is true?
   a. In most individuals, alcohol sharpens the responses of the brain and nervous system, enhancing sensation and perception.
   b. Moderate drinking may have a positive effect on the cardiorespiratory system.
   c. French researchers have found that drinking red wine with meals may have a positive effect on the digestive system.
   d. The leading alcohol-related cause of death is liver damage.

2. Racial and ethnic patterns related to alcohol use include which of the following?
   a. Asian American women tend to have higher rates of alcoholism than Asian American men.
   b. Alcohol-related deaths are highest as a percentage of population among Native Americans.
   c. White Americans tend to have higher rates of cirrhosis of the liver than African Americans or Native Americans.
   d. The Hispanic culture discourages men from drinking because heavy drinking indicates a lack of machismo.

3. Alcoholism
   a. is considered a chronic disease with genetic, psychosocial, and environment components.
   b. is characterized by a persistent lack of willpower.
   c. may be classified as either Type A, which affects people who are high-strung, or Type B, which affects people who are more mild mannered.
   d. is easily controlled by avoiding exposure to social situations where drinking is common.

4. Which of the following statements about alcohol abuse and dependence is *false?*
   a. Alcohol dependence involves a persistent craving for and an increased tolerance to alcohol.
   b. An individual may have a genetic predisposition for developing alcoholism.
   c. Alcoholics often abuse other psychoactive drugs.
   d. Alcohol abuse and alcohol dependence are different names for the same problem.

5. Health risks of alcoholism include all of the following *except*
   a. hypertension.   c. peptic ulcers.
   b. lung cancer.   d. hepatitis.

6. Which of the following statements about alcoholism treatment is true?
   a. Inpatient treatment has been shown to be more effective than outpatient treatment.
   b. Alcoholism can be cured by detoxifying or ridding the body of all traces of alcohol.
   c. Antabuse is a medication given to alcoholics with underlying mental disorders.

   d. A combination of medical, behavioral, and self-help approaches may be necessary to treat alcohol abuse and dependence.

7. Which of the following statements about drinking on college campuses is true?
   a. The federal government has a goal to reduce the binge-drinking rate among college students to 20 percent.
   b. The number of women who binge-drink has decreased.
   c. Because of peer pressure, students in fraternities and sororities tend to drink less than students in dormitories.
   d. Students who attend two-year institutions tend to binge-drink when alcohol is available.

8. Responsible drinking includes which of the following behaviors?
   a. Avoid eating while drinking because eating speeds up absorption of alcohol.
   b. Limit alcohol intake to no more than four drinks in an hour.
   c. Take aspirin while drinking to lower your risk of a heart attack.
   d. Socialize with individuals who limit their alcohol intake.

9. Which of these is a standard drink?
   a. a margarita
   b. a 12-oz regular beer
   c. a double martini
   d. a 16-oz can of malt liquor

10. An individual's response to alcohol depends on all of the following *except*
    a. the rate at which the drink is absorbed into the body's tissues.
    b. the blood alcohol concentration.
    c. socioeconomic status.
    d. gender and race.

Answers to these questions can be found on page 650.

Critical Thinking

1. Driving home from his high school graduation party, 18-year-old Rick has had too much to drink. As he crosses the dividing line on the two-lane road, the driver of an oncoming car—a young mother with two young children in the backseat—swerves to avoid an accident. She hits a concrete wall and dies instantly, but her children survive. Rick has no record of drunk driving. Should he go to prison? Is he guilty of manslaughter? How would you feel if you were the victim's husband? If you were Rick's friend?

2. Have you ever been around people who have been intoxicated when you have been sober? What did you think of their behavior? Were they fun to be around? Was the experience not particularly enjoyable, boring, or difficult in some way? Have you ever been intoxicated? How do you behave when you are drunk? Do you find the experience enjoyable?

What do the people around you think of your actions when you are drunk?

3. What effects has alcohol use had in your life? Try making a list of the positive and negative effects your own alcohol use has had. Be specific. If you continue to drink at your current rate, what positive and negative effects do you think it will have on your future? What effects have other people's drinking had on your life? List family members and friends who drink regularly and how their drinking has affected you.

Media Menu

CENGAGENOW™ Go to the CengageNOW for Health website at **www .cengage.com/sso** that will:
- Help you evaluate your knowledge of the material.
- Allow you to take an exam-prep quiz.
- Provide a Personalized Learning Plan targeting resources that address areas you should study.
- Coach you through identifying target goals for behavioral change and creating and monitoring your personal change plan throughout the semester.

Internet Connections

www.factsontap.org
This excellent site is geared to college students. Sections include Alcohol & Student Life, Alcohol & Sex, Alcohol & Your Body.

www.collegedrinkingprevention.gov
This website, sponsored by the National Institute of Alcohol Abuse and Alcoholism, focuses on the college alcohol culture with information for students, parents, college health administrators, and more. The site also features information about alcohol prevention, college alcohol policies, research topics, and factual information about the consequences of alcohol abuse and alcoholism.

www.al-anon.alateen.org
This site provides information and referrals to local Al-Anon and Alateen groups. It also includes a self-quiz to determine if you are affected by someone who has an alcohol problem.

www.nacoa.org
This association provides information about and for children of alcoholics. Their website contains numerous links to relevant support groups.

Key Terms

The terms listed are used on the page indicated. Definitions of the terms are in the Glossary at the end of the book.

absorption 393
alcohol abuse 399
alcohol dependence 400
alcoholism 401
binge drinking 383
blood-alcohol concentration (BAC) 391
delirium tremens (DTs) 403
detoxification 403
ethyl alcohol 389
fetal alcohol effects (FAE) 397
fetal alcohol syndrome (FAS) 399
predrinking 385
proof 391
relapse prevention 405

Chapter 13 - Tobacco Use, Misuse, and Abuse

1. The U.S. national health goal to reduce the number of adults smoking by the year 2010 is: (Pg. 412)
   - A. 5%
   - B. 12%
   - C. 15%
   - D. 24%

2. Which ethnic group of college students is least likely to smoke cigarettes? (Pg. 412)
   - A. African American
   - B. Hispanic
   - C. Asian
   - D. White

3. The number one reason why college students say they smoke is: (Pg. 413)
   - A. peer pressure
   - B. to reduce stress
   - C. to control their appetite
   - D. to help them concentrate

4. Of the top 20 global countries, which country has the highest number of male smokers? (Pg. 419)
   - A. U.S.A.
   - B. Canada
   - C. France
   - D. China

5. High nicotine intake in males can affect their blood circulation and cause: (Pg. 418)
   - A. chronic bronchitis
   - B. reduced flow of blood to the penis and cause erectile dysfunction
   - C. emphysema
   - D. allergies

6. With smoking cigarettes, young women are most concerned with: (Pg. 413)
   - A. nicotine dependence
   - B. developing a mental disorder
   - C. weight control
   - D. reducing stress

7. Women who smoke during their pregnancy increase their risk for: (Pg. 418)
   - A. smaller birth weight babies
   - B. miscarriage
   - C. birth defects such as cleft lip
   - D. all of the above

8. Which of the following is not a health effect of cigarette smoking on a young college-aged student who has been smoking for about four or five years now? (Pg. 421)
   - A. dulled taste buds
   - B. increased heart rate
   - C. decreased alertness
   - D. shortened breath

9. What is the condition which is worsened by smoking, when the bronchial tubes become inflamed and mucus production increases: (Pg. 423)
   - A. chronic bronchitis
   - B. asthma
   - C. emphysema
   - D. chronic obstructive lung disorder

10. A condition characterized by white patches inside the gums of the mouth from chewing tobacco users could lead to: (Pg. 425)

A. asthma
B. oral cancer
C. emphysema
D. periodontal disease

11. A skinny sweet-flavored cigarette becoming more popular with the younger crowd is: (Pg. 424)

A. clove cigarettes
B. bidis
C. smokeless tobacco
D. natural tobacco

12. The active ingredient in clove cigarettes that allows smokers to inhale more deeply and hold the smoke in their lungs longer is: (Pg. 424)

A. phenol
B. eugenol
C. nicotine
D. Zyban

13. Smokeless tobacco can cause: (Pg. 425)

A. heart rate to increase
B. to form sores and lead to mouth cancer
C. increased blood pressure
D. all of the above

14. The most effective way to stop tobacco smoking is to: (Pg. 426)

A. chew lots of gum
B. use hypnosis
C. be an active participant and take self responsibility to quit
D. undergo electric shock treatments every time one tries to light up

15. Tori is working with a counselor to quit smoking. Her counselor pairs the act of smoking with noxious stimuli, such as smoking rapidly. What technique is he having Tori use? (Pg. 427)

A. aversion therapy
B. self control therapy
C. nicotine withdrawal
D. rapid smoke technique

16. Mainstream smoke is the smoke that a smoker: (Pg. 430)

A. exhales out of the mouth and nostrils
B. inhales through the mouth
C. the smoke that nonsmokers are breathing in
D. the smoke that is given off while sitting in the ashtray

17. Environmental tobacco smoke is also known as: (Pg. 430)

A. primary smoke
B. mainstream smoke
C. secondhand smoke
D. sidestream smoke

18. Children who breathe environmental tobacco smoke around their smoking parent are at an increased risk of all the following except: (Pg. 431- 432)

A. bronchitis
B. asthma
C. obesity
D. heart disease

Andrea didn't really want her first cigarette. Her tent mate at camp had snatched one from a counselor's pack, and the two of them had climbed to a remote rock to share it. Andrea hated everything about her first drag: the taste, the smell, the horrible burning in her throat and lungs. But she loved feeling more grown-up and sophisticated than other seventh graders. By the time she reached high school, Andrea would sneak off to smoke with friends at least once a week. By graduation, she was smoking daily.

Tobacco Use, Misuse, and Abuse

As a college freshman, Andrea discovered that she was part of an unpopular minority. Even though her dorm didn't ban smoking, her roommate declared their room a smoke-free zone. Her college didn't allow smoking in any classrooms or public areas. And many of her new friends reacted as if smoking was a sign of impaired intelligence. Andrea has decided to quit, but she's discovered that nicotine dependence is very difficult to overcome. "I just wish I'd never started smoking in the first place," she says.

Despite overwhelming evidence of tobacco's dangers, smoking remains widespread. Some 12 million cigarettes are smoked around the world every minute of every day. An estimated 6.3 trillion cigarettes are produced annually—more than 900 cigarettes for every man, woman, and child on the planet.[1]

This chapter discusses smoking around the world, in America, and on campus. It provides information on the effects of tobacco on the body, tobacco dependence, quitting smoking, smokeless tobacco, and environmental tobacco smoke. This information may help you to breathe easier today—and may help ensure cleaner air for others to breathe tomorrow.

After studying the material in this chapter, you should be able to

- **Describe** today's tobacco smokers and the common reasons why they smoke.
- **Provide** an overview of smokers in the United States and around the globe, and **explain** the common reasons they smoke.
- **Discuss** several of the gender-specific health effects of smoking.
- **Discuss** the health problems that can be prevented by quitting smoking.
- **Identify** the different types of tobacco products.
- **Discuss** several recommended ways to quit smoking.
- **Describe** the health effects of environmental, or secondhand, tobacco smoke.
- **Assess** the health risks you may have experienced as a result of your own or others' use of tobacco.

Log on to CengageNOW for Health at **www.cengage.com/sso** to find your Behavior Change Planner and to explore self-assessments, interactive tutorials, and practice quizzes.zes.

411

Smoking in America

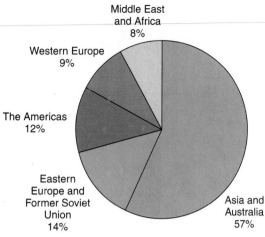

Figure 13.1 World Cigarette Consumption by Region, 2007

Source: The Tobacco Atlas, www.tobaccoatlas.org

The total number of smokers is increasing as the world population continues to climb. Male smoking is declining slowly, but female smoking, especially in some developing countries, is increasing. Although cigarettes are expensive in the poorest countries, their citizens are the heaviest smokers. (See Figure 13.1.)[2]

Despite widespread awareness of the dangers of tobacco, smoking continues to kill more people than AIDS, alcohol, drug abuse, car crashes, murders, suicides, and fires combined. The worldwide death toll is 6 million people a year and is expected to climb to 8 million by 2030. (See Health on a Budget, p. 413.)

According to the Centers for Disease Control and Prevention (CDC), slightly less than 20 percent of American adults—some 43 million men and women—smoke.[3] The more and the longer they smoke, the greater their risks of heart disease, respiratory problems, several types of cancer, and a shortened lifespan. An estimated 400,000 individuals die prematurely in the United States due to tobacco use each year.[4]

 The drop in smoking in the overall population still falls short of the national health objective of reducing cigarette smoking among adults to 12 percent by 2010. (See Figure 13.2.) However, some groups have met this goal. They include women with undergraduate or graduate degrees, men with graduate degrees, Hispanic and Asian women, people over age 65, and the state of Utah.[5] Native Americans have the highest smoking rates, while Asians and Hispanics have the lowest. Individuals with undergraduate and graduate degrees are least likely to smoke.

There are now more former smokers than active smokers in the United States, and more than half the population lives where smoking is prohibited in workplaces.

Tobacco Use on Campus

About one in every four to five students currently smoke, but a majority have never smoked. (See Reality Check, p. 413.) Many students who had never tried smoking may experiment with cigarettes in college. However, eight in ten college smokers started smoking before age 18. They report smoking on twice as many days and smoke nearly four times as many cigarettes as those who began smoking at an older age.[6]

White students have the highest smoking rates, followed by Hispanic, Asian, and African American students. Although black students are least likely to smoke, more are doing so than in the past. Smoking rates remain consistently lower at predominantly black colleges and universities, however.[7] About equal percentages of college men and women smoke although women are somewhat more likely than men to report smoking daily.[8]

Many college students say they smoke as a way of managing depression or stress. (See Figure 13.3.) Studies consistently link smoking with depression and low life satisfaction. Smokers are significantly more likely to have higher levels of perceived stress than nonsmokers. In one study, students who had been diagnosed or treated for depression were seven times as likely as other students to use tobacco. The more depressed students are, the more likely they are to smoke. In a recent study, student smokers low in depressive symptoms smoked less than one pack of cigarettes a week, while those high in depressive symptoms smoked more than two packs a week. Depressed students may use nicotine as a form of self-medication.[9]

 Male students who smoke are more likely to say that smoking makes them feel more masculine and less anxious. More than half of female smokers feel that smoking helps them control their weight, although only 3 percent say it is their primary reason for smoking. Overweight female students are more likely to smoke to lose weight and to see weight gain as a barrier to quitting.

Students can and do change their smoking behavior. In one study, over the course of four years of college, about half of students who smoked every few days, every few weeks, or every few months quit, as did 13 percent of daily smokers. More than a quarter of daily smokers cut back. On the other hand, 12 percent of nonsmokers took up the habit, and most daily smokers continued to smoke through the end of college.[10]

Social Smoking

 Some college students who smoke say they are "social smokers" who average less than one cigarette a day and smoke mainly in the company of others. On the positive side, social smokers smoke less often and less intensely than other smokers and are less dependent on tobacco. However, they are still jeopardizing their health. The more they smoke, the greater the health risks they face. Even smokers who don't inhale or nonsmokers who breathe in secondhand smoke are at increased risk for negative health effects.

 In research studies, smoking less than a pack a week of cigarettes has proved to damage the lining of blood vessels and to increase the risk of heart disease as well as of cancer. In women taking birth control pills, even a few cigarettes a week can increase the likelihood of heart disease, blood clots, stroke, liver cancer, and gallbladder disease. Pregnant women who smoke only occasionally still run a higher risk of giving birth to unhealthy babies. Another risk is addiction. Social smokers are less motivated to quit and make fewer attempts to do so. Many end up smoking more cigarettes for many more years than they intended.

HEALTH ON A BUDGET

The Toll of Tobacco

Whether or not you smoke, you indirectly pay the price of tobacco use around the world:

Global economic cost	$500 billion
U.S. economic cost	$193 billion
Annual global number of tobacco-caused deaths	6 million
Annual number of premature deaths due to tobacco in the U.S.	443,000
Property damage in fires caused by smoking, globally	$27 billion
Injuries in fires caused by smoking, globally	60,000
Deaths in fires caused by smoking, globally	17,300
Deaths caused by secondhand smoke in the U.S.	3,000

Sources: Tobacco Atlas, www.tobaccoatlas.org; "State Specific Prevalence and Trends in Adults Cigarette Smoking," *Morbidity and Mortality Weekly Report,* CDC, Vol. 68, No. 9, March 13, 2009, pp. 221–228.

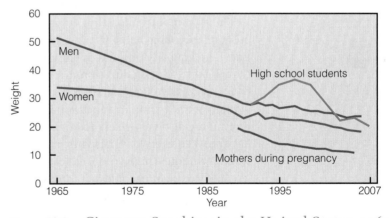

Figure 13.2 Cigarette Smoking in the United States, 1965–2007

Sources: CDC/NCHS, *Health, United States, 2008,* Figure 6. Data from the National Health Interview Survey, Youth Risk Behavior Survey, National Vital Statistics System.

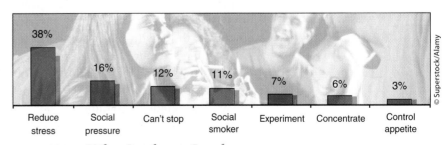

Figure 13.3 Why Students Smoke

Source: From *Wasting the Best and the Brightest: Substance Abuse at America's Colleges and Universities.* New York: National Center on Addiction and Substance Abuse (CASA) at Columbia University, March 2007.

College Tobacco–Control Policies

A growing number of colleges are stamping out smoking on campus. More than 140 schools are completely smoke-free; an additional 30 have banned smoking everywhere but in designated outdoor areas. At least 500 campuses have smoke-free policies in residential housing.[11]

Several national health organizations, including the American College Health Association and the National Center on Addiction and Substance Abuse, have recommended that colleges ban smoking in and around all campus buildings, including student housing, and prohibit the sale, advertisement, and promotion of tobacco products on campus. Universities that have banned smoking from designated residence halls report decreased damage to the buildings, increased retention of students, and improved enforcement of marijuana policies. In general, schools in the West have done the most to implement tobacco policies. Those in the South, particularly in the major tobacco-growing states, have done the least.

Why People Start Smoking

  Most people are aware that an enormous health risk is associated with smoking, but many don't know exactly what that risk is or how it might affect them.

The two main factors linked with the onset of a smoking habit are age and education. The majority of white men with less than a high school education are current or former daily cigarette smokers. White women with a similar educational background are also very likely to smoke or to have smoked every day. Hispanic men and women without a high school education are less likely to be or become daily smokers.

The following factors are associated with reasons for smoking.

Limited Education

People who have graduated from college are much less likely to smoke than high school graduates; those with fewer than 12 years of education are more likely to smoke. An individual with 8 years or less of education is 11 times more likely to smoke than someone with postgraduate training.

Underestimation of Risks

Young people who think the health risks of smoking are fairly low are more likely than their peers to start smoking. In a two-year study, teenagers who thought they had little chance of developing either short-term problems—such as a higher risk of colds or a chronic cough—or long-term problems—such as heart disease, cancer, and respiratory diseases—were three to four times more likely to start smoking.[12]

Adolescent Experimentation and Rebellion

For teenagers, smoking may be a coping mechanism for dealing with boredom and frustration; a marker of the transition into high school or college; a bid for adult status; a way of gaining admission to a peer group; or a way to have fun, reduce stress, or boost energy. The teenagers most likely to begin smoking are those least likely to seek help when their emotional needs are not met. They might smoke as a means of gaining social acceptance or to self-medicate when they feel helpless, lonely, or depressed. Depressed teens are more susceptible to cigarette ads than their counterparts. For example, they are more likely to have a favorite cigarette ad or own clothing with cigarette logos.

Stress

In studies that have analyzed the impact of life stressors, depression, emotional support, marital status, and income, researchers have concluded that an individual with a high stress level is approximately 15 times more likely to be a smoker than a person with low stress. About half of smokers identify workplace stress as a key factor in their smoking behavior.

Parental Role Models

Children who start smoking are 50 percent more likely than youngsters who don't smoke to have at least one smoker in their family. A mother who smokes seems a particularly strong influence on making smoking seem acceptable. The majority of youngsters who smoke say that their parents also smoke and are aware of their own tobacco use.

Addiction

Nicotine addiction is as strong or stronger than addiction to drugs such as cocaine and heroin. The first symptoms of nicotine addiction can begin within a few days of starting to smoke and after just a few cigarettes, particularly in teenagers. Smoking a single cigarette before age 11 increases the odds of becoming dependent on nicotine. (See Self Survey: "Are You Addicted to Nicotine?" on page 434.)

Mental Disorders

The percentage of smokers jumps to more than 90 percent among those with alcoholism and other addictions, 85 percent among schizophrenia patients, and 80 percent among depressed patients. The relationship between depression and smoking is complex. Smokers are more likely to be depressed, while adults who are depressed are 40 to 50 percent more likely to smoke than adults who are not depressed. Research has identified biological connections between smoking and depression, suggesting a biological similarity between substance use and depressive disorders.

Genetics

Researchers speculate that genes may account for about 50 percent of smoking

behavior, with environment playing an equally important role. Studies have shown that identical twins, who have the same genes, are more likely to have matching smoking profiles than fraternal twins. If one identical twin is a heavy smoker, the other is also likely to be; if one smokes only occasionally, so does the other.

According to NIDA research, genetic factors play a more significant role for initiation of smoking in women than in men, but they play a less significant role in smoking persistence for women.

Social smoking has negative short- and long-term health effects and can lead to dependence.

Smoking has become more inconvenient, expensive, and socially unacceptable, but many smokers still light up.

Weight Control

  Concern about weight is a significant risk factor for smoking among young women. Daily smokers are two to four times more likely to fast, use diet pills, and purge to control their weight than nonsmokers. Although black girls smoke at substantially lower rates than white girls, the common factor in predicting daily smoking among all girls, regardless of race, is concern with weight.

Aggressive Marketing

Cigarette companies spend billions of dollars each year on advertisements and promotional campaigns, with manufacturers targeting ads especially at teens, minorities, and the poor. Many ads create an association between cigarettes and alcohol, linking the act of smoking with lifestyles that involve drinking—a combination that public health officials describe as "alarming" because of the health risks posed by these two behaviors.

The tobacco industry markets smoking to men by promoting it as a masculine habit linked to health, happiness, fitness, wealth, power, and virility. In reality, smoking leads to sickness, premature death, sexual impotence, and infertility.[13]

Tobacco companies market smoking to girls and women using "female-only" cigarette brands that are long, slim, low-tar, packaged in brightly colored packs, and sometimes mentholated and/or candy-flavored. Their ads feature seductive images of vitality, slimness, freedom, sophistication, and sexual allure. In reality, smoking causes reproductive damage, disease, and death.[14]

Cigarette ads project an image of smokers as young, healthy, stylish, and sexy. In reality, smoking leads to sickness, premature death, and sexual difficulties.

Why People Keep Smoking

Whatever the reasons for lighting up that first cigarette, very different factors keep cigarettes burning pack after pack, year after year. In national polls, 7 in 10 smokers say that they want to quit but can't. The reason isn't a lack of willpower. Medical scientists have recognized tobacco dependence as an addictive disorder that may be more powerful than heroin dependence and that may affect more than 90 percent of all smokers.

Pleasure

According to the American Cancer Society, 9 in 10 regular smokers find smoking pleasurable. Nicotine—the addictive ingredient in tobacco—is the reason. Researchers have shown that nicotine reinforces and strengthens the desire to smoke by acting on brain chemicals that influence feelings of well-being. This drug also can improve memory, help in performing certain tasks, reduce anxiety, dampen hunger, and increase pain tolerance.

Mental Disorders

Individuals with mental disorders are twice as likely to smoke as others, and people with mental illness may account for nearly one-half of the tobacco market in the United States. Heavy smoking also is linked with an almost elevenfold risk of anxiety disorders in early adulthood.

Smokers with a history of depression are about half as likely to quit as others. Even after a recovery from major depression, smokers often continue to report some symptoms of depression. Smokers who are depressed tend to smoke more cigarettes than other smokers, are less successful in their efforts to stop smoking, and are more prone to depression after quitting. The longer people smoke, the more likely they are to develop symptoms of depression and anxiety.

Fear of Weight Gain

Smokers burn up an extra 100 calories a day—the equivalent of walking a mile—probably because nicotine increases metabolic rate. Once they start smoking, many individuals say they cannot quit because they fear they'll gain weight. The CDC estimates that women who stop smoking gain an average of 8 pounds, while men put on an average of 6 pounds. One in eight women and one in ten men who stop smoking put on 29 pounds or more. The reasons for this weight gain include nicotine's effects on metabolism as well as emotional and behavioral factors, such as the habit of frequently putting something into one's mouth. Yet as a health risk, smoking a pack and a half to two packs a day is a greater danger than carrying 60 pounds of extra weight.

Weight gain for smokers who quit is not inevitable. Aerobic exercise helps increase metabolic rate, and limiting alcohol and foods high in sugar and fat can help smokers control their weight as they give up cigarettes.

Dependence

Nicotine has a much more powerful hold on smokers than alcohol does on drinkers. Whereas about 10 percent of alcohol users lose control of their intake of alcohol and become alcoholics, as many as 80 percent of all heavy smokers have tried to cut down on or quit smoking but cannot overcome their dependence.

 About 8 percent of full-time college students meet the diagnostic criteria for past-30-day nicotine dependence, much lower than the rate of the general population (15 percent).[15]

Nicotine causes dependence by at least three means:

- It provides a strong sensation of pleasure.
- It leads to fairly severe discomfort during withdrawal.
- It stimulates cravings long after obvious withdrawal symptoms have passed.

Few drugs act as quickly on the brain as nicotine does. It travels through the bloodstream to the brain in seven seconds—half the time it takes for heroin injected into a blood vessel to reach the brain. And a pack-a-day smoker gets 200 hits of nicotine a day—73,000 a year.

After a few years of smoking, the most powerful incentive for continuing to smoke is to avoid the discomfort of withdrawal. Generally, 10 cigarettes a day will prevent withdrawal effects. For many who smoke heavily, signs of withdrawal, including changes in mood and performance, occur within two hours after smoking their last cigarette. Smokeless tobacco users also get constant doses of nicotine. However, absorption of nicotine by the lungs is more likely to lead to dependence than absorption through the linings of the nose and mouth. As with other drugs of abuse, continued nicotine intake results in tolerance (the need for more of a drug to maintain the same effect), which is why only 2 percent of all smokers smoke just a few cigarettes a day, or smoke only occasionally.

Use of Other Substances

Many smokers also drink or use drugs. According to the Addiction Research Foundation in Canada, tobacco smokers say cigarettes are harder to abandon than other drugs, even when they find them less pleasurable than their preferred drug of abuse. Individuals who drink excessively also find their cigarette habit a hard one to break.

Smoking, Gender, and Race

  Almost 1 billion men in the world smoke— about 35 percent of men in developed countries and 50 percent of men in developing countries. (See Figure 13.4.) Male smoking rates are slowly declining, but tobacco still kills about 5 million men every year. In general, higher-educated men are abandoning tobacco addiction, while poorer, less-educated men continue to smoke.[16]

High nicotine intake may affect male hormones, including testosterone. Smoking also can reduce blood flow to the penis, impairing a man's sexual performance and increasing the likelihood of erectile dysfunction.

Smoking is a risk factor for developing rheumatoid arthritis for men, but not for women. Women who smoke are more likely to develop osteoporosis, a bone weakening disease. On average, girls who begin smoking during adolescence continue smoking for 20 years, four years longer than boys. Women are at greater risk for developing smoking-related illnesses compared with men who smoke the same amount. Lung cancer now claims more women's lives than breast cancer. As discussed later in this chapter, both active and passive smoking increase a woman's risk of breast cancer.[17] In men, cigarette smoking increases the risk of aggressive prostate cancer.

About 250 million women in the world are daily smokers—22 percent of women in developed countries and 9 percent of women in low- and middle-resource countries. Cigarette smoking among women is declining in the United States, but in several southern, central, and eastern European countries, cigarette smoking rates among women are either stable or increasing.

According to the U.S. Surgeon General, women account for 39 percent of smoking-related deaths each year, a proportion that has doubled since 1965. Each year, American women lose an estimated 2.1 million years of life due to premature deaths attributable to smoking. If she smokes, a woman's annual risk of dying more than doubles after age 45 compared with a woman who has never smoked.

Smoking directly affects women's reproductive organs and processes. Women who smoke are less fertile and experience menopause one or two years earlier than women who don't smoke. Smoking also greatly increases the possible risks associated with taking oral contraceptives.

Women who smoke during pregnancy increase their risk of miscarriage and pregnancy complications, including bleeding, premature delivery, and birth defects such as cleft lip or palate. Smoking narrows the blood vessels and reduces blood flow to the fetus, resulting in lower birth weight, shorter length, smaller head circumference, and possibly lower IQ.[18] Youngsters whose mothers smoked during pregnancy also tend to have problems with hyperactivity, inattention, and impulsivity. Some of these behavior problems persist through the teenage years and even into adulthood. At ages 16 to 18, children exposed to prenatal smoking have higher rates of conduct disorder, substance use, and depression than others.

Cigarette smoking is a major cause of disease and death in all population groups. However, tobacco use varies within and among racial and ethnic minority groups. Among adults, Native Americans and Alaska Natives have the highest rates of tobacco use. African American and Southeast Asian men also have a high smoking rate. Asian American and Hispanic women have the lowest rates of smoking. Tobacco

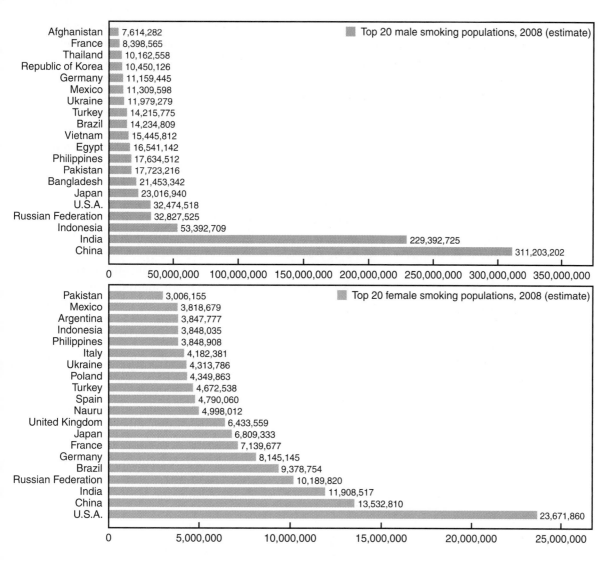

Figure 13.4 Number of Smokers by Country

Source: The Tobacco Atlas, www.tobaccoatlas.org.

use is significantly higher among white college students than among Hispanic, African American, and Asian American students.

Tobacco is the substance most abused by Hispanic youth, whose smoking rates have soared in the last ten years. In general, smoking rates among Hispanic adults increase as they adopt the values, beliefs, and norms of American culture. Recent declines in the prevalence of smoking have been greater among Hispanic men with at least a high school education than among those with less education.

Tobacco's Immediate Effects

Tobacco, an herb that can be smoked or chewed, directly affects the brain. While its primary active ingredient is nicotine, tobacco smoke contains almost 400 other compounds and chemicals, including gases, liquids, particles, tar, carbon monoxide, cadmium, pyridine, nitrogen dioxide, ammonia, benzene, phenol, acrolein, hydrogen cyanide, formaldehyde, and hydrogen sulfide.

How Nicotine Works

A colorless, oily compound, **nicotine** is poisonous in concentrated amounts. If you inhale while smoking, 90 percent of the nicotine in the smoke is absorbed into your body. Even if you draw smoke only into your mouth and not into your lungs, you still absorb 25 to 30 percent of the nicotine. The FDA has concluded that nicotine is a dangerous, addictive drug that should be regulated. Yet in recent years tobacco companies have increased the levels of addictive nicotine by an average of 1.6 percent per year.

Faster than an injection, smoking speeds nicotine to the brain in seconds (Figure 13.5). Nicotine affects the brain in much the same way as cocaine, opiates, and amphetamines, triggering the release of dopamine, a neurotransmitter associated with pleasure and addiction, as well as other messenger chemicals. Because nicotine acts on some of the same brain regions stimulated by interactions with loved ones, smokers subconsciously come to regard cigarettes as a friend that they turn to when they're stressed, sad, or mad.

Nicotine may enhance smokers' performance on some tasks but leaves other mental skills unchanged.[19] Nicotine also acts as a sedative. How often you smoke and how you smoke determine nicotine's effect on you. If you're a regular smoker, nicotine will generally stimulate you at first, then tranquilize you. Shallow puffs tend to increase alertness because low doses of nicotine facilitate the release of the neurotransmitter *acetylcholine*, which makes the smoker feel alert. Deep drags, on the other hand, relax the smoker because high doses of nicotine block the flow of acetylcholine.

Nicotine stimulates the adrenal glands to produce adrenaline, a hormone that increases blood pressure, speeds up the heart rate by 15 to 20 beats a minute, and constricts blood vessels (especially in the skin). Nicotine also inhibits the formation of urine, dampens hunger, irritates the membranes in the mouth and throat, and dulls the taste buds so foods don't taste as good as they would otherwise.

Nicotine withdrawal usually begins within hours. Symptoms include craving, irritability, anxiety, restlessness, and increased appetite.

Tar and Carbon Monoxide

As it burns, tobacco produces **tar,** a thick, sticky dark fluid made up of several hundred different chemicals—many of them poisonous, some of them *carcinogenic* (enhancing the growth of cancerous cells). As you inhale tobacco smoke, tar and other particles settle in the forks of the branchlike bronchial tubes in your lungs, where precancerous changes are apt to occur. In addition, tar and smoke damage the mucus and the cilia in the bronchial tubes, which normally remove irritating foreign materials from your lungs.

Smoke from cigarettes, cigars, and pipes also contains **carbon monoxide,** the deadly gas that comes out of the exhaust pipes of cars, in levels 400 times those considered safe in industry. Carbon monoxide interferes with the ability of the hemoglobin in the blood to carry oxygen, impairs normal functioning of the nervous system, and is at least partly responsible for the increased risk of heart attacks and strokes in smokers.

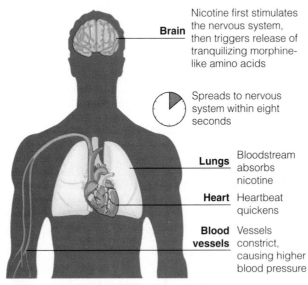

Brain — Nicotine first stimulates the nervous system, then triggers release of tranquilizing morphine-like amino acids

Spreads to nervous system within eight seconds

Lungs — Bloodstream absorbs nicotine

Heart — Heartbeat quickens

Blood vessels — Vessels constrict, causing higher blood pressure

Figure 13.5   The Immediate Effects of Nicotine on the Body

The primary active ingredient in tobacco is nicotine, a fast-acting and potent drug.

Sources: American Cancer Society, National Cancer Institute.

Health Effects of Cigarette Smoking

Figure 13.6 shows a summary of the physiological effects of tobacco and the other chemicals in tobacco smoke. If you're a smoker who inhales deeply and started smoking before the age of 15, you're trading a minute of future life for every minute you now spend smoking. Smoking's effect on your chance of dying is similar to adding five to ten years to your age. A 55-year-old man or woman who smokes has about the same risk of dying in the next decade as a 65-year-old who never smoked. Smoking is responsible for 64 percent of deaths in current smokers and 28 percent in past smokers.[20] (See Figure 13.7 on projected smoking deaths.)

A cigarette smoker is 10 times more likely to develop lung cancer than a nonsmoker and 20 times more likely to have a heart attack. Daily smokers also are more likely to have suicidal thoughts or attempt suicide, although the reasons are not clear (see Chapter 4).

Health Effects on Students

Although little research has focused specifically on college students, young people who smoke are less physically fit and suffer diminished lung function and growth. Young smokers frequently report symptoms such as wheezing, shortness of breath, coughing, and increased phlegm. They also are more susceptible to respiratory diseases. Young smokers are three times more likely to have consulted a doctor or mental health professional because of an emotional or psychological problem and almost twice as likely to develop symptoms of depression. Frequent smoking also has been linked to panic attacks and panic disorder in young people.

Long-term health consequences of smoking in young adulthood include dental problems, lung disorders (including asthma, chronic bronchitis, and emphysema), heart disease, and cancer. Young women who smoke may

nicotine   The addictive substance in tobacco; one of the most toxic of all poisons.

tar   A thick, sticky dark fluid produced by the burning of tobacco, made up of several hundred different chemicals, many of them poisonous, some of them carcinogenic.

carbon monoxide   A colorless, odorless gas produced by the burning of gasoline or tobacco; displaces oxygen in the hemoglobin molecules of red blood cells.

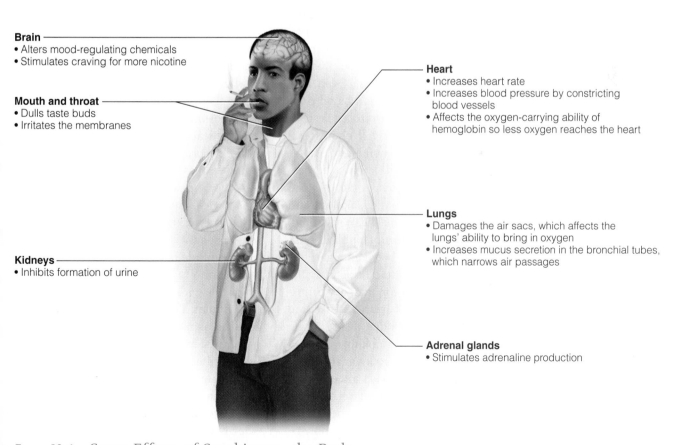

Brain
• Alters mood-regulating chemicals
• Stimulates craving for more nicotine

Mouth and throat
• Dulls taste buds
• Irritates the membranes

Kidneys
• Inhibits formation of urine

Heart
• Increases heart rate
• Increases blood pressure by constricting blood vessels
• Affects the oxygen-carrying ability of hemoglobin so less oxygen reaches the heart

Lungs
• Damages the air sacs, which affects the lungs' ability to bring in oxygen
• Increases mucus secretion in the bronchial tubes, which narrows air passages

Adrenal glands
• Stimulates adrenaline production

Figure 13.6   Some Effects of Smoking on the Body
Smoking harms the respiratory system and the cardiorespiratory system. The leading cause of death for smokers is heart attack.

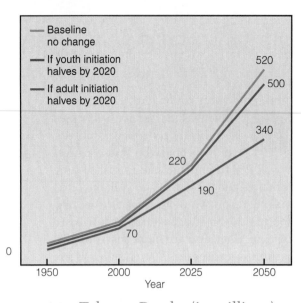

Figure 13.7 Tobacco Deaths (in millions)

Unless current smokers quit, smoking deaths will rise dramatically over the next 50 years.

Source: The Tobacco Atlas, www.tobaccoatlas.org.

develop menstrual problems, including irregular periods and painful cramps. If they use oral contraceptives, they are at increased risk of heart disease or stroke.

Heart Disease and Stroke

The toxic chemicals in tobacco signal the heart to beat faster and harder. Blood vessels constrict, forcing blood to travel through a narrower space. Blood pressure increases—temporarily at first. Over time, smokers develop chronic high blood pressure. Smoking increases harmful cholesterol (LDL) and lowers beneficial cholesterol (HDL). It also leads to the buildup of plaque, or fatty deposits within the arteries; hardening of the arteries; and greater risk of blood clots. Both current and former smokers ran a higher risk for an abnormal heart rhythm.[21]

Although a great deal of publicity has been given to the link between cigarettes and lung cancer, heart attack is actually the leading cause of death for smokers. Smoking doubles the risk of heart disease and increases the risk of sudden death two to four times. The effect of smoking on risk of heart attack is greater in younger smokers.

Smokers who suffer heart attacks have only a 50 percent chance of recovering. Smokers have a 70 percent higher death rate from heart disease than nonsmokers, and those who smoke heavily have a 200 percent higher death rate.

 The federal Office of the Surgeon General blames cigarettes for one of every ten deaths attributable to heart disease. Smoking is more dangerous than the two most notorious risk factors for heart disease: high blood pressure and high cholesterol. If smoking is combined with one of these, the chances of heart attack are four times greater. Women who smoke and use oral contraceptives have a ten times higher risk of suffering heart attacks than women who do neither.

In addition to contributing to heart attacks, cigarette smoking increases the risk of stroke two to three times in men and women, even after other risk factors are taken into account.

Even people who have smoked for decades can reduce their risk of heart attack if they quit smoking. However, studies indicate some irreversible damage to blood vessels. Progression of atherosclerosis (hardening of the arteries) among former smokers continues at a faster pace than among those who never smoked.

Lung Cancer

Smoking is linked to at least ten different cancers and accounts for 30 percent of all deaths from cancer. Smoking is the cause of more than 80 percent of all cases of lung cancer. The more people smoke, the longer they smoke, and the earlier they start smoking, the more likely they are to develop lung cancer.

Smoking causes about 130,000 lung cancer deaths each year. Smokers of two or more packs a day have lung cancer mortality rates 15 to 25 times greater than nonsmokers. If smokers stop smoking before cancer has started, their lung tissue tends to repair itself, even if there were already precancerous changes.

Chemicals in cigarette smoke and other environmental pollutants switch on a particular gene in the lung cells of some individuals. This gene produces an enzyme that helps manufacture powerful carcinogens, which set the stage for cancer. The gene seems more likely to be activated in some people than in others, and people with this gene are at much higher risk of developing lung cancer. However, smokers without the gene still remain at risk, because other chemicals and genes also may be involved in the development of lung cancer.

Smokers who are depressed are more likely to get cancer than nondepressed smokers. Although researchers don't know exactly how smoking and depression may work together to increase the risk of cancer, one possibility is that stress and depression cause biological changes that lower immunity, such as a decline in natural killer cells that fight off tumors.

Respiratory Diseases

Smoking quickly impairs the respiratory system, including the cough reflex, a vital protective response. Even some teenage smokers show signs of respiratory difficulty—breathlessness, chronic cough, excess phlegm production—when compared with nonsmokers of the same age. Cigarette smokers are up to 18 times more likely than nonsmokers to die of noncancerous diseases of the lungs.

Cigarette smoking is the major cause of chronic obstructive pulmonary disease (COPD), which includes emphysema and chronic bronchitis. COPD is characterized by progressive limitation of the flow of air into and out of the lungs. In emphysema, the limitation of air flow is the result of disease changes in the lung tissue, affecting the bronchioles (the smallest air passages) and the walls of the alveoli (the tiny air sacs of the lung). Eventually, many of the air sacs are destroyed, and the lungs become much less able to bring in oxygen and remove carbon dioxide. As a result, the heart has to work harder to deliver oxygen to all organs of the body.

In chronic bronchitis, the bronchial tubes in the lungs become inflamed, thickening the walls of the bronchi, and the production of mucus increases. The result is a narrowing of the air passages. Smoking is more dangerous than any form of air pollution, at least for most Americans, but exposure to both air pollution and cigarettes is particularly harmful.

© Arthur Glauberman/Photo Researchers, Inc.

Healthy nonsmoker's lung (left) and smoker's lung (right). Healthy lungs are pink, with a smooth but porous texture. A smoker's lungs show obvious signs of impairment. Bronchial tubes are inflamed, air passages are constricted, and tar coats the bronchial tubes.

Other Smoking-Related Problems

Smokers are more likely than nonsmokers to develop gum disease, and they lose significantly more teeth. Even those who quit have worse gum problems than people who never smoked at all. Smoking may also contribute to the loss of teeth and teeth-supporting bone, even in individuals with good oral hygiene.

Cigarette smoking is associated with stomach and duodenal ulcers; mouth, throat, and other types of cancer; and cirrhosis of the liver. Smoking may worsen the symptoms or complications of allergies, diabetes, hypertension, peptic ulcers, and disorders of the lungs or blood vessels. Some men who smoke ten cigarettes or more a day may experience erectile dysfunction. Cigarette smokers also tend to miss work one-third more often than nonsmokers, primarily because of respiratory illnesses. In addition, each year cigarette-ignited fires claim thousands of lives.

Smoking is an independent risk factor for high-frequency hearing loss and also adds to the danger of hearing loss for those exposed to noise. Cigarette smoking also may increase the likelihood of anxiety, panic attacks, and social phobias.

Other Forms of Tobacco

Two percent of Americans smoke cigars; 2 percent use smokeless tobacco. Ingesting tobacco may be less deadly than smoking cigarettes, but it is dangerous. Smoking cigars, clove cigarettes, and pipes and chewing or sucking on smokeless tobacco all put the user at risk of cancer of the lip, tongue, mouth, and throat, as well as other diseases and ailments. Despite claims of lower risk, "safer" cigarettes still jeopardize smokers' health. (See "Consumer Alert," p. 431.)

Cigars

  Cigar use has declined in the last few years. However, after cigarettes, cigars are the tobacco product most widely used by college students. About 16 percent of college men (and 4 percent of women) smoke cigars. White and African American students are more likely to smoke cigars than Hispanic or Asian American students.[22]

Cigar smoking is as dangerous as cigarette smoking even though cigar smokers do not inhale. Cigars can cause cancer of the lung and the digestive tract. The risk of death related to cigars approaches that of cigarettes, depending on the number of cigars smoked and the amount of cigar smoke inhaled. Cigar smoking can lead to nicotine addiction, even if the smoke is not inhaled. The nicotine in the smoke from a single cigar can vary from an amount roughly equivalent to that in a single cigarette to that in a pack or more of cigarettes.

Clove Cigarettes

Sweeteners have long been mixed with tobacco, and clove, a spice, is the latest ingredient to be added to the recipe for cigarettes. Clove cigarettes typically contain two-thirds tobacco and one-third clove. Consumers of these cigarettes are primarily teenagers and young adults.

Many users believe that clove cigarettes are safer because they contain less tobacco, but this isn't necessarily the case. The CDC reports that people who smoke clove cigarettes may be at risk of serious lung injury.

Clove cigarettes deliver twice as much nicotine, tar, and carbon monoxide as moderate-tar American brands. Eugenol, the active ingredient in cloves (which dentists have used as an anesthetic for years), deadens sensation in the throat, allowing smokers to inhale more deeply and hold smoke in their lungs for a longer time. Chemical relatives of eugenol can produce the kind of damage to cells that may lead to cancer.

Bidis

Skinny, sweet-flavored cigarettes called **bidis** (pronounced "beedees") have become a smoking fad among teens and young adults. For centuries, bidis were popular in India, where they are known as the poor man's cigarette and sell for less than five cents a pack. They look strikingly like clove cigarettes or marijuana joints and are available in flavors like grape, strawberry, and mandarin orange. Bidis are legal for adults and even minors in some states and are sold on the Internet as well as in stores.

Although bidis contain less tobacco than regular cigarettes, their unprocessed tobacco is more potent. Smoke from bidis has about three times as much nicotine and carbon monoxide and five times as much tar as smoke from regular filtered cigarettes. Because bidis are wrapped in nonporous brownish leaves, they don't burn as easily as cigarettes, and smokers have to inhale harder and more often to keep them lit. In one study, smoking a single bidi required 28 puffs, compared to 9 puffs for cigarettes.

Pipes

Many cigarette smokers switch to pipes to reduce their risk of health problems. But former cigarette smokers may continue to inhale, even though pipe smoke is more irritating to the respiratory system than cigarette smoke. People who have smoked only pipes and who do not inhale are much less likely to develop lung and heart disease than cigarette smokers. However, they are as likely as cigarette smokers to develop—and die of—cancer of the mouth, larynx, throat, and esophagus.

Smokeless Tobacco

An estimated 3 percent of adults in the United States use smokeless tobacco products (sometimes called "spit").[23] Use of chewing tobacco by teenage boys, particularly in rural areas, has surged 30 percent in the last decade.[24] About 9 percent of college men (and 0.4 percent of women) are smokeless tobacco users.[25] These substances include snuff, finely ground tobacco that can be sniffed or placed inside the cheek and sucked, and chewing tobacco, tobacco leaves mixed with flavoring agents such as molasses. With both, nicotine is absorbed through the mucous membranes of the nose or mouth.

Smokeless tobacco causes a user's heart rate, blood pressure, and epinephrine (adrenaline) levels to jump. In addition, it can cause cancer and noncancerous oral conditions and lead to nicotine addiction and dependence. Smokeless tobacco users are more likely than nonusers to become cigarette smokers.

Powerful carcinogens in smokeless tobacco include nitrosamines, polycyclic aromatic hydrocarbons, and radiation-emitting polonium. Its use can lead to the development of white patches on the mucous membranes of the mouth, particularly on the site where the tobacco is placed. Most lesions of the mouth lining that result from the use of smokeless tobacco dissipate six weeks after the use of the tobacco product is stopped. However, when first found, about 5 percent of these lesions are cancerous or exhibit changes that progress to cancer within ten years if not properly treated. Cancers of the lip, pharynx, larynx, and esophagus have all been linked to smokeless tobacco.

Nicotine replacement with gum or patches decreases cravings for smokeless tobacco and helps with short-term abstinence. However, it does not improve long-term abstinence. Behavioral approaches are more effective for long-term quitting.

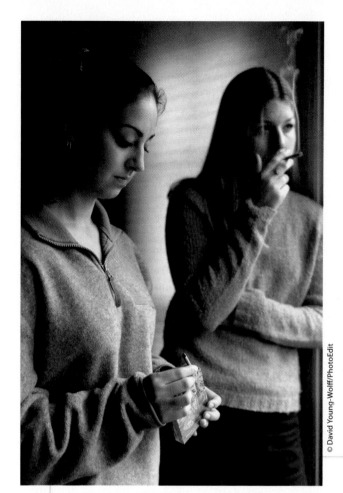

The smoke produced by bidis—skinny cigarettes—can contain higher concentrations of toxic chemicals than the smoke from regular cigarettes.

Quitting

The U.S. Public Health Service's most recent guidelines for treating tobacco use and dependence recognize tobacco dependence as "a chronic disease that often requires repeated intervention and multiple attempts to quit. Effective treatments exist, however, that can significantly increase rates of long-term abstinence."[26]

More than 70 percent of the 45 million smokers in the United States say they want to quit; approximately 44 percent try to quit each year. Yet only 4 to 7 percent succeed in any given year.[27] (See "Butt Out" in Making Change Happen, p. 427, and in *Labs for IPC.*)

 About half of whites who have smoked were able to kick the habit, compared with 45 percent of Asian Americans, 43 percent of Hispanics, and 37 percent of African Americans. Men and women with college and graduate degrees were much more likely to quit successfully than high school dropouts. Quitting eliminates the excess risk of dying from heart disease fairly quickly; after 20 smoke-free years the risk of smoking-related cancers drops to that of someone who never smoked.[28]

Compared with men, women seem to have a higher behavioral dependence on

bidis Skinny, sweet-flavored cigarettes.

cigarettes. For them, wearing a nicotine patch or chewing nicotine gum does not substitute for the "hand-to-mouth" behaviors associated with smoking, such as lighting a cigarette, inhaling, and handling the cigarette. Some investigators have found that women are more likely to quit successfully when they receive a combination of nicotine replacement and the use of a device like a nicotine inhaler to substitute for smoking behaviors.

While counseling and medication are each beneficial, the combination is more effective than either alone. In a study of community college students, a computer-assisted interactive smoking cessation program helped 17 percent stop.[29] One campus-based program that employed peer facilitators to help smokers quit and avoid relapse reported a success rate of 88 percent. Being "in the group" was the single most powerful contributor to quitting, and participants said their sense of connectedness helped them quit and stay smoke-free.

Nicotine withdrawal symptoms can behave like characters in a bad horror movie: Just when you think you've killed them, they're back with a vengeance. In recent studies, some people who tried to quit smoking reported a small improvement in withdrawal symptoms over two weeks, but then their symptoms leveled off and persisted. Others found that their symptoms intensified rather than lessened over time. For reasons scientists cannot yet explain, former smokers who start smoking again put their lungs at even greater jeopardy than smokers who never quit.

Once a former smoker takes a single puff, the odds of a relapse are 80 to 85 percent. Smokers are most likely to quit in the third, fourth, or fifth attempt. But thanks to new products and programs, it may be easier now than ever before to become an ex-smoker.

Quitting on Your Own

More than 90 percent of former smokers quit on their own—by throwing away all their cigarettes, by gradually cutting down, or by first switching to a less potent brand. One characteristic of successful quitters is that they see themselves as active participants in health maintenance and take personal responsibility for their own health. Physically active smokers have greater success quitting, possibly because participating in one healthy behavior, such as exercise, leads to adoption of other positive behaviors.[30] Often they experiment with a variety of strategies, such as learning relaxation techniques. In women, exercise has proved especially effective for quitting and avoiding weight gain. Making a home a smoke-free zone also increases a smoker's likelihood of successfully quitting.

Virtual Support

Electronic communications via cell phones, e-mails, text-messages, blogs, and social networking sites may be particularly effective in helping young smokers quit. In the few research studies that have been done, these approaches generally resulted in higher quit rates—but only if continued over time.[31]

Stop-Smoking Groups

Joining a support group doubles your chances of quitting for good. The American Cancer Society's FreshStart program runs about 1,500 stop-smoking clinics, each with about 8 to 18 members meeting for eight two-hour sessions over four weeks. Instructors explain the risks of smoking, encourage individuals to think about why they smoke, and suggest ways of unlearning their smoking habit. A quitting day is set for the third or fourth session.

The American Lung Association's Freedom from Smoking program consists of eight one- to two-hour sessions over seven weeks. The approach is similar to the American Cancer Society's, but smokers keep diaries and team up with buddies. Ex-smokers serve as advisers on quitting day. Both groups estimate that 27 or 28 percent of their participants successfully stop smoking.

Stop-smoking classes are also available through science departments and student health services on many college campuses, as well as through community public health departments. The Seventh-Day Adventists sponsor a four-week Breathe Free Plan, in which smokers commit themselves to clean living (no smoking, alcohol, tea, or coffee, along with a balanced diet and regular exercise).

Butt Out

Stained teeth. Bad breath. Premature wrinkles. Gum disease. Yellow fingernails. No one starts smoking to acquire any of these, but they come with the territory—along with far more serious health consequences. Maybe you don't think of yourself as a smoker because you only smoke at parties, or during finals, or with particular friends. Maybe you've cut back or are thinking about quitting.

If you smoke at all—a cigarette a week or a pack a day, in social settings or anywhere you can—do the "Butt Out" lab in *Labs for IPC*. There is nothing more important that you can do for yourself, your health, and your future than to quit.

Get Real
In this stage you answer a series of questions in your *IPC Journal,* including the following:

- Describe your smoking style:
  - Where do you smoke?
  - When do you smoke?
  - With whom do you smoke?
  - How do you smoke (light one cigarette after another, smoke between sips of coffee or beer, smoke before meals to kill your appetite, etc.)?

You also write a story called "My Smoking History," using only the past tense and the phrase "chose to smoke" rather than the word "smoked."

Get Ready
In this stage, you list all the reasons you decided to quit. For example:
- No more coughing.

- No more complaints from my partner about how I smell or taste.
- Save money.

You print out your list, and read it at the beginning and end of every day. You also read pages 425 to 430 in this chapter and decide on a quit plan. You check out any campus-based programs and make the necessary appointments and arrangements . . .

Get Going
You start the morning by saying, "I am not a smoker." Be sure to repeat this mantra morning and night and as often as possible during the day. Make this statement even if you are tapering down your tobacco use and continuing to smoke. In time you will find it easier not to smoke because you see yourself as a nonsmoker.

Additional steps include:
- Staying out of smoking zones.
- Dealing with nicotine withdrawal.
- Talking back to yourself when a rationalization for smoking pops into your mind. For example, if you think, "You've got to die of something," your response would be, "I don't have to get a terrible disease and die years ahead of my time in pain."

Lock It In
Staying quit is the final, and most important, stage of the butt-out process. This stage provides proven strategies, including the following:
- **Rehearse.** If you used to smoke at parties, visualize yourself going to the party with a nonsmoker friend. See yourself steering away from the smokers outside. Visualize yourself saying, "No, thank you. I don't smoke . . ."

Many businesses sponsor smoking-cessation programs for employees, which generally follow the approaches of professional groups. Motivation may be even higher in these programs than in programs outside the workplace because some companies offer attractive incentives to participants, such as lower rates on their health insurance.

Some smoking-cessation programs rely primarily on **aversion therapy,** which provides a negative experience every time a smoker has a cigarette. This may involve taking drugs that make tobacco smoke taste unpleasant, undergoing electric shocks, having smoke blown at you, or rapid smoking (the inhaling of smoke every six seconds until you're dizzy or nauseated).

Nicotine Anonymous, a nonprofit organization based on the 12 steps to recovery developed by Alcoholics Anonymous, acknowledges the power of nicotine and provides support to help smokers, chewers, and dippers live free of nicotine. New members are encouraged to abstain from using nicotine "one day at a time" and to attend meetings regularly. In addition to local meetings, NicA offers online support and networking, which puts people in touch with others in their region who share their desire to quit using nicotine.

Nicotine Replacement Therapy (NRT)
This approach uses a variety of products that supply low doses of nicotine in a way that allows smokers to taper off gradually over a period of months. Nicotine replacement therapies include nonprescription products (nicotine gum, lozenges, and nicotine

aversion therapy A treatment that attempts to help a person overcome a dependence or bad habit by making the person feel disgusted or repulsed by that habit.

patches) and prescription products (nicotine nasal spray and nicotine inhaler). The nasal spray, dispensed from a pump bottle, delivers nicotine to the nasal membranes and reaches the bloodstream faster than any other nicotine replacement therapy product. The inhaler delivers nicotine into the mouth and enters the bloodstream much more slowly than the nicotine in cigarettes.

Smokers who use NRT are 1.5 to 2 times more likely to quit. Because nicotine is a powerful, addictive substance, using nicotine replacements for a prolonged period is not advised. Pregnant women and individuals with heart disease shouldn't use them.

The most effective approaches combine medication—nicotine patches or Zyban, for instance—with psychological intervention. Each doubles a person's chance of quitting successfully.

Nicotine replacement therapy has proved more beneficial for men than for women—particularly with higher doses of nicotine. Men who receive more nicotine achieve a higher quit rate than men getting lower doses.

For women, the nicotine "dose" does not have an impact on successful quitting. They are no more likely to stop smoking with high doses than with lower ones, indicating that they may be less dependent on nicotine than men.

Nicotine Gum

Nicotine gum (now available in generics as well) contains a nicotine resin that's gradually released as the gum is chewed. Absorbed through the mucous membrane of the mouth, the nicotine doesn't produce the same rush as a deeply inhaled drag on a cigarette. However, the gum maintains enough nicotine in the blood to diminish withdrawal symptoms.

Although this gum is lightly spiced to mask nicotine's bitterness, many users say that it takes several days to become accustomed to its unusual taste. Its side effects include mild indigestion, sore jaws, nausea, heartburn, and stomachache. Also, because nicotine gum is heavier than regular chewing gum, it may loosen fillings or cause problems with dentures. Drinking coffee or other beverages may block absorption of the nicotine in the gum; individuals trying to quit smoking shouldn't ingest any substance immediately before or while chewing nicotine gum.

Most people use nicotine gum as a temporary crutch and gradually taper off until they can stop chewing it relatively painlessly. However, 5 to 10 percent of users transfer their dependence from cigarettes to the gum. When they stop using nicotine gum, they experience withdrawal symptoms, although the symptoms tend to be milder than those prompted by quitting cigarettes. Intensive counseling to teach smokers coping methods can greatly increase success rates.

Nicotine Patches

Nicotine transdermal delivery system products, or patches, provide nicotine, their only active ingredient, via a patch attached to the skin by an adhesive. Like nicotine gum, the nicotine patch minimizes withdrawal symptoms, such as intense craving for cigarettes. Nicotine patches help nearly 20 percent of smokers quit entirely after six weeks, compared with 7 percent on a placebo patch. Some insurance programs pay for patch therapy. Nicotine patches, which cost between $3.25 and $4 each, are replaced daily during therapy programs that run between 6 and 16 weeks. There is no evidence that continuing their use for more than 8 weeks provides added benefit.

Some patches deliver nicotine around the clock and others for just 16 hours (during waking hours). Those most likely to benefit from nicotine patch therapy are people who smoke more than a pack a day, are highly motivated to quit, and participate in counseling programs. While using the patch, 37 to 77 percent of people are able to abstain from smoking. When combined with counseling, the patch can be about twice as effective as a placebo, enabling 26 percent of smokers to abstain for six months.

Patch wearers who smoke or use more than one patch at a time can experience a nicotine overdose; some users have even suffered heart attacks. Occasional side effects include redness, itching, or swelling at the site of the patch application; insomnia; dry mouth; and nervousness.

Nicotine Inhaler

Available only by prescription, the Nicotine Inhaler consists of a mouthpiece and a cartridge containing

Nictotine gum, when chewed, gradually releases a nicotine resin and helps some smokers break their habit.

© AJPhoto/Photo Researchers, Inc.

a nicotine-impregnated plug. The smoker inhales through the mouthpiece, using either shallow or deep puffs. The inhaled air becomes saturated with nicotine, which is absorbed mainly through the tissues of the mouth. The inhaler releases less nicotine per puff than a cigarette and does not contain a cigarette's harmful tars, carbon monoxide, and smoke. Treatment is recommended for 3 months with a gradual reduction over the next 6 to 12 weeks. Total treatment should not exceed 6 months.

Medications

Another alternative to the patch is *bupropion*, a drug initially developed to treat depression, that is marketed in a slow-release form for nicotine addiction as Zyban. In studies that have combined Zyban with nicotine replacement and counseling, 40 to 60 percent of those treated have remained smoke-free for at least a year after completing the program. This success rate is much higher than the 10 to 26 percent reported among smokers who try to quit by using nicotine replacement alone. The combination of Zyban and nicotine replacement also prevented the initial weight gain that often accompanies quitting. Other medications used to treat nicotine addiction are varenicline (Chantix) clonidine, mecamylamine, and buspirone. However, varenicline has been linked with an increased risk of suicidal thoughts and behavior.[32]

Other Ways to Quit

Hypnosis may help some people quit smoking. Hypnotherapists use their techniques to create an atmosphere of strict attention and give smokers in a mild trance positive suggestions for breaking their cigarette habit.

Acupuncture, in which a circular needle or staple is inserted in the flap in front of the opening to the ear, has also had some success. When smokers feel withdrawal symptoms, they gently move the needle or staple, which may increase the production of calming chemicals in the brain.

Since 1976, a November day has been set aside in the United States for the annual Great American Smoke-Out, an idea promoted by the American Cancer Society to encourage smokers to give up cigarettes for 24 hours. As many as 36 percent of American smokers have given up cigarettes on Smoke-Out Day; about 5 to 6 percent have quit permanently; 15 percent reduced smoking for extended periods. In addition, the World Health Organization has established World No-Tobacco Days in May to call on nations to urge tobacco users to abstain for at least one day and perhaps quit for good.

Quitting and the Risks Associated with Smoking

Not smoking another cigarette is a gift to your body and your life. (See Table 13.1.) It is not a guarantee that there will be no consequences of the cigarettes you've already smoked.

Within a year of quitting, an ex-smoker's risk of heart disease drops to half that of active smokers. After 15 years, it approaches that of people who've never smoked. This is great news because the risk of dying prematurely from heart disease is far greater than that of dying from cancer.

The risk of lung cancer from smoking fades more slowly, perhaps because of permanent DNA damage to lung cells. Even 10 to 15 years after quitting, an ex-smoker is several times more likely to die of lung cancer than someone who has never smoked. Former smokers are also more vulnerable

A nicotine patch releases nicotine through the skin in measured amounts, which are gradually decreased over time.

> ## TABLE 13.1

Why Quit?

Quitting is the smartest choice a smoker can make—and keeps paying off far into the future. Consider these facts:

- **20 minutes after quitting:** Your heart rate and blood pressure drop.

- **12 hours after quitting:** The carbon monoxide level in your blood drops to normal.

- **2 weeks to 3 months after quitting:** Your circulation improves and your lung function increases.

- **1 to 9 months after quitting:** Coughing and shortness of breath decrease; cilia (tiny hairlike structures that move mucus out of the lungs) regain normal function, increasing the ability to handle mucus, clean the lungs, and reduce the risk of infection.

- **1 year after quitting:** Your excess risk of coronary heart disease is half that of a smoker's.

- **5 years after quitting:** Your stroke risk is reduced to that of a nonsmoker.

- **10 years after quitting:** The lung cancer death rate is about half that of a continuing smoker's. Your risk of cancer of the mouth, throat, esophagus, bladder, cervix, and pancreas also decreases.

- **15 years after quitting:** Your risk of coronary heart disease is that of a nonsmoker's.

Source: American Cancer Society.

to the effects of secondhand smoke in the workplace, even if they haven't lit up for the last ten years.

Does the lung cancer risk ever go away? That may depend partly on how old you are when you quit. Women who quit before age 30 are no more likely to die from lung cancer than those who never smoked. However, a study of American veterans started in the 1950s showed that, even 40 years later, former smokers had a 50 percent greater chance of dying from lung cancer than lifetime nonsmokers.

While quitting sooner is better than later, later is better than never. Even smokers who quit in their sixties significantly reduce their lung cancer risk—and add several years to their life expectancy.

Environmental Tobacco Smoke

Maybe you don't smoke—never have, never will. That doesn't mean you don't have to worry about the dangers of smoking, especially if you live or work with people who smoke. **Environmental tobacco smoke,** or secondhand cigarette smoke, the most hazardous form of indoor air pollution, ranks behind cigarette smoking and alcohol as the third-leading preventable cause of death.

On average, a smoker inhales what is known as **mainstream smoke** eight or nine times with each cigarette, for a total of about 24 seconds. However, the cigarette burns for about 12 minutes, and everyone in the room (including the smoker) breathes in what is known as **sidestream smoke.**

According to the American Lung Association, incomplete combustion from the lower temperatures of a smoldering cigarette makes sidestream smoke dirtier and chemically different from mainstream smoke. It has twice as much tar and nicotine, five times as much carbon monoxide, and 50 times as much ammonia. And because the particles in sidestream smoke are small, this mixture of irritating gases and carcinogenic tar reaches deeper into the lungs and poses a greater threat to infants and children. If you're a nonsmoker sitting next to someone smoking seven cigarettes an hour, even in a ventilated room, you'll take in almost twice the maximum amount of carbon monoxide set for air pollution in industry—and it will take hours for the carbon monoxide to leave your body.

Even a little secondhand smoke is dangerous. As a cancer-causing agent, secondhand smoke may be twice as dangerous as radon gas and more than a hundred times more hazardous than outdoor pollutants regulated by federal law. Secondhand smoke also increases the sick leave rates among employees.

Health Effects of Secondhand Smoke

As Figure 13.8 shows, environmental tobacco smoke is both dangerous and deadly. A proven culprit in the development of lung cancer, it leads to an estimated 3,000 deaths among adult nonsmokers every year. The Surgeon General estimates that living with a smoker increases a nonsmoker's chances of developing lung cancer by 20 to 30 percent.

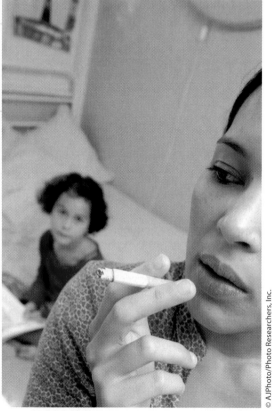

Secondhand smoke is the most common and hazardous form of indoor air pollution.

© AJPhoto/Photo Researchers, Inc.

	Adults	Children
Sufficient Evidence	Coronary artery disease Lung cancer Reproductive effects in women	Middle ear disease Respiratory symptoms, e.g. cough, wheeze Impaired lung function SIDS (sudden infant death syndrome) Lower respiratory illness, including infections Low birth weight
Suggestive Evidence	Stroke Nasal sinus cancer Breast cancer Atherosclerosis Chronic obstructive pulmonary disease, chronic respiratory symptoms, asthma, impaired lung function Preterm delivery	Brain tumors Lymphoma Leukemia

Smoking late in pregnancy can endanger the physical and intellectual development of the unborn child.

Figure 13.8 Harm Caused by Secondhand Smoke

Source: The Tobacco Atlas, www.tobaccoatlas.org.

Secondhand smoke also may increase the risk of breast cancer in women; cancer of the nasal sinus cavity and of the pharynx in adults; and leukemia, lymphoma, and brain tumors in children.

Exposure to tobacco smoke irritates the airways and contributes to respiratory diseases such as asthma. Because of its toxic effects on the heart and blood vessels, it may increase the risk of heart disease by an estimated 25 to 30 percent. In the United States secondhand smoke is thought to cause about 46,000 heart disease deaths a year.[33] According to a recent study, people exposed to secondhand smoke may face a significantly greater risk of developing Alzheimer's disease or other dementias.[34]

Children are particularly vulnerable to secondhand smoke, beginning before birth.[35] Prenatal exposure to tobacco can have significant effects that may extend from infancy into adulthood. A mother's smoking during pregnancy affects a child's growth, cognitive development, and behavior both before and after birth. Birthweight decreases in direct proportion to the

CONSUMER**ALERT**

"Safer" Cigarettes

Tobacco companies are producing low-tar and "lower-risk" cigarettes that they claim reduce secondhand smoke or have fewer carcinogens and less nicotine. These brands claim to use genetic engineering or a chemical process to remove major carcinogens.

Facts to Know

- Low-tar, "lite" cigarettes impair blood flow just as severely as regular cigarettes.
- So-called safer cigarettes may actually lead to increased addiction. In one experiment, smokers puffed on their own brand and then on a so-called safer cigarette brand called Advance. While Advance cigarettes supposedly contain less of a type of cancer-causing substance called nitrosamines, they delivered 25 percent more nicotine into the blood than the smokers' own brands.
- Other cigarettes deliver less nicotine and boost smokers' heart rates and carbon monoxide levels less than traditional cigarettes. However, they aren't as satisfying to smokers, who may smoke more of them.

Steps to Take

- Don't believe claims that any cigarette is safe or "safer."
- Do the truly safe thing: Stop smoking.

environmental tobacco smoke Secondhand cigarette smoke; the third-leading preventable cause of death.

mainstream smoke The smoke inhaled directly by smoking a cigarette.

sidestream smoke The smoke emitted by a burning cigarette and breathed by everyone in a closed room, including the smoker; contains more tar and nicotine than mainstream smoke.

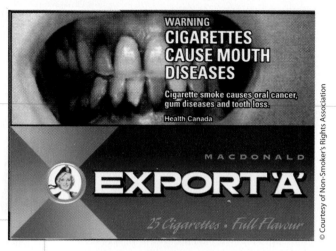

Graphic warning labels on cigarette packages in Canada have proven effective in discouraging smoking.

number of cigarettes smoked. The babies of teenage mothers who smoke have lower birthweight, length, head circumference, and chest circumference. As they grow, children of smokers tend to be shorter and weigh less than children of nonsmokers.

Even if their mothers don't smoke, children exposed to secondhand smoke before birth also are likely to weigh less and to perform more poorly on tests of speech, language skills, intelligence, and visual-spatial abilities and to develop behavior problems. These youngsters perform at a level between that of children of active smokers and children of nonsmokers.

Exposure to smoke after birth increases the risk of sudden infant death syndrome (SIDS) and is associated with lower IQ scores and deficits in cognitive development.

Children who breathe environmental tobacco smoke suffer from more asthma, wheezing, and bronchitis than children in smoke-free homes. They also face increased risk of lung cancer, heart disease, and stroke. African American children may be more susceptible to the toxins in secondhand smoke.

The negative effects of early exposure to environmental tobacco smoke persist even after youngsters leave home. In recent research at Ohio State University, college students who grew up in a smokers' household had higher resting heart rates and blood pressure at rest and during psychological stress than those who grew up in smoke-free homes. Teen exposure to cigarette smoke increases the risk of metabolic syndrome (discussed in Chapter 14).

Tobacco Control Policies

More than three decades after U.S. government health authorities began to warn of the dangers of cigarette smoking, tobacco remains a politically hot topic. However, a majority of people support tobacco control strategies, including creation of smoke-free environments, an increase in cigarette excise taxes, more funds to prevent people from smoking and to help smokers quit, and restriction of youth access to tobacco. (See Point/Counterpoint.)

The Family Smoking Prevention and Tobacco Control Act, signed into law in 2009, allows the FDA to forbid advertising geared toward children, to lower the amount of nicotine in tobacco products, to ban sweetened cigarettes that appeal to young people, and to prohibit labels like "light" and "low tar."

Policy initiatives, such as bans on smoking in public places, have proven beneficial for smokers and everyone in their vicinity. Nonsmokers are exposed to less secondhand smoke, while smokers tend to smoke less and are more likely to quit. In regions where smoking bans have been mandated by law, employees, customers, and business owners report high compliance and satisfaction with the results.[36] Since smoking was banned in clubs and restaurants in New

POINT COUNTERPOINT *Are Smokers Victims of Discrimination?*

POINT
State and federal civil rights laws prevent discrimination based on age, race, color, gender, marital status, national origin, weight, height, and religion. No-smoking bans in public and private places violate the rights of smokers and encourage discriminatory treatment of the victims of nicotine dependence.

COUNTERPOINT
As science has conclusively shown, tobacco is hazardous to nonsmokers as well as smokers. No one has the right to jeopardize the health of others. Nicotine dependence may be very difficult to break, but individuals who chose to start smoking must face all the consequences, including restrictions on where they can light up.

YOUR VIEW
Should smokers be singled out for exclusion from certain places? Are they a threat to public health? Do you smoke or not? If you do, how do you feel about smoking restrictions? If not, how do you feel when someone lights up next to you? Do you ever ask smokers to move or put out their cigarettes? Do you feel you have a right to do so?

Chapter - 14   Preventing Major Disease

1. **Which of the following cardio metabolic risk factors would one not be able to control: (Pg. 440- 441)**
   A. physical inactivity
   B. being too heavy
   C. genetic disposition to heart disease
   D. tobacco use

2. **Cardio metabolic health refers to: (Pg. 440)**
   A. heart functions
   B. basal metabolism issues
   C. diabetes control
   D. a combination of cardio and biochemical functions in the body

3. **Metabolic syndrome increases the chance to developing which of the following diseases: (Pg. 440)**
   A. diabetes
   B. stroke
   C. heart attack
   D. any of the above

4. **Juvenile onset diabetes is classified as: (Pg. 447)**
   A. prediabetes
   B. Type 1 diabetes
   C. Type 2 diabetes
   D. gestational diabetes

5. **All of the following except one are considered early symptoms of Type 2 diabetes: (Pg. 448)**
   A. increased thirst
   B. blurred vision
   C. angina chest pains
   D. slow healing sores and infections

6. **When your physician tells you that you have hypertension, the doctor is referring to: (Pg. 449)**
   A. high cholesterol
   B. high level of tension and stress
   C. slow heart rate
   D. high blood pressure

7. **The fatty deposits which line the inside of our arteries and causes the constricted blood flow to increase our blood pressure is known as: (Pg. 450)**
   A. cholesterol
   B. plaque
   C. calcium deposits
   D. sodium chloride salts

8. **Which of the following food would be a culprit to causing high blood pressure? (Pg. 452)**
   A. eating too many fruits and vegetables
   B. sugars and sweets
   C. high salty junk foods
   D. dairy products

9. **What is the medical term for thickening or hardening of the arteries? (Pg. 461)**
   A. myocardial infarction
   B. atherosclerosis
   C. arrhythmia
   D. cerebral hemorrhage

10. **The cholesterol type that is considered to be the 'good' kind to help lower your risk of heart disease is the: (Pg. 452- 453)**
    (A. LDL
    B. triglycerides
    C. HDL
    D. plaque

11. **All of the following are effective strategies for lowering cholesterol levels except: (Pg. 453- 454)**
    A. medication
    B. physical activity
    C. daily glass of wine consumption
    D. weight management

12. **The chambers of the heart that receive the blood are called: (Pg. 455)**
    A. ventricles
    B. the aorta
    C. atrium
    D. vena cava

13. **The single biggest risk factor for developing cardiovascular disease is: (Pg. 441)**
    A. smoking
    B. obesity
    C. heredity
    D. physical inactivity

14. **The one issue that can be most damaging to male cardiovascular health is: (Pg. 457)**
    A. diabetes
    B. borderline cholesterol
    C. anger and hostility
    D. lack of physical exercise

15. **The feelings of pain and tightness a man may feel when there is a sudden drop in the oxygen levels to the heart is known as: (Pg. 462)**
    A. myocardial infarction
    B. angina pectoris
    C. arteriosclerosis
    D. cerebral vascular blockage

16. **Uncle Roy complains that his eyes are getting blurred, he can't seem to stand up and his face feels distorted along with his speech. Your uncle may be suffering from a(n): (Pg. 464)**
    A. heart attack
    B. stroke
    C. insulin attack
    D. heart arrhythmia

17. **A tumor that is known to be non-cancerous is said to be: (Pg 467)**
    A. neoplastic
    B. malignant
    C. benign
    D. cured

18. **When cancer cells have been said to metastasized, this means that: (Pg. 467)**
    A. the cancer is reducing and shrinking in size
    B. the cells have become benign in their growth
    C. the cancer cells have infiltrated to the heart muscle
    D. the cancer cells have spread to other body organs

19. **The type of cancer that begins to grow in the epithelial tissues of the body is known as: (Pg. 471)**
    A. sarcoma
    B. basal cell cancer
    C. carcinoma
    D. lymphoma

20. **An example of a lymphoma is: (Pg. 471)**
    A. cancer in the breast tissue of a woman
    B. blood cancer in a child
    C. skin cancer
    D. cancer of the lymph nodes under the armpits of a man

Jarryd never forgot the terror he felt when his dad had his first heart attack. Only ten, he couldn't understand why this towering giant of a man had fallen to the ground, his face twisted in pain, his fist pressed against his chest. His father seemed different when he came home from the hospital, as if something had gone out of him. But his face would still light up with an impish grin, especially when he'd sneak a cigarette and wink at Jarryd so he wouldn't tell his mother. The second heart attack came four years later. This time Jarryd's dad didn't come home.

Preventing Major Disease

Jarryd promised his mother that he'd take better care of his heart. He wouldn't smoke; he'd watch his blood pressure and weight; he'd keep tabs on his diet; he'd exercise regularly. Jarryd didn't forget these promises as time passed. But like many college students, he felt invincible. He was shocked when a sports physical revealed that his blood pressure was high and his levels of the most dangerous type of cholesterol were elevated. But he also felt lucky: "I got my wake-up call," he explains. "And I'm not going to ignore it."

As Jarryd realizes, it's never too soon, or too late, to start protecting your health and your future. Whether or not you will get a serious disease at some time in your life may seem to be a matter of odds. Genetic tendencies, environmental factors, and luck affect your chances of having to face many health threats. However, often you can prevent or delay major illnesses, such as heart disease, for years, even decades.

The time to start protecting your health is now. People mistakenly think of heart disease, cancer, and other disorders as illnesses of middle and old age. But the events leading up to these diseases often begin in childhood, progress in adolescence, and become a health threat to men in their thirties and forties and to women in their forties and fifties. This chapter provides the information about the risk factors, silent dangers, and medical advances that can improve your chances of a healthier, longer life.

- **Define** cardiometabolic health, and **list** actions for lowering cardiometabolic risk.
- **Explain** the disease process of diabetes mellitus, the precursors to and types of diabetes, and **describe** the early symptoms and treatment for this disease.
- **Define** hypertension, and **discuss** why it is dangerous and ways to prevent it.
- **Describe** the types of cholesterol that compose your lipoprotein profile and the effects of each on cardiometabolic health.
- **Explain** how the heart functions, and **define** a myocardial infarction.
- **Define** stroke and **describe** its major risk factors.
- **Discuss** the most common types of cancer, and **describe** the treatments for each.
- **List** your cardiometabolic and cancer risk factors.

Image Source Black/Jupiterimages

Log on to CengageNOW for Health at **www.cengage.com/sso** to find your Behavior Change Planner and to explore self-assessments, interactive tutorials, and practice quizzes.

The Power of Prevention

Young people often feel immune to serious diseases, but illness can strike anyone. Regardless of your age, being in tune with your body is one of the best ways to safeguard your health.

More Americans are developing chronic illnesses such as diabetes and high blood pressure, often having more than three such conditions at a time—a financial as well as a physiological burden.[1] Many chronic problems begin early in life. An estimated one in four college students already has at least one risk factor, such as excess weight or physical inactivity, that increases the risk of conditions affecting the heart and metabolism. The habits you develop now—regular exercise, sensible eating, responsible drinking—can keep you healthy for decades to come.

Deaths from the two major killers of Americans—cancer and heart disease—have dropped sharply in recent decades. According to an analysis of the decline in heart-related mortality, preventive steps to reduce the risk of disease were responsible for 44 percent of the decrease.[2] Despite the gains that have been made, more people are still dying of illnesses than should be, many at young ages. Two in three deaths could be delayed and one in three hospitalizations could be avoided by basic preventive steps, such as weight management, not smoking, and regular screenings. (See Reality Check, p. 443.)

Your Cardiometabolic Health

In recent years medical scientists have focused on the complex connections between various risk factors, symptoms, and diseases. Physical inactivity, for instance, increases the risk of obesity, which in turn leads to greater risk of many diseases. This new awareness has led to a focus on **cardiometabolic** health. "Cardio" refers to the heart and blood vessels of the cardiovascular system; "metabolic," to the biochemical processes involved in the body's functioning.

Cardiometabolic Risk Factors

Specific risk factors determine your cardiometabolic health. Once you understand your risk, you can start making changes to lower your odds of developing metabolic syndrome, diabetes, and heart disease. Although you may have no signs of these illnesses, you may have at least one cardiometabolic risk factor. This alone increases the likelihood of having others. The more cardiometabolic risk factors you have, the greater risk you face of developing a serious health problem. However, you can reduce most cardiometabolic risk factors by making healthy changes in your lifestyle. (See Health on a Budget, p. 441.)

Risk Factors You Can Control The choices you make and the habits you follow can have a significant impact on whether or not you remain healthy. Avoid the following potential risks for the sake of your cardiometabolic health.

Overweight/Obesity Excess weight has emerged as an increasingly common and dangerous cardiometabolic risk factor in both men and women. BMI and measurement of waist circumference, discussed in Chapter 5, are good indicators of increased risk.

Waist Circumference As discussed in Chapter 5, apple-shaped people who carry most of their excess weight around their waists are at greater risk of cardiometabolic conditions than are pear-shaped individuals who carry most of their excess weight below their waist. The more visceral (abdominal) fat that you have, the more resistant your body's cells become to the effects of your own insulin. A waist measurement of more than 40 inches in men and more than 35 inches in women indicates increased health risks. A "pot belly" raises risk even when a person's weight is normal.

Physical Inactivity   As discussed in Chapter 5, about one-quarter of U.S. adults are sedentary and another third are not active enough to reach a healthy level of fitness. The risk for cardiometabolic conditions is higher for people who are inactive compared with those who engage in regular physical activity.

Fitness may be more important than overweight or obesity per se for women's cardiometabolic risk. A minimum of 30 minutes a day of moderate activity at least five days a week, can lift a woman from the "low-fitness category" and lessen her cardiometabolic risk.

The greater the exercise "dose," the more benefits it yields. In studies that compared individuals of different fitness levels, the least fit were at much greater risk of dying. In men, more rigorous exercise, such as jogging, produces greater protection against heart disease and boosts longevity.

Tobacco Use   Smoking may be the single most significant risk factor for cardiometabolic conditions. Each year smoking causes more than 250,000 deaths from cardiovascular disease—far more than it causes from cancer and lung disease. Smokers who have heart attacks are more likely to die from them than are nonsmokers. Smoking is the major risk factor for *peripheral arterial disease,* in which the vessels that carry blood to the leg and arm muscles become hardened and clogged.

Both active and passive smoking accelerate the process by which arteries become clogged and increase the risk of heart attacks and strokes. Overall, nonsmokers exposed to environmental tobacco smoke are at a 25 percent higher relative risk of developing coronary heart disease than nonsmokers not exposed to environmental tobacco smoke.

High Blood Glucose   As discussed in greater detail on page 445, your stomach and digestive system break down the food you eat into glucose, a type of sugar. The hormone insulin acts like a key, letting glucose into cells and providing energy. "Insulin resistant" cells no longer respond well to insulin, and then glucose, unable to enter the cells, builds up in the bloodstream. Frequent thirst, blurry vision, weakness, unexplained weight loss, or unusual hunger can be signs of high blood glucose. A simple blood test will tell you if your glucose levels are too high. Here is what the readings mean:

Healthy blood glucose	Under 100
Prediabetes	100–125
Diabetes	More than 125

High Blood Pressure (Hypertension)   Blood pressure is a result of the contractions of the heart muscle, which pumps blood through

cardiometabolic   Referring to the heart and to the biochemical processes involved in the body's functioning.

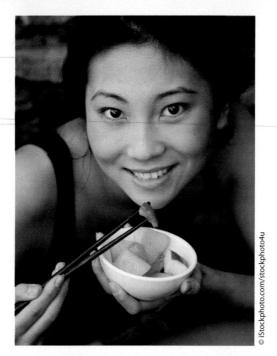

You can do something today to prevent heart disease in your future. Eat some fruit.

systolic blood pressure Highest blood pressure when the heart contracts.

diastolic blood pressure Lowest blood pressure between contractions of the heart.

hypertension High blood pressure occurring when the blood exerts excessive pressure against the arterial walls.

cholesterol An organic substance found in animal fats; linked to cardiovascular disease, particularly atherosclerosis.

lipoprotein A compound in blood that is made up of proteins and fat; a high-density lipoprotein (HDL) picks up excess cholesterol in the blood; a low-density lipoprotein (LDL) carries more cholesterol and deposits it on the walls of arteries.

triglyceride A fat that flows through the blood after meals and is linked to increased risk of coronary artery disease.

your body, and the resistance of the walls of the vessels through which the blood flows. Each time your heart beats, your blood pressure goes up and down within a certain range. It's highest when the heart contracts; this is called **systolic blood pressure.** It's lowest between contractions; this is called **diastolic blood pressure.** A blood pressure reading consists of the systolic measurement "over" the diastolic measurement, recorded in millimeters of mercury (mm Hg).

High blood pressure, or **hypertension,** occurs when the artery walls become constricted so that the force exerted as the blood flows through them is greater than it should be. Physicians see blood pressure as a continuum: The higher the reading, the greater the risk of stroke and heart disease.

As a result of the increased work in pumping blood, the heart muscle of a person with hypertension can become stronger and also stiffer. This stiffness increases resistance to filling up with blood between beats, which can cause shortness of breath with exertion. Hypertension can also act on the kidney arteries, which can lead to kidney failure in some cases. In addition, hypertension accelerates the development of plaque buildup within the arteries. Especially when combined with obesity, smoking, high cholesterol levels, or diabetes, hypertension increases the risks of cardiovascular problems several times. However, you can control high blood pressure through diet,

exercise, and if necessary, medication. (See page 451.)

Lipoprotein Levels **Cholesterol** is a fatty substance found in certain foods and also manufactured by the body. The measurement of cholesterol in the blood is one of the most reliable indicators of the formation of plaque, the sludgelike substance that builds up on the inner walls of arteries. You can lower blood cholesterol levels by cutting back on high-fat foods and exercising more, thereby reducing the risk of a heart attack.

Lipoproteins are compounds in the blood that are made up of proteins and fat. The different types are classified by their size or density. The heaviest are *high-density lipoproteins,* or HDLs, which have the highest proportion of protein. These "good guys," as some cardiologists refer to them, pick up excess cholesterol in the blood and carry it back to the liver for removal from the body. An HDL level of 40 mg/dL or lower substantially increases the risk of heart disease. (Cholesterol levels are measured in milligrams of cholesterol per deciliter of blood—mg/dL.) The average HDL for men is about 45 mg/dL; for women, it is about 55 mg/dL.

Low-density lipoproteins, or (LDLs), and very low-density lipoproteins (VLDLs) carry more cholesterol than HDLs and deposit it on the walls of arteries—they're the "bad guys." The higher your LDL cholesterol, the greater your risk for heart disease. If you are at high risk of heart disease, any level of LDL higher than 100 mg/dL may increase your danger.

Triglycerides are fats that flow through the blood after meals and have been linked to increased risk of coronary artery disease, especially in women. Triglyceride levels tend to be highest in those whose diets are high in calories, sugar, alcohol, and refined starches. High levels of these fats may increase the risk of obesity, and cutting back on these foods can reduce high triglyceride levels.

Figure 14.1 summarizes the factors to ask your doctor about at your next checkup.

Risk Factors You Can't Control

Family History Certain cardiometabolic risk factors, such as abnormally high blood levels of lipids, can be passed down from generation to generation. Although you can't rewrite your family history, individuals with an inherited vulnerability can lower the danger by changing the risk factors within their control. Your cardiometabolic health depends to a great extent on your behavior, including the decisions you make about the foods you eat or the decision not to smoke.

Race and Ethnicity Cardiometabolic risk 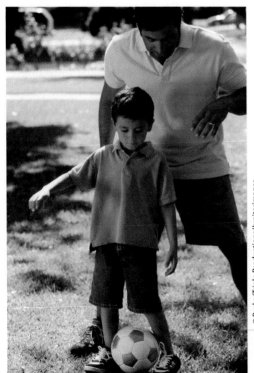 factors occur at higher rates among ethnic minority populations such as African Americans, Hispanic Americans, and Native Americans. For reasons that aren't entirely clear, people of some races are more likely to develop diabetes. Blacks and Hispanics have double the rate for whites. The incidence is even higher among American Indians. Among the Pima Indians of Arizona, half of all adults have type 2 diabetes, one of the highest rates of diabetes in the world. Nearly four in every ten black adults have cardiovascular disease. Among Hispanic Americans, nearly three in ten have cardiovascular disease.

African Americans are twice as likely to develop high blood pressure as whites. African Americans also suffer strokes at an earlier age and of greater severity. Poverty may be an unrecognized risk factor for members of this minority group, who are

✓ REALITYCHECK

- *How many college students have had their blood pressure checked within the last two years?*
- *How many have had their cholesterol checked within the last five years?*
- *How many college women performed a breast self-exam in the last month?*
- *How many college men performed a testicular self-exam in the last month?*
- *How many college students use sunscreen every day?*

Answers on next page.

less likely to receive medical treatments or undergo corrective surgery. Family history, lifestyle, diet, and stress may also play a role, starting early in life. However, researchers have found no single explanation for why African American youngsters, like their parents, tend to have higher blood pressure than white children.

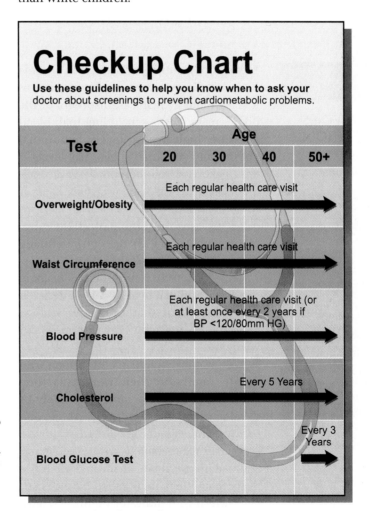

Figure 14.1 Checkup Chart
Adapted from CheckUpAmerica.org.

© Burke/Triolo Productions/Jupiterimages

A child's risk of heart disease later in life depends on many factors, including family history, diet, and physical activity.

PART 2: *Just the Facts*
- **89** *percent of college students have had their blood pressure checked within the last two years.*
- **45** *percent of college students have had their cholesterol checked within the last five years.*
- **41** *percent of college women performed a self-exam in the last month.*
- **41** *percent of college men performed a testicular self-exam in the last month.*
- **19** *percent of college students use sunscreen every day.*

Source: American College Health Association. *American College Health Association National College Health Assessment Reference Group Executive Summary Fall 2008.* Baltimore: American College Health Association, 2009.

 Black women are twice as likely as white women to suffer heart attacks and to die from heart disease. Common cardiometabolic risk factors—high blood pressure, diabetes, and high cholesterol—account for this increased jeopardy. In addition, black women are less likely to receive common medications, such as cholesterol-lowering drugs, to lower their risk.

Age Cardiometabolic risk factors increase as people get older, especially past the age of 45. This may be because many individuals tend to exercise less, lose muscle mass, and gain weight as they age. However, cardiometabolic conditions are also increasing dramatically among younger people.

Metabolic Syndrome

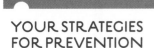

YOUR STRATEGIES FOR PREVENTION

How to Overcome Metabolic Syndrome

The following steps have proved effective in reversing metabolic syndrome and reducing the risks associated with it:

- Eat a low-fat, low-calorie diet.
- Engage in a regular moderate exercise, such as walking, almost every day.
- Reduce your body weight by 5 to 7 percent.
- If these strategies don't work for you, talk to your doctor about taking a glucose-lowering medication.

Metabolic syndrome, once called Syndrome X or insulin-resistant syndrome, is not a disease but a cluster of disorders of the body's metabolism—including high blood pressure, high insulin levels, abdominal obesity, and abnormal cholesterol levels—that make a person more likely to develop diabetes, heart disease, or stroke. Each of these conditions is by itself a risk factor for other diseases. In combination, they dramatically boost the chances of potentially life-threatening illnesses.

This dangerous syndrome has become so widespread that health officials describe it as an epidemic that affects one in four Americans, especially Hispanic men and women.

College-age men and women who maintain their weight as they get older are much less likely to develop metabolic syndrome. About one in four undergraduates already has one risk factor for metabolic syndrome. Young adults with metabolic syndrome are more likely than others their age to have thicker neck arteries, an indicator of atherosclerosis, the buildup of fatty plaques in arteries. Because retired professional football players have increased rates of metabolic syndrome and atherosclerosis, health professionals

have called for regular screening of athletes, beginning in high school and college.[3] "Bulking up" to play positions such as lineman may account for a heightened risk of heart problems later in life.[4]

As discussed in Chapter 6, drinking more than one soft drink (diet or regular) a day increases the risk of metabolic syndrome. Losing 7 to 10 percent of your initial body weight may reverse the symptoms of metabolic syndrome.

Three or more of the following characteristics indicate metabolic syndrome:

- **A larger-than-normal waist measurement**—40 inches or more in men and 35 inches or more in women (for Asians and individuals with a genetic predisposition to diabetes, 37 to 39 inches in men and 31 to 35 inches in women).
- **A higher-than-normal triglyceride level**—150 mg/dL or more.
- **A lower-than-normal high-density lipoprotein (HDL) level**—less than 40 mg/dL in men or 50 mg/dL in women.
- **A higher-than-normal blood pressure**—130 mm Hg systole over 85 mm Hg diastole (130/85), or higher.
- **A higher-than-normal fasting blood sugar**—110 mg/dL or higher.

People with three factors of metabolic syndrome are nearly twice as likely to have a heart attack or stroke and more than three times more likely to develop heart disease than those with none.

 Men with four or five characteristics of the syndrome have nearly four times the risk of heart attack or stroke and more than 24 times the risk of diabetes.

Insulin Resistance and Prediabetes

In a healthy body, the digestive system breaks food down into glucose, which then travels in the bloodstream to cells throughout the body. As the blood glucose level rises after a meal, the pancreas releases insulin to help cells take in the glucose. Insulin resistance is a condition in which the body produces insulin but does not use it properly.

When muscle, fat, and liver cells do not respond properly to insulin, the pancreas tries to keep up with the increased demand for insulin by producing more, but eventually it cannot. Excess glucose builds up in the bloodstream, setting the stage for diabetes. Many people with insulin resistance have high levels of both glucose and insulin circulating in their blood at the same time.

Insulin resistance increases the chance of developing type 2 diabetes and heart disease. Excess weight and lack of physical activity, along with genetic factors, contribute to insulin resistance.

Prediabetes—sometimes called impaired fasting glucose or impaired glucose tolerance—is a condition in which blood glucose levels are higher than normal but not high enough for a diagnosis of diabetes. According to federal estimates, about one in four U.S. adults aged 20 years or older—or 57 million people—has prediabetes.

Risk Factors for Prediabetes and Diabetes

Several factors—some of which you can control—increase your risk for prediabetes and diabetes.

- Overweight or obese.
- Age 45 or older.
- Physically inactive.
- Parent or sibling with diabetes.
- Family background that is African American, Alaska Native, American Indian, Asian American, Hispanic/ Latino, or Pacific Islander.
- Giving birth to a baby weighing more than nine pounds or being diagnosed with diabetes during pregnancy.
- High blood pressure—140/90 or above—or being treated for high blood pressure.
- HDL, or "good," cholesterol level below 35 mg/dL or a triglyceride level above 250 mg/dL.
- Polycystic ovary syndrome, also called PCOS.
- Impaired fasting glucose (IFG) or impairing glucose tolerance (IGT) on previous testing.
- Other conditions associated with insulin resistance, such as severe obesity.
- History of cardiovascular disease.

Insulin resistance and prediabetes usually do not cause symptoms. Some people develop dark rings or patches of skin on the neck, elbows, knees, knuckles, and armpits. Most people with prediabetes develop type 2 diabetes (discussed in the following pages) within 10 years, unless they lose at least five percent of their body weight by making changes in their diet and level of physical activity.

Long-term damage to the body, especially the heart and circulatory system, may occur during prediabetes. If people with prediabetes take action to manage their blood glucose, they can delay or prevent these harmful effects. Diets rich in cereal fiber, magnesium, calcium, and Vitamin D may help. Lifestyle changes also have shown promise.

metabolic syndrome A cluster of disorders of the body's metabolism that make diabetes, heart disease, or stroke more likely.

Diabetes Mellitus

About 13 percent of people in the United States have **diabetes mellitus,** a disease in which the body doesn't produce or respond properly to insulin.[5] In those with diabetes, the pancreas, which produces insulin (the hormone that regulates carbohydrate and fat metabolism) doesn't function as it should. When the pancreas either stops producing insulin or doesn't produce sufficient insulin to meet the body's needs, almost every body system can be damaged. (See Figure 14.2.)

The prevalence of diabetes has nearly doubled in the last three decades, and health experts describe it as a global epidemic. About 6.3 percent of Americans have diabetes; a third are not aware that they have it because certain types develop insidiously with no visible symptoms.

Diabetes shortens life expectancy by an average of 8 years—7.8 years for men, 8.4 years for women. The risk of premature death among people with diabetes is about twice that of people without the disease. Obesity, diabetes, and heart disease also can work together to speed dementia and other brain disorders, such as cognitive impairment.[6] According to the American Diabetes Association, the total economic cost of diabetes is more than $132 billion a year. Diabetes accounts for $1 of every $10 spent on health care in the United States. An estimated 48 million Americans may develop diabetes by 2050.

Understanding Diabetes

Glucose is the primary form of sugar that the body cells use for energy. When a person without diabetes eats a meal, the level of glucose in the blood rises, triggering the production and release of insulin by special cell clusters in the pancreas. Insulin enhances the movement of glucose into various body cells, bringing down the level of glucose in the blood. In those who have diabetes, however, insulin secretion is either nonexistent or deficient. Without sufficient insulin, the glucose in the blood is unable to enter most body cells, so the cells' energy needs aren't met. The levels of glucose in the blood rise higher and higher after each meal. This unused glucose eventually passes through the kidneys, which are unable to process the excessive glucose, and out of the body in urine.

Deprived of the fuel it needs, the body begins to break down stored fat as a source of energy. This process produces weak acids, called ketones. A buildup of ketones leads to ketoacidosis, an upheaval in the body's chemical balance that brings on nausea,

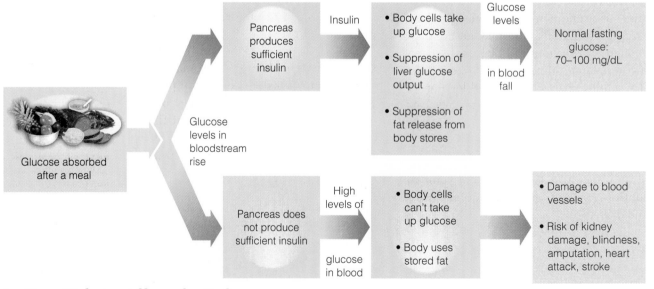

Figure 14.2 How Diabetes Affects the Body

Diabetes affects almost every organ system of the body in complex and often subtle ways.

vomiting, abdominal pain, lethargy, and drowsiness. Severe ketoacidosis can lead to coma and eventual death.

Before the development of insulin injections, diabetes was a fatal illness. Today diabetics can have normal lifespans. However, diabetes still can lead to devastating complications. Uncontrolled glucose levels slowly damage blood vessels throughout the body; thus, individuals who become diabetic early in life may face devastating complications even before they reach middle age. Diabetes is the number one cause of blindness, nontraumatic amputations, and kidney failure, and diabetes increases by two or three times the risk of heart attack or stroke.

 Diabetic women who become pregnant face higher risks of miscarriage and babies with serious birth defects; however, precise control of blood sugar levels before conception and in early pregnancy can lower the likelihood of these problems.

Types of Diabetes Diabetes includes several conditions in which the body has difficulty controlling levels of glucose in the bloodstream. After an overnight fast, most people have blood glucose levels between 70 and 100 milligrams of glucose per deciliter of blood (mg/dL). This is considered normal. If your fasting blood glucose level is between 101 and 125 mg/dL, you have prediabetes. If your fasting blood glucose is consistently 126 mg/dL or higher, you have diabetes.

- **Type 1 diabetes.** In this form of diabetes (once called juvenile-onset or insulin-dependent diabetes), the body's immune system attacks the insulin-producing beta cells in the pancreas and destroys them. The pancreas then produces little or no insulin and therefore blood glucose cannot enter the cells to be used for energy. Type 1 diabetes develops most often in young people but can appear in adults. Individuals with type 1 diabetes require insulin therapy because their own bodies no longer supply this vital hormone.

- **Type 2 diabetes.** In type 2 diabetes (once called adult-onset or non-insulin-dependent diabetes), either the pancreas does not make enough insulin or the body is unable to use insulin correctly.

Type 2 diabetes is becoming more common in children and teenagers because of the increase in obesity in the young.[7]

- **Gestational diabetes.** Women who get diabetes while they are pregnant are more likely to have a family history of diabetes, especially on their mothers' side; they are at greater risk of developing diabetes later in life.

Although type 1 and type 2 diabetes have different causes, two factors are important in both: an inherited predisposition to the disease and something in the environment that triggers diabetes. Genes alone are not enough. In most cases of type 1 diabetes, people need to inherit risk factors from both parents and to experience some environmental trigger, which might involve prenatal nutrition, a virus, or an unknown agent.

 In type 2 diabetes, family history is one of the strongest risk factors for getting the disease, but only in Westernized countries. African Americans, Mexican Americans, and Native Americans have the highest rates, but people who live in less developed nations tend not to get type 2 diabetes, no matter how high their genetic risk.

Excess weight, especially around the waistline, is the major and most controllable risk factor for type 2 diabetes.[8] Losing weight greatly reduces this risk and, in individuals with the disease, can help get blood sugar under control. Researchers also have found a complex relationship between depression and type 2 diabetes. Individuals with depressive symptoms are somewhat more likely to develop the disorder, while people being treated for type 2 diabetes have higher odds of becoming depressed.

Diabetes Signs and Symptoms About a third of individuals with type 2 diabetes do not realize they have the illness. If you have risk factors for the disease, watch for the following warning signs:

- **Increased thirst and frequent urination.** Excess glucose circulating in your body draws water from your tissues, making you feel dehydrated. Drinking water and other beverages to quench thirst leads to more frequent urination.

diabetes mellitus A disease in which the inadequate production of insulin leads to failure of the body tissues to break down carbohydrates at a normal rate.

The Diabetes Prevention Program (DPP), a landmark study sponsored by the National Institutes of Health, found that people at increased risk for type 2 diabetes can prevent or delay the onset of the disease by taking the following steps:

- Exercise 30 minutes on at least five days of the week.
- If you're overweight or obese, lose weight. Aim to lose 5 to 7 percent of your initial weight.
- Eat a diet rich in complex carbohydrates (bread and other starches) and high-fiber foods, and low in sodium and fat.
- Eat fruits and vegetables that are rich in anti-oxidants, substances that prevent oxygen damage to cells.
- If your doctor advises, take medications, such as metformin (Glucophage), to help lower your blood sugar.

- **Flu-like symptoms.** Type 2 diabetes can sometimes feel like a viral illness, with such symptoms as extreme fatigue and weakness. When glucose, your body's main fuel, doesn't reach cells, you may feel tired and weak.

- **Weight loss or weight gain.** Because your body is trying to compensate for lost fluids and glucose, you may eat more than usual and gain weight, or the opposite may occur. Although eating more than normal, you may lose weight because your muscle tissues don't get enough glucose to generate growth and energy.

- **Blurred vision.** High levels of blood glucose pull fluid from body tissues, including the lenses of the eyes, which affects ability to focus. Vision should improve with treatment of diabetes.

- **Slow-healing sores or frequent infections.** Diabetes affects the body's ability to heal and fight infection. Bladder and vaginal infections can be a particular problem for women.

- **Nerve damage (neuropathy).** Excess blood glucose can damage the small blood vessels to your nerves, leading to symptoms such as tingling and loss of sensation in hands and feet.

- **Red, swollen, tender gums.** Diabetes increases the risk of infection in your gums and in the bones that hold your teeth in place.

Detecting Diabetes

To identify individuals with this disease as early as possible, the American Diabetes Association now recommends screening every three years for all men and women beginning at age 45. The American College of Endocrinology recommends screening at age 30 for individuals at risk, including those who are overweight, sedentary, have a family history of diabetes, or have high blood pressure or heart disease.

Tests that can detect diabetes include:

- **Random blood sugar test.** Because you don't necessarily fast for this test, your blood glucose may be high because you've just eaten. Even so, it shouldn't be higher than 200 mg/dL.

- **Fasting blood glucose test.** In general, glucose is lowest after an overnight fast. That's why the preferred way to test your blood sugar is after you've fasted overnight or for at least eight hours.

- **Glucose challenge test.** Often used to screen pregnant women for gestational diabetes, this test measures glucose before drinking eight ounces of an extremely sweet liquid after fasting for six hours, then every hour for a three-hour period. If your blood sugar rises more than expected and doesn't return to normal by the third hour, you likely have diabetes.

Diabetes Management

Unlike many other medical conditions, patients must take charge of their diabetes and monitor their blood glucose regularly to prevent or delay the serious complications of the disease. Diabetes educators teach patients a new set of ABCs: Manage your **A**1c (blood glucose or sugar), **B**lood pressure, and **C**holesterol:

- **A** is for the *A1c test.* This test measures the amount of glucose attached to hemoglobin molecules, the iron-rich molecules in red blood cells that deliver oxygen to the body. The higher your blood glucose levels, the more hemoglobin molecules you will have with glucose attached—and the greater the risk of damage to eyes, kidneys, and feet. In general, the life cycle of a red blood cell is 75 to 90 days, which is why the A1c test shows average blood glucose levels for the past two to three months. The American Diabetes Association recommends a goal for A1c of less than 7 percent. The American College of Endocrinology recommends a goal of 6.5 percent. (Normal A1c levels are below 6.) Individuals with diabetes should have their A1c levels checked at least twice a year.

- **B** is for *blood pressure.* As discussed on page 451, the goal for most people is 115/75. High blood pressure can cause heart attack, stroke, and kidney disease.

- **C** is for *cholesterol.* The LDL goal for most people is less than 160 mg/dL (see Table 14.2 on page 453). Bad cholesterol, or LDL, can build up and clog your blood vessels.

Treatment The goal for diabetics is to keep blood sugar levels as stable as possible to prevent complications, such as kidney damage.[9] Home glucose monitoring, including new continuous glucose monitors, allows diabetics to check their blood sugar levels as many times a day as necessary and to adjust their diet or insulin doses as appropriate.

Types of insulin differ in how long it takes to start working after injection (onset), when it works hardest (peak), and how long it lasts in the body (duration). Individuals with diabetes may use different types in various combinations, depending on time of day and timing of meals. New insulin inhalers offer an alternative to injections for those with type 2 diabetes.

Those with type 1 diabetes require daily doses of insulin via injections, an insulin infusion pump, or oral medication. Those with type 2 diabetes often can control their disease through a well-balanced diet, exercise, and weight management. However, insulin therapy may be needed to keep blood glucose levels near normal or normal, thereby reducing the risk of damage to the eyes, nerves, and kidneys. New medications help control weight and lower blood pressure and cholesterol.

Medical advances hold out bright hopes for diabetics. Laser surgery, for instance, is saving eyesight. Bypass operations are helping restore blood flow to the heart and feet. Dialysis machines and kidney and pancreas transplants save many lives.

Can Diabetes Be Cured?

In most cases, diabetes requires lifelong management and treatment. However, a cure for some patients no longer seems impossible.[10] About 400 to 500 pancreas transplants are performed in the United States every year; when successful they normalize glucose levels, thereby curing diabetes. However, only about half of these transplants continue to function for ten years.

Gastric bypass surgery (which limits the amount of food a person can ingest) for extremely obese individuals has led to lasting remission of diabetes, sometimes even before a patient loses weight. (See Chapter 6.) Scientists do not yet know how bypass surgery "cures" diabetes, but it may affect chemicals involved in insulin resistance. Some surgeons are advocating this approach for all diabetics with body mass indexes (BMIs) over 50; others, as an option for those with BMIs over 35.[11]

Among other promising approaches are the use of stem cells to "rejuvenate" the pancreas, antibodies to block the autoimmune response of type 1 diabetes, and a more sophisticated artificial pancreas to monitor and manage glucose levels.[12]

An insulin pump delivers insulin to the body 24 hours a day through a thin plastic tube inserted just under the skin, usually on the abdomen.

Hypertension

Blood pressure refers to the force of blood against the walls of arteries. When blood pressure remains elevated over time—a condition called hypertension—it forces the heart to pump harder than is healthy. Because the heart must force blood into arteries that are offering increased resistance to blood flow, the left side of the heart becomes enlarged. If untreated, high blood pressure can cause a variety of cardiovascular complications, including heart attack and stroke—two of the three leading causes of death among U.S. adults—as well as kidney failure and blindness (Figure 14.3).

In a young person even mild hypertension can cause organs such as the heart, brain, and kidneys to start to deteriorate. By age 50 or 60, the damage may be irreversible.

Who Is at Risk?

The World Health Organization estimates that hypertension causes one in every eight deaths globally, making it the third leading killer in the world. In the United States, high blood pressure is responsible for about a third of cardiovascular problems like heart

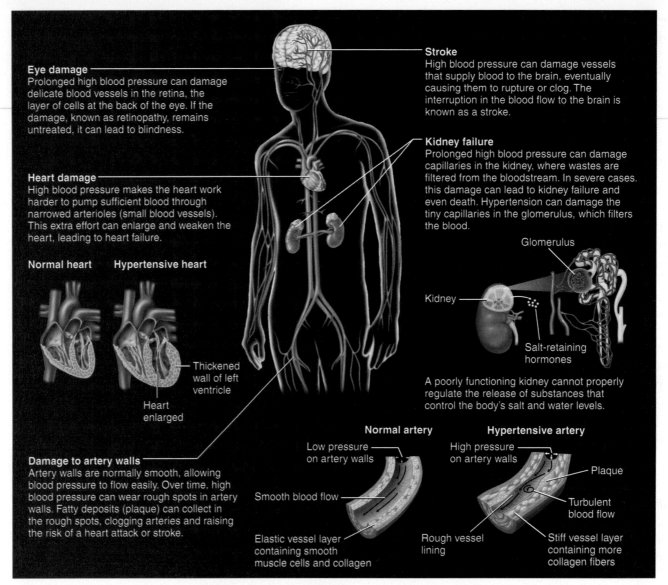

Eye damage
Prolonged high blood pressure can damage delicate blood vessels in the retina, the layer of cells at the back of the eye. If the damage, known as retinopathy, remains untreated, it can lead to blindness.

Stroke
High blood pressure can damage vessels that supply blood to the brain, eventually causing them to rupture or clog. The interruption in the blood flow to the brain is known as a stroke.

Kidney failure
Prolonged high blood pressure can damage capillaries in the kidney, where wastes are filtered from the bloodstream. In severe cases, this damage can lead to kidney failure and even death. Hypertension can damage the tiny capillaries in the glomerulus, which filters the blood.

Heart damage
High blood pressure makes the heart work harder to pump sufficient blood through narrowed arterioles (small blood vessels). This extra effort can enlarge and weaken the heart, leading to heart failure.

Glomerulus

Kidney

Salt-retaining hormones

Normal heart   **Hypertensive heart**

A poorly functioning kidney cannot properly regulate the release of substances that control the body's salt and water levels.

Thickened wall of left ventricle

Heart enlarged

Normal artery   **Hypertensive artery**

Low pressure on artery walls

High pressure on artery walls

Plaque

Damage to artery walls
Artery walls are normally smooth, allowing blood pressure to flow easily. Over time, high blood pressure can wear rough spots in artery walls. Fatty deposits (plaque) can collect in the rough spots, clogging arteries and raising the risk of a heart attack or stroke.

Smooth blood flow

Turbulent blood flow

Elastic vessel layer containing smooth muscle cells and collagen

Rough vessel lining

Stiff vessel layer containing more collagen fibers

Figure 14.3 Consequences of High Blood Pressure
If left untreated, elevated blood pressure can damage blood vessels in several areas of the body and lead to serious health problems.

attack or stroke and a quarter of all premature deaths.

 About a third of adults age 18 and older in the United States—some 65 million men and women—have high blood pressure. Blood pressure has increased among children and adolescents as well as adults, with the highest rates among black and Mexican American children. The primary culprit is the increase in obesity in the young. No one knows why African Americans are more vulnerable, although some speculate that overweight or dietary factors may contribute.

Different races also suffer different consequences of high blood pressure. An African American with the same elevated blood pressure reading as a Caucasian faces a greater risk of stroke, heart disease, and kidney problems.

Family history also plays a role. "If you study healthy college students with normal blood pressures, those who have one parent with hypertension will have blood pressure that's a little higher than average," notes Rose Marie Robertson, M.D., of the American Heart Association. "If two parents have high blood pressure, their levels will be a little higher, and they're destined to go higher still. If your parents have high blood pressure, have yours checked regularly."[13]

Men and women are equally likely to develop hypertension, but in women blood pressure tends to rise around the time of menopause. Half of all women over age 45 have hypertension.

> ## TABLE 14.1

What Your Blood Pressure Reading Means

Normal Results

In adults, the systolic pressure should be less than 120 mmHg and the diastolic pressure should be less than 80 mmHg.

What Abnormal Results Mean

Prehypertension
Top number is consistently 120 to 139 or the bottom number reads 80 to 89.

Stage 1: Mild hypertension
Top number is consistently 140 to 159 or the bottom number reads 90 to 99.

Stage 2: Moderate-to-severe hypertension
Top number is consistently 160 or over or the bottom number reads 100 or over.

Low blood pressure (hypotension)
Top number reading lower than 90 or pressure 25 mHg lower than usual.

Blood pressure readings may be affected by many different conditions, including cardiovascular disorders, neurological conditions, kidney and urological disorders, psychological factors such as stress, anger, or fear, various medications and "white coat hypertension," which may occur if the medical visit itself produces extreme anxiety.

Source: National Institute of Medicine National Institutes of Health.

© iStockphoto.com/Simone van den Berg

For individuals who smoke, are overweight, don't exercise, or have high cholesterol levels, hypertension multiplies the risk of heart disease and stroke. Overweight people with high blood pressure have twice the risk of dying of a heart attack or stroke as those with normal blood pressure. At ultrahigh risk are people with diabetes or kidney disease.

What Is a Healthy Blood Pressure?

Current guidelines (Table 14.1) categorize a reading of 120-139/80-89 as **prehypertension,** a condition that is likely to worsen in time. A healthy reading is 115/75 mm Hg. Once blood pressure rises above this threshold, the risk of cardiovascular disease may increase.

 In healthy adults, blood pressure screening should begin at age 21, with repeat evaluations at least every two years, or more often depending on your current health, medical history, and risk factors for cardiovascular disease. According to the National College Health Assessment survey, about nine in ten students have done so. (See Reality Check, p. 443.)

To get an accurate blood pressure reading, you should visit the doctor's office at least twice and have your blood pressure taken two or more times while you're seated. The average of those measurements determines how your blood pressure is classified.

The current guidelines classify hypertension into two categories:

- **Stage 1.** This consists of a systolic pressure ranging from 140 to 159 or a diastolic pressure ranging from 90 to 99.
- **Stage 2.** The most severe form of hypertension occurs with a systolic pressure of 160 or higher or a diastolic reading of 100 or higher.

Only one of the numbers—the top or bottom—needs to be high to meet these criteria. In people over age 50, systolic pressure is more important than diastolic. If it rises to 140 mm Hg or higher, doctors advise treatment regardless of the diastolic pressure.

Lowering High Blood Pressure

Lifestyle changes are a first-line weapon in the fight against high blood pressure. Rather than making a single change, a combination of behavioral changes, including losing weight, eating heart-healthy foods, reducing sodium, and exercising more, yields the best results.

High intake of folate, a B vitamin, can significantly reduce the risk of hypertension. In a study of women under age 35, those who consumed the most folate had one-third the risk of developing high blood pressure as those consuming very little. Among the approaches that have not proved effective are dietary supplements, such as calcium, magnesium, potassium, and fish oil.

The National Heart, Lung and Blood Institute has developed what is known as the

prehypertension A condition of slightly elevated blood pressure, which is likely to worsen in time.

- **Get moving.** Regular exercise can lower blood pressure by 10 points, prevent the onset of high blood pressure, or let you reduce your dosage of blood pressure medications.
- **Eat your way** to better blood pressure. Choose more fruits, vegetables, low-fat dairy products, whole grains, poultry, fish, and nuts. Cut down on red meat, sweets, sugar-containing beverages, and saturated fat and cholesterol.
- **Lose ten.** Shedding 10 percent of your current weight—or even 10 pounds—can make a big difference.
- **Don't smoke.** A single cigarette can cause a 20-point spike in systolic blood pressure. Don't light up. See Chapter 13 for tips on quitting.
- **Hold the salt.** If you're salt sensitive, you may be spiking your blood pressure as you spice your food.
- **Stick with your medications.** If your doctor has prescribed medication to lower your blood pressure, take it conscientiously. Your future health may depend on it.

DASH diet. Following DASH, which stands for Dietary Approaches to Stop Hypertension, has proved as effective as drug therapy in lowering blood pressure. An additional benefit: The DASH diet also lowers harmful blood fats, including cholesterol and low-density lipoprotein, and the amino acid homocysteine (one of the new suspects in heart disease risk).

Too much sodium and too little potassium boost blood pressure in people who are sensitive to salt. The American Medical Association is calling for food makers and restaurants to cut the sodium content of food by 50 percent by 2016. For a healthful diet, aim for less than 1.5 grams of sodium a day, and at least 4.7 grams of potassium. The lower the amount of sodium in the diet, the lower the blood pressure for both those with and those without hypertension and for both genders and all racial and ethnic groups. However, reducing dietary sodium has an even greater effect on blood pressure in blacks than whites, and in women than men.

Medications   Making healthy lifestyle modifications can help reduce Stage 1 hypertension, but most people also require a medication. Drugs for lowering blood pressure come in a range of regimens (once a day to several times a day) with a range of effects on other conditions, interactions with other drugs, and potential side effects. Some of the medicines used to treat high blood pressure are:

- Alpha blockers.
- Angiotensin-converting enzyme (ACE) inhibitors.
- Angiotension receptor blockers (ARBs).
- Beta-blockers.
- Calcium channel blockers.
- Central alpha agonists.
- Diuretics.
- Renin inhibitors, including aliskiren (Tekturna).
- Vasodilators.

If your blood pressure is very high, you may need additional medications. Those with Stage 2 hypertension typically need at least two types of high blood pressure medications (antihypertensives) to reduce blood pressure to a safer level. The goal for most people with hypertension is to reduce blood pressure to below 140/90 mm Hg.

About 20 to 30 percent of people with high blood pressure have "resistant hypertension," which means that their blood pressure remains elevated despite taking three medications to lower it. In addition to medical conditions and certain medications, lifestyle factors, including excess weight, salt intake, and alcohol consumption, can contribute to this problem. New guidelines from the American Heart Association recommend weight loss, reduced salt, and decreased alcohol.[14]

Only about one-third of people with hypertension have it effectively controlled—below 140/90 mm Hg. Reducing systolic blood pressure 12 mm Hg for 10 years can prevent 1 death in every 11 people treated for hypertension. In those with existing cardiovascular disease or organ damage, such as kidney disease, that reduction has an even bigger benefit, preventing 1 death in every 9 people treated.

Your Lipoprotein Profile

Medical science has changed the way it views and targets the blood fats that endanger the healthy heart. In the past, the focus was primarily on total cholesterol in the blood. The higher this number was, the greater the risk of heart disease. The NHLBI's National Cholesterol Education Program has recommended more comprehensive testing, called a *lipoprotein* profile, for all individuals age 20 or older.

This blood test, which should be performed after a 9- to 12-hour fast and repeated at least once every five years, provides readings of:

- **Total cholesterol.**
- **LDL (bad) cholesterol**, the main culprit in the buildup of plaque within the arteries.

- **HDL (good or _healthy_) cholesterol,** which helps prevent cholesterol buildup.
- **Triglycerides,** the blood fats released into the bloodstream after a meal.

What Is a Healthy Cholesterol Reading?

Total cholesterol is the sum of all the cholesterol in your blood. Less than 200 mg/dL total cholesterol is ideal, and 200–239 mg/dL is borderline-high. Total cholesterol above 240 mg/dL is high and doubles your risk of heart disease. However, total cholesterol is not the only crucial number you should know. Because LDL increases your risk for heart disease, you always should find out your LDL level. Even if your total cholesterol is higher than 200, you may not be at high risk for a heart attack. Some people—such as women before menopause and young, active men who have no other risk factors—may have high HDL cholesterol and desirable LDL levels. Ask your doctor to interpret your results so you both know your numbers and understand what they mean. (See Table 14.2.)

HDL, good cholesterol, also is important, particularly in women. Federal guidelines define an HDL reading of less than 40 mg/dL as a major risk factor for developing heart disease. HDL levels of 60 mg/dL or more are protective and lower the risk of heart disease.

Triglycerides, the free-floating molecules that transport fats in the bloodstream, ideally should be below 150 mg/dL. Individuals with readings of 150 to 199 mg/dL, considered borderline, as well as those with higher readings, may benefit from weight control, physical activity, and, if necessary, medication.

Lowering Cholesterol

According to federal guidelines, about one in five Americans may require treatment to lower his or her cholesterol level. However, nearly half of people who need cholesterol treatment, which can reduce the risk of heart disease by 30 percent over five years, don't get it. The National Cholesterol Education Program (NCEP) estimates that some 36 million Americans should be watching their diet and exercising more. Another 65 million should be taking cholesterol-lowering

TABLE 14.2

Interpreting Your Lipoprotein Profile

Total Cholesterol Level	Category
Less than 200 mg/dL	Desirable level that puts you at lower risk for coronary heart disease. A cholesterol level of 200 mg/dL or higher raises your risk.
200 to 239 mg/dL	Borderline high
240 mg/dL and above	High blood cholesterol. A person with this level has more than twice the risk of coronary heart disease as someone whose cholesterol is below 200 mg/dL.

HDL Cholesterol Level	Category
Less than 40 mg/dL (for men)	
Less than 50 mg/dL (for women)	Low HDL cholesterol. A major risk factor for heart disease.
60 mg/dL and above	High HDL cholesterol. An HDL of 60 mg/dL and above is considered protective against heart disease.

LDL Cholesterol Level	Category
Less than 100 mg/dL	Optimal
100 to 129 mg/dL	Near or above optimal
130 to 159 mg/dL	Borderline high
160 to 189 mg/dL	High
190 mg/dL and above	Very high

Your LDL cholesterol goal depends on how many other risk factors you have.

- If you don't have coronary heart disease or diabetes and have one or no risk factors, your LDL goal is less than 160 mg/dL.
- If you don't have coronary heart disease or diabetes and have two or more risk factors, your LDL goal is less than 130 mg/dL.
- If you do have coronary heart disease or diabetes, your LDL goal is less than 100 mg/dL.

Triglyceride Level	Category
Less than 150 mg/d	Normal
150–199 mg/dL	Borderline high
200–499 mg/dL	High
500 mg/dL or above	Very high

Source: National Cholesterol Education Program (NCEP) and American Heart Association. Adapted from http://www.americanheart.org/presenter.jhtml?identifier54500.

drugs. Depending on your lipoprotein profile and an assessment of other risk factors, your physician may recommend that you take steps to lower your LDL cholesterol.

Lifestyle Changes Some individuals with elevated cholesterol can improve their lipoprotein profile with lifestyle changes:

- **Dietary changes.** In the past, dietary changes produced relatively modest improvements compared to the effects of medications, which can cut cholesterol by as much as 35 percent. However, a diet consisting of cholesterol-lowering foods, including nuts, soy, oats, and plant sterols (in margarine

- Go to your primary health-care provider to get a lipoprotein profile. Although cholesterol tests at shopping malls or health fairs can help identify people at risk, the analyzers are often not certified technicians, and the readings may be inaccurate.

- Ask about accuracy. Find out if the lab is using the National Institutes of Health standards, and ask about the lab's margin for error (which should be less than 5 percent).

- Fast beforehand. Cholesterol tests are most accurate after a 9- to 14-hour fast. Women may not want to get tested at the end of their menstrual cycles, when minor elevations in cholesterol levels occur because of lower estrogen levels. Cholesterol levels can also rise 5 to 10 percent during periods of stress. Reschedule the test if you come down with an intestinal flu because the viral infection could interfere with the absorption of food and thus with cholesterol levels. Let your doctor know if you're taking any drugs. Common medications, including birth control pills and hypertension drugs, can affect cholesterol levels.

- Sit down before allowing blood to be drawn or your finger to be pricked. Don't let a technician squeeze blood from your finger, which forces fluid from cells, diluting the blood sample and possibly leading to a falsely low reading.

and green leafy vegetables), reduced LDL cholesterol by about 30 percent. An added benefit: a reduction in C-reactive protein, discussed later in this chapter. Researchers are recommending this diet as an effective first treatment for individuals with high cholesterol levels, particularly when coupled with exercise and weight loss.

- **Weight management.** For individuals who are overweight, losing weight can help lower LDL. This is especially true for those with high triglyceride levels and/or low HDL levels and those who have a large waist measurement (more than 40 inches for a man and more than 35 inches for a woman).

- **Physical activity.** Regular activity can help lower LDL, lower blood pressure, reduce triglycerides, and particularly important, raise HDL. Again, these benefits are especially important for those with high triglyceride levels or large waist measurements.

Lifestyle changes can lower harmful LDL levels by 5 to 10 percent. However, a greater reduction of 30 to 40 percent requires either intensive lifestyle changes, including an extremely low-fat diet, or the addition of cholesterol-lowering medication.

Medications The last decade has seen a revolution in treatment for high cholesterol, thanks to a new class of drugs called statins—better known by brand names such as Lipitor, Mevacor, Pravachol, and Zocor. These medications can cut the risk of dying of a heart attack by as much as 40 percent. Initially tested in men, statins have proved equally beneficial for women, including those whose cholesterol levels rise after menopause.

Statins also protect patients who have not had a heart attack but are at high risk for developing cardiovascular disease because of high cholesterol or other risk factors. Large-scale studies indicate that statins protect against heart attacks and strokes even in older adults without known cardiovascular disease or diabetes and with low cholesterol—if these patients also have high levels of CRP or C-reactive protein (discussed on p. 457).[15]

Statins work in the liver to block production of cholesterol. When the liver can't make cholesterol, it draws LDL cholesterol from the blood to use as raw material. This means that less LDL is available to trigger or promote the artery-clogging process known as atherosclerosis. Statins also appear to stabilize cholesterol-filled deposits in artery walls and to cool down inflammation. Long-term therapy with statins reduces the risk for death, heart attack, and stroke among people with heart disease, even when LDL levels are not elevated. The lower the LDL, the lower the risk.

Cardiovascular (Heart) Disease

In the United States, death rates from cardiovascular disease have dropped by 60 percent since 1950, one of the major U.S. health achievements of the twentieth century. The medical advances described in this chapter have contributed to this decline, but much of the credit goes to lifestyle changes, such as quitting smoking and making dietary changes that lower blood pressure and cholesterol levels.

Yet we still have a long way to go to keep the hearts of all Americans healthy. Nearly 2,600 Americans die of heart disease every day—that's one every 34 seconds. More than 64 million Americans have heart disease. Each year an estimated 1 million Americans suffer a heart attack; nearly half of them die.

How the Heart Works

The heart is a hollow, muscular organ with four chambers that serve as two pumps (see Figure 14.4). It is about the size of a clenched fist. Each pump consists of a pair of chambers formed of muscles. The upper two—each called an **atrium**—receive blood, which then flows through valves into the lower two chambers, the **ventricles,** which contract to pump blood out into the arteries through a second set of valves. A thick wall divides the right side of the heart from the left side; even though the two sides are separated, they contract at almost the same time. Contraction of the ventricles is called **systole;** the period of relaxation between contractions is called **diastole.** The heart valves, located at the entrance and exit of the ventricular chambers, have flaps that open and close to allow blood to flow through the chambers of the heart.

The *myocardium* (heart muscle) consists of branching fibers that enable the heart to contract, or beat, between 60 and 80 times per minute, or about 100,000 times a day. With each beat, the heart pumps about 2 ounces of blood. This may not sound like much, but it adds up to nearly 5 quarts of blood pumped by the heart in one minute, or about 75 gallons per hour.

The heart is surrounded by the *pericardium*, which consists of two layers of a tough membrane. The space between the two contains a lubricating fluid that allows the heart muscle to move freely. The *endocardium* is a smooth membrane lining the inside of the heart and its valves.

Blood circulates through the body by means of the pumping action of the heart, as shown in Figure 14.5. The right ventricle (on your own right side) pumps blood, via the *pulmonary arteries*, to the lungs, where it picks up oxygen (a gas essential to the body's cells) and gives off carbon dioxide (a waste product of metabolism). The blood returns from the lungs via the *pulmonary veins* to the left side of the heart, which pumps it, via the **aorta**, to the arteries in the rest of the body.

The arteries divide into smaller and smaller branches and finally into **capillaries**, the smallest blood vessels of all (only slightly larger in diameter than a single red blood cell). The blood within the capillaries supplies oxygen and nutrients to the cells of the tissues and takes up various waste products. Blood returns to the heart via the veins: The blood from the upper body (except the lungs) drains into the heart through the *superior vena cava*, while blood from the lower body returns via the *inferior vena cava*.

(a)

(b)

Figure 14.4 The Healthy Heart

(a) The heart muscle is nourished by blood from the coronary arteries, which arise from the aorta. (b) The cross section shows the four chambers and the myocardium, the muscle that does the heart's work. The pericardium is the outer covering of the heart.

The workings of this remarkable pump affect your entire body. If the flow of blood to or through the heart or to the rest of the body is reduced, or if a disturbance occurs in the small bundle of highly specialized cells in the heart that generate electrical impulses to control heartbeats, the result may at first be too subtle to notice. However, without diagnosis and treatment, these changes could develop into a life-threatening problem.

Perhaps the biggest breakthrough in the field of cardiology has been not a test or a treatment but a realization: Heart disease

atrium (plural **atria**) Either of the two upper chambers of the heart, which receive blood from the veins.

ventricle Either of the two lower chambers of the heart, which pump blood out of the heart and into the arteries.

systole The contraction phase of the cardiac cycle.

diastole The period between contractions in the cardiac cycle, during which the heart relaxes and dilates as it fills with blood.

aorta The main artery of the body, arising from the left ventricle of the heart.

capillary A minute blood vessel that connects an artery to a vein.

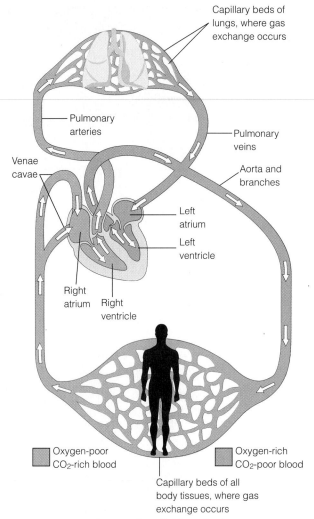

Capillary beds of lungs, where gas exchange occurs

Pulmonary arteries

Pulmonary veins

Venae cavae

Aorta and branches

Left atrium

Left ventricle

Right atrium

Right ventricle

☐ Oxygen-poor CO₂-rich blood

☐ Oxygen-rich CO₂-poor blood

Capillary beds of all body tissues, where gas exchange occurs

Figure 14.5 The Path of Blood Flow

Blood is pumped from the right ventricle into the pulmonary arteries, which lead to the lungs, where gas exchange (oxygen for carbon dioxide) occurs. Oxygenated blood returning from the lungs drains into the left atrium and is then pumped into the left ventricle, which sends the blood into the aorta and its branches. The oxygenated blood flows through the arteries, which extend to all parts of the body. Again, gas exchange occurs in the body tissues; this time oxygen is "dropped of" and carbon dioxide "picked up."

is not inevitable. We can keep our hearts healthy for as long as we live, but the process of doing so must start early and continue throughout life.

Heart Risks on Campus

 Many people, including college students and other young adults, are unaware of habits and conditions that put their hearts at risk. Many undergraduates view heart disease as mainly a problem for white men and underestimate the risks for women and ethnic groups. Students rate their own knowledge of heart disease as lower than that of sexually transmitted infections and psychological disorders. Yet heart disease is the third-leading cause of death among adults age 25 to 44. Diabetes, family history, and other risk factors increase their likelihood of heart disease.

Young athletes face special risks. Each year seemingly healthy teens or young adults die suddenly on playing fields and courts. The culprit in one of every three cases of sudden cardiac death in young athletes is a silent condition called hypertrophic cardiomyopathy (HCM), an excessive thickness of the heart muscle. Because of HCM, the heart is more prone to dangerous heart irregularities.

Hearts and Minds: Psychological Risk Factors

How you respond to everyday sources of stress can affect your heart as well as your overall health. While you may not be able to control the sources of stress, you can change how you habitually respond to it.

Researchers classify psychological risk factors for heart disease into three categories: chronic, episodic, and acute. Chronic factors, such as job strain or lack of social support, play an important role in the buildup of artery-clogging plaque and may increase blood pressure. Even feeling that life has treated you unfairly boosts a person's chance of having a heart attack.

Episodic factors, such as depression, can last from several weeks to two years and may lead to the creation of "unstable" plaque, which is more likely to break off and block a blood vessel within the heart. Short-term or acute psychological risk factors, such as an angry outburst, can directly trigger a heart attack in people with underlying heart disease.

These factors may act alone or combine and exert different effects at different ages and stages of life. They may influence behaviors such as smoking, diet, alcohol consumption, and physical activity, as well as directly cause changes in physiology.

Depression Depression and heart disease often occur together. People with heart disease are more likely to be depressed, and some seemingly healthy people with depression are at greater risk of heart problems. Depressed women younger than age 60 are more likely to suffer a heart attack than those who do not suffer from depression. After a heart attack, depression is common in both men and women, but physicians are less likely to recognize and treat depression in women.

Patients who suffer heart attacks and develop clinical depression have higher rates of complications and an increased risk of dying from another heart attack or other heart problems. People who are physically healthy with no risk factors for heart disease but who are prone to anger, hostility, and mild depression have higher levels of C-reactive protein, a substance linked to increased risk of heart disease.

Anger and Hostility

Anger and hostility have both short- and long-term consequences for the heart, particularly for men. In general the angriest men are three times more likely to develop heart disease than the most placid ones. Hostility more than doubles the risk of recurrent heart attacks in men (but not women). Research has linked hostility to increased cardiac risk factors, to decreased survival in men with coronary artery disease below the age of 61, to an increased risk of heart attack in men with metabolic syndrome, and to an increased risk of abnormal heart rhythms. Adults whose spouses rate them high in "antagonism"—a tendency to be argumentative, competitive, or cold—are more likely to have calcium buildup in their heart arteries.

Angry young men may be putting their future heart health in jeopardy. In a study that tracked more than 1,000 physicians for 36 years and took into account other physical and psychological risk factors, the angriest young men were six times more likely to suffer heart attacks by 55 and three times more likely to develop any form of cardiovascular disease. (See "Taming a Toxic Temper" in Making Change Happen, p. 458, and in *Labs for IPC.*)

How does hostility harm the heart? Anger triggers a surge in stress hormones that can provoke abnormal and potentially lethal heart rhythms and activates platelets, the tiny blood cells that trigger blood clotting. High levels of anger can also trigger a

Hostility in men of any age can increase their risk of heart attacks and heart disease later in life.

spasm in a coronary artery, which results in the additional narrowing of a partially blocked blood vessel.

In women, anger and hostility do not always lead to heart troubles. However, women who outwardly express anger may be at increased risk if they also have other risk factors for heart disease, such as diabetes or unhealthy levels of lipoproteins.

Personality Types

In addition to stress, anger, and depression, other psychological traits can increase the risk of heart disease. Based on more than a decade of research, Dutch scientists have identified a "Type D" (for distressed) personality type. Type D people tend to be anxious, self-conscious, irritable, insecure, negative, and go to great lengths not to say or do anything that others might not like. In the Dutch study, almost four times as many Type D individuals as others in cardiac rehabilitation programs died within an eight-year period.

In the past, other personality types have been linked to disease, for example, hard-charging, hostile Type As to heart disease and conflict-avoiding, emotion-suppressing Type Cs to cancer. However, these traits have not proved to be significant risk factors for these illnesses.

Other Risk Factors

Inflammation and C-Reactive Protein

Inflammation—the process by which the body responds to fever, injury, or infection—plays an essential role in healing and recovering from infection. However, chronic low-grade inflammation may contribute to atherosclerosis and set the stage for heart

Taming a Toxic Temper

Are you a hothead? Do you lose it, blow up, explode, go ballistic, have a fit? The terms we use for getting angry reveal its dangers. Anger is a bomb, and if you have a short fuse, you and everyone around you are in harm's way. In the long run, chronic rage puts your life at risk—especially if you're an angry young male. In a study that tracked more than 1,000 physicians for 36 years, the angriest young men were six times more likely to suffer heart attacks by 55 and three times more likely to develop any form of cardiovascular disease. Anger and hostility also threaten the hearts of women with other cardiac risk factors.

"Taming a Toxic Temper" in *Labs for IPC* shows you how to recognize the earliest signs of anger and analyze the situations that trigger your anger—so you can handle them, change the ways in which you respond, and keep in mind the consequences of an angry outburst. It is important that you, not your temper, be in control of your life. Here's a preview.

Get Real
In this stage you test your temper by answering 14 questions, including the following:
- Do people describe you as hotheaded?
- Do you get so annoyed when someone tries to get ahead of you in a line that you confront the person?
- Do you get so angry you forget what you're thinking?
- Did you ever become so angry with someone that you felt as if you would explode?

After reviewing your answers, you rate your temper on a scale of 1 (tranquil) to 10 (red-hot). You also review your anger history by describing the five worst rage explosions of your life and listing all of the negative consequences of your anger and outbursts.

Get Ready
Preparation primarily involves setting aside time to practice anger-reduction exercises you learn and writing journal entries.

Get Going
Taming your temper is a six-step process. You learn one step each week, and each week add a new one. Here's a sampling of the first one:

WEEK 1. Tune into your cues. To control your anger, you must be mindful and sensitive to subtle cues that you are becoming angry *as early as possible.* What is the earliest sign of anger you experience in your body . . . ?
- Do you clench your fists?
- Do you tighten your jaw?
- Do you feel heat?

Whenever you feel the first sensation, look for something subtle that comes before it—a thought, perhaps, or a perception of something about another person that does not set right with you. The earlier you sense that something is beginning to make you angry, the greater the opportunity . . .
The other five steps are:
- **Identify your triggers.**
- **Talk yourself down.**
- **Rely on anger-reducers.**
- **Develop better coping tools.**
- **Take it to the street.**

Lock It In
You continue to monitor your anger levels, triggers, and cues daily and continue to rehearse in real life, by deliberately putting yourself in circumstances that used to set off angry outbursts. Let someone take the last bagel even though you were obviously reaching for it. Stand next to the student talking loudly on her cell phone. . . .

attacks, strokes, and other forms of cardiovascular disease. The most common triggers of inflammation are smoking, lack of exercise, high-fat and high-calorie meals, and highly processed foods.

C-reactive protein (CRP), produced in the liver, rises whenever the body responds to inflammation. As scientists recognized the role of inflammation in heart disease, they developed the high-sensitivity CRP test (hsCRP), which detects coronary artery inflammation by measuring small changes in CRP. Several investigations have shown that CRP can predict heart disease before

any other risk factors become evident, particularly in women. Individuals with the highest CRP levels are two to seven times more likely to develop heart disease than those with the lowest levels (see Table 14-3). High concentrations of CRP also may predict greater risk of sudden death. The test seems most useful in combination with a lipoprotein profile and assessments of other blood components.

CRP also may indicate a higher risk for cancer. Individuals with high CRP levels are thus at high risk not only for heart disease but also for cancer. Cancer patients with the highest CRP levels are more likely to die early than are others.[16]

Various strategies can reduce CRP levels. These include lifestyle changes (healthful diet, exercise, weight control, and not smoking) and medications (aspirin and, as needed, drugs to lower cholesterol and blood pressure).

Homocysteine

High levels of *homocysteine*—an amino acid in the blood—have been linked to a greater risk of heart disease and stroke. Homocysteine may have an effect on atherosclerosis by damaging the inner lining of arteries and promoting blood clots. Several clinical trials are under way to test whether lowering homocysteine will reduce the risk of heart disease.

Illegal Drugs

Illegal drugs pose many dangers—one of the most serious is their potentially deadly impact on the cardiovascular system. Ecstasy, amphetamines, and cocaine can cause a sudden rise in blood pressure, heart rate, and contractions of the left ventricle (the pumping chamber) of the heart, which can increase the risk of a heart attack.

The hallucinogens lysergic acid diethylamide (LSD) and psilocybin (psychoactive mushrooms) also have the potential for triggering irregular heartbeats and heart attacks, although less serious cardiac complications, such as a temporary rise in blood pressure, are more common. Morphine and heroin, which account for almost half of drug-related deaths, can lower blood pressure and affect the heart rate. Inhalants can produce fatal heartbeat irregularities. Marijuana, the most widely used illegal drug among young adults, can affect blood pressure and heart rate, but it is not known whether it can trigger a heart attack.

Bacterial Infection

Certain bacteria may indeed put the heart at risk. *Streptococcus sanguis,* the bacterium found in dental plaque, has been implicated in the buildup of atherosclerotic plaque. Individuals with periodontal disease are at increased risk of heart disease and stroke. Regular brushing, flossing, and dental visits can reduce this danger.

Another common bacterium, *Chlamydia pneumoniae,* long linked to respiratory infections, also may threaten the heart. Individuals with high levels of antibodies to this bacteria are more likely to suffer a heart-related problem. Researchers have reported that antibiotics, taken to treat common infections, may protect against first-time heart attacks. A national clinical trial to determine whether antibiotics can reduce the risk of heart attack and stroke is under way.

The Heart of a Woman

Many people still think of heart disease as a "guy problem." Men do have a higher incidence of cardiovascular problems than women before age 45. Although women develop heart problems later in life, by about age 65, their risk is about the same as men's. Heart disease, which now kills one in four women in the United States, is the largest single cause of death of women worldwide. American women are four to six times more likely to die of heart disease than of breast cancer.

According to the American Heart Association, all women with at least one major cardiometabolic risk factor are at risk for heart disease. Nine in ten women may meet this standard. Many women don't get a proper diagnosis because they have a form of heart disease that doesn't show up on the usual diagnostic tests. In women with *vascular dysfunction,* the blood vessels—both the large coronary arteries and the small microvessels—supplying the heart do not expand properly to accommodate increased blood flow. Standard diagnostic procedures, including stress tests and coronary angiograms, do not reveal this condition. However, newer tests, including ultrasound of the blood vessels, can reveal heart problems that angiograms fail to pick up.

Because research has long focused on men, it also is not clear if women benefit equally from standard therapies. Aspirin, for instance, lowers the risk of heart attack in men of all ages, but not in women under age 65 (although it does reduce their stroke risk). In women over 65, however, aspirin reduces both strokes and heart attacks.

> ### TABLE 14.3
>
> **C-Reactive Protein (CRP) Levels and Cardiovascular Risk**
>
> | CRP (milligrams per Liter) | Level of Cardiovascular Risk |
> | --- | --- |
> | Less than 0.5 mg/L | Lowest |
> | Less than 1q mg/L | Low |
> | 1–3 mg/L | Moderate |
> | Greater than 3 mg/L | High (risk doubles) |

- Don't smoke.
- Eat a diet rich in fruit and vegetables.
- Increase your daily servings of whole grains and bran-containing foods.
- Switch from saturated fats and/or trans fats to olive oil, which has potent anti-inflammatory properties.
- Avoid highly refined carbohydrates (white bread, white rice, French fries, sugar-laden soda, etc.), which increase levels of inflammatory messengers called cytokines. Instead, eat whole grains, which dampen cytokine production.
- Munch on walnuts, peanuts, almonds, and other nuts and seeds that ease inflammation.
- Spice up your food with herbs and spices such as turmeric, ginger, garlic, basil, pepper, and many others with anti-inflammatory properties.

Women are less likely to survive heart attacks than men, perhaps because they don't seek or receive treatment as soon as men. That's why women need to know the early signs and symptoms of female heart disease:

- Tiredness, even after getting adequate sleep.
- Trouble breathing.
- Trouble sleeping.
- Feeling sick to the stomach.
- Feeling scared or nervous.
- New or worse headaches.
- An ache in the chest.
- Feeling "heavy" or "tight" in the chest.
- A burning feeling in the chest.
- Pain in the back, between the shoulders.
- Pain or tightness in the chest that spreads to the jaw, neck, shoulders, ear, or the inside of the arms.
- Pain in the belly, above the belly button.

Researchers long believed that postmenopausal hormone therapy (HT) protected women from heart disease. However, more recent large-scale studies have shown little, if any, benefit. In fact, in older women HT increases the risk of cardiovascular problems and blood clots. However, women in their 50s who take estrogen therapy have lower levels of dangerous calcium deposits in their arteries, suggesting that supplemental estrogen for younger women with menopausal symptoms may benefit their hearts.

In light of these inconclusive and contradictory results, the AHA guidelines recommend against use of hormone therapy simply to prevent heart disease. They also recommend not using antioxidant supplements or folic acid, which have proven ineffective.

Aspirin and the Heart

Daily low-dose aspirin has been recommended as a preventive step for men at high risk of cardiovascular disease because it reduces the stickiness of platelets (cells that cause blood clotting). This lowers the risk of blood clots, which can block a blood vessel and trigger a heart attack or stroke. Several research studies have demonstrated an association between aspirin use and reductions in heart attacks in men. However, while aspirin lowers the likelihood of heart attack, it may slightly increase stroke risk.

According to new recommendations from the U.S. Preventive Services Task Force, people should consider various factors including age, gender, diabetes, blood pressure, cholesterol levels, smoking, and risk of gastrointestinal bleeding before deciding to use aspirin. The more risk factors they have, the more likely they are to benefit from aspirin.

The Task Force recommends that men between the ages of 45 and 79 should use aspirin to reduce their risk for heart attacks when the benefits outweigh the harm from potential gastrointestinal bleeding. Women between ages 55 and 70 should use aspirin to reduce their risk for ischemic stroke when the benefits outweigh the risk from gastrointestinal bleeding. The Task Force recommends against aspirin use in men under age 45 or women under age 55 because heart attacks and strokes are less likely in these age groups.[17]

Aspirin can produce side effects, including gastrointestinal bleeding, allergic reactions, and peptic ulcers. However, the very low doses recommended for heart disease prevention generally do not cause serious problems. Aspirin is not advised for people taking anticlotting medication, who have stomach ulcers, or who have kidney or liver disease. Some individuals are aspirin-resistant and do not benefit from its protective effects.

Researchers are testing a "polypill," a single pill that contains a statin, three blood pressure medications, and aspirin to see if this combination might best reduce the risk of heart attack, stroke, and other cardiovascular problems.[18]

Crises of the Heart

Coronary Artery Disease

The general term for any impairment of blood flow through the blood vessels, often referred to as "hardening of the arteries," is **arteriosclerosis.** The most common form is **atherosclerosis,** a disease of the lining of the arteries in which **plaque**—deposits of fat, fibrin (a clotting material), cholesterol, other cell parts, and calcium—narrows the artery channels. Twenty-first century research has revealed that inflammation also plays a crucial role.

Atherosclerosis This process begins when LDL cholesterol penetrates the wall of an artery. Ideally, HDL cholesterol carries the cholesterol out of the artery wall to the liver for disposal. However, if LDL accumulates, the artery responds by releasing chemical messengers called cytokines, which trigger active inflammation in the artery wall. T-lymphocytes and macrophages, specialized white blood cells that are part of the body's defensive immune system, move from the bloodstream into the artery and engulf the LDL. As they ingest the LDL, the macrophages enlarge and become foam cells, which rupture, releasing cholesterol into the artery wall, where the cycle of damage begins again. In response, the smooth muscle cells in the artery wall create a fibrous cap over the inflamed area (Figure 14.6).

These hard-capped plaques are dangerous: They narrow arteries, reduce the flow of blood, and produce angina (chest pain). However, the usual culprits in heart attacks are smaller, softer plaques that can rupture. As the body responds with clotting factors, platelets, and blood cells, a blood clot, or thrombus, forms on the disrupted plaque's surface. The clot ultimately blocks the artery and kills heart muscle cells. Similar clots can block blood flow to the brain and lead to other complications, including kidney failure and circulation problems in the legs and feet.

Unclogging the Arteries Reversing the buildup of plaque inside the arteries is possible with cholesterol-lowering drugs and a low-fat diet. A strict program of dietary and lifestyle change without any medication, developed by Dean Ornish, M.D., of the University of California, San Francisco, also has proved effective in reversing coronary artery disease. The following are the key elements of this approach:

- **A very low-fat, vegetarian diet,** including nonfat dairy products and egg whites, keeping fat intake to below 8 percent of total calories consumed. Ornish's recommended diet allows no meat, poultry, fish, butter, cheese, ice cream, or any form of oil.

arteriosclerosis Any of a number of chronic diseases characterized by degeneration of the arteries and hardening and thickening of arterial walls.

atheriosclerosis A form of arteriosclerosis in which fatty substances (plaque) are deposited on the inner walls of arteries.

plaque The sludgelike substance that builds up on the inner walls of arteries.

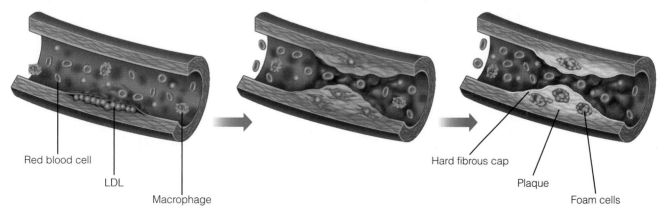

Red blood cell

LDL

Macrophage

Hard fibrous cap

Plaque

Foam cells

Figure 14.6 How Atherosclerosis Happens

LDL cholesterol penetrates an artery wall, and the accumulation of LDL cholesterol triggers an inflammation. Macrophages engulf the LDL and become foam cells. The artery wall creates a fibrous cap over this plaque, and the artery is narrowed. If the plaque ruptures, blood clots can block blood flow to the heart or to the brain.

- **Moderate exercise,** consisting of an hour of aerobic activity three times a week. Walking is recommended because more rigorous exercise might be dangerous for heart patients, who may develop increased risk of blood clots, irregular heartbeats, or coronary artery spasms during exertion.

- **Stress counseling.** Ornish's patients learn how the body's stress response can cause a rapid heartbeat and narrowing of the arteries, and how stress reduction can reduce cholesterol levels.

- **An hour a day of yoga, meditation, breathing, and progressive relaxation.** Some patients use visualization, for instance, imagining their arteries being cleared by a tunneling machine.

Angina Pectoris A temporary drop in the supply of oxygen to the heart tissue causes feelings of pain or discomfort in the chest known as **angina pectoris.** Some people suffer angina only when the demands on their hearts increase, such as during exercise or when under stress. Many people have angina for years and yet never suffer a heart attack; in some, the angina even disappears. However, angina should be considered a warning of danger if it becomes more severe or more frequent, occurs with less activity or exertion, begins to waken a person from a sound sleep at night, persists for more than ten to fifteen minutes, or causes unusual perspiration.

Heart Attack (Myocardial Infarction)

Each year, about 1.5 million Americans suffer a heart attack. About 500,000 die. Half of the deaths occur within an hour of the start of symptoms and before the person reaches the hospital. The medical name for a heart attack, or coronary, is **myocardial infarction (MI).** The *myocardium* is the cardiac muscle layer of the wall of the heart. It receives its blood supply, and thus its oxygen and other nutrients, from the coronary arteries. If an artery is blocked by a clot or plaque, or by a spasm, the myocardial cells do not get sufficient oxygen, and the portion of the myocardium deprived of its blood supply begins to die.

Although such an attack may seem sudden, usually it has been building up for years, particularly if the person has ignored risk factors and early warning signs. According to research, 80 to 90 percent of those who develop heart disease and 95 percent of those who suffer a fatal heart attack have at least one major risk factor.

Is It a Heart Attack? If they experience the following symptoms, individuals should seek immediate medical care and take an aspirin (325 milligrams) to keep the blood clot in a coronary artery from getting any bigger:

- A tight ache, heavy, squeezing pain, or discomfort in the center of the chest, which may last for 30 minutes or more and is not relieved by rest.
- Chest pain that radiates to the shoulder, arm, neck, back, or jaw.
- Anxiety.
- Sweating or cold, clammy skin.
- Nausea and vomiting.
- Shortness of breath.
- Dizziness, fainting, or loss of consciousness.

As noted on page460, women often experience heart attacks differently than men. In the month before an attack, many report unusual fatigue and disturbed sleep. Far fewer women than men experience chest pain. More common symptoms are shortness of breath, weakness and fatigue, a clammy sweat, dizziness, and nausea.

If you're with someone who's exhibiting the classic signs of heart attack, and if they last for two minutes or more, act at once. Expect the person to deny the possibility of anything as serious as a heart attack, but insist on taking prompt action.

Time is of the essence when a heart attack occurs. If you develop symptoms or if you're with someone who does, call 911 immediately. The sooner emergency personnel get to a heart attack victim and administer cardiac life support, the greater the odds of survival. Yet according to the American Heart Association, most patients wait three hours after the initial symptoms begin before seeking help. By that time, half of the affected heart muscle may already be lost.

Cardiac Arrest Cardiac arrest occurs when the heart stops beating. If circulation isn't restored within four or five minutes, the brain shuts down completely, and the person dies. **Cardiopulmonary resuscitation (CPR)** is an emergency procedure for a person whose heart has stopped or who is no longer breathing. CPR can maintain circulation and breathing until emergency medical help arrives.

The combination of mouth-to-mouth "rescue" breathing and chest compressions performed by individuals trained in CPR is the most effective method. However, according to the most recent research, chest compressions or "hands-only" CPR, which does not require extensive training, also can keep blood circulating until emergency help arrives. (For video instructions on hands-on CPR, go to: http://handsonlycpr.eisenberginc .com/)

Automated external defibrillators (AEDs), portable computerized devices, can actually restart a heart with a lethal rhythm (ventricular fibrillation) or that is not beating at all. The machines, widely available on airplanes and in public places like stadiums and terminals, also can be purchased by individuals. Written and voice instructions allow lay people as well as trained professionals to use them in case of emergency. A combination of CPR and defibrillation boosts the survival rate much higher than from CPR alone.

Saving Hearts State-of-the-art treatments for heart attacks include clot-dissolving drugs, early administration of medications to thin the blood, intravenous nitroglycerin, and in some cases, a beta-blocker (which blocks many of the effects of adrenaline in the body, particularly its stimulating impact on the heart).

Percutaneous transluminal coronary angioplasty (PTCA), also called balloon angioplasty, is the most often performed heart operation. Less costly and less risky than bypass surgery, PTCA opens blood vessels in the heart that are narrowed but not completely blocked. PTCA involves a precise, time-consuming technique called *cardiac catheterization*—the threading of a narrow tube or catheter through an artery to the heart. An X-ray taken with a special dye injected into the arteries reveals the location and extent of a blockage. By inflating a tiny balloon at the tip of the catheter, physicians can break up the clog and widen the narrowed artery. When they deflate the balloon, circulation is restored. Stents can help prevent balloon-opened arteries from clogging again.

A *coronary bypass* is a procedure in which an artery from the patient's leg or chest wall is grafted onto a coronary artery to detour blood around the blocked area. Each year hundreds of thousands of coronary bypasses are performed in the United States; about 1 to 5 percent of these patients die as a result of surgical complications. Surgery or angioplasty to improve blood flow in patients with moderate to severe levels of blood flow restriction to the heart reduces the risk of cardiac death more than drugs alone.

Stroke

 When the blood supply to a portion of the brain is blocked, a cerebrovascular accident, or **stroke,** occurs. More than a quarter of those who have strokes are under age 65. About two-thirds of the 750,000 strokes that occur every year in the United States strike women. However, before age 85, men experience more strokes. Nonetheless, women of every age fare worse than men in the prevention, diagnosis, treatment, and outcome of stroke. An estimated 20 percent of stroke victims die within three months; 50 to 60 percent are disabled. About half of those who have a stroke are partially paralyzed on one side of their body; between a quarter and a half are partially or completely dependent on others for daily living; a third become depressed; a fifth cannot walk. Quick treatment with a clot-busting drug at a hospital can reduce the chance of disability after a stroke, but few people recognize the signs of a stroke and seek medical care within three hours of the first symptoms.

angina pectoris A severe, suffocating chest pain caused by a brief lack of oxygen to the heart.

myocardial infarction (MI) A condition characterized by the dying of tissue areas in the myocardium, caused by interruption of the blood supply to those areas; the medical name for a heart attack.

cardiopulmonary resuscitation (CPR) A method of artificial stimulation of the heart and lungs; a combination of mouth-to-mouth breathing and chest compression.

Prompt treatment can stop a stroke in its tracks—but only with prompt treatment. Researchers have found that the following steps can identify facial weakness, arm weakness, and speech problems, all signs of a stroke:

- Ask the individual to smile.
- Ask him or her to raise both arms.
- Ask the person to speak a simple sentence, such as "It is sunny out today."

If he or she has trouble with any of these tasks, call 911 immediately and describe the symptoms to the dispatcher.

Strokes rank third, after heart disease and cancer, as a cause of death in this country. Worldwide, stroke is second only to heart disease as a cause of death. After decades of steady decline, the number of strokes per year has begun to rise. The main reasons seem to be that more people in the United States are living longer, advanced medical care is allowing more people to survive heart disease, and doctors are better able to diagnose and detect strokes. Yet 80 percent of strokes are preventable, and key risk factors can be modified through either lifestyle changes or drugs. The most important steps are treating hypertension, not smoking, managing diabetes, lowering cholesterol, and taking aspirin, which reduces stroke risk in women, but not men.

Drinking coffee or tea may lower the risk of a stroke. In studies that followed thousands of men and women, the more coffee the adults drank, the less likely they were to have either a stroke or a mini-stroke. In a study of more than 80,000 women who didn't smoke, those who drank four or more cups a day had a 20 percent lower stroke risk. Tea drinkers also may benefit. In one study, those who drank three cups a day had a 21 percent lower risk of stroke than those who sipped less than a cup daily. Scientists are searching for an explanation for why these beverages may benefit the brain.[19]

Risk Factors

Risk factors for stroke, like those for heart disease, include some that can't be changed (such as gender, race, and age) and some that can be controlled:

- **Gender.** Men have a greater risk of stroke than women.[20] However, women are at increased risk at times of marked hormonal changes, particularly pregnancy and childbirth. Past studies have shown an association between oral contraceptive use and stroke, particularly in women over age 35 who smoke. The newer low-dose oral contraceptives have not shown an increased stroke risk among women ages 18 to 44. Early menopause (before age 42) may double a woman's stroke risk.[21]

- **Race.** The incidence of strokes is two to three times greater in blacks than

 whites in the same communities. Hispanics also are more likely to develop hemorrhagic strokes than whites.

- **Age.** A person's risk of stroke more than doubles every decade after age 55.

- **Hypertension.** Detection and treatment of high blood pressure are the best means of stroke prevention.

- **High red blood cell count.** A moderate to marked increase in the number of a person's red blood cells increases the risk of stroke.

- **Heart disease.** Heart problems can interfere with the flow of blood to the brain; clots that form in the heart can travel to the brain, where they may clog an artery.

- **Blood fats.** Although the standard advice from cardiologists is to lower harmful LDL levels, what may be more important to lower stroke risk is an increase in the levels of protective HDL.

- **Diabetes mellitus.** Diabetics have a higher incidence of stroke than nondiabetics.

- **Estrogen therapy.** In the Women's Health Initiative—a series of clinical trials of hormone therapy for postmenopausal women—estrogen-only therapy significantly increased the risk of stroke.

- **A diet high in fat and sodium.** Individuals consuming the largest amounts of fatty foods and sodium are at much greater risk then those eating low-fat, low-salt diets.

Causes of Stroke

There are two types of stroke: *ischemic stroke,* which is the result of a blockage that disrupts blood flow to the brain, and *hemorrhagic stroke,* which occurs when blood vessels rupture. One of the most common causes of ischemic stroke is the blockage of a brain artery by a thrombus, or blood clot—a *cerebral thrombosis.* Clots generally form around deposits sticking out from the arterial wall. Sometimes a wandering blood clot (embolus), carried in the bloodstream, becomes wedged in one of the cerebral arteries. This is called a *cerebral embolism,* and it can completely plug up a cerebral artery.

In hemorrhagic stroke, a diseased artery in the brain floods the surrounding tissue with blood. The cells nourished by the artery are deprived of blood and can't function, and the blood from the artery forms a clot that may interfere with brain function. This is most likely to occur if the patient suffers from a combination of hypertension and atherosclerosis. Hemorrhage (bleeding) may also be caused by a head injury or by the bursting of an aneurysm, a blood-filled pouch that balloons out from a weak spot in the wall of an artery.

Brain tissue, like heart muscle, begins to die if deprived of oxygen, which may then cause difficulty speaking and walking, and loss of memory. These effects may be slight or severe, temporary or permanent, depending on how widespread the damage and whether other areas of the brain can take over the function of the damaged area. About 30 percent of stroke survivors develop dementia, a disorder that robs a person of memory and other intellectual abilities. (See Figure 14.7.)

Silent Strokes

As many as one in ten middle-aged adults may suffer a "silent" stroke, known as a "silent cerebral infarct," that does not produce clear symptoms but causes damage within the brain. According to new research, silent strokes may be at least five times more common than full-blown strokes in people under age 65 and are not uncommon in those younger than 50. The parts of the brain affected by the stroke may not involve motion or speech, but silent strokes can affect mood or memory.

Doctors note that mild strokes are not really silent but "whisper," causing very subtle symptoms that people might ignore. However, on tests of mental and physical functioning, individuals who've had very mild strokes suffer clear impairments. Even if they do not cause symptoms, brain imaging techniques such as MRIs can detect their effects.[22] The best medical advice: know the warning signs of a stroke and seek immediate treatment.[23]

Transient Ischemic Attacks (TIAs)

Sometimes a person will suffer **transient ischemic attacks (TIAs)**, "little strokes" that cause minimal damage but serve as warning signs of a potentially more severe stroke. One of three people who suffer TIAs will have a stroke during the following five years if they don't get treatment. The two major types of TIAs are:

- **Transient monocular blindness.** Blurring, a blackout or whiteout of vision, a sense of a shade coming down, or another visual disturbance in one eye.
- **Transient hemispheral attack.** Diminished blood flow to one side of the brain, causing numbness or weakness of one arm, leg, or side of the face, or problems speaking or thinking.

Many TIAs are caused by a narrowing of blood vessels in the neck (carotid arteries) because of a buildup of plaque. Specialists can diagnose this problem by feeling and listening to the arteries, by ultrasound, by measuring the pressure or circulation rate from the carotid arteries to the eyes, or by arterial angiography (injection of a dye into the arteries as X-rays are taken), a procedure that can be either dangerous, even deadly, or lifesaving.

Surgery to widen the carotid arteries may be recommended for individuals under age 60 with significant narrowing (50 to 80 percent or more). For other patients, aspirin and other drugs that make platelets less sticky and interfere with clotting may be effective.

Treatments for Strokes

Daily low-dose aspirin cuts in half the risk of strokes caused by abnormal heartbeats, which strike 75,000 Americans each year. Extremely rapid beating of the heart's upper chambers causes blood clots to form; they may enter the bloodstream and travel to the brain, where they can get stuck and choke off the blood supply. In the past, the only way to prevent such strokes was regular use of a medication called warfarin, which inhibits blood clotting and therefore increases the risk of severe bleeding. However, aspirin proved as effective as warfarin—without that dangerous side effect.

For patients who suffer a thrombotic stroke, thrombolytic drugs such as tissue-type plasminogen activator (tPA) can restore

stroke A cerebrovascular event in which the blood supply to a portion of the brain is blocked.

transient ischemic attack (TIA) A cerebrovascular event in which the blood supply to a portion of the brain is blocked temporarily; repeated attacks are predictors of more severe strokes.

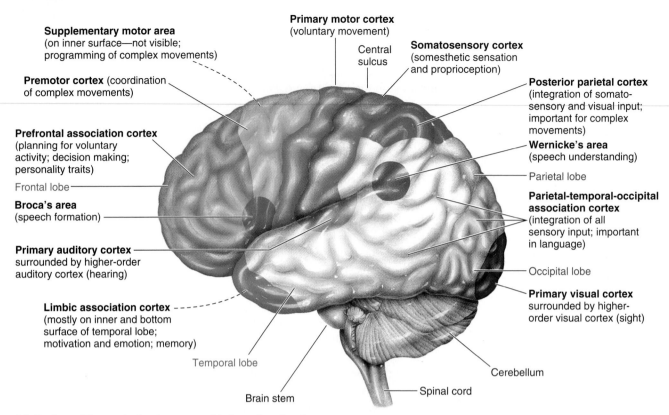

Supplementary motor area (on inner surface—not visible; programming of complex movements)

Premotor cortex (coordination of complex movements)

Prefrontal association cortex (planning for voluntary activity; decision making; personality traits)

Frontal lobe

Broca's area (speech formation)

Primary auditory cortex surrounded by higher-order auditory cortex (hearing)

Limbic association cortex (mostly on inner and bottom surface of temporal lobe; motivation and emotion; memory)

Temporal lobe

Brain stem

Primary motor cortex (voluntary movement)

Central sulcus

Somatosensory cortex (somesthetic sensation and proprioception)

Posterior parietal cortex (integration of somatosensory and visual input; important for complex movements)

Wernicke's area (speech understanding)

Parietal lobe

Parietal-temporal-occipital association cortex (integration of all sensory input; important in language)

Occipital lobe

Primary visual cortex surrounded by higher-order visual cortex (sight)

Cerebellum

Spinal cord

(a) Regions of the cerebral cortex responsible for various functions

HEARING

SEEING

SPEAKING

THINKING

MAX

MIN

(b) Regions of increased blood flow during different tasks

Figure 14.7 The Effects of Stroke on the Brain

brain blood flow and save blood cells. Other medications called heparinoids can reduce the blood's tendency to clot. For thrombolytic drugs to be effective, they must be administered within three hours after the stroke; heparinoids must be given within 24 hours. People who get to a hospital within an hour of having the first symptoms of a stroke are twice as likely to receive tPa.[24] However, the average person does not seek help for 22 hours or longer.

Men are more likely than women to receive clot-busting drugs.[25]

Cancer

Cancer is overtaking heart disease as the world's leading cause of death. According to the World Health Organization, cancer's toll is expected to double by 2020 and nearly triple by 2030, with the most severe impact on low- and middle-income countries. The global incidence of cancer is expected to rise 1 percent every year, with larger increases in China, Russia, and India. The factors contributing to increased cancer risk in these countries include population growth and adoption of Western style lifestyles, including more tobacco use and higher-fat diets.[26]

Many of the more than half a million deaths caused by cancer each year in the United States could be prevented. A third of cancers are related to smoking; another third, to obesity, poor diet, and lack of exercise.

Understanding Cancer

The uncontrolled growth and spread of abnormal cells causes cancer. Normal cells follow the code of instructions embedded in DNA (the body's genetic material); cancer cells do not. Think of the DNA within the nucleus of a cell as a computer program that controls the cell's functioning, including its ability to grow and reproduce itself. If this program or its operation is altered, the cell goes out of control. The nucleus no longer regulates growth. The abnormal cell divides to create other abnormal cells, which again divide, eventually forming *neoplasms* (new formations), or tumors.

Tumors can be either benign (slightly abnormal, not considered life-threatening) or malignant (cancerous). The only way to determine whether a tumor is benign is by microscopic examination of its cells. Cancer cells have larger nuclei than the cells in benign tumors; they vary more in shape and size; and they divide more often. In general, one billion cancer cells need to have formed before a cancer can be detected. This is the number of cells in a tumor that measures one centimeter (about a third of an inch.)[27]

At one time cancer was thought to be a single disease that attacked different parts of the body. Now scientists believe that cancer comes in countless forms, each with a genetically determined molecular "fingerprint" that indicates how deadly it is. With this understanding, doctors can identify how aggressively a tumor should be treated.

Without treatment, cancer cells continue to grow, crowding out and replacing healthy cells. This process is called **infiltration**, or invasion. Cancer cells may also **metastasize**, or spread to other parts of the body via the bloodstream or lymphatic system

infiltration A gradual penetration or invasion.

metastasize To spread to other parts of the body via the bloodstream or lymphatic system.

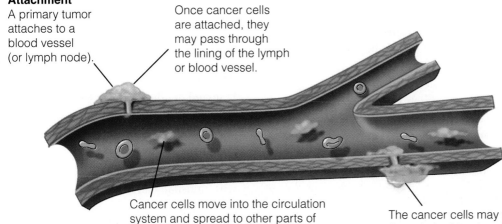

Attachment
A primary tumor attaches to a blood vessel (or lymph node).

Once cancer cells are attached, they may pass through the lining of the lymph or blood vessel.

Cancer cells move into the circulation system and spread to other parts of the body, colonizing other organs. This traveling and reproducing is called metastasizing.

The cancer cells may then move through the blood and lymph system to form a secondary tumor, or metastasis, at another site in the body.

Figure 14.8 Metastasis, or Spread of Cancer
Cancer cells can travel through the blood vessels to spread to other organs or through the lymphatic system to form secondary tumors.

(Figure 14.8). For many cancers, as many as 60 percent of patients may have metastases (which may be too small to be felt or seen without a microscope) at the time of diagnosis. Early detection and treatment result in the highest rate of cure.

Risk Factors for Cancer

According to the American Cancer Society, 1.4 million individuals are diagnosed with cancer each year; about 559,000 die of it. The five-year survival rate for all cancer is 66 percent, up from 50 percent three decades ago.

Cancer strikes individuals at all social, economic, and educational levels. However, not everyone receives a prompt diagnosis and equal high-quality care. Those who lack health insurance or whose policies do not cover all the costs of treatments often face delays in detecting a cancer and in beginning treatment. (See Community Focus, p. 470.)

Since the occurrence of cancer increases over time, most cases affect adults who are middle-aged or older. In the United States, men have a one in two lifetime risk of developing cancer; for women, the risk is one in three (Figure 14.9).

The term **relative risk** compares the risk of developing cancer in people with a certain exposure or trait to the risk in those who do not have this exposure or trait. Smokers, for instance, have a ten-times-greater relative risk of developing lung cancer than nonsmokers. Most relative risks are smaller. For example, women who have a first-degree (mother, sister, or daughter) family history of breast cancer have about a twofold increased risk of developing breast cancer compared with women who do not have a family history of the disease. This means that they are about twice as likely to develop breast cancer.

About 108 million Americans have a history of cancer.[28] Medical experts recommend that cancer survivors exercise regularly, eat at least five servings of fruits and vegetables daily, and not smoke. However, only a small minority—5 percent in one study—are following all three recommendations.[29]

Heredity An estimated 13 to 14 million Americans may be at risk of a hereditary cancer. In hereditary cancers, such as retinoblastoma (an eye cancer that strikes young children) or certain colon cancers, a specific cancer-causing gene is passed down from generation to generation. The odds of any child with one affected parent inheriting this gene and developing the cancer are 50–50.

Other people are born with genes that make them susceptible to having certain cells grow and divide uncontrollably, which may contribute to cancer development. The most well-known are mutations of the BRCA gene, linked with increased risk of breast, colon, and ovarian cancer.

Genetic tests can identify some individuals who are born with an increased susceptibility to cancer. By spotting a mutated gene in an individual, doctors can sometimes detect cancer years earlier through increased cancer screening. The most likely sites for inherited cancers to develop are the breast, brain, blood, muscles, bones, and adrenal glands. (See Point/Counterpoint, p. 471.)

The telltale signs of inherited cancers include:

- **Early development.** Genetic forms of certain diseases strike earlier than noninherited cancers. For example, the average age of women diagnosed with breast cancer is 62. But if breast cancer is inherited, the average age at diagnosis is 44, an 18-year difference.

- **Family history.** Anyone with a close relative (mother, father, sibling, child) with cancer has about three times the usual chance of getting the same type of cancer.

- **Multiple targets.** The same type of hereditary cancer often strikes more than once—in both breasts or both kidneys, for instance, or in two separate parts of the same organ.

- **Unusual gender pattern.** Genes may be responsible for cancers that generally don't strike a certain gender—for example, breast cancer in a man.

- **Cancer family syndrome.** Some families, with unusually large numbers of relatives affected by cancer, seem clearly cancer-prone. For instance, in Lynch syndrome (a form of colon cancer), more than 20 percent of the family members in at least two generations develop cancer of both the colon and the endometrium.

Estimated New Cases*		Estimated Deaths	
Male	**Female**	**Male**	**Female**
Prostate 218,890 (29%)	Breast 178,480 (26%)	Lung & bronchus 89,510 (31%)	Lung & bronchus 70,880 (26%)
Lung & bronchus 114,760 (15%)	Lung & bronchus 98,620 (15%)	Prostate 27,050 (9%)	Breast 40,460 (15%)
Colon & rectum 79,130 (10%)	Colon & rectum 74,630 (11%)	Colon & rectum 26,000 (9%)	Colon & rectum 26,180 (10%)
Urinary bladder 50,040 (7%)	Uterine corpus 39,080 (6%)	Pancreas 16,840 (6%)	Pancreas 16,530 (6%)
Non-Hodgkin lymphoma 34,200 (4%)	Non-Hodgkin lymphoma 28,990 (4%)	Leukemia 12,320 (4%)	Ovary 15,280 (6%)
Melanoma of the skin 33,910 (4%)	Melanoma of the skin 26,030 (4%)	Liver & intrahepatic bile duct 11,280 (4%)	Leukemia 9,470 (4%)
Kidney and renal pelvis 31,590 (4%)	Thyroid 25,480 (4%)	Esophagus 10,900 (4%)	Non-Hodgkin lymphoma 9,060 (3%)
Leukemia 24,800 (3%)	Ovary 22,430 (3%)	Urinary bladder 9,630 (3%)	Uterine corpus 7,400 (3%)
Oral cavity & pharynx 24,180 (3%)	Kidney and renal pelvis 19,600 (3%)	Non-Hodgkin lymphoma 9,600 (3%)	Brain & other nervous system 5,590 (2%)
Pancreas 18,830 (2%)	Leukemia 19,440 (3%)	Kidney & renal pelvis 8,080 (3%)	Liver and intrahepatic bile duct 5,500 (2%)
All Sites 766,860 (100%)	All sites 678,060 (100%)	All sites 289,550 (100%)	All sites 270,100 (100%)

* Excludes basal and squamous cell skin cancers and in situ carcinoma except urinary bladder.

Figure 14.9 Sex Differences in Cancer Rates and Deaths
© 2008, American Cancer Society, Inc., Surveillance Research.

Racial and Ethnic Groups More cases of cancer occur in African Americans than in any other racial or ethnic group.[30] Blacks are 30 percent more likely to die of cancer than are whites. African American women have the highest incidence of colorectal and lung cancers of any ethnic group, while black men have the highest rates of prostate, colorectal, and lung cancer. African Americans also have higher rates of incidence and deaths from other cancers, including those of the mouth, throat, esophagus, stomach, pancreas, and larynx.

Cancer rates also vary in other racial and ethnic groups. Hispanics have a six times lower risk of developing melanoma than Caucasians, yet tend to have a worse prognosis than Caucasians when they do develop this skin cancer. The incidence of female breast cancer is highest among white women and lowest among Native American women. Cervical cancer is most common in Hispanic women.

Asian Americans, both those born in the United States and immigrants, generally have lower cancer rates than other ethnic groups. Vietnamese men have much higher rates of liver cancer than whites, while Korean men and women are much more likely to develop stomach cancer. Compared with other Asian Americans, Chinese and Vietnamese women have higher rates of lung cancer. Asian Americans who have lived in the United States the longest are likely to develop the cancers that are most common here, such as breast and colon cancer, although at lower rates than whites.

Obesity Long recognized as threats to cardiovascular health, overweight and obesity

relative risk The risk of developing cancer in persons with a certain exposure or trait compared to the risk in persons who do not have the same exposure or trait.

COMMUNITY FOCUS *Who Can Afford to Get Sick?*

PROBLEM When Michelle Morse, a 20-year-old New Hampshire undergraduate, was diagnosed with advanced colon cancer, her doctors recommended that she cut back her class schedule during chemotherapy. However, her family's health insurance would not cover her if she were not a full-time student. And so Michelle was forced to carry a full course load during ten months of aggressive treatment. Michelle died after graduating in 2005, and her mother lobbied for legislation to protect other college students from losing their insurance if they become ill. "Michelle's Law," already enacted in New Hampshire, is now before the U.S. Congress.

Cases like Michelle's are rare, but problems affording quality care for serious illness are not. Young adults between the age of 18 and 24 are most likely to be uninsured, often because they do not have full-time jobs or their employers do not provide health insurance. But almost everyone, including those with coverage, faces the risk of being "underinsured" in the event of a major illness. ("Underinsured" refers to anyone who would have to spend more than 10 percent of the family income on out-of-pocket medical expenses for a catastrophic illness.)

Often insurance policies place limits on services and charge high deductibles and co-payments. As a result many patients with serious illnesses cannot get the timely, lifesaving treatments they need. According to the American Cancer Society, one in five people with insurance uses all or most of his or her savings because of the financial cost of dealing with cancer. Even if you are young and healthy, you cannot afford not to think about what might happen to you or your family if you developed a major disease.

BECOME INFORMED

- Learn about the serious medical consequences of not having health insurance. According to a recent report from the American Cancer Society, the uninsured are less likely to receive recommended cancer screening tests, are more likely to be diagnosed with later stage disease, and have lower survival rates than those with private insurance.
- Look into the details of your insurance coverage. If you have your own policy, read it carefully. Make note of co-payments, excluded services, and "caps" on reimbursements for health services. To find out more about getting and keeping health insurance in your state, click on **www.healthinsuranceinfo.net/** for user-friendly guides prepared by the Georgetown University Health Policy Institute.
- Check into low- or no-cost health resources in your area. Does your campus provide free blood pressure checks or other screenings at the student health center? Are there campus or local health fairs where you can get free information and assessments? Contact local chapters of the American Cancer Society and the American Heart Association to find out what services they offer.

BECOME INVOLVED

- Support Michelle's Law. If approved by the U.S. Congress, it would allow full-time college students covered under their parents' policies to take up to 12 months of medical leave. The website **www.michelleslaw.com** provides background and contact information for all senators and representatives. E-mail yours today.
- Help low-income, inner-city, and minority women get free mammograms. All you have to do is click on the Breast Cancer Site at **www.thebreastcancersite.com/click-ToGive/home.faces? siteId=2.** Its sponsors provide funding for mammograms at clinics throughout the United States. Click every day to sustain this important service.
- Join up. Become a volunteer for a group such the American Cancer Society Cancer Action Network (**www.acscan.org**). You can simply make yourself available on an as-needed basis to help with e-mail campaigns for specific legislation, or you can commit to regular participation in fund-raisers, political rallies, and other events.

may play a role in an estimated 90,000 cancer deaths each year. According to American Cancer Society researchers who examined the relationship between body mass index (BMI) and risk of dying from cancer, 14 percent of cancer deaths in men and 20 percent of cancer deaths in women may stem from excess weight.

The higher an individual's BMI, the greater the likelihood of dying of cancer. An unhealthy body weight increases the risk of many types of cancer, including breast (in postmenopausal women), colon and rectum, kidney, cervix, ovary, uterus, esophagus, gallbladder, stomach (in men), liver, pancreas, prostate, non-Hodgkin's lymphoma, and multiple myeloma.

The degree to which extra pounds affect cancer risk varies by site. Obesity elevates the risk of esophageal cancer fivefold; increases the risk of breast or uterine cancer by two to four times; and boosts the risk for colon cancer by 35 percent to twofold.

Infectious Agents Worldwide, an estimated 17 percent of cancers can be attributed to infection. In economically developing countries, infections cause or contribute to 26 percent of cancers. In developed countries, they play a role in 7 percent of new cases of cancer.

Among the cancers that have been linked with infectious agents are human papilloma virus (HPV) with cervical cancer and *Helicobacter pylori* with stomach cancer. Viruses have been implicated in certain leukemias (cancers of the blood system) and lymphomas (cancers of the lymphatic system), cancers of the nose and pharynx, liver cancer, and cervical cancer. (See Chapter 16 for details on the human papilloma virus.) Human immune deficiency virus (HIV) can lead to certain lymphomas and leukemias and to a type of cancer called Kaposi's sarcoma.

Generally, the presence of a bacterium or a virus per se is not enough to cause cancer. A predisposing environment and other cofactors—most still unknown—are needed for cancer development and growth.

Common Types of Cancer

Cancer refers to a group of more than a hundred diseases characterized by abnormal cell growth. Although all cancers have similar characteristics, each is distinct. Some cancers are relatively simple to cure, whereas others are more threatening and mysterious. The earlier any cancer is found, the easier it is to treat and the better the patient's chances of survival.

Cancers are classified according to the type of cell and the organ in which they originate, such as the following:

- **Carcinoma,** the most common kind, which starts in the epithelium, the layers of cells that cover the body's surface or line internal organs and glands.

- **Sarcoma,** which forms in the supporting, or connective, tissues of the body: bones, muscles, blood vessels.

- **Leukemia,** which begins in the blood-forming tissues: bone marrow, lymph nodes, and the spleen.

- **Lymphoma,** which arises in the cells of the lymph system, the network that filters out impurities.

Skin Cancer One of every five Americans can expect to develop skin cancer in their lifetimes. Once scientists thought exposure to the B range of ultraviolet light (UVB), the wavelength of light responsible for sunburn, posed the greatest danger. However, longer-wavelength UVA, which penetrates deeper into the skin, also plays a major role in skin cancers. An estimated 80 percent of total lifetime sun exposure occurs during childhood, so sun protection is especially important in youngsters. Tanning salons and sunlamps also increase the risk of skin cancer because they produce ultraviolet radiation. A half-hour dose of radiation from a sunlamp can be equivalent to the amount you'd get from an entire day in the sun. Often skin damage is invisible to the naked eye but shows up under special diagnostic lights.

 Young adults spend the most time in the sun and also frequent tanning salons. Even when they perceive the seriousness of skin cancer, college students—particularly women—describe suntanned skin as attractive, healthy, and athletic-looking and view the benefits of getting a suntan as outweighing the risks of skin cancer or premature aging. Some students actually become addicted to tanning.[31] (See Consumer Alert, p. 473.) However, a CDC report concluded

that indoor tanning is "simply not safe" and causes sunburn, infection, eye damage, and increased risk of skin cancer.

The most common skin cancers are *basal cell* (involving the base of the epidermis, the top level of the skin) and *squamous cell* (involving cells in the epidermis). Their incidence is increasing among men and women under the age of 40. Long-term exposure to the sun is the biggest risk factor for these cancers.

Every year more than 5 million Americans develop skin lesions known as actinic keratoses (AKs), rough red or brown scaly patches that develop in the upper layer of the skin, usually on the face, lower lip, bald scalp, neck, back of the hands, and forearms. Forty percent of squamous cell carcinomas, the second leading cause of skin cancer deaths, begin as AKs. Treatments include surgical removal, cryosurgery (freezing the skin), electrodesiccation (heat generated by an electric current), topical chemotherapy, and removal with lasers, chemical peels, or dermabrasion.

Smoking and exposure to certain hydrocarbons in asphalt, coal tar, and pitch may increase the risk of squamous cell skin cancer. Other risk factors include occupational exposure to carcinogens and inherited skin disorders, such as xeroderma pigmentosum and familial atypical multiple-mole melanoma.

YOUR STRATEGIES FOR PREVENTION

Seven Warning Signs of Cancer

If you note any of the following seven warning signs, immediately schedule an appointment with your doctor:

- Change in bowel or bladder habits.
- A sore that doesn't heal.
- Unusual bleeding or discharge.
- Thickening or lump in the breast, testis, or elsewhere.
- Indigestion or difficulty swallowing.
- Obvious change in a wart or mole.
- Nagging cough or hoarseness.

New ultraviolet scanning technology can reveal skin damage that may not be visible to the naked eye.

Malignant *melanoma*, the deadliest type of skin cancer, causes 1 to 2 percent of all cancer deaths. During the 1930s, the lifetime risk of melanoma was about 1 in 1,500. Today it is 1 in 75. This increase in risk is due mostly to overexposure to UV radiation. The use of a tanning bed ten times or more a year doubles the risk for individuals over age 30.

Both the amount and the intensity of lifetime sun exposure play key roles in determining risk for melanoma. People living in areas where the sun's ultraviolet rays reach Earth with extra intensity, such as tropical or high-altitude regions, are at increased risk. Although melanoma occurs more often among people over 40, it is increasing in younger people, particularly those who had severe sunburns in childhood. The rate of increase in melanoma also has risen more in men (4.6 percent a year) than in women (3.2 percent). Men are more likely than women to be diagnosed with melanoma after age 40.

Individuals with any of the following characteristics are at increased risk:

- Fair skin, light eyes, or fair hair.

- A tendency to develop freckles and to burn instead of tan.

- A history of childhood sunburn or intermittent, intense sun exposure.

- A personal or family history of melanoma.

- A large number of nevi, or moles (200 or more, or 50 or more if under age 20), or dysplastic (atypical) moles.

Detection   The most common predictor for melanoma is a change in an existing mole or development of a new and changing pigmented mole. The most important early indicators are change in color, an increase in diameter, and changes in the borders of a mole (Figure 14.10). An increase in height signals a corresponding growth in depth under the skin. Itching in a new or long-standing mole also should not be ignored.

Treatment   If caught early, melanoma is highly curable, usually with surgery alone. Once it has spread, chemotherapy with a single drug or a combination can temporarily shrink tumors in some people. However, the five-year survival rate for metastatic melanoma is only 14 percent.

Breast Cancer   Every 3 minutes, a woman in the United States learns that she has breast cancer. Every 12 minutes, a woman dies of breast cancer. Many women misjudge their own likelihood of developing breast cancer, either overestimating or underestimating their susceptibility. In a national poll, 1 in every 10 surveyed considered herself at no risk at all. This is never the case. Every woman is at risk for breast cancer simply because she's female.

However, not all women's risks are equal. The National Cancer Institute (NCI) has developed a computerized Breast Cancer Risk Assessment Tool, based on data from more than 280,000 women, that allows a woman to sit down with her doctor and discuss her own odds of developing breast cancer within the next five years and over her entire lifetime.

The most common risk factors include the following:

- **Age.** As shown in Figure 14.11 on p. 474, at 25, a woman's chance of developing breast cancer is 1 in 19,608; by age 45, it has increased to 1 in 93; by 65, it is 1 in 17. The mean age at which women are diagnosed is 63.

- **Family history.** The overwhelming majority of breast cancers—90 to 95 percent—are not due to strong genetic factors. However, having a first-degree relative—mother, sister, or daughter—with breast cancer does increase risk, and if the relative developed breast cancer before menopause, the cancer is more likely to be hereditary.

- **Long menstrual history.** Women who had their first period before age 12 are at greater risk than women who began menstruating later. The reason is that the more menstrual cycles a woman has, the longer her exposure to estrogen, a hormone known to increase breast cancer danger. For similar reasons, childless women, who menstruate continuously for several decades, are also at greater risk. Neither miscarriage nor induced abortion increases the risk of breast cancer.

© Sion Touhig/Getty Images

Are You Addicted to Tanning?

You know that exposure to ultraviolet rays increases your risk of developing skin cancer, but maybe you still can't stay out of the sun or a tanning booth. Why?

Facts to Know

- Researchers theorize that repetitive tanning behavior may be the result of a kind of addiction.[32]
- Texas beachgoers, asked questions about their tanning habits, gave replies similar to those who gamble or drink compulsively.

Steps to Take

- Test your risk of "ultraviolet light (UVL) dependency" by taking the CAGE screening testing for addictive behavior.

- Ask yourself the following questions;
  - **C**ut: Ever felt you ought to cut down on your behavior?
  - **A**nnoyed: Have people annoyed you by criticizing your behavior?
  - **G**uilt: Ever felt bad or guilty about your behavior?
  - **E**ye Opener: Ever engaged in your behavior to steady your nerves in the morning?

Answering yes to two of the CAGE questions is a strong indication for an addictive behavior; answering yes to three confirms it.

- **Age at birth of first child.** An early pregnancy—in a woman's teens or twenties—changes the actual maturation of breast cells and decreases risk. But if a woman has her first child in her forties, precancerous cells may actually flourish with the high hormone levels of the pregnancy.

- **Breast biopsies.** Even if laboratory analysis finds no precancerous abnormalities, women who require such tests are more likely to develop breast cancer. Fibrocystic breast disease, a term often used for "lumpy" breasts, is not a risk factor.

- **Race and ethnicity.** Breast cancer rates are lower in Hispanic and Asian American populations than in whites and in African American women. Caucasian women over 40 have the highest incidence rate for breast cancer in this country, but African American women at every age have a greater likelihood of dying from breast cancer.

    BRCA1 mutations indicate a higher risk of aggressive forms of breast cancer and of ovarian cancer.[33] Hispanic women, particularly those of Mexican descent, are more likely than white or black women to have hereditary forms of cancer. Screening for the BRCA1 mutations could lead to earlier diagnosis and more effective treatment.[34] In Asian American women a diet low in meat and starches and high in legumes has been linked with a reduced risk of breast cancer.[35]

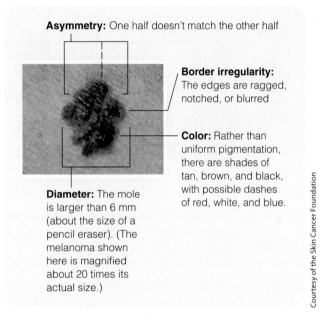

Asymmetry: One half doesn't match the other half

Border irregularity: The edges are ragged, notched, or blurred

Color: Rather than uniform pigmentation, there are shades of tan, brown, and black, with possible dashes of red, white, and blue.

Diameter: The mole is larger than 6 mm (about the size of a pencil eraser). (The melanoma shown here is magnified about 20 times its actual size.)

Courtesy of the Skin Cancer Foundation

Figure 14.10   ABCD: The Warning Signs of Melanoma

An estimated 95 percent of cases of melanoma arise from an existing mole. A normal mole is usually round or oval, less than 6 millimeters (about 1/4 inch) in diameter, and evenly colored (black, brown, or tan). Seek prompt evaluation of any moles that change in ways shown in the photo.

Source: American Academy of Dermatology. All rights reserved.

- **Occupation.** Based on two decades of following more than a million women, Swedish researchers have developed a list of jobs linked with a high risk of breast cancer. These include pharmacists, certain types of teachers, schoolmasters, systems analysts and programmers, telephone operators, telegraph and radio operators, metal platers and coaters, and beauticians.

YOUR STRATEGIES FOR PREVENTION

How to Save Your Skin

- Once a month, stand in front of a full-length mirror to examine your front and back, and your left and right sides with your arms raised. Check the backs of your legs, the tops and soles of your feet, and the surfaces between your toes. Use a hand mirror to check the back of your neck, behind your ears, and your scalp.

- Watch for changes in the size, color, number, and thickness of moles. Suspicious moles are likely to be asymmetrical (one half doesn't match the other), with ragged, notched, or blurred edges. Also look for any signs of darkly pigmented growth, oozing, scaliness, bleeding, or a change in sensation, itchiness, tenderness, or pain.

- Don't put too much faith in sunscreens. Wearing sunscreen (with a sun protection factor, or SPF, of at least 15) is good, but protective clothing is better—and staying in the shade is best. Check your shadow. One simple guideline for reducing the risk of skin cancer is avoiding the sun anytime your shadow is shorter than you are. According to the National Cancer Institute (NCI), this shadow method—based on the principle that the closer the sun comes to being directly overhead, the stronger its ultraviolet rays—works for any location and at any time of year.

- Check for photosensitivity. If you are taking any drugs, ask your doctor or pharmacist to see if the medication could make you more sensitive to sun damage. Be especially cautious about sun exposure if you have been using a synthetic preparation derived from vitamin A (Retin A) as an acne or anti-wrinkle treatment; it can increase your susceptibility.

- Use extra caution near water, snow, and sand since they reflect the damaging rays of the sun and increase the risk of sunburn. Wear protective clothing, such as a wide-brimmed cap or hat, whenever possible.

- **Alcohol.** Women's risk of breast cancer increases with the amount of alcohol they drink. Those who take two or more drinks per day are 40 percent more likely to develop breast cancer than women who don't drink at all. For a nondrinking woman, the lifetime risk of breast cancer by age 80 is 1 in 11. For heavy drinkers it's about 1 in 7, regardless of race, education, family history, use of hormone therapy, or other risk factors.

- **Hormone therapy (HT).** Several studies confirm an increased risk with a combination of estrogen and progestin, particularly in women who use combination HT for five years or longer. Women taking combination HT are more likely to have abnormal mammograms requiring further testing and to be diagnosed at a more advanced stage of breast

By age 25	1 in 19,608
By age 30	1 in 2,525
By age 35	1 in 622
By age 40	1 in 217
By age 45	1 in 93
By age 50	1 in 50
By age 55	1 in 33
By age 60	1 in 24
By age 65	1 in 17
By age 70	1 in 14
By age 75	1 in 11
By age 80	1 in 10
By age 85	1 in 9
Ever	1 in 8

Figure 14.11 A Woman's Risk of Developing Breast Cancer

Source: Surveillance Program, National Cancer Institute.

cancer. The risk persisted for at least three years after women discontinued combination hormone therapy.[36] Women taking only estrogen for shorter periods did not have an elevated rate of breast cancer, but their risk increased significantly after 15 years of use. In African American women, estrogen use has been linked to higher breast cancer risk, particularly in leaner women.

- **Obesity.** Excess weight, particularly after menopause, increases the risk of getting breast cancer. Overweight women, both pre- and postmenopausal, with breast cancer are more likely to die of their disease.

- **Sedentary lifestyle.** According to the World Health Organization, regular physical activity may cut the risk of developing breast cancer by 20 to 40 percent, regardless of a woman's menopausal status or the type or intensity of the activity. The reason may be that exercise lowers levels of circulating ovarian hormones.

Detection   Doctors have long advised women to perform monthly breast self-exams (BSEs) after their periods (Figure 14.12). In its newest guidelines, the American Cancer Society now describes BSE as "an option" for women starting in their twenties and urges all women to report any breast changes promptly. It recommends a breast exam by a trained practitioner every three years for women in their twenties and thirties and every year for women 40 and over and a yearly mammogram for all women, starting at age 40.

The best tool for early detection is the diagnostic X-ray exam called **mammography**. Women whose breast cancer is detected by screening mammography have a significantly better prognosis than those whose cancer is found another way—even if the cancer has already spread to their lymph nodes. A likely reason is that mammography can detect tumors that are both slower growing and less biologically lethal than others.

Magnetic Resonance Imaging may be more accurate than mammography for detecting early forms of breast cancer before they progress to more aggressive forms. The

1. Lie flat on your back. Place a pillow or towel under one shoulder, and raise that arm over your head. With the opposite hand, you'll feel with the pads, not the fingertips, of the three middle fingers, for lumps or any change in the texture of the breast or skin.

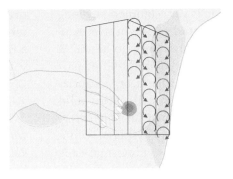

2. The area you'll examine is from your collarbone to your bra line and from your breastbone to the center of your armpit. Imagine the area divided into vertical strips. Using small circular motions (the size of a dime), move your fingers up and down the strips. Apply light, medium, and deep pressure to examine each spot. Repeat this same process for your other breast.

3. Gently squeeze the nipple of each breast between your thumb and index finger. Any discharge, clear or bloody, should be reported to your doctor immediately.

Figure 14.12   Breast Self-Exam
The best time to examine your breasts is after your menstrual period every month.

American Cancer Society now recommends MRI screening for women with a strong family history of breast or ovarian cancer and those who have been treated for Hodgkin's disease. Women who've had cancer in one breast or those with extremely dense breasts may also benefit.

Treatment   Breast cancer can be treated with surgery, radiation, and drugs (chemotherapy and hormonal therapy). Doctors may use one of these options or a combination, depending on the type and location of the cancer and whether the disease has spread.

Most women undergo some type of surgery. **Lumpectomy,** or breast-conserving surgery, removes only the cancerous tissue and a surrounding margin of normal tissue. A modified radical **mastectomy** includes the entire breast and some of the underarm lymph nodes. Removing underarm lymph nodes is important to determine if the cancer has spread, but a technique called sentinel node biopsy allows physicians to pinpoint the first lymph node into which a tumor drains (the sentinel node) and remove only the nodes most likely to contain cancer cells.

Radiation therapy is treatment with high-energy rays or particles to destroy cancer. In almost all cases, lumpectomy is followed by six to seven weeks of radiation. Chemotherapy is used to reach cancer cells that may have spread beyond the breast—in many cases even if no cancer is detected in the lymph nodes after surgery.

The use of drugs such as tamoxifen and aromatase inhibitors, in addition to standard chemotherapy, can significantly lower the risk of recurrence.

Cervical Cancer   Cervical cancer, the second most common cancer in women worldwide, claims 250,000 lives every year. Approximately 85 percent of these deaths occur in developing countries where women do not have access to effective cervical cancer screening. An estimated 11,000 cases of invasive cervical cancer are diagnosed in the United States every year. The highest incidence rate occurs among Vietnamese women; Alaskan Native, Korean, and Hispanic women also have higher rates than the national average. The mortality rate for African American women is more than twice that of whites, largely because of a high number of deaths among older black women.

Women are at higher risk for cervical cancer if they engaged in sexual activity before the age of 16 or have had multiple sexual partners (more than five in a lifetime). Genital herpes, smoking, and secondhand smoke increase the danger. However, as numerous studies have conclusively demonstrated in the last two decades, human papilloma virus (HPV) infection is the primary risk factor for cervical cancer.

mammography   A diagnostic X-ray exam used to detect breast cancer.

lumpectomy   The surgical removal of a breast tumor and its surrounding tissue.

mastectomy   The surgical removal of an entire breast.

HPV infection is very common in young women. In some studies one in five sexually active women under age 30 has HPV. However, only about 13 of the hundred-plus types of HPV cause dysplasia, or precancerous changes in cervical cells. Most mild cases go away on their own, but some progress to moderate or severe dysplasia within two to four years. These abnormal cells could develop into cervical cancer, usually over a period of more than 10 years.

Screening for HPV and Cervical Cancer In the past the Pap test, a sampling of cervical cells, was the standard screening test for cervical cancer. Many physicians, including those in college health centers, have been moving away from the recommendation to perform an initial Pap test at the time of first sexual activity to doing so three years after a young woman becomes sexually active or at age 21, whichever comes first, and to test for HPV if a Pap smear is unclear or abnormal (see Table 14.4).[37]

Several new screening tests, including HPV DNA testing, have proven more sensitive and yield fewer false positives than the Pap smear alone. Health professionals are still doing research to determine the best way to combine HPV and Pap tests. According to some studies, HPV testing can safely be used for primary screening of women over age 30.[38] However, other researchers recommend HPV testing first, followed by a Pap smear. In one study in which women with normal Pap smears were given a HPV DNA test within a year, researchers detected 30 percent more cases of cervical cancer.[39]

HPV is very common among college women. In one survey of students whose Pap smears were abnormal, half tested positive for HPV. Doctors may simply monitor patients with such results, since many cases of dysplasia clear up on their own in healthy young women. However, they may recommend a colposcopy, a direct examination of the genital area with a special lighted microscope called a colposcope that magnifies the surface of the cervix and vagina. The combination of the two tests results in fewer false positives and a more accurate diagnosis.[40]

Ovarian Cancer Ovarian cancer is the leading cause of death from gynecological cancers. Risk factors include a family history of ovarian cancer; personal history of breast cancer; obesity; infertility (because the abnormality that interferes with conception may also play a role in cancer development); and low levels of transferase, an enzyme involved in the metabolism of dairy foods. Often women develop no obvious symptoms until the advanced stages, although they may experience painless swelling of the abdomen, irregular bleeding, lower abdominal pain, digestive and urinary abnormalities, fatigue, backache, bloating, and weight gain. Ovarian cancer may be diagnosed by pelvic examination, ultrasound, MRI, computed tomography, or PET (positron emission tomography) scan.

Testicular Cancer In the last 20 years the incidence of testicular cancer has risen 51 percent in the United States—from 3.61 to 5.44 per 100,000. It is not clear why testicular cancer is on the rise, although researchers speculate that changing environmental or socioeconomic risk factors could have a role. Chronic use of marijuana increases the risk of an especially aggressive form of testicular cancer.[41] Testicular cancer occurs mostly among young men between the ages of 18 and 35, who are not normally at risk of cancer. At highest risk are men with an undescended testicle (a condition that is almost always corrected in childhood

> ### TABLE 14.4

What Your Pap Test Results Mean

A Pap test may come back as "normal," "unclear," or "abnormal."

Normal

A normal (or "negative") result means that no cell changes were found on the cervix.

Unclear

It is common for test results to come back unclear. Doctors may use other words to describe this result such as *inconclusive*, or *ASC-US*. These all mean the same thing: that some cervical cells *could* be abnormal, perhaps because of an infection. An HPV test will indicate if the changes are related to HPV.

Abnormal

An abnormal result means that cell changes were found on the cervix. This usually does not indicate cervical cancer.

Abnormal changes on your cervix are likely caused by HPV. The changes may be minor (low-grade) or serious (high-grade). Most of the time, minor changes go back to normal on their own. But more serious changes can turn into cancer if the cells are not removed. The more serious changes are often called "pre-cancer" because they are not yet cancer but could turn into cancer over time.

to prevent this danger). To detect possibly cancerous growths, men should perform monthly testicular self-exams, as shown in Figure 14.13.

Often the first sign of this cancer is a slight enlargement of one testicle. There also may be a change in the way it feels when touched. Sometimes men with testicular cancer report a dull ache in the lower abdomen or groin, along with a sense of heaviness or sluggishness. Lumps on the testicles also may indicate cancer.

A man who notices any abnormality should consult a physician. If a lump is indeed present, a surgical biopsy is necessary to find out if it is cancerous. If the biopsy is positive, a series of tests generally is needed to determine whether the disease has spread.

Treatment for testicular cancer generally involves surgical removal of the diseased testis, sometimes along with radiation therapy, chemotherapy, and the removal of nearby lymph nodes. The remaining testicle is capable of maintaining a man's sexual potency and fertility. Only in rare cases is removal of both testicles necessary. Testosterone injections following such surgery can maintain potency. The chance for a cure is very high if testicular cancer is spotted early.

Colon and Rectal Cancer
Colon and rectal, or colorectal, cancer is the third most common cancer and accounts for 10 percent of cancer deaths. Most cases occur after age 50. Both age and gender influence the risk of colon cancer. Older individuals and men are more likely to develop polyps (nonmalignant growths that may turn cancerous at some point) and tumors in the colon than young people and women.

Risk factors include age (over 50), personal or family history of colon and rectal cancer, polyps in the colon or rectum, ulcerative colitis, smoking, alcohol consumption, prolonged high consumption of red and processed meat, high-fat or low-fiber diet, and inadequate intake of fruits and vegetables. In the landmark Women's Health Initiative trials, a low-fat diet did not reduce the risk of colon and rectal cancer in postmenopausal women. Low doses of aspirin or other non-steroidal anti-inflammatory drugs appear to reduce the risk of precancerous polyps that can lead to colon and rectal cancer.[42]

Figure 14.13

Testicular Self-Exam

The best time to examine your testicles is after a hot bath or shower, when the scrotum is most relaxed. Place your index and middle fingers under each testicle and the thumb on top, and roll the testicle between the thumb and fingers. If you feel a small, hard, usually painless lump or swelling, or anything unusual, consult a urologist.

Current guidelines recommend a screening colonoscopy beginning at age 50, earlier for those at higher risk based on personal, family, or medical history. The initial screening is crucial because it detects the largest, most dangerous polyps, which can then be removed.

Early signs of colorectal cancer are bleeding from the rectum, blood in the stool, or a change in bowel habits. Treatment may involve surgery, radiation therapy, and/or chemotherapy.

Prostate Cancer
After skin cancer, prostate cancer is the most common form of cancer in American men. The risk of prostate cancer is 1 in 6; the risk of death due to metastatic prostate cancer is 1 in 30. More than a quarter of men diagnosed with cancer have prostate cancer. The disease strikes African American men more often than white; Asian and American Indian men are affected less often.

The risk of prostate cancer increases with age, family history, exposure to the heavy metal cadmium, high number of sexual partners, and history of frequent sexually transmitted infections. A diet high in saturated fat may be a risk factor. An inherited predisposition may account for 5 to 10 percent of cases. A purported link between vasectomy and prostate cancer has been disproved. Statin drugs, commonly prescribed to lower cholesterol, also may lower the risk of prostate cancer.

The development of a simple annual screening test that measures levels of a protein called prostate-specific antigen

(PSA) in the blood has revolutionized the diagnosis of prostate cancer. PSA testing is recommended for men at high risk (African Americans and men with close relatives with prostate cancer) starting at age 45 and for all men at age 50. It remains controversial, however. Some claim that PSA testing saves lives; others, that it leads to unnecessary and potentially harmful treatments. Annual screening has not reduced deaths from the disease in older men and new guidelines recommend against screening for men age 75 or older. There is insufficient evidence to assess the balance of benefits and risks in younger men.[43]

Treatment may include hormones, chemotherapy, a low-fat diet, and radiation. About 60,000 men undergo radical prostate surgery in the United States every year. The five-year survival rate has increased from 67 percent to 99 percent over the past 20 years.

Other Major Illnesses

Other noninfectious diseases have a debilitating effect on many people. But most of the diseases discussed in this section can be controlled, if not cured.

Epilepsy and Seizure Disorders

About 10 percent of all Americans will have at least one seizure at some time. Between 0.5 and 1 percent of all Americans have recurrent seizures. Derived from the Greek word for seizure, **epilepsy** is the term used to refer to a variety of neurological disorders characterized by sudden attacks (seizures) of violent muscle contractions and unconsciousness. Epilepsy is rarely fatal; the primary danger to life is to suffer an attack while driving or swimming.

Seizures can be major, referred to as *grand mal*; minor, referred to as *petit mal;* or psychomotor. In a grand-mal seizure, the person loses consciousness, falls to the ground, and experiences convulsive body movements. Petit-mal seizures are brief, characterized by a loss of consciousness for 10 to 30 seconds, by eye or muscle flutterings, and occasionally by a loss of muscle tone. About 90 percent of all epileptics have grand-mal seizures; 40 percent suffer both petit-mal and grand-mal seizures. The frequency of attacks defines the severity of the epilepsy. Diagnosis is based on a history of recurring attacks and a study of the brain's electrical activity, called an electroencephalogram (EEG).

About half of all cases of epilepsy have no known cause and are therefore classified as *idiopathic.* Others stem from conditions that affect the brain, such as trauma, tumors, congenital malformations, or inflammation of the membranes covering the brain. *Idiopathic* epilepsy usually begins between the ages of 2 and 14. Seizures before age 2 are usually related to developmental defects, birth injuries, or a metabolic disease affecting the brain. (Fever-induced convulsions are not related to epilepsy.) Seizures after age 14 are generally symptoms of brain disease or injury.

Seizure disorders don't reflect or affect intellectual or psychological soundness; people who suffer from them have normal intelligence. Therapy with anticonvulsant drugs can control seizures in most people, and once seizures are under control, epileptics can live full, normal lives by continuing to take their medications.

If you're with a person who suffers a grand-mal seizure, make sure he or she isn't injured during the attack. Don't try to restrain the person or interfere with his or her movements, and don't try to force anything into the person's mouth.

The bacterium *Helicobacter pylori* has flagella that enable it to tunnel beneath the protective layer coating the stomach lining.

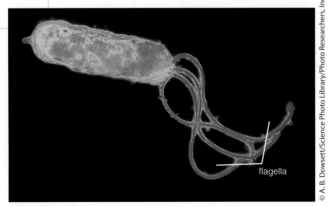

flagella

© A. B. Dowsett/Science Photo Library/Photo Researchers, Inc.

Asthma

Asthma is a disease characterized by constriction of the breathing passages. As with allergy, asthma rates have skyrocketed in the last two decades. Approximately 20 million Americans have asthma. Asthma-related problems account for more than half a million hospital stays each year and 14 deaths each day in the United States, according to the Asthma and Allergy Foundation of America.

 Asthma is more common among inner-city residents and blacks. The disease disproportionately affects African Americans. A black man in New York City is 11 times more likely to die from asthma than other men in the city.

While asthma is not always linked to allergy, the two are related. Among people with asthma, 90 percent of the children, 70 percent of young adults, and 50 percent of older adults also have allergies. According to epidemiologic research, 23 percent of youngsters diagnosed with allergies by age 1 develop asthma by age 6. Of those diagnosed after age 1, 13 percent eventually become asthmatic. Symptoms include wheezing, coughing, shortness of breath, and chest tightness. If the symptoms are untreated or undertreated, they can worsen and damage the lungs. Oral contraceptives increase the risk in some women.[44]

 The number of people with asthma continues to increase into adulthood. However, as shown by a study that followed college students for 23 years, most report that their symptoms improve or disappear.

Over the last decade advances in asthma medications and tools have significantly improved management of this disease. Inhaled corticosteroids, long-acting bronchodilators (such as Advair), and leukotriene receptor antagonists (such as Singulair) have proven particularly helpful in controlling symptoms and preventing serious attacks that would require treatment with oral steroids.[45]

Ulcers

Open sores, often more than an inch wide, that develop in the lining of the stomach or the duodenum (the first part of the small intestine) are called **ulcers.** They are caused by excessive acidic digestive juices. The major symptom is a burning pain felt throughout the upper abdomen. The pain may come and go, lasting up to three hours. It may begin either right after eating or several hours later.

 One in five men and one in ten women get ulcers of the stomach or duodenum, but the number of ulcers is declining. Risk factors include heavy use of cigarettes, alcohol, or caffeine; the ingestion of large amounts of painkillers that contain aspirin or ibuprofen; and advanced age. Bleeding is not common but may be dangerous, even life-threatening. An untreated stomach ulcer can lead to serious weight loss and anemia.

Researchers have identified a bacterium, *Helicobacter pylori*, that may infect the digestive system and set the stage for ulcers. According to various studies, most ulcer patients carry this organism. One theory is that infection leads to an inflammation of the stomach lining called gastritis, which increases vulnerability to other stressors, such as smoking, alcohol, or anxiety. Treatment with antibiotics leads to improvement in most patients.

Conventional therapy for ulcers includes self-help measures, such as avoiding aspirin; eating small, frequent meals; taking antacids; and not smoking or drinking alcohol or caffeine. Drugs such as cimetidine, ranitidine, and sucralfate can reduce the amount of acid produced by the stomach and relieve ulcer symptoms.

epilepsy A variety of neurological disorders characterized by sudden attacks (seizures) of violent muscle contractions and unconsciousness.

asthma A disease or allergic response characterized by bronchial spasms and difficult breathing.

ulcer A lesion in, or an erosion of, the mucous membrane of an organ.

You may not be able to control every risk factor in your life or environment, but you can protect yourself from the obvious ones.

- **Don't smoke.** There's no bigger favor you can do for your heart or your lungs—your entire body.

- **Cut down on saturated fats and cholesterol.** This can help prevent high blood cholesterol levels, obesity, and heart disease.

- **Watch your weight.** Even relatively modest gains can have a big effect on your risk of heart disease. Overweight and obesity are associated with increased risks for cancers at several sites: breast (among post-menopausal women), colon, endometrium, esophagus (adenocarcinoma), and kidney.

- **Get moving.** Regular exercise can help lower your blood pressure, lower LDL, and reduce triglycerides.

- **Lower your stress levels.** If too much stress is a problem in your life, try the relaxation techniques described in Chapter 3.

- **Get your blood pressure checked regularly.** Knowing your numbers can alert you to a potential problem long before you develop any symptoms.

- **Avoid excessive exposure to ultraviolet light.** If you spend a lot of time outside, protect your skin by using sunscreen and wearing long-sleeve shirts and a hat. Also, wear sunglasses to protect your eyes. Don't purposely put yourself at risk by binge-sunbathing or by using sunlamps.

- **Control your alcohol intake.** The risk of cancers of the mouth, pharynx, larynx, esophagus, liver, and breast increases substantially with intake of more than two drinks per day for men or one drink for women.

- **Be alert to changes in your body.** You know your body's rhythms and appearance better than anyone else, and only you will know if certain things aren't right. Changes in bowel habits, skin changes, unusual lumps or discharges—anything out of the ordinary—may be clues that require further medical investigation.

SELF SURVEY Are You At Risk of Cancer?

Answer the following questions:

1. Do you protect your skin from overexposure to the sun? _____
2. Do you abstain from smoking or using tobacco in any form? _____
3. If you're over 40 or if family members have had colon cancer, do you get routine digital rectal exams? _____
4. Do you eat a balanced diet that includes the recommended daily value for vitamins A, B, and C? _____
5. If you're a woman, do you have regular Pap tests and pelvic exams? _____
6. If you're a man over 40, do you get regular prostate exams? _____
7. If you have burn scars or a history of chronic skin infections, do you get regular checkups? _____
8. Do you avoid smoked, salted, pickled, and high-nitrite foods? _____
9. If your job exposes you to asbestos, radiation, cadmium, or other environmental hazards, do you get regular checkups? _____
10. Do you limit your consumption of alcohol? _____
11. Do you avoid using tanning salons or home sunlamps? _____
12. If you're a woman, do you examine your breasts every month for lumps? _____
13. Do you eat plenty of vegetables and other sources of fiber? _____
14. If you're a man, do you perform regular testicular self-exams? _____
15. Do you wear protective sunglasses in sunlight? _____
16. Do you follow a low-fat diet? _____
17. Do you know the cancer warning signs? _____

Scoring

If you answered no to any of the questions, your risk for developing various kinds of cancer may be increased.

Your Health Action Plan for Detecting Cancer

Site	Recommendation
Breast	• Yearly mammograms are recommended starting at age 40. The age at which screening should be stopped should be individualized by considering the potential risks and benefits of screening in the context of overall health status and longevity. • Clinical breast exam should be part of a periodic health exam, about every 3 years for women in their twenties and thirties, and every year for women 40 and older. • Women should know how their breasts normally feel and report any breast change promptly to their health care providers. Breast self-exam is an option for women starting in their twenties. • Women at increased risk (e.g., family history, genetic tendency, past breast cancer) should talk with their doctors about the benefits and limitations of starting mammography screening earlier, having additional tests (i.e., breast ultrasound and MRI), or having more frequent exams.
Colon and Rectum	Beginning at age 50, men and women should begin screening with one of the examination schedules that follow: • A fecal occult blood test (FOBT) or fecal immunochemical test (FIT) every year. • A flexible sigmoidoscopy (FSIG) every 5 years. • Annual FOBT or FIT and flexible sigmoidoscopy every 5 years.* • A double-contrast barium enema every 5 years. • A colonoscopy every 10 years.
Prostate	The PSA test and the digital rectal examination should be offered annually, beginning at age 50, to men who have a life expectancy of at least 10 years. Men at high risk (African American men and men with a strong family history of one or more first-degree relatives diagnosed with prostate cancer at an early age) should begin testing at age 45. For both men at average risk and high risk, information should be provided about what is known and what is uncertain about the benefits and limitations of early detection and treatment of prostate cancer so that they can make an informed decision about testing.

Site	Recommendation
Uterus	**Cervix:** Screening should begin approximately 3 years after a woman begins having vaginal intercourse, but no later than 21 years of age. Screening should be done every year with regular Pap tests or every 2 years using liquid-based tests. At or after age 30, women who have had three normal test results in a row may get screened every 2 to 3 years. Alternatively, cervical cancer screening with human papilloma virus (HPV) DNA testing and conventional or liquid-based cytology could be performed every 3 years. However, doctors may suggest that a woman get screened more often if she has certain risk factors, such as HIV infection or a weak immune system. Women 70 years and older who have had three or more consecutive normal Pap tests in the last 10 years may choose to stop cervical cancer screening. Screening after total hysterectomy (with removal of the cervix) is not necessary unless the surgery was done as a treatment for cervical cancer. **Endometrium:** The American Cancer Society recommends that at the time of menopause all women should be informed about the risks and symptoms of endometrial cancer, and strongly encouraged to report any unexpected bleeding or spotting to their physicians. Annual screening for endometrial cancer with endometrial biopsy beginning at age 35 should be offered to women with or at risk for hereditary nonpolyposis colon cancer (HNPCC).
Cancer-Related Checkup	For individuals undergoing periodic health examinations, a cancer-related checkup should include health counseling, and, depending on a person's age and gender, might include examinations for cancers of the thyroid, oral cavity, skin, lymph nodes, testes, and ovaries, as well as for some nonmalignant diseases.

*Combined testing is preferred over either annual FOBT or FIT, or FSIG every 5 years, alone. People who are at moderate or high risk for colorectal cancer should talk with a doctor about a different testing schedule.

CENGAGENOW™ If you want to write your own goals for lowering your risk for major diseases, go to the Wellness Journal at CengageNOW for Health: **www.cengage.com/sso.**

Source: American Cancer Society, Cancer Facts and Figures-2007. © 2007 American Cancer Society, Inc. **www.cancer.org.** Reprinted with permission.

MAKING THIS CHAPTER WORK FOR YOU

Review Questions

1. The heart
   a. has four chambers, which are responsible for pumping blood into the veins for circulation through the body.
   b. pumps blood first to the lungs where it picks up oxygen and discards carbon dioxide.
   c. beats about 10,000 times and pumps about 75 gallons of blood per day.
   d. has specialized cells that generate electrical signals to control the amount of blood that circulates through the body.

2. A heart attack
   a. occurs when the myocardium receives an excessive amount of blood from the coronary arteries.
   b. is typically suffered by individuals who have irregular episodes of atherosclerosis.
   c. can be treated successfully up to four hours after the event.
   d. occurs when the myocardial cells are deprived of oxygen-carrying blood, causing them to die.

3. You can protect yourself from certain types of cancer by
   a. not smoking.
   b. avoiding people who have had cancer.
   c. wearing sunscreen with an SPF of less than 15.
   d. using condoms during sexual intercourse.

4. Which of the following statements about skin cancer is true?
   a. Individuals with a large number of moles are at decreased risk for melanoma.
   b. The most serious type of skin cancer is squamous cell carcinoma.
   c. The safest way to get a tan and avoid skin cancer is to use tanning salons and sunlamps instead of sunbathing in direct sunlight.
   d. Individuals with a history of childhood sunburn are at increased risk for melanoma.

5. A woman's risk of developing breast cancer increases if
   a. she is Caucasian over the age of 40.
   b. she had her first child when in her teens or twenties.
   c. her husband's mother had breast cancer.
   d. she began menstruating when she was 15 or 16.

6. Prostate cancer
   a. occurs mostly among men between the ages of 18 and 35.
   b. is usually more aggressive in white men.
   c. has a low survival rate.
   d. can be detected through a screening test that measures the levels of prostate-specific antigen in the blood.

7. You can control all of these cardiometabolic risk factors *except*
   a. lipoprotein levels.
   b. high blood glucose.
   c. family history.
   d. overweight.

8. Which of the following statements about diabetes mellitus is *false*?
   a. Individuals with type 2 diabetes can often control the disease without taking insulin.
   b. The incidence of diabetes has decreased in the last decade, especially among African Americans, Native Americans, and Latinos.
   c. Individuals with diabetes must measure the levels of glucose in their blood to ensure that it does not rise to unsafe levels.
   d. Untreated or uncontrolled diabetes can lead to coma and eventual death.

9. Hypertension
   a. is diagnosed when blood pressure is consistently lower than 130/85 mm Hg.
   b. may be treated with dietary changes, which include eating low-fat foods and avoiding sodium.
   c. can cause fatty deposits to collect on the artery walls.
   d. usually does not respond to medication, especially in severe cases.

10. In your lipoprotein profile, having a high level of this blood element is a good thing.
    a. HDL cholesterol
    b. LDL cholesterol
    c. C-reactive protein
    d. triglyceride

Answers to these questions can be found on page 650.

Critical Thinking

1. Have you had your blood pressure checked lately? If your reading was high, what steps are you now taking to help reduce your blood pressure?

2. Have you had a lipoprotein profile lately? Do you think it's necessary for you to obtain one? If your reading was/is borderline or high, what lifestyle changes can you make to help control your cholesterol level?

3. Do you have family members who have had cancer? Were these individuals at risk for cancer because of specific environmental factors, such as long-term exposure to tobacco smoke? If no particular cause was identified, what other factors could have triggered their diseases? Are you concerned that you might have inherited a genetic predisposition to any particular type of cancer because of your family history?

4. A friend of yours, Karen, discovered a small lump in her breast during a routine self-examination. When she mentions it, you ask if she has seen a doctor. She tells you that she hasn't had time to schedule an appointment; besides, she says, she's not sure it's really the kind of lump one has to worry about. It's clear to you that Karen is in denial and procrastinating about seeing a doctor. What advice would you give her?

Media Menu

Internet Connections

www.diabetes.org

Here you will find the latest information on both type 1 and type 2 diabetes mellitus, including suggestions regarding diet and exercise. The online bookstore features meal planning guides, cookbooks, and self-care guides. Type in your zip code to find community resources.

www.americanheart.org

This comprehensive site features a searchable database of all major cardiovascular diseases, plus information on healthy lifestyles, current research, CPR, cardiac warning signs, risk awareness, low-cholesterol diets, and family health. The interactive Heart Profilers® provides personalized information about treatment options for common cardiovascular conditions such as hypertension, heart failure, and cholesterol.

www.fi.edu/biosci/heart.html

This interesting site, developed by the Franklin Institute of Science, provides an interactive multimedia tour of the heart, as well as statistics, resources, links, and information on how to monitor your heart's health by becoming aware of your vital signs.

www.cdc.gov/cancer/

This site, sponsored by the Centers for Disease Control and Prevention (CDC), features current information on cancer of the breast, cervix, prostate, skin, and colon. The site also provides monthly spotlights on specific cancers, as well as links to the National Comprehensive Cancer Control Program and the National Program of Cancer Registries.

Key Terms

The terms listed are used on the page indicated. Definitions of the terms are in the Glossary at the end of the book.

angina pectoris 463
aorta 455
arteriosclerosis 461
asthma 479
atherosclerosis 461
atrium 455
capillary 455
cardiometabolic 441
cardiopulmonary
   resuscitation (CPR) 463
cholesterol 442
diabetes mellitus 447
diastole 455
diastolic blood pressure 442
epilepsy 479
hypertension 442
infiltration 467
lipoprotein 442
lumpectomy 475
mammography 475
mastectomy 475
metabolic syndrome 445
metastasize 467
myocardial infarction (MI) 463
plaque 461
prehypertension 451
relative risk 469
stroke 465
systole 455
systolic blood pressure 442
transient ischemic attack (TIA) 465
triglyceride 442
ulcer 479
ventricle 455

Chapter 15 - Avoiding Infectious Diseases

1. An organism that can cause disease in the human body is known as a: (pg 486)
   - A. host
   - B. pathogen
   - C. vector
   - D. bacterium

2. The biological or physical vehicle that transfers the organism to a host represents: (pg 486)
   - A. pathogen
   - B. virus
   - C. vector
   - D. carrier

3. The most plentiful of all organisms are: (pg 487)
   - A. bacteria
   - B. mold
   - C. viruses
   - D. mosquitoes

4. All of the following except one are ways that microorganisms get around to infect the human body: (pg 488)
   - A. water
   - B. insects
   - C. toilet seats
   - D. food

5. Where do many invading pathogens get taken to in the body to be destroyed? (pg 489)
   - A. spleen
   - B. red blood cells
   - C. bone marrow
   - D. lymph nodes

6. Receiving a vaccine to protect oneself from a serious infectious disease is known as: (pg 490)
   - A. passive immunity
   - B. active immunity
   - C. immune efficiency
   - D. immunotherapy

7. Which of the following is not an effective strategy for preventing the common cold? (pg 497)
   - A. frequent handwashing
   - B. exercising daily
   - C. avoiding stress overload
   - D. using a handkerchief instead of disposal tissues

8. The incubation of an organism inside your body is the time: (pg 488)
   - A. between the first exposure to the organism to the first symptom
   - B. when you are most contagious to other people
   - C. the body's immune system kicks in to fight off the invading organisms from spreading
   - D. the disease has died off and recovery begins

9. The difference between an adenovirus and a rhinovirus is: (pg 496)
   - A. adenoviruses occur more in the spring months of the year
   - B. rhinoviruses are usually lower respiratory with coughing and bronchitis
   - C. rhinoviruses tend to be in the fall and cause more nasal type colds
   - D. rhinoviruses occur more during the cold winter months

10. Sally has a bad runny nose cold and sneezing. She should look for a cold medicine that is a(n): (pg 497)
   - A. expectorant
   - B. pain reliever
   - C. cough suppressant
   - D. antihistamine

11. **Inflammation is usually characterized by: (pg 491)**
    A. pale clammy skin with perspiration
    B. redness and swelling at wound site
    C. high fevers and delirium
    D. blotches on the skin

12. **Meningitis, whether the bacterial or viral species, causes 1/3 of the illness among which population group ? (pg 499)**
    A. newborn babies
    B. young children
    C. late teens through college-aged students
    D. senior citizens

13. **Even if you patronize a legal body art studio to have a piercing or tattoo placed on your body and it is done in a sanitary manner, it is still possible to pick up diseases like: (p 501)**
    A. Herpes
    B. Hepatitis B
    C. Hepatitis A
    D. Group A Strep infection

14. **The greatest danger from having contracted mononucleosis is: (pg 502)**
    A. never being able to kiss another person again
    B. rupturing the spleen from physical activity
    C. developing tuberculosis as a secondary infection
    D. developing mumps of the salivary glands

15. **Lyme disease is caused by the parasite: (pg 506)**
    A. mosquito
    B. rats
    C. ticks
    D. fleas

16. **What other acute infectious disease claims more lives besides pneumonia? (pg 503)**
    A. mononucleosis
    B. strep infection
    C. meningitis
    D. tuberculosis

17. **The pending avian or swine flu is expected to cause a pandemic. This means that: (pg 509)**
    A. outbreaks will only be sporadic in different places
    B. widespread illness will affect many people in the United States only
    C. widespread illness will affect many people globally
    D. the bird population will be the first to succumb to the viral attack

18. **In which Pandemic Phase would increased and sustained mass spread of the virus among the population be identified as? (pg 509)**
    A. pandemic period phase 6
    B. interpandemic period phase 1
    C. pandemic alert period phase 3
    D. pandemic alert phase 5

19. **Which of the following statements is true to protect yourself from infectious diseases? (pg 514)**
    A. immunizations are only important to receive as an infant and not necessary in adult life
    B. hand washing is a very useful means of protection against seasonal influenza
    C. reducing your stress level doesn't do anything to protect yourself from illness
    D. it is not necessary to wash fruits and vegetables prior to consuming

20. **All of the following are important health action plans to take to minimize your chance of contracting a serious infectious disease for which of the following: (pg 514)**
    A. avoid eating fatty foods
    B. use a cloth handkerchief rather than paper tissues
    C. wash your hands frequently
    D. stay away from large crowds during the flu season

Zach shrugged off the headache and sore throat he woke up with and rushed to class. During the lecture he started shivering. When he got up to leave, his legs felt shaky, and it hurt to walk. His entire body seemed stiff. Back in his dorm, Zach collapsed onto his bed. He felt feverish. His head throbbed. He started vomiting. Dark blotches broke out on his forehead, arms, and legs.

That evening his resident advisor drove Zach to the emergency room. The pain in his legs was excruciating, but his blood pressure was so low that the doctors

Avoiding Infectious Diseases

couldn't give him pain medication. A spinal tap revealed that Zach had bacterial meningitis, a potentially deadly infection that causes swelling in the brain and spinal cord. Intensive treatment saved Zach's life, although he suffered hearing loss and severe nerve damage that required months of rehabilitation. Zach considers himself lucky. Bacterial meningitis can strike so unexpectedly and worsen so quickly that it can kill a healthy young person within days.

Throughout history, infectious diseases have claimed more lives than any military conflict or natural disaster. Although modern medicine has won many victories against the agents of infection, we remain vulnerable to a host of infectious illnesses. Drug-resistant strains of tuberculosis and *Staphylococcus* bacteria challenge current therapies. New infectious diseases such as swine flu are emerging and traveling around the world. Agents of infection also can be used as weapons of war and terrorism.

This chapter is a lesson in self-defense against all forms of infection. The information it provides can help you boost your defenses, recognize and avoid enemies, shield yourself from infections, and realize when to seek help.

After studying the material in this chapter, you should be able to

- **Explain** how the different agents of infection spread disease.
- **Describe** how your body protects itself from infectious disease.
- **List** ways to protect yourself from catching a cold or the flu and ways to feel better if you do catch one.
- **Name** and **describe** some common infectious diseases.
- **Explain** pandemic and **describe** the levels of alert.
- **Name** the infectious diseases for which you are most at risk, and **list** your strategies for avoiding them.

Log on to CengageNOW for Health at **www.cengage.com/sso** to find your Behavior Change Planner and to explore self-assessments, interactive tutorials, and practice quizzes.

Understanding Infection

(a)

(b)

(c)

(d)

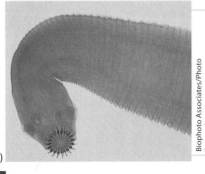

(e)

© Purdue University Photo/Rossmann Lab

© Dr. David Chase/Phototake

© E. GUEHO/Photo Researchers, Inc.

Professors P.M. Motta & F.M. Magliocca/ Photo Researchers, Inc

Biophoto Associates/Photo Researchers, Inc.

We live in a sea of microbes. Most of them don't threaten our health or survival; some, such as the bacteria that inhabit our intestines, are actually beneficial. Yet in the course of history, disease-causing microorganisms have claimed millions of lives. The twentieth century brought the conquest of infectious killers such as cholera and scarlet fever. Although modern science has won many victories against the agents of infection, infectious illnesses remain a serious health threat.

Infection is a complex process, triggered by various **pathogens** (disease-causing organisms) and countered by the body's own defenders. Physicians explain infection in terms of a **host** (either a person or a population) that contacts one or more agents in an environment. A **vector**—a biological or physical vehicle that carries the agent to the host—provides the means of transmission.

Agents of Infection

The types of microbes that can cause infection are viruses, bacteria, fungi, protozoa, and helminths (parasitic worms).

Viruses The tiniest pathogens—**viruses**—are also the toughest; they consist of a bit of nucleic acid (DNA or RNA,

Examples of the major categories of organisms that cause disease in humans. Except for the helminthes (parasitic worms), pathogens are microorganisms that can be seen only with the aid of a microscope. (a) Viruses: common cold, (b) Bacteria: syphilis, (c) Fungi: athlete's foot fungus, (d) Protozoa: Giardia lamblia, (e) Helminths: tapeworm.

but never both) within a protein coat. Unable to reproduce on its own, a virus takes over a body cell's reproductive machinery and instructs it to produce new viral particles, which are then released to enter other cells. The common cold, the flu, herpes, hepatitis, and AIDS are viral diseases.

The most common viruses are these types:

- **Rhinoviruses and adenoviruses**, which get into the mucous membranes and cause upper respiratory tract infections and colds.

- **Coronaviruses**, named for their corona, or halo-like appearance, are second only to rhinoviruses in causing the common cold and other respiratory infections. A coronavirus is the cause of severe acute respiratory syndrome (SARS).

- **Influenza viruses**, which can change their outer protein coats so dramatically that individuals resistant to one strain cannot fight off a new one. (See page 508 for a discussion of the H1N1 (swine flu) virus.)

- **Herpes viruses**, which take up permanent residence in the cells and periodically flare up.

- **Papilloma viruses**, which cause few symptoms in women and almost none in men but may be responsible, at least in part, for a rise in the incidence of cervical cancer among younger women.

- **Hepatitis viruses**, which cause several forms of liver infection, ranging from mild to life-threatening.

- **Slow viruses**, which give no early indication of their presence but can produce fatal illnesses within a few years.

- **Retroviruses**, which are named for their backward (retro) sequence of genetic replication compared to other viruses. One retrovirus, human immunodeficiency virus (HIV), causes acquired immune deficiency syndrome (AIDS).

- **Filoviruses**, which resemble threads and are extremely lethal.

The problem in fighting viruses is that it's difficult to find drugs that harm the virus and not the cell it has commandeered. **Antibiotics** (drugs that inhibit or kill bacteria) have no effect on viruses. **Antiviral drugs** don't completely eradicate a viral infection, although they can decrease its severity and duration. Because viruses multiply very quickly, antiviral drugs are most effective when taken before an infection develops or in its early stages.

Bacteria Simple one-celled organisms, **bacteria** are the most plentiful microorganisms as well as the most pathogenic. Most kinds of bacteria don't cause disease; some, like certain strains of *Escherichia coli* that aid in digestion, play important roles within our bodies. Even friendly bacteria, however, can get out of hand and cause acne, urinary tract infections, vaginal infections, and other problems.

Bacteria harm the body by releasing either enzymes that digest body cells or toxins that produce the specific effects of such diseases as diphtheria or toxic shock syndrome. In self-defense, the body produces specific proteins (called *antibodies)* that attack and inactivate the invaders. Tuberculosis, tetanus, gonorrhea, scarlet fever, and diphtheria are examples of bacterial diseases.

Because bacteria are sufficiently different from the cells that make up our bodies, antibiotics can kill them without harming our cells. Antibiotics work only against specific types of bacteria. If your doctor thinks you have a bacterial infection, tests of your blood, pus, sputum, urine, or stool can identify the particular bacterial strain.

Fungi Single-celled or multicelled organisms, **fungi** consist of threadlike fibers and reproductive spores. Fungi lack chlorophyll and must obtain their food from organic material, which may include human tissue. Fungi release enzymes that digest cells and are most likely to attack hair-covered areas of the body, including the scalp, beard, groin, and external ear canals. They also cause athlete's foot. Treatment consists of antifungal drugs.

Protozoa These single-celled, microscopic animals release enzymes and toxins that destroy cells or interfere with their function. Diseases caused by **protozoa** are not a major health problem in this country, primarily because of public health measures. Around the world, however, some 2.24 billion people (more than 40 percent of the world's population) are at risk for acquiring malaria—a protozoan-caused disease. Up to 3 million die from this disease annually. Many more come down with amoebic dysentery. Treatment for protozoa-caused diseases consists of general medical care to relieve the symptoms, replacement of lost blood or fluids, and drugs that kill the specific protozoan.

The most common disease caused by protozoa in the United States is *giardiasis,* an intestinal infection caused by microorganisms in human and animal feces. It has become a threat at day-care centers, as well as among campers and hikers who drink contaminated water. Symptoms include nausea, lack of appetite, gas, diarrhea, fatigue, abdominal cramps, and bloating. Many people recover in a month or two without treatment. However, in some cases the microbe causes recurring attacks over many years. Giardiasis can be life-threatening in small children and the elderly, who are especially prone to severe dehydration from diarrhea. Treatment usually consists of antibiotics.

Helminths (Parasitic Worms) Small parasitic worms that attack specific tissues or organs and compete with the host for nutrients are called **helminths.** One major worldwide health problem is *schistosomiasis,* a disease caused by a parasitic worm, the fluke, that burrows through the skin and enters the circulatory system. Infection with another helminth, the tapeworm, may be contracted from eating undercooked beef, pork, or fish containing larval forms of the tapeworm. Helminthic diseases are treated with appropriate medications.

How Infections Spread

The major *vectors*, or means of transmission, for infectious disease are animals and insects, people, food, and water.

Animals and Insects Disease can be transmitted by house pets, livestock, birds, and wild animals. Insects also spread a variety

pathogen A microorganism that produces disease.

host A person or population that contracts one or more pathogenic agents in an environment.

vector A biological or physical vehicle that carries the agent of infection to the host.

virus A submicroscopic infectious agent; the most primitive form of life.

antibiotics Substances produced by microorganisms, or synthetic agents, that are toxic to bacteria.

antiviral drug A substance that decreases the severity and duration of a viral infection if taken prior to or soon after onset of the infection.

bacteria (singular, **bacterium**) One-celled microscopic organisms; the most plentiful pathogens.

fungi (singular, **fungus**) Organisms that reproduce by means of spores.

protozoa Microscopic animals made up of one cell or a group of similar cells.

helminth A parasitic roundworm or flatworm.

of diseases. The housefly may spread dysentery, diarrhea, typhoid fever, or trachoma (an eye disease rare in the United States but common in other parts of the world). Other insects, including mosquitoes, ticks, mites, fleas, and lice, can transmit such diseases as malaria, yellow fever, encephalitis, dengue fever (a growing threat in Mexico), and Lyme disease.

New threats in the United States include West Nile virus (WNV), which can be spread to humans by mosquitoes that bite infected birds, and monkeypox virus, carried by various animals, including prairie dogs. Concern has grown about avian influenza, or bird flu, which has spread to wild and domestic birds around the world. H1N1 (swine) flu, which can be transmitted between humans and pigs, appeared as a threat in 2009. (These illnesses are discussed later in this chapter.)

People The people you're closest to can transmit pathogens through the air, through touch, or through sexual contact. To avoid infection, stay out of range of anyone who's coughing, sniffling, or sneezing, and don't share food or dishes. Carefully wash your dishes, utensils, and hands, and abstain from sex or make self-protective decisions about sexual partners. (See Chapter 16 on Sexually Transmitted Infections.)

Food Every year foodborne illnesses strike millions of Americans, sometimes with fatal consequences. Bacteria account for two-thirds of foodborne infections, and thousands of suspected cases of infection with *Escherichia coli* bacteria in undercooked or inadequately washed food have been reported. (See Chapter 6 for more on *E. coli* outbreaks.)

Every year as many as 4 million Americans have a bout with *Salmonella* bacteria, which have been found in about a third of all poultry sold in the United States. These infections can be serious enough to require hospitalization and can lead to arthritis, neurological problems, and even death. Consumers can greatly reduce the number of salmonella infections by proper handling, cooking, and refrigeration of poultry (see Chapter 6).

Water Waterborne diseases, such as typhoid fever and cholera, are still widespread in less developed areas of the world. They have been rare in the United States, although outbreaks caused by inadequate water purification have occurred.

The Process of Infection

If someone infected with the flu sits next to you on a bus and coughs or sneezes, tiny viral particles may travel into your nose and mouth. Immediately, the virus finds or creates an opening in the wall of a cell, and the process of infection begins. During the **incubation period,** the time between invasion and the first symptom, you're unaware of the pathogen multiplying inside you. In some diseases, incubation may go on for months, even years; for most, it lasts several days or weeks.

The early stage of the battle between your body and the invaders is called the *prodromal period*. As infected cells die, they release chemicals that help block the invasion. Other chemicals, such as *histamines,* cause blood vessels to dilate, thus allowing more blood to reach the battleground. During all of this, you feel mild, generalized symptoms, such as headache, irritability, and discomfort. You're also highly contagious. At the height of the battle—the typical illness period—you cough, sneeze, sniffle, ache, feel feverish, and lose your appetite.

Recovery begins when the body's forces gain the advantage. With time, the body destroys the last of the invaders and heals itself. However, the body is not able to develop long-lasting immunity to certain viruses, such as colds, flu, or HIV.

Who Is at Highest Risk?

Like human bullies, the viruses responsible for the most common infectious illnesses tend to pick on those least capable of fighting back. Among the most vulnerable are the following groups:

- **Children and their families.** Youngsters get up to a dozen colds annually; adults average two a year. When a flu epidemic hits a community, about 40 percent of school-age boys and girls get sick, compared with only 5 to 10 percent of adults. But parents get up to six times as many colds as other adults.

- **The elderly.** Statistically, fewer older men and women are likely to catch a cold or flu, yet when they do, they face greater danger than the rest of the population. People over 65 who get the flu have a one in ten chance of being hospitalized for pneumonia or other respiratory problems, and a one in fifty chance of dying from the disease.
- **The chronically ill.** Lifelong diseases, such as diabetes, kidney disease, or sickle-cell anemia, decrease an individual's ability to fend off infections. Individuals taking medications that suppress the immune system, such as steroids, are more vulnerable to infections, as are those with medical conditions that impair immunity, such as infection with HIV.
- **Smokers and those with respiratory problems.** Smokers are a high-risk group for respiratory infections and serious complications, such as pneumonia. Chronic breathing disorders, such as asthma and emphysema, also greatly increase the risk of respiratory infections.
- **Those who live or work in close contact with someone sick.** Health-care workers who treat high-risk patients, nursing home residents, and others living in close quarters—such as students in dormitories—face greater odds of catching others' colds and flus.
- **Residents or workers in poorly ventilated buildings.** Building technology has helped spread certain airborne illnesses, such as tuberculosis, via recirculated air. Indoor air quality can be closely linked with disease transmission in winter, when people spend a great deal of time in tightly sealed rooms.

How Your Body Protects Itself

Various parts of your body safeguard you against infectious diseases by providing **immunity,** or protection, from these health threats. Your skin, when unbroken, keeps out most potential invaders. Your tears, sweat, skin oils, saliva, and mucus contain chemicals that can kill bacteria. Cilia, the tiny hairs lining your respiratory passages, move mucus, which traps inhaled bacteria, viruses, dust, and foreign matter, to the back of the throat, where it is swallowed; the digestive system then destroys the invaders.

When these protective mechanisms can't keep you infection-free, your body's immune system, which is on constant alert for foreign substances that might threaten the body, swings into action. The immune system includes structures of the lymphatic system—the spleen, thymus gland, lymph nodes, and lymph vessels—that help filter impurities from the body (Figure 15.1). The **lymph nodes,** or glands, are small tissue masses in which some protective cells are stored. If pathogens invade your body, many of them are carried to the lymph nodes to be destroyed. This is why your lymph nodes often feel swollen when you have a cold or the flu.

More than a dozen different types of white blood cells (lymphocytes) are concentrated in the organs of the lymphatic system or patrol the entire body by way of the blood and lymph vessels. Some of these white blood cells are generalists and some are specialists. The generalists include *macrophages*, which are large scavenger cells with insatiable appetites for foreign cells, diseased and run-down red blood cells, and other biological debris (Figure 15.2 on p. 491). The specialists are the *B cells* and *T cells*, which respond to specific invaders.

An *antigen* is any substance the white blood cells recognize as foreign. B cells create antibodies, which are proteins that bind to antigens and mark them for destruction by other white blood cells. Antigens are specific to the pathogen, and the antibody to a particular antigen binds only to that antigen (Figure 15.2). Once the human

incubation period The time between a pathogen's entrance into the body and the first symptom.

immunity Protection from infectious diseases.

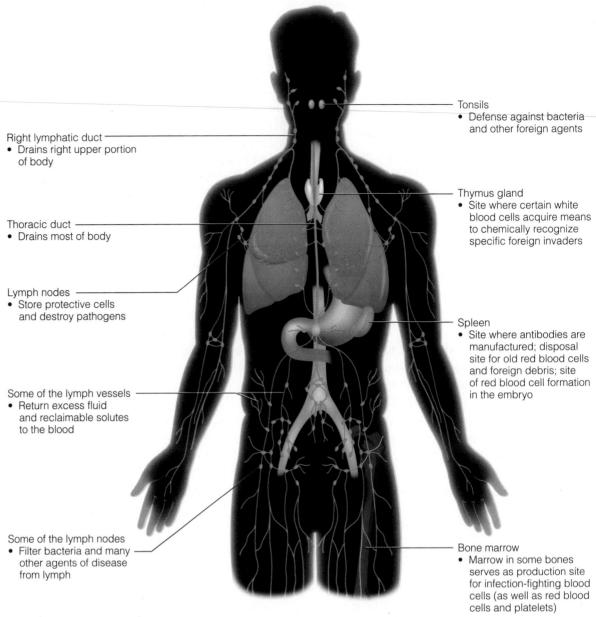

Right lymphatic duct
- Drains right upper portion of body

Thoracic duct
- Drains most of body

Lymph nodes
- Store protective cells and destroy pathogens

Some of the lymph vessels
- Return excess fluid and reclaimable solutes to the blood

Some of the lymph nodes
- Filter bacteria and many other agents of disease from lymph

Tonsils
- Defense against bacteria and other foreign agents

Thymus gland
- Site where certain white blood cells acquire means to chemically recognize specific foreign invaders

Spleen
- Site where antibodies are manufactured; disposal site for old red blood cells and foreign debris; site of red blood cell formation in the embryo

Bone marrow
- Marrow in some bones serves as production site for infection-fighting blood cells (as well as red blood cells and platelets)

Figure 15.1   The Human Lymphatic System and Its Functions
The lymphatic system helps filter impurities from the body.

body produces antibodies against a specific antigen—the mumps virus, for instance—you're protected against that antigen for life. If you're again exposed to mumps, the antibodies previously produced prevent another episode of the disease.

But you don't have to suffer through an illness to acquire immunity. Inoculation with a vaccine containing synthetic or weakened antigens can give you the same protection. The type of long-lasting immunity in which the body makes its own antibodies to a pathogen is called *active immunity*. Immunity produced by the injection of **gamma globulin**, the antibody-containing part of the blood from another person or animal that has developed antibodies to a disease, is called *passive immunity*.

Immune Response

Attacked by pathogens, the body musters its forces and fights. Sometimes the invasion is handled like a minor border skirmish; other times a full-scale battle is waged throughout the body. Together, the immune cells work like an internal police force. When an antigen enters the body, the T cells aided by macrophages engage in combat with the

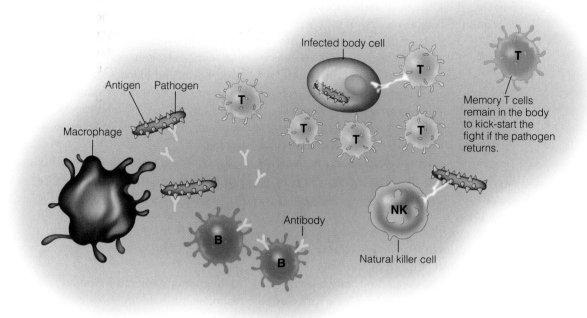

Figure 15.2 The Immune Response

Some T cells can kill infected body cells. B cells churn out antibodies to tag pathogens for destruction by macrophages and other white blood cells.

invader. Certain T cells (cytotoxic T cells) can destroy infected body cells or tumor cells by "touch-killing." Meanwhile, the B cells churn out antibodies, which rush to the scene and join in the fray. Also busy at surveillance are natural killer cells that, like the elite forces of a SWAT team, seek out and destroy viruses and cancer cells (Figure 15.2).

If the microbes establish a foothold, the blood supply to the area increases, bringing oxygen and nutrients to the fighting cells. Tissue fluids, as well as antibacterial and antitoxic proteins, accumulate. You may develop redness, swelling, local warmth, and pain—the signs of **inflammation.**

Chronic low-grade inflammation increases by twofold to fourfold the levels of cytokines, substances secreted by certain immune cells, in the bloodstream. These elevated levels serve as inflammatory markers that have emerged as major players in the development of several major diseases, including atherosclerosis, hypertension, and other cardiovascular disorders, insulin resistance, metabolic syndrome, type 2 diabetes, and cancer. Recent research has linked chronic inflammation with depression as well.[1] Medical scientists are continuing to investigate the role of inflammatory markers and to identify ways to reduce elevated levels. In a number of studies, vigorous exercise, including cycling, running, swimming, and resistance training, did reduce markers of inflammation. The impact of these markers on disease risk and progression is not yet clear.

Systemic Disease As more tissue is destroyed, a cavity, or **abscess,** forms and fills with fluid, battling cells, and dead white blood cells (pus). If the invaders aren't killed or inactivated, the pathogens are able to spread into the bloodstream and cause what is known as **systemic disease.**

Some people have an **immune deficiency**—either inborn or acquired. A very few children are born without an effective immune system; their lives can be endangered by any infection. Although still experimental, therapy to implant a missing or healthy gene may offer new hope for a normal life.

Immunity and Stress

Whenever we confront a crisis, large or small, our bodies produce powerful hormones that provide extra energy. However,

lymph nodes Small tissue masses in which some immune cells are stored.

gamma globulin The antibody-containing portion of the blood fluid (plasma).

inflammation A localized response by the body to tissue injury, characterized by swelling and the dilation of the blood vessels.

this stress response dampens immunity, reducing the number of some key immune cells and the responsiveness of others.

 As discussed in Chapter 3, stressful experiences in childhood can have a long-term effect on health.[2] Students' stress and mental health affects their susceptibility to infections. In an analysis of ACHA data on more than 47,000 undergraduates, those who did not report depression, anxiety, or exhaustion were least likely to develop an acute infectious illness (bronchitis, ear infection, sinus infection, or strep throat). The more exhausted students said they were, the greater their probability of coming down with an infection.[3]

Stress affects the body's immune system in different ways, depending on two factors: the controllability or uncontrollability of the stressor and the mental effort required to cope with the stress. An uncontrollable stressor that lasts longer than 15 minutes may interfere with cytokine interleukin-6, which plays an essential role in activating the immune defenses. Uncontrollable stressors also produce high levels of the hormone cortisol, which suppresses immune system functioning. The mental efforts required to cope with high-level stressors produce only brief immune changes that appear to have little consequence for health. However, stress has been shown to slow pro-inflammatory cytokine production, which is essential for healing.

Immunity and Gender

 When the flu hits a household, the last one left standing is likely to be Mom. The female immune system responds more vigorously to common infections, offering extra protection against viruses, bacteria, and parasites.

The genders also differ in their vulnerability to allergies and autoimmune disorders. Although both men and women frequently develop allergies, allergic women are twice as likely to experience potentially fatal anaphylactic shock. A woman's robust immune system also is more likely to overreact and turn on her own organs and tissues. On average, three of four people with autoimmune disorders, such as multiple sclerosis, Hashimoto's thyroiditis, and scleroderma, are women.

Why are there such large gender differences in susceptibility? Scientists believe that the sex hormones have a great impact on immunity. Through a woman's childbearing years, estrogen, which protects heart, bone, brain, and blood vessels, also bolsters the immune system's response to certain infectious agents. Women produce greater numbers of antibodies when exposed to an antigen.

In contrast, testosterone may suppress this response—possibly to prevent attacks on sperm cells, which might otherwise be mistaken as alien invaders. When the testes are removed from mice and guinea pigs, their immune systems become more active.

Pregnancy dampens a woman's immune response, probably to ensure that her natural protectors don't attack the fetus as a foreign invader. This impact is so great that pregnant women with transplanted kidneys may require lower doses of drugs to prevent organ rejection. Pregnant women with multiple sclerosis and rheumatoid arthritis typically experience decreased symptoms during the nine months of gestation, then return to their prepregnancy state after giving birth. Oral contraceptives also can diminish symptoms of multiple sclerosis and rheumatoid arthritis. Neither pregnancy nor birth control pills has such an impact on lupus.

Immune Disorders

Sometimes our immune system overreacts to certain substances, mistakes the body's own tissues for enemies, or doesn't react adequately. The result is immune disorders such as allergies and autoimmune disorders.

Allergies An **allergy** represents a hypersensitivity to a substance in the environment or diet that does not bother most other people. More than half of Americans between ages 6 and 59 are sensitive to one or more allergens. Allergies consistently rate as one of the top health problems among college students. In one study, almost half of college students reported a problem with allergies in the previous year. Allergies are the sixth leading cause of chronic disease and cost the U.S. health-care system approximately $18 billion annually.

Among the substances that trigger allergic reactions are:

- Pollen.
- Dust mites.
- Mold spores.
- Pet dander.
- Food (discussed in Chapter 6).
- Insect stings.
- Medicine.

In an allergic reaction, the immune system reacts as if it were defending the body against germs such as bacteria and viruses. When an allergic person first comes into contact with an allergen, the immune system generates large amounts of a type of antibody called immunoglobulin E or IgE. Each IgE antibody is specific for one particular substance, such as a particular pollen. The next time the allergen encounters its specific IgE, it attaches to it like a key fitting into a lock. This signals the cell to produce or release powerful chemicals like histamine that cause inflammation and the symptoms of allergy. The most common are:

- Runny or clogged nose.
- Sneezing.
- Coughing.
- Itching eyes, nose, and throat.
- Eye irritation.

Allergy sufferers run annual tabs of up to $2 billion in doctor visits, diagnostic tests, prescriptions, and decreased productivity. Every year allergies account for more than 10 million workdays missed; every day they keep 10,000 children out of school.

Thanks to treatment breakthroughs, allergy sufferers no longer have to choose between feeling better or feeling alert. Treatment options include nonsedating oral medications, nasal sprays, and **immunotherapy,** which consists of a series of injections of small but increasing doses of an allergen.

Autoimmune Disorders Sometimes the body's defenses go awry, and the immune system declares war on the cells, tissues, or organs it normally protects. **Autoimmune disorders** rank among the top ten killers and disablers of American adults, particularly women. They strike about three times as many women as men, possibly because of the effects of female hormones on the immune system. Women are most vulnerable in the prime of life, during their reproductive years. (See Table 15.1.)

Some autoimmune disorders directly damage a single organ, as happens with Addison's disease, which targets the adrenal glands, or Crohn's disease, which affects the gastrointestinal tract. Other autoimmune disorders attack multiple organs. Systemic lupus erythematosus, for instance, can affect the skin, joints, kidneys, heart, brain, and red blood cells.

For many people with autoimmune disorders, the biggest challenge is finding out what's wrong. Early symptoms, such as low-grade fever or achiness, often wax and wane and are dismissed or misdiagnosed by doctors. New blood tests for lupus and multiple sclerosis are promising faster, more accurate diagnoses, but for many autoimmune disorders, there are no conclusive laboratory tests.

Patients should keep a detailed record of when symptoms start, recur, flare, or subside, and seek a specialist—a rheumatologist, dermatologist, immunologist, or gastroenterologist, depending on symptoms—who has expertise in autoimmune disorders. New treatments are revolutionizing treatments for many autoimmune disorders, including rheumatoid arthritis.

abscess A localized accumulation of pus and disintegrating tissue.

systemic disease A pathologic condition that spreads throughout the body.

immune deficiency Partial or complete inability of the immune system to respond to pathogens.

allergy A hypersensitivity to a particular substance in one's environment or diet.

immunotherapy A series of injections of small but increasing doses of an allergen, used to treat allergies.

autoimmune disorder Resulting from the attack on body tissue by an immune system that fails to recognize the tissue as self.

Immunization for Adults

One of the great success stories of modern medicine has been the development of vaccines that provide protection against many infectious diseases. Immunization has reduced cases of measles, mumps, tetanus, whooping cough, and other life-threatening illnesses by more than 95 percent. Nonetheless some parents remain reluctant

TABLE 15.1

Autoimmune Disorders

Disorder	Characteristics	Prevalence in Women vs. Men	Common Symptoms
Systemic lupus erythematosus (Lupus)	A chronic autoimmune disorder that can affect any tissue or organ system, including the joints, kidneys, heart, lungs, brain, blood, or skin.	9:1	Achy joints; frequent fever of 100°F or higher; anemia; fatigue; arthritis; skin rash; butterfly-shaped rash across cheek and nose; hair loss.
Graves' disease	A thyroid condition characterized by an overactive thyroid gland, which produces too much thyroid hormone.	7:1	Nervousness and irritability; weight loss; fast/irregular heart rate; heat intolerance/increased perspiration; increased appetite; sleep disturbances (such as insomnia); muscle weakness; trembling hands; irregular menstrual periods; exophthalmos (bulging eyes); appearance of a goiter (a swelling in the neck caused by enlargement of the thyroid gland).
Scleroderma	Proliferation of immune cells that produce scar tissue in the skin, some internal organs, and small blood vessels.	3:1	Reynaud's phenomenon, a condition characterized by decreased blood flow, usually to the fingers, and often brought on by cold temperatures; swelling and puffiness of the fingers or hands, followed by skin thickening a few months later; skin ulcers on the fingers; joint stiffness in the hands; sore throat; diarrhea.
Rheumatoid arthritis	Develops when the immune system attacks the synovium (the membranes that surround joints) causing inflammation, which gradually destroys cartilage, making movement of the joints painful and difficult. May also affect muscles, lungs, and liver.	2.5:1	Inflamed, swollen, and tender joints that may eventually become deformed; weakness or loss of function of joints; morning stiffness, fatigue, or general sense of malaise. Often affects joints in a symmetrical pattern: If one knee or hand is affected, usually the other one also is impaired.
Multiple sclerosis	Occurs when the immune system attacks the myelin sheath—the fatty insulation surrounding nerve cells in the brain and spinal cord. The myelin sheath enables high-speed transmission of messages between these centers and the rest of the body; gradually, as scar tissue develops in different areas of myelin, nerve messages are disrupted, affecting the body in a variety of ways.	2:1	Fatigue; short-term memory problems; temporary weakness, tingling, or paralysis in one or more limbs; loss of coordination or unsteady gait; balance problems; swallowing; any or all symptoms may appear and then subside, then appear again, weeks, months, or years later.

Sources: American Autoimmune Related Diseases Association, Inc.; American Diabetes Association; American Thyroid Association; Lupus Foundation of America; National Graves' Disease Foundation; National Institute of Diabetes and Digestive and Kidney Diseases; National Institute of Arthritis and Musculoskeletal and Skin Diseases; National Multiple Sclerosis Society.

to vaccinate their children. (See Point/Counterpoint.)

However, according to a recent government survey, adult immunization rates are "unacceptably low," and many people are unaware of the threat of infectious diseases. In the survey, only 2 percent of 18- to 64-year-olds are immunized against tetanus-diphtheria-whooping cough; just about 10 percent of women age 18 to 26 are immunized against HPV.[4]

Although many people think that vaccines are only for children, they remain an important part of protection throughout life. Table 15.2 lists the vaccines recommended for college students and Figure 15.3 shows the recommended adult immunization schedule. (See Reality Check, p. 499.)

One increased risk for adults is pertussis, or whooping cough, which has been steadily increasing. Because immunity typically wanes five to ten years after vaccination, adolescents and young adults are at risk. With the development of safer new vaccines, the CDC is recommending a "Tdap" (tetanus, diphtheria, and pertussis) booster vaccination every ten years for everyone aged 19 to 64. Immunity against measles also may wane; check with your doctor about a booster.

TABLE 15.2

Vaccines Recommended for College Students

Tetanus-Diphtheria-Pertussis (Tdap) vaccine

Meningococcal vaccine*

HPV vaccine series

Hepatitis A vaccine series

Hepatitis B vaccine series

Polio vaccine series

Measles-Mumps-Rubella (MMR) vaccine series

Varicella (chicken pox) vaccine series

Influenza vaccine

Pneumococcal polysaccharide (PPV) vaccine

*Recommended for previously unvaccinated college freshmen living in dormitories.

© Bob Pardue/Alamy

POINT COUNTERPOINT *To Vaccinate or Not to Vaccinate*

POINT
The vaccines given from birth to adolescence save 33,000 lives, prevent 14 million infections, and save $10 billion in medical costs. Unvaccinated children—about 2 to 3 percent of youngsters in the United States—are vulnerable to life-threatening diseases that could jeopardize others. By requiring immunizations of all schoolchildren, the government protects not just an individual child's well-being, but the health and safety of the community.

COUNTERPOINT
Despite scientific evidence that vaccines do not cause autism or other disorders, some parents remain convinced that vaccines have the potential to harm. These parents argue that they have the right to put their child's welfare first and that the government should not ban unvaccinated youngsters from schools. Some would like to choose which immunizations to give their child rather than the full complement currently required for all children.

YOUR VIEW
Do you think health officials should put the public good above any risk vaccines might pose to an individual child? Do you think parents are protecting or jeopardizing their children's health by refusing vaccinations? Have you received all the vaccinations recommended for college students (see Figure 15.3)? If not, why not?

Vaccine	19–26 years	27–49 years	50–59 years	60–64 years	≥ 65 years
Tetanus, diphtheria, pertussis [Td/Tdap]	Substitute 1-time dose of Tdap for Td booster; then boost with TD every 10 yrs				Td booster every 10 yrs
Human papillomavirus (HPV)	3 doses (females)				
Measles, mumps, rubella (MMR)	1 or 2 doses		1 dose		
Varicella (chicken pox)	2 doses				
Influenza	1 dose annually		1 dose annually		
Pneumococcal (polysaccharide)	1–2 doses				1 dose
Hepatitis A	2 doses				
Hepatitis B	3 doses				
Meningococcal	1 or more doses				
Zoster				1 dose	

For all persons in this category who meet the age requirements and who lack evidence of immunity

Recommended if some other risk factor is present (e.g., on the basis of medical, occupational, lifestyle, or other indications)

Figure 15.3 Recommended Adult Immunization, United States, 2009

Source: Centers for Disease Control and Prevention.

Common Cold

There are more than 200 distinct cold viruses. Although in a single season you may develop a temporary immunity to one or two, you may then be hit by a third. Americans come down with 1 billion colds annually.

Every year, about 25 million cold sufferers in the United States visit their family doctors with uncomplicated upper respiratory infections. The common cold results in about 20 million days of absence from work and 22 million days of absence from school.

 College and university students are at increased risk for colds and influenza-like illnesses. In one study that followed more than 3,000 students from fall to spring, 9 in 10 had at least one cold or flu-like illness. Colds can strike in any season, but different cold viruses are more common at different times of years. Rhinoviruses cause most spring, summer, and early fall colds and tend to cause more symptoms above the neck (stuffy nose, headache, runny eyes). Adenoviruses, parainfluenza viruses, coronaviruses, influenza viruses, and others that strike in the winter are more likely to get into the trachea and bronchi (the breathing passages) and cause more fever and bronchitis.

Cold viruses spread by coughs, sneezes, and touch. Cold sufferers who sneeze and then touch a doorknob or countertop leave a trail of highly contagious viruses behind them. The best preventive tactics are frequent hand washing, replacing toothbrushes regularly, exercising regularly, and avoiding stress overload.

A lack of sleep can increase your odds of getting a cold. People who get less than seven hours of sleep a night are three times more likely to catch a cold. Those who sleep poorly are five times more susceptible.[5] (See Making Change Happen, p. 498, and "Sleep Power" in *Labs for IPC*.)

High levels of stress increase the risk of becoming infected by respiratory viruses and developing cold symptoms. People who feel unable to deal with everyday stresses have an exaggerated immune reaction that may intensify cold or flu symptoms once they've contracted a virus. Those with a positive emotional outlook are less vulnerable.

Although colds and sore throats—a frequent cold symptom—are caused by viruses, many people seek treatment with antibiotics, which are effective only against bacteria. Unless you're coughing up green or foul yellow mucus (signs of a secondary bacterial infection), antibiotics won't help. They have no effect against viruses and may make your body more resistant to such medications when you develop a bacterial infection in the future. An estimated 5 to 17 percent of sore throats in adults are caused by bacteria (*Group A streptococci*). For effective treatments, see Health on a Budget.

Excess prescribing for antibiotics accounts for more than half of all prescriptions and costs more than $700 million a year. In addition to their costs, antibiotics may increase risks to users and their contacts. An increasing number of studies show that antibiotics foster the growth of one or more strains of antibiotic-resistant bacteria for at least two to six months inside the person taking the pills—who can pass on this drug-resistant bug to family, roommates, and others.

According to a recent review of 30 published studies, taking vitamin C every day does not ward off the common cold or shorten its length or severity. However, some people might indeed benefit—those exposed to short bouts of extreme physical exercise or cold temperatures. Tests of high-dose vitamin C after the onset of cold symptoms showed no consistent effect on either the length of a cold or the severity of its symptoms.

The latest findings on *Echinacea* are more positive. According to a new review of previous studies, the herbal supplement can cut the chances of catching a cold by more than half and shorten the duration of a cold by an average of 1.4 days. The combination

Washing your hands often with soap and hot water for 15 to 20 seconds will help protect you from germs. When soap and water are not available, you can use alcohol-based disposable hand wipes or gel sanitizers. If using gel, rub your hands until the gel is dry; the alcohol in the gel kills the germs.

© Corbis

Caring for Your Cold

Fortunately, the most effective treatments for a cold are inexpensive—or even free:

- **Drink plenty of fluids,** particularly warm ones. Warmth is important because the aptly named "cold" viruses replicate at lower temperatures. Hot soups and drinks (particularly those with a touch of something pungent, like lemon or ginger) raise body temperature and help clear the nose. Tea may enhance the immune system.
- **Get plenty of rest.** Taking it easy reduces demands on the body, which helps speed recovery.
- **Do not take antibiotics.** They are ineffective against colds and flu.
- **Do not take aspirin or acetaminophen** (Tylenol), which may suppress the antibodies the body produces to fight cold viruses and increase symptoms such as stuffiness. Children, teenagers, and young adults should never take aspirin for a cold or flu because of the danger of Reye's syndrome, a potentially deadly disorder that can cause convulsions, coma, swelling of the brain, and kidney damage. A better alternative for achiness is ibuprofen (brand names include Motrin, Advil, and Nuprin), which doesn't seem to affect immune response.
- **Choose the right medicines for your symptoms.**

If you want to:	Choose medicine with:
Unclog a stuffy nose	Nasal decongestant
Quiet a cough	Cough suppressant
Loosen mucus so that you can cough it up	Expectorant
Stop runny nose and sneezing	Antihistamine
Ease fever, headaches, minor aches and pains	Pain reliever (analgesic)

- **Know when to call your doctor.**
  You usually do not have to call a doctor right away if you have signs of a cold or flu. But be sure to call in these situations:
  - Your symptoms get worse.
  - Your symptoms last a long time.
  - After feeling a little better, you show signs of a more serious problem. Some of these signs are a sick-to-your-stomach feeling, vomiting, high fever, shaking, chills, chest pain, or coughing with thick, yellow-green mucus.

YOUR STRATEGIES FOR PREVENTION

How to Avoid Getting a Cold

- Avoid people with colds when possible.
- Sneeze or cough into a tissue and then throw the tissue away.
- Clean surfaces you touch with a germ-killing disinfectant.
- Don't touch your nose, eyes, or mouth. Germs can enter your body easily by these paths.
- Wash your hands often. Use hot water and lather up, covering the back of your hands as well as your fingers and palms. Scrub for at least 15 seconds—about the time it takes to sing one chorus of "Happy Birthday to You."
- Don't switch to alcohol-based hand sanitizers. While they are handy when you can't get to a sink, they must come into contact with all surfaces of your hands in order to be effective. Even then, they cleanse no better than plain soap and water.
- Dry your hands thoroughly. Wet hands are more likely to spread germs than dry ones.

of vitamin C and *Echinacea* may be even more effective. In the studies, the herbal supplement reduced the risk of catching a cold by 58 percent, while the combination of *Echinacea* and vitamin C reduced cold incidence by 86 percent.

Influenza

Although similar to a cold, **influenza**—or the flu—causes more severe symptoms that last longer. Every year 10 to 20 percent of Americans develop influenza, more than 200,000 are hospitalized, and 36,000 die.

Flu viruses, transmitted by coughs, sneezes, laughs, and even normal conversation, are extraordinarily contagious, particularly in the first three days of the disease. The usual incubation period is two days, but symptoms can hit hard and fast. Two varieties of viruses—influenza A and influenza B—cause most flus.

The CDC has set priorities for individuals who should get a flu shot because they are at higher risk for flu complications, such as heart disease, diabetes, and asthma. They are:

- **Individuals age 65 years and older,** with and without chronic health conditions.
- **Residents of long-term care facilities.**
- **Persons with higher risk of flu complications** because of underlying medical conditions.

Sleep Power

Sleep, as decades of research have shown, has the power to keep you well. Without adequate sleep, your immune system weakens, your heart becomes more vulnerable, and your risk of diabetes, obesity, and other illnesses increases. Unfortunately, college students can be notoriously poor sleepers. Many keep irregular schedules, bolt high-caffeine energy drinks, and pull all-nighters. However, if you want to tap into the power of sleep instead of searching for shortcuts or substitutes, "Sleep Power" in *Labs for IPC* can help. Here's a preview.

Get Real

In this stage, you test your rest by completing a sleep log for a week and recording information such as how much sleep you got and how sleepy you were morning, afternoon, and evening. You also assess your "sleep smarts" by indicating which of ten statements apply to you, including the following:

- I get up at the same time most weekdays.   _____
- I never drink caffeinated beverages after 6:00 p.m.   _____
- I don't take long naps, especially in the evening.   _____

Get Ready

As part of your preparation, you assess your sleep environment by answering questions such as:

- Where do you sleep? In a dorm room with one or more roommates? In your room at your parents' house? In an apartment?
- What is the state of your bed? The mattress may be old, but do you have a comfortable pillow? Are the sheets clean?

Get Going

In this stage you find eight strategies for better sleeping and greater energy. Here is our favorite:

- **Power Nap.** A short nap of about 15 to 20 minutes can boost mood, motivation, and performance, and lower stress as well as improve memory and learning. As researchers have demonstrated, you can train yourself to take efficient daytime naps. Here are some basic guidelines:

- Try a nap in the late morning or just after lunch.
- In the hour or two before your nap, avoid caffeine or foods that are heavy in fat and sugar.

If you don't have time or can't find a place for a power nap, try the following:

- **A mini-nap.** Just 5 to 15 minutes of sleep can increase alertness and stamina.
- **A micro-nap.** Rather than struggling to keep your eyes open, give yourself 2 to 5 minutes of rest, which has proven effective in overcoming sleepiness.
- **A nano-nap.** Just 10 to 20 seconds of releasing all thoughts and tension from your body provides a breather for your brain.

Lock It In

You audit your sleep and sleepiness and use the information to make the most of your "down time."

- **Children age 6 months to 18 years.**
- **Pregnant women.**
- **Health-care personnel** who provide direct patient care.
- **Household contacts and caregivers** of children under 6 months.

In older individuals, flu shots may offer significant protection against strokes, heart disease, and illnesses similar to the flu.[6] The only individuals who should steer clear are those allergic to eggs, since the inactivated flu viruses are grown in chick embryos.

Vaccination with the live, nasal-spray flu vaccine (FluMist®) is an option for healthy people aged 5 to 49 years who are not pregnant. The spray represents a particular advantage for children since more than 30 percent of youngsters get the flu, but most don't receive a flu shot. However, its recipients are likely to have more health-care visits related to flu and pneumonia than those given standard flu shots.[7]

For those who don't get vaccinated, antiviral drugs, which must be taken within 36 to 48 hours of the first flu symptom, have provided the next best line of defense. Two of the oldest of these medications, amantadine and rimantadine, which work only against the type A flu virus, are no longer effective, possibly because the flu virus has mutated and become resistant. Two newer agents, Tamiflu (oseltamivir) and Relenza (zanamivir), fight both type A and type B influenza.

 Flu shots are now advised for almost everyone, but the majority of college health centers report vaccinating fewer than 20 percent of their students. Those living in dormitories are at higher risk of influenza than those in nondormitory settings. The specific aspects of dormitory life that increase the risk of flu symptoms include the number of roommates and the presence/absence of carpeting. Students living in "triples," with three beds to a room; those sleeping in the same room with a roommate in a double; and those with uncarpeted floors have higher rates of flu symptoms, such as fever, sore throat, and fatigue.

Meningitis

Meningitis, or invasive meningococcal disease, attacks the membranes around the brain and spinal cord and can result in hearing loss, kidney failure, and permanent brain damage. One of the most common types is caused by the bacterium *Neisseria meningitis.* Viral meningitis is typically less severe.

Most common in the first year of life, the incidence of bacterial meningitis rises in young people between ages 15 and 24. Adolescents and young adults account for nearly 30 percent of all cases of meningitis in the United States. If not treated early, meningitis can lead to death or permanent disabilities. One in five of those who survive suffers from long-term side effects, such as brain damage, hearing loss, seizures, or limb amputation. Fatality rates are five times higher among 15- to 24-year-olds.

 Each year 100 to 125 cases of meningitis occur on college campuses. An estimated 5 to 15 students die as a result. One in five survivors suffers long-term side effects. Individuals living in crowded living situations, such as dormitories, sleep-away camps, and barracks, are at increased risk.

Meningitis spreads through the exchange of respiratory droplets, which can come from sharing a drink, cigarette, or silverware; kissing; coughing; or sneezing. Even inhaling secondhand smoke can infect you with the disease.

Preventing Meningitis

Vaccination protects against four of the five most common types of meningococcal bacteria. These four strains cause more than 80 percent of cases in adolescents and young adults. As with other immunizations, minor reactions may occur. These include pain and swelling at the injection site, headache, fatigue, or a vague sense of discomfort. The incidence of life-threatening meningitis has declined substantially since the vaccine was developed.[8]

The CDC and other major health organizations, such as the American College Health Association, recommend routine vaccination with a new type of meningococcal vaccine, which provides longer-lasting protection than the previous type. However, vaccinations are not advisable for everyone.

Recognizing Meningitis

The early symptoms of meningitis may be mild and resemble symptoms of flu or other less severe infections. Bacterial meningitis symptoms may develop within hours; viral meningitis symptoms may develop quickly or over several days. Fever, headache, and neck stiffness are the hallmark symptoms of meningitis. Not all symptoms may appear, but they can progress very quickly, killing an otherwise healthy person in 48 hours or less, so it is critical to seek medical attention quickly.

The most common symptoms of meningitis are:

• Sudden high fever.

• Severe, persistent headache.

• Neck stiffness and pain that makes it difficult to touch the chin to the chest.

• Nausea and vomiting, sometimes along with diarrhea.

influenza Any type of fairly common, highly contagious viral diseases.

meningitis An extremely serious, potentially fatal illness that attacks the membranes around the brain and spinal cord; caused by the bacterium *Neisseria meningitis.*

Who should be vaccinated:

• All children when they turn 11 or 12 or when they enter high school, if they have not been previously vaccinated.

• College freshmen living in dorms.

• Military recruits.

• People who may have been exposed to meningitis during an outbreak.

Who should not get vaccinated or should wait:

• Anyone who has had a severe, life-threatening reaction or allergy to any vaccine component.

• Anyone who is moderately or severely ill at the time of the scheduled immunization.

• Anyone who had ever had Guillain-Barre syndrome (a neurological disorder).

• Pregnant women.

• Confusion and disorientation (acting "goofy").

• Drowsiness or sluggishness.

• Eye pain or sensitivity to bright light.

• Pain or weakness in the muscles or joints.

Other possible signs and symptoms include:

• Abnormal skin color.

• Stomach cramps.

• Ice-cold hands and feet.

• Dizziness.

• Reddish or brownish skin rash or purple spots.

• Numbness and tingling.

• Seizures.

When to Seek Medical Care

If two or more of the symptoms of meningitis appear at the same time or if the symptoms are very severe or appear suddenly, seek medical care right away. If a red rash appears along with fever, see if the rash disappears when a glass is pressed against it. If it does not, this could be a sign of blood infection, which is a medical emergency. Call 911 without delay. Other symptoms that might require emergency treatment include loss of consciousness, seizures, muscle weakness, or sudden severe dementia.

A new rapid test can determine the presence of viral meningitis in just 2.5 hours. Because it can help quickly distinguish between viral and bacterial meningitis, the test could help reduce the unnecessary use of antibiotics. About one in ten people who get meningitis dies from it. Of those who survive, another 11 to 19 percent lose fingers, arms, or legs, become deaf, have problems with their nervous systems, or suffer seizures, strokes, or brain damage.[9] Thus it is critical to seek medical care for this infection. A new concern is the emergence of the first U.S. cases of bacterial meningitis resistant to a widely used antibiotic.[10]

Hepatitis

An estimated 500,000 Americans contract hepatitis each year. At least five different viruses, referred to as **hepatitis** A, B, C, Delta, and E, can cause this inflammation of the liver. Newly identified viruses also may be responsible for some cases of what is called "non-A, non-B" hepatitis. Thanks largely to effective vaccines, rates of hepatitis A and hepatitis B infections have declined to their lowest rates in decades. Although there is no vaccine for hepatitis C, its incidence also has declined significantly.

All forms of hepatitis target the liver, the body's largest internal organ. Symptoms include headaches, fever, fatigue, stiff or aching joints, nausea, vomiting, and diarrhea. The liver becomes enlarged and tender to the touch; sometimes the yellowish tinge of jaundice develops. Treatment consists of rest, a high-protein diet, and the avoidance of alcohol and drugs that may stress the liver. Alpha interferon, a protein that boosts immunity and prevents viruses from replicating, may be used for some forms.

Most people begin to feel better after two or three weeks of rest, although fatigue and other symptoms can linger. As many as 10 percent of those infected with hepatitis B and up to two-thirds of those with hepatitis C become carriers of the virus for several years or even life. Some have persistent inflammation of the liver, which may cause mild or severe symptoms and increase the risk of liver cancer.

Hepatitis A

Hepatitis A, a less serious form, is generally transmitted by poor sanitation, primarily fecal contamination of food or water, and is less common in industrialized nations than in developing countries. As many as 30 percent of individuals in the United States show evidence of past infection with the virus. Among those at highest risk in the United States are children and staff at day-care centers, residents of institutions for the mentally handicapped, sanitation workers, and workers who handle primates such as monkeys. Gamma globulin can provide short-term immunity; vaccines against hepatitis A have been approved by the FDA. The CDC recommends routine immunization against hepatitis A in states with high rates, as well as for travelers to countries where hepatitis A is common, men who have sex with men, and persons who use illegal drugs.

Hepatitis B

Hepatitis B, a potentially fatal disease transmitted through the blood and other bodily fluids, infects an estimated 400,000 people around the world each year. Once spread mainly by contaminated tattoo needles, needles shared by drug users, or transfusions of contaminated blood, hepatitis B is now transmitted mostly through sexual contact. It can cause chronic liver infection, cirrhosis, and liver cancer. Medications for hepatitis B often must be taken long-term, or the disease comes back even stronger.

Hepatitis B is a particular threat to young people; 75 percent of new cases are diagnosed in those between ages 15 to 39. They usually contract hepatitis B through high-risk behaviors such as multiple sex partners and use of injected drugs. Athletes in contact sports, such as wrestling and football, may transmit the hepatitis B virus in sweat. With the discovery that HBV is more common in athletes than had been suspected, health experts are calling for mandatory HBV testing and vaccination against hepatitis B for all athletes.

Individuals who have tattoos or body piercing may also be at risk if procedures are not done under regulated conditions. At highest risk are male homosexuals, heterosexuals with multiple sex partners, health-care workers with frequent contact with blood, injection drug users, and infants born to infected mothers. Vaccination can prevent hepatitis B and is recommended for all newborns.

Hepatitis C

Hepatitis C virus (HCV) is four times as widespread as HIV, infecting about 2 percent of Americans. A simple blood test can show if you are infected with HCV. However, few of the estimated 3 to 4 million carriers in the United States realize they are infected. Of those infected with HCV, 80 percent have no symptoms.

The risk factors for HCV infection are blood transfusion or organ transplant before 1992, exposure to infected blood, illegal drug use, tattoos, or body piercing. If you choose to have a body piercing, avoid piercing guns, and make certain that the piercing equipment has been sterilized (see Consumer Alert). Hepatitis C virus is not spread by casual contact, such as hugging, kissing, or sharing food utensils. There is controversy over whether HCV can be transmitted sexually.

About three-quarters of those infected with HCV develop chronic or long-term hepatitis. About one-quarter develop progressive, irreversible liver damage, with scar tissue (cirrhosis) gradually replacing healthy liver tissue. Hepatitis C also increases the risk of a rare form of liver cancer.[11] If the liver no longer functions adequately, a patient may require liver transplantation. Hepatitis C infection also increases the risk of non-Hodgkin's lymphoma by up to 30 percent.

The most common treatment for hepatitis C is a combination of interferon, which stops the virus from making copies of itself, and ribavirin, an antiviral medication. The treatment lasts for 6 to 12 months and can be extremely difficult to endure.

Getting a tattoo or a piercing can pose health risks, including bacterial infection and hepatitis.

hepatitis An inflammation and/or infection of the liver caused by a virus, often accompanied by jaundice.

The Perils of Piercing

"Body art"—tattoos and piercings—has become increasingly widespread. In a national sampling of 500 men and women between age 18 and 50, 24 percent had tattoos. In surveys of college students, higher percentages have reported permanent tattoos or body piercing. As many as one in five individuals with body piercing may suffer medical complications. In a British study, almost half of tongue piercings resulted in infections and other problems.

Facts to Know

- With no state or federal regulations of "body artists," unsafe tattooing and piercing practices can put consumers in danger. In one survey of "skin-penetration operators," only half said that they followed governmental guidelines for infection control.
- Epidemiologists have identified tattooing as a strong, independent risk factor for testing positive for hepatitis C virus (HCV) but not for development of acute hepatitis. In other words, individuals for tattoos may acquire HCV but may not develop symptoms themselves.
- Even so-called temporary tattooing with henna is not without risk. Dermatologists have reported an increasing number of skin reactions. Piercings of the tongue, lips, or cheeks present different dangers, including recessed gums; loose, chipped, or fractured teeth; pain; infection; inflammation; nerve damage; and tooth loss.

- You may think you're safe if you go to a licensed tattoo or piercing salon. However, there are no formal schools, no certification requirements, and no diplomas for these practitioners. In many states it is possible to get a license without the benefit of any kind of training.

Steps to Take

- **Ask to see certification that the autoclave—a high-temperature pressure cooker used for medical instruments—has been sterilized.**
- **Make sure the artist is wearing standard medical latex gloves.**
- **Find out if the artist is vaccinated for hepatitis B.** Can he or she show you proof, such as a doctor's record, of vaccination?
- **Make sure the artist uses only new sterile needles.**
- **Make sure the artist doesn't "double-dip."** The ink should be new, used on only one client—you.
- **If you require prophylactic antibiotics for dental cleanings or other procedures, do not get a tattoo.** Consumers with rheumatic heart disease and other conditions that increase their risk of infections have died as a result of bacterial infection contracted from a tattoo.

Epstein–Barr Virus and Infectious Mononucleosis

Epstein-Barr virus (EBV), a member of the herpes virus family, infects most people at some time in their lives. As many as 95 percent of American adults between ages 35 and 45 have been infected. When infected in childhood, boys and girls usually show no or very mild symptoms. However, when infection with EBV occurs during adolescence or young adulthood, it causes infectious mononucleosis 35 to 50 percent of the time.[12]

You can get **mononucleosis** through kissing—or any other form of close contact. "Mono" is a viral disease that targets people 15 to 24 years old. Its symptoms include a sore throat, headache, fever, nausea, and prolonged weakness. The spleen is swollen and the lymph nodes are enlarged. You may also develop jaundice or a skin rash similar to rubella (German measles).

The major symptoms usually disappear within two to three weeks, but weakness, fatigue, and often depression may linger for at least two more weeks. The greatest danger is from physical activity that might rupture the spleen, resulting in internal bleeding. The liver may also become inflamed. A blood test can determine whether you have mono. However, there's no specific treatment other than rest.

Chronic Fatigue Syndrome (CFS)

More than a million Americans have the array of symptoms known as **chronic fatigue syndrome (CFS).** CFS is a complex disorder characterized by profound fatigue that does not improve with bed rest and that may get worse with physical or mental activity. Other symptoms include weakness, muscle pain, impaired memory or concentration, insomnia, and postexertion fatigue that lasts for more than 24 hours. Symptoms can persist for years. CFS affects four times as many women as men.

Diagnosis of CFS remains difficult, although numerous studies have found significant immune abnormalities, such as high levels of certain immune cells (B lymphocytes and cytokines) that act as if they were constantly battling a viral infection. There is no known cure, but a combination of therapies can help relieve symptoms.

Herpes Gladiatorum (Mat Herpes, Wrestler's Herpes, Mat Pox)

Herpes gladiatorum is a skin infection caused by the herpes simplex type 1 virus and spread by direct skin-to-skin contact. It most commonly occurs among wrestlers, judo players, or other athletes who have with very close skin contact with each other.

Within a few days of infection, some people develop a sore throat, swollen lymph nodes, fever, or tingling on the skin. *Herpes gladiatorum* lesions appear as a cluster of blisters on the face, extremities, or trunk. Generally, lesions appear within eight days after exposure to an infected person, but they may take longer to emerge. All wrestlers with skin sores or lesions should see a physician for evaluation and should not participate in practice or competition until their lesions have healed.

Herpes gladiatorum infections can recur. The virus can "hide out" in the nerves and reactivate later, causing another infection. Generally, recurrent infections are less severe and don't last as long. However, a recurring infection is just as contagious as the original infection, so the same precautions are needed to prevent infecting others.[13]

mononucleosis   An infectious viral disease characterized by an excess of white blood cells in the blood, fever, bodily discomfort, a sore throat, and kidney and liver complications.

chronic fatigue syndrome (CFS)   A cluster of symptoms whose cause is not yet known; a primary symptom is debilitating fatigue.

tuberculosis (TB)   A highly infectious bacterial disease that primarily affects the lungs and is often fatal.

Tuberculosis

A bacterial infection of the lungs that was once the nation's leading killer, **tuberculosis (TB)** still claims the lives of more people than any acute infectious disease other than pneumonia (Figure 15.4). About 30 percent of the world's population is infected with the TB organism, although not all develop active disease. In the United States, immigration from countries where TB is common, poverty, homelessness, alcoholism and drug abuse, the HIV/AIDS epidemic, and the emergence of resistant strains of TB account for most new cases of TB. Approximately 15 million Americans have the disease.

Although TB is most prevalent among high-risk groups, the overall danger increases as more people develop active disease because TB is highly contagious. TB outbreaks have occurred throughout the country in hospitals, nursing homes, prisons, and office buildings,

When someone with active tuberculosis exhales, coughs, or sneezes, TB bacteria are expelled in tiny airborne droplets that others may inhale.

The TB bacteria lodge mainly in the lungs, where they slowly multiply, creating patches, then cavities.

Other parts of the lung are affected, including the bronchi and the lining of the lung.

If untreated, TB can eventually spread to and damage the brain, bone, eyes, liver and kidneys, spine, and skin.

Figure 15.4 How Tuberculosis Spreads
If untreated, TB can eventually spread to and damage the brain, bone, eyes, liver, kidneys, spine, and skin.

where inadequate ventilation increases the risk of infection.

Symptoms vary, depending on the organs that are infected. They include fever and sweating (particularly at night), unexplained weight loss, loss of appetite, fatigue, persistent cough that may produce bloody sputum, and difficulty breathing or chest pain when breathing.

Most TB patients recover completely after six months of taking a combination of three different medicines. Drug-resistant forms of the tuberculosis microorganism strike mostly patients who start drug treatment but don't follow through with it. Because they don't take enough of the medication to kill all the TB bacteria in their system, those that survive become resistant. Even with full treatment, the risk of dying from drug-resistant tuberculosis is 50 percent. HIV infection greatly increases susceptibility to infection with TB and the risk of dying if infected with treatment-resistant forms. Fortunately, a combination of two drugs approved for treating other infections has proven effective against normal and resistant strains of TB.[14]

If you think you may have been exposed to TB or if you develop suspicious symptoms (loss of appetite and weight, low-grade fever, fatigue, chills, night sweats, coughing), see your doctor for a TB test. This consists of an injection just under the skin. The area of the arm where the test was administered should be checked by a health-care professional to determine the presence of the TB bacteria; further tests confirm the diagnosis. If the skin test is positive, indicating that TB is present, you'll be monitored with yearly chest X-rays. You may also require treatment, which usually requires three to four antibiotics taken daily for at least 6 to 9 months.

Group A and Group B Strep Infection

Sore throats are common winter complaints, but those caused by group A streptococcus bacteria—*strep throats*—are more than a trivial threat. If not treated promptly with antibiotics, strep bacteria can travel to the kidneys, the liver, or the heart, where they can cause rheumatic fever—an inflammation of the heart that can cause weakness, shortness of breath, joint pain, and an abnormal heartbeat. In recent years clusters of rheumatic fever have sprung up in

several major cities. The best way to prevent further increases in rheumatic fever and heart disease is accurate diagnosis and thorough treatment of strep throat.[15] Rapid new diagnostic tests can identify strep within minutes. If the test is positive, treatment with penicillin or a similar antibiotic is indicated. Brief treatment (five days) with Omnicef, a newer antibiotic, has proved as effective as ten days of oral penicillin.

Toxic streptococcal shock syndrome, or toxic strep, is an invasive form of the disease in which strep gains access to the blood and causes a drop in blood pressure, a very high fever, and the production of exotoxins (substances that can attack various organs, such as the kidneys, heart, or in rare cases, flesh). Toxic strep is rather rare and usually doesn't occur with strep throats. Prompt treatment is critical.

 Group B streptococcus (GBS), the leading cause of life-threatening perinatal infections in the United States, is primarily a threat to newborns. Because some 15 to 40 percent of pregnant women carry GBS but have no symptoms, the American Academy of Pediatrics has called for universal screening of expectant mothers. Each year 12,000 newborns are infected, most of them during childbirth; more than 1,600 die; and another 1,600 suffer permanent brain damage from meningitis. Women at high risk of infecting their newborns with GBS are those who have premature labor, early rupture of their amniotic membranes, fever, and a high group B strep count before or during pregnancy, or who have previously borne an infant infected with GBS. Also at risk are diabetics, low-income women, and those under age 20.

Toxic Shock Syndrome

 As discussed in Chapter 9, toxic shock syndrome (TSS) is a potentially deadly disease associated with the use of tampons, particularly high-absorbency types. It is caused by *Staphylococcus aureus* and group A *Streptococcus pyogenes* bacteria that release toxins (poisonous waste products) into the bloodstream. Symptoms include a high fever; a rash that leads to peeling of the skin on the fingers, toes, palms, and soles; dizziness; dangerously low blood pressure; and abnormalities in several organ systems (the digestive tract and the kidneys) and in the muscles and blood.

In addition to women who use high-absorbency tampons, or leave their tampons in too long, those who have given birth within the preceding six to eight weeks are at greater risk. Children (including newborns), men, and postmenopausal women also have developed TSS, which usually has been traced to bacteria in skin abscesses, boils, cuts, or postsurgical wounds.

Without prompt treatment, TSS can cause severe and permanent damage, including muscle weakness, partial paralysis, amnesia, disorientation, an inability to concentrate, and impaired lung and kidney function. Sometimes toxic shock weakens the blood vessels, increasing the risk of heart problems. Victims can enter the life-threatening crisis called shock, in which blood flow throughout the body is inadequate to sustain life. Treatment usually consists of immediate hospitalization, intravenous administration of fluids, medications to raise blood pressure, and powerful antibiotics; intravenous administration of immunoglobins that attack the toxins produced by these bacteria may also be beneficial.

The "Superbug" Threat: MRSA

For decades most strains of the bacterium *Staphylococcus aureus* responded to treatment with penicillin. When the bacterium became resistant to penicillin, physicians switched to a newer antibiotic, methicillin. Within a year the first case of methicillin-resistant *S. aureus* (MRSA) was detected. This "superbug," which fights off traditional antibiotics, has become a major health threat.

One in three healthy people carry *S. aureus* bacteria on their skin. Of these as

Hospitals can be dangerous places. MRSA spreads from patient to patient when hand washing is inadequate or when gloves or equipment are contaminated.

©YASSER AL-ZAYYAT/AFP/Getty Images

many as 1 in 100 may be carrying MRSA. In medical terms, these individuals are "colonized" but not infected. For infection to occur, MRSA must enter the body through an accidental injury such as a scrape or burn or via a deliberate break in the skin such as a surgical incision.

The rate of MRSA infections is highest in hospitals and health-care facilities, but MRSA also can develop among sports teams, child-care attendees, and prison inmates.

MRSA spreads by touch. In health-care settings, it can spread from patient to patient through contact with doctors and nurses with unwashed hands or contaminated gloves or contact with unsterile medical equipment. Health advocates are calling for increased screening of patients for MRSA, isolating and treating MRSA carriers, more conscientious hand washing, and more diligent use of gowns, gloves, and masks to prevent transmission of MRSA.[16]

Outside of hospitals, community-associated MRSA (CA-MRSA) is a growing threat that can occur in people without any established risks, including college students, who often live in close quarters and participate in contact sports such as football, wrestling, and fencing.[17] Commonsense health precautions can lower your risk.

According to CDC estimates, some 94,000 American get serious MRSA infections each year, and nearly 19,000 die.[18] The number of these infections has decreased significantly in hospital intensive care units since 2001.[19] Among the simple steps responsible for this decline are closer monitoring of hand washing, better means of disinfecting rooms, and improved tracking of patients as they transfer from one hospital or room to another.[20]

Who Is at Highest Risk?

People at high risk of becoming infected with MRSA are those in close contact with carriers, as hospital patients are. MRSA poses the greatest danger to individuals who have:

- A weakened immune system.
- A preexisting infection.
- Open wounds, cuts, or burns.
- Other types of wounds, such as skin breaks from an intravenous drug line.
- Undergone surgery.
- Taken antibiotics recently or for a long period.

Also at greatest risk are:

- Athletes in contact sports.
- Elderly individuals
- Premature or newborn babies.

The Dangers of MRSA Infections

MRSA bacteria can infiltrate a range of tissues and body systems causing problems such as wound infections, deep abscesses, lung infections, and blood poisoning, which can be fatal. Because of its antibiotic resistance, MRSA is difficult, but not impossible, to treat. Most strains of the bacteria are responding to newer antibiotics.

Insect- and Animal-Borne Infections

Common insects and animals, including ticks and mosquitoes, can transmit dangerous infections, among them Lyme disease and West Nile virus.

Lyme Disease

Lyme disease, a bacterial infection, is spread by ixodid ticks that carry a particular bacterium—the spirochete *Borrelia burgdorferi.* An

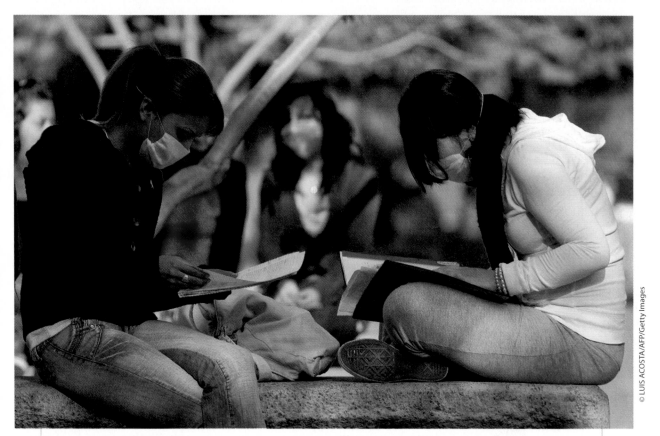

Although many people try to protect themselves by wearing face masks, there is no evidence that they lower the risk of infection in open spaces.

© LUIS ACOSTA/AFP/Getty Images

Bioterror Threats

Americans have learned firsthand that certain infectious agents can be used as weapons of terrorism and war. Bioterror agents, such as anthrax and, potentially, smallpox, botulism, and tularemia, have been added to the ranks of emerging infectious diseases.

Anthrax Anthrax, which is found naturally in wild and farm animals, can also be produced in a laboratory. The disease is spread through exposure to anthrax spores, not through exposure to an infected person.

Smallpox Smallpox is a serious, contagious, and sometimes fatal infectious disease. Smallpox was eradicated decades ago after a successful worldwide vaccination program. The last case of smallpox in the United States was in 1949. The last naturally occurring case in the world was in Somalia in 1977. There is no treatment, and up to 30 percent of those infected with smallpox die.

Because of fear that terrorists might use smallpox as a biological weapon, the U.S. government has stockpiled enough vaccine to inoculate everyone in the event of an emergency. Most individuals vaccinated before 1972, when mandated smallpox immunization ended in the United States, retain some immunity for many years, some for up to 75 years. However, half of all Americans have never received the smallpox vaccine, and many scientists believe protection wanes over time for those who did. Those vaccinated in the past can safely be revaccinated for optimum protection. An Institute of Medicine committee has recommended against vaccinating the entire population at this time.

Botulism Botulism is a muscle-paralyzing disease caused by a toxin made by the bacterium *Clostridium botulinum*. Botulinum toxin is among the most lethal substances known, and it can kill within 24 hours. Botulism causes muscle weakness and eventual paralysis that starts at the top of the body and works its way down. The disease kills by paralyzing muscles used to breathe. The CDC and some state health departments keep an antidote to botulinum toxin in storage. Treatment includes taking the antidote and possibly using a ventilator for breathing until the toxin works its way out of the system.

Tularemia Tularemia is an illness that normally infects wild animals, such as rabbits and squirrels. Humans can acquire the illness by coming in contact with the blood or body fluids of infected animals, from the bite of a fly or tick that carries blood from an infected animal, or from contaminated food or water. As a biological weapon, tularemia-causing bacteria could be dispersed through the air to be inhaled.

Reproductive and Urinary Tract Infections

Reproductive and urinary tract infections are very common. Many are not spread exclusively by sexual contact, so they are not classified as sexually transmitted diseases.

Vaginal Infections

 Vaginal complaints account for approximately 10 million medical office visits a year. The most common are trichomoniasis, candidiasis, and bacterial vaginosis (Table 15.3).

Protozoa (*Trichomonas vaginalis*) that live in the vagina can multiply rapidly, causing itching, burning, and discharge—all symptoms of **trichomoniasis**. Male carriers usually have no symptoms, although some may develop urethritis or an inflammation of the prostate and seminal vesicles. Anyone with this infection should be screened for syphilis, gonorrhea, chlamydia, and HIV. Sexual partners must be treated with oral medication (metronidazole, trade name Flagyl), even if they have no symptoms, to prevent reinfection.

Populations of a yeast called *Candida albicans*—normal inhabitants of the mouth, digestive tract, and vagina—are usually held in check. Under certain conditions, however (such as poor nutrition, stress, or antibiotic use), the microbes multiply, causing burning, itching, and a whitish discharge, and producing what is commonly known as a yeast infection. Common sites for **candidiasis**, which is also called *moniliasis*, are the vagina, vulva, penis, and mouth.

The women most likely to test positive for candidiasis have never been pregnant, use condoms for birth control, have sexual intercourse more than four times a month, and have taken antibiotics in the previous 15 to 30 days. Vaginal medications, such as GyneLotrimin and Monistat, are nonprescription drugs that provide effective treatment. Women should keep the genital area dry and wear cotton underwear.

Male sexual partners may be advised to wear condoms during outbreaks of candidiasis.

Bacterial vaginosis is characterized by alterations in the microorganisms that live in the vagina, including depletion of certain bacteria and overgrowth of others. It typically causes a white or gray vaginal discharge with a distinctive fishy odor similar to that of trichomoniasis. Its underlying cause is unknown, although it occurs most frequently in women with multiple sex partners. Long-term dangers include pelvic inflammatory disease and pregnancy complications. Metronidazole, either in the form of a pill or a vaginal gel, is the primary treatment. According to CDC guidelines, treatment for male sex partners appears to be of little benefit, but some health practitioners recommend treatment for both partners in cases of recurrent infections. Antibiotic therapy may help prevent an infected woman from acquiring an STI.

Urinary Tract Infections

A urinary tract infection (UTI) can be present in any of the three parts of the urinary tract: the urethra, the bladder, or the kidneys.

TABLE 15.3

Common Reproductive Tract Infections

Infection	Transmission	Symptoms	Treatment
Bacterial vaginosis	Most common causative agent, *Gardnerella vaginalis* bacterium, sometimes transmitted through coitus	Women: Fishy- or musty-smelling thin discharge, like flour paste in consistency and usually gray Men: Mostly asymptomatic	Metronidazole (Flagyl) by mouth or intravaginal applications of topical metronidazole gel or clindamycin cream
Candidiasis (yeast infection)	*Candida albicans* fungus may accelerate growth when the chemical balance of the vagina is disturbed; also transmitted through sexual interaction	Women: White, "cheesy" discharge; irritation of vaginal and vulval tissues	Vaginal suppositories or topical cream, such as clotrimazol (GyneLotrimin) and miconazole (Monistat), or oral fluconazole
Trichomoniasis	Protozoan parasite *Trichomonas vaginalis,* usually passed through genital sexual contact	Women: White or yellow vaginal discharge with an unpleasant odor; sore and irritated vulva Men: No symptoms	Metronidazol (Flagyl) for both women and men

An infection involving the urethra is known as **urethritis.** If the bladder is also infected, it's called **cystitis.** If it reaches the kidneys, it's called *pyelonephritis.*

An estimated 40 percent of women report having had a UTI at some point in their lives. Three times as many women as men develop UTIs, probably for anatomical reasons. A woman's urethra is only 1.5 inches long; a man's is 6 inches. Therefore, bacteria, the major cause of UTIs, have a shorter distance to travel to infect a woman's bladder and kidneys. About one-fourth to one-third of all women between ages 20 and 40 develop UTIs, and 80 percent of those who experience one infection develop recurrences.

Conditions that can set the stage for UTIs include irritation and swelling of the urethra or bladder as a result of pregnancy, bike riding, irritants (such as bubble bath, douches, or a diaphragm), urinary stones, enlargement of the prostate gland in men, vaginitis, and stress. Early diagnosis is critical because infection can spread to the kidneys and, if unchecked, result in kidney failure. Symptoms include frequent, burning, or painful urination; chills; fever; fatigue; and blood in the urine.

Recurrent UTIs, a frequent problem among young women, have been linked with a genetic predisposition, sexual intercourse, and the use of diaphragms.

trichomoniasis An infection of the protozoan *Trichomonas vaginalis;* females experience vaginal burning, itching, and discharge, but male carriers may be asymptomatic.

candidiasis An infection of the yeast *Candida albicans,* commonly occurring in the vagina, vulva, penis, and mouth and causing burning, itching, and a whitish discharge.

bacterial vaginosis A vaginal infection caused by overgrowth and depletion of various microorganisms living in the vagina, resulting in a malodorous white or gray vaginal discharge.

urethritis Infection of the urethra.

cystitis Infection of the urinary bladder.

LEARN IT   LIVE IT   The Best Defense

Microorganisms such as bacteria and viruses greatly outnumber humans on the planet. Yet despite their vast numbers, relatively few invade, multiply, and cause illness in people. Many microorganisms, such as those living in your intestine, actually play a role in keeping you healthy. The goal isn't to wipe out all microbes but to recognize those with a potential to harm us and take steps to defend ourselves.

The three steps to infection protection are:

- **Immunizations.** Keep track of the vaccinations you've received and the dates you received them. Check with your doctor about any booster shots you may require. Get a tetanus booster every five years (an easy way not to forget: get one every time you celebrate a birthday ending in a 5 or 0, such as 25 and 30). Get your flu

shot or spray. As discussed in the following chapter, if you're a woman and have not been vaccinated against human papilloma virus (HPV), talk to your doctor about the potential benefits for you.

- **Good health habits.** Take this chapter's Self Survey to check your infection protection IQ. Identify the areas where you may need to boost your defenses, and follow the guidelines in Your Health Action Plan.

- **Prompt treatment.** The early symptoms of many infectious diseases are similar. Yes, it may just be a bad cold or the flu, but you can't rule out the possibility of a more deadly threat, such as bacterial meningitis. Don't ignore severe or persistent symptoms.

Check the items that apply to you.

_____ I wash my hands with soap and water after I use the restroom.
_____ I wash my hands with soap and water before I eat.
_____ Before and after using exercise equipment, I wipe the handles.
_____ I wash my hands with soap and water after working out with weights or exercise equipment at a gym.
_____ I avoid contact with people who are coughing and sneezing.
_____ I wash my hands with soap and water more often during the cold and flu season.
_____ All of my vaccinations are current.
_____ I eat at least 3 balanced meals a day.
_____ I get 6 to 8 hours of sleep at night.
_____ I use relaxation techniques to lower my stress level.
_____ I do not smoke.
_____ I do not drink or keep alcohol consumption to a minimum.
_____ I do not use drugs of any kind, including steroids.
_____ I throw leftovers out after 3 days.
_____ I wash fruits and vegetables before eating.
_____ I check expiration dates on food items.
_____ I apply insect spray (containing DEET) when I am outdoors.
_____ I wear long-sleeved clothing and long pants when hiking.
_____ I check myself for ticks after a hike.

Scoring

Add up your checkmarks, and look for patterns in your protective behaviors. Are you conscientious about exercise and sleep, but careless about washing your hands or wiping down gym equipment? Do you protect yourself against food infections (discussed in Chapter 6) but not against sexually transmitted infections (discussed in Chapter 16)? Identify the aspects of infection protection that need the most work, and start practicing the defensive behaviors that will lower your risk.

Your Health Action Plan for Infection Protection

Some day medical science may develop vaccines or other means of providing total protection against infectious diseases. Until then your best defense is to take commonsense steps to promote well-being and reduce the risks of infection. Here are some basic principles of self-defense:

- **Eat a balanced diet** to be sure you get essential vitamins and minerals. Severe deficiencies in vitamins B_6, B_{12}, and folic acid impair immunity. Keep up your iron and zinc intake. Iron influences the number and vigor of certain immune cells, whereas zinc is crucial for cell repair. Too little vitamin C also may increase susceptibility to infectious diseases.
- **Avoid fatty foods.** A low-fat diet can increase the activity of immune cells that hunt down and knock out cells infected with viruses.
- **Get enough sleep.** Without adequate rest, your immune system cannot maintain and renew itself.
- **Exercise regularly.** Aerobic exercise stimulates the production of an immune-system booster called interleukin-2.
- **Don't smoke.** Smoking decreases the levels of some immune cells and increases susceptibility to respiratory infections.
- **Control your alcohol intake.** Heavy drinking interferes with normal immune responses and lowers the number of defender cells.

- **Wash your hands frequently** with hot water and soap. In a public restroom, use a paper towel to turn off the faucet after you wash your hands, and avoid touching the doorknob. Wash objects used by someone with a cold.
- **Don't share food, drinks, silverware, glasses,** and other objects that may carry infectious microbes.
- **Spend as little time as possible in crowds** during cold and flu season, especially closed places, such as elevators and airplanes. When out, keep your distance from sneezers and coughers.
- **Don't touch your eyes, mouth, and nose,** especially after being with someone who has cold symptoms.
- **Use tissues** rather than cloth handkerchiefs, which may harbor viruses for hours or days.
- **Avoid irritating air pollutants** whenever possible.

CENGAGENOW If you want to write your own goals for preventing infectious diseases, go to the Wellness Journal at CengageNOW for Health at **www.cengage.com/sso.**

Review Questions

1. Which of the following statements about the common cold and influenza is *true*?
   a. Influenza is just a more severe form of the common cold.
   b. Aspirin should be avoided by children and young adults who have a cold or influenza.
   c. The flu vaccine is also effective against most of the viruses that cause the common cold.
   d. Antibiotics are appropriate treatments for colds but not for influenza.

2. The meningitis vaccination
   a. is recommended for all college freshmen.
   b. protects against four of the five most common types of meningococcal bacteria.
   c. also protects against gonorrhea.
   d. may cause minor reactions such as fever or hives.

3. Hepatitis B
   a. is spread mainly through contaminated needles.
   b. infects mostly middle-aged people.
   c. does not have a preventive vaccine.
   d. can be spread in the sweat of athletes.

4. Which statement about methicillin-resistant *Staphylococcus aureus* (MRSA) is *false*?
   a. MRSA can be spread by doctors in a hospital.
   b. MRSA can be spread by athletes playing contact sports.
   c. MRSA is carried on the skin of as many as 1 in 100 people.
   d. MRSA can cause lung infections.

5. Which of the following statements is *true*?
   a. Lyme disease is a bacterial infection transmitted by ticks.
   b. West Nile virus is transmitted to humans by birds.
   c. West Nile virus is the most commonly reported vector-borne infectious disease in the United States.
   d. Avian flu has been transmitted from human to human.

6. Which statement about reproductive and urinary tract infections is *false*?
   a. Yeast infections can be treated with nonprescription drugs.
   b. Symptoms of UTIs include burning urination, chills, fever, and blood in the urine
   c. Three times as many women as men develop UTIs.
   d. Bacterial vaginosis usually causes a vaginal discharge with a rotten-egg odor.

7. Public health officials define a pandemic as
   a. a sudden rise in the incidence of a particular disease.
   b. an atypically large number of people in a region suffering from the same disease.
   c. a high proportion of the population over a wide geographic area suffering from the same disease.
   d. more than 25 percent the world's population suffering from the same disease.

8. Which of the following statements is true?
   a. The Lyme disease vaccine stimulates the immune system to produce antibodies against the bacterium *Borrelia burgdorferi*.
   b. West Nile virus is transmitted to humans by birds.
   c. West Nile virus is the most commonly reported vector-borne infectious disease in the United States.
   d. Avian flu has been transmitted from human to human.

9. Which of the following statements about specific infectious diseases is *false*?
   a. Symptoms of SARS include high fever, coughing, headache, and chills.
   b. Anthrax can be found in wild and farm animals.
   c. Hepatitis A is usually transmitted through contaminated needles, transfusions, and sexual contact.
   d. College freshmen are at higher risk for contracting meningitis than the general population of young people between the ages of 18 and 23.

10. Which statement about reproductive and urinary tract infections is *false*?
    a. Yeast infections can be treated with nonprescription drugs.
    b. Symptoms of UTIs include burning urination, chills, fever, and blood in the urine.
    c. Three times as many women as men develop UTIs.
    d. Bacterial vaginosis usually causes a vaginal discharge with a rotten-egg odor.

Answers to these questions can be found on page 650.

Critical Thinking

1. Prior to reading this chapter, describe what you did to avoid contracting infectious disease. Now that you have read the chapter, will you be making any changes in your practices? Briefly explain the convenience, advantages, and disadvantages of each practice that you have and/or will be using to prevent infection.

2. At the pharmacy, the shelves are full of medications for cold and flu. How do you sort through them? Do you get recommendations from family and friends? Do you study the labels? Do you keep track of what works for you?

3. Did you get vaccinated for meningitis? Why or why not? Where did you get your information on the disease and the vaccine, and how did you make your decision?

Media Menu

CENGAGENOW™ Go to the CengageNOW for Health website at **www.cengage.com/sso** that will:
- Help you evaluate your knowledge of the material.
- Allow you to take an exam-prep quiz.
- Provide a Personalized Learning Plan targeting resources that address areas you should study.
- Coach you through identifying target goals for behavioral change and creating and monitoring your personal change plan throughout the semester.

Internet Connections

www.immunize.org
This site features comprehensive vaccination information for children, adolescents, and adults.

www3.niaid.nih.gov
This institute is part of the National Institutes for Health. Its website provides information about current research and includes fact sheets about all manner of topics related to allergies and infectious diseases.

www.cdc.gov/ncidod
This comprehensive site, sponsored by the Centers for Disease Control and Prevention (CDC), features an infectious disease index, news on emerging infectious diseases, and a section for travelers.

Key Terms

The terms listed are used on the page indicated. Definitions of the terms are in the Glossary at the end of the book.

abscess 493
allergy 493
antibiotics 487
antiviral drug 487
autoimmune disorder 493
bacteria 487
bacterial vaginosis 513
candidiasis 513
chronic fatigue syndrome (CFS) 503
cystitis 513
fungi 487
gamma globulin 491
helminth 487
hepatitis 501
host 487
immune deficiency 493
immunity 489
immunotherapy 493
incubation period 489
inflammation 491
influenza 499
Lyme disease 507
lymph nodes 491
meningitis 499
mononucleosis 503
pathogen 487
protozoa 487
systemic disease 493
trichomoniasis 513
tuberculosis (TB) 503
urethritis 513
vector 487
virus 487

Chapter - 16 Lowering Your Risks of Sexually Transmitted infections

1. **The ABCs of safer sex refer to: (pg 520 - 521)**
    - A. Abstaining from sex, being faithful, and using a Condom
    - B. not flossing or brushing your teeth before having oral sex
    - C. practicing monogamy with each other
    - D. all of the above

2. **Which of the following would not be an example of a low-risk non-insertive type of sexual activity? (pg 525)**
    - A. outercourse
    - B. masturbation
    - C. waginal intercourse without condom
    - D. petting & fondling

3. **The most risky unprotected sexual activity for the greatest chance to become infected with the HIV virus is: (pg 525)**
    - A. oral sex
    - B. vaginal sex
    - C. anal sex
    - D. heavy deep throat kissing

4. **Sexually transmitted infections are most likely to spread via: (pg 522)**
    - A. where there is a break in the outer skin
    - B. fragile inner skin of the anus or vagina
    - C. direct transmission where barrier protection did not take place
    - D. all of the above

5. **The most common STI in the U.S. is: (pg 526)**
    - A. gonorrhea
    - B. Chlamydia
    - C. human papiloma virus
    - D. herpes simplex

6. **Herpes simplex type 1 is typically associated with: (pg 528)**
    - A. genital herpes on vagina or penis
    - B. skin around the face
    - C. the anal region
    - D. the lips and around the mouth

7. **Chlamydia STI tends to infect which ethic group much more than other groups? (pg 530)**
    - A. Whites
    - B. Asians
    - C. African Americans
    - D. Native Americans

8. **Which of the following STIs is also known as "the clap"? (pg 532)**
    - A. syphilis
    - B. herpes simplex
    - C. gonorrhea
    - D. Chlamydia

9. **Which STI shows symptoms of a white milky discharge from the penis along with a painful burning sensation when urinating? (pg 532)**
    - A. pelvic inflammatory disease
    - B. HPV
    - C. syphilis
    - D. gonorrhea

10. **The stage of syphilis that typically has pinkish or whitish small rashes on the skin or palms of the hand is: (pg 534)**
    - A. primary syphilis
    - B. secondary syphilis
    - C. latent stage syphilis
    - D. tertiary syphilis

11. **Pubic lice lay eggs in the hairy regions of the body are called: (pg 535)**
    A. larvae   C. nits
    B. pustules   D. cells

12. **With the rampant growth of sexually transmitted infections (STIs) in this country, STIs are now considered to be in the top _____ most frequently reportable diseases. (pg 523)**
    A. 5   C. 20
    B. 10   D. 100

13. **College-aged students account for about what percentage of contracting STIs? (pg 523)**
    A. 25%   C. 50%
    B. 33%   D. 66%

14. **When it comes to sexually transmitted infections in women, they are more likely to: (pg 524)**
    A. develop asymptomatic symptoms of an STI
    B. contract a STI more so than a male partner would
    C. develop sterility from unknown STIs being properly diagnosed
    D. all of the above

15. **Antibiotic medicines cannot be used to destroy which type of STI? (pg 529)**
    A. gonorrhea   C. syphilis
    B. herpes   D. Chlamydia

16. **During which stage of syphilis does a chancre develop? (pg 534)**
    A. primary   C. latent
    B. secondary   d. teritary

17. **A newer form of helping people to fight their HIV infection is by: (pg 540)**
    A. reducing their viral load
    B. reducing the protective T-cells
    C. taking mega doses of vitamin C
    D. administering the HIV vaccine

18. **HIV tests used to determine if one has developed HIV look for: (pg 539)**
    A. HIV viral cells   C. number of white blood cells
    B. antibodies   D. mutations in the cells

19. **All but one are true statements regarding the sexual transmission of the HIV virus: (pg 538)**
    A. causal contact does spread the HIV virus
    B. the HIV virus is very difficult to get
    C. oral sex can lead to HIV transmission
    D. no cases of HIV from heavy French kissing have been reported

20. **Which of the following is not an important aspect of reviewing your sexual history to assess for health risks? (pg 541)**
    A. respecting your partner and your decisions to engage in sex or not
    B. carrying two condoms with you in case one breaks or is defective
    C. abstinence means affection can still happen with your partner
    D. it is not your partner's business to know that you have an STI as you don't want to jeopardize your relationship

2

There's something I have to tell you." Anise knew, just by the sound of her boyfriend's voice, that the "something" wasn't good news.

"My herpes is back."

Stunned, Anise tried to absorb all the information packed into this short sentence: She'd had no idea that the man she'd been sleeping with for several months had a sexually transmitted infection (STI). How did he get it? What else hadn't he told

Lowering Your Risk of Sexually Transmitted Infections

her about his past? What did he mean that it was "back"? Could she have caught it? And, finally, she asked the all-too-human question: How could this have happened to me?

By their very nature, infectious diseases take people by surprise. Some of today's most common and dangerous infectious illnesses spread primarily through sexual contact, and their incidence has skyrocketed. The federal government estimates that 65 million Americans have a sexually transmitted infection (STI). These diseases cannot be prevented in the laboratory. Only you, by your behavior, can prevent and control them.

All human beings are sexual from birth to death. Whether you are male or female, single or married, straight, gay, lesbian, bisexual, or transgender, sexuality is a normal, natural part of your life. You are just as responsible for your sexual health as for any other aspect of your well-being. To safeguard your sexual health, you need to be aware of and protect yourself from sexually transmitted infections and diseases.

After studying the material in this chapter, you should be able to

- **Recite** the ABCs of safer sex, **and explain** some specific steps for safeguarding sexual health.
- **Describe** the methods of STI transmission.
- **Name** the sexually transmitted infections, and **describe** the symptoms and treatment for each.
- **Define** HIV infection, **list** five facts about sexual transmission of HIV, and **name** strategies for reducing the risk of HIV infection.
- **Review** your sexual history, **assess** the risks you have taken in the past, and **describe** your strategies for the future.

© William B. Plowman/Stringer/Getty Images

The ABCs of Safer Sex

Making smart, healthy choices about sex is the key to preventing sexual illnesses. (See the lab on "The Sexiness of Safer Sex" in *Making Change Happen*, p. 521, and *Labs for IPC*.) As you will discover in this chapter, there are many specific steps to take to safeguard your sexual health. However, the three key fundamentals are as simple as A, B, C.

A Is for Abstain

Abstinence from vaginal and anal intercourse and oral sex is free, available to everyone, extremely effective at preventing both pregnancy and sexually transmitted infections, and has no medical or hormonal side effects. If you decide to abstain only from vaginal or anal penetration, remember that other sexual activity such as oral sex can also expose you to STIs. If you have oral sex, make it safer by using effective barrier methods such as condoms or latex dental dams. (A dental dam is a square piece of latex that can be stretched across the vulva or anus to prevent the transmission of STI.) In the absence of barrier methods, men should avoid ejaculating in their partners' mouths. Also,

- Be aware of sores and discharge or unpleasant odors from your partner's genitals. These are signs to avoid oral sex.
- Don't floss or brush teeth before oral sex. It might tear the lining of the mouth, increasing exposure to viruses.
- Avoid aggressive and deep thrusting in oral sex, which can damage throat tissues and increase susceptibility for throat-based gonorrhea, herpes, and abrasions.
- Remember that oral sex can transmit various STIs, including HPV, herpes, gonorrhea, syphilis, and HIV.

B Is for Be Faithful

For men and women who are sexually active, a mutually faithful sexual relationship with just one healthy partner is the safest option. Women and men in a committed relationship don't need to worry about getting sexually transmitted infections if:

- Neither partner ever had sex with anyone else.
- Neither partner ever shared needles.
- Neither partner currently has or ever had an STI.

If these criteria fail to apply, two partners should be sure that neither has an STI before giving up on safer-sex practices. Some infections, like HIV, may take years to develop symptoms. The only way to know is by testing.

Of course, a committed relationship remains safe only as long as both partners remain committed. Most women who get HIV from having sex think they are their sex partners' only lover and never suspect that their partners' other lovers are men or women with HIV.

Abstain, Be faithful, or use Condoms. Following the ABC's of safer sex doesn't mean you can't have an intimate, loving relationship.

© iStockphoto.com/Aldo Murillo

The Sexiness of Safer Sex

Protecting yourself and your partner doesn't take anything away from the quality of your sex life In fact, it makes it better. Sex involves more than two *bodies;* it involves, engages, and delights two *people.* Protection doesn't mean less affection. You can still have an intimate relationship with someone, and you can still enjoy the pleasures of being together. Safer sex is still sexy—and certainly far sexier than nagging worries about infections that could jeopardize your future sex life. If you're sexually active, read through "The Sexiness of Safer Sex" in *Labs for IPC.* Even if you're not, read through this preview.

Get Real

In this stage you rate your sexual safety skills by answering twelve questions, including the following:

- How well do you know your partner(s)? Did you share each other's sexual histories before having sex? Is your partner always open about everything with you? Does your partner keep secrets from you?
- How do you protect yourself and a partner from STIs and, if you are heterosexual, pregnancy?
- Do you use this form of protection every time you have sex?

You also read through a list of sexual behaviors, and check any you've engage in with someone whose sexual history and HIV status you did not know. The list includes safe behaviors, such as computer or phone sex, possibly safe ones such as intercourse with a condom, and unsafe ones, such as intercourse without a condom. On the basis of your answers, you rate your sexual safety skills on a scale from 1 (no risk) to 10 (highest risk). You also get checked for STIs, even if you have no symptoms . . .

Get Ready

To prepare, you inform yourself by reading this chapter and going to authoritative websites such as http://www.ashastad.org/ (American Social Health Association) . . .

Get Going

You do one of six exercises in this stage every week. Here is an example:

- **Condom Sense.** Talk with your partner about using a condom before having sex. Don't let embarrassment put your health at risk. Visualize the conversation, and practice the following rebuttals:

Don't you trust me?	Trust isn't the point. People can have an STI and not realize it. OR: I trust you but I don't know your last partner. How can I trust that person?
Condoms interrupt us just when things are getting hot.	Now if we put it on together.
I don't have a condom with me.	I do.
But I love you.	Then you'll help us to protect ourselves.
Just this once.	Once is all it takes . . .

Lock It In

Make your sexual health a priority. Bring up questions related to STIs with your doctor. If you're a woman under age 26, discuss the pros and cons of getting an HPV vaccination. And be prepared. If you are sexually active and not in an exclusive relationship with a healthy partner, carry condoms with you . . .

C Is for Condoms

Condoms are the only contraceptive that helps prevent both pregnancy and STIs when used properly and consistently. Male condoms reduce the risk of transmission of an STI by 50 to 80 percent. They are more effective against STIs transmitted by bodily fluids (chlamydia, gonorrhea, HIV, etc.) than those transmitted by skin-to-skin contact (HPV, syphilis, herpes, chancroid).[1] Inexpensive and widely available in pharmacies, supermarkets, and convenience stores, condoms don't require a doctor visit or a prescription.

Most physicians recommend prelubricated, American-made latex or polyurethane condoms. Check the package for FDA approval. Also check the expiration (Exp) or manufacture (MFG) date on the box or individual package to see until when it is safe to use the condom. Make sure the package and the condom appear in good condition. If the package does not state that the condoms are meant to prevent disease, they may not provide adequate protection even if they are the most expensive ones on the shelf.

Condoms can deteriorate if not stored properly since they are affected by both heat and light. Don't use a condom that has been stored in your back pocket, your wallet, or the glove compartment of your car. Keep fresh condoms handy at all times. If a condom feels sticky or very dry don't use it; the packaging has probably been damaged.

Although it can be awkward to bring up the subject of condoms, don't let your embarrassment put your health at risk. Discuss using a condom before having sex; don't wait until you're on the brink of a sexual encounter.

See Chapter 10 for instructions on how to put on a condom. Here are some additional guidelines:

- **Use a new condom** each and every time you engage in any form of intercourse.
- **Do not use spermicide containing nonoxynol-9.** According to recent research, nonoxynol-9 without condoms is ineffective against HIV transmission. Even with condoms, it does not protect women from the bacteria that cause gonorrhea and chlamydia.
- **If a condom fails** during vaginal or anal intercourse, remove it carefully. If you continue sexual activity, replace it with a new condom.

Sexually Transmitted Infections and Diseases

In medical terms **sexually transmitted infection (STI)** refers to the presence of an infectious agent that can be passed from one sexual partner to another. In public health this term is replacing **sexually transmitted disease (STD)** because sexual infections can be—and often are—transmitted by people who do not have symptoms.

STIs occur in all animals (and even plants) that reproduce sexually. Some people view sexual infections in moral terms. By attaching stigma and shame to STIs, these individuals may not seek treatment and thereby jeopardize their sexual health. However, embarrassment should never justify putting your health at risk.

Remember, STIs can:

- Last a lifetime.
- Put stress on relationships.
- Cause serious medical complications.
- Impair fertility.
- Cause birth defects.
- Lead to major illness and death.

According to the CDC, STDs cost the U.S. health-care system an estimated $15.3 billion annually.[2]

Although each STI is distinct, they are all transmitted mainly through:

- Direct sexual contact with someone's symptoms (like genital ulcers) or sexual

contact with someone's infected semen, vaginal fluids, blood, and other body fluids.

- Sharing contaminated needles through injectable drug use.
- Maternal transfer (mother to fetus during pregnancy or childbirth).

All STI pathogens like dark, warm, moist body surfaces, particularly the mucous membranes that line the reproductive organs; they hate light, cold, and dryness. Figure 16.1 shows how STIs in body fluids spread from person to person and how a barrier can help prevent their entry.

Table 16.1 on p. 524 lists the common STIs, their transmission, symptoms, and treatment. It is possible to catch or have more than one STI at a time. Curing one doesn't necessarily cure another, and treatments don't prevent another bout with the same STI.

Many STIs, including early HIV infection and gonorrhea in women, may not cause any symptoms. As a result, infected individuals may continue their usual sexual activity without realizing that they're jeopardizing another's well-being.

STIs in Society

More Americans are infected with STIs now than at any other time in history. (See Reality Check, p. 525.) According to the Institute of Medicine, the odds of acquiring an STI during a lifetime are one in four. STIs are among the top ten most frequently reported diseases in the United States. The major cause of preventable sterility in America, STIs have tripled the rate of ectopic (tubal) pregnancies, which can be fatal if not detected early. STI complications, including miscarriage, premature delivery, and uterine infections after delivery, annually affect more than 100,000 women.

 STIs do not strike the races or genders equally. Gonorrhea is 19 times more common among blacks than whites, *chlamydia* is 8 times more common, and syphilis 7 times more common. The two most frequently reported STIs, *chlamydia* and gonorrhea, infect many more women than men. The reason may be that male-to-female transmission occurs more readily than female-to-male transmission. Black women ages 15 to 19 have the highest rates of both chlamydia and gonorrhea.[3]

Infection with an STI greatly increases the risk of HIV transmission (discussed later in this chapter). The incidence of STIs is highest in 16- to 24-year-olds—particularly older teenagers—and homosexual men. Others affected by STIs include unborn and newborn children who can "catch" potentially life-threatening infections in the womb or during birth.

Around the world, some 50 million cases of curable STIs occur each year (not including HIV and herpes). Almost 700,000 people are infected every day with one of the over 20 STIs tracked by world health officials. STIs are much more widespread in developing nations because of lack of adequate health standards, prevention practices, and access to treatment.

STIs on Campus

About 19 million new STIs occur each year in the United States.[4] Young people under age 25 account for nearly half.[5] A quarter of teenage girls, according to a recent survey, have at least one STI; the two most common are HPV and chlamydia.[6] Among the girls who reported ever having sex, the prevalence of STIs was 40 percent.[7]

The college years are a prime time for contracting STIs. According to a recent survey, 86 percent of undergraduates are sexually active, but only about half reported using a condom the last time they had vaginal intercourse or using one mostly or always within the last 30 days; for anal intercourse, the percentage fell to about 27 percent; for oral sex, 4 percent. Two-thirds (67 percent) have never been tested for HIV infection. In the National College Health Assessment, infection with human papilloma virus (HPV) was the most commonly reported STI on campus; 2.4 percent of students said they had HPV in the past school year. Genital herpes, reported by 1.0 percent, ranked second, while 0.9 percent of students had chlamydia and 0.3 percent had pelvic inflammatory disease.[8]

Contracting STIs may increase the risk of being infected with HIV. Because college students have more opportunities to have different sexual partners and may use drugs and alcohol more often before sex, they are at greater risk.

Colleges and universities vary in the STI services offered, including screening, diagnosis, and treatment. According to a recent survey, about half of students attend a school where STI screening is available.[9] About half of colleges and universities make condoms available to students—some free in an open display, some free on request, and some for a fee or in vending machines. Larger schools, those with health centers, and those with on-campus housing are more likely to provide STI education and services.

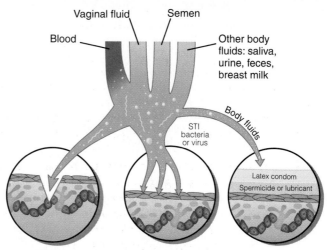

Tough outer skin covers the outside of your body, including hands and lips. Viruses and bacteria enter when skin is chapped or through a hangnail, cut, scrape, sore, or needle puncture.

Fragile inner skin lines the inside of your vagina or penis, anus, and mouth. Viruses and bacteria can enter through microscopic tears in the skin during sexual contact that involves movement or that lacks lubrication.

Barrier protection Latex condoms prevent your partner's body fluids from entering your body. Spermicides kill many STI microbes and reduce friction so condoms are less likely to break.

Figure 16.1 How STIs Spread
Most STIs are spread by viruses or bacteria carried in certain body fluids

sexually transmitted infection (STI) The presence in the human body of an infectious agent that can be passed from one sexual partner to another.

sexually transmitted disease (STD) A disease that is caused by a sexually transmitted infection that produces symptoms.

) TABLE 16.1

Common Sexually Transmitted Infections (STIs): Mode of Transmission, Symptoms, and Treatment

STI	Transmission	Signs and Symptoms	Treatment
Human papilloma virus (HPV) (genital warts) (p. 526)	Spread primarily through vaginal, anal, or oral sex	Cauliflowerlike growths in genital and rectal areas	Removal of lesions by laser surgery or chemicals
Herpes simplex (p. 528)	Genital herpes virus (HSV-2) transmitted by vaginal, anal, or oral sex. Oral herpes virus (HSV-1) transmitted primarily by kissing.	Small, painful red bumps (papules) to the genital region (genital herpes) or mouth (oral herpes). The papules become painful blisters that eventually rupture to form wet, open sores.	No known cure. Treatment may reduce symptoms; acyclovir, famcyclovir, or valacyclovir promote healing and suppress recurrent outbreaks.
Chlamydia (p. 530)	*Chlamydia trachomatis* bacterium transmitted primarily through sexual contact (can also be spread by fingers from one body site to another)	Men: Watery discharge; pain when urinating Women: Usually asymptomatic; sometimes a similar discharge to men's; leading cause of pelvic inflammatory disease (PID)	Antibiotics: doxycycline, azithromycin, ofloxacin, levofloxacin
Gonorrhea ("clap") (p. 532)	*Neisseria gonorrhoeae* bacterium ("gonococcus") spread through genital, oral-genital, or genital-anal contact	Men: Pus discharge from urethra; burning during urination Women: Usually asymptomatic; can lead to PID and sterility in both men and women	Antibiotics: cephalosporins (ceftriaxone or cefixime)
Nongonococcal urethritis (NGU) (p. 533)	Bacteria, most commonly transmitted through sexual intercourse	Men: Discharge from the penis and irritation during urination Women: Mild discharge of pus from the vagina but often no symptoms	A single dose of azithromycin or doxycycline for seven days
Syphilis (p. 533)	*Treponema pallidum* bacterium ("spirochete") transmitted from open lesions during genital, oral-genital, or genital-anal contact	Primary: Chancre Secondary: Rash Latent: Asymptomatic Late: Irreversible damage to central nervous system, cardiovascular system	Penicillin or other antibiotic
Chancroid (p. 535)	*Haemophilus ducrevi* bacterium transmitted by sexual interaction	Men: Painful irregular chancre on penis Women: Chancre on labia	Tetracycline
Pubic lice ("crabs") (p. 535)	*Phthirus pubis* spread easily through body contact or through shared clothing or bedding	Persistent itching; visible lice often located in public hair or other body hairs	1% permethrin cream for body areas; 1% lindane shampoo for hair
HIV/AIDS (p. 536)	HIV transmitted in blood and semen, primarily through sexual contact or needle sharing among injection drug users	Asymptomatic at first; opportunistic infections	Combination of three or more antiretroviral drugs (termed highly active antiretroviral therapies, or HAART) plus other specific treatment for opportunistic infections and tumors

STIs and Gender

 Both men and women can develop STIs, but their risks are not the same. Here is some gender-specific information.

If You Are a Woman

- Keep in mind that your risk of getting an infection is greater than a man's. STIs can be transmitted through breaks in the mucous membranes, and women have more mucosal area exposed and experience more trauma to these tissues during sexual activity than men.

- Don't think you don't have to worry just because you have no symptoms.

Symptoms of STIs also tend to be more "silent" in women, so they often go undetected and untreated, leading to potentially serious complications. For instance, pelvic inflammatory disease has no symptoms but puts you at risk of infertility and ectopic pregnancy.

- At your checkup talk to your doctor about whether you should be tested for sexually transmitted infections. You need to ask for these tests, or else they won't be done.

If You Are a Man

- Involve your partner. Men are more likely to avoid common errors, such as removing condoms before sexual contact ends or slippage during withdrawal, when both partners mutually decide on their use.[10]

- After potential exposure to an STI, give yourself a little extra protection by urinating and washing your genitals with an antibacterial soap.

- At your checkup talk to your doctor about whether you should be tested for sexually transmitted infections. You need to ask for these tests, or else they won't be done.

STI Risk Factors and Risk Continuums

Various factors put young people at risk of STIs, including:

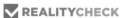 **REALITYCHECK** ....

- *What are a person's odds of acquiring an STI in the course of a lifetime?* ____
- *What percent of sexually active women acquire HPV by age 50?* ____
- *What percent of young people aged 15 to 24 have been infected with the herpes virus?* ____

Answers on next page.

- **Feelings of invulnerability,** which lead to risk-taking behavior. Even when they are well informed of the risks, adolescents and young adults may remain unconvinced that anything bad can or will happen to them.

- **Multiple partners.** Figure 16.2 illustrates how STI risks increase as relationships become less familiar and exclusive.

RELATIONSHIPS

Low risk

Celibacy/Abstinence

Monogamy
  lifetime
  less than lifetime
  (with negative STI/HIV tests)

  less than lifetime
  (with no tests)

A few well-known partners

Multiple well-known partners

A few anonymous partners

Multiple anonymous partners

High risk

BEHAVIORS

Noninsertive

Kissing/Making out
Petting/Fondling
Masturbation
Sex toy use
Outercourse

Insertive and protected
(condoms, other barriers)

Cunnilingus
Fellatio
Vaginal intercourse (i)
Vaginal intercourse (r)
Anal intercourse (i)
Anal intercourse (r)

Insertive and
not protected
(withdrawal)

Fellatio
Cunnilingus
Anilingus
Vaginal intercourse (i)
Vaginal intercourse (r)
Anal intercourse (i)
Anal intercourse (r)

Insertive, not protected,
including ejaculation

Fellatio
Vaginal intercourse (r)
Anal intercourse (r)

i = insertive partner
r = receptive partner

Figure 16.2 Continuum of Risk for Sexual Relationships and Behaviors

STI risks increase as relationships become less familiar and exclusive and as sexual activities become unprotected and receptive.

In surveys of students, a significant number report having had four or more sexual partners during their lifetime.

- **Failure to use condoms.** Among those who reported having had sexual intercourse in the previous three months, fewer than half of the students reported condom use.

Students who'd had four or more sexual partners were significantly less likely to use condoms than those who'd had fewer partners.

- **Substance abuse.** Individuals who drink or use drugs are more likely to engage in sexually risky behaviors, including sex with partners whose health status and history they do not know, and unprotected intercourse.

Rate your own sexual health risk by taking this chapter's Self Survey on page 541.

Human Papilloma Virus

Human papilloma virus (HPV) is the most common sexually transmitted infection in the United States. Most people who become infected with HPV do not have any symptoms, and the infection clears on its own. However, HPV infection can cause cervical cancer in women and genital warts and other types of cancers in both sexes.

The biggest risk factor for HPV infection in men is a large number of lifetime sex partners. Men who've had more than 16 sex partners have about three times the HPV risk of those with fewer sex partners and are nearly ten times more likely to contract a potentially cancer-causing strain. Once infected, men who have been circumcised are more likely to have their immune systems "clear" the virus. Medical scientists do not know how circumcision may protect against persistent infection.[11]

Of the 100 or more different strains, or types, of HPV, approximately 40 are sexually transmitted. Condoms provide only limited protection. Some "high-risk" HPV strains may lead to cancer of the cervix, vulva, vagina, anus, or penis. If transmitted via oral sex, they increase the risk of mouth and throat cancers. In a recent study, individuals with HPV infections were 32 times more likely to develop such cancers. The risk increases along with the number of oral sex partners.

The "low-risk" types of HPV may cause changes in cervical cells that cause Pap test abnormalities or genital warts. Genital warts are single or multiple growths or bumps, sometimes shaped like cauliflower, that appear in the genital area.

Incidence

Approximately 20 million people in the United States are currently infected with HPV, and 6.2 million Americans get a new HPV infection each year. Worldwide there are more than 440 million individuals with HPV infection. As many as 80 percent of sexually active women acquire HPV by age 50.[12]

Young women who engage in sexual intercourse at an early age are more likely than those with later sexual debuts to become infected with HPV. Their risk also increases if they have multiple sexual partners or a history of a sexually transmitted infection, use drugs, or have partners with multiple sexual partners.

College-age women are among those at greatest risk of acquiring HPV infection. In various studies conducted in college health centers, 10 to 46 percent of female students (mean age 20 to 22) had positive HPV tests.

Among women age 14 to 65 screened for cervical cancer, almost one in four tested positive for HPV. Over half of the women younger than 30 who had abnormal (although not clearly cancerous) cells on their Pap smear had HPV infection.[13] About a third of women with HPV acquire the infection within the year following first intercourse. In a recent study, almost half of young women with just one male partner developed HPV over a three-year period. The probability of HPV infection increased with partners who had at least two previous sex partners.[14]

College students' awareness of HPV and their potential risk is very low. In one study, both sexes saw themselves as not susceptible to HPV. Male students were more likely than female students to think that only women could acquire HPV. In another report, even women with adequate to high levels of knowledge about HPV did not take steps such as using condoms or having regular Pap tests to protect themselves.

The HPV Vaccine Gardasil, the first vaccine developed to prevent cervical cancer, targets four HPV types that together cause 70 percent of cervical cancers and 90 percent of genital warts.[15] It does not protect against all HPV types that cause cervical cancer. Gardasil is most effective when given before first sexual contact and exposure to HPV. In girls and women who have never been infected with HPV, the vaccine can prevent almost all cases of disease caused by the four targeted types of HPV, including cancers of the genitals, cervix, and anus. In women with prior infection—with the HPV strains targeted by the vaccine, other strains, or both—Gardasil's efficacy falls from almost 100 percent to as low as 17 percent.

The CDC has recommended HPV vaccination for all girls before they turn 13, and some states are considering mandatory immunization. However, there is continuing controversy over the timing and need for universal vaccination. (See Consumer Alert, page 528.)

A male vaccine is being tested. In a study of college men, those most willing to be vaccinated were primarily concerned about safeguarding their own sexual health rather than reducing their female partners' cervical cancer risk.[16]

Human papillomavirus, which causes genital warts, is the most common viral STI.

Signs and Symptoms

Most people with HPV infection do not know they are infected. The virus lives in the skin or mucous membranes and usually cause no symptoms. Some people get visible genital warts or have precancerous changes in the cervix, vulva, anus, or penis. After contact with an infected individual, genital warts may appear within three weeks to eighteen months, with an average period of about three months.

 HPV infection may invade the urethra and cause urinary obstruction and bleeding. It greatly increases a woman's risk of developing a precancerous condition called cervical *intraepithelial neoplasia*, which can lead to cervical cancer. Adolescent girls infected the HPV appear to be particularly vulnerable to developing cervical cancer. It is not known if HPV itself causes cancer or acts in conjunction with cofactors (such as other infections, smoking, or suppressed immunity). A woman's risk of cervical cancer is strongly related to the number of her partner's current and lifetime female partners. Women are five to eleven times as likely to get cervical cancer

human papilloma virus (HPV) A pathogen that causes genital warts and increases the risk of cervical cancer.

Should You Get the HPV Vaccine?

Some states are considering legislation to make HPV vaccination mandatory for all girls because the vaccine is most effective when given before a girl becomes sexually active. Some religious groups oppose mandatory immunization because they feel that vaccinating girls against an STI gives them the wrong message about sexual responsibility. Consumer advocates worry about the unknown long-term effects. Others feel that the decision should be made privately by parents in consultation with their pediatricians.

Facts to Know

- The HPV vaccine, Gardasil, which consists of three shots given over a six-month period, has been extensively tested in thousands of young women worldwide and is considered safe. However, the longest study so far has lasted only five years, so long-term effects are not known.
- Gardasil confers immunity for at least five years, abut no one yet knows whether a booster shot or shots will be necessary.
- The most common side effects are pain at the injection site and fever. There have been cases of tingling, numbness, and loss of sensation in young girls receiving the vaccine.

Steps to Take

- Talk with your doctor if you are under age 26 and have not yet been vaccinated.
- Check with your insurance provider. Gardasil costs about $120 per shot, or $360 for the three-shot series. Most insurance companies cover recommended vaccines, but since this one is new, yours may or may not.
- Do *not* get the HPV vaccine if you:
  - are older than 26 (the vaccine is still being tested in women in this age group).
  - are pregnant.
  - have ever had a life-threatening allergic reaction to any component of HPV vaccine.
  - are moderately to severely ill at the time of vaccination.

if their steady sex partner has had 20 or more previous partners.

Most HPV infections are asymptomatic in men, who may unwittingly increase their partners' risk. Men who test positive for HPV typically report significantly more sex partners than those who do not. HPV may also cause genital warts in men and increase the risk of cancer of the penis. People with visible genital warts also may have asymptomatic or subclinical HPV infections that are extremely difficult to treat.

Diagnosis and Treatment

Most women are diagnosed with HPV after an abnormal Pap test or HPV DNA test. The results of HPV DNA testing can help health-care providers decide if treatment is necessary to prevent or treat cervical cancer. (See Chapter 14 for a discussion of cervical cancer.) Warning signs for cervical cancer include irregular bleeding or unusual vaginal discharge. Precancerous cervical cells can be destroyed by laser surgery or freezing during a visit to a doctor's office.

No form of therapy has been shown to completely eradicate HPV, nor has any single treatment been uniformly effective in removing warts or preventing their recurrence. CDC guidelines suggest treatments that focus on the removal of visible warts—laser therapy cryotherapy (freezing), and topical applications of podofilox, podophyllin, or trichloroacetic acid—and then eradication of the virus. At least 20 to 30 percent of treated individuals experience recurrence.

Genital Herpes

Herpes (from the Greek word that means *to creep)* collectively describes some of the most common viral infections in humans. Characteristically, **herpes simplex** causes blisters on the skin or mucous membranes.

Herpes simplex exists in several varieties. *Herpes simplex virus 1 (HSV-1)* can be transmitted by kissing and generally causes cold sores and fever blisters around the mouth. *Herpes simplex virus 2 (HSV-2)* is sexually transmitted and may cause blisters on the penis, inside the vagina, on the cervix, in the public area, on the buttocks, on the thighs, or in the mouth and throat (transmitted via oral sex).

HSV transmission occurs through close contact with mucous membranes or abraded skin. Condoms help prevent infection but aren't foolproof. When herpes sores are present, the infected person is highly contagious and should avoid bringing the lesions into contact with someone else's body through touching, sexual interaction, or kissing.

Individuals without any obvious symptoms shed the virus subclinically, whether or not they have lesions. Most people with herpes contract it from partners who were not aware of any symptoms or of their own contagiousness.

The herpes virus is present in genital secretions even when patients do not notice any signs of the disease, and people infected with genital herpes can spread it even between flare-ups when they have no symptoms. There is growing evidence that genital herpes promotes the spread of HIV.

A newborn can be infected with genital herpes while passing through the birth canal, and the frequency of mother-to-infant transmission seems to be increasing. Most infected infants develop typical skin sores, which can be cultured to confirm a herpes diagnosis. Some physicians recommend treatment with acyclovir. Because of the risk of severe damage and possible death, caesarean delivery may be advised for a woman with active herpes lesions.

Incidence

Genital herpes has skyrocketed during the last three decades, yet only a minority of infections with HSV-2 are recognized by those infected. About 40 percent of new cases of genital herpes occur in young people aged 15 to 24. An estimated 45 million young adults in this age range—an estimated one in five adolescents and adults—have been infected. About one in four women and one in eight men carries the herpes virus.[17]

Signs and Symptoms

Most people with genital herpes have no symptoms or very mild symptoms that go unnoticed or are not recognized as a sign of infection. The most common is a cluster of blistery sores, usually on the vagina, vulva, cervix, penis, buttocks, or anus. They may last several weeks and go away. They may return in weeks, months, or years.

Other symptoms include: blisters, burning feelings if urine flows over sores, inability to urinate if severe swelling of sores blocks the urethra, itching and pain in the infected area. Severe first episodes of herpes may also cause swollen, tender lymph glands in the groin, throat, and under the arms, fever, chills, headache, and achy flu-like feelings.

The virus that causes herpes never entirely goes away; it retreats to nerves near the lower spinal cord, where it remains for the life of the host. Herpes sores can return without warning weeks, months, or even years after their first occurrence, often during menstruation or times of stress, or with sudden changes in body temperature. Of those who experience HSV recurrence, 10 to 35 percent do so frequently—that is, about six or more times a year. In most people, attacks diminish in frequency and severity over time. Herpes, like other STIs, can trigger feelings of shame, guilt, and depression. It also may make people more susceptible to HIV infection.[18]

Diagnosis and Treatment

Standard methods of diagnosing genital herpes in women, which rely primarily on physical examination and viral cultures, may miss as many as two-thirds of all cases. Blood tests are more effective in detecting unrecognized infections with HSV-2.

The three antiviral medications approved for the treatment of genital herpes are:

- *Acyclovir.* The oldest antiviral medication for herpes, acyclovir is sold as a generic drug and under the brand name Zovirax®. Available as an ointment and pill, acyclovir has been shown to be safe in persons who have used it continuously (every day) for as long as 10 years.

- *Valacyclovir.* Sold as Valtrex®, this medication delivers acyclovir more efficiently so that the body absorbs more of the drug and medication can be taken fewer times during the day.

(a) Herpes simplex virus (HSV-1) as a mouth sore; (b) Herpes simplex virus (HSV-2) as a genital sore.

herpes simplex A condition caused by one of the herpes viruses and characterized by lesions of the skin or mucous membranes; herpes simplex virus 2 is sexually transmitted and causes genital blisters or sores.

- *Famciclovir.* Sold as Famvir®, this drug utilizes penciclovir as its active ingredient to stop HSV. Like valacyclovir, it is well absorb, persists for a long time in the body, and can be taken less frequently than acyclovir.

These antiviral medications are prescribed for initial and recurrent episodes of herpes. In episodic therapy, a person begins taking medication at the first sign of recurrence and continues for several days to hasten the healing or prevent a full outbreak from occurring. In suppressive therapy, people with genital herpes take antiviral medication daily to prevent symptoms. For individuals who have frequent recurrences (six or more per year), suppressive therapy can reduce the number of outbreaks by at least 75 percent. Suppressive therapy may also reduce asymptomatic shedding of HSV.

Various treatments—compresses made with cold water, skim milk, or warm salt water; ice packs; or a mild anesthetic cream—can relieve discomfort. Herpes sufferers should avoid heat, hot baths, or nylon underwear. Some physicians have used laser therapy to vaporize the lesions. Clinical trials of an experimental vaccine to protect people from herpes infections are underway.

Chlamydia

The most widespread sexually transmitted bacterium in the United States is *Chlamydia trachomatis,* which causes more than a million cases of **chlamydia** each year, a number that continues to rise.[19] Almost half of reported cases occur among sexually active young adults between age 15 and 24.[20] The use of condoms with spermicide can reduce, but not eliminate, the risk of chlamydial infection.

Incidence

A record number of Americans—some 1.1 million, or 1 in 25 young Americans—are infected with chlamydia.[21] Chlamydia is six times more prevalent in young black adults than in young white adults. Women have three times the rate of chlamydia as men.[22] Chlamydial infections are more common in younger than in older women, and they also occur more often in both men and women with gonorrhea.

In a study of almost 800 students who volunteered for screening at ten southern colleges, nearly 10 percent tested positive for chlamydia, with higher rates among black women than white women. Younger students also were more likely to be infected than older ones, possibly because they are more likely to have unprotected intercourse, to engage in sex with multiple partners, and to have partners at higher risk for STDs.[23]

Those at greatest risk of chlamydial infection are individuals 25 years old or younger who engage in sex with more than one new partner within a two-month period and women who use birth control pills or other nonbarrier contraceptive methods. The U.S. Preventive Services Task Force recommends regular screening for chlamydia for all sexually active women under age 25 and for older women with multiple sexual partners, a history of STIs, or inconsistent use of condoms.

Signs and Symptoms

As many as 75 percent of women and 50 percent of men with chlamydia have no symptoms or symptoms so mild that they don't seek medical attention. Without treatment, up to 40 percent of cases of chlamydia can lead to pelvic inflammatory disease, a serious infection of the woman's fallopian tubes that also can damage the ovaries and uterus. Also, women infected with chlamydia may have three to five times the risk of getting infected with HIV if exposed. Babies exposed to chlamydia in the birth canal during delivery can be born with pneumonia or with an eye infection called conjunctivitis, both of which can be dangerous unless treated early with antibiotics. Symptomless women who are screened and treated for chlamydial infection are almost 60 percent less likely than unscreened women to develop pelvic inflammatory disease. Chlamydia may also be linked to cervical cancer.

When women have symptoms of chlamydia they may experience

- Abdominal pain.
- Abnormal vaginal discharge.
- Bleeding between menstrual periods.
- Cervical or rectal inflammation.
- Low-grade fever.
- Yellowish discharge from the cervix that may have a foul odor.
- Vaginal bleeding after intercourse.
- Painful intercourse.
- Painful urination.
- The urge to urinate more than usual.

When men have symptoms of chlamydia, they may experience

- Pain or burning while urinating.
- Pus or watery or milky discharge from the penis.
- Swollen or tender testicles.
- Rectal inflammation.

Men often don't take these symptoms seriously because the symptoms may appear only early in the day and can be very mild.

Chlamydia, which can spread from a man's urethra to his testicles, can also cause a condition called epididymitis, which can cause sterility. Symptoms include fever, swelling, and extreme pain in the scrotum. Six percent of men with epididymitis develop reactive arthritis, which causes swelling and pain in the joints and can progress and become disabling.

In women and men, chlamydia may cause the rectum to itch and bleed. It can also result in a discharge and diarrhea. If it infects the eyes, it may cause redness, itching, and a discharge. If it infects the throat, it may cause soreness.

Diagnosis and Treatment

Various antibiotics kill *Chlamydia*. Some are taken in a single dose; others over several days. Both partners must be treated to avoid reinfections.

The CDC, in its most recent guidelines, recommends that all women with chlamydia be rescreened three to four months after treatment is completed. The reason is that reinfection, which often happens because a patient's sex partners were not treated, increases the risk of pelvic inflammatory disease and other complications. Immediately treating the partners of people infected with gonorrhea or chlamydia can reduce rates of recurrence of these infections.

A baby exposed to chlamydial infection in the birth canal during delivery may develop an eye infection. Symptoms include a bloody discharge and swollen eyelids.

Pelvic Inflammatory Disease (PID)

Infection of a woman's fallopian tubes or uterus, called **pelvic inflammatory disease (PID)**, is not actually an STI, but rather a complication of STIs. Ten to 20 percent of initial episodes of PID lead to scarring and obstruction of the fallopian tubes severe enough to cause infertility. Other long-term complications are ectopic pregnancy and chronic pelvic pain. Smoking also may increase the likelihood of PID. Two bacteria—*Gonococcus* (the culprit in gonorrhea) and *Chlamydia*—are responsible for one-half to one-third of all cases of PID. Other organisms are responsible for the remaining cases.

Several studies have shown that women with PID are more likely to have used douches than those without the disease. Consistent condom use may decrease PID risk.

Incidence

About one in every seven women of reproductive age has PID; half of all adult women may have had it. Each year, about 1 million new cases are reported.[24]

Most cases of PID occur among women under age 25 who are sexually active. *Gonococcus*-caused cases tend to affect poor women; those caused by *Chlamydia* range across all income levels. One-half to one-third of all cases are transmitted sexually, and others have been traced to some IUDs that are no longer on the market.

chlamydia A sexually transmitted infection caused by the bacterium *Chlamydia trachomatis,* often asymptomatic in women, but sometimes characterized by urinary pain; if undetected and untreated, may result in pelvic inflammatory disease (PID).

pelvic inflammatory disease (PID) An inflammation of the internal female genital tract, characterized by abdominal pain, fever, and tenderness of the cervix.

Signs and Symptoms

PID is a silent disease that in half of all cases produces no noticeable symptoms as it progresses and causes scarring of the fallopian tubes. Experts are encouraging women with mild symptoms, such as abdominal pain or tenderness, to seek medical evaluation and are encouraging physicians to test these patients for infections.

Other symptoms include fever, vaginal discharge that may have a foul odor, painful intercourse or urination, irregular menstrual bleeding, and, rarely, pain in the right upper abdomen.

Diagnosis and Treatment

Urine testing is a cost-effective method of detecting gonorrhea and chlamydia in young women and can prevent development of PID. For women with symptoms, a pelvic ultrasound can show whether fallopian tubes are enlarged or an abscess is present. Magnetic resonance imaging (MRI) also can establish a diagnosis of PID and detect other diseases that may be responsible for the symptoms. Treatment consists of antibiotic therapy, usually with at least two antibiotics effective against a wide range of bacteria. A woman's sex partner(s) also should be treated to decrease the risk of reinfection, even if they have no symptoms. PID causes an estimated 15 to 30 percent of all cases of infertility every year and about half of all cases of ectopic pregnancy.

Gonorrhea

Gonorrhea (sometimes called "the clap" in street language) is one of the most common STIs in the United States.

Incidence

 After steady declines from the 1970s to the late 1990s, gonorrhea infections rose in the mid-2000s and have remained stable. However, this rate—118.9 cases per 100,000 population—greatly exceeds the Healthy People 2010 goal of 19 cases per 100,000.[25] As with chlamydia, gonorrhea rates are higher in women, particularly those between ages 15 and 24, than in men. Sexual contact, including oral sex, is the primary means of transmission.

Signs and Symptoms

Most men who have gonorrhea know it. Thick, yellow-white pus oozes from the penis and urination causes a burning sensation. These symptoms usually develop two to nine days after the sexual contact that infected them. Men have a good reason to seek help: It hurts too much not to.

In men, untreated gonorrhea can spread to the prostate gland, testicles, bladder, and kidneys. Among the serious complications are urinary obstruction and sterility caused by blockage of the vas deferens (the excretory duct of the testis).

Women also may experience discharge and burning on urination. However, as many as eight out of ten infected women have no symptoms.

Gonococcus, the bacterium that causes gonorrhea, can live in the vagina, cervix, and fallopian tubes for months, even years, and continue to infect the woman's sexual partners. Approximately 5 percent of sexually active American women have positive gonorrhea cultures but are unaware that they are silent carriers.

If left untreated in men or women, gonorrhea spreads through the urinary-genital tract. In women, the inflammation travels from the vagina and cervix, through the uterus, to the fallopian tubes and ovaries. The pain and fever are similar to those caused by stomach upset, so a woman may dismiss the symptoms. Eventually these symptoms diminish, even though the disease spreads to the entire pelvis. Pus may ooze from the fallopian tubes or ovaries into the peritoneum (the lining of the abdominal cavity), sometimes causing serious inflammation. However, this, too, can subside in a few weeks.

Gonorrhea, the leading cause of sterility in women, can cause PID. In pregnant women, gonorrhea becomes a threat to the newborn. It can infect the infant's external genitals and can cause a serious form of conjunctivitis. As a preventive step, newborns may have penicillin dropped into their eyes at birth.

In both sexes, gonorrhea can develop into a serious, even fatal, bloodborne infection that can cause arthritis in the joints, attack the heart muscle and lining, cause meningitis, and attack the skin and other organs.

Diagnosis and Treatment

Although a blood test has been developed for detecting gonorrhea, the tried-and-true method of diagnosis is still a microscopic analysis of cultures from the male's urethra, the female's cervix, and the throat and anus of both sexes.

Because gonorrhea often occurs along with chlamydia, practitioners often prescribe an agent effective against both, such as ofloxacin. Fluoroquinolones are no longer advised for use in its treatment. The cephalosporin antibiotics are now the recommended treatment. Antibiotics taken for other reasons may not affect or cure gonorrhea, because of their dosage or type. And you can't develop immunity to gonorrhea; within days of recovering from one case, you can catch another.

A cloudy discharge is symptomatic of gonorrhea.

Nongonococcal Urethritis (NGU)

The term **nongonococcal urethritis (NGU)** refers to any inflammation of the urethra that is not caused by gonorrhea. NGU is the most common STI in men, accounting for 4 to 6 million visits to a physician every year. Three microorganisms—*Chlamydia trachomatis, Ureaplasma urealyticum,* and *Mycoplasma genitalium*—are the primary causes; the usual means of transmission is sexual intercourse. Other infectious agents, such as fungi or bacteria, allergic reactions to vaginal secretions, or irritation by soaps or contraceptive foams or gels also may lead to NGU.

In the United States, NGU is more common in men than gonococcal urethritis.

The symptoms in men are similar to those of gonorrhea, including discharge from the penis (usually less than with gonorrhea) and mild burning during urination. Women frequently develop no symptoms or very mild itching, burning during urination, or discharge. Symptoms usually disappear after two or three weeks, but the infection may persist and cause cervicitis or PID in women and, in men, may spread to the prostate, epididymis, or both. Treatment usually consists of doxycycline or azithromycin and should be given to both sexual partners.

gonorrhea A sexually transmitted infection caused by the bacterium *Neisseria gonorrhoeae*; symptoms include discharge from the penis; women are generally asymptomatic.

nongonococcal urethritis (NGU) Inflammation of the urethra caused by organisms other than the *Gonococcus* bacterium.

syphilis A sexually transmitted infection caused by the bacterium *Treponema pallidum* and characterized by early sores, a latent period, and a final period of life-threatening symptoms, including brain damage and heart failure.

Syphilis

A corkscrew-shaped, spiral bacterium called *Treponema pallidum* causes **syphilis**. This frail microbe dies in seconds if dried or chilled but grows quickly in the warm, moist tissues of the body, particularly in the mucous membranes of the genital tract. Entering the body through any tiny break in the skin, the germ burrows its way into the bloodstream. Sexual contact, including oral sex or intercourse, is a primary means of transmission. Genital ulcers caused by syphilis may increase the risk of HIV infection, while individuals with HIV may be more likely to develop syphilis.

Incidence

The rate of syphilis in the United States declined by about 90 percent from 1990 through 2000, but has increased every year since, mostly in men. However, syphilis has also been rising in women for the last three years.[26]

Signs and Symptoms

Syphilis has clearly identifiable stages:

- **Primary syphilis.** The first sign of syphilis is a lesion, or *chancre* (pronounced "shanker"), an open lump or crater the size of a dime or smaller, teeming with bacteria. The incubation period before its appearance ranges from 10 to 90 days; three to four weeks is average. The chancre appears exactly where the bacteria entered the body: in the mouth, throat, vagina, rectum, or penis. Any contact with the chancre is likely to result in infection.

- **Secondary syphilis.** Anywhere from 1 to 12 months after the chancre's appearance, secondary-stage symptoms may appear. Some people have no symptoms. Others develop a skin rash or a small, flat rash in moist regions on the skin; whitish patches on the mucous membranes of the mouth or throat; temporary baldness; low-grade fever; headache; swollen glands; or large, moist sores around the mouth and genitals. These sores are loaded with bacteria; contact with them, through kissing or intercourse, may transmit the infection. Symptoms may last for several days or several months. Even without treatment, symptoms eventually disappear as the syphilis microbes go into hiding.

- **Late and latent syphilis.** Although there are no signs or symptoms, no sores or rashes at this stage, the bacteria are invading various organs inside the body, including the heart and brain. For two to four years, there may be recurring infectious and highly contagious lesions of the skin or mucous membranes. However, syphilis loses its infectiousness as it progresses: After the first two years, a person rarely transmits syphilis through intercourse.

After four years, even congenital syphilis is rarely transmitted. Until this stage of the disease, however, a pregnant woman can pass syphilis to her unborn child. If the fetus is infected in its fourth month or earlier, it may be disfigured or even die. If infected late in pregnancy, the child may show no signs of infection for months or years after birth, but may then become disabled with the symptoms of tertiary syphilis.

- **Tertiary syphilis.** Ten to 20 years after the beginning of the latent stage, the most serious symptoms of syphilis emerge, generally in the organs in which the bacteria settled during latency. Syphilis that has progressed to this stage has become increasingly rare. Victims of tertiary syphilis may die of a ruptured aorta or of other heart damage, or may have progressive brain or spinal cord damage, eventually leading to blindness, insanity, or paralysis. About a third of those who are not treated during the first three stages of syphilis enter the tertiary stage later in life.

Diagnosis and Treatment

Health experts are urging screening with a blood test for syphilis for everyone who seeks treatment for an STI, especially adolescents; for everyone using illegal drugs; and for the partners of these two groups. They also recommend that anyone diagnosed with syphilis be screened for other STIs and be counseled about voluntary testing for HIV.

Penicillin is the drug of choice for treating primary, secondary, and latent syphilis. The earlier treatment begins, the more effective it is. Those allergic to penicillin may be treated with doxycycline, ceftriaxone, or erythromycin. An added danger of not getting treatment for syphilis is an increased risk of HIV transmission.

Chancroid

A **chancroid** is a soft, painful sore or localized infection caused by the bacterium *Haemophilus ducrevi* and usually acquired through sexual contact. Half of the cases heal by themselves. In other cases, the infection may spread to the lymph glands near the chancroid, where large amounts of pus can accumulate and destroy much of the local tissue. The incidence of this STI, widely prevalent in Africa and tropical and semitropical regions, is rapidly increasing in the United States, with outbreaks in several states, including Louisiana, Texas, and New York. Chancroids, which may increase susceptibility to HIV infection, are believed to be a major factor in the heterosexual spread of HIV. This infection is treated with antibiotics (ceftriaxone, azithromycin, or erythromycin) and can be prevented by keeping the genitals clean and washing them with soap and water in case of possible exposure.

Pubic Lice and Scabies

These infections are sometimes, but not always, transmitted sexually. *Pubic lice* (or "crabs") are usually found in the pubic hair, although they can migrate to any hairy areas of the body. Lice lay eggs called nits that attach to the base of the hair shaft. Irritation from the lice may produce intense itching. Scratching to relieve the itching can produce sores. *Scabies* is caused by a mite that burrows under the skin, where they lay eggs that hatch and undergo many changes in the course of their life cycle, producing great discomfort, including intense itching.

Lice and scabies are treated with applications of permethrin cream and lindane shampoo to all the areas of the body where there are concentrations of body hair (genitals, armpits, scalp). You must repeat treatment in seven days to kill any newly developed adults. You must also wash or dry-clean clothing and bedding.

Actual size

A pubic louse, or "crab."

© E. Gray/Photo Researchers, Inc.

Trichomoniasis

An estimated 7.4 million new cases of this common curable STI our each year in men and women. The cause is a single-celled protozoan parasite *Trichomonas vaginalis,* transmitted by vaginal intercourse or vulva-to-vulva contact with an infected partner. Women can acquire this disease from male or female partners; men usually contract it only from infected women.

Most men have no signs or symptoms; some experience irritation inside the penis, mild discharge, or slight burning on urination or ejaculation. Some women develop a frothy, yellow-green vaginal discharge with a strong odor and may experience discomfort during intercourse and urination as well as genital itching and irritation. This inflammation may increase a woman's

chancroid A soft, painful sore or localized infection usually acquired through sexual contact.

susceptibility to HIV if she is exposed to the virus.

Diagnosis is based on a physical examination and a laboratory test. Treatment consists of a single dose of oral medication, either metronidazole or tinidazole. If untreated, an infected man, even if he has never had symptoms or if his symptoms have gone away, can continue to infect or reinfect partners.[27]

HIV and AIDS

Thirty years ago, no one knew about **human immunodeficiency virus (HIV).** No one had ever heard of **acquired immune deficiency syndrome (AIDS).** Once seen as an epidemic affecting primarily gay men and injection drug users, AIDS has taken on a very different form. Today, heterosexuals in developing countries have the highest rates of infection and mortality. And HIV infection continues to spread, doubling at an estimated rate of every ten years.

Incidence

  About 39.4 million people worldwide are infected with HIV; 15,000 more individuals are infected every day. Every nine-and-a-half minutes another person becomes infected in the United States. AIDS now claims about 3 million lives—more than half children—around the world each year. About 36,300 new HIV infections occur in the United States—a number much higher than previous estimates because of improved technology for reporting cases.

Annual transmission rates fell from higher than 30 percent a year during the early 1980s to below 6 percent from 1991 through 2006. The most recent estimate was 5 percent. These data suggest that most HIV-infected people (at least 95 percent, are not spreading the disease.[28]

Yet even though the rate of new infections is falling, the prevalence has risen because of earlier detection and because, thanks to better treatment, more people with HIV/AIDS are living longer. In some areas, such as Washington, DC, 3 percent of people over age 12 (three times the rate classified as an epidemic) are infected with HIV. Among black men, 6.5 percent are infected.[29]

Men who have sex with men account for slightly more than half of new cases (53 percent), while heterosexuals account for 31 percent and injection drug users for 12 percent.

Infection rates among blacks are seven times as high as for white and almost three times as high as for Hispanics. Homosexual and bisexual men, particularly those who are young or nonwhite and living in metropolitan areas, are at particularly high risk. The percentage of individuals who acquired HIV through heterosexual contact has increased. Many heterosexuals are not aware of their partner's HIV status and may not see themselves as being at risk of HIV infection. About a fifth of the HIV-infected individuals in the United States have not been diagnosed. (See Figure 16.3.)

African Americans and Hispanics account for a disproportionate share of new AIDS diagnoses. Almost half of all those living with HIV/AIDS in the United States are African American (Figure 16.4). The AIDS case rate per 100,000 people is 9.5 times that of whites. African Americans are less likely to survive after a diagnosis of AIDS than other ethnic or racial groups. HIV/AIDS is the third-leading cause of death among African Americans between ages 25 and 34 and the sixth leading cause of death for whites and Hispanics in this age group.

HIV/AIDS is seen as a threat to men, but 27 percent of new HIV infections in the United States occur among women. About a quarter of Americans living with HIV/AIDS are women. Nonwhite women, particularly African Americans, have been hardest hit. While African American women make up just 13 percent of the female population of the United States, they account for 67 percent of newly diagnosed female cases. HIV/AIDS is most prevalent among women in their childbearing years.

Reducing the Risk of HIV Transmission

HIV/AIDS can be so frightening that some people have exaggerated its dangers, whereas others understate them. The fact is that although no one is immune to HIV, you can reduce the risk if you abstain from sexual activity or remain in a monogamous relationship with an uninfected partner, and do not inject drugs. (See Health on a Budget, p. 539.)

If you're not in a long-term monogamous relationship with a partner you're sure is safe, and you're not willing to abstain from sex, there are things you can do to lower your risk of HIV infection. Remember that the risk of HIV transmission depends on sexual behavior, not sexual orientation. Among young men, the prevalence and frequency of sexual risk behaviors are similar regardless of sexual orientation, ethnicity, or age. Homosexual, heterosexual, and bisexual individuals all need to know about the kinds of sexual activity that increase their risk.

Sexual Transmission Here's what you should know about sexual transmission of HIV:

- Casual contact does *not* spread HIV infection. You cannot get HIV infection from drinking from a water fountain, contact with a toilet seat, or touching an infected person.

- Compared to other viruses, HIV is extremely difficult to get.

- HIV can live in blood, semen, vaginal fluids, and breast milk.

- Many chemicals, including household bleach, alcohol, and hydrogen peroxide, can inactivate HIV.

- In studies of family members sharing dishes, food, clothing, and frequent hugs with people with HIV infection or AIDS, those who have contracted the virus have shared razor blades, toothbrushes, or had other means of blood contact.

- You cannot tell visually whether a potential sexual partner has HIV. A blood test is needed to detect the antibodies that the body produces to fight HIV, thus indicating infection. As noted in Chapter 15, circumcision greatly

reduces the risk for HIV infection.

- HIV can be spread in semen and vaginal fluids during a single instance of anal, vaginal, or oral sexual contact between heterosexuals, bisexuals, or homosexuals. The risk increases with the number of sexual encounters with an infected partner.

- Teenage girls may be particularly vulnerable to HIV infection because the immature cervix is easily infected.

- Anal intercourse is an extremely high-risk behavior because HIV can enter the bloodstream through tiny breaks in the lining of the rectum. HIV transmission is much more likely to occur during unprotected anal intercourse than vaginal intercourse.

- Other behaviors that increase the risk of HIV infection include having multiple sexual partners, engaging in sex without condoms or virus-killing spermicides, sexual contact with persons known to be at high risk (for example, prostitutes or injection drug users), and sharing

human immunodeficiency virus (HIV) A type of virus that causes a spectrum of health problems, ranging from a symptomless infection to changes in the immune system, to the development of life-threatening diseases because of impaired immunity.

acquired immune deficiency syndrome (AIDS) The final stages of HIV infection, characterized by a variety of severe illnesses and decreased levels of certain immune cells.

Figure 16.3 HIV/AIDS in America: A Statistical Snapshot

Number of people living with HIV/AIDS:	1.1 million
Annual number of new HIV infections:	56,300
Cumulative number of AIDS deaths:	583,298
Percent of people infected with HIV who do not know it:	21 percent
Percent of women among those with new infections:	27 percent
Percent of people under age 30 among those with new infections:	34 percent

Source: "The HIV/AIDS Epidemic in the United States." *HIV/AIDS Policy Fact Sheet*, Kaiser Family Foundation, February 2009. www.kff.org.

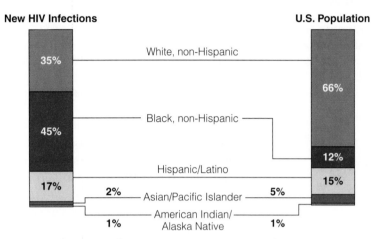

Figure 16.4 Racial Disparities in HIV Infection

Source: "The HIV/AIDS Epidemic in the United States." *HIV/AIDS Policy Fact Sheet*, Kaiser Family Foundation, February 2009. www.kff.org.

POINT

Individuals diagnosed with an STI that could cause serious, even life-threatening illness, such as HIV, should abstain from sex or inform any potential sex partner of their condition. If they fail to do so, they should face legal prosecution for endangering the health of another person. The penalties in cases involving HIV should be severe.

COUNTERPOINT

Failing to inform a potential sexual partner of an STI is morally wrong. However, many circumstances, such as drinking, can interfere with clear communication. As long as two people mutually consent to sex, failure to disclose should not be viewed as a crime.

YOUR VIEW

Do you think individuals who jeopardize their partners' health by not informing them of an STI deserve punishment? Or is it the responsibility of every person engaging in sexual activity to ask about a potential partner's history and insist on safer-sex practices? How would you feel if you found out after the fact that a partner has an STI and that you may be infected?

injection equipment for drugs.

- Individuals are at greater risk if they have an active sexual infection. Sexually transmitted infections, such as herpes, gonorrhea, and syphilis, facilitate transmission of HIV during vaginal or anal intercourse.

- No cases of HIV transmission by deep (French) kissing have been reported, but it could happen. Studies have found blood in the saliva of healthy people after kissing; other lab studies have found HIV in saliva. Social (dry) kissing is safe.

- Oral sex can lead to HIV transmission. The virus in any semen that enters the mouth could make its way into the bloodstream through tiny nicks or sores in the mouth. A man's risk in performing oral sex on a woman is smaller because an infected woman's genital fluids have much lower concentrations of HIV than does semen.

- HIV infection is not widespread among lesbians, although there have been documented cases of possible female-to-female HIV transmission. However, in each instance, one partner had had sex with a bisexual man or male injection drug user or had injected drugs herself.

Federal health officials fear that a new generation may not be using adequate safer-sex precautions, because they have grown complacent about the dangers of HIV/AIDS. Efforts to prevent sexual transmission of HIV have taken a new focus: counseling those who already have HIV in an attempt to get them to stop spreading it. Those who knowingly transmit HIV may face legal prosecution. (See Point/Counterpoint.)

Nonsexual Transmission Efforts to prevent nonsexual forms of HIV transmission have been very effective. Screening the blood supply has reduced the rate of transfusion-associated HIV transmission by 99.9 percent. Treatment with antiretroviral drugs during pregnancy and birth has reduced transmission to newborns by about 90 percent in optimal conditions. Among drug users in some settings, programs that combine addiction treatment and needle exchange reduced the incidence of HIV infection by 30 percent.

Signs and Symptoms

HIV infection refers to a spectrum of health problems that results from immunologic abnormalities caused by the virus when it enters the bloodstream. In theory, the body may be able to resist infection by HIV. In reality, in almost all cases, HIV destroys the cell-mediated immune system, particularly the CD4+ T-lymphocytes (also called *T4 helper cells)*. The result is greatly increased susceptibility to various cancers and opportunistic infections (infections that take hold because of the reduced effectiveness of the immune system).

HIV triggers a state of all-out war within the immune system. Almost immediately following infection with HIV, the immune system responds aggressively by manufacturing enormous numbers of CD4+ cells. It eventually is overwhelmed, however, as the viral particles continue to replicate, or multiply. The intense war between HIV and the immune system indicates that the virus itself, not a breakdown in the immune system, is responsible for disease progression.

Shortly after becoming infected with HIV, individuals may experience a few days of flu-like symptoms, which most ignore or attribute to other viruses. Some people develop a more severe mononucleosis-type syndrome. After this stage, individuals may not develop any signs or symptoms of disease for a period ranging from weeks to more than 12 years.

HIV symptoms, which tend to increase in severity and number the longer the virus is in the body, may include any of the following:

- Swollen lymph nodes.
- Fever, chills, and night sweats.
- Diarrhea.
- Weight loss.
- Coughing and shortness of breath.
- Persistent tiredness.
- Skin sores.
- Blurred vision and headaches.
- Development of other infections, such as certain kinds of pneumonia.

HIV infection is associated with a variety of HIV-related diseases, including different cancers and dangerous infections including tuberculosis. HIV-infected individuals may develop persistent generalized lymphadenopathy, enlargement of the lymph nodes at two or more different sites in the body. This condition typically persists for more than three months without any other illness to explain its occurrence. Diminished mental function may appear before other symptoms. Tests conducted on infected but apparently healthy men have revealed impaired coordination, problems in thinking, or abnormal brain scans. Psychological problems, including depression, anxiety, and stress, occur "in epidemic proportions" in individuals with HIV, according to recent research, and can affect their behavior (such as taking steps to prevent transmitting the virus) and treatment outcome.[30]

Diagnosing and Treatment

HIV Testing One in five Americans infected with HIV doesn't know it.[31] Anyone receiving routine medical care and testing can be screened for HIV without giving specific informed consent. The goal is to identify the estimated 250,000 Americans who have undiagnosed HIV.

All HIV tests measure antibodies, cells produced by the body to fight HIV infection. A negative test indicates no exposure to HIV. It can take three to six months for the body to produce the telltale antibodies, however, so a negative result may not be accurate, depending on the timing of the test.

HIV testing can be either confidential or anonymous. In confidential testing, a person's name is recorded along with the test results, which are made available to medical personnel and in 32 states, the state health department. In anonymous testing, no name is associated with the test results. Anonymous testing is available in 39 states.

The only home HIV test approved by the FDA, Home Access, is available in drug stores or online for $40 to $50. An individual draws a blood sample by pricking a finger and sends it to a laboratory along with a personal identification number. Results are given over the phone by a trained counselor, usually within several days.

Newly developed blood tests can determine how recently a person was infected with HIV and distinguish between long-standing infections and those contracted within the previous four to six months.

Recognizing AIDS A diagnosis of AIDS applies to anyone with HIV whose immune system is severely impaired, as indicated by a CD4+ count of less than 200 cells per cubic millimeter of blood, compared to normal CD4+ cell counts in healthy people not infected with HIV of 800 to 1,200 per cubic millimeter of blood. In addition, AIDS is diagnosed in persons with HIV infection who experience recurrent pneumonia, invasive cervical cancer, or pulmonary tuberculosis.

People with AIDS also may experience persistent fever, diarrhea that persists for more than one month, or involuntary weight loss of more than 10 percent of

Electron micrograph of a white blood cell being attacked by HIV (*light blue particles*), the virus that causes AIDS.

Lennart Nilsson © Boehringer Ingelheim International GmbH

normal body weight. Neurological disease—including dementia (confusion and impaired thinking) and other problems with thinking, speaking, movement, or sensation—may occur. Secondary infectious diseases that may develop in people with AIDS include *Pneumocystis carinii* pneumonia, tuberculosis, or oral candidiasis (thrush). Secondary cancers associated with HIV infection include Kaposi's sarcoma and cancer of the cervix.

Treating HIV/AIDS New forms of therapy have been remarkably effective in boosting levels of protective T cells and reducing *viral load*—the amount of HIV in the bloodstream. Starting HIV treatment early, before a patient's immune system is badly weakened, can dramatically improve survival.[32] People with high viral loads are more likely to progress rapidly to AIDS than people with low levels of the virus.

The current "gold-standard" approach to combating HIV is known as HAART (highly active antiretroviral therapies), which dramatically reduces viral load even though it does not eradicate the virus. This complex regimen uses one of 250 different combinations of three or more antiretroviral drugs. Since the development of HAART, the number of deaths among persons with AIDS in the United States has declined by 70 percent, and the number of those living with AIDS has risen.

Because HAART can drastically lower viral load, there is some evidence that it also may reduce the risk of infectiousness of HIV-positive individuals. Fearing that this could lead to unsafe sex, researchers did a meta-analysis of HAART recipients and found no increased sexual risk behavior. Even when HIV levels are undetectable, they note, this does not mean the infected person is "cured," nor does it eliminate the possibility of transmitting HIV.

In the last few years, several new drugs have become available, and many of these antiretroviral agents can be taken just once or twice a day. New antiretroviral agents and new types of drugs are currently in clinical trials. Work is also continuing toward an HIV vaccine. As more effective therapies have emerged, there has been a major shift in attitude: Physicians are more optimistic about long-term treatments, and hope is replacing despair as more individuals are living productive lives with HIV.

Breakthrough drugs are indeed allowing HIV-infected people to live longer. However, new dangers have emerged. Up to 15 percent of new HIV cases in the country may stem from drug-resistant strains of the virus. "Superinfection" with more than one strain of HIV seems more common than previously thought. As a result, HIV-infected people who initially were doing well without drugs may become ill after contracting a second strain of the AIDS virus. Experimental vaccines against HIV have not proven successful in clinical trials.

LEARN IT LIVE IT Protecting Your Sexual Health

As with other aspects of your well-being, your sexual health depends on your choices and behaviors. Here are some basic guidelines:

- **Talk first.** Get to know your partner. Before having sex, establish a committed relationship that allows trust and open communication. You should be able to discuss past sexual histories and any previous STIs or IV drug use. You should not feel coerced or forced into having sex.

- **Stay sober.** Alcohol and drugs impair your judgment, make it harder to communicate clearly, and can lead to forgetting or failing to use condoms properly.

- **Be honest.** If you have an STI, like HPV or herpes, advise any prospective sexual partner. Allow him or her to de-

cide what to do. If you mutually agree on engaging in sexual activity, use latex condoms and other protective measures.

- **Don't feel you have to have sex** for fear of hurting someone's feelings or fear of being the "only one" who isn't doing it. If you don't want to have sex, be honest, discuss the reasons behind your decision with your partner, and stay true to you.

- **Respect** everyone's right to make his or her own personal decision—including yours. There is no perfect point in a relationship where sex has to happen. If your partner tells you that he or she is not ready to have sex, respect this decision, discuss the reasons behind it, and be supportive.

- **Be prepared for a sex emergency.** Consider carrying two condoms with you just in case one breaks or tears. Both men and women are equally responsible for preventing STIs, and both should carry condoms.

- **Abstinence doesn't mean less affection.** Practicing abstinence—the most effective way to protect against STIs—

doesn't mean you can't have an intimate relationship with someone. It just means you don't have vaginal or anal intercourse or oral sex.

- **Make your sexual health a priority.** Whether you are having sex or not, both men and women need regular check-ups to make sure they are sexually healthy.

SELF SURVEY   Assessing Your STI Risk

This Self Survey looks at your risk of acquiring or transmitting any sexually transmitted infection.

STI Quiz

1. **True** or **False:** A person can have an STI and not know it.
2. **True** or **False:** It is normal for women to have some vaginal discharge.
3. **True** or **False:** Once you have had an STI and have been cured, you can't get it again.
4. **True** or **False:** HIV is mainly present in semen, blood, vaginal secretions, and breast milk.
5. **True** or **False:** Chlamydia and gonorrhea can cause pelvic inflammatory disease.
6. **True** or **False:** A pregnant woman who has an STI can pass the disease on to her baby.
7. **True** or **False:** Most STIs go away without treatment, if people wait long enough.
8. **True** or **False:** STIs that aren't cured early can cause sterility.
9. **True** or **False:** Birth control pills offer excellent protection from STIs.
10. **True** or **False:** Condoms can help prevent the spread of STIs.
11. **True** or **False:** If you know your partner, you can't get an STI.
12. **True** or **False:** Chlamydia is the most common bacterial STI.
13. **True** or **False:** A sexually active woman should get an annual Pap test from her doctor.

Answers

1. **True** Some of the most common symptoms of an STI infection include abnormal discharge, painful urination, burning, and itching or tingling in the genital area, but it is important to remember that many women and men who have an STI often do not experience any symptoms at all. Chlamydia, for example, often has no symptoms.

2. **True** Normal vaginal discharge has several purposes: cleaning and moistening the vagina and helping to prevent and fight infections. Although it's normal for the color, texture, and amount of vaginal fluids to vary throughout a woman's menstrual cycle, some changes in discharge may indicate a problem.

    If you think you may have a problem, you should see a doctor as soon as possible. First, though, it helps to learn some of the differences between what is normal and abnormal vaginal discharge for you.

3. **False** Having an STI and being cured from it does not mean that your body now has a built-in immunity to the bacteria that causes the infection. You must protect yourself from becoming infected again by using a condom. Remember, it is your body!

4. **True** Although small traces of HIV can be found in tears, saliva, urine, and perspiration, extensive studies have shown that there is not enough of the virus or the virus is not strong enough to be transmitted. Only blood, semen, vaginal secretions, and breast milk have been proven to transmit the HIV virus and hepatitis B. HIV cannot be passed on by casual contact.

5. **True** Many different organisms can cause PID, but most cases are associated with gonorrhea and genital chlamydial infections, two very common STIs. Scientists have found that bacteria normally present in small numbers in the vagina and cervix also may play a role.

6. **True** STIs can be passed from a pregnant woman to the baby before, during, or after the baby's birth. Some STIs (like syphilis) cross the placenta and infect the baby while it is in the uterus (womb). Other STIs (like gonorrhea, chlamydia, hepatitis B, and genital herpes) can be transmitted from the mother to the baby during delivery as the baby passes through the birth canal. HIV can cross the placenta during pregnancy, infect the baby during the birth process, and unlike most other STIs, can infect the baby through breastfeeding.

7. **False** Even if symptoms appear to go away, the infected person will still have the infection and is able to pass the infection on to others until he/she gets treatment. STIs that aren't cured early can cause sterility.

8. **True** If the fallopian tubes are blocked at one or both ends, the egg can't travel through the tubes into the uterus. Blocked tubes may result from pelvic inflammatory disease, which is often caused by untreated STIs.

9. **False** The birth control pill does not protect against sexually transmitted infections. For those having sex, condoms must always be used along with birth control pills to protect against STIs. Abstinence (the decision to not have sex) is the only method that always prevents pregnancy and sexually transmitted infections.

10. **True** Most condoms are made of latex. Those made of lambskin may offer less protection against some sexually transmitted infections, including HIV, so use of latex condoms is recommended. For people who may have an allergic skin reaction to latex, both male and female condoms made of polyurethane are available.

    When properly used, latex and plastic condoms are effective against most STIs. Condoms do not protect against infections spread from sores on the skin not covered by a condom (such as the base of the penis or scrotum).

11. **False** As stated in question number 1, a person can have an STI and not know it. If they can't tell, how can you?

12. **True** The U.S. Centers for Disease Control and Prevention estimates that more than 4 million new cases of chlamydia occur each year. The highest rates of chlamydial infection are in 15- to 19-year-old adolescents regardless of demographics or location.

13. **True** The Pap test is a way to find cell changes on the cervix. Abnormal cells may lead to cancer, so having a Pap test can find and treat them early, before they have time to progress to cancer.

Although Pap tests do not test for STIs, some STIs such as HPV (human papillomavirus infection) can cause abnormal Pap test results. Certain types of HPV are linked to cancer in both women and men.

Source: Material taken from The Bacchus Network™ Website, smartersex .org.

Your Health Action Plan for Coping with STIs

What to Do If You Have an STI

- If you suspect that you have an STI, don't feel too embarrassed to get help through a physician's office or a clinic. Treatment relieves discomfort, prevents complications, and halts the spread of the disease.
- Following diagnosis, take oral medication (which may be given instead of or in addition to shots) exactly as prescribed.
- Try to figure out from whom you got the STI. Be sure to inform that person, who may not be aware of the problem.
- If you have an STI, never deceive a prospective partner about it. Tell the truth—simply and clearly. Be sure your partner understands exactly what you have and what the risks are.

Telling a Partner You Have an STI

Even though the conversation can be awkward and embarrassing, you need to talk honestly about any STI that you may have been exposed to or contracted. What you don't say can be hazardous to your partner's health. Here are some guidelines:

- **Talk before you become intimate.** A good way to start is simply by saying, *"There is something we need to talk over first."*
- **Be honest.** Don't downplay any potential risks.
- **Don't blame.** Even if you suspect that your partner was the source of your infection, focus on the need for medical attention.
- **Be sensitive to your partner's feelings.** Anger and resentment are common reactions when someone feels at risk. Try to listen without becoming defensive.
- **Seek medical attention.** Do not engage in sexual intimacies until you obtain a doctor's assurance that you are no longer contagious.

Source: Bacchus and Gamma Peer Education Network, www.smartersex .org.

CENGAGENOW™ If you want to write your own goals for preventing STIs, go to the Wellness Journal at CengageNOW for Health at **www.cengage. com/sso.**

MAKING THIS CHAPTER WORK FOR YOU

Review Questions

1. Chlamydial infections
   a. are caused by a virus.
   b. can cause eye infections in men.
   c. usually display no symptoms in women.
   d. are more common in older women.

2. Which statement is *true*?
   a. Gonorrhea is mostly symptomless in men.
   b. Secondary syphilis usually occurs 10 to 20 years after the latent stage.
   c. Pubic lice can be killed with regular shampoo.
   d. African Americans account for a disproportionate share of new AIDS diagnoses.

3. Which of the following statements about HIV transmission is *true*?
   a. Individuals are not at risk for HIV if they are being treated for chlamydia or gonorrhea.
   b. HIV can be transmitted between lesbians.
   c. Heterosexual men who do not practice safe sex are at less risk for contracting HIV than homosexual men who do practice safe sex.
   d. HIV cannot be spread in a single instance of sexual intercourse.

4. A person with AIDS
   a. has a low viral load and a high number of T4 helper cells.
   b. can no longer pass HIV to a sexual partner.
   c. may suffer from secondary infectious diseases and cancers.
   d. will not respond to treatment.

5. Sexually transmitted infections
   a. are the major cause of preventable sterility in the United States.
   b. are declining in incidence on college campuses.
   c. have declined in incidence in developing nations due to improving health standards.
   d. do not increase the risk of being infected with HIV.

6. Viral agents cause all of the following STIs *except*
   a. herpes.
   b. genital warts.
   c. HIV.
   d. chlamydia.

7. Jake is sexually active but doesn't want to use a condom. His other choices to protect himself against STIs include all of these *except*
   a. abstinence.
   b. a sexual relationship with a longtime friend.

c. a sexual relationship with one STI-free partner.

d. masturbation only.

8. Which of these activities cannot transmit an STI?
   a. having oral sex
   b. hugging
   c. sharing a needle with a fellow athlete using steroids
   d. sharing a razor

9. Which statement about HPV infection is *false*?
   a. HPV cannot be transmitted through oral sex.
   b. HPV increases a woman's risk of developing cervical cancer.
   c. HPV causes genital warts.
   d. HPV increases a man's risk of cancer of the penis.

10. The herpes simplex virus HSV-2
    a. cannot be transmitted through oral sex.
    b. cannot be transmitted if a condom is used.
    c. can be transmitted even when the infected person shows no symptoms.
    d. can be permanently killed with antiviral medications.

Answers to these questions can be found on page 650.

Critical Thinking

1. Your friend Shayla recently broke up after a five-year relationship with her first boyfriend. How would you counsel Shayla on re-entering the dating scene and becoming intimate with a new partner?

2. Tad has told his girlfriend, Kylie, that he has never taken any sexual risks. But when she suggested that they get tested for STIs, he became furious and refused. Now Kylie says she doesn't know what to believe. Could Tad be telling the truth, or is he hiding something? If he is telling the truth, why is Tad so upset? Kylie doesn't want to take any risks, but she doesn't want to lose him either. What would you advise her to say or do? What would you advise Tad to say or do?

3. Have you ever dated someone with an STI? If so, when did you find out about it? How did you feel? Did it affect your sex life? In what way?

4. Any time a person has a blood test, an HIV screening can be performed without asking permission. Do you see this as a violation of privacy or as a good public health practice? Explain.

CENGAGENOW™ Go to the CengageNOW for Health website at **www .cengage.com/sso** that will:
- Help you evaluate your knowledge of the material.
- Allow you to take an exam-prep quiz.
- Provide a Personalized Learning Plan targeting resources that address areas you should study.
- Coach you through identifying target goals for behavioral change and creating and monitoring your personal change plan throughout the semester.

Internet Connections

www.cdc.gov/std
www.cdc.gov/hiv
These sites at the CDC feature current information, fact sheets, treatment guides, surveillance, and statistics on sexually transmitted infections and HIV/AIDS.

www3.niaid.nih.gov/research/topics/STI/
This site, which is part of the National Institutes of Health, features research on STIs, including basic and clinical research and activities related to vaccine development.

http://hivinsite.ucsf.edu
This site, sponsored by the University of California San Francisco School of Medicine, provides statistics, education, prevention, and new developments related to HIV/AIDS.

Key Terms

The terms listed are used on the page indicated. Definitions of the terms are in the Glossary at the end of the book.

acquired immune deficiency syndrome (AIDS) 537
chanchroid 535
chlamydia 531
gonorrhea 533
herpes simplex 529
human immunodeficiency virus (HIV) 537
human papilloma virus (HPV) 527
nongonococcal urethritis (NGU) 533
pelvic inflammatory disease (PID) 531
sexually transmitted disease (STD) 523
sexually transmitted infection (STI) 523
syphilis 533

Chapter 17 - Getting Quality Traditional and Nontraditional Health Care

1. **Personalizing one's health refers to which of the following? (pg 546)**

    A. tailoring a test or treatment to a specific patient

    B. the patient takes responsibility for his or her own health issues

    C. alerting the doctor to potential health threats or concerns

    D. all of the above

2. **When looking for reliable online medical advice, you should be wary or suspicious of: (pg 557)**
    A. ridiculous medical claims being made
    B. a person who 'claims' to be a doctor
    C. pushing hard the company's products or services
    D. all of the above one should be leery of

3. **When performing your own temperature check to determine if you have a fever, a fever would be indicative when you temperature begins to be above: (pg 549)**
    A. 96 degrees F
    B. 98.9 degrees F
    C. 100 degrees F
    D. 101. 9 degrees F

4. **Which of the following would not be an example of self care vital signs? (pg 549)**
    A. taking your blood pressure
    B. taking your temperature
    C. drawing blood to determine your level of cholesterol
    D. checking your pulse

5. **A medical test that your doctor runs on you to record the electrical activity of your heart is called: (pg 553)**
    A. urinalysis
    B. electrocardiogram
    C. echocardiogram
    D. chest x-ray

6. **The health related information collected during an interview with the patient by the health care provider is known as: (pg 552)**
    A. evidence based medicine
    B. integrative medicine
    C. medical history
    D. primary care analysis

7. **Which of the following would most likely lead to periodontitis? (pg 549)**
    A. having halitosis bad breath
    B. eating too many sugary sweets and chewing gum
    C. not flossing the gums
    D. irregular brushing of the teeth

8. **The inflammation that attacks the gums of the mouth to cause teeth problems is caused by: (pg 549)**
    A. gingivitis
    B. sugar
    C. herpes
    D. plaque

9. **A patient must legally give consent for hospitalization or surgery. This is known as: (pg 554)**
    A. health care directive
    B. informed consent
    C. notice of privacy practice
    D. conformity standards

10. **Chiropractic care is an example of which CAM? (pg 559)**
    A. mind-body connection
    B. energy therapies
    C. biological-based therapy
    D. manipulative and body-based methods

11. **Of all the various types of complementary and alternative medicines (CAM), which is considered to be the most commonly used? (pg 561)**
    A. chiropractic
    B. acupuncture
    C. prayer
    D. homeopathy

12. **Using magnet therapy is an example of which CAM category? (pg 559)**
    A. biologically-based treatment
    B. manipulative methods
    C. energy-based methods
    D. mind-body connections

13. **Which type of alternative medical system emphasizes the restoration of health rather than curing the disease? (pg 560)**
    A. homeopathic
    B. chiropractic
    C. naturopathic
    D. ayurvedic

14. **The Chinese art of inserting fine needles at various points of the skin that fall along the pathways of energy is known as: (pg 559 -560)**
    A. iridology
    B. reflexology
    C. acupuncture
    D. acupressure

15. **The alternative treatment based on the theory that human illnesses are sometimes caused by subluxation is known as: (pg 562)**
    A. chiropractic
    B. iridology
    C. quackery
    D. acupuncture

16. **Designing medical care based on outcomes refers to what type of medical practice? (pg 553)**
    A. diagnostic testing
    B. evidence-based medicine
    C. retrospective medicine based on one's past medical history
    D. results of absence of treatment for a medical condition

17. **A doctor who uses a holistic approach to medical treatment on a patient is using what type of approach? (p 557)**
    A. traditional western medicine approach
    B. getting to the root of the medical ailment
    C. using an approach compromising of not only body, but of the mind and spirit as well
    D. unconventional treatments

18. **Integrative medicine uses a combination of: (pg 559)**
    A. different kinds of drugs and medicines to treat the illness
    B. alternative and allopathic treatments
    C. two different alternative treatments
    D. mind and body medicine

Long after she immigrated to the United States from India, Tapu's grandmother refused to go to Western doctors. She preferred practitioners who used the herbs and techniques she had relied on in her homeland. Tapu's father, an American-trained physician, would argue with his mother-in-law about what he considered her old-fashioned views. As a doctor's son, Tapu grew up believing in the superiority of Western medicine.

In his sophomore year at college, Tapu found out that he needed oral surgery. To his surprise, the oral surgeon suggested an alternative method of controlling

Getting Quality Traditional and Nontraditional Health Care

postoperative pain: acupuncture. "My dad's never going to approve," he said. "And he's the one who's still paying my medical bills." The doctor referred Tapu—and his father—to recent studies conducted by National Institute of Health researchers on acupuncture's efficacy in relieving postsurgical pain. After doing more research online, Tapu agreed to try acupuncture following his operation.

Like Tapu, millions of Americans are turning to complementary and alternative medicine (CAM), a term that includes a broad range of healing philosophies, approaches, and therapies not traditionally taught in medical schools or provided in hospitals. But consumers are learning that they have to be just as savvy—and skeptical—about these therapies and practitioners as they are with any other form of health care.

By describing most of today's many health-care choices, this chapter, particularly "Health Assurance" in Making Change Happen and *Labs for IPC*, will help you take greater responsibility for your personal well-being. Whether you are monitoring your blood pressure, taking medication, or deciding whether to try an alternative therapy, you need to gather information, ask questions, weigh advantages and disadvantages, and take charge of your health. The reason: No one cares more about your health than you and no one will do more to promote your well-being.

After studying the material in this chapter, you should be able to

- **List** ways of participating in your own health care.
- **Discuss** strategies for self-care.
- **Describe** common medical exam procedures and medical tests.
- **Identify** strategies for maintaining good oral health.
- **List** your rights as a medical consumer.
- **Describe** the different types of complementary and alternative therapies and **explain** what research has shown about their effectiveness.
- **Compare** and **contrast** the different types of health-care practitioners and health-care facilities.
- **Describe** how you can get the best information from your next medical exam.

Log on to CengageNOW for Health at **www.cengage.com/sso** to find your Behavior Change Planner and to explore self-assessments, interactive tutorials, and practice quizzes.

Getting Quality Health Care

Quality matters in health care perhaps more than anywhere because your life may depend on it. Yet the quality of health care varies greatly in this country. Some physicians, some hospitals, some health-care plans do a better job of helping people stay healthy or get better if they become ill. At one time, patients simply put their faith in physicians and assumed that they knew best and would make the correct medical decisions. Today health care has become far more complex and impersonal. Increasingly, doctors as well as consumer advocates insist that patients need to take responsibility for their own care. Rather than assuming that health-care providers will do whatever is necessary and appropriate, you must take the initiative to ensure that you get quality care.[1]

Quality begins with you. By learning how to maintain your health, evaluate medical information, and spot early signs of a problem, you're more likely to get the best possible care—and to keep down your medical bills. Self-care means head-to-toe maintenance, including good oral care, appropriate screening tests, knowing your medical rights, and understanding the health-care system.

Chances are that you've tried—or will try—alternative therapies. Many use a "whole-person" approach that addresses all the dimensions of health. You need to be just as savvy a consumer when considering a complementary or alternative treatment as you would with a more mainstream one. You also need to continue your best healthy practices throughout your life so you can function at your best for as long as possible. But your future begins with the healthy choices you make today and every day.

Personalizing Your Health Care

You can learn about your future health risks by asking your parents, grandparents, uncles, and aunts about any medical conditions they may have.

Thanks to advances in genomics (the study of the entire set of human genes), physicians are tailoring tests and treatments to individual patients. "Personalized" medicine can alert your doctor to potential threats that might be prevented, delayed, or detected at an earlier, more treatable stage and, if you do develop a disease, pinpoint the mediations that will do the most good and cause the least harm.

But "personalizing" health care is also a personal responsibility. You can take charge of your own health by compiling a family health history and informing yourself about risks related to your gender, race, and ethnicity.

Your Family Health History
Someday a DNA scan from a single drop of blood may tell you the diseases you're most likely to develop. A family history can do the same—now.

Mapping your family medical history can help identify health risks you may face in the future. One way of charting your health history is to draw a medical family "tree" that includes your parents and siblings (who

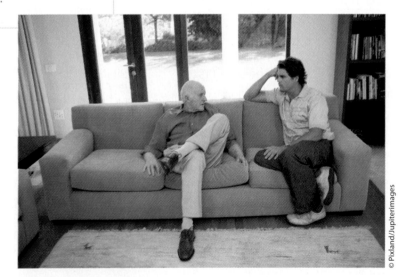

© Pixland/Jupiterimages

Health Assurance

You—your resources, your common sense, your choices, your feelings of self-efficacy and self-worth—determine how long and how well you live. Nothing and no one else has a greater impact on your health than you. Knowledge about health and health care is indeed power, but information alone isn't enough. Action is the key. The habits you form now, the decisions you make while in college, will affect you for decades to come. "Health Assurance" in *Labs for IPC* can equip you with the basic skills and tools you need to ensure and assure yourself of a healthy future. Here's a preview.

Get Real

In this stage you evaluate your sense of self-efficacy (discussed in Chapter 1) for your health by answering True or False to ten questions, including the following:

- I can avoid getting sick by taking care of myself. _____
- Most people do not realize how much circumstances contribute to their illnesses. _____
- The only way to protect my health is to do what my doctor tells me to do. _____

You also evaluate how well you are taking care of yourself by answering 16 questions, including the following:

- Have you had your blood glucose checked? (This is a test for prediabetes and diabetes.)
- Do you check your entire body for changes in moles and other early signs of skin cancer at least once a year?
- Do you wear a helmet when you ride a bicycle or motorcycle?

Based on your answers, you rate your conscientiousness in taking care of your health on a scale of 1 (whatever happens happens) to 10 (ever vigilant).

Get Ready

You get ready for the exercises in this lab by gathering information on your health and family history and scheduling medical appointments.

Get Going

You create your personal health record as both an electronic file and a hard-copy file that includes basic information such as:

- Dates and results of tests and screenings.
- Major illnesses and surgeries, with dates.
- A list of your medicines, dosages, and how long you've taken them.

You also assemble your family history, including all major illnesses and tendencies toward conditions such as allergies or migraines.

Every week you select a personally relevant topic, such as high blood pressure or diabetes, based on your personal or family medical history, and research it. You also prepare for your next doctor's visit by following directions for what to ask; what to tell; what to do if you get a diagnosis; what to do if you need a lab test, an X-ray, or another kind of test; what to do if you receive a prescription for a new medicine; and how to follow up.

Lock It In

To maintain your health, you give yourself a checkup every week, recording any new health problems.

You also keep up with health news, particularly any conditions that affect you or your family.

---

share half your genes), as well as grandparents, uncles, aunts, and cousins. Depending on how much information you're able to obtain for each relative, your medical family tree can include health issues each family member has faced, including illnesses with a hereditary component, such as high blood pressure, diabetes, some cancers, and certain psychiatric disorders. Although having a relative with a certain disease may increase your risk, your likelihood of ending up with the same condition also depends on your health habits, such as diet and exercise. Knowing now that you're at risk can motivate you to change any unhealthy behaviors. Realizing that you have a relative with, say, colon cancer could mean that you should start screening tests ten years before others

because you're at risk of developing a tumor at an earlier age.

For guidance on creating a family history, check these websites: **www.mayoclinic.com** or **www.ashg.org/genetics/ashg/educ/007 .shtml.**

Men and Women as Health-Care Consumers

 The genders differ significantly in the way they use health-care services in the United States. Women see doctors more often than men, take more prescription drugs, are hospitalized more, and control the spending of three of every four health-care dollars. In a national telephone poll, 76 percent of American women—but only 60 percent of men—said

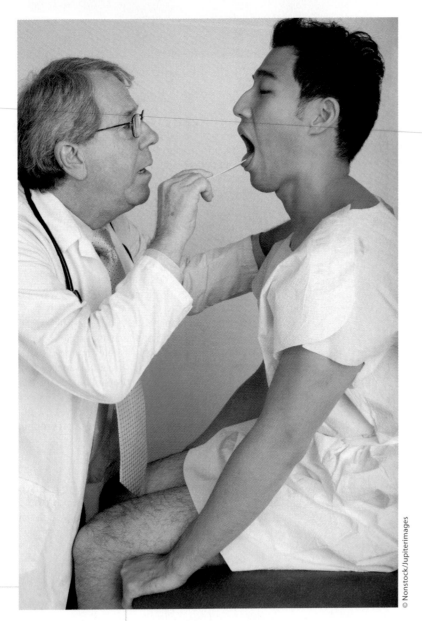

Regular check-ups are equally important for both sexes, but men often put off seeing a physician until symptoms become too serious to ignore.

© Nonstock/Jupiterimages

One reason men die earlier than women is because of the length of time they wait to go for treatment.

The genders also differ in the symptoms and syndromes they develop. For instance, men are more prone to back problems, muscle sprains and strains, allergies, insomnia, and digestive problems. Men develop heart disease about a decade earlier in life than women. More men develop ulcers and hernias; women are more likely to get gallbladder disease and irritable bowel syndrome. An estimated 3 to 6 percent of men suffer from migraines, compared with 15 to 17 percent of women. Yet women and men spend similar proportions of their lifetimes—about 81 percent—free of disability. For men, whose lifespans are shorter, this translates into an average of 58.8 years; for women, 63.9 years.

Self-Care

Most people do treat themselves. You probably prescribe aspirin for a headache, chicken soup or orange juice for a cold, or a weekend trip to unwind from stress. At the very least, you should know what your **vital signs** are and how they compare against normal readings (Figure 17.1).

Once a thermometer was the only self-testing equipment found in most American homes. Now hundreds of home tests are available to help consumers monitor everything from fertility to blood pressure to cholesterol levels (Table 17.1). More convenient and less expensive than a visit to a clinic or doctor's office, the new tests are generally as accurate as those administered by a professional.

Self-care also can mean getting involved in the self-help movement, which has grown into a major national trend. An estimated 20 million people participate in self-help support groups. Millions of others join virtual support communities online.

Oral Health

Oral health involves more than healthy teeth—it refers to the entire mouth, including all the structures that allow us to talk, bite, chew, taste, swallow, smile, scream, or scowl. Oral health is a critical part of overall health. Research has revealed links between

they had had a health exam in the last 12 months.

Many experts believe that the need for birth control and reproductive health services gets women into the habit of making regular visits to health-care professionals, primarily gynecologists. There are no comparable specialists for men, who tend to visit urologists, specialists in male reproductive organs, only when they develop problems. Men also are conditioned to take a stoic, tough-it-out attitude to early symptoms of a disease.

Men feel they are not allowed to manifest illness unless it's overt, says family practitioner Martin Miner, M.D., who has conducted research on men and health care.

TABLE 17.1

Home Health Tests: A Consumer's Guide

Type of Test	What It Does
Pregnancy	Determines if a woman is pregnant by detecting the presence of human chorionic gonodatropin in urine. Considered 99 percent accurate.
Fertility	Measures levels of luteinizing hormone (LH), which rise 24 to 36 hours before a woman conceives. Can help women increase their odds of conceiving.
Blood pressure	Measures blood pressure by means of an automatically inflating armband or a cuff for the finger or wrist; helps people taking hypertension medication or suffering from high blood pressure to monitor their condition.
Cholesterol	Checks cholesterol in blood from a finger prick; good for anyone concerned about cholesterol.
Colon cancer	Screening test to detect hidden blood in stool; recommended for anyone over 40 or concerned about colorectal disease.
Urinary tract infection	Diagnoses infection by screening for certain white blood cells in urine; advised for women who get frequent UTIs and whose doctors will prescribe antibiotics without a visit.
HIV infection	Detects antibodies to HIV in a blood sample sent anonymously to a lab. Controversial because no face-to-face counseling is available for those who test positive.

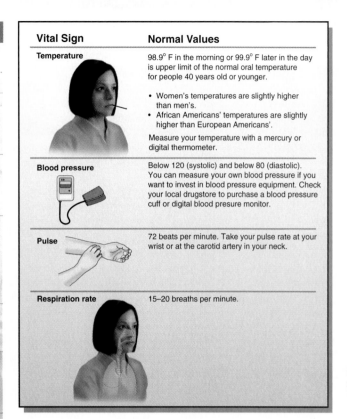

Vital Sign	Normal Values
Temperature	98.9° F in the morning or 99.9° F later in the day is upper limit of the normal oral temperature for people 40 years old or younger. • Women's temperatures are slightly higher than men's. • African Americans' temperatures are slightly higher than European Americans'. Measure your temperature with a mercury or digital thermometer.
Blood pressure	Below 120 (systolic) and below 80 (diastolic). You can measure your own blood pressure if you want to invest in blood pressure equipment. Check your local drugstore to purchase a blood pressure cuff or digital blood presure monitor.
Pulse	72 beats per minute. Take your pulse rate at your wrist or at the carotid artery in your neck.
Respiration rate	15–20 breaths per minute.

Figure 17.1 Take Your Own Vital Signs

© bilderlounge/Jupiterimages

chronic oral infection and heart and lung diseases, stroke, low birthweight, premature births, and diabetes.

Poor oral health can lead to a variety of health problems. People with gum disease are at higher risk for developing heart disease, stroke, uncontrolled diabetes, preterm births, and respiratory disease. One recent study found an increased risk of pancreatic cancer in individuals who had experienced tooth loss.

Thanks to fluoridated water and toothpaste and improved dental care, Americans' oral health is better than in the past. However, without good self-care, you probably will lose some teeth to decay and gum disease. The best way to prevent such problems is through proper and regular brushing and flossing.

Gum, or periodontal, **disease** is an inflammation that attacks the gum and bone that hold your teeth in place. The culprit is **plaque,** the sticky film of bacteria that forms on teeth. More than 300 species of bacteria live under the gum line, and about half a dozen have been linked to serious gum problems. The early stage of gum disease is called **gingivitis.** If untreated, it develops into a more serious form known as **periodontitis,** in which plaque moves down the tooth to the roots, which then become infected. In advanced periodontitis, the infection destroys the bone and fibers that hold teeth in place.

Symptoms of gum disease include bleeding during brushing or flossing, redness and puffiness of gums, tenderness or pain, persistent bad breath or a bad taste in the mouth, receding gums, shifted or loosened teeth, and changes in the way your teeth fit together when you bite. New treatments, which offer an alternative to traditional gum surgery, include a single antibiotic injection or the implant of a small antibiotic chip in the periodontal pockets to promote healing.

vital signs Measurements of physiological functioning; specifically, temperature, blood pressure, pulse rate, and respiration rate.

gum disease Inflammation of the gum and bones that hold teeth in place.

plaque The sticky film of bacteria that forms on teeth.

gingivitis Inflammation of the gums.

periodontitis Severe gum disease in which the tooth root becomes infected.

YOUR STRATEGIES FOR PREVENTION

How to Take Care of Your Mouth

- Brush your teeth every morning and every night. Oral bacteria reach their highest count during sleep because fluids in the mouth accumulate. Nighttime cleaning reduces the bacterial population; morning cleaning lets you reduce the buildup.

- Use a toothpaste that has the American Dental Association (ADA) seal of acceptance and a toothbrush with soft, rounded bristles. Replace your toothbrush every three months.

- Hold the brush at a 45-degree angle from your gums. Pay particular attention to the space between your teeth and gums, especially on the inside, toward your tongue. Brush for two to five minutes. Don't brush too vigorously. If you scrub as hard as you can, you may damage your teeth and gums. Abrasion—a problem for more than half of American adults—erodes tooth surfaces, weakens teeth, and increases sensitivity to hot and cold foods. There is some evidence that

- powered toothbrushes are better at removing plaque and reducing the risk of gum disease than are ordinary manual toothbrushes.

- Because brushing can't reach plaque and food trapped between teeth, daily flossing is essential. Using waxed or unwaxed floss, start behind the upper and lower molars at one side of your mouth and work toward the other side.

- See your dentist twice a year for routine cleaning and examination. Your dentist should take a complete medical history from you and update it every six months, examine your mouth for signs of cancer, and thoroughly outline all treatment options.

- Make sure that everyone who works on the inside of your mouth wears a mask and rubber gloves to reduce the risk of disease transmission (that is, bacterial and viral infections, such as hepatitis, herpes, and HIV).

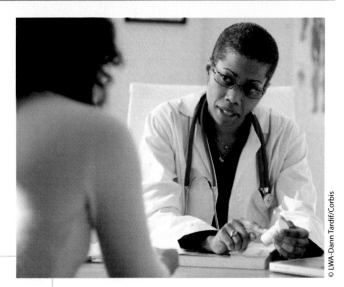

© LWA-Dann Tardif/Corbis

Take charge of your health by educating yourself and asking your doctor questions about your health and treatments.

Taking care of your mouth isn't important only for dental health: It may affect how long you live. Gingivitis and periodontitis trigger an inflammatory response that causes the arteries to swell, which leads to a constriction of blood flow that can increase the incidence of cardiovascular disease. Periodontal disease also leads to a higher white blood cell count, an indicator that the

immune system is under increased stress. The good news: You can prevent these problems by flossing daily and brushing your teeth and your tongue (to get rid of bacteria that can cause gum disease and bad breath).

The Doctor–Patient Partnership

Once the family doctor was indeed part of the family. The family doctor brought babies into the world, shepherded them through childhood, comforted and counseled them, stood by their bedside in their darkest hours. Patients entrusted the doctor with their cares, their confidences, their very lives. Dramatic breakthroughs in diagnosing and treating illness shifted the focus in medicine from the family physician to the specialist, from basic caring to high-tech medical care. Patients today are more likely to be cured of a vast array of illnesses than were patients a century ago. However, they often complain of insensitive, uncaring physicians who focus on their diseases rather than on them as individuals.

As more physicians have joined managed-care organizations (discussed later in this chapter), which emphasize efficiency, they sometimes feel pressure to see more patients a day, to spend less time with each, and to discourage expensive tests and treatments.

Because physicians have less time and less autonomy, patients today must do more. Your first step should be learning more about your body, any medical conditions or problems you develop, and your options for treatment. You can find a great deal of information via computer online services, patient advocacy and support organizations (see the Hales Health Almanac at the end of this book for listings), and libraries.

This information can help you know what questions to ask and how to evaluate what your doctor says. But you have to be willing to speak up. Busy doctors give patients less than a minute on average during a routine visit to say what's bothering them before they interrupt. This doesn't mean your doctor isn't interested, but it does mean that you have to develop good communication skills so you can tell physicians what they need to know to help you.

Choosing a Primary Care Physician

Why does a healthy young adult need a doctor? To stay healthy as long as possible. At some point in early adulthood, you should establish a relationship with a physician who will do basic screening tests (Table 17.2), record your family history, and help you prevent problems down the road. The primary care physicians who are playing increasingly important roles in American health care include family practitioners, general internists, and pediatricians.

 Obstetrician-gynecologists serve as the primary providers of health care for more than half of all women. If you're a woman and your gynecologist is the only physician you see, make sure that he or she performs other tests—such as measuring your blood pressure—in addition to a pelvic and breast exam. If you develop other symptoms or health concerns, ask for an appropriate referral.

 At college health centers, clinics, and some health-care organizations, consumers may be assigned to a primary physician or restricted to certain doctors. Even if your choices are limited, don't suspend your critical judgment. If your assigned physician does not listen to your concerns or is not providing adequate care, you can—and should—request another physician. Your rapport with your primary physician and the feelings of mutual trust and respect that develop between you can have as much of an impact on your well-being as your doctor's technical expertise.

One key to making the health-care system work for you lies in choosing a good physician. After seeing your primary care

TABLE 17.2

Screening Tests and Recommendations

Anemia
Beginning in adolescence, all nonpregnant women should be screened every five to ten years until menopause.

Clinical Breast Exam/Mammogram
Women age 20 to 39 should receive a clinical breast exam every three years. Women age 40 and older should receive an annual clinical breast exam and a mammogram.

Cervical Cancer Screening (Pap Smear)
Three years after first sexual intercourse or by age 21, whichever comes first, until age 30, women should receive an annual Pap smear. After age 30, the screening rate may decrease. See "Your Health Action Plan for Early Detection of Cancer" in Chapter 14.

Cholesterol and Lipids
Adults over age 20 should have a lipoprotein panel test every five years.

Colorectal Cancer Screening
Adults age 50 and older should receive an annual fecal occult blood test and colonoscopy every ten years.

Type 2 Diabetes
Beginning at age 45, adults should have a fasting blood glucose test every three years.

Hypertension Screening
Adults age 18 and older should have an annual blood pressure (BP) check. If the BP is less than 130/85, it should be checked every two years. If the blood pressure is between 130–139/85–89, it should be checked annually. After age 60, blood pressure should be checked annually.

Osteoporosis
Women age 65 and older should have a baseline bone mineral density test. To reduce the risk of fractures, women should increase dietary calcium and vitamin D, perform weight-bearing exercise, stop smoking, and moderate alcohol intake.

Prostate Cancer Screening
Men age 50 and older should discuss potential benefits and known harms of screening with PSA and digital rectal exam.

Skin Cancer Screening
Adults should receive an annual skin exam.

Visual Exam
Adults age 18 to 40 should have a complete visual examination every two to three years; age 41 to 60, every two years; and age 61 and older, every year.

- **Prepare in advance.** Write down your questions, organize them in a logical fashion, and select the top ten queries you want answered. Make a copy of all your questions to review and leave with your doctor.
- **Ask about a "question hour."** Many health-care practitioners set aside a specific time of day for patients with call-in questions. Find out if your college health center offers this service. Does a nurse field all calls? Can you get specific advice?
- **Go online.** Many doctors' offices answer queries by email. Ask your doctor if you can email follow-up questions or progress reports on how you're feeling.
- **Interrupt the interrupter.** If you're having difficulty explaining what's wrong, say so. If your doctor tries to put words in your mouth, say, "Please just listen so I can tell you the whole story without getting sidetracked."

physician, ask yourself the following questions to evaluate the quality of care you are getting.

- Did your physician take a comprehensive history? Was the physical examination thorough?
- Did your physician explain what he or she was doing during the exam?
- Did he or she spend enough time with you?
- Did you feel free to ask questions? Did your physician give you straight answers? Did he or she reassure you when you were worried?
- Does your physician seem willing to admit that he or she doesn't know the answers to some questions?
- Does your physician hesitate to refer you to a specialist even when you have a complex problem that warrants such care?

Look back at your answers. If they make you feel uneasy, have a talk with your physician. Or find a physician or a health plan that provides better service.

Your Medical Exam

Although analysts have not found evidence that an annual screening physical is warranted for healthy adults, primary care physicians feel differently. In a recent survey about two-thirds agreed that an annual physical examination is necessary. The benefits, as doctors see them, include time to counsel patients about preventive health services, detection of underlying illnesses before symptoms develop, and improved patient-physician relationships.

Your physician will want a past **medical history,** including major illnesses, surgery, and treatments. Report any allergies you have, particularly to drugs, and the medications you take, including aspirin, antacids, sleeping pills, oral contraceptives, and recreational drugs, even if illegal. Your physician may also want to know about topics you consider private, such as sexually transmitted infections. Remember that he or she needs all this information to provide you with comprehensive treatment. Note, too, that a physician must report certain information—for example, certain

sexually transmitted diseases—to health authorities.

After the physician has asked you questions about your complaints, medical history, and lifestyle, he or she will probably perform the standard tests described below. During the examination, point out any pains, lumps, or skin growths you've noticed. If you feel pain when the physician palpates (feels) any part of your body, say so.

- **Head.** Using a flashlightlike instrument called an *ophthalmoscope,* the physician will look at the lens, retina, and blood vessels of your eyes. He or she also will examine your ears, mouth, tongue, teeth, and gums.
- **Neck.** Feeling around your neck, the physician will check for enlarged lymph glands (a sign of infection), for lumps in the thyroid gland, and for warning signs of stroke in the neck arteries.
- **Chest.** With a *stethoscope,* the physician will listen to the sounds made by your heart, to detect heart murmurs and irregular contractions, and by your lungs, to detect asthma or emphysema. By tapping on your chest and back with his or her fingers, the physician can tell the size and shape of your heart, which may reveal some forms of heart disease, and whether any fluid has collected in your lungs. The physician will also check for abnormal lumps in a woman's breasts.
- **Abdomen.** Here the physician uses his or her fingers to probe for tender spots and malformations of the liver and other organs, which may reveal signs of alcoholism, hepatitis, or hernias.
- **Rectum and genitals.** With a gloved hand, the physician can feel in the rectum for growths and hemorrhoids. A rectal examination can also reveal enlargement of the male's prostate gland. The physician will check male testicles and spermatic cords for abnormalities.
- **Pelvic examination.** During a pelvic examination, a woman lies on her back, with her heels in stirrups at the end of the examining table

and her legs spread out to the sides. The physician inspects the labia, clitoris, and vaginal opening. Using two gloved, lubricated fingers, the physician will check for abnormalities in the vagina, uterus, fallopian tubes, and ovaries. Many physicians will also perform a rectal or rectovaginal (one finger in the rectum and one in the vagina) examination. A nurse or other health-care worker should be present throughout the exam.

The *speculum* is a medical instrument that spreads the walls of the vagina so that the inside can be seen. As discussed in Chapters 15 and 16, doctors are using HPV tests as well as the conventional **Pap smear** to screen for cervical cancer.

- **Extremities.** The physician may check your knees and other joints for reflexes, which can indicate nerve disorders, and look for tremors in outstretched hands or in the face. The color, elasticity, and wetness or dryness of your skin can alert him or her to nutritional problems, or can indicate diabetes or skin cancer. Hair and nails can give indications of internal health, such as blood disorders. Swelling of the ankles can be an indication of heart, kidney, or liver disease.

- **Pulse and blood pressure.** Your physician may check your pulse in various places, looking for signs of poor circulation. The rhythm and speed of the heart may also signal diseases of the heart or thyroid gland. High blood pressure can be an early warning sign of possible heart attack, stroke, or kidney damage.

Medical Tests

Besides the diagnostic tests just listed, the physician may order some laboratory and other tests, including the following:

- **Chest X-ray.** A chest X-ray can reveal abnormalities of the heart and lungs; if you're a smoker, the physician may insist on one.

- **Electrocardiogram.** The *electrocardiogram*, performed while you're at rest, records the electrical activity of your heart. It can show irregularities in heart rhythm or muscle damage, as well as hardening of the arteries.

- **Urinalysis.** Your urine may be analyzed by a medical laboratory. If sugar (glucose) is found in your urine, your physician may order a separate blood test to check for diabetes. The presence of blood cells may indicate infection of the bladder or kidneys. Abnormal amounts of albumin (protein) in the urine may also suggest kidney disease.

- **Blood tests.** The physician or laboratory technician may draw blood to do a blood cell count. An excess of white blood cells may indicate an infection or, occasionally, leukemia. A deficiency of red blood cells may indicate anemia. Your blood also may be analyzed to measure the levels of its various components. High levels of glucose can indicate diabetes, and high levels of uric acid may mean gout or kidney stones. Your lipoprotein profile may indicate cardiac risk (see Chapter 14).

See the Hales Health Almanac found on the companion website for a comprehensive guide to medical tests.

Evidence-Based Medicine

One of the ways in which physicians are working to improve the quality of care is by basing diagnostic testing and treatments on solid evidence produced by rigorous research studies (usually randomized controlled trials). Evidence-based medicine is not an entirely new concept of medical care but a methodical approach that establishes a solid and conscientious scientific basis for decision making about health care. Evidence-based medicine pays particular attention to **outcomes,** that is, the impact that a specific medication or treatment has on a patient's condition, overall health, and quality of life.

Outcomes research is designed to answer questions such as: Is treatment better or worse than no treatment? Is one treatment better than another? If a treatment is effective, is a little just as good as a lot? Does quality of life change because of treatment? Are the benefits of treatment worth the cost or the risks to the patient?

Studies of outcomes look at how patients fared with or without a specific treatment, the costs involved, and the impact of undergoing or not undergoing treatment in terms

medical history The health-related information collected during the interview of a client by a health-care professional.

Pap smear A test in which cells removed from the cervix are examined under a microscope for signs of cancer; also called a Pap test.

outcomes The ultimate impacts of particular treatments or absence of treatment.

The value of medical care depends not just on health care professionals, but on you:

- **If you receive a diagnosis,** make sure you understand what may be wrong with you, as well as which medications you are taking and why.
- **When your doctor writes you a prescription,** make sure you can read it and know why and how you are to take the medication.
- **Ask for information about your medicines** in terms you can understand, including explanations of possible interactions with other drugs or dietary supplements and potential side effects.
- **If you must undergo surgery** and you can choose a hospital, select one at which many patients have had the procedure or surgery you need.
- **Speak up if you have questions or concerns.** Ask a family member or friend to be your advocate and speak up for you if you can't.

of the patients' quality of life. Outcomes research can help determine which of several therapies or approaches provides the best results at the most reasonable costs.

When you are diagnosed with a health problem, ask your doctor if your treatment is based on the latest evidence and clinical guidelines. The National Guideline Clearinghouse provides a comprehensive database of evidence-based clinical practice guidelines for many common health problems, available at **www.guideline.gov.**

Preventing Medical Errors

More people die from medical errors than from motor vehicle accidents, breast cancer, or AIDS.[2] Medical errors occur when a planned part of medical care doesn't work properly or when the wrong plan was used in the first place. They can happen anywhere in the health-care system, from doctors' offices to pharmacies to hospitals to patients' homes. They may involve medications, diagnoses, tests, lab equipment, surgery, or infection. They are most likely to occur when doctors and patients have problems communicating.

Your best defense against medical errors is information. "Questions are the answer," is the theme of a prevention campaign by the Agency for Healthcare Research and Quality.[3] Your questions can keep you safe and ensure you get quality health care. See Health on a Budget.

Asserting Your Medical Rights

As a consumer, you have basic rights that help ensure that you know about any potential dangers, receive competent diagnosis and treatment, and retain control and dignity in your interactions with health-care professionals. Many hospitals publish a patient's bill of rights, including your rights to know whether a procedure is experimental; to refuse to undergo a specific treatment; to designate someone else to make decisions about your care if and when you cannot; and to leave the hospital, even against your physician's advice.

You have the right to be treated with respect and dignity, including being called "Mr." or "Ms." or whatever you wish, rather than by your first name. Make clear your preferences. If you feel that health-care professionals are being condescending or inconsiderate, say so—in the same tone and manner that you would like others to use with you. If you're hospitalized, find out if there's a patient advocate or representative at your hospital. These individuals can help you communicate with physicians, make any special arrangements, and get answers to questions or complaints.

Your Right to Information

By law, a patient must give consent for hospitalization, surgery, and other major treatments. **Informed consent** is a right, not a privilege. Use this right to its fullest. Ask questions. Seek other opinions. Make sure that your expectations are realistic and that you understand the potential risks, as well as the possible benefits, of a prospective treatment.

Your Right to Privacy and Access to Medical Records

Your medical records are your property. You have the right to see them whenever you choose and to limit who else can see them. Federal standards protecting the privacy of patients' medical information guarantee patients access to their medical records, give them more control over how personal health information is disclosed, and limit the ways that health plans, pharmacies, and hospitals can use personal medical information.

Key provisions include:

- **Access to medical records.** As a patient, you should be able to see and obtain copies of your medical records and request corrections if there are errors. Health-care providers must provide these within 30 days; they may charge for the cost of copying and mailing records.

- **Notice of privacy practices.** Your providers must inform you of how they use personal medical information. Doctors, nurses, and other providers may not disclose information for purposes not related to your health care.

- **Prohibition on marketing.** Pharmacies, health plans, and others must obtain specific authorization before disclosing patient information for marketing.

- **Confidentiality.** Patients can request that doctors take reasonable steps to ensure confidential communications, such as calling a cell phone rather than home or office.

Your Right to Quality Health Care

The essence of a *malpractice* suit is the claim that the physician failed to meet the standard of quality care required of a reasonably skilled and careful medical doctor. Although physicians don't have to guarantee good results to their patients and aren't held liable for unavoidable errors, they are required to use the same care and judgment in treatment that other physicians in the same specialty would use under similar circumstances. To protect themselves financially, physicians, particularly those in surgical specialties who are most likely to be sued, pay tens of thousands of dollars a year in malpractice insurance premiums. Some of this cost is passed on to patients.

Most lawsuits are based on negligence and assert that a physician failed to render diagnosis and treatment with appropriate professional knowledge and skill. Other cases are brought for failure to provide information, obtain consent, or respect a patient's confidentiality. However, analysis of malpractice cases has shown that, in 70 to 80 percent, a doctor's attitude and inability to communicate effectively— by devaluing patients' views, delivering information poorly, failing to understand patients' perspectives, or displaying an air of superiority—also played a role.

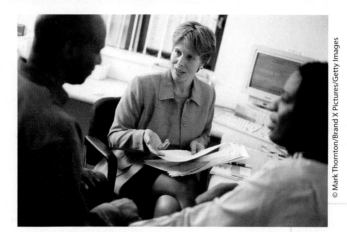

© Mark Thornton/Brand X Pictures/Getty Images

In the hospital, you can discuss the patient's rights and other individual concerns with a patient advocate.

Elective Treatments

As medical technology has developed new options, millions of Americans are trying elective procedures and products that are not medically necessary but that promise to enhance health or appearance. Some are new alternatives for correcting common problems, such as poor vision, while others offer the promise of looking younger or more attractive.

informed consent Permission (to undergo or receive a medical procedure or treatment) given voluntarily, with full knowledge and understanding of the procedure—or treatment and its possible consequences.

You are probably NOT a good candidate for refractive surgery if:

- **You are not a risk taker.** Certain complications are unavoidable in a percentage of patients, and there are no long-term data available for current procedures.

- **Cost is an issue.** Most medical insurance will not pay for refractive surgery. Although the cost is coming down, it is still significant.

- **You required a change in your contact lens or glasses prescription in the past year.** This is called refractive instability. Patients who are in their early twenties or younger, whose hormones are fluctuating due to disease such as diabetes, who are pregnant or breastfeeding, or who are taking medications that may cause fluctuations in vision are more likely to have refractive instability and should discuss the possible additional risks with their doctor.

- **You have a disease or are on medications that may affect wound healing.** Certain conditions, such as autoimmune diseases and diabetes, and some medications may prevent proper healing after a refractive procedure.

- **You actively participate in contact sports.** If you participate in boxing, wrestling, martial arts, or other activities in which blows to the face and eyes are a normal occurrence, LASIK is probably not right for you.

- **You are under 18.** Currently, no lasers are approved for LASIK on persons under the age of 18.

- **It will jeopardize your career.** Some jobs, including certain military assignments, prohibit refractive procedures.

Source: Food and Drug Administration, www.fda.gov/cdrh/LASIK/when.htm.

Vision Surgery

Millions of people in the United States have undergone laser surgery to correct their vision. In LASIK (laser-assisted in situ keratomileusis), the most common technique, a surgeon uses a razorlike instrument to lift a flap of the cornea—the clear stiff outer layer over the colored iris—and then reshapes the exposed area using a laser. The surgery alters the way the eye focuses light, correcting nearsightedness, farsightedness, and some astigmatism. Laser surgery cannot make an aging eye's lens flexible again to improve close-up vision in middle-aged adults. Numbing eye drops make the treatment painless, although burning and scratchiness are normal for a couple of hours afterward. An estimated 10 to 30 percent of patients require additional surgery, or "enhancements," to sharpen their vision. Other complications include glare, sensitivity to bright lights, and poor night vision.

Prices have fallen, but ophthalmologists have warned consumers that some laser surgery centers have cut corners to cut prices, such as hiring inexperienced surgeons or using optometrists or technicians rather than MDs for pre- and postoperative checkups. A qualified eye surgeon should have a record of 100 or more LASIK procedures and at least 25 enhancements—but no more than 20 percent of his or her patients should require enhancements. Ideally, the surgeon should also be the one doing your pre- and postprocedure checks.

Cosmetic Surgery

Approximately 11 million cosmetic treatments are performed every year.[4] About a quarter of those undergoing plastic surgery are between the ages of 18 and 29. The number of teenagers opting for cosmetic procedures—primarily liposuction, nose reshaping, and breast augmentation—is increasing. Nonsurgical cosmetic procedures such as injections of synthetic collagen and botulinum toxin (Botox®) also have become more popular. Health insurance rarely covers cosmetic procedures, which can run into the tens of thousands of dollars.

The most common cosmetic operation is liposuction, the removal of fatty tissue by means of a vacuum device. It can be performed on many areas of the body, from sagging jowls to midsection "love handles" or "muffin tops." The doctor first flushes the target area with a solution of lidocaine (a local anesthetic with a numbing effect), saline, and epinephrine (a drug that reduces bleeding by constricting blood vessels). Inserting a hollow wandlike cannula under the skin, the doctor breaks up fatty deposits and suctions them, along with other body fluids, with a vacuum device.

Risks and complications include infection, numbness, bleeding, discoloration, lumpiness, and, if too much tissue is removed without proper cautions, potentially fatal complications. The American Society of Plastic and Reconstructive Surgeons estimates the mortality rate is one in 5,000 liposuction patients. Several states are considering legislation to tighten restrictions on training and credentialing doctors who perform liposuction.

Breast augmentation is another cosmetic procedure. The Institute of Medicine, after reviewing all available evidence, has reported that there appears to be no link between breast implants and autoimmune disease, connective tissue disorders, or cancer. However, today's surgeons use

Health Hoaxes

Every year millions of Americans go searching for medical miracles that never happen. In all, they spend more than $10 billion on medical **quackery**, unproven health products and services. Those who lose only money are the lucky ones. Many also waste precious time, during which their conditions worsen. Some suffer needless pain, along with crushed expectations.

Facts to Know

Promoters of fraudulent health products often use similar claims and practices to trick consumers into buying their products. Be suspicious when you see:

- Claims that a product is a "scientific breakthrough," "miraculous cure," "secret ingredient," or "ancient remedy."
- Claims that the product is an effective cure for a wide range of ailments. No product can cure multiple conditions or diseases.
- Claims that use impressive-sounding medical terms. They're often covering up a lack of good science.
- Undocumented case histories of people who've had amazing results. It's too easy to make them up. And even if true, they can't be generalized to the entire population. Anecdotes are not a substitute for valid science.
- Claims that the product is available from only one source and payment is required in advance.
- Claims of a "money-back" guarantee.
- Websites that fail to list the company's name, physical address, phone number, or other contact information.

Steps to Take

To keep from risking your life on false hope, follow these guidelines:

- Arm yourself with up-to-date information about your condition or disease from appropriate organizations, such as the American Cancer Society or the Arthritis Foundation, which keep track of unproven and ineffective methods of treatment.
- Ask for a written explanation of what a treatment does and why it works, evidence supporting all claims (not just testimonials), and published reports of the studies, including specifics on numbers treated, doses, and side effects. Be skeptical of self-styled "holistic practitioners," treatments supported by crusading groups, and endorsements from self-proclaimed experts or authorities.
- Don't part with your money quickly. Insurance companies won't reimburse for unproven therapies.
- Don't discontinue your current treatment without your physician's approval. Many physicians encourage supportive therapies—such as relaxation exercises, meditation, or visualization—as a supplement to standard treatments.

Source: Federal Trade Commission, www.ftc.gov/bcp/consumer.shtm.

---

implants filled with a saltwater solution. Patients still face possible complications, including rupture, scarring, infection, and leaking or hardening of their implants.

Getting Quality Nontraditional Health Care

Complementary and alternative medicine (CAM) refers to various medical and health care systems, practices, and products that are not considered part of conventional medicine because there is not yet sufficient proof of their safety and effectiveness. CAM's varied healing philosophies, approaches, and therapies include preventive techniques designed to delay or prevent serious health problems before they start and **holistic** methods that focus on the whole person and the physical, mental, emotional, and spiritual aspects of well-being. Some approaches are based on the same physiological principles as traditional Western methods; others, such as acupuncture, are based on different healing systems. The most commonly used are nonvitamin, nonmineral, natural products (such as fish or omega 3 oil and echinacea) and deep breathing exercises. (See Table 17.3.)

Most people who choose CAM want to improve their overall health and well-being

quackery Medical fakery; unproven practices claiming to cure diseases or solve health problems.

complementary and alternative medicine (CAM) A term used to apply to all health-care approaches, practices, and treatments not widely taught in medical schools, not generally used in hospitals, and not usually reimbursed by medical insurance companies.

holistic An approach to medicine that takes into account body, mind, emotions, and spirit.

TABLE 17.3

10 Most Common CAM Therapies among Adults

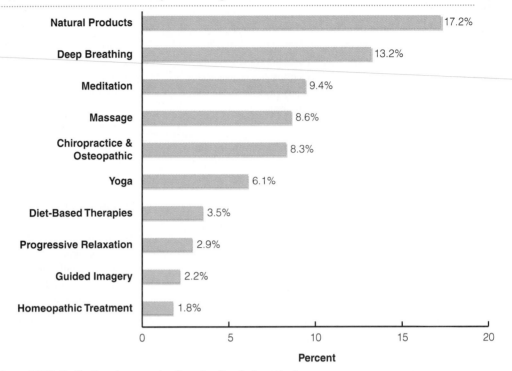

Natural Products — 17.2%
Deep Breathing — 13.2%
Meditation — 9.4%
Massage — 8.6%
Chiropractice & Osteopathic — 8.3%
Yoga — 6.1%
Diet-Based Therapies — 3.5%
Progressive Relaxation — 2.9%
Guided Imagery — 2.2%
Homeopathic Treatment — 1.8%

Percent

Source: *NIH MedlinePlus Magazine*, www.n/m.nih.gov/medlineplus/magazine/.

or to relieve the symptoms associated with chronic or terminal illnesses or the side effects of conventional treatments for such diseases. Some are seeking a transformational experience that changes their worldview or want greater control over their health. The overwhelming majority of patients use CAM as a complement to rather than a substitute for conventional care.[5]

The list of available CAM treatment changes constantly as treatments that are proven safe and effective become adopted into conventional health care and as new approaches to health care emerge. Federally funded research into CAM began in the 1990s, but many health practitioners are not familiar with the latest findings.[6] Informed consent remains an issue because there are no widespread standards for disclosing risks, discussing alternatives, and assessing potential benefits.[7]

About 25 percent of the scientific reviews of various CAM approaches that have been done in recent years have found sufficient evidence to conclude that that certain therapies are effective for certain conditions.

These include:

- Acupuncture and yoga for back pain.
- Acupuncture for knee pain.
- Acupuncture for insomnia.
- Acupuncture for nausea and vomiting, whether the cause is pregnancy, cancer chemotherapy, or post-surgery.
- Hypnosis for hot flashes in breast cancer survivors.[8]

Acupuncture and, to a lesser extent, massage therapy are now included among the recommended therapies for treating back pain in guidelines released by the American College of Physicians and the American Pain Society.[9]

Who Uses CAM

According to recent surveys, about four in ten adults in the United States report use of CAM therapy in the previous twelve months. The most frequent reasons are back pain or other problems, head or chest colds, neck pain or problems, joint pain or stiffness, and anxiety or depression. Individuals with cancer, cardiovascular diseases, and lung disorders also are likely to try CAM.[10] Not all CAM users have health problems. About one fifth of adults with no health conditions and a quarter of those who had not visited a doctor in the past 12 months used CAM therapies.

About one in nine children has used CAM, including natural products, chiropractic or osteopathic manipulation, deep breathing exercises, yoga, and homeopathic remedies.[11] Youngsters whose parents use CAM are much more likely to receive CAM treatments than those whose parents do not.[12] For both adults and children, individuals worried about costs were more likely to delay conventional care and try CAM.

The populations most likely to use CAM are:

- Women.
- Adults between ages 30 and 69.
- Adults with higher levels of education.
- Individuals who are physically active during their leisure time.
- People who have existing medical conditions or made frequent medical visits in the prior year.
- Residents of Western states.
- Former smokers.
- People with private health insurance (for those under age 65).

 CAM use is more prevalent among American Indian or Alaska Native adults (50 percent) and white adults (43 percent) than Asian adults (40 percent) or black adults (26 percent). Among Hispanics, Mexicans are less likely to use CAM than Puerto Rican, Mexican American, Dominican, and Central or South American adults.[13] CAM is more widely used in many other countries. In Germany, for instance, 82 percent of patients use CAM treatments, with acupuncture, massage, and relaxation techniques the most widely used.[14]

Some states have mandated health insurance coverage for CAM therapies, which also are becoming more common in Canada and Europe. Many medical schools now include training in CAM in their curricula. **Integrative medicine,** which combines selected elements of both conventional and alternative medicine in a comprehensive approach to diagnosis and treatment, has gained greater acceptance within the medical community.

Types of CAM

The National Center for Complementary and Alternative Medicine (NCCAM) has classified CAM therapies into five categories (Figure 17.2).

- **Alternative medical systems.**
- **Mind-body medicine.**
- **Biologically based therapies.**
- **Manipulative and body-based methods.**
- **Energy therapies.**

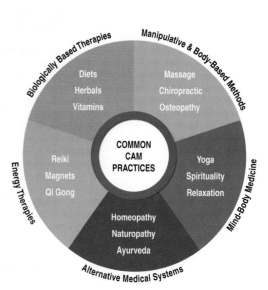

Figure 17.2 The Five Categories of CAM
Source: NCCAM, http://nccam.nih.gov.

Alternative Medical Systems Systems of theory and practice other than traditional Western medicine are included in this group. They include acupuncture, Eastern medicine, t'ai chi, external and internal qi, Ayurvedic medicine, naturopathy, and unconventional Western systems, such as homeopathy and orthomolecular medicine.

Acupuncture is an ancient Chinese form of medicine, based on the philosophy that a cycle of energy circulating through the body controls health. Pain and disease are the result of a disturbance in the energy flow, which can be corrected by inserting long, thin needles at specific points along longitudinal lines, or *meridians*, throughout the body. Each point controls a different corresponding part of the body. Once inserted, the needles are rotated gently back and forth or charged with a small electric current for a short time. Western scientists aren't sure exactly how acupuncture works, but some believe that the needles alter the functioning of the nervous system.

Over the past 10 years, federal studies have looked at acupuncture's effect on specific health conditions and how it affects the brain and nervous system; the neurological properties of meridians and acupuncture points; and methods for improving the quality of acupuncture research.

integrative medicine An approach that combines traditional medicine with alternative/complementary therapies.

acupuncture A Chinese medical practice of puncturing the body with needles inserted at specific points to relieve pain or cure disease.

The ancient Chinese practice of acupuncture produces healing through the insertion and manipulation of needles at specific points, or meridians, throughout the body.

Ayurveda A traditional Indian medical treatment involving meditation, exercise, herbal medications, and nutrition.

homeopathy A system of medical practice that treats a disease by administering dosages of substances that would in healthy persons produce symptoms similar to those of the disease.

naturopathy An alternative system of treatment of disease that emphasizes the use of natural remedies such as sun, water, heat, and air. Therapies may include dietary changes, steam baths, and exercise.

herbal medicine
An ancient form of medical treatment using substances derived from trees, flowers, ferns, seaweeds, and lichens to treat disease.

Recent studies have found that acupuncture:

- Helps alleviate nausea in cancer patients undergoing chemotherapy.

- Relieves pain and improves function for some people with osteoarthritis of the knee and complements standard medical care.

- Helps in treating chronic lower back pain.

- Can be useful in treatment of posttraumatic stress disorder (PTSD) symptoms.

- May improve pregnancy rates following in vitro fertilization (IVF).

- May or may not be of value for many other conditions, including irritable bowel syndrome and some neurologic disorders.[15]

Considered alternative in this country, **Ayurveda** is a traditional form of medical treatment in India, where it has evolved over thousands of years. Its basic premise is that illness stems from incorrect mental attitudes, diet, and posture. Practitioners use a discipline of exercise, meditation, herbal medication, and proper nutrition to cope with such stress-induced conditions as hypertension, the desire to smoke, and obesity.

Homeopathy is based on three fundamental principles: like cures like; treatment must always be individualized; and less is more—the idea that increasing dilution (and lowering the dosage) can increase efficacy. By administering doses of animal, vegetable, or mineral substances to a large number of

healthy people to see if they all develop the same symptoms, homeopaths determine which substances may be given, in small quantities, to alleviate the symptoms. Some of these substances are the same as those used in conventional medicine: nitroglycerin for certain heart conditions, for example, although the dose is minuscule.

Naturopathy emphasizes natural remedies, such as sun, water, heat, and air, as the best treatments for disease. Therapies might include dietary changes (such as more vegetables and no salt or stimulants), steam baths, and exercise. Some naturopathic physicians (who are not MDs) work closely with medical doctors in helping patients.

Mind-Body Medicine Mind-body medicine uses techniques designed to enhance the mind's capacity to affect bodily function and symptoms. Some techniques that were considered alternative in the past have become mainstream (for example, patient support groups and cognitive-behavioral therapy). Other mind-body approaches are still considered CAM, including meditation, prayer (see Chapter 2), yoga, t'ai chi, visual imagery, mental healing, and therapies that use creative outlets such as art, music, or dance. About 30 percent of Americans report using relaxation techniques and imagery, biofeedback, and hypnosis; 50 percent use prayer.

The physical and emotional risks of using mind-body interventions are minimal. Although we need much more research on how these approaches work and when to apply them most effectively, there is considerable evidence that mind-body interventions have positive effects on psychological functioning and quality of life and may be particularly helpful for patients coping with chronic illnesses.

Mind-body approaches definitely have won some acceptance in modern medical care. Techniques such as hypnosis have proved helpful in reducing discomfort and complications during and after various surgical procedures and in relieving hot flashes in breast cancer survivors.[16] With *biofeedback* (discussed in Chapter 3), people can learn to control usually involuntary functions, such as circulation to the hands and feet, tension in the jaws, and heartbeat rates. Biofeedback has been used to treat dozens of ailments, including asthma, epilepsy, pain, and Raynaud's disease (a condition in which the fingers become painful and white when exposed to cold). Many health insurers now cover biofeedback treatments.

Creative *visualization* (also discussed in Chapter 3) helps patients heal, including some diagnosed as terminally ill with cancer. Other patients use visualization to create a clear idea of what they want to achieve, whether the goal is weight loss or relaxation.

Biologically Based Therapies

Biologically based CAM therapies use substances such as herbs, foods, and vitamins. They include **herbal medicine** (botanical medicine or phytotherapy), the use of individual herbs or combinations; special diet therapies, such as macrobiotics, Ornish, Atkins, and high fiber; orthomolecular medicine (use of nutritional and food supplements for preventive or therapeutic purposes); and use of other products (such as shark cartilage) and procedures applied in an unconventional manner.

In the last ten years, sales of herbal supplements have skyrocketed by 100 percent, but most people don't consider evidence-based indications before trying them. According to recent research, two-thirds of people who use herbs do not do so in accordance with scientific guidelines. Although more than 1,500 different preparations are on the U.S. market, just a few single-herb preparations account for about half the sales in the United States: echinacea, garlic, ginkgo biloba, ginseng, kava, St. John's wort, and valerian. Unlike medications, herbal products are exempt from the FDA's regulatory scrutiny. The ingredients and the potency of active ingredients can vary from batch to batch.

Rigorous research studies are producing the first scientific evidence on the safety and efficacy of herbal supplements. Their benefits generally have proved modest (Table 17.4). Echinacea may cut the risk and severity of a cold. However, garlic has shown no effect on cholesterol. Other agents, such as saw palmetto, produce slight benefits but far less than available medications.

Most of the herbs tested have proved generally safe, although side effects such as headache and nausea can occur. However, some herbs can cause serious, even fatal dangers. Echinacea may cause liver damage if taken in combination with anabolic steroids. Several widely used herbs, including ginger, garlic, and ginkgo biloba, are dangerous if taken prior to surgery.

The FDA has prohibited the sale of dietary supplements containing ephedra, which was linked with dozens of deaths and more than 1,000 adverse reactions. It has issued warnings on other potentially dangerous herbs, including chaparral, comfrey, yohimbe, lobelia, germander, willow bark, jin bu huan, and products containing magnolia or stephania.

Manipulative and Body–Based Methods

CAM therapies based on manipulation and/or movement of the body are divided into three subcategories:

- **Chiropractic medicine.**
- **Massage therapy and body work** (including osteopathic manipulation, Swedish massage, Alexander technique,

Prayer is the most commonly used of the CAM therapies.

© Brand X Pictures/Jupiterimages

You should never decide on any treatment—traditional or CAM—without fully evaluating it. Here are some key questions to ask:

- **Is it safe?** Be particularly wary of unregulated products.

- **Is it effective?** Check the website of the National Center for CAM: **http://nccam.nih.gov.**

- **Will it interact with other medicines or conventional treatments?** Many widely used alternative remedies can interact with prescription medications in dangerous ways.

- **Is the practitioner qualified?** Find out if your state licenses practitioners who provide acupuncture, chiropractic services, naturopathy, herbal medicine, homeopathy, and other treatments.

- **What has been the experience of others?** Talk to people who have used CAM for a similar problem, both recently and in the past.

- **Can you talk openly and easily with the practitioner?** You should feel comfortable asking questions and confident in the answers you receive. And the practitioner's office should put you at ease.

- **What are the costs?** Many CAM services are not covered by HMOs or health insurers.

TABLE 17.4

Evidence-Based Evaluations of Herbal Supplements

Herb	Evidence
Saw palmetto	Reduces an enlarged prostate, but the effect is small compared with prescription medication
Ginseng	Improves energy of cancer patients
Echinacea and vitamin C	Cut risk of cold in half
Kava	May reduce anxiety, but can cause liver damage
Ginkgo biloba	No improvement in memory or thinking in the healthy elderly, but a small benefit for patients with dementia
Garlic	Not effective in lowering cholesterol
Black cohosh	No more effective than placebo for hot flashes; long-term effects unknown

© David Young-Wolff/PhotoEdit, Inc.

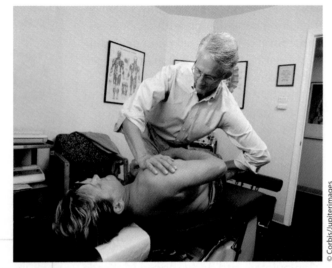

© Corbis/Jupiterimages

Chiropractic medicine is among the popular manipulative forms of CAM.

reflexology, Pilates, acupressure, and rolfing).

- **Unconventional physical therapies** (including colonics, hydrotherapy, and light and color therapies).

Chiropractic is a treatment method based on the theory that many human diseases are caused by misalignment of the spine (subluxation). Chiropractors are licensed in all 50 states, but chiropractic is considered a mainstream therapy by some and a form of CAM by others. Significant research in the last ten years has demonstrated its efficacy for acute lower-back pain. NIH is funding research on other potential benefits, including headaches, asthma, middle ear inflammation, menstrual cramps, and arthritis.

Chiropractors, who emphasize wellness and healing without drugs or surgery, may use X-rays and magnetic resonance imaging (MRI) as well as orthopedic, neurological, and manual examinations in making diagnoses. However, chiropractic treatment consists solely of the manipulation of misaligned discs that may be putting pressure on nerve tissue and affecting other parts of the body. Many HMOs offer chiropractic services, which are the most widely used alternative treatment among managed care patients.

Energy Therapies Various approaches focus on energy fields believed to exist in and around the body. Some use external energy sources, such as electromagnetic fields. Magnets are marketed to relieve pain but there is little scientific evidence of their efficacy. Others, such as therapeutic touch, use a therapist's healing energy to repair imbalances in an individual's biofield.

The Health-Care System

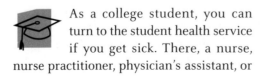

As a college student, you can turn to the student health service if you get sick. There, a nurse, nurse practitioner, physician's assistant, or medical doctor may evaluate your symptoms and provide basic care. However, you may rely on a primary care physician in your hometown to perform regular checkups or manage a chronic condition like asthma. If you're injured in an accident, you probably will be treated at the nearest emergency room. If you become seriously ill and require highly specialized care, you may have to go to a university-affiliated medical center to receive state-of-the-art treatment.

Students can often continue their health-care coverage under their parents' policy until the age of 23. However, if a parent belongs to an HMO with a local network of providers, the student may not be covered for anything outside the plan's service area except emergency care. A more open plan, like a preferred provider organization, may allow students to see doctors near school, but the costs may be high.

Most colleges offer some type of health insurance plan, with the student health center acting as the primary care provider. Many schools require enrollment if the student is not covered under any other plan. Check the plan carefully. Physicals, gynecological visits, and other preventive care may not be covered. College plans also may not cover preexisting conditions, such as asthma.

Health-Care Practitioners

Fewer than 10 percent of health-care practitioners are physicians; other types of health professionals are assuming more important roles in delivering primary, or basic, health services. As a consumer, you should be aware of the range and special skills of the most common types of health-care providers.

Physicians A medical doctor (M.D.) trained in American medical schools usually takes at least three years of premedical college courses (with an emphasis on biology, chemistry, and physics) and then completes four (but sometimes three or five) years of medical school. The first two years of medical school are devoted to the study of human anatomy, embryology, pharmacology, and similar basic subjects. During the last two years, students work directly with physicians in hospitals. Medical students who pass a series of national board examinations then enter a one-year internship in a hospital, followed by another two to five years of residency (depending on their specialty), which

leads to certification in a particular field, or specialty.

About 500,000 of the nation's 700,000 physicians are specialists or subspecialists, who focus on a specific part of the body, organ system, type of disease, or type of treatment. Traditionally, they have had greater status and earned much larger incomes than primary care physicians—family practitioners, pediatricians, and internists—who provide preventive care, regular checkups, and routine treatments of uncomplicated medical conditions. However, changes in health policy (such as increases in Medicare payments to primary care physicians) and in the delivery of services have given a more prominent role to primary care physicians. They now often function as "gatekeepers" who decide whether a patient needs to see a medical specialist.

Nurses A registered nurse (RN) graduates from a school of nursing approved by a state board and passes a state board examination. RNs may have a bachelor's or an associate degree and may specialize in certain areas, such as intensive care or nurse-midwifery. Nurse practitioners, RNs with advanced training and experience, may run community clinics or provide screening and preventive care at group medical practices. Some have independent practices.

Licensed practical nurses (LPNs), also called licensed vocational nurses, are licensed by the state. After graduating from state-approved schools of practical nursing, they must take a board exam. They work under the supervision of RNs or physicians. Certified nursing assistants (CNAs), nursing aides, and orderlies assist registered and practical nurses in providing services directly related to the comfort and well-being of hospitalized patients.

Specialized and Allied-Health Practitioners More than 60 types of health practitioners work with physicians and nurses in providing medical services. Some, such as *occupational therapists*, have at least a bachelor's degree. Allied-health professionals may specialize in a variety of fields. *Clinical psychologists* have graduate degrees and provide a wide range of mental health

chiropractic A method of treating disease, primarily through manipulating the bones and joints to restore normal nerve function.

services but don't prescribe medications—as do *psychiatrists. Optometrists,* trained in special schools of optometry, diagnose visual abnormalities and prescribe lenses or visual aids; however, they don't prescribe drugs, diagnose or treat eye diseases, or perform surgery—functions performed by *ophthalmologists. Podiatrists* are specially trained, licensed health-care professionals who specialize in problems of the feet.

Dentists   Most dental students earn a bachelor's degree and then complete two more years of training in the basic sciences and two years of clinical work before graduating with a degree of D.D.S. or D.M.D. (Doctor of Dental Surgery or Doctor of Medical Dentistry). To qualify for a license, graduates must pass both a written and a clinical examination. Dentists may work in general practice or choose a specialty, such as orthodontics (straightening teeth).

Chiropractors   Chiropractors hold the degree of Doctor of Chiropractic (D.C.), which signifies that they have had two years of college-level training, plus four years in a health-care school specializing in chiropractic, described earlier in this chapter.

Health-Care Facilities

As a prospective patient, you can choose from various options: a physician's office, a clinic, an emergency room, or a hospital. Most **primary care**—also referred to as ambulatory or outpatient care—is provided by a physician in an office, emergency room, or clinic. *Secondary care* usually is provided by specialists or subspecialists in either an outpatient or inpatient (hospital)

setting. *Tertiary care,* available at university-affiliated hospitals and regional referral centers, includes special procedures such as kidney dialysis, open-heart surgery, and organ transplants.

College Health Centers   The American College Health Association estimates that 1,500 institutions of higher learning provide direct health services. Student health centers, initially developed by departments of physical education and hygiene, range in size from small dispensaries staffed by nurses to large-scale, multispecialty clinics that provide both inpatient and outpatient care and are fully accredited by the Joint Commission on Accreditation of Healthcare Organizations. Some serve only students; others provide services for faculty, staff, and family members.

On some campuses, health educators work with the student health centers to provide counseling on such topics as nutrition; tobacco, drug, and alcohol abuse; exercise and fitness; sexuality; and contraception. Some college health centers provide psychological counseling, as well as dental, pharmacy, and optometric services. Some campuses also provide sports-medicine services for student athletes. Services are paid for by various combinations of prepaid health fees, general university funds, fee-for-service charges, and health-insurance reimbursements.

Outpatient Treatment Centers   Increasingly, procedures that once required hospitalization, such as simple surgery, are being performed at outpatient centers, which may be freestanding or affiliated with a medical center. Patients have any necessary tests performed beforehand, undergo surgery or receive treatment, and return home after a few hours to recuperate. Outpatient centers can handle many common surgical procedures, including cataract removal, tonsillectomy, breast biopsy, dilation and curettage (D and C), vasectomy, and face-lifts.

Without the high overhead costs of a hospital, outpatient surgery costs run only about 30 to 50 percent of standard hospital fees. Today, 70 percent of hospitals do outpatient, or "in-and-out," surgery. To cut health-care costs, insurance companies are encouraging, or in some cases requiring,

Student health centers on campus offer a variety of services , usually including basic medical care as well as counseling on health-related issues.

© AP IMAGES

their policyholders to choose outpatient surgery. However, operations requiring prolonged general anesthesia or extensive postoperative care still must be performed on an inpatient basis.

Freestanding emergency or urgent-care centers (those not part of a hospital) claim that they deliver high-quality medical treatment with maximum convenience in minimal time. Rather than going to crowded hospital emergency rooms when they slice a finger in the kitchen, patients can go to a freestanding emergency center and receive prompt attention.

Hospitals and Medical Centers Different types of hospitals offer different types of care. The most common type of hospital is the *private,* or *community, hospital,* which may be run on a profit or a nonprofit basis, generally contains 50 to 400 beds, and provides more personalized care than public hospitals do. The quality of care individual patients receive depends mostly on the physicians themselves. *Public hospitals* include city, county, public health service, military, and Veterans Administration hospitals. The quality of patient care depends on the overall quality of the institution.

Of the more than 6,500 hospitals nationwide, about 300 are major *academic medical centers* or *teaching hospitals.* Affiliated with medical schools, they generally provide the most up-to-date and experienced care, because staff physicians must stay current in order to teach their students. These centers, with the best equipment, researchers, and resources, offer high-technology care—at a price. The cost of treatment at all teaching hospitals averages approximately 20 percent higher than at nonteaching hospitals. At major teaching hospitals with large graduate training programs for physicians and other health providers, the costs are as much as 45 percent higher than those at nonteaching hospitals.

The Joint Commission on the Accreditation of Healthcare Organizations (JCAH) reviews all hospitals every three years. Eighty percent of hospitals qualify for JCAH accreditation. If you have to enter a hospital and your health insurance or plan allows a choice, try to find out as much as you can about the alternatives available to you:

- Talk to your physician about a hospital and why he or she recommends it.
- As a cost-cutting strategy, many hospitals have cut back on the use of registered nurses. Check with the local nursing association about the ratio of patients to nurses, and the ratio of RNs to LPNs.
- Find out room rates and charges for ancillary services, including tests, lab work, X-rays, and medications. Check with your health plan to see whether you need preapproval for any of these costs and ask what you will be expected to pay.
- Ask how many times in the past year the hospital has performed the procedure recommended for you, and what the success and complication rates have been. Ask about the hospital's nosocomial (hospital-caused) infection rate and accident rate. You also have the right to information on the number and types of malpractice claims filed against a hospital.
- If possible, go on a tour of the hospital. Does the setting seem comfortable? Is the staff courteous? Does the hospital seem clean and efficiently run?

Emergency Services Hospital emergency rooms should be used only in a true emergency. Most are overwhelmed, understaffed, and underfinanced—particularly in big cities. Patients usually see a different physician each time; he or she deals with the main complaints but doesn't have time for a full examination. Extensive tests and procedures are difficult to arrange in an emergency room, and patients who don't have truly urgent problems may have to wait for a long time. Emergency-room fees are higher than those for standard office visits and are not always covered by medical insurance.

Inpatient Care Inpatient hospital care remains the most expensive form of health care. Health-insurance companies and health-care plans (described on pages 567–568) often demand a second opinion or make their own evaluation before approving coverage of an

primary care Ambulatory or outpatient care provided by a physician in an office, emergency room, or clinic.

elective, or nonemergency, hospital admission. As another means of controlling costs, health insurers (including Medicare) may limit hospital stays or pay for hospital care on the basis of **diagnostic-related groups,** or **DRGs.** Under this system, hospitals are paid according to a patient's diagnosis—for example, a set number of dollars for every appendectomy. If the hospital can treat and discharge patients more quickly than the national average for that DRG, it makes money. On the other hand, if a patient develops unexpected complications or is slow to recover, the hospital loses money.

Because hospital stays are shorter than in the past, patients often leave "quicker and sicker"—after a shorter stay and not as far along in their recovery. Nevertheless, the benefits of shorter hospital stays, including reduced risk of infection and more rapid resumption of normal life activities, may outweigh the slightly increased risks associated with early discharge.

Home Health Care With hospitals discharging patients sooner, **home health care**—the provision of equipment and services to patients in the home to restore or maintain comfort, function, and health—has become a major industry. Advances in technology have made it possible for treatments once administered only in hospitals—such as kidney dialysis, chemotherapy, and traction—to be performed at home at 10 to 40 percent of the cost. The physician's house call, once considered an anachronism, has also come back in fashion. According to various surveys, the majority of primary care physicians will see patients in their homes.

Hospital discharge planners usually arrange home health care for patients who've been hospitalized. Families can also contact health aides, nurses, and other needed professionals on their own. According to the Health Insurance Association of America, most private insurance policies offer some coverage for these home health-care costs.

Paying for Health Care

Health-care spending in the United States has soared to $2.2 trillion—$7,421 per man, woman, and child. Although the rate of growth in health-care spending has been declining in the last few years, it still remains higher than overall inflation. This has led to added cost pressures on private and public insurers and on patients and to a national debate on health care reform and insurance.[17]

Many individuals with insurance are covered under an employer-based plan (options offered and partially funded by their employer). Individual health insurance coverage, though more costly, can be obtained through some companies. Uninsured persons depend on their own ability to pay, their qualifying for government insurance, or the care that physicians and institutions donate to those unable to pay.

Your health plan affects many things, including:

- **Who** will care for you (doctors and other health-care providers), and how much choice you will have.
- **What** kind of care you will receive (for example, which preventive services are covered).
- **Where** you will receive your care (which hospitals, for example).
- **When** you will receive your care (will you receive it when you need it).
- **How** you will be cared for (the quality of care you receive).
- **How much** you will pay.

Managed Care Managed care has become the predominant form of health care in the United States. Managed-care organizations, which take various forms, deliver care through a network of physicians, hospitals, and other health-care professionals who agree to provide their services at fixed or discounted rates. Nine in ten physicians in the United States have contracted with managed-care companies.

Consumers in a managed-care group must follow certain procedures in advance of seeking care (for example, getting prior approval for a test or treatment) and must abide by a limit on reimbursement for certain services. Some procedures may be deemed unnecessary and not be covered at all. Patients who choose to see a physician who is not a participating member of

Cutting-edge technology, such as this so-called "brain bucket MRI," may make it possible to diagnose disease earlier and to target treatments more precisely.

Courtesy of Lawrence Wald, PhD.

the medical-insurance coverage group may have to pay the entire fee themselves.

Managed-care plans have been criticized for pressuring providers to "undertreat" patients—for example, sending them home from the hospital too soon or denying them costly tests or treatments. Members have complained of long waits, the need to switch primary physicians if their doctor leaves the plan, difficulty getting approval for needed services, and a sense that providers pay more attention to the bottom line than to the health needs of their patients.

As dissatisfaction with managed care has grown, consumers have demanded more choice of physicians, direct access to specialists, and the ability to go "out of network." In response to patients' complaints, many states have approved "patient protection acts" or "comprehensive consumer bills of rights."

According to the National Committee for Quality Assurance, managed-care plans have shown improvement in the delivery of care, but health-care costs continue to rise. As a result, employers are cutting back coverage and asking employees to shoulder more of the burden of their health care in the belief that consumers will seek more efficient care when they are required to pay more out of pocket.

Health Maintenance Organizations (HMOs)

Health maintenance organizations, or **HMOs,** are managed-care plans that emphasize routine care and prevention by providing complete medical services in exchange for a predetermined monthly payment. In a *group-model HMO,* physicians provide care in offices at a clinic run by the HMO. In an *individual practice association (IPA),* or network HMO, independent physicians provide services in their own offices. HMOs generally pay a fixed amount per patient to a physician or hospital, regardless of the type and number of services actually provided. This is called *capitation.*

Members of HMOs pay a regular, preset fee that usually includes diagnostic tests, routine physical exams, and vaccinations as well as treatment of illnesses. HMOs usually do not require a deductible, and copayments for medications or services are small. The primary drawback of standard HMOs is that the consumer is limited to a particular health-care facility and staff.

Preferred Provider Organizations   In a **preferred provider organization (PPO),** a third party—a union, an insurance company, or a self-insured business—contracts with a group of physicians and hospitals to treat members at a discount. PPO members may choose any physician within the network, and usually pay a 10 percent copayment for care within the system and a higher percentage (20 to 30 percent) for care elsewhere. PPOs generally require prior approval for expensive tests or major procedures.

A *point-of-service* (POS) plan is a PPO that permits patients to use physicians outside the network. Consumers pay the difference between the preferred provider's discounted fee and the outside physician's fee. A *gatekeeper* plan requires members to choose a primary physician, as in an HMO, who must approve all referrals to specialists.

When deciding on an HMO or PPO, use these questions as a guide:

- How many doctors can I choose from?
- Is the network made up of private or group practice physicians?
- Which doctors are accepting new patients?
- Can I change my primary care physician?
- What is the procedure for referrals to specialists?
- How easy is it to get an appointment?
- How far in advance must routine visits be scheduled?
- What arrangements are there for handling emergency care?
- What health-care services are offered?
- Are there limits on medical tests, surgery, or other services?
- What if I want or need a special service that is not covered?
- Which hospitals are used?

diagnostic-related group (DRG) A category of conditions requiring hospitalization for which the cost of care has been determined prior to a client's hospitalization.

home health care   Provision of medical services and equipment to patients in the home to restore or maintain comfort, function, and health.

managed care   Health-care services and reimbursement predetermined by third-party insurers.

health maintenance organization (HMO)   An organization that provides health services on a fixed-contract basis.

preferred provider organization (PPO)   A group of physicians contracted to provide health care to members at a discounted price.

PART 2: *Just the Facts*
- **23** *percent of men ages 18–19 are uninsured.*
- **39** *percent of men ages 20–24 are uninsured.*
- **34** *percent of men ages 25–29 are uninsured.*
- **18** *percent of women ages 18–19 are uninsured.*
- **28** *percent of women ages 20–24 are uninsured.*
- **25** *percent of women ages 25–29 are uninsured.*

Source: CDC/NCHS. *Health United States 2008.* Figure 38. Data from the National Health Interview Survey.

- What happens if I'm out of town and need medical attention?

- What is the yearly total for monthly premiums?

- Are there any copayments? For which services and how much?

Government–Financed Insurance Plans

The government, through programs like Medicare and Medicaid, funds 45 percent of total U.S. health spending. Under Medicare, the federal government pays 80 percent of most medical bills, after a deductible fee, for people over age 65. Medicare also offers options for coverage of prescription medications.

Medicaid, a federal and state insurance plan that protects people with very low or no incomes, is the chief source of coverage for the unemployed. However, many unemployed Americans don't qualify because their family incomes are above the poverty line. Publicly insured patients are more likely than those with private insurance to receive inadequate care and to experience adverse health outcomes.

The Uninsured

The United States is the only industrialized nation that does not have national health insurance. More Americans lack health insurance coverage than a decade ago—an estimated 47 million. Many more experience temporary lapses in coverage or are underinsured, meaning that they don't have adequate coverage and are less likely to receive preventive care or routine check-ups. Uninsured individuals who experience a change in health caused by an injury or a new chronic condition have more difficulty obtaining recommended care and are more likely to suffer a greater decline in short-term health.

Racial and ethnic minorities are much more likely to be uninsured than white Americans. More than a third of the Hispanic population and over a quarter of Native Americans are uninsured, compared to 12 percent of whites. The uninsured rates among African Americans and Asian Americans are also much higher than among whites. Nearly one-third of the uninsured are Hispanic, despite the fact that Hispanics make up just 13 percent of the population. This disparity results from several factors, including citizenship issues and language barriers.

Young adults, 18 to 24 years of age, are more likely than any other age group to be uninsured. Of Americans between the ages of 18 and 24 years, almost a third are without medical insurance. (See Reality Check, p. 567.)

A committee of the Institute of Medicine (IOM), after years of exhaustive study, has urged federal leaders to provide health insurance for everyone living in the United States. The consequences of being uninsured, the IOM concluded, include "worse health and earlier death," including 18,000 deaths every year. It proposed that coverage be universal (for all residents, not just citizens), continuous, affordable, sustainable, and provided in such a way as to promote access to high-quality care.

POINT COUNTERPOINT *Who Should Pay for Insurance?*

POINT
Almost one in five Americans—including many families and young adults—has no health insurance. Unable to pay for routine care, they are at risk of developing serious illnesses that will cost far more to treat than to prevent. It is in society's best interest to make health care available to all, regardless of ability to pay.

COUNTERPOINT
The costs of providing universal health coverage are too great. Taxpayers who obtain health coverage through jobs or who pay independently should not bear the additional burden of underwriting care for those who cannot afford it.

YOUR VIEW
Do you think the nation has a responsibility to ensure that all citizens get health-care insurance? Or should health insurance be a personal responsibility? Who pays for your health care? Who will pay after you graduate from college? What will you do if you can't afford health insurance?

You can do more to safeguard and enhance your well-being than any health-care provider. Here are some recommendations to keep in mind:

- **Trust your instincts.** You know your body better than anyone else. If something is bothering you, it deserves medical attention. Don't let your health-care provider—or your health plan administrator—dismiss it without a thorough evaluation.

- **Do your homework.** Go to the library or online and find authoritative articles that describe what you're experiencing. The more you know about possible causes of your symptoms, the more likely you are to be taken seriously.

- **Find a good primary care physician who listens carefully and responds to your concerns.** Look for a family doctor or general internist who takes a careful history, performs a thorough exam, and listens and responds to your concerns.

- **See your doctor regularly.** If you're in your twenties or thirties, you may not need an annual exam, but it's important to get checkups at least every two or three years so you and your doctor can get to know each other and develop a trusting, mutually respectful relationship.

- **Get a second opinion.** If you are uncertain of whether to undergo treatment or which therapy is best, see another physician and listen carefully for any doubts or hesitation about what you're considering.

- **Seek support.** Patient support and advocacy groups can offer emotional support, information on many common problems, and referral to knowledgeable physicians.

- **If your doctor cannot or will not respond to your concerns, get another one.** Regardless of your health coverage, you have the right to replace a physician who is not meeting your health-care needs.

- **Speak up.** If you don't understand, ask. If you feel that you're not being taken seriously or being treated with respect, say so. Sometimes the only difference between being a patient or becoming a victim is making sure your needs and rights are not forgotten or overlooked.

- **Bring your own advocate.** If you become intimidated or anxious talking to physicians, ask a friend to accompany you, to ask questions on your behalf and to take notes.

SELF SURVEY Are You a Savvy Health-Care Consumer?

1. You want a second opinion, but your doctor dismisses your request for other physicians' names as unnecessary. What do you do?
   a. Assume that he or she is right and you would merely be wasting time.
   b. Suspect that your physician has something to hide and immediately switch doctors.
   c. Contact your health plan and request a second opinion.

2. As soon as you enter your doctor's office, you get tongue-tied. When you try to find the words to describe what's wrong, your physician keeps interrupting. When giving advice, your doctor uses such technical language that you can't understand what it means. What do you do?
   a. Prepare better for your next appointment.
   b. Pretend that you understand what your doctor is talking about.
   c. Decide you'd be better off with someone who specializes in complementary/alternative therapies and seems less intimidating.

3. You feel like you're running on empty, tired all the time, worn to the bone. A friend suggests some herbal supplements that promise to boost energy and restore vitality. What do you do?
   a. Immediately start taking them.
   b. Say that you think herbs are for cooking.
   c. Find out as much as you can about the herbal compounds and ask your doctor if they're safe and effective.

4. Your hometown physician's office won't give you a copy of your medical records to take with you to college. What do you do?
   a. Hope you won't need them and head off without your records.
   b. Threaten to sue.
   c. Politely ask the office administrator to tell you the particular law or statute that bars you from your records.

5. Your doctor has been treating you for an infection for three weeks, and you don't seem to be getting any better. What do you do?
   a. Talk to your doctor, by phone or in person, and say, "This doesn't seem to be working. Is there anything else we can try?"
   b. Stop taking the antibiotic.
   c. Try an herbal remedy that your roommate recommends.

6. Your doctor suggests a cutting-edge treatment for your condition, but your health plan or HMO refuses to pay for it. What do you do?
   a. Try to get a loan to cover the costs.
   b. Settle for whatever treatment options are covered.
   c. Challenge your health plan.

7. You call for an appointment with your doctor and are told nothing is available for four months. What do you do?
   a. Take whatever time you can get whenever you can get it.
   b. Explain your condition to the nurse or receptionist, detailing any symptoms and pain you're experiencing.
   c. Give up and decide you don't need to see a doctor at all.

8. Even though you've been doing sit-ups faithfully, your waist still looks flabby. When you see an ad for waist-whittling liposuction, What do you do?
   a. Call for an appointment.
   b. Talk to a health-care professional about a total fitness program that may help you lose excess pounds.
   c. Carefully research the risks and costs of the procedure.

9. You have a condition that you do not want anyone to know about, including your health insurer and any potential employer. What do you do?
   a. Use a false name.
   b. Give your physician a written request for confidentiality about this condition.
   c. Seek help outside the health-care system.

10. Your doctor suggests a biopsy of a funny-looking mole that's sprouted on your nose. Rather than using a laboratory that specializes in skin analysis, your HMO requires that all samples be sent to a general lab, where results may not be as precise. What do you do?
   a. Ask your doctor to request that a specialty pathologist at the general lab perform the analysis.
   b. Hope that in your case, the general lab will do a good-enough job.
   c. Threaten to change HMOs.

Answers
1: c; 2: a; 3: c; 4: c; 5: a; 6: c; 7: b; 8: b and c; 9: b; 10: a

Your Health Action Plan for Protecting Yourself from Medical Mistakes and Misdeeds

Just as physicians practice "defensive" medicine to protect themselves from legal liability, today's patients should take preventive steps to defend themselves from potentially harmful health services.

The Whats, Whys, and Hows of Medical Testing

- Before undergoing any test, find out why you need it. Get a specific answer, not a "just in case" or "for your peace of mind." If you've had the test before, could the earlier results be used? Would a follow-up exam be just as helpful?

- Get some practical information as well: Should you do specific things before the test (such as not eat for a specified period)? How long will the test take? What will the test feel like? Will you need help getting home afterward?

- Check out the risks. Any invasive test—one that penetrates the body with a needle, tube, or viewing instrument—involves some risk of infection, bleeding, or tissue damage. Tests involving radiation also present risks, and some people develop allergic reactions to the materials used in testing.

- Get information on the laboratory that will be evaluating the test. Ask how often false positives or false negatives occur. (False positives are abnormal results indicating that you have a particular condition when you really don't; false negatives indicate that you don't have a particular condition when you really do.) Find out about civil or criminal negligence suits filed against the laboratory on charges such as failing to diagnose cervical cancer because of incorrect reading of Pap smears.

- You'll also want to know what happens when the test indicates a problem: Will the test be repeated? Will a different test be performed? Will treatment begin immediately? Could any medications you're taking (including nonprescription drugs, like aspirin) affect the testing procedures or results?

- If you have a test, don't assume that no news is good news. Check back to get the results.

CENGAGENOW If you want to write your own goals for getting quality medical care or using CAM, go to the Wellness Journal at CengageNOW for Health at **www.cengage.com/sso**.

MAKING THIS CHAPTER WORK FOR YOU

Review Questions

1. Periodontal disease
   a. results from poor eating habits.
   b. can lead to cardiovascular problems.
   c. in its early stage can be prevented by brushing alone.
   d. is caused by a variety of bacteria and viruses.

2. During a medical exam, your doctor will
   a. check your cardiovascular system by listening to your heart and feeling your neck arteries.
   b. check your lungs by probing for tender spots and malformations.
   c. look into your eyes to see if you have vision problems that require glasses or contact lenses.
   d. evaluate your joints by tapping on the knees and elbows.

3. Informed consent means that
   a. the patient has informed the doctor of his or her symptoms and has consented to treatment.
   b. the physician has informed the patient about the treatment to be given and has consented to administer the treatment.
   c. the patient has informed the doctor of his or her symptoms, and the doctor has consented to administer treatment.
   d. the physician has informed the patient about the treatment to be given, and the patient has consented to the treatment.

4. Patients have all the following rights *except* the right
   a. to access their medical records.
   b. to medical care that meets accepted standards of quality.
   c. to donate a body part for compensation.
   d. to leave the hospital against their physician's advice.

5. People use complementary and alternative therapies
   a. to spend less money on health care.
   b. to take an active role in their own treatment.
   c. to show their disdain for the medical establishment.
   d. to take more prescription drugs.

6. Which statement is *false?*
   a. Acupuncture has been shown to control nausea in patients after surgery.
   b. Chiropractic has been shown to relieve acute lower-back pain.
   c. People can learn to control involuntary functions through biofeedback.
   d. Naturopathy is based on the premise that like cures like.

7. Which of the following statements about the health-care system is *true?*
   a. Primary care is usually provided by specialists in a hospital.
   b. Nurses can perform some surgical procedures once they are board certified.
   c. Most hospitals in the United States are teaching hospitals and affiliated with medical schools.

d. The length of hospital stays may be determined by a patient's diagnosis rather than the person's pace of recovery.

8. Managed care features all of the following *except*
   a. health maintenance organizations.
   b. a fee-for-service system of insurance.
   c. preferred provider organizations.
   d. limitations on reimbursement for certain health services.

9. Personalizing health care—tailoring medical care to individual patients—may include all the following *except*
   a. DNA testing.
   b. mapping a family medical history.
   c. taking into account gender and ethnic background.
   d. taking into account economic status.

10. Which of the following is *not* a common form of CAM therapy?
    a. taking multivitamins.
    b. meditation.
    c. massage.
    d. using guided imagery.

Answers to these questions can be found on page 650.

Critical Thinking

1. Think about an experience you've had with a traditional medical practitioner. How did you feel during the physical examination? Did you trust the practitioner? Were you comfortable with the level of communication? Evaluate your experience and give your opinion of the value of the checkup.

2. Have you used any complementary or alternative approaches to health care? If so, were you satisfied with the results? How did your experience with the CAM therapist compare with your most recent experience with a traditional medical practitioner? Do you feel confident that you know the difference between alternative care and quackery?

3. Jocelyn has been experiencing a great deal of fatigue and frequent headaches for the past couple of months. She doesn't have health insurance and doesn't want to spend money on a doctor visit. So she did some research on the Internet about ways to relieve her symptoms and was considering taking a couple of herbal supplements that were touted as potential treatments. If she asked you for your advice, what would you tell her? Do you think that self-care is appropriate in this situation?

Media Menu

CENGAGENOW Go to the CengageNOW for Health website at **www .cengage.com/sso** that will:
- Help you evaluate your knowledge of the material.
- Allow you to take an exam-prep quiz.
- Provide a Personalized Learning Plan targeting resources that address areas you should study.
- Coach you through identifying target goals for behavioral change and creating and monitoring your personal change plan throughout the semester.

Internet Connections

www.health.gov/nhic/
This excellent site, sponsored by the National Health Information Center (NHIC) of the U.S. Office of Disease Prevention and Health Promotion, is a health information referral service providing health professionals and consumers with a database of various health organizations. The site provides a searchable database, publications, and a list of toll-free numbers for health information.

http://nccam.nih.gov
This National Institutes of Health site features a variety of fact sheets on alternative therapies and dietary supplements, research, current news, and databases for the public as well as for practitioners.

www.medicinenet.com
This comprehensive site is written for the consumer by board-certified physicians and contains medical news, a directory of procedures, a medical dictionary, a pharmacy, and first aid information. You can use the information at MedicineNet.com to prepare for a doctor visit, learn about a diagnosis, or understand a prescribed treatment or procedure.

www.fda.gov
In addition to providing information on regulation and legislation relating to food and drugs, the FDA website offers information on strategies for evaluating health products and services.

www.odsw.od.nih.gov/Health_Information/Health_Information.aspx
Health information on dietary supplements, including vitamins and minerals.

Key Terms

The terms listed are used on the page indicated. Definitions of the terms are in the Glossary at the end of the book.

acupuncture 559
Ayurveda 560
chiropractic 563
complementary and alternative medicine (CAM) 557
diagnostic-related groups (DRGs) 567
gingivitis 549
gum disease 549
health maintenance organization (HMO) 567
herbal medicine 560
holistic 557
home health care 567
homeopathy 560
informed consent 555
integrative medicine 559
managed care 567
medical history 553
naturopathy 560
outcomes 553
Pap smear 553
periodontitis 549
plaque 549
preferred provider organization (PPO) 567
primary care 565
quackery 557
vital signs 549

Chapter 18 - Protecting Yourself from Injury, Violence, & Victimization

1. The leading cause of accidents leading to death among college-aged young people is: (pg 576)
   A. suicide
   B. murder
   C. automobile accidents
   D. acute alcohol poisoning

2. Unintentional accidents refer to: (pg 576)
   A. murder
   B. rape
   C. trips and falls
   D. violence

3. All of the following are risk factors for an accident except: (pg 576)
   A. feeling stressed out
   B. under the influence of alcohol
   C. wearing your seat belt
   D. driving on a raining wet road surface

4. Defensive driving includes all but the following: (pg 577 – 578)
   A. keeping awake by playing music or allowing for some fresh air
   B. drive more slowly when the weather or roads become bad
   C. talking on your cell phone to pass the time from becoming bored
   D. be alert for the other driver and anticipate their moves

5. The most effective means of reducing traffic fatalities while driving your vehicle is: (pg 578)
   A. install safety glass on the windshield
   B. wearing your seatbelt all the time
   C. keeping both hands on the steering wheel
   D. deactivate the airbag so it does not become a distraction

6. The most common injury associated with motorcycle or bicycle riding is: (pg 580)
   A. falls resulting in broken limbs
   B. wind or sunburn from air and sun exposure
   C. head trauma
   D. frostbite when it is cold

7. All of the following except one are good strategies to employ when confronted with road rage while driving: (pg 579)
   A. don't let other drivers annoy you
   B. drive faster and pass annoying drivers in other cars
   C. be courteous to other drivers even if they are not polite to you
   D. never retaliate to other driver who has cut you off

8. 'Inattention blindness' while driving refers to: (pg 579)
   A. the blind spot not shown in the rear or side view mirror to show passing cars
   from behind you
   B. listening to the radio while driving
   C. not knowing the way on a strange road you are driving on
   D. talking on your cell phone

9. What is the most common type of crime or violence found on college campuses? (pg 584)
   A. hate and bias crimes
   B. mass murders
   C. victimization violence
   D. hazing incidents

10. Which of the following should be avoided to prevent one of the leading causes of serious automobile accidents among young people: (pg 578)
   A. don't use your cell phone while driving
   B. don't drive while intoxicated (drunk)
   C. car convertible tops should be kept closed to avoid windy distractions
   D. make sure your air bags are properly installed and useable

11. Which of the following is not an example of sexual harassment? (pg 587)
    A. displaying pornography to classmates
    B. making sexual obscenities to the opposite sex
    C. rape
    D. stalking someone and making cat calls or whistling

12. Any form of unwanted sexual attention defines: (pg 587)
    A. sexual assault
    B. nonvolitional sex
    C. domestic violence
    D. sexual harassment

13. When Tashika began her new job with all male coworkers, her supervisor told her that he enjoyed having an attractive woman in his office and winked at her. His comment would be construed as: (pg 587)
    A. sexual coercion
    B. sexual harassment
    C. sexual assault
    D. sexual battering

14. Forced sexual activity is the same as: (pg 588)
    A. rape
    B. sexual coercion
    C. sexual abuse
    D. sexual harassment

15. Rape by a man known to the victim which did not involve physical beating nor the use of a weapon is called: (pg 589)
    A. aggravated rape
    B. acquaintance rape
    C. anger rape
    D. sexual harassment

16. When a man is raping a woman to gain a 'power trip' or the upper hand over a woman, this is known as: (pg 589)
    A. anger rape
    B. power rape
    C. statutory rape
    D. sadistic rape

17. What is the main reason why so few college women will report a sexual or abusive incident to the police? (pg 592)
    A. that the incident was not serious enough
    B. unaware the incident was a crime worth reporting
    C. not wanting to tell anyone for fear of humiliation
    D. all are reasons why women do not report their victimization to the police but should

18. Which type of sexual violence scars takes longer for a woman to recover or heal from? (pg 592)
    A. social innuendoes that the woman is a whore and likes sex
    B. psychological scars from the traumatic experience of being violated
    C. physical wounds from forced vaginal penetration
    D. spiritual low self esteem resulting from feelings of being punished by God

19. What are some positive things a woman can do to protect herself from unwanted sexual advances or social violence aimed at her? (pg 591)
    A. take a self-defense class to learn about self protection
    B. using a buddy system at night when walking
    C. avoid giving a man misleading messages or engaging in sexual teasing
    D. all of the above are safety measures to initiate to keep a woman safer

20. Which of the following would be a good thing to include in your personal safety action plan while in school to keep you safe from sexual or social violence? (pg 594 - 595)
    A. always keep your dorm room locked when absent
    B. share your schedule with parents and close network of buddies and roommates
    C. survey your campus buildings and grounds at night to see where potential danger spots might be
    D. all of the above are prudent things to do for your personal safety

This can't be happening to me!" This was the phrase that first ran through Parker's mind when the car swerved out of control. He kept repeating it to himself as he heard the sickening sound of metal hitting metal and felt a terrible crushing pain shoot up through his legs. Later at the hospital, when he woke up after surgery, it was his first thought. And all through the long months of rehabilitation, on the days when he thought life would never go back to normal, he'd try to tell himself that this too couldn't be happening to him.

Protecting Yourself from Injury, Violence, and Victimization

Most young people think the same way. Accidents, injuries, assaults, crimes—all seem like things that happen only to other people, only in other places. But no one, regardless of how young, healthy, or strong, is immune from danger. The risks to college students include alcohol-associated injuries and illnesses, traffic accidents, and physical and sexual assaults.

Recognizing the threat of intentional and unintentional injury is the first step to ensuring your personal safety. You may think that the risk of something bad happening is simply a matter of chance, of being in the wrong place at the wrong time. That's not the case. Certain behaviors, such as using alcohol or drugs or not buckling your seat belt, greatly increase the risk of harm.

Ultimately, you have more control over your safety than anyone or anything else in your life. (See Making Change Happen, p. 575, and "Your Guardian Angel" in *Labs for IPC*.)

This chapter is a primer in self-protection that could help safeguard—perhaps even save—your life. Included are recommendations for commonsense safety on the road, at home, and at work. This chapter also explores other serious threats to personal safety in our society: violence and sexual victimization.

After studying the material in this chapter, you should be able to

- **List** and **explain** factors that increase the likelihood of an accident.
- **Name** four key factors in driving safely.
- **Describe** three ways of improving personal safety on campus.
- **Define** sexual victimization, sexual harassment, stalking, and sexual coercion.
- **List** the different types of rape, and **describe** recommended actions for preventing rape.
- **Explain** the consequences of sexual violence.
- **Assess** your risk of sexual or social violence, and **make a plan** to lower that risk.

Log on to CengageNOW for Health at **www.cengage.com/sso** to find your Behavior Change Planner and to explore self-assessments, interactive tutorials, and practice quizzes.

573

Personal Safety

 The major threat to the lives of college students isn't illness but injury. Almost 75 percent of deaths among Americans 15 to 24 years old are caused by "unintentional injuries" (a term public health officials prefer), suicides, and homicides. Accidents, especially motor vehicle crashes, kill more college-age men and women than all other causes combined; the greatest number of lives lost to accidents is among those 25 years of age.[1]

Life can never be risk-free, but you can do more than anyone else to avoid unnecessary hazards and to maximize your ability to cope with potentially dangerous situations. According to research on survivors of various types of disasters, those who respond well in a crisis tend to have three underlying psychological attributes:

- They believe that they can influence events. (Refer back to the discussion of self-efficacy in Chapter 1.)

- They are able to find meaningful purpose in turmoil and trauma. (See the discussion on spirituality in Chapter 2.)

- They know that they can learn from both positive and negative experiences. (See Chapter 3, "The School of Life," in *IPC.*)[2]

As discussed in Making Change Happen, you can improve both your awareness of potential risks and your ability to minimize danger.

Unintentional Injury: Why Accidents Happen

Some of the many factors that influence an individual's risk of accident or injury are these:

- **Age.** Injury is the leading cause of death during the first four decades of life in the United States. Every day more than 2,000 children and teenagers die from an injury that could have been prevented. The five most common causes of unintentional injury are road traffic injuries, drowning, burns, falls, and poisoning.[3] Most victims of fatal accidents are males. Feeling full of life and energy, they may take dangerous risks because they think they're invulnerable.

- **Alcohol.** An estimated 40 percent of Americans are involved in an alcohol-related accident sometime during their lives. Alcohol plays a role in about a quarter of fatal motor vehicle accidents and half of fatal motorcycle crashes.

- **Stress.** When we're tense and anxious, we all pay less attention to what we're doing. One common result is an increase in accidents. If you find yourself having a series of small mishaps or near-misses, do something to lower your stress level, rather than wait for something more harmful to happen (see Chapter 3). When facing danger, take deep, controlled, regular breaths—a technique first-responders learn in their training.

- **Situational Factors.** Some situations—such as driving on a curvy, wet road in a car with worn tires—are so inherently dangerous that they greatly increase the odds of an accident. But even when there's greater risk, you can lower the danger: For instance, you can make sure your tires and brakes are in good condition.

- **Thrill Seeking.** To some people, activities that others might find terrifying—such as skydiving or parachute jumping—are stimulating. These thrill seekers may have lower than normal levels of the brain chemicals that regulate excitement. Because the stress of potentially hazardous sports may increase the levels of these chemicals, they feel pleasantly aroused rather than scared.

Accidents can happen to anyone at any time, so it's important that you be prepared.

Safe Driving

With more drivers and more vehicles on the roads than ever before, accidents kill

Your Guardian Angel

In a world full of many potential dangers, we all need someone to watch over us and keep us safe from harm. Whether or not you believe in guardian angels, there is always someone who—better than any other—can look out for you. That person is you.

"Your Guardian Angel" in *Labs for IPC* provides a comprehensive personal security program, based on the Stages of Change, discussed in Chapter 1 of this text and in *IPC*. By systematically working through this lab, you will come to value yourself so much that you avoid unwise risks, and you will consistently take the necessary measures to safeguard your physical and psychological well-being. Here's a preview.

Get Real

In this stage, you assess your values by ranking the importance of seven dimensions of safety on a scale of 0 to 100. Try these two examples:

- physical safety, protection of life and limbs from accidents and injury _____
- safety in intimate situations _____

You then do a self-appraisal of your risk awareness by assigning a numerical score to 15 behaviors, including these:

- If someone behaves strangely, I move away and keep my distance. _____
- I do not let people "guilt" me into situations that I do not want to be in. _____
- I am careful to observe people long and well before allowing them an intimate position in my life. _____

You also rate your accident prevention skills on the road, at home, out and about, and on a date. Here are just three of the 42 skills covered in the lab:

- Do you always wear a seat belt? _____
- Do you never lend your keys or ID to anyone? _____
- Do you never leave a party, concert, or bar with someone you just met or don't know well? _____

Get Ready

The next stage includes five steps to prepare for change. Here is the first:

- Decide in which areas of your life you are going to put special focus on being a better guardian angel to yourself. Choose at least three, but do not limit yourself to these.

Get Going

This is the stage where you start taking action with concrete steps that you incorporate into your daily life. Here is one example:

- **Become more mindful.** For the first four weeks of this lab, once a week survey the risk factors in a familiar or unfamiliar environment. For example, if you have heard about a new club or bar, take someone along with you and scope out the place. Or go to a campus event and see what risks might formerly have escaped your attention. . .

Lock It In

You never outgrow your need for a guardian angel. That's why it's important to know how to steer clear of danger by taking steps such as the following:

- **Watch over yourself.** At the end of each week, identify any circumstances under which you might have put yourself in harm's way—consciously or not. In your *IPC Journal,* write about how you perceived the possible risks to yourself at the time and how you see them now . . .

---

more than 41,000 people a year and injure some 2.5 million.[4] An average of 117 people die every day in motor vehicle crashes—approximately one every twelve minutes.[5] Alcohol use is a factor in about 40 percent of these crashes; speeding, in about one-third. Rollovers caused by drivers who lose control of their vehicles kill about 25 people daily. Crashes involving teen drivers result in about 25 fatalities each day.

College students aren't necessarily safer drivers than others their age. According to national data, full-time college students drink and drive more often than part-time students and other young adults, but they also are more likely to wear seat belts while driving and riding in cars. How can you increase your odds of staying safe on the road? Some key factors are staying sober and alert, using your seat belt, making sure your vehicle has working air bags, and controlling road rage. The number one culprit in car crashes is distraction—whether by chatting on the phone, fiddling with a CD player, or eating.

Stay Sober and Alert The number of fatalities caused by drunk driving, particularly among young people, has dropped. The National Highway Traffic Safety Administration (NHTSA) attributes this decline to increases in the drinking age, to educational programs aimed at reducing nighttime driving by teens, to the formation of Students Against Destructive Decisions (SADD, originally called Students Against Drunk Driving) and similar groups, and to changes in state laws that lowered the legal blood-alcohol concentration level for drivers under age 21 (some states have zero tolerance blood-alcohol level [BAC] for drivers under 21).

Falling asleep at the wheel is second only to alcohol as a cause of serious motor vehicle accidents. About half of drivers in the United States drive while drowsy. Nearly 14 million have fallen asleep at the wheel in the past year, according to the National Sleep Foundation. Men and young adults between the ages of 18 and 29 are at the highest risk for driving while drowsy or falling asleep at the wheel.

Buckle Up   Seat belt use has reached an all-time high, with three in four Americans buckling up. States with seat belt laws have even higher rates of use: 80 percent. However, young people are less likely to use seat belts. Men between ages 19 and 29 are least likely to wear seat belts while driving or riding in a car. By official estimates, two-thirds of 15- to 20-year-olds killed in motor vehicle accidents were not wearing seat belts.

Seat belts save an estimated 9,500 lives in the United States each year. When lap-shoulder belts are used properly, they reduce the risk of fatal injury to front-seat passengers by 45 percent and the risk of moderate to critical injury by 50 percent. Because an unrestrained passenger can injure others during a crash, the risk of death is lowest when all occupants wear seat belts, according to federal analysts. Seat belt use by everyone in a car may prevent about one in six deaths that might otherwise occur in a crash.

Check for Air Bags   An air bag, either with or without a seat belt, has proved the most effective means of preventing adult death, somewhat more so for women than for men. The combination of airbags and seat belts affords the best protection against spine fractures; an airbag alone decreases this risk but to a lesser extent.[6]

Because there is controversy over the potential hazard air bags pose to children, the American Academy of Pediatrics recommends that children be placed in the backseat, whether or not the car is equipped with a passenger air bag.

Rein in Road Rage   The emotional outbursts known as road rage are a factor in as many as two-thirds of all fatal car crashes and one-third of nonfatal accidents, according to the NHTSA. Psychologist Arnold Nerenberg of Whittier, California, a specialist in motorway mayhem, estimates 1.78 billion episodes of road rage occur each year, resulting in more than 28,000 deaths and 1 million injuries.[7]

Some strategies for reducing road rage include the following:

- **Lower the stress in your life.** Take a few moments to breathe deeply and relax your shoulders before putting the key in the ignition.

- **Consciously decide not to let other drivers get to you.** Decide that whatever happens, it's not going to make your blood pressure go up.

- **Slow down.** If you're going five or ten miles over the speed limit, you won't have the time you need to react to anything that happens.

- **Modify bad driving habits one at a time.** If you tend to tailgate slow drivers, spend a week driving at twice your usual following distance. If you're a habitual horn honker, silence yourself.

Even a (crash) dummy knows that it's smart to buckle up whenever you get into a vehicle.

© Steve Hathaway/Workbook Stock/Jupiterimages

- **Be courteous—even if other drivers aren't.** Don't dawdle in the passing lane. Never tailgate or switch lanes without signaling. Don't use your horn or high beams unless absolutely necessary.

- **Never retaliate.** Whatever another driver does, keep your cool. Count to ten. Take a deep breath. If you yell or gesture at someone who's upset with you, the conflict may well escalate.

- **If you do something stupid, show that you're sorry.** On its website, the AAA Foundation for Traffic Safety solicited suggestions for automotive apologies. The most popular: slapping yourself on your forehead or the top of your head to indicate that you know you goofed. Such gestures can soothe a miffed motorist—and make the roads a slightly safer place for all of us.

Use Cell Phones Safely

According to recent surveys, most drivers—approximately seven in ten of those interviewed—talk on cell phones while driving, while about one in five sends and receives text messages.[8] In some states, it is now illegal to talk or text on a cell phone while driving, and drivers who do so can be ticketed and fined.

Driver inattention is responsible for 25 to 30 percent of crashes. Drivers are most likely to be distracted by common activities, such as reaching for an item in the glove compartment or talking to passengers. However, motorists who use cell phones while driving are four times as likely to get into crashes serious enough to injure themselves. Even if the cell phone is a hands-free model, using it while driving is as dangerous as driving drunk. The reason is that talking or texting while driving distracts the brain as well as the eyes—much more so than talking to another person in the vehicle. Conversation on any type of phone disrupts a driver's attention to the visual environment, leading to what researchers call "inattention blindness," the inability to recognize objects encountered in the driver's visual field. This form of cognitive impairment may distract drivers for up to two minutes after the phone conversation has ended. Phone conversations have proven more distracting than those between drivers and passengers, who tend to slow down or stop speaking as driving conditions change and often alert drivers to potential dangers.[9] Cell phone use also can endanger others. In a recent study, drivers talking on cell phones were more likely to hit, injure, and kill pedestrians.[10]

Here are some tips for safer cell phone use:

- Find out if cell phone use while driving is legal in your state.

- Do not dial new calls until you're stopped or in a safe low-traffic environment.

- Keep calls short, less than one or two minutes.

- When you're on the phone, avoid difficult maneuvers, such as changing lanes, that require a lot of attention.

- Have a passenger send or receive calls.

- Invest in a hands-free model, especially if you use your phone regularly. While the cognitive distraction is the same, it helps to avoid the mechanical distraction.

YOUR STRATEGIES FOR PREVENTION

What to Do in an Emergency

Life-threatening situations rarely happen more than once or twice in any person's life. When they do, you must think and act quickly to prevent disastrous consequences.

- **Stop, look, and listen.** Your immediate response to an emergency may be overwhelming fear and anxiety. Take several deep breaths. Start by assessing the circumstances. Look for any possible dangers to you or the victim, such as a live electrical wire or a fire. Listen for sounds, such as a cry for help or a siren. Don't attempt rescue techniques, such as cardiopulmonary resuscitation (CPR), unless you're trained.

- **Don't wait for symptoms to go away or get worse.** If you suspect that someone is having a heart attack or stroke, or has ingested something poisonous, *phone for help immediately.* A delay could jeopardize the person's life.

- **Don't move a victim.** The person may have a broken neck or back, and attempting to move him or her could cause extensive damage or even death.

- **Don't drive.** Even if the hospital is just ten minutes away, you're better off waiting for a well-equipped ambulance with trained paramedics who can deliver emergency care on the spot.

- **Don't do too much.** Often well-intentioned good Samaritans make injuries worse by trying to tie tourniquets, wash cuts, or splint broken limbs. Also, don't give an injured person anything to eat or drink.

- **At home, keep a supply of basic first-aid items in a convenient place.** Beyond the emergency number 911, make sure that telephone numbers for your doctor and neighbors are handy.

Any form of distraction, including talking on a cell phone, can put you and others at risk.

reading and thinking. It can also cause personality changes and psychiatric problems, such as depression, anxiety, uncontrollable mood swings, and anger. Complete recovery from head trauma can take four to six years, and the costs can be staggering. Head injury can also result in permanent disability, coma, and death. To prevent head trauma, motorcycle helmets are required in most states. They reduce the risk of head injury by about 69 percent and death by around 42 percent.[11]

More than 80 million people ride bicycles. Each year, bicycle crashes kill about 700 of these individuals and send 450,000 to 587,000 to emergency rooms. Men are more likely to suffer cycling injuries. Head injury is the cause of 75 percent of bicycle crash deaths. (See Consumer Alert.)

According to a national survey, 50 percent of all bicycle riders in the United States regularly wear bike helmets—43 percent every time they ride and 7 percent more than half the time. Wearing a helmet can reduce head injuries and deaths by an estimated 29 to 90 percent, depending on the type of helmet.

Safe Cycling

Per vehicle mile, motorcyclists are 35 times more likely to die in a crash than passenger car occupants. The most common motorcycle injury is head trauma, which can lead to physical disability, including paralysis and general weakness, as well as problems

CONSUMER ALERT

Bicycle Helmet Heads-Up

When will you fall off your bike? According to the Bicycle Helmet Safety Institute, the average careful bike rider can expect to crash about every 4,500 miles.

Facts to Know
- Bike helmets can prevent 85 percent of cyclists' head injuries, which cause 75 percent of bicycle-related deaths.
- Even a low-speed fall on a bicycle path can result in a head injury.
- Laws in 22 states and at least 192 localities require helmets.

Steps to Take
- Always look inside a helmet for a Consumer Product Safety Commission (CPSC) sticker before purchasing.

- Check the fit. The helmet should sit level on your head, touching all around, comfortably snug but not tight. The helmet should not move more than about an inch in either direction, regardless of how hard you tug at it.
- Pick a bright color for visibility. Avoid dark colors, thin straps, or a rigid visor that could snag in a fall.
- Look for a smooth plastic outer shell, not one with alternating strips of plastic and foam.
- Watch out for excessive vents, which put less protective foam in contact with your head in a crash.

Safety at Work

The workplace is second only to the home as the most frequent site of accidents. The industries with the highest fatality rates are mining; transportation, communication, and public utilities; construction; and agriculture, forestry, and fishing. Whatever your job, find out about potential hazards and learn the proper safety regulations. (Chapter

© David Papazian Photography Inc./Brand X Pictures/ Jupiterimages

19 discusses some potential environmental hazards at work, including noise and toxic substances.)

According to a report by the National Research Council and Institute of Medicine, annually about one million workers suffer musculoskeletal disorders of the lower back and upper extremities as a result of their "particular jobs and working conditions— including heavy lifting, repetitive and forceful motions, and stressful working conditions." Many can be prevented.

Computers and Your Health

As computers have become part of daily life for everyone from preschoolers to seniors, health professionals have learned a great deal about potential health problems, including repetitive motion injuries and vision-related difficulties.

Repetitive Motion Injuries **Repetitive motion injuries (RMIs)** have surpassed back and neck injuries as the number one claim for workers compensation injuries. Repeated motions—such as the hand and arm movements made while using a computer keyboard—all day, every day, can result in muscle and tendon strain and inflammation. About 20 percent of people with pain, tingling, or numbness in the hands may have carpal tunnel syndrome, an overuse injury caused by repetitive motions in the hands and wrists. Symptoms include pain, swelling, and numbness and weakness in the hands or the arms. If these problems are identified early, permanent damage can generally be avoided by altering the work environment and allowing for more breaks during the day.

The slope and height of a computer keyboard can affect the likelihood of repetitive motion injuries. If you work at a computer, good posture and correct positioning of the computer screen and keyboard can help prevent repetitive motion injuries, eyestrain, and back strain (Figure 18.1). Here are some additional tips:

- Place the keyboard so that your elbows are bent at a 90° angle and you don't have to bend your wrists to type.
- Use a chair that provides ample back support. Keep your thighs parallel to the floor and your feet on the floor. If your feet don't reach the floor, use a footrest.

The screen should be at eye level (22–26 inches higher than your seat).

Position the keyboard so that your elbows are bent at a 90° angle and your hands and wrists are straight.

Sit straight in your chair; for extra back support, place a rolled-up towel behind you.

Keep your hands and wrists relaxed.

Figure 18.1
Safe Computing
By paying attention to your posture and your computer's position, you can help protect yourself from repetitive motion injury, back strain, and eyestrain.

- If you experience neck strain, place a document holder next to your screen so that you can view the materials more easily.
- Every 15 minutes take a 30-second break, stretch your arms, and walk around the office. Take a 15-minute break at least once every two hours.

Vision Problems **Computer vision syndrome** is a condition marked by tired and sore eyes, blurred vision, headaches, and neck, shoulder, and back pain. The American Optometric Association estimates that it afflicts nearly 90 percent of workers who use computers and also is common among children and students of all ages. The symptoms result from repeatedly stressing some aspect of the visual system, but they often disappear as soon as the person stops working at the computer.

The eye focuses on a computer image differently from the way it focuses on a printed one. The pixels that appear on a computer screen, unlike printed characters, are bright in the center and gradually fade away into the background color. This makes it difficult for the eye to sustain focus. Optometrists have developed a specific method, called a PRIO examination, that simulates how the eye responds to pixels on a computer screen. It can determine the need and proper prescription for computer-only eyeglasses.

repetitive motion injury (RMI) Inflammation of or damage to a part of the body due to repetition of the same movements.
computer vision syndrome A condition caused by computer use marked by tired and sore eyes, blurred vision, headaches, and neck, shoulder, and back pain.

Safety at Home

Every year home accidents cause nearly 25 million injuries. Over 30 percent of fatal injuries to adolescents occur in the home.[12] According to a recent study of home safety, households tend to be safe in some ways but not in others. In the survey, many homes had smoke detectors, but more than 90 percent did not have carbon monoxide detectors, 29 percent had unlocked firearms on the premises, and 21 percent had exposed electrical cords.[13] Poison poses the greatest threat, causing more than 17,000 deaths every year. Half a million children swallow poisonous materials each year; 90 percent are under age 5. Adults may also be poisoned by mistakenly taking someone else's prescription drugs or taking medicines in the dark and swallowing the wrong one. In most cities, you can call a poison control center for advice.

Falls of all kinds are the second leading cause of death from unintentional injury in the United States. High heels or worn footgear, poor lighting, slippery or uneven walkways, broken stairs and handrails, loose or worn rugs, and objects left where people walk all increase the likelihood of a slip.

You can prevent fires by making sure that the three ingredients of fire—fuel, a heat source, and oxygen—don't get a chance to mix. Almost anything can act as fuel for fire, including paper, wood, and flammable liquids such as oils, gasoline, and some paints.

A heat source can be a spark from a lighted match, a pilot light, or an electrical wire. Oxygen is necessary for the chemical reaction between the fuel and heat source that causes combustion.

If a fire starts and it's small, you may be able to put it out with a portable fire extinguisher before it spreads. However, if the fire does get out of control, you might have only two to five minutes to get out of the house or building alive. A fire-escape plan can save time and lives. Sketch a plan of your house, apartment building, dormitory, or fraternity or sorority house. Identify two ways out of each room or apartment. Make sure everyone is familiar with these escape routes. Designate an area outside where all family members or dorm residents should meet after escaping from a fire.

 In a national survey, 67 percent of colleges had at least one dorm without a sprinkler system. If a fire breaks out in your dorm room, get out as quickly as possible, but don't run. Before opening a room door, place your hand on it. If it's hot, don't open it. If the door feels cool, open it slightly to check for smoke; if there's none, leave by your planned escape route. If you're on an upper floor and your escape routes are blocked, open a window (top and bottom, if possible) and wait or signal from the window for help. Never try to use an elevator in a fire.

Which Gender Is at Greater Risk?

Just like illness, injury doesn't discriminate against either gender. Both men and women can find themselves in harm's way—but for different reasons. Here are some gender differences in vulnerability:

- Men are ten times more likely to die of an occupational injury than women.

- Males are most often the victims and the perpetrators of homicides in the United States. In about 68 percent of cases reported by the Bureau of Justice Statistics, both the offender and the victim were male.

- Overall, men are 3.6 times more likely than women to be murdered and 9 times more likely to commit murder. Both men and women are more likely to kill or attempt to kill male victims than female victims.

- Men are more likely than women to be assaulted as adults.
- The genders also differ in their fear of crime. In a recent study, women—but not men—tended to become less apprehensive and to feel less vulnerable as they became older. Increased income correlated with higher levels of fear for men but lower levels for women.[14]

Living in a Dangerous World

The World Health Organization (WHO) defines violence as "the intentional use of physical force or power, threatened or actual, against oneself, another person, or a group or community, that either results in, or has a high likelihood of resulting in, injury, death, psychological harm, maldevelopment, or deprivation." A simpler way of putting it is that "violence is anything you wouldn't want someone to do to you."[15] Although anyone is capable of violent crime, being aware of certain behaviors in a person may keep you safer.

After more than a decade of declining rates, violent crime in the United States seems to be increasing. Guns are the second-leading cause of injury-related death in the United States after car accidents. About 260 Americans are injured by firearms every day; one-third die from their wounds. Gun violence annually takes the lives of nearly 30,000 Americans. The cost of hospital treatment for the victims of violence (including attempted suicide and murder, fights, rapes, and assaults) exceeds $2.3 billion a year.[16]

 Although men commit nine times more violent crimes than women, the rates are getting closer. Individuals with mental illness are somewhat more likely to become violent and to be the victims of violent crimes.

There are ethnic and racial differences in patterns of violence. African Americans are at greater risk of victimization by violent crime than whites or persons of other racial groupings. Hispanics are at greater risk of violent victimization than non-Hispanics. There is little difference between white women and nonwhite women in rape, physical assault, or stalking. Native American and Alaska Native women are significantly more likely than white women or African American women to report being raped. Mixed-race women also have a significantly higher incidence of rape than white women. Native American and Alaska Native men report significantly more physical assaults than Asian and Pacific Islander men.

Crime and Violence on Campus

According to the Bureau of Justice, college students are victims of almost half a million violent crimes a year, including assault, robbery, sexual assault, and rape. While this number may seem high, the overall violent crime rate has dropped from 88 to 41 victimizations per 1,000 students in the last decade.[17] You can take steps to lower your risk—at little or no financial cost. (See Health on a Budget, p. 582.)

College students ages 18 to 24 are less likely to be victims of violent crime, including robbery and assault, than nonstudents of the same age. More than half (58 percent) of crimes against students are committed by strangers. More than nine in ten occur off campus, most often in an open area or street, on public transportation, in a place of business, or at a private home. In about two-thirds of the crimes, no weapon is involved. Most off-campus crimes occur at night,

---

YOUR STRATEGIES FOR PREVENTION

How to Recognize Potentially Violent People

Trust your gut. If you feel uneasy or sense danger, there may well be good reason. Be wary if a person exhibits:

- Frequent loss of temper, physical fighting, serious damage to property.
- Increased use of drugs or alcohol.
- Extreme impatience, irritation, agitation.
- Fascination with weapons and violent movies, newspaper stories, Internet sites, television programs, and radio shows.
- Threatening, blaming, defensive, or argumentative behavior.
- Feelings of rejection or isolation, withdrawal from others.
- Unusual interest in obtaining or using weapons, especially guns.

while on-campus crimes are more frequent in the day.[18]

Male college students are twice as likely to be victims of overall violence as female students. White undergraduates have higher rates of violent victimization than students of other races. Simple assault accounts for two-thirds of violent crimes against students; sexual assault or rape account for around 6 percent.[19]

A study of a random sample of college students found a strong relationship between substance use and sexual and physical victimization of college students. College women were more likely to report sexual violence associated with most forms of substance use, while college men were more likely to be victims of physical violence.[20]

About three in four campus crimes are never reported to the police. The main reasons students give for not reporting crimes are that they are too minor or private or they are not certain that it was a crime. Individuals also may be too ashamed or emotionally overwhelmed to contact authorities.

According to researchers, only 2 percent of victimized college women report crimes to the police. The most frequent reason for not reporting sexual and physical incidents is that they didn't seem serious enough. However, women who were sexually victimized also felt ashamed, feared that they would be held responsible, or didn't want anyone to know what happened. Nonwhite women were significantly more likely than white women to say that they did not report an incident to the police because they thought they

would be blamed or because they did not want the police involved.[21]

The Jeanne Clery Disclosure of Campus Security Policy and Campus Crime Statistics Act, originally known as the Student Right-to-Know and Campus Security Act, requires colleges to publish annual crime statistics for their campuses. However, the act excludes certain offenses, such as theft, threats, harassment, and vandalism, so the picture it presents may not be complete. The most recent crime statistics for the nation's colleges, universities, and career schools are posted on the Internet at http://ope.ed.gov/security. How safe is your school? Take the Self Survey: "How Safe Is Your School?" on page 591.

Campuses have implemented dozens of programs to halt violence, and many have proven effective.[22] One school used a poster campaign to raise awareness of dating violence.[23] Others have designed sexual violence prevention programs for members of fraternities, sororities, and intercollegiate athletic teams.[24] (See Community Focus, p. 584.) Many have established codes of conduct barring the use of alcohol and drugs, fighting, and sexual harassment, and have instituted policies requiring suspension or expulsion for students who violate this code.

Hazing

Hazing refers to any activity that humiliates, degrades, or poses a risk of emotional or physical harm for the sake of joining a group or maintaining full status in that group. This behavior may occur in fraternities and sororities, athletic teams, or other campus organizations. Its forms include verbal ridicule and abuse, forced consumption of alcohol or ingestion of vile substances, sexual violation, sleep deprivation, paddling, beating, burning, or branding.

Among the initial findings of the government-sponsored National Study of Student Hazing are the following:[25]

- Many students come to college having experienced hazing in high school.
- Many students who experience specific hazing behaviors do not think they have been hazed.
- Hazing activities occur across a wide range of student groups, including athletics, fraternities/sororities, recreation

and sports clubs, bands, and performing arts organizations.

- More than two-thirds of students are aware of hazing behaviors in student groups on campus.
- Advisors and coaches are often aware of and/or involved in student hazing.

More schools are requiring all campus organizations to ban hazing and to inform new members of this policy. Do you know if your school has an antihazing policy? Are you aware of hazing in any groups you belong to or might consider joining?

Hate or Bias Crimes

 Recent years have seen the emergence of violent crimes motivated by hatred of a particular person's (or group of persons') race, ethnicity, religion, sexual orientation, or political values.

More than half of hate or bias crimes on campus are motivated by race. Twenty percent of students, faculty, and staff surveyed fear for their physical safety because of their sexual orientation or gender identity.[26] These crimes can take the form of graffiti; verbal slurs; bombings; threatening notes, e-mails, or phone calls; and physical attacks. They often generate fear and intimidation in large groups of students, undermining health, academic work, and the basic security of a campus.

Shootings, Murders, and Assaults

Shootings of students and faculty have occurred at several campuses in recent years. However, like murder and manslaughter, they remain uncommon. There are about 3,000 aggravated assaults—an attack with a weapon or one that causes serious injury—each year. Weapons were involved in about a third of violent college crimes. Firearms were used in 9 percent of all violent crimes and 8 percent of assaults. (See Point/Counterpoint.)

Campus shootings have a psychological impact on students on other campuses as well. In a study of students at a school in the same geographical area, the most common reaction was greater caution in social settings.[27]

The American College Health Association, in its most recent "Campus Violence White

Does your campus have regular security patrols, surveillance cameras, or late-night escorts? Have you taken advantage of these services?

Paper," has recommended various strategies to keep campuses safe, including:

- Enforcing codes of conduct.
- Tougher sanctions, including expulsion, for serious misconduct.
- Zero-tolerance policies for campus violence.
- Building a sense of community.
- Screening out students who pose a real threat.

hazing Any activity that humiliates, degrades, or poses a risk of emotional or physical harm for the sake of joining a group or maintaining full status in that group.

PROBLEM Campus life may in many ways seem idyllic, but violent crimes, including murders, aggravated assaults, sexual assaults, rapes, and robberies, can and do occur. In 80 percent of campus crimes, students are both perpetrators and victims. Alcohol is involved more than 90 percent of the time.

Colleges and universities, parents' and advocacy groups, and students are taking steps to make campuses safer, and their efforts are paying off. Here is what you can do to safeguard yourself and others at your school.

BECOME INFORMED

- Go to Security on Campus, Inc. at **http://campussafety.org** for an overview of the history of the fight for safer campuses, legal milestones, and current initiatives.
- Educate yourself about violence against women at websites such as Students Active for Ending Rape (**www.safercampus.org**), which offers a free PDF guide to action called "Change Happens."
- How safe is your campus? You have the right to know. By law all colleges and universities that receive federal funding must distribute an annual report on their security and law enforcement policies, crime prevention activities, procedures for reporting crimes on campus, and certain crime statistics.

BECOME INVOLVED

- Organize a campaign to build awareness by means such as posters and articles in the campus newspaper. Set up a campus blog to monitor safety on campus. Find other ideas at **http://www.safer campus.org/blog/**.
- Sign up for a self-defense class. Follow-up studies of college women have found that self-defense training increased their sense of control over their life as well as their confidence, security, independence, and physical prowess.
- Find out if your school or community offers preventive programs such as Men Against Violence, which confronts male students' conception of manhood and appropriate gender roles to reduce their likelihood of physical or sexual violence.
- Remember that alcohol is involved in nine in every ten campus crimes and sexual assaults. Pay attention to what you drink, how much you drink—and whether anyone else has access to your drink.

- Warning students about criminal activity at orientation, through the campus newspaper, in residence halls, and through campus Internet communications devices.[28]

Consequences of Campus Violence

The toll of crime and violence at colleges and universities is high. Violence can cripple as well as claim lives. Moreover, the victims of violent crime often suffer lasting psychological and emotional effects. Some victims take a leave of absence or transfer to another school. Those who remain in school may have problems concentrating, studying, and attending classes, and may avoid academic and social activities. Some develop clinical symptoms that affect their mental and physical health (see Chapter 2).

Sexual Victimization and Violence

Sexual victimization refers to any situation in which a person is deprived of free choice and forced to comply with sexual acts. This is not only a woman's issue; in fact, men also are victimized. In recent years, researchers have come to view acts of sexual victimization along a continuum, ranging from street hassling, stalking, and obscene telephone calls to rape, battering, and incest. Sexual violence has its roots in social attitudes and beliefs that demean women and condone aggression. According to international research, much sexual violence takes place within families, marriage, and dating relationships. In many settings, rape is a culturally approved strategy to control and discipline women. In these places, laws and policies to improve women's status are critical to ending sexual coercion.

Sexual Harassment

All forms of **sexual harassment** or unwanted sexual attention—from the display of pornographic photos to the use of sexual obscenities to a demand for sex by anyone in a position of power or authority—are illegal.

 Nearly two-thirds of students experience sexual harassment at some point during college, including nearly one-third of first-year students, according to a recent research report on campus sexual harassment. Nearly one-third of students say they have experienced physical harassment, such as being touched, grabbed, or pinched in a sexual way. Sexual comments and jokes are the most common form of harassment. More than half of female students and nearly half of male students say they have experienced this type of harassment. Lesbian, gay, bisexual, and transgender (LGBT) students are more likely than heterosexual students to be sexually harassed.

 Sexual harassment takes an especially heavy toll on female students, who often feel upset, self-conscious, embarrassed, or angry. Men are much less likely to admit to being very or somewhat upset. A third of harassed college women say they felt afraid; one-fifth say they were disappointed in their college experience as a result of sexual harassment.

About half of college men and a third of women admit that they have sexually harassed someone on campus. Private college students are more likely than their public college peers to have ever done so. Students at large schools (population of 10,000 or more) are more likely than students at small schools with fewer than 5,000 students to say they have experienced sexual harassment. The most common rationale for harassment is "I thought it was funny." Harassment occurs in dorms or student housing as well as outside on campus grounds and in classrooms or lecture halls.

If you encounter sexual harassment as a student, report it to the department chair or dean. If you don't receive an adequate response to your complaint, talk with the campus representatives who handle matters involving affirmative action or civil rights. Federal guidelines prevent any discrimination against you in terms of grades or the loss of a job or scholarship if you report harassment. Schools that do not take measures to remedy harassment could lose federal funds.

Stalking

 The "willful, repeated, and malicious following, harassing, or threatening of another person," as **stalking** is defined, is common on college campuses—perhaps more so than in the general population. About a fifth of college women report being watched, followed, or spied on or receiving unsolicited e-mails. Most college women know their stalkers. About half are acquaintances; a high percentage of these are classmates, boyfriends, or ex-boyfriends. In one study, about half of the women said they had not sought help from anyone. Those who did seek assistance

turned to friends, parents, residence hall advisors, or police.[29]

 College students may be targeted for several reasons. Simply because they are young and still learning how to manage complex social relationships, some individuals may not recognize their behavior as stalking or even as disturbing. In addition, college students tend to live close to each other and to have flexible schedules and large amounts of unsupervised time.

Stalking is not a benign behavior and can result in emotional or psychological distress, physical harm, or sexual assault. By some estimates, 10 percent of stalking incidents result in forced or attempted sexual contact. The most common consequence is psychological, with victims reporting emotional or psychological distress.

Dating Violence

Actual or threatened physical or sexual violence or psychological and emotional abuse of a current or former dating partner is a form of violence. It can occur between heterosexual, homosexual, or bisexual partners.

 Violence in dating relationships is common on campuses around the world. In the International Dating Violence study, which surveyed 15,927 college students in 22 locations, 30 percent had physically assaulted a dating partner in the previous 12 months. The proportion of students who reported being the victims

sexual harassment Uninvited and unwanted sexual attention.
stalking The willful, repeated, and malicious following of another person.

POINT
According to the American College Health Association, 8 percent of college students keep a weapon on campus. Many contend that guns have no place on campus, and schools often ban all firearms. Advocates of gun control view the presence of guns as increasing the danger to their owners and to others.

COUNTERPOINT
Although violent crime remains uncommon on campuses, some students argue that they need a gun for self-defense. Opponents of gun control contended that if students were allowed to carry weapons on campus, they might be able to defend themselves in case of an armed attack.

YOUR VIEW
Gun control is one of the most controversial topics in our society. Do you think weapons should be banned from college campuses? Or do you believe that every American, on or off campus, should have the right to own a gun?

of a physical assault ranged from 14 to 39 percent. India, Korea, New Zealand, Germany, Greece, Russia, the United Kingdom, the United States, and Canada had consistently high rates of assault, injury, and sexual coercion, while Israel, Australia, Belgium, Sweden, and Switzerland had lower rates.[30]

In the United States, one in seven college student couples reported at least one episode of male-to-female violence in the preceding 12 months. In dating relationships, 39 percent of college women and 33 percent of men reported being a victim of violence from their dating partners. (See Reality Check, p. 587.)

Such behavior may start even before college. Based on a national sample, about 400,000 adolescents—roughly 2 percent—have experienced serious forms of dating violence.[31] A study of African American and Latino teens found even higher levels. Seven percent of the young couples reported physical aggression; 27 percent reported psychological abuse.[32]

In research on students at American universities, a larger percentage of women than men assault a dating partner by, for example, throwing something that could hurt at a partner, pushing, shoving, grabbing, or slapping. However, the rates of perpetrating an assault resulting in an injury, as well as being a victim of an assault that resulted in an injury, are overwhelmingly higher for males.

The percentage of students who say they coerced a partner into sex in the previous 12 months is about 20 percent, while 24 percent of students report being victims of sexual coercion. Rates of sexual coercion—for example, making a partner have sex without a condom or insisting on sex when a partner did not want to—were higher for men than women.

In addition to physical injury, victims of violence in their intimate relationships are at increased risk of posttraumatic stress disorder (PTSD), depression, and suicidal thoughts. Women exposed to acute or previous domestic violence are more likely than other women to have made suicide attempts. In general, suicide attempt rates among battered women are high, ranging from 20 to 26 percent.

Nonvolitional Sex and Sexual Coercion

Nonvolitional sex is sexual behavior that violates a person's right to choose when and with whom to have sex and what sexual behaviors to engage in. The more extreme forms of this behavior include sexual coercion or forced sex, rape, childhood sexual abuse, and violence against people with nonconventional sexual identities. Other forms, such as engaging in sex to keep one's partner or to pass as heterosexual, are so common that many think of them as normal.

Sexual coercion can take many forms, including exerting peer pressure, taking advantage of one's desire for popularity, threatening an end to a relationship, getting someone intoxicated, stimulating a partner against his or her wishes, or insinuating an obligation based on the time or money one has expended. Men may feel that they need to live up to the sexual stereotype of taking advantage of every opportunity for sex. Women are far more likely than men to encounter physical force.

Many schools are alerting incoming female students about what researchers call "the red zone," a period of time early in one's first undergraduate year when women are at particularly high risk for unwanted sexual experiences. One university defines the red zone more precisely as "the time period between freshman move-in and fall break wherein there is a particularly high risk of victimization." Unwanted touching and attempted intercourse are the most common behaviors reported, although researchers also have documented sexual assaults and rapes.[33]

Rape

Rape refers to sexual intercourse with an unconsenting partner under actual or threatened force. Sexual intercourse between a male over the age of 16 and a female under the age of consent (which ranges from 12 to 21 in different states) is called *statutory rape.* In *acquaintance rape,* or *date rape,* the victim knows the rapist. In *stranger rape,* the rapist is an unknown assailant. Both acquaintance and stranger rapes are serious crimes that can have a devastating impact on their victims.

All states now recognize as rape the assault of a victim who is incapable of giving consent because of alcohol or other substances. However, many women who experience a sexual encounter that meets this legal definition do not label it as a rape or even as sexual victimization. Compared with stranger rapes, these assaults are typically less violent and involve less force by the assailant, less resistance by the victim, and less injury to her. Yet women who do not acknowledge an unwanted sexual experience as rape nonetheless suffer psychological consequences, including distress and other trauma symptoms.[34]

Over the course of five years (the national average for a college career), including summers and vacations, one of every four or five female students is raped. In a single academic year, 2.7 percent of coeds are raped—35 rapes for every 1,000 women. According to the U.S. Department of Justice, a campus with 6,000 coeds averages one rape a day every day for the entire school year.

In nine surveys of male university students, between 3 and 6 percent had been raped by other men; up to 25 percent had been sexually assaulted. Like female rape victims, male victims suffer long-term psychological problems and physical injuries, and are at risk of contracting a sexually transmitted infection.

For many years, the victims of rape were blamed for doing something to bring on the attack. However, researchers have shown that women are raped because they encounter sexually aggressive men, not because they look or act a certain way. Although no woman is immune to attack, many rape victims are children or adolescents.

Women who successfully escape rape attempts do so by resisting verbally and physically, usually by yelling and fleeing. Women who use forceful verbal or physical resistance (screaming, hitting, kicking, biting, and running) are more likely to avoid rape than women who try pleading, crying, or offering no resistance.

Types of Rape

Although rape has long been viewed as an act of violence and domination, recent studies indicate that not all rapes fit into a single pattern. Within the broad category of rape are specific, but not mutually exclusive, subcategories of the crime, including anger rape, power rape, sadistic rape, gang rape, and sexual gratification rape.

Anger rape, usually on a total stranger, is motivated by hatred and a desire for revenge for the rejection the rapist feels he's suffered from women. Anger rapists often harbor long-standing hostility toward women, use far more physical violence than is needed for submission, and usually don't find the rape sexually gratifying.

Power rape is a generally premeditated attack motivated by a desire to dominate and control another person. Power rapists, unable to deal with stress and their sense of failure, may rape to regain a sense of power. They use only as much force as needed to make their victims submit and may find the rape sexually gratifying, even though that's not their primary motive.

Sadistic rape is a premeditated assault that often involves bondage, torture, or sexual abuse. Sadistic rapists find power and anger sexually arousing and may subject victims to rituals of humiliation or torture. They're often preoccupied with violent pornography; their motives are more complex and difficult to understand than those of other types of rapists.

Gang rape involves three or more rapists. Men in close groups that drink and party together—such as fraternities or athletic teams—are more likely to participate in such assaults. The reasons may go beyond aggression and sexual gratification to the excitement and camaraderie the men feel while sharing the experience.

✔ REALITYCHECK

• What percentage of U.S. college students report assaulting their partner in a dating relationship?
Men _____   Women _____
• What percentage report being the victims of violence in a dating relationship?
Men _____   Women _____
• What percentage of college students report coercing a partner into having sex?
Men _____   Women _____
• What percentage of college students report being coerced into sex by a partner?
Men _____   Women _____

Answers on next page.

nonvolitional sex Sexual behavior that violates a person's right to choose when and with whom to have sex and what sexual behaviors to engage in.

sexual coercion Sexual activity forced upon a person by the exertion of psychological pressure by another person.

rape Sexual penetration of a female or a male by means of intimidation, force, or fraud.

PART 2: *Just the Facts*
- *33 percent of college men and 29 percent of college women report assaulting a dating partner.*
- *28 percent of men and 35 percent of women report being the victims of violence in a dating relationship.*
- *36 percent of college men and 25 percent of college women report coercing a partner into having sex.*
- *34 percent of college men and 31 percent of college women report being coerced into having sex by a partner.*

Source: Chan, K. L., et al. "Prevalence of Dating Partner Violence and Suicidal Ideation Among Male and Female University Students Worldwide." *Journal of Midwifery and Women's Health*, Vol. 53, No. 6, 2008, pp. 529–537.

young age, earlier and more frequent than usual childhood sexual experiences (both forced and voluntary), hostility toward women, irresponsibility, lack of social consciousness, and a need for dominance over sexual partners.

- **Situational variables (what happens during the date).** Men who initiate a date, pay all expenses, and provide transportation are more likely to be sexually aggressive, perhaps because they feel they can call all the shots.

- **Rape-tolerant attitudes.** As several studies have confirmed, college men hold more rape-tolerant attitudes than do college women. For example, college men are significantly more likely than college women to agree with statements such as, "Some women ask to be raped and may enjoy it" and "If a woman says 'no' to having sex, she means 'maybe' or even 'yes.'"

  Some social groups, such as fraternities and athletic teams, may encourage the use of alcohol; reinforce stereotypes about masculinity; and emphasize violence, force, and competition. The group's shared values, including an acceptance of sexual coercion, may keep individuals from questioning their behavior.

- **Drinking.** Alcohol use is one of the strongest predictors of acquaintance rape. Men who've been drinking may not react to subtle signals, may misinterpret a woman's behavior as a come-on, and may feel more sexually aroused. At the same time, drinking may impair a woman's ability to effectively communicate her wishes and to cope with a man's aggressiveness.

- **Date rape drugs.** Drugs such as Rohypnol (flunitrazepam) and GHB (gamma hydroxybutyrate) have been implicated in cases of acquaintance, or date, rape. Since both drugs are odorless and tasteless, victims have no way of knowing their drink has been tampered with. The subsequent loss of memory leaves victims with no explanation for where they've been or what's happened.

  Rohypnol—which can cause impaired motor skills and judgment, lack of inhibitions, dizziness, confusion,

Sexual gratification rape is usually an impulsive attack by someone willing to use physical coercion for the sake of sex. These rapists generally use no more force than needed to get a partner to submit and may stop the attack if it becomes clear they'll have to use extreme violence to overcome resistance. Many acquaintance rapes fit into this category.

Acquaintance, or Date, Rape The same factors that lead to other forms of sexual victimization can set the stage for date rape. Socialization into an aggressive role, acceptance of rape myths, and a view that force is justified in certain situations increase the likelihood of a man's committing date rape. Other factors can also play a role, including the following:

- **Personality and early sexual experiences.** Certain factors may predispose individuals to sexual aggression, including first sexual experience at a very

Acquaintance rape and alcohol use are very closely linked. Both men and women may find their judgment impaired or their communications unclear as a result of drinking,.

© Masterfile

lethargy, very low blood pressure, coma, and death—has been outlawed in the United States. Deaths also have been attributed to GHB overdoses.

 College women often aren't aware of the possibility that their drinks may be tampered with or that they may have been given a date-rape drug. In one study, female undergraduates did not perceive any risk in leaving their drinks unattended. Even if they started feeling ill at a party, many did not suspect that a date-rape drug could be the cause. The victims of prior assaults were slower at picking up on and responding to potentially dangerous dating situations, possibly because they feel that personal risks are unavoidable and beyond their control.[35]

- **Gender differences in interpreting sexual cues.** In research comparing college men and women, the men typically overestimated the woman's sexual availability and interest, seeing friendliness, revealing clothing, and attractiveness as deliberately seductive. In one study of date rape, the men reported feeling "led on," in part because their female partners seemed to be dressed more suggestively than usual.

Stranger Rape   Rape prevention consists primarily of making it as difficult as possible for a rapist to make you his victim:

- Don't advertise that you're a woman living alone. Use initials on your mailbox. Install and use secure locks on doors and windows, changing door locks after losing keys or moving into a new residence.

- Don't open your door to strangers. If a repairman or public official is at your door, ask him to identify himself and call his office to verify that he is a reputable person on legitimate business.

- Lock your car when it is parked, and drive with locked car doors. Should your car break down, attach a white cloth to the antenna and lock yourself in. If someone other than a uniformed officer stops to offer help, ask this person to call the police or a garage but do not open your locked car door.

YOUR STRATEGIES FOR PREVENTION
How to Avoid Date Rape

According to data from the U.S. Bureau of Justice, nine in ten reported rapes and sexual assaults in the United States involve a single offender with whom the victim had a prior relationship.

Both women and men report having been forced into sexual activity by someone they know. Many college students are in the age group most likely to face this threat: women aged 16 to 25 and men under 25. Women are most vulnerable and men are most likely to commit assaults during their senior year of high school and their first year of college.

Women who describe incidents of sexual coercion that meet the legal definition of rape often don't label it as such. They may have a preconceived notion that true rape consists of a blitzlike attack by a stranger. Or they may blame themselves for getting into a situation in which they couldn't escape. They may feel some genuine concern for others who would be devastated if they knew the truth (for example, if the rapist were the brother of a good friend or the son of a neighbor).

Here are strategies that can lower your risk of being involved in a date rape:

For Men:
- Remember that it's okay not to "score" on a date.
- Don't assume that a sexy dress or casual flirting is an invitation to sex.
- Be aware of your partner's actions. If she pulls away or tries to get up, understand that she's sending you a message—one you should acknowledge and respect.
- Restrict drinking, drug use, or other behaviors (such as hanging out with a group known to be sexually aggressive in certain situations) that could affect your judgment and ability to act responsibly.
- Think of the way you'd want your sister or a close female friend to be treated by her date. Behave in the same manner.

For Women:
- If the man pays for all expenses, he may think he's justified in using force to get "what he paid for." If you cover some of the costs, he may be less aggressive.
- Back away from a man who pressures you into other activities you don't want to engage in on a date, such as chugging beer or drag racing with his friends.
- Avoid misleading messages and avoid behavior that may be interpreted as sexual teasing. Don't tell him to stop touching you, talk for a few minutes, and then resume petting.
- Despite your clearly stated intentions, if your date behaves in a sexually coercive manner, use a strategy of escalating forcefulness—direct refusal, vehement verbal refusal, and if necessary, physical force.
- Avoid using alcohol or other drugs when you definitely do not wish to be sexually intimate with your date.

- Avoid dark and deserted areas, and be aware of the surroundings where you're walking. Should a driver ask for directions when you're a pedestrian, avoid approaching his car. Instead, call out your reply from a safe distance.

- Have house or car keys in hand as you approach the door. Check the back seat before getting into your car.

- Carry a device for making a loud noise, like a whistle or, even better, a pint-sized compressed air horn available in many sporting goods and boat supply stores. Sound the noise alarm at the first sign of danger.

Male Nonconsensual Sex and Rape No one knows how common male rape is because men are less likely to report such assaults than women. Researchers estimate that the victims in about 10 percent of acquaintance rape cases are men. These hidden victims often keep silent because of embarrassment, shame, or humiliation, as well as their own feelings and fears about homosexuality and conforming to conventional sex roles.

Although many people think men who rape other men are always homosexuals, most male rapists consider themselves to be heterosexual. Young boys aren't the only victims. The average age of male rape victims is 24. Rape is a serious problem in prison, where men may experience brutal assaults by men who usually resume sexual relations with women once they're released.

Impact of Rape Rape-related injuries include unexplained vaginal discharge, bleeding, infections, multiple bruises, and fractured ribs. Victims of sexual violence often develop chronic symptoms, such as headaches, backaches, high blood pressure, sleep disorders, pelvic pain, and sexual fertility problems. But sexual violence has both a physical and a psychological impact. The psychological scars of a sexual assault take a long time to heal. Therapists have linked sexual victimization with hopelessness, low self-esteem, high levels of self-criticism, and self-defeating relationships. An estimated 30 to 50 percent of

women develop posttraumatic stress disorder (see Chapter 3) following a rape. Many do not seek counseling until a year or more after an attack, when their symptoms have intensified or become chronic.

Acquaintance rape may cause fewer physical injuries but greater psychological torment. Often too ashamed to tell anyone what happened, victims may suffer alone, without skilled therapists or sympathetic friends to reassure them. Women raped by acquaintances blame themselves more, see themselves less positively, question their judgment, have greater difficulty trusting others, and have higher levels of psychological distress. Nightmares, anxiety, and flashbacks are common. The women may avoid others, become less capable of protecting themselves, and continue to be haunted by sexual violence for years. A therapist can help these victims begin the slow process of healing.

What to Do in Case of Rape Fewer than 5 percent of college rapes are reported. Women who are raped should call a friend or a rape crisis center. A rape victim should not bathe or change her clothes before calling. Semen, hair, and material under her fingernails or on her apparel all may be useful in identifying the man who raped her.

A rape victim who chooses to go to a doctor or hospital should remember that she may not necessarily have to talk to police. However, a doctor can collect the necessary evidence, which will then be available if she later decides to report the rape to police. All rape victims should talk with a doctor or health-care worker about testing and treatment for sexually transmitted infections and postintercourse conception.

Even an unsuccessful rape attempt should be reported because the information a woman may provide about the attack—the assaulter's physical characteristics, voice, clothes, car, even an unusual smell—may prevent another woman from being raped.

Counseling from a trained professional can help ease the trauma suffered by a rape victim.

© Geri Engberg/The Image Works

As their numbers have grown and their anguish has been recognized, the victims of violence have received greater attention. Hundreds of shelters for battered wives and their children have been set up across the country. They offer physical and psychological treatment and a haven where women can begin to rebuild their shattered self-esteem, as well as their daily lives. Rape counseling and crisis centers on college campuses and in the community provide various forms of assistance to victims of rape. In many cities, the telephone directory lists hot lines and resources. More than 400 victims' advocacy groups have been set up across the country to advise those hurt by crime. Support organizations help many survivors deal with the emotional aftermath of their experiences.

Sometimes well-intentioned friends and relatives add to the stress felt by the victims of violence. Here's how to offer comfort without implying criticism:

- **Don't try to deny that it happened.** Although it may be hard to talk about—or even listen to—what happened, the reality of the event must not be ignored. Denial makes victims doubt their own experience and question themselves at a time when they crave reassurance.

- **Don't pressure the victim to talk—or not to talk.** Some individuals need to go over every detail of what happened, again and again, until they work out their feelings of outrage and become ready to get on with their lives. Others find going into details too humiliating. Let the victim set the tone and limits for disclosure. Don't pry or prod.

- **Don't blame the victim.** Even when no one doubts that the victim is completely innocent, individuals may be plagued by regrets and self-accusation: Why didn't I lock the windows? Why did I park on that dark street? Any second-guessing or implied criticism adds to this burden of blame and shame.

- **Don't try to rush the victim to leave the past behind and get on with his or her life.** Recovery from any traumatic event takes time, and only the victim knows the appropriate pace. If, however, months pass without any lessening of symptoms or improvement in day-to-day functioning, family members and friends shouldn't hesitate to recommend that their loved one see a mental health professional..

SELF SURVEY · How Safe Is Your School?

Residence Hall Security

YES	NO	
—	—	Single-sex residence halls
—	—	Coed residence halls
—	—	Freshman residence halls
—	—	Substance-free residence halls
—	—	Senior residence halls
—	—	Alcohol prohibited
—	—	Drugs prohibited
—	—	Propped door alarms
—	—	Coed bathrooms
—	—	Card swipe—like hotels—for exterior and interior residence hall rooms
—	—	Patented keys
—	—	Standard keys
—	—	Automatic locked doors
—	—	Propped doors
—	—	Doors locked at night
—	—	Doors never locked
—	—	Doors always locked
—	—	Guards on duty 24 hours/day
—	—	Guards on duty at night
—	—	Apartments on campus
—	—	Fire sprinklers
—	—	Peep hole in room door
—	—	Dead bolt on room door
—	—	Safety chain on room door
—	—	Bath in room
—	—	Bathrooms down hallway
—	—	Single-sex bathrooms kept locked
—	—	Floors locked—all floors
—	—	Secure windows—all floors
—	—	Panic alarms in rooms

Visitors

YES	NO	
—	—	Phone/intercom at entrance
—	—	Leave ID with guard
—	—	Guest passes with guard
—	—	Sign in guests with guard

Security Patrols in Residence Halls

YES	NO	
—	—	By police nightly
—	—	By security nightly
—	—	By students—RA or equivalent
—	—	By no one

Roommate Conflicts

YES	NO	**Offending Roommate Quickly Transferred:**
—	—	For using illegal drugs
—	—	For having sex while roommate present
—	—	For binge/underage drinking
—	—	For noisy parties
—	—	For hate speech
—	—	For physical abuse or violence
—	—	For vandalism

Health Services

YES	NO	
—	—	Rape crisis center
—	—	Alcohol–drug counselors
—	—	Student AA meetings on campus

___	___	Peer education programming
___	___	Safety education programming
___	___	Alcohol and other drug programming
___	___	Support groups—depression, eating disorders, etc.
___	___	Wellness center
___	___	Women's center

Campus Security

YES	NO	
		Campus Security Force
___	___	Sworn police
___	___	Unsworn security
___	___	Security guards
___	___	Trained volunteer students
___	___	Arrest power
___	___	Patrolling day
___	___	Patrolling night
___	___	Carry firearms
___	___	Bicycle patrols
___	___	Surveillance cameras
___	___	Emergency phones in working condition
___	___	Escort services—24 hours
___	___	Shuttle services
___	___	Personal alarm devices

Parental Notification

YES	NO	
___	___	For suicide attempts
___	___	For depression
___	___	For alcohol poisoning
___	___	For DUI
___	___	For stalking
___	___	For acts of violence
___	___	For illegal drug use
___	___	For underage drinkers
___	___	For public drunkenness
___	___	For housing firearms
___	___	For sexual assault
___	___	For hate crimes or speech

___	___	For academic probation
___	___	For disciplinary probation
___	___	For residence hall violations
___	___	For off-campus citations

Campus Judicial System

YES	NO	
___	___	Releases results in hearings involving crimes of violence
___	___	Open campus judicial hearings
___	___	Reveals names of campus sex offenders

Get campus crime statistics from **www.ope.ed/gov/security** *or from your admissions office.*

Criminal Offenses

Murder	___
Forcible sex offenses	___
Nonforcible sex offenses	___
Robbery	___
Aggravated assault	___
Burglary	___
Arson	___
Motor vehicle theft	___
Hate crimes	___
Total criminal offenses	___
Per student crime ratio	___

Campus Arrests

Liquor law violations	___
Drug law violations	___
Weapons violations	___
Total Campus Arrests	___

Calculate campus crimes per thousand students and compare them with other schools. Also, attempt a balanced evaluation by combining your subjective impressions with any calculations.

Source: Security on Campus, Inc., www.securityoncampus.org.

Your Health Action Plan for Personal Safety on Campus

Fundamentals

- Freshmen should "respectfully decline" to have photo and personal information published for distribution to the campus community. Fraternities and upperclassmen have abused this type of publication to "target" naive freshmen.

- Study the campus and neighborhood with respect to routes between your residence and class/activities schedule. Know where emergency phones are located if you do not have a cell phone.

- Share your class/activities schedule with parents and a network of close friends, effectively creating a type of "buddy" system. Give network telephone numbers to your parents, advisors, and friends.

- Survey the campus, academic buildings, residence halls, and other facilities while classes are in session and after dark to see that buildings, walkways, quadrangles, and parking lots are adequately secured, lit, and patrolled. Are emergency phones, escorts, and shuttle services adequate?

- To gauge the social scene, drive down fraternity row on weekend nights and stroll through the student hangouts. Are people behaving responsibly, or does the situation seem reckless and potentially dangerous? Remember, alcohol and/or drug abuse is involved in about 90 percent of campus crime. Carefully evaluate off-campus student apartment complexes and fraternity houses if you plan to live off-campus.

Residence

- Doors and windows to your residence hall should be equipped with quality locking mechanisms. Room doors should be equipped with peep holes and deadbolts. Always lock them when you are absent. Do not loan out your key. Rekey locks when a key is lost or stolen.

- Card access systems are far superior to standard metal key and lock systems. Card access enables immediate lock changes when keys are lost, stolen, or when housing arrangements change. Most hotels and hospitals have changed to card access systems for safety reasons. Higher education institutions need to adopt similar safety features.

- Dormitories should have a central entrance/exit lobby where night-time access is monitored, as well as an outside telephone which visitors must use to gain access.

- Dormitory residents should insist that residential assistants and security patrols routinely check for propped doors—day and night.

- Know your neighbors and don't be reluctant to report illegal activities and suspicious loitering.

Off-Campus Residents

Off-campus residents should contact their student legal aid representative to draft leases that stipulate minimum standards of security and responsibility. Students and parents should also consult any "Neighborhood Watch" association active in the community or the municipal police regarding local crime rates.

Source: Reprinted with permission by Security on Campus, Inc., http://www .securityoncampus.org. Security on Campus assists victims of campus crime.

CENGAGENOW If you want to write your own goals for staying safe, go to the Wellness Journal at CengageNOW for Health: **www.cengage.com/ sso.**

MAKING THIS CHAPTER WORK FOR YOU

Review Questions

1. Signs of a potentially violent person include
   a. crying jags.
   b. heightened focus on schoolwork.
   c. frequent loss of temper.
   d. increased social activity.

2. Which of the following is *not* a safe-driving tip?
   a. Avoid driving at night for the first year after getting a license.
   b. Make sure your car has snow tires or chains before driving in hazardous snowy conditions.
   c. If riding with an intoxicated driver, keep talking to him so that he doesn't fall asleep at the wheel.
   d. Don't let packages or people obstruct the rear or side windows.

3. Which of the following statements about home safety is *true*?
   a. Falls pose the greatest threat of injury in the home, followed by poison.
   b. The three ingredients of fire are fuel, a heat source, and oxygen.
   c. The risk of falls is lowest in the elderly.
   d. If you're on the top floor of the dorm when a fire breaks out, get to the elevator quickly.

4. Which statement about violence on college campuses is *false?*
   a. Campus hazing often involves activities that would be called torture if perpetrated elsewhere.
   b. Most crimes against students occur on campus.
   c. Many campuses have codes of conduct on alcohol, drugs, and fighting.
   d. Crime statistics for colleges and universities are posted on the Internet.

5. Sexual victimization
   a. includes sexual harassment, sexual coercion, and rape.
   b. is gender-specific, affecting women who are violated emotionally or physically by men.
   c. is rare in academic environments such as college campuses.
   d. most commonly takes the form of physical assault and stalking.

6. You can avoid computer health hazards by
   a. positioning the monitor so that you are looking up at it.
   b. positioning the keyboard so that you don't have to bend your wrists to use it.
   c. sustaining focus on the screen with the PRIO method.
   d. taking a 15-minute break every 30 minutes.

7. Which of the following statements about rape is *true*?
   a. When a person is sexually attacked by a stranger, it is referred to as *rape*. When a person is sexually attacked by an acquaintance, it is referred to as *sexual coercion.*
   b. Statutory rape is defined as sexual intercourse initiated by a woman under the age of consent.
   c. Men who rape other men usually consider themselves heterosexuals.
   d. Women who flirt and dress provocatively are typically more willing to participate in aggressive sex than women who dress conservatively and do not flirt.

8. Seat belt use
   a. is optional if your car has air bags.
   b. is higher in teenage men than women.
   c. reduces the risk of serious injury by about 50 percent.
   d. is declining in the United States.

9. Ways to protect or prevent rape include which of the following?
   a. Use alcohol and drugs only in familiar surroundings.
   b. Take a self-defense class.
   c. To avoid angering a sexually aggressive person, become passive and quiet.
   d. Do not discuss your sexual limits on a first or second date because just talking about sex will encourage your date to think you are interested in a sexual relationship.

10. Which of the following factors affects an individual's risk of accident or injury?
    a. hunger level
    b. stress level
    c. amount of automobile insurance coverage
    d. knowledge of CPR

    Answers to these questions can be found on page 650.

Critical Thinking

1. Can you name two risk factors in your daily life that might increase the likelihood of accidental injury? What actions have you taken to keep yourself safe? Are there other risk factors you could minimize or eliminate? What might you do about them?

2. A friend of yours, Eric, frequently makes crude or derogatory comments about women. When you finally call him on this, his response is, "I didn't say anything wrong. I like women." What might you say to him?

Media Menu

CENGAGENOW™ Go to the CengageNOW for Health website at **www .cengage.com/sso** that will:
- Help you evaluate your knowledge of the material.
- Allow you to take an exam-prep quiz.
- Provide a personalized Learning Plan targeting resources that address areas you should study.
- Coach you through identifying target goals for behavioral change and creating and monitoring your personal change plan throughout the semester.

Internet Connections

www.rainn.org
This site provides great information from an organization fighting against rape, assault, and incest.

www.rapecrisis.com
This private nonprofit organization provides support to victims of sexual violence and their families, including a 24/7 crisis hotline and several advocacy programs.

www.nsc.org
The mission of the NSC is to educate and influence society to adopt safety, health, and environmental policies, practices, and procedures that prevent human suffering and economic losses arising from preventable causes.

www.safeyouth.org
This site is a gateway to resources for professionals, parents, youth, and individuals working to prevent and end violence committed by and against young people.

Key Terms

The terms listed are used on the page indicated. Definitions of the terms are in the Glossary at the end of the book.

computer vision syndrome 579
hazing 583
nonvolitional sex 587
rape 587
repetitive motion injury (RMI) 579
sexual coercion 587
sexual harassment 585
stalking 585

Chapter 19 - Creating a Healthier Environment

1. **Global warming has been a culprit in climatic changes such as all the following except for:** (pg 602)
   A. more hurricanes
   B. rising water temperatures
   C. thermal inversions
   D. plants getting taller

2. **One of the more serious after-effects of climate change that will promote more infectious disease outbreaks among humans will be:** (Pg. 603)
   A. more hardier flies that will contaminate more food supplies and cause food borne illnesses
   B. mosquito-born illnesses such as malaria and yellow fever
   C. coastal floods creating more mold problems in people's homes and causing severe fungi-type allergies
   D. growth of toxic weeds and plants causing skin rashes on people

3. **Climate change can affect all of the following health perils in our environment except for:** (pg 603)
   A. floods
   B. supply of fresh water
   C. population increases
   D. food availability

4. **Which component of air pollution is deemed to be the primary source of smog air pollution?** (pg 605)
   A. smog
   B. ozone
   C. particulate matter
   D. cigarette smoking

5. **What is meant by the 'greenhouse effect' that creates irregular climatic changes on the planet Earth?** (pg 602)
   A. it keeps the planet warm
   B. gases trap energy from the sun and bounce it back down to the earth
   C. the production of fossil fuels give off poisonous gases that destroy the outer atmosphere
   D. solar radiation passes through the clean atmosphere

6. **One way to increase sustainability with the environment is to use precycled materials which are:** (pg 606)
   A. substances made only of biodegradable plastics
   B. products packaged in recycled materials
   C. reusable containers
   D. materials which are compostable

7. **An example of a precycled material is:** (pg 606)
   A. recyclable containers to package eggs in
   B. throw away milk jugs
   C. glass containers that can be recycled
   D. boxes made out of paper pulp from trees

8. **Composting works by a method of:** (p 607)
   A. burying rotten foods into the ground
   B. burning trash at the landfill and reusing the remaining ashes
   C. recycling containers that originally stored fresh foods
   D. using organic products mixed with vegetation, whereby bacteria eat the organic material and turn it into a rich soil

9. **A hazardous form of indoor pollutant is considered to be:** (p 610 – 611)
   A. formaldehyde
   B. asbestos
   C. radon
   D. all of the above

10. **Which indoor pollutant is commonly found in building materials and can cause stinging eyes and burning lung irritation?** (pg 612)

   A. asbestos   C. formaldehyde
   B. lead   D. mercury

11. A radioactive odorless gas that can seep into basement walls and foundations to cause lung disease is: (pg 610)
     A. mold
     B. radon
     C. carbon monoxide
     D. ozone

12. Soon after Jack and Jill moved into their new house, they began experiencing respiratory problems, headaches, watery eyes, and rashes. One possible source of their problem appeared to be from the carpeting which could be emitting: (pg 612)
     A. radon
     B. ozone
     C. formaldehyde
     D. natural gas

13. A newer type of indoor pollutant created from a biological source is: (pg 61)
     A. bacteria
     B. dead cockroach larvae skins
     C. mold
     D. dust mites

14. An older type of material used in building construction that can cause serious lung problems is: (pg 613)
     A. asbestos
     B. plastic
     C. cement
     D. roofing tar

15. Identify where long term hearing loss may occur: (pg 619)
     A. in a restaurant
     B. at a concert
     C. on the job
     D. at airports

16. Decibels measure: (pg 618)
     A. volume of noise in a room
     B. intensity of sound
     C. range of sound frequencies
     D. ringing of the ears

17. Tinitus is a medical term for: (pg 619)
     A. ringing in the ears
     B. severe headaches from loud sounds
     C. middle ear infections
     D. conductive hearing loss

18. A whisper would be approximately how many decibels: (pg 619)
     A. 5
     B. 10
     C. 20
     D. 100

19. All of the following except one are good ways to protect your ears from hearing damage: (pg 620)
     A. wear foam ear plugs
     B. soundproof your living quarters with drapery or carpeting to reduce noise
     C. always keep the noise level up at home to drown out the outside noise
     D. reduce intake of aspirin which can aggravate the damage caused by loud noise

20. One of the following is not a good idea in protecting the planet: (pg 621)
     A. wash laundry in warm or cool water
     B. carry and use recyclable and reusable shopping bags
     C. ride a bicycle instead of driving the car when possible
     D. use a dishwasher instead of manually washing dishes to save on water

Until college Neri's commitment to the environment consisted of carrying the recyclables out to the curb every week. She opted to live in a "green" residence hall on campus because she liked the light, airy architecture, the plantings everywhere, and the opportunity to join a community of individuals committed to a shared cause. But as Neri learned more about energy sources and usage, living green became a way of life. She stopped buying plastic bottles of water, relied on natural light whenever possible, and switched to energy-efficient lightbulbs. Like a growing number of students, she joined an environmental action group whose

Creating a Healthier Environment

activities include planting trees, setting up recycling centers, and launching energy-conservation makeovers on campus.

Some describe the campaign to create a healthier environment and combat climate change as this generation's equivalent of the civil rights movement.[1] Without doubt these issues cannot be ignored. Although environmental concerns may seem so enormous that nothing any individual can do will have an effect, this is not the case. All of us, as citizens of the world, can help find solutions to the challenges confronting our planet. The first step is realizing that you have a personal responsibility for safeguarding the health of your environment and, thereby, your own well-being.

This chapter explores the complex interrelationships between your world and your well-being. It discusses major threats to the environment, including climate changes; atmospheric changes; air, water, and noise pollution; chemical risks; and radiation. You can find specific guidance on what you can do in Making Change Happen and "OurSpace" in *Labs for IPC*.

After studying the material in this chapter, you should be able to

- **Name** some of the direct and indirect health risks associated with climate change.
- Briefly **describe** the process by which greenhouse gases are formed.
- **Describe** three important paths to sustainability
- **Identify** the major indoor pollutants and one or more ways to reduce exposure.
- **Describe** three to five ways of protecting the ears from loud noise.
- **Write** a list of actions that you can take to protect the environment.

Log on to CengageNOW for Health at **www.cengage.com/sso** to find your Behavior Change Planner and to explore self-assessments, interactive tutorials, and practice quizzes.

597

MAKING CHANGE HAPPEN

Going Green

Environmental concerns may seem so enormous that you may think that nothing you do will have an effect. This is not the case. The world can be made better instead of worse. You have the power to make choices and changes that will protect the environment we all share.

The lab "OurSpace" in *Labs for IPC* provides a systematic approach to living a "greener" life. Based on the Stages of Change discussed in Chapter 1 of this text and in *IPC*, the lab provides a blueprint that will guide you as you make changes that will benefit you and your environment. Here's a preview:

Get Real

Before you know where you're going, you need to understand where you are. In this stage, you evaluate your environmental values by rating how important (on a scale of 0 to 100) each of 11 goals is to you, including:

- Slowing or stopping global warming. _____
- Improving air quality. _____

You record a second number for how involved you are with each item, with 0 representing not involved and 100 as involved in taking action as humanly possible.

You also assess how green your lifestyle is by checking which of 19 things you do regularly. These behaviors include:

- I buy products packaged simply in recycled or recyclable materials. _____
- I limit use of disposables such as paper napkins and plastic utensils. _____

Get Ready

Your next step is to prepare for change by following recommendations such as the following:

- **Check out campus resources.** Look for a local chapter of groups such as the Campus Climate Challenge, Student Environmental Action Coalition, or the Sierra Club. These organizations launch energy-conservation campaigns for their campuses, sponsor conferences, and so on. Download their calendars of scheduled activities for the term and get involved.

Get Going

This is the stage where you start taking action with concrete steps that you incorporate into your daily life. Here is an excerpt from the comprehensive six-week green makeover included in the lab.

- **Adopt a space.** Take personal responsibility for a piece of the planet. This could be part of a path you walk every day to class, the stairs outside your dorm or apartment building, a neglected flower bed on the quad, your bus stop, whatever. Check on it regularly, and . . .

Lock It In

Your planet is going to need your help for the rest of your life. That's why it's important to make your new environmentally friendly habits permanent. Here is an excerpt from one suggestion of how to do so:

- **Keep informed of environmental issues.** Americans are paying more attention to global warming and other environmental threats. Follow political discussions. Become familiar with the environmental positions of political candidates. Note which businesses are taking the initiative in fostering innovative, energy-saving programs. Be aware of . . .

The Environment and Your Health

Ours is a planet in peril. Glaciers are melting. Sea levels are rising. Forests are being destroyed. Droughts have become more frequent and more intense. Heat waves have killed tens of thousands of people. Hurricanes and floods have ravaged cities. Millions have died from the effects of air pollution and contaminated water.

The planet Earth—once taken for granted as a ball of rock and water that existed for our use for all time—is a single, fragile **ecosystem** (a community of organisms that share a physical and chemical environment). Our environment is a closed ecosystem, powered by the sun. The materials needed for the survival of this planet must be recycled over and over again. Increasingly, we're realizing just how important the health of this ecosystem is to our own well-being and survival.

The World Health Organization (WHO) has identified the three major environmental threats to health: unsafe water, sanitation, and hygiene; indoor air pollution from solid fuel use; and outdoor air pollution. Improving water, sanitation, hygiene, and indoor and outdoor air could prevent an estimated 4 million deaths a year and greatly reduce child mortality in the world's lowest-income countries.[2]

For good or for ill, we cannot separate our individual health from that of the environment in which we live. However, efforts to clean up the environment are paying off. According to a recent epidemiological study, the residents of cities that have improved the quality of their air have nearly five months added to their life expectancy.[3] The water we drink and the chemicals we use also have an impact on the quality of our lives. At the same time, the lifestyle choices we make, the products we use, the efforts we undertake to clean up a beach or save wetlands affect the quality of our environment. For some ideas on what you can do, see Community Focus, p. 601, and Health on a Budget.

ecosystem A community of organisms sharing a physical and chemical environment and interacting with each other.

HEALTH ON A BUDGET $

No- and Low-Cost Ways to "Green" Your Space

Whether you live in a dorm, apartment, or house, you can take simple, inexpensive steps to create a greener personal environment. Here are some ways to get started. (See Figure 19.1 for more ideas.)

- Buy furniture and household items secondhand, or recycle your parents' things. If you can't find everything you need in the attic or basement, try a website such as **http://www.freecycle.com**, where you can barter your way to greener furnishings.
- Choose recycled notebooks and printer paper and eco-friendly shampoos, conditioners, and lotions (found in local CO-OP stores).
- Rather than relying on air-conditioning or central heat, use a space heater or fan, depending on the season, to regulate the temperature around you.

- Buy a stainless steel or coated aluminum water bottle instead of using disposable bottles.
- Use green cleaning products like vinegar and baking soda instead of expensive and potentially harmful chemicals.
- Tote books and groceries in canvas bags rather than paper or plastic ones.
- Chip in with roommates or friends so you can buy in bulk, which saves money and requires less packaging.
- Don't throw anything out before asking yourself if it can be recycled, donated, or simply used in another way.

Aluminum water bottle

Space heater

Used desk chair

Recycle paper

Recycled notebooks

Second-hand clothing

Eco-friendly boxes

Canvas tote

Figure 19.1 Greening Your Space

Climate Change

The International Panel on Climate Change of the United Nations, made up of leading scientists from around the world, has reported with absolute certainty that the world's climate is changing in significant ways and will continue to do so in the foreseeable future. These experts predict an increase in extreme weather events (such as hurricanes and heat waves), greater weather variability, and rising water temperatures. The American Association for the Advancement of Science (AAAS) and other prestigious institutions around the world have issued warnings on the growing dangers of global climate change.[4]

Global Warming

Earth's average temperature increased about 1 degree in the 20th century to approximately 59 degrees, but the rate of warming in the last three decades has been three times the average rate since 1900. Seas have risen about six to eight feet globally over the last century and are rising at a higher rate.

Why is our planet getting warmer? Figure 19.2 shows the normal greenhouse effect:

Certain gases in Earth's atmosphere trap energy from the sun and retain heat somewhat like the glass panels of a greenhouse. These "greenhouse" gases include carbon dioxide, methane, and nitrous oxide. Human activities, scientists now say with 90 percent certainty, have increased the greenhouse gases in our atmosphere. We burn fossil fuels (oil, natural gas, coal) and wood products, which release carbon dioxide into the atmosphere. We produce coal, natural gas, and oil, which emit methane. Livestock and the decomposition of organic wastes also produce methane. Agricultural and industrial processes emit nitrous oxide. These emissions enhance the normal greenhouse effect, trapping more heat and raising the temperature of the atmosphere and Earth's surface.

After years of doubt and debate, most leading experts agree that the buildup of greenhouse gases is changing natural climate and weather patterns in new and potentially dangerous ways. Carbon dioxide levels are higher now than at any time in the past 800,000 years and, according to the AAAS, are "heading for levels not experienced for millions of years."[5]

Figure 19.2 The Greenhouse Effect

The normal greenhouse effect warms Earth to a hospitable temperature. An increase in greenhouse gases intensifies the greenhouse effect, trapping more heat and raising Earth's temperature.

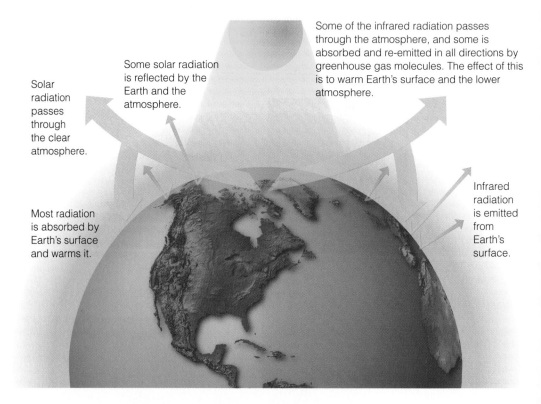

Some solar radiation is reflected by the Earth and the atmosphere.

Solar radiation passes through the clear atmosphere.

Some of the infrared radiation passes through the atmosphere, and some is absorbed and re-emitted in all directions by greenhouse gas molecules. The effect of this is to warm Earth's surface and the lower atmosphere.

Most radiation is absorbed by Earth's surface and warms it.

Infrared radiation is emitted from Earth's surface.

The Health Risks

No individual is immune to the effects of climate change. WHO estimates that climate change is already causing at least 150,000 excess deaths a year and that this number will climb to at least 300,000 annually by 2030.[6]

Climate change can imperil health directly—for example, as the result of floods or heat waves—and indirectly—by changing the patterns of infectious diseases, supplies of fresh water, and food availability. For example, as the planet continues to warm, infectious diseases—particularly mosquito-borne illnesses such as malaria, dengue fever, yellow fever, and encephalitis—may spread to more regions. Already in the United States, mosquitoes and other insects that carry diseases such as West Nile virus, Rocky Mountain spotted fever, and Lyme disease are spreading to areas once considered too cold for these insects to survive.

COMMUNITY FOCUS *Creating a Healthier World*

PROBLEM In recent decades college students, faculty, and administrators have taken the lead in the struggle to protect their planet and their future. Some schools are relying on wind and solar installations for more of their energy. Others offer "green dorms" where students can live an eco-friendly lifestyle. Many are replacing gas-guzzling campus vans with hybrids or other fuel-saving vehicles.

As global warming and energy independence have emerged as critical political issues, students have played an increasingly important role in campaigns for "green" candidates and against projects that threaten the local environment. College research teams, composed of professors and students, have taken on challenges such as finding sustainable sources of water for dry, highly populated cities such as Phoenix. More than 450 school presidents have signed the American College and University Presidents' Climate Commitment, which requires schools to have a plan to become carbon neutral—that is, to balance the amount of carbon released with the amount offset or sequestered.

What can you do? In addition to the ideas in Making Change Happen, p. 598, try these suggestions:

BECOME INFORMED

- Read a book or watch a documentary on environmental issues and practical solutions. Some possibilities include: *An Inconvenient Truth,* a book and film by Al Gore; *Who Killed the Electric Car?,* a documentary by Chris Paine; *The Green Book: The Everyday, Guide to Saving the Planet, One Simple Step at a Time,* by Elizabeth Rogers and Thomas Kostigen; and *It's Easy Being Green: A Handbook for Earth-Friendly Living,* by Crissy Trask.
- Keep up with environmental issues. Follow political discussions. Become familiar with the environmental positions of political candidates. Note which businesses are taking the initiative in fostering innovative, energy-saving programs. Be aware of campus policies and projects such as building more energy-efficient dorms and offices.
- Assess your own lifestyle. How green are your choices and behaviors? See "OurSpace" in *Labs for IPC* to examine your environmental values and develop a six-week "green makeover." Check out websites such as **www.thegreenguide.com** and **www.geocities.com/RainForest/Vines/4990/gglist.html.** (See also Health on a Budget, p. 599.)

BECOME INVOLVED

- Check out campus resources. Look for a local chapter of groups such as the Campus Climate Challenge, the Student Environmental Action Coalition, or the Sierra Club. These organizations set up recycling centers, launch energy-conservation campaigns for their campuses, sponsor conferences, and more. Find out how to contact environmental groups on campus, and download their calendars of scheduled activities.
- Work with student groups to organize fun eco-events on campus, such as a green film festival with movies like *Erin Brockovich* and *FernGully,* a "Trashion Show" with clothes made from recycled materials, or a "Recycle Mania" competition.
- Raise awareness—yours and others'. If you live in a dorm, residence hall, or fraternity or sorority, find out how much trash is being recycled—and how much could be.
- Put up a sign in the laundry room reminding residents to wash clothes in cold water rather than hot. Not only will you save power and cut your electricity bill, but your clothes won't show wear and tear as quickly.
- Make your voice heard. Write or e-mail your senators and representatives—the people who vote on pollution controls, the enforcement of safety regulations, and the preservation of forests and wildlife.

The Impact of Pollution

Any change in the air, water, or soil that could reduce its ability to support life is a form of *pollution*. Natural events, such as smoke from fires triggered by lightning, can cause pollution. However, most sources of pollution are man-made. There are now about ten times as many cars around the world as there were 50 years ago. The number of people living in cities has increased by more than a factor of four, and global energy consumption by nearly a factor of five.[7]

The effects of pollution depend on the concentration (amount per unit of air, water, or soil) of the **pollutant**, how long it remains in the environment, and its chemical nature. An *acute effect* is a severe, immediate reaction, usually after a single, large exposure. For example, pesticide poisoning can cause nausea and dizziness, even death. A *chronic effect* may take years to develop or may be a recurrent or continuous reaction, usually after repeated exposure. The development of cancer after repeated exposure to a pollutant such as asbestos is an example of a chronic effect.

Environmental agents that trigger changes, or *mutations*, in the genetic material (the DNA) of living cells are called **mutagens**. The changes that result can lead to the development of cancer. A substance or agent that causes cancer is a **carcinogen**: All carcinogens are mutagens; most mutagens are carcinogens. Furthermore, when a mutagen affects an egg or a sperm cell, its effects can be passed on to future generations. Mutagens that can cross the placenta of a pregnant woman and cause a spontaneous abortion or birth defects in the fetus are called *teratogens*.

Pollution is a hazard to all who breathe. Deaths caused by air pollution exceed those from motor vehicle injuries. Those with respiratory illnesses and other chronic health problems are at greatest risk during days when smog or allergen counts are high.[8] However, as a recent study showed, even healthy college students suffer impairments in their heart and circulatory systems as a result of urban air pollution.[9] The effects of carbon monoxide are much worse in smokers, who already have higher levels of the gas in their blood.

As carbon dioxide levels in the air rise due to the greenhouse effect, air quality will worsen. Gases found in polluted air—such as ozone, sulfur dioxide, and nitrogen dioxide—contribute to heart disease and worsen the health of individuals who already have heart conditions. Poor air quality also contributes to breathing difficulties and may be responsible for the dramatic increase in asthma in recent decades. Elevated carbon dioxide levels can trigger asthma attacks and allergies by increasing ragweed pollen. Greater carbon dioxide in the air also stimulates the growth of poison ivy and other nuisance plants.

Toxic substances in polluted air can enter the human body in three ways: through the skin, through the digestive system, and through the lungs. The combined interaction of two or more hazards can produce an effect greater than that of either one alone. Pollutants can affect an organ or organ system directly or indirectly.

Among the health problems that have been linked with pollution are the following:

- Headaches and dizziness.
- Eye irritation and impaired vision.
- Nasal discharge.
- Cough, shortness of breath, and sore throat.
- Constricted airways.
- Constriction of blood vessels and increased risk of heart disease.
- Chest pains and aggravation of the symptoms of colds, pneumonia, bronchial asthma, emphysema, chronic bronchitis, lung cancer, and other respiratory problems.
- Birth defects and reproductive problems.
- Nausea, vomiting, and stomach cancer.
- Allergy and asthma from diesel fumes in polluted air.

The Air You Breathe

Remember the last time you stood at a busy intersection as a bus or truck spewed brownish fumes in your face? Maybe your eyes stung, or your throat burned. But breathing polluted air can do more than irritate: It can take months or even years off your life. As pollutants destroy the hairlike cilia that remove irritants from the lungs, individuals may suffer chronic bronchitis, characterized by excessive mucus flow and continuous coughing. Emphysema may develop or worsen, as pollutants constrict the bronchial tubes and destroy the air sacs in the lungs, making breathing more difficult.

When air pollution levels are high, heart attacks, strokes, heart failure flare-ups, and lung troubles increase. Air contamination also has enduring effects on heart health and increases atherosclerosis and deaths due to heart disease. For the elderly and people with asthma or heart disease, polluted air can be life-threatening.[10] Even healthy individuals can be affected, particularly if they exercise outdoors during high-pollution periods.

Ozone

Ozone, the primary ingredient of smog air pollution, can impair the body's immune system and cause long-term lung damage. (Ozone in the upper atmosphere protects us by repelling harmful ultraviolet radiation from the sun, but ozone in the lower atmosphere is a harmful component of air pollution.) Automobiles also produce carbon monoxide, a colorless and odorless gas that diminishes the ability of red blood cells to carry oxygen. The resulting oxygen deficiency can affect breathing, hearing, and vision in humans and stunt the growth of plants and trees.

Several large investigations have confirmed that ozone at levels currently found in the United States can shorten lives. Even on days when ozone levels are below the national standard, the risk of premature death is greater in areas with higher levels. The individuals most vulnerable to the effects of ozone are children, senior citizens, people who work or exercise outdoors, those with a respiratory disease such as asthma, and "responders" who are otherwise healthy but respond intensely to ozone.

Ozone's other ill effects include shortness of breath, chest pain when inhaling deeply, wheezing, coughing, and increased susceptibility to respiratory infections. Studies of college freshmen who were lifelong residents of Los Angeles or the San Francisco Bay Area found that long exposure

pollutant A substance or agent in the environment, usually the by-product of human industry or activity, that is injurious to human, animal, or plant life.

mutagen An agent that causes alterations in the genetic material of living cells.

carcinogen A substance or agent that causes cancer.

ozone A form of oxygen that is a harmful component of air pollution.

© iStockphoto.com/Daniel Stein

to elevated ozone levels had reduced their "lung function," that is, their lungs' ability to work efficiently.

Particle Pollution

Scientists refer to the mix of very tiny solid and liquid particles in the air as *particle pollution*. The particles themselves can range in size from microscopic to one-tenth the diameter of a strand of hair. Our natural defenses help us to cough or sneeze large particles out of our bodies, but they don't keep out smaller particles, which get trapped in the lungs. The smallest ones pass through the lungs into the bloodstream.

Particle pollution damages the body in ways similar to cigarette smoking. Even short-term exposure can be deadly because particle pollution increases the risk of heart attacks and strokes, especially among the elderly and those with heart conditions. It also diminishes lung function, causes inflammation of lung tissue in young, healthy adults, increases the number and severity of asthma attacks, and increases mortality in infants and young children.

Living near highways or spending time in heavy traffic, whether driving or taking public transportation, may be especially dangerous. Several studies have found an increased risk of premature death in those who live, work, drive, or ride in high-traffic areas. Air pollution may permanently impair the capacity of the lungs of 10- to 18-year-olds who live within about a third of a mile of a freeway, limiting their ability to breathe for the rest of their lives and increasing their risk of serious lung diseases.[11]

Particle pollution—considered the most dangerous because it can be an immediate as well as a long-term threat to life—has increased in the eastern part of the United States but decreased in the West. Cities that have reduced particle pollution—such as Pittsburgh, Buffalo, Los Angeles, Indianapolis, and St. Louis—have reported gains in life expectancy of about five months.[12]

Working Toward Sustainability

More universities are developing programs to achieve **sustainability,** the use of as little as possible of resources that cannot be renewed. (See Point/Counterpoint, p. 607.) Innovative programs include "green" dorms and campaigns to reduce energy waste. Not all undergraduates share this concern, but higher numbers express commitment to environmental action than in the past. (See Reality Check, p. 607.)

Three important paths to sustainability are precycling, recycling, and composting. **Precycling** refers to buying products packaged in recycled materials. According to the consumer group Earthworks, packaging makes up a third of what people in the United States throw away. When you precycle, you consider how you're going to dispose of a product and the packaging materials before purchasing it. For example, you might choose eggs in recyclable cardboard packages, rather than in Styrofoam cartons, and look for juice and milk in refillable bottles.

Recycling—collecting, reprocessing, marketing, and reusing materials once considered trash—serves several important functions, including:

- **Preserving natural resources.** Reprocessing used materials to make new products and packaging reduces the consumption of natural resources. Recycling steel saves iron ore, coal, and limestone. Recycling newsprint, office paper, and mixed paper saves trees.

- **Saving energy.** Recycling used aluminum cans, for instance, requires only about 5 percent of the energy needed to produce aluminum. Recycling just one can save enough electricity to light a 100-watt bulb for 3 1/2 hours.

- **Reducing greenhouse gas emissions.** Recycling cuts these gases by decreasing the amount of energy used to produce and transport new products.

- **Decreasing the need for landfill storage** or **incineration**. Both are more costly and can contribute to air pollution.

Different communities take different approaches to recycling. Many provide regular curbside pickup of recyclables, and others have drop-off centers. Buyback centers pay for recyclables. In some places, reverse vending machines accept returned beverage containers and provide deposit refunds.

Discarded computers, other electronic devices, and printer cartridges also should be recycled, by donating them to schools or charitable organizations. "Tech trash" buried in landfills is creating a new hazard because trace amounts of potentially hazardous agents, such as lead and mercury, can leak into the ground and water. Find out if your campus has a program to recycle electronic devices.

With *composting*—which some people describe as nature's way of recycling—the benefits can be seen as close as your backyard. Organic products, such as leftover food and vegetable peels, are mixed with straw or other dry material and kept damp. Bacteria eat the organic material and turn it into a rich soil. Some people keep a compost pile (which should be stirred every few days) in their backyard; others take their organic garbage (including mowed grass and dead leaves) to community gardens or municipal composting sites.

✔ REALITYCHECK

- *What percentage of college freshmen say that "becoming involved in programs to clean up the environment" is essential or very important?* _____
- *Are women or men more committed to improving the environment?* _____

Answers on next page.

© Frank Whitney/Photographer's Choice/Getty Images

Renewable fuel sources, such as wind turbines, can provide more environmentally friendly alternative sources of energy. However, individual choices and behaviors also have an impact on the state of our world.

POINT COUNTERPOINT *Environmental Action 101*

POINT
A growing number of colleges and universities are designing innovative buildings and creating programs to reduce energy usage and conserve natural resources. Some, for instance, have bought alternative-fuel vehicles for campus transportation or installed solar panels to heat dormitories.

COUNTERPOINT
Institutions of higher education should focus on their mission of educating young people rather than committing resources to energy reduction. The government or corporations should take the lead in environmental innovation. Academics should primarily serve as consultants or advisors.

YOUR VIEW
Do you think students should support and participate in the search for innovative solutions to environmental problems? Should schools require students to limit their energy usage on campus?

sustainability A method of using a resource so that the resource is not depleted or permanently damaged.

precycling The use of products that are packaged in recycled or recyclable material.

recycling The processing or reuse of manufactured materials to reduce consumption of raw materials.

PART 2: *Just the Facts*

• **30** *percent of entering freshman say that "becoming involved in
programs to clean up the environment" is essential or very important.*

• *Slightly more women than men—32 percent compared to 27 percent—
say they are committed to improving the environment.*

Source: Pryor, John, et al. *The American Freshman: National Norms for Fall 2008.* Los Angeles: Higher Education Research Institute, UCLA, 2009.

CONSUMER**ALERT**

Change That Bulb!

What difference does a light bulb make?

Facts to Know

- A compact fluorescent bulb (CFL) gives off the same amount of light as a conventional bulb but uses only a quarter of the electricity.

- A CFL bulb that qualifies for the government's "Energy Star" symbol lasts about ten times longer and saves about $30 or more in electricity over a conventional bulb.

- If every American home replaced just one light bulb with CFL bulb, this simple step would save enough energy to light more than 3 million homes for a year, more than $600 million in annual energy costs, and prevent greenhouse gases equivalent to the emissions of more than 800,000 cars.

Steps to Take

- When shopping for a light bulb, look on the product packages for the "Energy Star" label and buy one labeled as equivalent to the incandescent bulb you are replacing.

- CFLs are made of glass and contain mercury; be careful when removing them from their packages and installing

them. Always screw and unscrew bulbs by their base (not the glass). Never forcefully twist the CFL into a light socket. (If one does break, follow the EPA guidelines for cleanup, available at **www.energystar. gov.**)

- When a CFL burns out, the EPA recommends disposing of it at a local recycling center. You can find one near you at **www.epa. gov/bulbrecycling** or **www.earth911.com.** Never put a CFL or any mercury-containing product in an incinerator or a trash bin.

© Katrina Wittkamp/Photodisc/Getty Images

The Water You Drink

Fears about the public water supply have led many Americans to turn off their taps. About two-thirds take steps to drink purer water, either by using filtration and distillation methods or by drinking bottled water. However, Consumers Union, a nonprofit advocacy group, maintains that the United States has the safest water supply in the world. The Environmental Protection Agency has set standards for some 80 contaminants. These include many toxic chemicals and heavy metals—including lead, mercury, cadmium, and chromium—that can cause kidney and nervous system damage and birth defects.

Each year the CDC reports an average of 7,400 cases of illness related to the water people drink. The most common culprits include parasites, bacteria, viruses, chemicals, and lead. Traces of prescription drugs also have been found in the water of some communities. Home filters can block certain pathogens that can cause diarrhea and other gastrointestinal problems, but they do not seem to remove most chemical contaminants.[13] If you decide to use a filter, clean it regularly to prevent a buildup of bacteria.

Is Bottled Better?

Consumers seem convinced that bottled water is purer than tap. The market for bottled water in the United States has been growing by 10 percent per year, making it second only to soft drinks as America's favorite beverage. On average we drink about 25 gallons of bottled water every year, compared to 51.5 gallons of soft drinks and 21 gallons of beer.[14]

However, medical researchers have not found a scientific reason to recommend bottled water over tap water. Nutritionists contend that even "vitamin" waters provide no additional benefits. (See Chapter 6 for more on water and other beverages.) Dentists report an increase in cavities among children and teenagers who drink bottled water rather than fluoridated tap water. An estimated 25 to 30 percent of bottled water sold in this country is, in fact, tap water, sometimes further treated and sometimes not. Despite images of mountain streams and glacier peaks on the labels, most comes from an urban water supply.[15]

Does bottled water taste better? In various taste tests, consumers sometimes rated water from particular types of plastic bottles as having an inferior taste, but the EPA has stated that variations in taste or smell do not necessarily mean unhealthy water. Is it safe to drink bottled water that's been stored for a long time or to drink from a partially consumed bottle? The best scientific answer is, "No one knows." Reliable data on such issues are very limited.

Portable Water Bottles

The simplest, safest, most ecofriendly water container is a glass. If you want to carry water with you, you have plenty of alternatives, but some portable drinking containers may pose risks to you or to the environment.

Most disposable water bottles are made with lightweight polyethylene terephthalate (PET). Reusing these bottles may pose some health dangers, although there is little scientific agreement on how serious these risks may be. Your mouth leaves a residue of bacteria when you drink from a bottle, and this may accumulate with repeated

© Terri Miller/E-Visual Communications, Inc.

use. Disposable bottles also pose a risk to the environment. The manufacture of the estimated 30 billion PET water bottles sold annually in the United States requires about 17 million barrels of oil. About 86 percent of these bottles become waste, which may take as long as 400 to 1,000 years to degrade.[16]

Many consumers have switched to harder bottles made with polycarbonate plastic (known by the brand name Nalgene). However, they contain bisphenol A (BPA), a synthetic hormone that mimics estrogen and may be released by hot fluids (including baby formula). Doctors recommend that concerned parents use alternatives such as glass bottles. It is not clear if small amounts of BPA pose any risk to adults.

Portable metal containers are another option. One popular brand is aluminum with a nontoxic liner; a second is simply made of stainless steel. A recent study—perhaps the first to study contamination of water with trace minerals leaching from such containers—found that the coated aluminum and stainless steel bottles are safe. However, pocket flasks, particularly those made of pewter, can leach potentially harmful amounts of trace metals into their watery contents.[17]

> Although there is little scientific agreement on the health risks of reusing disposable water bottles, the harm to the environment is clear. Choosing a reusable container is better for the environment.

Indoor Pollutants: The Inside Story

You may think of pollution as primarily a threat when you're outdoors, but people in industrialized societies spend more than 90 percent of their time inside buildings. Think of how much time you spend in your dorm, apartment, or home and in classrooms, dining halls, movie theatres, offices, stores, and shops. The quality of the air you breathe inside these places can have an even greater impact on your well-being than outdoor pollution.

Some sources—such as building materials and household products such as air fresheners—release pollutants more or less continuously. Other sources—such as tobacco smoke, solvents in cleaning products, and pesticides—can produce high levels of pollutants that remain in the air for long periods after their use.

The material on the following pages, based on the latest recommendations from the Environmental Protection Agency, can help protect you from invisible hazards in indoor air.[18]

Environmental Tobacco Smoke (ETS)

The mixture of smoke from the burning end of a cigarette, pipe, or cigar and a smoker's exhalations contains over 4,000 compounds, more than 40 of which are known to cause cancer in humans or animals. At greatest risk for the dangers of "passive smoking" or "secondhand smoke" are infants and young children and youngsters with asthma or other respiratory problems. (See Chapter 13 for a further discussion of the health risks of ETS.)

- **Sources:** Cigarette, pipe, and cigar smoking.
- **Health Effects:** Eye, nose, and throat irritation; headaches; lung cancer; may contribute to heart disease. In children,

increased risk of lower respiratory tract infections, such as bronchitis and pneumonia, and ear infections; build-up of fluid in the middle ear; increased severity and frequency of asthma episodes; decreased lung function.

- **Steps to Reduce Exposure:**
  - Do not smoke in your home or permit others to do so.
  - Do not smoke if children are present, particularly infants and toddlers.
  - If smoking indoors cannot be avoided, increase ventilation by opening windows.
  - Observe community restrictions on smoking. Most schools have banned smoking in dorms, classrooms, and other campus buildings. Do you know the policy of your school?

Radon

Colorless and odorless, radioactive radon gas enters homes through dirt floors, cracks in concrete walls and floors, floor drains, and sumps. When radon becomes trapped in buildings and concentrations build up indoors, exposure to the gas becomes a concern.

- **Sources:** Earth and rock beneath home; well water; building materials.
- **Health Effects:** No immediate symptoms. Exposure to high levels of radon increases the risk of lung cancer. The EPA estimates that radon causes from 7,000 to 30,000 lung cancer deaths each year. Smokers are at higher risk of developing radon-induced lung cancer.
- **Steps to Reduce Exposure:**
  - If you have any reason to suspect a radon problem in your home, you can buy inexpensive, do-it-yourself radon test kits online and in hardware stores. Look for ones that are state-certified or have met the requirements of a national radon proficiency program.
  - If testing reveals unsafe levels, contractors trained to fix radon problems can make changes to reduce the risk.
  - For more information on radon, contact your state radon office, or call 800-SOS-RADON.

Nonsmokers exposed to secondhand smoke, including children, face increased risk of developing lung cancer and heart disease.

Molds and Other Biological Contaminants

Bacteria, mildew, viruses, animal dander, cat saliva, house dust mites, cockroaches, and pollen can all pose a threat to health. One of the oldest and most widespread substances on Earth, mold—a type of fungus that decomposes organic matter and provides plants with nutrients—has emerged as a major health concern. Common molds include *Aspergillus, Penicillium,* and *Stachybotrys,* a slimy, dark green mold that has been blamed for infant deaths and various illnesses, from Alzheimer's disease to cancer, in adults that breathe in its spores. Faulty ventilation systems and airtight buildings have been implicated as contributing to the increased mold problem.

- **Sources:** Wet or moist walls, ceilings, carpets, and furniture; poorly maintained humidifiers, dehumidifiers, and air conditioners; bedding; household pets.

- **Health Effects:** Eye, nose, and throat irritation; shortness of breath; dizziness; lethargy; fever; digestive problems. Diseases like humidifier fever are associated with exposure to toxins that can grow in ventilation systems of large buildings. However, these diseases can also be traced to microorganisms in home heating and cooling systems and humidifiers. Children, the elderly, and people with breathing problems, allergies, and lung diseases are particularly susceptible to disease-causing biological agents in the indoor air.

- **Steps to Reduce Exposure:**

  - Use fans vented to outdoors in kitchens and bathrooms.

  - Clean cool mist and ultrasonic humidifiers in accordance with manufacturer's instructions and refill with clean water daily.

  - Empty water trays in air conditioners, dehumidifiers, and refrigerators frequently.

  - Keep your personal living space clean. No, your mother may not be checking on you, but regular cleaning reduces house dust mites, pollens, animal dander, and other allergy-causing agents.

Household Products

The liquids, foams, gels, and other materials you use to clean, disinfect, degrease, polish, wax, and preserve contain powerful chemicals that can pollute indoor air during and for long periods after their use. EPA researchers have found levels of about a dozen common organic pollutants to be two to five times higher inside homes than outside, regardless of whether the homes were located in rural or highly industrial areas.

- **Sources:** Paints, paint strippers, and other solvents; wood preservatives; aerosol sprays; cleansers and disinfectants; moth repellents and air fresheners; stored fuels and automotive products; hobby supplies; dry-cleaned clothing.

- **Health Effects:** Eye, nose, and throat irritation; headaches, loss of coordination, nausea; damage to liver, kidney, and central nervous system. Some organics can cause cancer in animals; some are suspected or known to cause cancer in humans.

- **Steps to Reduce Exposure:**

  - Follow instructions carefully. If the label says to use the product in a well-ventilated area, go outdoors or open windows to provide the maximum amount of outdoor air possible.

  - Never mix household care products unless so directed on the label.

Read the labels on common cleaning products, and follow instructions for use and storage to avoid possible health risks.

- Throw away partially full containers of old or unneeded chemicals, which can leak gases even when closed. Do not simply toss them in the garbage can. Find out if your local government or any organization in your community sponsors special days for the collection of toxic household wastes. If no such collection days are available, think about organizing one.

- Buy limited quantities. Purchase only as much as you will use right away.

- Keep to a minimum any exposure to emissions from products containing methylene chloride, such a paint strippers, adhesive removers, and aerosol spray paints. Methylene chloride is converted to carbon monoxide in the body and can cause symptoms associated with exposure to carbon monoxide.

Formaldehyde

Some indoor pollutants come from the very materials that buildings are made of and from the appliances inside them. Formaldehyde is commonly used in building materials, carpet backing, furniture, foam insulation, plywood, and particle board. This chemical can cause nausea, dizziness, headaches, heart palpitations, stinging eyes, and burning lungs. Formaldehyde gas, which is colorless and odorless, has been shown to cause cancer in animals. Most manufacturers have voluntarily quit using it, but many homes already contain materials made with urea-formaldehyde, which can seep into the air.

The rate at which products like pressed wood or textiles release formaldehyde can change. Formaldehyde emissions will generally decrease as products age. When the products are new, high indoor temperatures or humidity can cause increased release of formaldehyde from these products.

- **Sources:** Pressed wood products (hardwood plywood wall paneling, particle board, fiberboard) and furniture made with these pressed wood products; urea-formaldehyde foam insulation (UFFI); combustion sources and environmental tobacco smoke; durable press drapes, other textiles, and glues.

- **Health Effects:** Watery eyes, burning sensations in the eyes and throat, nausea, and difficulty in breathing. High concentrations may trigger attacks in people with asthma. Has been shown to cause cancer in animals and may cause cancer in humans.

- **Steps to Reduce Exposure:**
  - Use "exterior-grade" pressed wood products (lower-emitting because they contain phenol resins, not urea resins).
  - Use air conditioning and dehumidifiers to maintain moderate temperature and reduce humidity levels.
  - Increase ventilation, particularly after bringing new sources of formaldehyde into the home.
  - Always ask about the formaldehyde content of pressed wood products, including building materials, cabinetry, and furniture before you purchase them. For further information on formaldehyde and consumer products, call the EPA Toxic Substance Control Act (TSCA) assistance line (202-554-1404).

Pesticides

According to a recent survey, 75 percent of U.S. households used at least one pesticide product indoors during the past year. Products used most often are insecticides and disinfectants. Pesticides used in and around the home include products to control insects (insecticides), termites (termiticides), rodents (rodenticides), fungi (fungicides), and microbes (disinfectants). They are sold as sprays, liquids, sticks, powders, crystals, balls, and foggers.

The EPA requires manufacturers to put information on the label about when and how to use a pesticide. Remember that the "-cide" in pesticides means "to kill." Pesticides are also made up of ingredients that are used to carry the active agent. These carrier agents are called "inerts" because they are not toxic to the targeted pest; nevertheless, some inerts are capable of causing health problems.

- **Sources:** Products used to kill household pests or on lawns and gardens (if the product drifts or is tracked inside the house).

- **Health Effects:** High levels of certain pesticides can produce various symptoms, including headaches, dizziness, muscle twitching, weakness, tingling sensations, and nausea. They also might cause long-term damage to the liver and the central nervous system, as well as an increased risk of cancer.

- **Steps to Reduce Exposure:**

  - Follow instructions. It is illegal to use any pesticide in any manner inconsistent with the directions on its label.

  - Use only the pesticides approved for use by the general public and then only in recommended amounts; increasing the amount does not offer more protection. Ventilate the area well after pesticide use.

  - If possible, take plants and pets outside when applying pesticides to them.

  - Dispose of unwanted pesticides according to the directions on the label or on special household hazardous waste collection days.

  - Use nonchemical methods of pest control where possible.

  - Keep indoor spaces clean, dry, and well ventilated to avoid pest and odor problems.

  - Minimize exposure to moth repellents, which contain paradichlorobenzene, a chemical known to cause cancer in animals. If using mothballs, place them and the items to be protected in trunks or other containers that can be stored in areas such as attics and detached garages. Do not buy air fresheners that contain paradichlorobenzene.

Asbestos

This mineral fiber has been used commonly in a variety of building construction materials for insulation and as a fire-retardant. The government has banned several asbestos products, and manufacturers have also voluntarily limited use of asbestos. Today asbestos is most commonly found in older homes, pipe and furnace insulation materials, asbestos shingles, millboard, textured paints, and floor tiles.

- **Sources:** Deteriorating, damage, or disturbed insulation, fireproofing, acoustical materials, and floor tiles.

- **Health Effects:** Too small to be visible, the most dangerous asbestos fibers accumulate in the lungs and can cause lung cancer, mesothelioma (a cancer of the chest and abdominal linings), and asbestosis (irreversible lung scarring that can be fatal). Symptoms of these diseases do not show up until many years after exposure began. Smokers are at higher risk of developing asbestos-induced lung cancer.

- **Steps to Reduce Exposure:**

  - Leave undamaged asbestos material alone if it is not likely to be disturbed.

  - Use trained and qualified contractors for control measures that may disturb asbestos and for cleanup.

  - Follow proper procedures in replacing woodstove door gaskets that may contain asbestos.

Lead

People are exposed to lead, a long-recognized health threat, through air, drinking water, food, contaminated soil, deteriorating paint, and dust. Airborne lead enters the body when an individual breathes or swallows lead particles or dust. Before its risks were known, lead was used in paint, gasoline, water pipes, and many other products.

- **Source:** Lead-based paint; contaminated soil, dust, and drinking water.

- **Health Effects:** Lead affects practically all systems within the body. Lead at high levels can cause convulsions, coma, and even death. Lower levels of lead can cause adverse health effects on the central nervous system, kidney, and blood cells. Fetuses, infants, and children are more vulnerable to lead exposure than adults—lead is more easily absorbed into growing bodies and the tissues of small children are more sensitive to the damaging effects of lead. Children may have higher exposures since they are more likely to get lead dust on their hands and then put their fingers or other lead-contaminated objects into their mouths.

- **Steps to Reduce Exposure:**
  - Keep areas where children play as dust-free and clean as possible.
  - Leave lead-based paint undisturbed if it is in good condition; do not sand or burn off paint that may contain lead.
  - Do not remove lead paint yourself.
  - Do not bring lead dust into the home.
  - If your work or hobby involves lead, change clothes and use doormats before entering your home.
  - Eat a balanced diet, rich in calcium, iron, and vitamin C. High levels of ascorbic acid (vitamin C) have been associated with a lower rate of elevated blood lead levels.

Carbon Monoxide and Nitrogen Dioxide

Carbon monoxide (CO) gas—which is tasteless, odorless, colorless, and nonirritating—can be deadly. Produced by the incomplete combustion of fuel in space heaters, furnaces, water heaters, and engines, CO reduces the delivery of oxygen in the blood. Every year an estimated 10,000 Americans seek treatment for CO inhalation; at least 250 die because of this silent killer. Those most at risk are the chronically ill, the elderly, pregnant women, and infants.

- **Sources:** Unvented kerosene and gas space heaters; leaking chimneys and furnaces; back-drafting from furnaces, gas water heaters, woodstoves, and fireplaces; gas stoves; automobile exhaust from attached garages.
- **Health Effects:** At low concentrations, fatigue in healthy people and chest pain in people with heart disease. At higher concentrations, impaired vision and coordination; headaches; dizziness; confusion; nausea. Can cause flu-like symptoms that clear up after leaving home. Fatal at very high concentrations.

Another dangerous gas, nitrogen dioxide (NO_2), can reach very high levels if you use a natural gas or propane stove in a poorly ventilated kitchen. This gas may lead to respiratory illnesses. Pilot lights are a steady source of nitrogen dioxide; to reduce exposure, switch to spark ignition.

- **Sources:** Kerosene heaters, unvented gas stoves and heaters.
- **Health Effects:** Eye, nose, and throat irritation. May cause impaired lung function and increased respiratory infections in young children.
- **Steps to Reduce Exposure of Both CO and NO_2:**
  - Keep appliances properly adjusted.
  - Open flues when fireplaces are in use.
  - Do not idle a car inside the garage.

Chemical Risks

Various chemicals, including benzene, asbestos, and arsenic, have been shown to cause cancer in humans. Probable carcinogens include DDT and PCB. Risks can be greatly increased with simultaneous exposures to more than one carcinogen, for example, tobacco smoke and asbestos.[19]

According to the CDC, the levels of potentially harmful chemicals, including pesticides and lead, in Americans' blood have declined. Still, an estimated 50,000 to 70,000 U.S. workers die each year of chronic diseases related to past exposure to toxic substances, including lung cancer, bladder cancer, leukemia, lymphoma, chronic bronchitis, and disorders of the nervous system. **Endocrine disruptors,** chemicals that act as or interfere with human hormones, particularly estrogen, may pose a different threat. Scientists are investigating their impact on fertility, falling sperm counts, and cancers of the reproductive organs. Exposure to toxic chemicals causes about 3 percent of developmental defects.

Agricultural Pesticides

 High quantities of toxic chemical waste from unused or obsolete pesticides are posing a continuing and worsening threat to people and the environment in Eastern Europe, Africa, Asia, the Middle East, and Latin America. In the United States, the FDA estimates that 33 to 39 percent of our food supply contains residues of pesticides that may pose a long-term danger to our health. Scientists have detected traces of pesticides in groundwater in both urban and rural areas. Exposure to pesticides may pose a risk to pregnant women and their unborn children. Men whose jobs routinely expose them to pesticides may be at increased risk of prostate cancer. Parental exposure does not increase the likelihood of childhood brain cancer.

Chlorinated hydrocarbons include several high-risk substances—such as DDT, kepone, and chlordane—that have been restricted or banned because they may cause cancer, birth defects, neurological disorders, and damage to wildlife and the environment. They are extremely resistant to breakdown.

Organophosphates, including chemicals such as malathion, break down more rapidly than the chlorinated hydrocarbons. Most are highly toxic, causing cramps, confusion, diarrhea, vomiting, headaches, and breathing difficulties. Higher levels in the blood can lead to convulsions, paralysis, coma, and death.

Chemical Weapons

Terrorist threats include the possibility of the use of chemical weapons. Possible bioterror agents include poison gases, herbicides, and other types of chemical substances that can kill, maim, or temporarily incapacitate. Chemical agents can be dispersed as liquids, vapors, gases, and aerosols that attack nerves, blood, skin, or lungs. In contrast to biological weapons, chemical weapons can kill rapidly, often within hours or minutes, and sometimes with just a small drop. Possible protection against chemical

© Spencer Grant/PhotoEdit

weapons includes gas masks, shelters, and sealed suits and vehicles. Treatment and antidotes can sometimes help after exposure. If contaminated, you need to flush your eyes and skin immediately for at least five to ten minutes while awaiting emergency help.

Pesticides protect crops from harmful insects, plants, and fungi but may endanger human health.

Multiple Chemical Sensitivity

The proliferation of chemicals in modern society has led to an entirely new disease, **multiple chemical sensitivity (MCS),** also called environmentally triggered illness, universal allergy, or chemical AIDS. MCS was first described almost a half century ago when a Chicago allergist treated a number of patients who reported becoming ill after being exposed to various petrochemicals. Since that time, many more cases of MCS have been reported, yet there is no agreed-upon definition of the condition, no medical test that can diagnose it, and no proven treatment.

According to medical theory, people become chemically sensitive in a two-step process: First, they experience a major exposure to a chemical, such as a pesticide, a solvent, or a combustion product. The sensitized person then begins to react to low-level chemical exposures from ordinary substances, such as perfumes and tobacco smoke. Symptoms include a runny nose, breathing difficulties, memory problems, chest pain, depression, dizziness, fatigue, headache, inability to concentrate, nausea, aches and pains in muscles and joints, and heart palpitations.

endocrine disruptors Synthetic chemicals that interfere with the ways that hormones work in humans and wildlife.

chlorinated hydrocarbons Highly toxic pesticides, such as DDT and chlordane, that are extremely resistant to breakdown; may cause cancer, birth defects, neurological disorders, and damage to wildlife and the environment.

organophosphates Toxic pesticides that may cause cancer, birth defects, neurological disorders, and damage to wildlife and the environment.

multiple chemical sensitivity (MCS) A sensitivity to low-level chemical exposures from ordinary substances, such as perfumes and tobacco smoke, that results in physiological responses such as chest pain, depression, dizziness, fatigue, and nausea. Also known as environmentally triggered illness.

Invisible Threats

Among the unseen threats to health are various forms of *radiation*, energy radiated in the form of waves or particles.

Electromagnetic Fields

Any electrically charged conductor generates two kinds of invisible fields: electric and magnetic. Together they're called **electromagnetic fields (EMFs).** For years, these fields, produced by household appliances, home wiring, lighting fixtures, electric blankets, and overhead power lines, were considered harmless. However, epidemiological studies have revealed a link between exposure to high-voltage lines and cancer (especially leukemia, a blood cancer) in electrical workers and children.

Laboratory studies on animals have shown that alternating current, which changes strength and direction 60 times a second (and electrifies most of North America), emits EMFs that may interfere with the normal functioning of human cell membranes, which have their own electromagnetic fields. The result may be mood disorders, changes in circadian rhythms (our inner sense of time), miscarriage, developmental problems, or cancer. Researchers have documented increases in breast cancer deaths in women who worked as electrical engineers, electricians, or in other high-exposure jobs, and a link between EMF exposure and increased risk of leukemia and possibly brain cancer.

The National Institute of Environmental Health Sciences concluded that the evidence of a risk of cancer and other human disease from the electric and magnetic fields around power lines is "weak." This finding applies to the extremely low frequency electric and magnetic fields surrounding both the big power lines that distribute power and the smaller but closer electric lines in homes and appliances. However, the researchers also noted that EMF exposure "cannot be recognized as entirely safe."

Expectant mothers who often use electric blankets or heated water beds during winter have a higher miscarriage rate than nonusers. Babies conceived in the winter by electric blanket–users grow more slowly in the womb and tend to have a lower birthweight than others. Federal officials urge "prudent avoidance" of electric blankets for women who are pregnant or hoping to conceive.

Cell Phones

Since cellular phone service was introduced in the United States in 1984, mobile and handheld phones have become ubiquitous, and concern has grown about their possible health risks. The federal government sets upper exposure limits to electromagnetic energy from cell phones known as the specific absorption rate, or SAR. A phone emits the most radiation during a call, but it also emits small amounts periodically whenever it's turned on.

Can exposure to low levels of electromagnetic energy that the body absorbs from a cell phone be harmful? More than 70 research papers on the potentially harmful effects of cell phone use have raised concerns about cancer, neurological disorders,

Although laboratory studies on animals indicate that EMFs affect human cell membranes, research on humans has found only a weak connection between EMFs and disease.

© Tony Freeman/PhotoEdit

sleep problems, or headaches; others have shown no association or were inconclusive. The Food and Drug Administration (FDA) and Federal Communications Commission (FCC) have stated that "the available scientific evidence does not show that any health problems are associated with using wireless phones. There is no proof, however, that wireless phones are absolutely safe." Additional studies are underway.

Researchers have documented an increase in ear canal temperature with cell phone use, protein changes in human cells exposed to cell phone radiation, and an increased rate of benign brain tumors. Other research found no impact on the daily patterns of hormones secreted by the gonads, pituitary, or adrenal glands in men.[20] Some health experts have discouraged children from using cell phones largely because of concerns that their developing nervous systems may be especially vulnerable.

As discussed in Chapter 18, cell phones do pose one serious health risk. Drivers distracted by cell phones are more likely to get into accidents and to hit—and kill—pedestrians.[21]

Microwaves

Microwaves (extremely high frequency electromagnetic waves) increase the rate at which molecules vibrate; this vibration generates heat. There's no evidence that existing levels of microwave radiation encountered in the environment pose a health risk to people, and all home microwave ovens must meet safety standards for leakage.

A concern about the safety of microwave ovens stems from the chemicals in plastic wrapping and plastic containers used in microwave ovens. Chemicals may leak into food. In high concentrations, some of the chemicals (such as DEHA, which makes plastic more pliable) can cause cancer in mice. Consumers should be cautious about using clingy plastic wrap when reheating leftovers, and plastic-encased metal "heat susceptors" included in convenience foods such as popcorn and pizza. Although these materials seem safe when tested in conventional ovens at temperatures of 300° to 350° Fahrenheit, microwave ovens can boost temperatures to 500° Fahrenheit.

Ionizing Radiation

Radiation that possesses enough energy to separate electrons from their atoms, leaving charged ions, is called **ionizing radiation.** Its effects on health depend on many factors, including the amount, length of exposure, type, part of the body exposed, and the health and age of the individual.

We're surrounded by low-level ionizing radiation every day. Most comes from cosmic rays and radioactive minerals, which vary according to geography. (Denver has more than Atlanta, for instance, because of its altitude.) Man-made sources, including medical and dental X-rays, account for approximately 18 percent of the average person's lifetime exposure.

Radiation exposure in humans is measured in units called rads and rems. A *rad (radiation absorbed dose)* is a measure of the energy deposited by ionizing radiation when it's absorbed by an object. A *rem (roentgen equivalent man)* is a measure of the biological effect of ionizing radiation. Different types of radiation cause different amounts of damage. The rem measurement takes this into account. For X-rays, rads and rems are equivalent. A quantity of 1 rad or 1 rem is a substantial dose of radiation. Smaller doses are measured in *millirads (thousandths of a rad)* or *millirems (thousandths of a rem).* The average annual radiation exposure for a person in the United States is about one-tenth of a rem.

Diagnostic X-Rays The EPA estimates that 30 to 50 percent of the 700 million X-rays taken every year in the United States are unnecessary. However, doctors sometimes prescribe X-rays or newer imaging techniques involving radiation, such as CT scans, to protect themselves from malpractice suits, and hospitals benefit financially from the heavy use of X-ray equipment.

Dental X-rays involve little radiation, but many people receive so many so often that they're second only to chest examinations in frequency. Dentists typically obtain radiographs of all the teeth at the beginning of a patient's care, and again every three to five years. However, you can cut down on total X-rays by bringing previous films with you or having your dentist forward copies when you switch dentists.

electromagnetic fields (EMFs) The invisible electric and magnetic fields generated by an electrically charged conductor.

microwaves Extremely high frequency electromagnetic waves that increase the rate at which molecules vibrate, thereby generating heat.

ionizing radiation A form of energy emitted from atoms as they undergo internal change.

Always ask why an X-ray is being ordered. Don't give your consent unless there's a clear need. Keep a record of the date and location of every X-ray exam. Some of these X-rays may someday provide information that would make more X-rays unnecessary. Ask the radiologist to explain specifically how much radiation you'll be exposed to, and be sure to wear a protective leaded apron. There's no sense in refusing a needed medical X-ray just because you're afraid of the radiation exposure. Under certain circumstances, the benefits far outweigh the risks.

Irradiated Foods   The use of radiation on food, from either radioactive substances or devices that produce X-rays, is known as **irradiation.** It doesn't make the food radioactive—its primary benefit is to prolong the food's useful life. Like the heat in canning, irradiation can kill all the microorganisms that might grow in food; the sterilized food can then be stored for years in sealed containers at room temperature without spoiling. In addition, low-dose irradiation can inhibit the sprouting of vegetables such as potatoes and onions, and delay the ripening of some fruits, such as bananas, mangoes, tomatoes, pears, and avocados—cost-saving benefits of great appeal to the food industry.

Irradiated foods are believed to be safe to eat, and the federal government has approved their distribution. Most research has focused on low-dose irradiation to delay ripening and destroy insects. Nutritional studies have shown no significant decreases in the quality of the foods, but high-dose treatments may cause vitamin losses similar to those that occur during canning. It's also possible that the ionizing effect of radiation creates new compounds in foods that may be mutagenic or carcinogenic. In meats, irradiation proved less effective than cooking in destroying bacteria.

Your Hearing Health

Besides listening to the music at your next concert, tune into the noise level and how your ears are feeling.

Hearing loss is the third-most common chronic health problem, after high blood pressure and arthritis, among older Americans. Noise-induced hearing loss is the most frequent preventable disability. Nearly 22 million Americans between ages 20 and 69 have irreversibly damaged hearing because of excessive noise exposure.[22] Loud noises cause hearing loss in an estimated 10 million Americans every year. Only about one-fifth of the 28 million Americans suffering from hearing loss have sought professional help.

How Loud Is That Noise?

Loudness, or the intensity of a sound, is measured in **decibels (dB).** A whisper is 20 decibels; a conversation in a living room is about 50 decibels. On this scale, 50 isn't two and a half times louder than 20, but 1,000 times louder: Each 10-dB rise in the scale represents a tenfold increase in the intensity of the sound. Very loud but short bursts of sounds (such as gunshots and fireworks) and quieter but longer-lasting sounds (such as power tools) can induce hearing loss.

Sounds under 75 dB don't seem harmful. However, prolonged exposure to any sound over 85 dB (the equivalent of a power mower

© iStockphoto.com/Robert Kohlhuber

or food blender) or brief exposure to louder sounds can harm hearing. The noise level at rock concerts can reach 110 to 140 dB, about as loud as an air raid siren. Personal sound systems (boom boxes) can blast sounds of up to 115 dB. Cars with extremely loud music systems, known as boom cars, can produce an earsplitting 145 dB—louder than a jet engine or thunderclap (Figure 19.3).

Common "sound offenders" are nightclubs (with sustained levels of well over 100 decibels), restaurants (with levels of 80 to 96 decibels), and street traffic (80 decibels or more). However, even low-level office noise can undermine well-being and increase health risks.

Effects of Noise

Noise-induced hearing loss is 100 percent preventable—and irreversible. Hearing aids are the only treatment, but they do not correct the problem; they just amplify sound to compensate for hearing loss.

The healthy human ear can hear sounds within a wide range of frequencies (measured in hertz), from the low-frequency rumble of thunder at 50 hertz to the high-frequency overtones of a piccolo at nearly 20,000 hertz. High-frequency noise damages the delicate hair cells that serve as sound receptors in the inner ear. Damage first begins as a diminished sensitivity to frequencies around 4,000 hertz, the highest notes of a piano.

Early symptoms of hearing loss include difficulty understanding speech and *tinnitus* (ringing in the ears). Brief, very loud sounds, such as an explosion or gunfire, can produce immediate, severe, and permanent hearing loss. Longer exposure to less intense but still hazardous sounds, such as those common at work or in public places, can gradually impair hearing, often without the individual's awareness.

Decibels	Example	Zone
0	The softest sound a typical ear can hear	Safe
10 dB	Just audible	
20 dB	Watch ticking; leaves rustling	
30 dB	Soft whisper at 16 feet	
40 dB	Quiet office; suburban street (no traffic)	
50 dB	Interior of typical urban home; rushing stream	1,000 times louder than 20 dB
60 dB	Normal conversation; busy office	
70 dB	Vacuum cleaner at 10 feet; hair dryer	
80 dB	Alarm clock at 2 feet; loud music; average daily traffic	1,000 times louder than 50 dB
90 dB*	Motorcycle at 25 feet; jet 4 miles after takeoff	Risk of injury
100 dB*	Video arcade; loud factory; subway train	
110 dB*	Car horn at 3 feet; symphony orchestra; chain saw	1,000 times louder than 80 dB
120 dB	Jackhammer at 3 feet; boom box; nearby thunderclap	Injury
130 dB	Rock concert; jet engine at 100 feet	
140 dB	Jet engine nearby; amplified car stereo; firearms	1,000 times louder than 110 dB

Figure 19.3 Louder and Louder

The human ear perceives a 10-decibel increase as a doubling of loudness. Thus, the 100 decibels of a subway train sound much more than twice as loud as the 50 decibels of a rushing stream.

*Note: The maximum exposure allowed on the job by federal law, in hours per day: 90 decibels, 8 hours; 100 decibels, 2 hours; 110 decibels, 1/2 hour.

Conductive hearing loss, often caused by ear infections, cuts down on perception of low-pitched sounds. Sensorineural loss involves damage or destruction of the sensory cells in the inner ear that convert sound waves to nerve signals.

Noise can harm more than our ears: High-volume sound has been linked to high blood pressure and other stress-related problems that can lead to heart disease, insomnia, anxiety, headaches, colitis, and ulcers. Noise frays the nerves; people tend to be more anxious, irritable, and angry when their ears are constantly barraged with sound.

Ear canal
Ear bones (Ossicles)
Hearing canal (Cochlea)

Earbud insert headphone

Eardrum (Tympanic membrane)

irradiation Exposure to or treatment by some form of radiation.

decibel (dB) A unit for measuring the intensity of sounds.

Are Earbuds Hazardous to Hearing?

Although there is limited research, audiologists (who specialize in hearing problems) report seeing greater noise-induced hearing loss in young people. One probable culprit is extended use of earbuds, tiny earphones used with portable music players that deliver sound extremely close to the eardrum. Hearing loss can be temporary or permanent.

The dangers to your hearing depend on how loud the music is and how long you listen. Because personal music players have long-lasting rechargeable batteries, people—especially young ones—both listen for long periods and turn up the volume because they feel "low personal vulnerability" to hearing loss.[23] As long as the sound level is within safety levels (see Figure 19.3), you can listen as long as you'd like. If you listen to music so loud that someone else can hear it two or three feet away, it's too loud.

For safe listening, limit listening to a portable music player with earphones or earbuds at 60 percent of its potential volume to one hour a day. At the very least, take a five-minute break after an hour of listening and keep the volume low.

Ask yourself the following questions to determine if you should have your hearing checked:

- Do you frequently have to ask people to repeat themselves?
- Do you have difficulty hearing when someone speaks in a whisper?
- Do people complain that you turn up the volume too much when watching television or listening to music?

YOUR STRATEGIES FOR PREVENTION
How to Protect Your Ears

- If you must live or work in a noisy area, wear hearing protectors to prevent exposure to blasts of very loud noise. Don't think cotton or facial tissue stuck in your ears can protect you; foam or soft plastic earplugs are more effective. Wear them when operating lawn mowers, weed trimmers, or power tools.
- Give your ears some quiet time. Rather than turning up the volume on your personal music player to blot out noise, look for truly quiet environments, such as the library, where you can rest your ears and focus your mind.
- Soundproof your home by using draperies, carpets, and bulky furniture. Put rubber mats under washing machines, blenders, and other noisy appliances. Seal cracks around windows and doors.
- Beware of large doses of aspirin. Researchers have found that eight aspirin tablets a day can aggravate the damage caused by loud noise; twelve a day can cause ringing in the ears (tinnitus).
- Don't drink in noisy environments. Alcohol intensifies the impact of noise and increases the risk of lifelong hearing damage.
- When you hear a sudden loud noise, press your fingers against your ears. Limit your exposure to loud noise. Several brief periods of noise seem less damaging than one long exposure.

- Do you have difficulty following conversation in a noisy environment?
- Do you avoid groups of people because of hearing difficulty?
- Have your friends or family suggested you might have hearing loss?

LEARN IT LIVE IT Taking Care of Mother Earth

Environmental problems can seem so complex that you may think there's little you can do about them. That's not the case. This world can be made better instead of worse. The job isn't easy, and all of us have to do our part. Just as many diseases of the previous century have been eradicated, so in time we may be able to remove or reduce many environmental threats. Your future—and our planet's future—may depend on it.

- **Plant a tree.** Even a single tree helps absorb carbon dioxide and produces cooling that can reduce the need for air conditioning.

- **Limit your driving.** If you usually drive to campus, check out alternatives, such as carpooling and public or campus transportation.
- **Precycle.** Surf the web for sites that sell products made from recycled materials, Click on **http://www.ecomall.com/** for listings.
- **Save the juice.** Plug your appliances and e-gadgets, which drain electricity even when turned off, into a power strip. Whenever you leave, flicking off the switch effectively unplugs them.

- **Integrate a new "green" habit into your life every week.** Turn the thermostat down in winter and up in summer. Spend a few minutes less in the shower. Use both sides of printer paper. Once a week declare a "spare the air" day, and don't drive.

- **Avoid disposables.** Use a mug instead of a paper or Styrofoam cup, a sponge instead of a paper towel, a cloth napkin instead of a paper one.

- **Recycle.** Buy products made from recycled materials. Shop for used furniture or clothing. Don't throw away anything someone else may be able to use.

- **Be water wise.** Turn off the tap while you shave or brush your teeth. Install water-efficient faucets, toilets, and shower heads. Wash clothes in cold water. Drink tap rather than bottled water.

- **Cancel junk mail.** It consumes 100 million trees a year. To get off mailing lists, write: Direct Mail Association, Mail Preference Service, P.O. Box 9008, Farmingdale, NY 11735-9008.

- **Spare the seas.** If you live near the coast or are picnicking or hiking near the ocean, don't use plastic bags (which are often blown into the water) or plastic six-pack holders (which can get caught around the necks of sea birds).

SELF SURVEY Are You Doing Your Part for the Planet?

You may think that there is little you can do, as an individual, to save Earth. But everyday acts can add up and make a difference in helping or harming the planet on which we live.

	Almost Never	Sometimes	Always
1. Do you walk, cycle, carpool, or use public transportation as much as possible to get around?	____	____	____
2. Do you recycle?	____	____	____
3. Do you reuse plastic and paper bags?	____	____	____
4. Do you try to conserve water by not running the tap as you shampoo or brush your teeth?	____	____	____
5. Do you use products made of recycled materials?	____	____	____
6. Do you drive a car that gets good fuel mileage and has up-to-date emission control equipment?	____	____	____
7. Do you turn off lights, televisions, and appliances when you're not using them?	____	____	____
8. Do you avoid buying products that are elaborately packaged?	____	____	____
9. Do you use glass jars and waxed paper rather than plastic wrap for storing food?	____	____	____
10. Do you take brief showers rather than baths?	____	____	____
11. Do you use cloth towels and napkins rather than paper products?	____	____	____
12. When listening to music, do you keep the volume low?	____	____	____
13. Do you try to avoid any potential carcinogens, such as asbestos, mercury, or benzene?	____	____	____
14. Are you careful to dispose of hazardous materials (such as automobile oil or antifreeze) at appropriate sites?	____	____	____
15. Do you follow environmental issues in your community and write your state or federal representatives to support "green" legislation?	____	____	____

Count the number of items you've checked in each column. If you've circled 10 or more in the "always" column, you're definitely helping to make a difference. If you've mainly circled "sometimes," you're moving in the right direction, but you need to be more consistent and more conscientious. If you've circled 10 or more in the "never" column, carefully read this chapter and "Your Health Action Plan for Protecting the Planet" to find out what you can do.

Your Health Action Plan for Protecting the Planet

Simple steps can help save energy, lower carbon dioxide (CO_2) emissions, and cut down on energy costs. Here are some recommendations from the Environmental Defense and World Wildlife Fund:

- Wash laundry in warm or cold water, not hot. *Average annual CO_2 reduction: up to 500 pounds for two loads of laundry a week.*

- Buy products sold in the simplest possible packaging. Carry a tote bag or recycle shopping bags. *Average annual CO_2 reduction: 1,000 pounds because garbage is reduced 25 percent.*

- Switch from standard light bulbs to energy-efficient fluorescent ones. *Average annual CO_2 reduction: about 500 pounds per bulb.*

- Set room thermostats lower in winter and higher in summer. *Average annual CO_2 reduction: about 500 pounds for each two-degree reduction.*

- Run dishwashers only when full, and choose the energy-saving mode rather than the regular setting. *Average annual CO_2 reduction: 200 pounds.*

- Bike, carpool, or take mass transit whenever possible. *Average annual CO_2 reduction: 20 pounds for each gallon of gasoline saved.*

- Drive a car that gets high gas mileage and produces low emissions. Keep your speed at or below the speed limit.

- Keep your tires inflated and your engine tuned. Recycle old batteries and tires. (Most stores that sell new ones will take back old ones.)

- Turn off your engine if you're going to be stopped for more than a minute.

- Collect all fluids that you drain from your car (motor oil, antifreeze) and recycle or properly dispose of them.

CENGAGENOW If you want to write your own goals for working toward a healthy environment, go to the Wellness Journal at CengageNOW for Health: **www.cengage.com/sso**

Review Questions

1. Which of the following statements about climate change is *true*?
   a. Increasing carbon dioxide production will slow the progress of global warming.
   b. Most experts say that the buildup of greenhouse gases is changing natural climate and weather patterns.
   c. Climate change poses no health risks for humans in the next 20 years.
   d. Increasing tree cover and agricultural lands will contribute to global warming.

2. An example of the concept of sustainability is
   a. getting enough to eat at every meal.
   b. lowering the price of gas to 1990 levels.
   c. using wind power to generate electricity.
   d. maintaining our current levels of energy usage.

3. Mutagens
   a. are caused by birth defects.
   b. result in changes to the DNA of body cells.
   c. are agents that trigger changes in the DNA of body cells.
   d. are caused by repeated exposure to pollutants.

4. Drinking water safety
   a. may be compromised if your water comes from a well.
   b. is low in the United States because of chemical treatment.
   c. can be guaranteed by using bottled water, which is completely free of chemical contaminants.
   d. is measured by the cases of illness reported each year.

5. Threats to the environment include
   a. an open ecosystem.
   b. depletion of the oxygen layer.
   c. ecological processes.
   d. global warming.

6. Pesticide risks to health include
   a. reduced male fertility.
   b. higher incidence of childhood brain cancer if parents have been exposed.
   c. higher incidence of cancer and birth defects from chlorinated hydrocarbons such as DDT.
   d. higher incidence of diabetes.

7. One of the most important things you can do to help protect the environment is
   a. use as much water as possible to help lower the ocean water levels.
   b. recycle paper, bottles, cans, and unwanted food.
   c. avoid energy-depleting fluorescent bulbs.
   d. use plastic storage containers and plastic wrap to save trees from being cut down.

8. Precycling is
   a. planning ahead about recycling.
   b. buying products packaged in recycled material.
   c. removing excess packaging and leaving it in the store where an item was purchased.
   d. preparing to recycle.

9. You can protect your hearing by
   a. avoiding prolonged exposure to sounds under 75 decibels.
   b. using foam earplugs when operating noisy tools or attending rock concerts.
   c. limiting noise exposure to short bursts of loud sounds such as fireworks.
   d. drinking alcohol in noisy environments to mute the sounds.

10. Which of the following statements about air pollution is *false*?
    a. More than 80 percent of the people in the United States live in counties with unhealthy levels of ozone or particle pollution.
    b. Ozone in the upper atmosphere protects us from harmful ultraviolet radiation from the sun, but in the lower atmosphere, it is a harmful air pollutant.
    c. Air pollution can cause the same types of respiratory health problems as smoking.
    d. Particle pollution diminishes lung function and increases the severity of asthma attacks.

Answers to these questions can be found on page 650.

Critical Thinking

1. How do you contribute to environmental pollution? How might you change your habits to protect the environment?

2. An excerpt from a recent newspaper article stated, "Children living in a public housing project near a local refinery suffer from a high rate of asthma and allergies, and an environmental group says the plant may be to blame." The refinery has met all the local air quality standards, employs hundreds in the community, and pays substantial city taxes, which support police, fire, and social services. If you were a city council member, how would you balance health and environmental concerns with the need for industry in your community? What actions would you recommend in this particular situation?

3. In one Harris poll, 84 percent of Americans said that, given a choice between a high standard of living (but with hazardous air and water pollution and the depletion of natural resources) and a lower standard of living (but with clean air and drinking water), they would prefer clean air and drinking water and a lower standard of living. What about you? What exactly would you be willing to give up: air conditioning, convenience packaging and products, driving your own car rather than using public transportation? Do you think most people are willing to change their lifestyles to preserve the environment?

Media Menu

Internet Connections

www.envirolink.org
Envirolink is a nonprofit organization that brings together individuals and groups concerned about the environment and provides access to a wealth of online environmental resources.

www.seac.org
Since 1988, the Student Environmental Action Coalition has been empowering students and youth to fight for environmental and social justice in our schools and communities.

www.campusclimatechallenge.org
The Challenge leverages the power of young people to organize on college campuses and high schools across Canada and the United States to win 100% Clean Energy policies at their schools.

www.stopglobalwarming.org
This site is a nonpartisan effort to bring citizens together to declare that global warming is here now and that it is time to demand solutions.

www.cdc.gov/nceh/
This site, sponsored by the U.S. Centers for Disease Control and Prevention, features a searchable database as well as fact sheets and brochures on a variety of environmental topics, from emergency preparedness and public health tracking to environmental hazards and lead poisoning prevention.

Key Terms

The terms listed are used on the page indicated. Definitions of the terms are in the Glossary at the end of the book.

carcinogen 603
chlorinated hydrocarbons 613
decibel (dB) 617
ecosystem 599
electromagnetic fields (EMFs) 615
endocrine disruptors 613
ionizing radiation 615
irradiation 617
microwaves 615
multiple chemical sensitivity (MCS) 613
mutagen 603
organophosphates 613
ozone 603
pollutant 603
precycling 605
recycling 605
sustainability 605

Chapter 20 -   A Lifetime of Health

1. All of the following but one are benefits of physical exercise performed by older people: (pg 629)
   - A. reduced risks of falls
   - B. greater ability to live more independently
   - C. increased blood pressure from physical activity
   - D. improvement in mood and feelings

2. Typical loss of memory functions includes all of the following except: (pg 630)
   - A. recall of information
   - B. verbal intelligence
   - C. multitasking
   - D. remembering people's names

3. Individuals who have which of the following are said to have a higher level of cognitive functioning into old age: (pg 631)
   - A. higher education
   - B. musically inclined
   - C. artistically talented
   - D. active physical fitness lifestyle

4. A woman is considered to have reached her menopause when she has: (pg 631)
   - A. no menstrual periods for six months
   - B. no menstrual periods for twelve straight months
   - C. not had any irregular menstrual cycles for 1 year prior to her last period
   - D. higher levels of estrogen in her blood

5. Many older men at midlife begin to experience andropause which is characterized by: (pg 633)
   - A. harder and longer lasting erections during sexual activity
   - B. impaired virility due to decreases in testosterone production
   - C. constriction of the urethra by the prostate
   - D. hot flashes similar to what older women experience

6. The most common nutritional disorder in older people is: (pg 630)
   - A. heart disease
   - B. anorexia
   - C. vitamin deficiency
   - D. obesity

7. The top risk factor for someone to develop Alzheimer's disease is: (pg 634)
   - A. cigarette smoking
   - B. excessive alcohol abuse
   - C. obesity
   - D. age

8. Which of the following statements about aging is false? (pg 635)
   - A. muscle strengths in the 20s and then begins to deteriorate
   - B. bones and joints become more brittle and arthritic
   - C. digestive enzymes increase in production to aid in digestion
   - D. the body is less resistant in fighting off foreign pathogens

9. Which of the following is true about older people developing osteoporosis? (pg 636)
   - A. smaller petite women are more likely to develop osteoporosis
   - B. only women can develop osteoporosis
   - C. African American women have the highest incidence of osteoporosis
   - D. osteoporosis only begins after women have gone through their menopause

10. An advance directive that you may write when terminally ill or dying is to express your: (pg 637)
   - A. wishes on how your property should be divided upon your death
   - B. views on how you want to be buried after you die
   - C. needs for medical treatment in case of a medical crisis
   - D. request for someone to make medical decisions on your behalf when you are

not of sound mind

11. **An advance directive known as DNR stands for: (pg 638)**
    A. do not revive
    B. department of natural resources
    C. do not resuscitate
    D. dead not returnable

12. **If you were to suddenly die and did not have a last will made out to determine who will receive your possessions, this is known as: (pg 638)**
    A. death will
    B. intestate
    C. non-estate disposal
    D. holographic determination

13. **A will written in your own handwriting and unwitnessed is called a(n): (pg 638)**
    A. testator last wishes
    B. donor's will
    C. holographic will
    D. intestate will

14. **When there is no indication of brain functioning in a deceased victim, this is known as: (pg 641)**
    A. cellular death
    B. functional death
    C. spiritual death
    D. brain death

15. **All of the following are examples of medically defined death of an individual except: (pg 641)**
    A. spiritual death
    B. cellular death
    C. brain death
    D. functional death

16. **Predict what the first reaction would be of a patient who learns she has terminal cancer: (pg 642)**
    A. anger
    B. denial
    C. bargaining
    D. depression

17. **It is suggested that one of the most difficult stages of the dying process for the patient to endure through is the: (pg 642)**
    A. anger
    B. depression
    C. denial
    D. acceptance

18. **Some people who have undergone near-death experiences and reported an autoscopic happening were describing: (pg 644)**
    A. transitory feeling of fear or confusion
    B. hovering over their body and watching it be resuscitated
    C. the movement into another dimension
    D. seeing light at the end of a tunnel

19. **After Carol's husband died, she experienced a loss of appetite, an inability to sleep at night, and not able to concentrate. She is experiencing what is known as: (pg 647)**
    A. grief
    B. denial
    C. mourning
    D. depression

20. **When preparing for a medical crisis with a family member, it is wise to do which of the following: (pg 649)**
    A. involve the person's personal physician in decision making
    B. investigate alternative living situations
    C. focus on values and what is important to the family member
    D. all of the above

Verena didn't feel old until she enrolled in a college personal health course. Formal at first, the other students—young enough to be her children—started calling her "Mom." When the professor announced that the next week's topic would be aging, Verena beamed, "I'll be the expert!"

More of us can expect to say the same. In the United States, the number of people over age 65 is expected to increase from 12 to nearly 20 percent of the population—an estimated 71.5 million in 2030.[1]

A Lifetime of Health

Although **aging**—the characteristic pattern of normal life changes that occurs as humans, plants, and animals grow older—remains inevitable, you can do a great deal to influence the impact that the passage of time has on you. Whether you're in your teens, twenties, thirties, or older, now is the time to take the steps that will add healthy, active, productive years to your life.

This chapter provides a preview of the changes age brings, the steps you can take to age healthfully, and the ways you can make the most of all the years of your life.

Invariably, though, no one gets out of this life alive. Death is the natural completion of things, as much a part of the real world as life itself. In time we all lose people we cherish: grandparents, aunts and uncles, parents, friends, neighbors, coworkers, siblings. With each loss, part of us may seem to die, yet each loss also reaffirms how precious life is. (See Making Change Happen, p. 624, and "Finity" in *Labs for IPC*.)

This chapter explores the meaning of death, describes the process of dying, provides information on end-of-life issues, and offers advice on comforting the dying and helping their survivors.

> After studying the material in this chapter, you should be able to

- **List** the benefits that older Americans can gain from physical activity.
- **Name** three memory skills that diminish with age.
- **Discuss** the hormonal changes that occur in men and women at midlife.
- **Name** two challenges of aging and **discuss** their risk factors and possible ways of preventing them.
- **Explain** the purposes of advance directives.
- **Define** death and **explain** the stages of emotional reaction experienced in facing death.
- **Name** a chapter topic that affects someone in your family, and **discuss** how your knowledge and attitude on the topic have changed.

aging The characteristic pattern of normal life changes that occur as living things grow older.

Log on to CengageNOW for Health at **www.cengage.com/sso** to find your Behavior Change Planner and to explore self-assessments, interactive tutorials, and practice quizzes.

623

Finding Life's Meaning

If you're in your teens, twenties, or thirties, aging and death seem remote, even unimaginable. That's normal. But whatever your age, coming to terms with the stark reality that life is not infinite—that it must end—can give greater meaning to your days.

The lab "Finity" in *Labs for IPC,* based on the Stages of Change discussed in Chapter 1 of this text and in *IPC,* celebrates living as fully, as richly, as joyfully as possible. By making smart choices every day, you can do a great deal to ensure that you live longer. By making conscious, creative choices, you also can ensure that your life is more enjoyable, meaningful, and fulfilling.

Get Real

In this section, you take a comprehensive inventory of your life so far. You begin with the Satisfaction with Life Scale, a reliable indicator of how individuals perceive their personal happiness. Using a scale of 7 (strongly agree) to 1 (strongly disagree), you respond to five statements, including:

- In most ways my life is close to my ideal.
- If I could live my life over, I would change almost nothing.

You also answer yes or no to 23 questions about the last 24 hours of your life, including:

- Did you look at the sky?
- Did you taste something absolutely yummy?
- Did you make someone smile?

Social psychology has identified the key components of a fulfilling, happy, high-quality life. You can see how yours compares by assessing:

- Your close relationships.
- Your sense of spirituality or a higher purpose.
- Your positive qualities.
- Your engagement with a passionate pursuit—for family, work, sport, or other experiences—that adds great satisfaction to your life.

Get Ready

In this section you block out time for the experiential exercises this lab requires in the action stage.

Get Going

You review a list of 25 adjectives, including descriptives such as:

- Cheerful.
- Mean-spirited.
- Hard-working.
- Whiny.

You pick one adjective that you want to describe you (or one that you want to erase from any description of you), and weave appropriate behaviors into your actions that day. You work with a "signature behavior" that you'd like to have associated with you.

- You make up a life list of the things you want to do before you die and do a series of imaginative and creative activities with goals you'd like to accomplish, experiences you'd like to have, things you don't want to regret . . .
- In your *IPC Journal* you develop an outline for your life—past, present, and future—with . . .

Lock It In

Living a life fully requires paying attention each and every day. In this section, you develop and deepen simple practices to ensure that you do so, such as:

- **Make your day.** Record in your *IPC Journal* the nicest thing that happened. It might be as small as a bus driver's hearty hello or a "Well done!" on an assignment, or as big as making a team, acing a final exam, or hearing a longed-for "I love you."

The Aging of America

About one in eight Americans—approximately 12 percent of the population—is over age 65. With millions of baby boomers reaching retirement age, one in every five Americans will be older than 65 by the year 2030. (See Figure 20.1.)[2]

 Older Americans are as diverse as other segments of our population. About one in five (19 percent) comes from a minority group.

The largest percentage of these are African American (9 percent) or Hispanic (6 percent). Asians or Pacific Islanders make up about 3 percent of older Americans.[3]

About three in four older Americans describe their health as good or better. Older African Americans, American Indians/Alaska Natives, and Hispanics are less likely to say they are in top health than are whites. Most older people have at least one chronic condition; many have several health problems. Women report more arthritis; men, more heart disease and cancer.[4]

How Long Can You Expect to Live?

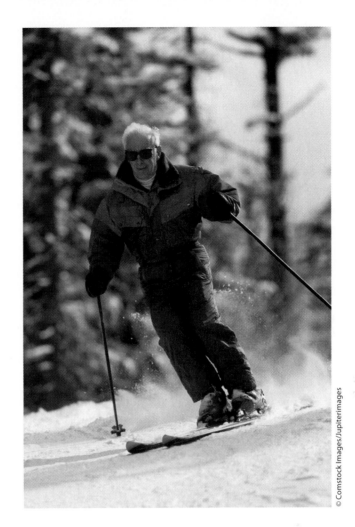

The answer depends on you. Statistically, you're likely to live longer than your parents or grandparents. Life expectancy has been increasing steadily over the last century, reaching an all-time high in the United States of 77.6 years. According to the National Center for Health Statistics, life expectancy for American women now stands at 80.4 years; for men, it is a record high of 75.2 years.

Researchers are identifying certain markers, such as the length of the telomere (the segment of DNA that occurs at the ends of chromosomes) in white blood cells, that may predict how well individuals are aging and how long they might live.[5] However, contrary to common belief, heredity doesn't determine how long you'll live or how well you'll age. Genes, as studies of identical twins have revealed, influence only about 30 percent of the rate and ways in which we age.

© Comstock Images/Jupiterimages

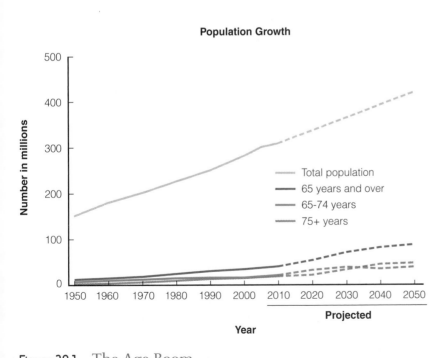

Figure 20.1 The Age Boom

The baby boomers (those born between 1946 and 1964) will start turning 65 in 2011, and the number of older people will increase dramatically. The older population in 2030 is projected to be twice as large as in 2000.

The Longevity Gender Gap

Women's lifespans average 5 to 10 percent longer than men's. No one knows exactly why. This longevity gender gap has been shrinking since 1990 and now stands at 5.2 years. Women in other developed nations—Australia, Canada, France, Greece, Italy, Japan, the Netherlands, Norway, Spain, Sweden, Switzerland—live up to two years longer than those in the United States and about seven years longer than men. In the former Soviet Union, life expectancy for females is 13 years longer than for males.

Why do men die sooner? The female edge may begin at conception with the extra X chromosome, which provides a backup for defects on the X gene and a double dose of the genetic factors that regulate the immune system. In addition, the female hormone estrogen bolsters immunity and protects heart, bone, brain, and blood vessels.

In some cancers, estrogen may somehow protect against distant metastases.

In contrast, testosterone may dampen the immune response in males—possibly to prevent attacks on sperm cells that might otherwise be mistaken as alien invaders. When the testes are removed from mice and guinea pigs, their immune systems become more active. In men, lessened immunity may lower resistance to cancer as well as infectious disease.

Testosterone also has been implicated in men's risk of heart disease and stroke. Originally designed to equip men with an instantaneous burst of power—essential for survival in Stone Age times—this potent male hormone may surge so intensely that it wreaks havoc throughout the cardiovascular system.

Males also die more often as a result of intentional and nonintentional injury. Overall, men are three times more likely than women to die in accidents, mainly in cars and on the job. Men also are four times more likely to die violently. Nine in ten murderers and eight in ten murder victims are men.

Successful Aging

Americans are living better as well as longer. Disability decreased steadily through the 1980s and 1990s, and the rate of improvement is accelerating. Nursing home use has fallen. Senior citizens are healthier and more independent.

According to research on "exceptional longevity" (survival to at least age 90), the key factors to living long and well are maintaining a healthy lifestyle (including regular exercise, weight management, and no smoking) and avoiding or delaying chronic illnesses.[6] Among the growing number of "centenarians" who live past their hundredth birthday, two-thirds did not develop age-related conditions such as diabetes, dementia, heart disease, osteoporosis, Parkinson's disease, or stroke until age 85 or older. In one recent study of this age group, the men who made it to the century mark had significantly better mental and physical functioning than women their age.[7]

When surveyed, about half of Americans age 65 to 69 say, "These are the best years of my life." Many people in their seventies and eighties agree. Sixty percent of older black and 57 percent of older Hispanic respondents say these are their best years. When asked about the keys to a meaningful and vital life, older adults rate having family and friends and taking care of their health as most important, followed by spiritual life. (See Reality Check, p. 627.)

Physical Activity: It's Never Too Late

The effects of ongoing activity are so profound that gerontologists sometimes refer to exercise as "the closest thing to an anti-aging pill." Exercise slows many changes associated with advancing age, such as loss of lean muscle tissue, increase in body fat, and decreased work capacity.[8]

The benefits of exercise extend to both men and women. In one recent study of healthy older men, regular exercise was associated with a nearly 30 percent lower mortality rate. In a study of overweight, postmenopausal women, exercise improved physical and mental well-being—and the more the women exercised, the greater the improvements in their quality of life.[9] In other research on Canadian women older than 65, those who took part in regular aerobic activity had higher scores of cognitive function than their sedentary peers.[10] The bottom line: What you *don't* do may matter more than what you do.

No one is ever too old to get in shape. The American College of Sports Medicine encourages seniors to engage in the full range of physical activities, including aerobic conditioning. With regular conditioning, 60-year-olds can regain the fitness they had at age 40 to 45. Adults over the age of 72 who exercise more and smoke less than their peers are most likely to enjoy long, healthy, and happy lives, according to a study that followed 1,000 seniors for nine years.

Exercise lowers the risk of diabetes, heart disease, and stroke in the elderly—and greatly improves general health.[11] Male and female runners over age 50 have much lower rates of disability and much lower health-care expenses than less active seniors. Even less-intense activities, such as gardening, dancing, and brisk walking, can delay chronic physical disability and cognitive decline.

According to the U.S. surgeon general, physical activity offers older Americans additional benefits, including the following:

- Greater ability to live independently.
- Reduced risk of falling and fracturing bones.
- Lower risk of dying from coronary heart disease and of developing high blood pressure, colon cancer, and diabetes.
- Reduced blood pressure in some people with hypertension.
- Fewer symptoms of anxiety and depression.
- Improvements in mood and feelings of well-being.

Despite these potential benefits, many seniors are not active. By age 75, about one in three men and one in two women engage in no physical activity. Yet even sedentary individuals in their eighties and nineties

✓ REALITYCHECK

- *Do you think the following statements are true or false?*
- *Happiness usually peaks in young adulthood and declines throughout life.* _____
- *The happiest Americans are older than age 50.* _____

Answers on next page.

© Deddeda/Design Pics/Jupiterimages

Age is partly a matter of attitude and zest for life.

can participate in an exercise program—and gain significant benefits.

At any age, staying fit doesn't have to be expensive. (See Health on a Budget.) Older adults who take part in low-cost fitness programs offered by YMCAs or senior centers have shown significant improvement in their daily functioning and lower risk of becoming disabled.[12]

The American College of Sports Medicine and American Heart Association recommend developing a fitness plan with a health professional to manage risks and take health conditions into account. Its basics should consist of:

- Moderately intense aerobic exercise 30 minutes a day, five days a week

  or

- Vigorously intense aerobic exercise 20 minutes a day, three days a week

  and

- 8 to 10 strength-training exercise, with 10 to 15 repetitions of each exercise, two or three times a week

  and

- balance exercises.

PART 2: *Just the Facts*
- **False.** *Happiness typically declines through adolescence and young adulthood, reaching its lowest point in a person's forties.*
- **True.** *Both women and men report greater happiness after age 50 and continue to do so until extreme old age.*

Sources: Based on the British Household Panel Survey, conducted by Andrew Oswald, Institute of Education, University of London. Several American studies have confirmed the same pattern of happiness increasing with age.

HEALTH ON A BUDGET

"Buy" Yourself a Longer Life

You don't need money for the only antiaging program that has been proven to add years to life expectancy. All you have to do is follow four basic steps:

- **Keep your arteries young.** If your arteries are clear and healthy, you're more likely to have a healthy heart and a sharper brain and less likely to develop high blood pressure, high cholesterol, kidney problems, and memory impairment. For your arteries' sake, exercise regularly, avoid high-fat foods, watch your weight, and find ways to manage daily stress (see Chapter 3).
- **Avoid illness.** Most individuals who live to celebrate their hundredth birthday don't suffer from chronic diseases. Defend yourself by eating a healthy diet, not smoking, avoiding weight gain in middle age, recognizing and treating conditions like high blood pressure and elevated cholesterol, and keeping up with immunizations.
- **Stay strong.** As landmark studies with frail nursing home residents in their eighties and nineties have shown, strength training at any age builds muscle and bone, speeds up metabolic rate, improves sleep and mobility, boosts the spirit, and enhances self-confidence.
- **Maintain your zest for living.** Just as with muscles, the best advice to keep your brain strong is "use it or lose it." Keep challenging yourself, asking questions, and pursuing new passions. Individuals who are optimistic, sociable, and happy generally outlive their more pessimistic, grumpier peers.

Nutrition and Obesity

The most common nutritional disorder in older persons is obesity. Overweight men and women over age 65 face higher risk of diabetes, heart disease, stroke, and other health problems, including arthritis.

Many elderly people who live independently do not get adequate amounts of one or more essential nutrients. The reasons are many: limited income, difficulty getting to stores, chronic illness, medications that interfere with the metabolism of nutrients, problems chewing or digesting, poor appetite, inactivity, illness, depression. Nutritionists urge the elderly, like other Americans, to concentrate on eating healthful foods; many also recommend daily nutritional supplements, which may provide the added benefit of improving cognitive function in healthy people over 65.

The Aging Brain

Scientists used to think that the aging brain, once worn out, could never be fixed. Now they know that the brain can and does repair itself. When neurons (brain cells) die, the surrounding cells develop "fingers" to fill the gaps and establish new connections, or synapses, between surviving neurons. Although self-repair occurs more quickly in young brains, the process continues in older brains. Even victims of Alzheimer's disease, the most devastating form of senility, have enough healthy cells in the diseased brain to regrow synapses. Scientists hope to develop drugs that someday may help the brain repair itself.

Mental ability does not decline along with physical vigor. Researchers have been able to reverse the supposedly normal intellectual declines of 60- to 80-year-olds by tutoring them in problem solving. Reaction time, intellectual speed and efficiency, nonverbal intelligence, and maximum work rate for short periods may diminish by age 75. However, understanding, vocabulary, ability to remember key information, and verbal intelligence remain about the same.

 Aspirin, even at low doses, appears to prevent declines in key areas of the brain, according to brain-imaging studies.[13] However, long-term use of low-dose aspirin did not lead to improved thinking, memory, and other cognitive skills in women over age 65 participating in the landmark Women's Health Study.[14] In other research, nonsteroidal anti-inflammatory drugs (NSAIDs) failed to prevent Alzheimer's disease in older men and women with a family history of the disorder.[15] A recent study found that the herbal supplement ginkgo biloba also has no clear-cut benefit in preventing memory problems.[16]

Memory According to data from a National Institute of Aging survey, memory loss and cognitive problems are becoming less common among older Americans. The reasons may be that today's seniors have more formal education, higher economic status, and better health care for problems such as high blood pressure and high cholesterol that can jeopardize brain function.[17]

Higher education does not prevent cognitive decline over time, according to recent research, but schooling does yield an advantage. Individuals with more education continue to have a higher level of cognitive functioning into old age so they remain independent for a longer period.[18] There is growing evidence that using your brain as you age—by reading, playing games, solving crossword puzzles, and doing crafts such as pottery or quilting—greatly decreases the risk of memory loss.[19]

Women at Midlife

(a) PET scan of a 20-year-old brain

(b) PET scan of an 80-year-old brain

© Alzheimer's Disease Education & Referral Center (both)

In the next two decades some 40 million American women will end their reproductive years. "The primary misconception is that this is a terrible time when all women suffer horrible symptoms," says Sherry Sherman, M.D., project officer for the National Institute of Aging's Study of Women Across the Nation, which has followed 3,300 women through midlife since 1996. "When you look at healthy women in the community in terms of what actually affects their lives, their periods stop. That's it."[20]

Perimenopause   While the average age of **menopause**—defined as the complete cessation of menstrual periods for 12 consecutive months—is 51.5, a woman's reproductive system begins changing more than a decade earlier. "The change of life starts in our thirties with irregular menstrual cycles and then heats up in our forties with hot flashes and night sweats," says psychiatrist Marsha Speller, M.D., author of *The Menopause Answer Book.*[21]

For many women, **perimenopause**—the four-to-ten-year span before a woman's last period—is more baffling and bothersome than the years after. During this time the egg cells, or oocytes, in a woman's ovaries start to senesce or die off at a faster rate. Eventually, the number of egg cells drops to a tiny fraction of the estimated 2 million packed into her ovaries at birth. Trying to coax some of the remaining oocytes to ripen, the pituitary gland churns out extra follicle-stimulating hormone (FSH). This surge is the earliest harbinger of menopause, occurring six to ten years before a woman's final periods. Eventually, the other menstrual messenger, luteinizing hormone (LH), also increases, but at a slower rate.

These hormonal shifts can trigger an array of symptoms. The most common is night sweats (a *subdromal hot flash,*

in medical terms), which can be intense enough to disrupt sleep. The drop in estrogen levels also may cause hot flashes (bursts of perspiration that last from a few seconds to 15 minutes).

A woman's habits and health history also have an impact. Women with a lifelong history of depression are more likely to experience early perimenopause. The fluctuating hormones of perimenopause may increase depressive symptoms even in women who have never had previous depressions. Smokers experience more symptoms at an earlier age than nonsmokers. Heavier women also have more severe symptoms.

Menopause   About 10 to 15 percent of women breeze through this transition with only trivial symptoms. Another 10 to 15 percent are virtually disabled. The majority fall somewhere in between these extremes. Women who undergo surgical or medical menopause (the result of removal of their ovaries or chemotherapy) often experience abrupt symptoms, including flushing, sweating, sleeplessness, early morning awakenings, involuntary urination, changes in libido, mood swings, perception of memory loss, and changes in cognitive function.

 Race and ethnicity profoundly affect women's experience. African American women report more hot flashes and night sweats but have more positive attitudes toward menopause. Japanese and Chinese women experience more muscle stiffness and fewer hot flashes but view menopause more negatively. Hispanic women reach menopause a year or two earlier than Caucasian women; Asian women, a year or two later.

In these PET scans, the red and yellow show greater neuron activity in the young adult. The brain of the older person shows less activity and more dark areas, indicating that the fluid-filled ventricles have grown larger. Recent research shows, however, that older brains do repair themselves.

menopause   The complete cessation of ovulation and menstruation for 12 consecutive months.

perimenopause   The period from a woman's first irregular cycles to her last menstruation.

Dwindling levels of estrogen subtly affect many aspects of a woman's health, from her mouth (where dryness, unusual tastes, burning, and gum problems can develop) to her skin (which may become drier, itchier, and overly sensitive to touch). With less estrogen to block them, a woman's androgens, or male hormones, may have a greater impact, causing acne, hair loss, and according to some anecdotal reports, surges in sexual appetite. (Other women, however, report a drop in sexual desire.)

At the same time, a woman's clitoris, vulva, and vaginal lining begin to shrivel, sometimes resulting in pain or bleeding during intercourse. Since the thinner genital tissues are less effective in keeping out bacteria and other pathogens, urinary tract infections may become more common. Some women develop breast or ovarian cysts, which usually go away on their own. Eventually, a woman's ovaries don't respond at all to her pituitary hormones. After the last ovulatory cycle, progesterone is no longer secreted, and estrogen levels decrease rapidly. A woman's testosterone level also falls.

In the United States, the average woman who reaches menopause has a life expectancy of about 30 more years. However, she faces risks of various diseases, including an increased risk of obesity, metabolic syndrome, heart disease, stroke, and breast cancer. Women can reduce these risks by exercise, good nutrition, and weight control both before and after menopause.

"Exercise is the best thing a woman can do for herself at midlife," says JoAnn Pinkerton, M.D., of the National Women's Health Resource Center. "It improves your heart function so you have less chance of heart disease. It improves your cognition so you think better. It decreases your risk of breast cancer. It helps your mood. It lessens the likelihood of depression. It increases energy and protects your bones."[22] In a recent study, walking proved effective in easing anxiety, boosting mood, and improving the quality of life of women during menopause.[23]

Hormone Therapy   Hormone therapy (**HT**) was long believed to prevent heart disease and strokes and help women live longer. But medical thinking on HT, particularly a combination of estrogen and progestin, has changed completely in recent years.[24] HT is no longer recommended for reasons other than short-term relief of symptoms such as hot flashes and night sweats.

The Women's Health Initiative (WHI)—a series of clinical trials begun in 1991 on postmenopausal women—halted its study of combination estrogen/progestin therapy in July 2002 and its study of estrogen-only therapy in 2004 because of safety concerns. Combination therapy slightly increased the risk of breast cancer, heart disease, blood clots, and stroke.[25]

The timing of hormone therapy influences the potential risks. Women who take HT around the time of menopause are at much less risk of blood clots and heart disease than those who begin therapy at later ages. According to the most recent analysis of the WHI data, women who take only estrogen for less than seven years have a lower breast cancer risk. After that period of time, they face a small elevated risk (0.1 percent).[26] Increasingly, women and their doctors are opting for treatments that are safer, can be taken at lower doses, can be administered via different routes (such as sprays), and do not include progesterone.

The increased risk of breast cancer continues for at least five years after discontinuing hormone therapy. Combined hormone therapy also increases the likelihood of abnormal mammograms and breast biopsies and may make it more difficult to diagnose breast cancer. Breast cancer survivors taking hormone therapy for menopausal symptoms also face an increased risk of cancer recurrence.[27]

Both estrogen therapy and estrogen-progestin therapy increase the risk of stroke in postmenopausal women. Neither has proven effective in preventing dementia or cognitive decline. Hormonal therapy does reduce the risk of postmenopausal osteoporosis, but its risks and benefits need to be weighed against those of other available treatments. Women who stop hormonal therapy have about a 50 percent chance that their menopausal symptoms will recur, regardless of their age or how long they used HT. In controlled trials, black cohosh, the most popular herbal treatment, either alone or with other herbs, proved no more effective than placebo in relieving hot flashes and other menopause symptoms. In a controlled trial, acupuncture also fails to provide reliable relief of menopausal hot flashes.

Men at Midlife

 Although men don't experience the dramatic hormonal upheaval that women do, they do experience a decline by as much as 30 to 40 percent in their primary sex hormone, testosterone, between the ages of 48 and 70. This change, sometimes called *andropause*, may cause a range of symptoms, including decreased muscle mass, greater body fat, loss of bone density, flagging energy, lowered fertility, and impaired virility. Some researchers are experimenting with testosterone supplements now available in various forms, including under-the-skin implants, transdermal patches, and gel.[28] In tests with young men, testosterone has increased lean body mass and decrease body fat—at least temporarily. However, other researchers warn that, particularly in older men, excess testosterone might raise the risk of prostate cancer and heart disease.

After age 40, the prostate gland, which surrounds the urethra at the base of the bladder, enlarges. This condition, called *benign prostatic hypertrophy*, occurs in every man. By age 50, half of all men have some enlargement of the gland; after 70, three-quarters do. As it expands, the prostate tends to pinch the urethra, decreasing urinary flow and creating a sense of urinary urgency, particularly at night. Other warning signs of prostate problems include difficult urination, blood in the urine, painful ejaculation, or constant lower-back pain.

Medical treatments for benign prostate hypertrophy include drugs that improve urine flow and reduce obstruction of the bladder outlet as well as medications that partially shrink the enlarged prostate by lowering the level of the major male hormone inside the prostate. In some cases, surgical treatment is necessary.

Sexuality and Aging

Health and sexuality interact in various ways as we age. When they are healthy and have a willing partner, a substantial number of older men remain sexually active. The fittest men and women report more frequent sexual activity.

Other research has found a relationship between sex and longevity. A Swedish study found that men, but not women, who had discontinued intercourse had higher death rates. A study of the entire male population of a small Welsh town found that the sexually active men had half the mortality of the inactive group. In a Duke University study, longevity in women correlated with enjoyment of sexual intercourse, rather than with its frequency.

Aging does cause some changes in sexual response: Women produce less vaginal lubrication. An older man needs more time to achieve an erection or orgasm and to attain another erection after ejaculating. Both men and women experience fewer contractions during orgasm. However, none of these changes reduce sexual pleasure or desire.

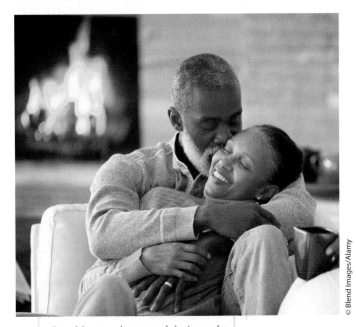

© Blend Images/Alamy

For older couples, sexual desire and pleasure can be enhanced by years of intimacy and affection.

hormone therapy (HT) The use of supplemental hormones during and after menopause.

The Challenges of Age

No matter how well we eat, exercise, and take care of ourselves, some physical changes are inevitable as we age. (See Consumer Alert, p. 634.) Figure 20.2 shows some of these changes, but most of them are not debilitating, and people can remain active and vital into extreme old age. Aging brains and bodies do become vulnerable to diseases like Alzheimer's and osteoporosis. Other common life problems, such as depression, substance misuse, and safe driving, become more challenging as we age.

Alzheimer's Disease

About 15 percent of older Americans lose previous mental capabilities, a brain disorder called **dementia.** Sixty percent of these—an estimated 2.4 to 4.5 million—suffer from the type of dementia called **Alzheimer's disease,** a progressive deterioration of brain cells and mental capacity.

Age is the top risk factor for Alzheimer's. Someone in America develops Alzheimer's every 72 seconds; by 2050 the rate will increase to every 33 seconds. The percentage of people with Alzheimer's doubles for every five-year age group beyond 65. By age 85, nearly half of men and women have Alzheimer's. A person with the disease typically lives eight years after the onset of symptoms, but some live as long as 20 years. Some 7.7 million older Americans will develop Alzheimer's by 2030. The greatest increase will be among people age 85 and older.

People who parents have been diagnosed with Alzheimer's disease or dementia may be more likely to experience memory loss themselves in middle age. Scientists have identified nine genes that make people more likely to develop Alzheimer's, including a variation in the receptor gene for vitamin D. Because of a link between low levels of this vitamin and dementia, researchers had suspected such an association.[29]

Women are more likely to develop Alzheimer's than men, and women with Alzheimer's perform significantly worse than men in various visual, spatial, and memory tests. Initiating hormone therapy after age 60 increases the risk of Alzheimer's disease.

Health habits, such as smoking and drinking, can affect the risk of developing dementia. According to recent research, heavy smokers and drinkers develop Alzheimer's several years earlier than those who do not.[30] Weight and body composition also have an effect. According to a study that followed middle-aged Americans for several decades, "belly fat" (discussed in Chapter 5) triples the risk of dementia later in life.[31]

Figure 20.2 The Effects of Aging on the Body

Hair and nails Hair often turns gray and thins out. Men may go bald. Fingernails can thicken.

Brain The brain shrinks, but it is not known if that affects mental functions.

The senses The sensitivity of hearing, sight, taste, and smell can all decline with age.

Skin Wrinkles occur as the skin thins and the underlying fat shrinks, and age spots often develop.

Glands and hormones Levels of many hormones drop, or the body becomes less responsive to them.

Muscles Strength usually peaks in the twenties, then declines.

Immune system The body becomes less able to resist some pathogens.

Heart and blood vessels Cardiovascular problems become more common. The heart grows less efficient; buildup within arteries decreases oxygen and nutrients to cells.

Breasts Tissue degenerates after menopause, and breasts sag.

Lungs Lung capacity drops; risk of bronchitis and pneumonia grows.

Kidneys and urinary tract The kidneys become less efficient. The bladder can't hold as much, so urination is more frequent.

Digestive system Digestion slows down as the secretion of digestive enzymes decreases.

Reproductive system Women go through menopause, and testosterone levels drop for men.

Bones and joints Wear and tear can lead to arthritic joints, and osteoporosis is common, especially in women.

Psychological, nutritional, and environmental factors also may affect the risk of Alzheimer's. Older people who are active, outgoing, and relaxed are less likely to develop dementia than their more sedentary, solitary, and uptight peers, according to research on the link between personality traits, lifestyle, and Alzheimer's.[32]

Middle-aged coffee drinkers also are at lower risk. In a recent epidemiological study, men and women who drank three to five cups of coffee per day in middle age were two-thirds less likely than those who drank none to develop dementia.[33] (See Chapter 11 for a discussion of other health benefits of coffee, including lower rates of Parkinson's and diabetes.)

Electromagnetic fields may pose an invisible threat. Older people living in close range of major power lines are at increased risk of dying from Alzheimer's disease or senile dementia.[34]

The early signs of dementia—insomnia, irritability, increased sensitivity to alcohol and other drugs, and decreased energy and tolerance of frustration—are usually subtle and insidious. Diagnosis requires a comprehensive assessment of an individual's medical history, physical health, and mental status, often involving brain scans and a variety of other tests.

Cholesterol-lowering statin drugs, discussed in Chapter 14, can reduce the risk of Alzheimer's, regardless of the medication used or the person's genetic risk for the disease.[35] Vitamin C or vitamin E, once touted as possible memory preservers, have not proven to lower the risk of dementia or Alzheimer's in older adults.[36]

Even though medical science cannot restore a brain that is in the process of being destroyed by an organic brain disease like Alzheimer's, medications can control

dementia Deterioration of mental capability.

Alzheimer's disease A progressive deterioration of intellectual powers due to physiological changes within the brain; symptoms include diminishing ability to concentrate and reason, disorientation, depression, apathy, and paranoia.

difficult behavioral symptoms and enhance or partially restore cognitive ability. Often physicians find other medical or psychiatric problems, such as depression, in these patients; recognizing and treating these conditions can have a dramatic impact.

The FDA has approved several prescription drugs for people with mild to moderate dementia, including Aricept, Exelon, Reminyl, and Mamenda. None has proven superior to the others.[37]

Osteoporosis

Another age-related disease is *osteoporosis*, a condition in which losses in bone density become so severe that a bone will break with even slight trauma or injury. A chronic disease, osteoporosis is silent for years or decades before a fracture occurs. Each year more than a third of Americans aged 65 and older experience a fall and nearly 16,000 die as a result of their injuries. Even a low-trauma fracture increases the risk of dying during the subsequent five years, while a hip fracture heightens this risk for ten years.[38]

Women, who have smaller skeletons, are more vulnerable than men; in extreme cases, their spines may become so fragile that just bending causes severe pain. But although commonly seen as an illness of women, osteoporosis occurs frequently in men. One in every two women and one in four men over 50 will have an osteoporosis-related fracture in their lifetimes.

(a)

(b)

The effect of osteoporosis on bone density. **(a)** Normal bone tissue. **(b)** After the onset of osteoporosis, bones lose density and become hollow and brittle.

Risk Factors   Osteoporosis doesn't begin in old age. The bone weakness that increases the risk of osteoporosis may actually begin before birth. Infants undernourished in the womb are small when born, remain smaller than their age peers at age 1, have low bone mass at 25, and have an increased risk of fractures in late adulthood. Other risk factors include:

CONSUMER**ALERT**

Can You Really Turn Back Time?

Americans spend billions of dollars on products that promise to make them look or feel younger. Are they getting their money's worth?

Facts to Know

- Over-the-counter skin products have little effect because fine lines, pigmentation, and other age-related changes occur in the skin's deeper layers.

- Herbs like gingko biloba do not improve memory or slow the onset of Alzheimer's.

- "Antiaging" vitamins and supplements do not protect the aging brain and heart and may contain preservatives and other chemicals that can trigger allergic reactions.

Steps to Take

- Read the claims carefully. Watch out for qualifying words like "aim to" and "designed to."

- Watch out for pseudoscientific language, such as "clinically shown to." Where? By whom? Remember that the gold standard of science is a randomized, double-blind clinical trial, performed by qualified researchers (usually affiliated with a university or teaching hospital) who have no financial stake in the outcome.

- Don't believe testimonials. The model in the "after" photograph may indeed look younger, thinner, and better than in the "before" shot, but that may be the result of airbrushing or professional lighting.

- **Age.** Risk increases as you grow older.
- **Being female.** Women have less bone tissue than do men and tend to experience a rapid loss of bone in the first few years after menopause.
- **Body size.** Small, thin-boned women are at greatest risk.
- **Ethnicity.** White and Asian women are at highest risk.

- **Family history.** Having parents with a history of osteoporosis as well as fractures in adulthood can place you at increased risk.
- **Sex hormones.** Abnormal absence of menstrual periods (amenorrhea) or menopause can increase risk.
- **Anorexia.**
- **Lifetime diet low in calcium and vitamin D.**

Preparing for Medical Crises and the End of Life

Throughout this book, we have stressed the ways in which you can determine how well and how long you live. You can also make decisions about the end of your life. When facing a serious, potentially life-threatening illness, people typically have practical, realistic goals, such as maintaining their quality of life, remaining independent, being comfortable, and providing for their families.[39]

 Various racial and ethnic groups have different preferences for their end-of-life wishes. Many Arab Americans prefer not to go to nursing homes as they near the end of their lives, while many African Americans are comfortable with nursing homes and hospitals. Hispanic individuals express strong concerns about dying with dignity. Many white people don't want their families to take care of them, although they—like members of most other racial and ethnic groups—want their families nearby as they live out their last days.

Advance Directives

All states and the District of Columbia have laws authorizing the use of **advance directives** to specify the kind of medical treatment individuals want in case of a medical crisis. These documents are important because, without clear indications of a person's preferences, hospitals and other institutions often make decisions on an individual's behalf, particularly if family members are not available or disagree among themselves.

The two most common advance directives are health-care proxies and living wills. Each state has different legal requirements for these forms. You can find state-specific forms at **www.caringinfo.org.** Once the forms are completed, make copies of your advance directives and give them to anyone who might have input in decisions on your behalf. Also give copies to your physician or health-care organization and ask that they be made part of your medical record.

Health-Care Proxy A *health-care proxy* is an advance directive that gives someone else the power to make health decisions on your behalf. This advance directive is also called Medical Power of Attorney or Health-Care Power of Attorney. People typically name a relative or close friend as their agent. Let family and friends know that you have completed a health-care proxy. Tell your primary physician, but you should not designate your doctor as your agent. Many states prohibit this. Even when allowed, it is not a good idea because your doctor's primary responsibility is to administer care.

Living Will Individuals can use a **living will** (also called health-care directive or physician's directive) to indicate whether they

advance directives Documents that specify an individual's preferences regarding treatment in a medical crisis.

living will An advance directive providing instructions for the use of life-sustaining procedures in the event of terminal illness or injury.

want or don't want all possible medical treatments and technology used to prolong their lives. Living wills are most effective when they focus on priorities and goals, not so much on how to achieve them.

Most states recognize living wills as legally binding, and a growing number of health-care professionals and facilities offer patients help in drafting living wills. Figure 20.3 shows a physician's directive for Texas and notes where state laws may differ.

The Five Wishes An innovative document called "Five Wishes" helps the aged, the seriously ill, their loved ones, and caregivers prepare for medical crises. Written with the help of the American Bar Association's Commission on the Legal Problems of the Elderly, the Five Wishes document has a health-care proxy, a health-care directive, and three other "wishes." Persons using this document can specify:

- Which person they want to make health-care decisions for them when they are no longer able to do so.
- Which kinds of medical treatments they do or don't want.
- How comfortable they want to be made.
- How they want people to treat them.
- What they want loved ones to know.

The Five Wishes document (at **www.aging-withdignity.org**) is legally valid in 38 states. Churches, synagogues, hospices, hospitals, physicians, social service agencies, and employers also are distributing the document to help people plan for their own care or that of aging parents.

DNR Order You can also sign an advance directive specifying that you want to be allowed to die naturally—you do not want to be resuscitated in case your heart stops beating. **Do-not-resuscitate (DNR)** orders apply mainly to hospitalized, terminally ill patients and must be signed by a physician. However, in some states, it is possible to complete a *nonhospital DNR* form that specifies an individual's wish not to be resuscitated at home. Patients in the final stages of advanced cancer or AIDS may choose to use such forms to protect their rights in case paramedics are called to their home.

Holographic Wills Perhaps you think that only wealthy or older people need to write wills. However, if you're married, have children, or own property, you should either hire a lawyer to draw up a will or at least write a **holographic will** yourself, specifying who should inherit your possessions. If you die *intestate* (without a will), the state will make these decisions for you. Even a modest estate can be tied up in court for a long period of time, depriving family members of money when they need it most.

A holographic will is a handwritten (not typed) statement that some states will recognize. You can:

- **Name a family member or friend** as the executor, the person who sees that your wishes are carried out.
- **List the things you own** and to whom you want them to go; include addresses and telephone numbers, if possible.
- **Select a guardian for your children** (if any), presumably someone whose ideas about raising children are similar to your own. Be sure that any named guardians are willing and able to accept this responsibility before writing them into your will.
- **Specify any funeral arrangements.**

Be sure to keep the will in a safe place, where your executor, family members, or closest beneficiary can find it quickly and easily; tell them where it is.

Ethical Dilemmas

Modern medicine can do more to delay or defy death than was once thought possible. However, the ability to sustain life in patients with no hope of recovery has created wrenching medical and moral dilemmas. Increasingly, lawyers, ethicists, and consumer advocates are arguing that health-care providers must recognize a fundamental right of patients: the right to die.

Health economists, noting that more than half of U.S. health-care dollars are spent in the last year of life, have questioned "heroic" measures to prolong the life of chronically ill elderly patients or those with fatal diseases. Policies on such aggressive measures vary from hospital to hospital and state to state; often medical staff are not aware of patients' wishes.

do-not-resuscitate (DNR) An advance directive expressing an individual's preference that resuscitation efforts not be made during a medical crisis.

holographic will A will wholly in the handwriting of its author.

DIRECTIVE TO PHYSICIANS
For Persons 18 Years of Age and Over

I, _____, recognize that the best health care is based upon a partnership of trust and communication with my physician. My physician and I will make health care decisions together as long as I am of sound mind and able to make my wishes known. If there comes a time that I am unable to make medical decisions about myself because of illness or injury, I direct that the following treatment preferences be honored:

If, in the judgment of my physician, I am suffering with a terminal condition from which I am expected to die within six months, even with available life-sustaining treatment provided in accordance with prevailing standards of medical care:

_____ I request that all treatments other than those needed to keep me comfortable be discontinued or withheld and my physician allow me to die as gently as possible; OR

_____ I request that I be kept alive in this terminal condition using available life-sustaining treatment (THIS SELECTION DOES NOT APPLY TO HOSPICE CARE).

If, in the judgment of my physician, I am suffering with an irreversible condition so that I cannot care for myself or make decisions for myself and am expected to die without life-sustaining treatment provided in accordance with prevailing standards of care:

_____ I request that all treatments other than those needed to keep me comfortable be discontinued or withheld and my physician allow me to die as gently as possible; OR

_____ I request that I be kept alive in this irreversible condition using available life-sustaining treatment (THIS SELECTION DOES NOT APPLY TO HOSPICE CARE).

Additional requests: (After discussion with your physician, you may wish to consider listing particular treatments in this space that you do or do not want in specific circumstances, such as artificial nutrition and fluids, intravenous antibiotics, etc. Be sure to state whether you do or do not want the particular treatment).

After signing this DIRECTIVE, if my representative or I elect hospice care, I understand and agree that only those treatments needed to keep me comfortable would be provided and I would not be given available life-sustaining treatments.

If I do not have a Medical Power of Attorney and I am unable to make my wishes known, I designate the following person(s) to make treatment decisions with my physician compatible with my personal values.

Name _____

Address _____

Name _____

Address _____

(If a Medical Power of Attorney has been executed, then an agent already has been named and you should not list additional names in this document.)

If the above persons are not available, or if I have not designated a spokesperson, I understand that a spokesperson will be chosen for me following standards specified in the laws of Texas. If, in the judgment of my physician, my death is imminent within minutes to hours, even with the use of all available medical treatment provided within the prevailing standard of care, I acknowledge that all treatments may be withheld or removed except those needed to maintain my comfort.

I understand that under Texas law this Directive has no effect if I have been diagnosed as pregnant. This DIRECTIVE will remain in effect until I revoke it. No other person may do so. I understand that I may revoke this DIRECTIVE at any time.

I understand the full import of this DIRECTIVE and I am emotionally and mentally competent to make this DIRECTIVE.

Signed _____

City, County, and State of Residence _____

Date _____

Two competent witnesses must sign below, acknowledging your signature. The witness designated as "Witness 1" may not be a person designated to make a treatment decision for the patient and may not be related to the patient by blood or marriage. The witness may not be entitled to any part of the estate and may not have a claim against the estate of the patient. The witness may not be the attending physician or an employee of the attending physician. If this witness is an employee of the health care facility in which the patient is being cared for, this witness may not be involved in providing direct patient care to the patient. This witness may not be an officer, director, partner, or business office employee of the health care facility in which the patient is being cared for or of any parent organization of the health care facility.

Witness 1 _____

Witness 2 _____

TEXAS LAW DOES NOT REQUIRE THIS DIRECTIVE TO BE NOTARIZED.

Figure 20.3 Preparing a Physician's Directive

Source: A Guide to the Living Will, *Hippocrates* (May/June, 1988).

POINT

As in some highly publicized cases, families often face an agonizing decision. As the result of an accident or devastating illness, a loved one cannot breathe without mechanical assistance. Without respiratory support, the person will die. With it, the individual may live for many years in what doctors call a vegetative state. In such a case, the family has the right to pull the plug.

COUNTERPOINT

If the individual has not made his or her preferences known, no one has the right to cut off life-sustaining medical support. The government should protect every patient's right to live rather than allowing families to withdraw care.

YOUR VIEW

What do you think is the right thing to do in a case like this? What would be your choice if the life at stake were your own? Your parent's? Your child's?

UNIFORM DONOR CARD

OF _____
Print or type name of donor

In the hope that I may help others, I hereby make this anatomical gift, if medically acceptable, to take effect upon my death. The words and marks below indicate my desires.

I give   (a)_____   any needed organs or parts
I give   (b)_____   only the following organs or parts

_____
Specifiy the organ(s) or part(s)

for the purposes of transplantation, therapy, medical research, or education.

Figure 20.4 Example of a Uniform Donor Card

Some health-care facilities require that staff members try to resuscitate any patient whose heart stops unless a do-not-resuscitate (DNR) order has been written, usually with the family's permission.

Families may demand aggressive medical care near the end of life on the basis of religious grounds, such as a conviction that every moment of life is a gift from God worth preserving at any cost. However, doctors are not obliged to provide a treatment they consider medically inappropriate or inhumane simply because of the family's religious beliefs. Ideally, doctors and family members, perhaps with the aid of a chaplain, work together to reach a consensus on the appropriate limits to life-sustaining treatment.

Another major ethical concern is the fate of an estimated 5,000 to 10,000 unconscious Americans who are being kept alive by artificial means. Some are in a **coma**, a state of total unconsciousness. They may have no sense of where they are, no memory, and no experience of pain. Others are in a **persistent vegetative state**, in which they're awake and yet unaware. They open their eyes; their brain waves show the characteristic patterns of waking and sleep. They can usually breathe on their own after a few weeks on artificial respiration; they can cough; the pupils of their eyes respond to light; but they do not respond to pain. (See Point/Counterpoint.)

The Gift of Life

If you're at least 18 years old, you can fill out a donor card (Figure 20.4), agreeing to designate, in the event of your death, any organs or tissues needed for transplantation. Corneas may help a blind person see, for example. Kidneys, or even a heart, may be transplanted. The donation takes effect upon your death and is a generous way of giving others the possibilities for life that you have had yourself. The card should be filled out and signed; some must be signed in the presence of two witnesses. Attach the donor card to the back of your driver's license or I.D. card. (Whole-body donations may require other arrangements.)

The reasons for becoming an organ donor or agreeing to donate a loved one's organs are complex. Older men and women generally have higher donation rates. Families often base their decision on a loved one's explicit desire either to donate organs or not. Concerns about disfigurement and feelings of emotional exhaustion also play a role.

Death and Dying

Some 2.4 million people die in the United States each year. Although most are older, death occurs in all age groups. The causes of death vary with both age and gender. Among those under age 35, intentional and nonintentional injury are the primary causes of death. Among older Americans, cancer and heart disease are the top killers. In fact, cancer, heart disease, and stroke continue to claim the most lives around the world. Men typically die at a younger age than women. College-age individuals are most likely to die as a result of accidents or assaults.

Defining Death

In our society, death isn't a part of everyday life, as it once was. Because machines can now keep alive people who, in the past, would have died, the definition of death has become more complex. Death has been broken down into the following categories:

- **Functional death.** The end of all vital functions, such as heartbeat and respiration.

- **Cellular death.** The gradual death of body cells after the heart stops beating. If placed in a tissue culture or, as is the case with various organs, transplanted to another body, some cells can remain alive indefinitely.

- **Death.** The moment when the heart stops beating.

- **Brain death.** The end of all brain activity, indicated by an absence of electrical activity (confirmed by an electroencephalogram, or EEG) and a lack of reflexes. The notion of brain death is bound up with what we consider to be the actual person, or self. The destruction of a person's brain means that his or her personality no longer exists; the lower brain centers controlling respiration and circulation no longer function.

- **Spiritual death.** The moment when the soul, as defined by many religions, leaves the body.

When does a person actually die? The traditional legal definition of death is failure of the lungs or heart to function. However, because respiration and circulation can be maintained by artificial means, most states have declared that an individual is considered dead only when the brain, including the brain stem, completely stops functioning. Brain-death laws prohibit a medical staff from "pulling the plug" if there is any hope of sustaining life.

Denying Death

Most of us don't quite believe that we're going to die. A reasonable amount of denial helps us focus on the day-to-day realities of living. However, excessive denial can be life-threatening. Some drivers, for instance, refuse to buckle their seat belts because they refuse to acknowledge that a drunk driver might collide with them. Similarly, cigarette smokers deny that lung cancer will ever strike them, and people who eat high-fat meals deny that they'll ever suffer a heart attack.

One important factor in denial is the nature of the threat. It's easy to believe that death is at hand when someone's pointing a gun at you; it's much harder to think that cigarette smoking might cause your death 20 or 30 years down the road. The late Elisabeth Kübler-Ross, a psychiatrist who extensively studied the process of dying, described the downside of denying death in *Death: The Final Stage of Growth:*

> It is the denial of death that is partially responsible for people living empty, purposeless lives; for when you live as if you'll live forever, it becomes too easy to postpone the things you know that you must do. You live your life in preparation for tomorrow or in the remembrance of yesterday—and meanwhile, each today is lost. In contrast, when you fully understand that each day you awaken could be the last you have, you take the time that day to grow, to become more of who you really are, to reach out to other human beings.[40]

Emotional Responses to Dying

Kübler-Ross identified five typical stages of reaction that a person goes through when facing death (Figure 20.5).

coma A state of total unconsciousness.

persistent vegetative state A state of being awake and capable of reacting to physical stimuli, such as light, while being unaware of pain or other environmental stimuli.

Figure 20.5

Kübler-Ross's Five Stages of Adjustment to Facing Death

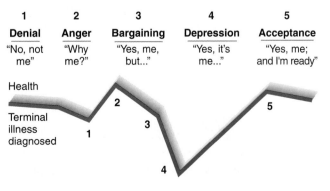

1	2	3	4	5
Denial	**Anger**	**Bargaining**	**Depression**	**Acceptance**
"No, not me"	"Why me?"	"Yes, me, but..."	"Yes, it's me..."	"Yes, me; and I'm ready"

Health

Terminal illness diagnosed

1. **Denial ("No, not me").** At first knowledge that death is coming, a terminally ill patient rejects the news. The denial overcomes the initial shock and allows the person to begin to gather together his or her resources. Denial, at this point, is a healthy defense mechanism. It can become distressful, however, if it's reinforced by the relatives and friends of the dying patient.

2. **Anger ("Why me?").** In the second stage, the dying person begins to feel resentment and rage regarding imminent death. The anger may be directed at God or at the patient's family and caregivers, who can do little but try to endure any expressions of anger, provide comfort, and help the patient on to the next stage.

3. **Bargaining ("Yes, me, but . . .").** In this stage, a patient may try to bargain, usually with God, for a way to reverse or at least postpone dying. The patient may promise, in exchange for recovery, to do good works or to see family members more often. Alternatively, the patient may say, "Let me live long enough to see my grandchild born" or "to see the spring again."

4. **Depression ("Yes, it's me").** In the fourth stage, the patient gradually realizes the full consequences of his or her condition. This may begin as grieving for health that has been lost and then become anticipatory grieving for the loss that is to come of friends, loved ones, and life itself. This stage is perhaps the most difficult: The dying person should not be left alone during this period. Neither should loved ones try to cheer up the patient, who must be allowed to grieve.

5. **Acceptance ("Yes, me; and I'm ready").** In this last stage, the person has accepted the reality of death: The moment looms as neither frightening nor painful, neither sad nor happy—only inevitable. The person who waits for the end of life may ask to see fewer visitors, to separate from other people, or perhaps to turn to just one person for support.

Several stages may occur at the same time and some may happen out of sequence.

Each stage may take days or only hours or minutes. Throughout, denial may come back to assert itself unexpectedly, and hope for a medical breakthrough or a miraculous recovery is forever present.

Some experts dispute Kübler-Ross's basic five-stage theory as too simplistic and argue that not all people go through such well-defined stages in the dying process. The way a person faces death is often a mirror of the way he or she has faced other major stresses in life: Those who have had the most trouble adjusting to other crises will have the most trouble adjusting to the news of their impending death.

An individual's will to live can postpone death for a while. In a study of elderly Chinese women, researchers found that their death rate decreased before and during a holiday during which the senior women in a household play a central role; it increased after the celebration. A similar temporary drop occurs among Jews at the time of Passover. However, different events may have different effects. The prospect of an upcoming birthday postpones death in women but hastens it in men. The will to live typically fluctuates in terminal patients, varying along with depression, anxiety, shortness of breath, and a sense of well-being.

The family of a dying person experiences a spectrum of often wrenching emotions. Family members, too, may deny the verdict of death, rage at the doctors and nurses who can't do more to save their loved one, bargain with God to give up their own health if necessary, sink into helplessness and depression, and finally accept the reality of their anticipated loss. Dying can be seen from different perspectives. The Renz model, for example, views it as a process of maturation consisting of pretransition, transition, and posttransition. The initial response is an upsurge of emotions, including anger, grief, feelings of personal emptiness, and despair. These may emerge again and again.

However, as patients confront reality, they eventually can "let go and let be." As one researcher observed, "There is happiness and well-being in the midst of illness. In the course of the dying process spiritual experiences of such intensity often happen more than just once. After a shorter or longer struggle, patients reach a new mental state, a gift of grace beyond human endeavor and power."[41]

How We Die

Life can end in very different ways. Sudden death, by accident or murder, for instance, brings an abrupt end to life in individuals who may have been in optimal health. A terminal illness, such as an aggressive and fatal cancer, can lead to a steep drop in functioning prior to death. When organs such as the kidneys fail, a patient's well-being tends to plummet and then recover but in a downward pattern. The frailty of old age leads to a gradual decline to ever lower levels of functioning and eventual death.

Most people who have a fatal or **terminal illness** prefer to know the truth about their health and chances for recovery. Even when they're not officially informed by a doctor or relative, most fatally ill people know or strongly suspect that they're dying. Dying people usually make it clear whether they want to talk about death and to what extent. The most frequent concern is how much time is left. Usually physicians can give only a rough estimate, such as "several weeks or months."

A "Good" Death

As life expectancy has increased and high-technology interventions have multiplied, many health-care professionals as well as citizens and social organizations have begun to demand a better way of caring for those who are dying. The Center to Improve Care of the Dying, in Washington, DC, has set goals for reintegrating dying within living, thus enhancing the prospect for growth at the end of life. These experts talk of "dying well," "living while dying," and "physician-assisted living." They aim to change our way of thinking about dying so that we view the end of life as a time of love and reconciliation, and transcendence of suffering.

Physicians who care for the dying are being urged to do all that they can to eliminate pain. They are encouraged not to withhold opioid drugs, such as morphine, simply out of fear of addiction. More efforts are being made for patients to be taken care of at home, with appropriate support and well-informed guidance.

Various psychological factors can affect those at risk of dying. Elderly people who lack hope in the future are much more likely to die within the next few years. Researchers speculate that hopelessness may lead to biochemical and nervous system abnormalities or that hopeless individuals may not eat well, take medications as prescribed, or follow a doctor's recommendations.

Spirituality plays a major role. In various surveys, many patients say they want their doctors and nurses to address their spiritual concerns. In one survey, even 45 percent of nonreligious patients thought physicians should inquire politely about patients' spiritual needs. However, some worry that such queries may be inappropriate or detract from a doctor's primary mission.

Caregiving

When someone becomes terminally ill, a woman—usually the patient's wife, daughter, or sister—is most likely to provide day-to-day care, often for periods longer than a year. Caregiving takes a different toll on men and women. In one study of adult daughters and husbands caring for terminally ill breast cancer patients, the daughters experienced more symptoms of anxiety and depression and greater family strain.

The impact of caregiving continues even after the death of an ill spouse. In one study, the health of older caregivers who had experienced strain prior to a spouse's death did not deteriorate. They showed no increase in depressive symptoms or use of antidepressant drugs and did not lose weight. Those who had not been caregivers were more likely to experience depression and weight loss.

Hospice: Caring When Curing Isn't Possible

A **hospice** is a homelike health-care facility or program that helps dying men and women who can afford such care to live their final days to the fullest, as free as possible from disabling pain and mental anguish.

terminal illness An illness in which death is inevitable.

hospice A homelike health-care facility or program committed to supportive care for terminally ill people.

Race and ethnicity affect the use of hospice. In a study of patients over age 65 (and all covered by Medicare) with terminal cancer, Asian American and black patients were less likely to enroll in a hospice program than whites and Hispanics. They also were more likely to be hospitalized in an intensive care unit at least twice during their last month of life.[42]

Hospice workers generally work in teams, usually consisting of a nurse, physician, social worker, chaplain, and trained volunteers. Other professionals, such as a physical therapist, may join the team when needed. These workers provide the comfort, support, and care dying patients need until they do die.

Hospice programs offer a combination of medical and emotional care that involves not only the patient but also the family members or others concerned with caring for the patient. Most hospice patients have life expectancies of six months or less and are no longer receiving treatments aimed at curing their diseases. When someone is available to provide care, patients remain in their own homes. Hospice nurses regularly visit all home patients and are available around the clock.

For patients requiring care that the family cannot provide, round-the-clock care is available at the hospice facility. Unlike a traditional hospital, where the focus is on diagnosis, cure, and treatment, a hospice works to make what is left of life pain-free and comfortable. Visiting hours for relatives and friends are flexible, with no restrictions on visits by children and grandchildren. Hospice services are covered, in full or in part, by most major insurance companies.

Near-Death Experiences

Reports of near-death experiences have grown, thanks largely to advances in emergency medical care. Most are remarkably similar, whether they occur in children or adults, whether they're the result of accidents or illnesses, even whether the individuals actually are near death or only think they are. Some individuals who have survived a close brush with death report **autoscopy** (watching, from several feet in the air, resuscitation attempts on their own bodies) or **transcendence** (the sense of passing into a foreign region or dimension). Some see light, often at the end of a tunnel. Their vision seems clearer; their hearing, sharper. Some recall scenes from their lives or feel the presence of loved ones who have died. Many report profound feelings of joy, calm, and peace. Fewer than 1 percent of those who've reported near-death experiences described them as frightening or distressing, although a larger number recall transitory feelings of fear or confusion.

Many near-death experiences occur in individuals who've been sedated or given other medications; however, many others do not. Several studies have shown that individuals who received medication or anesthesia were actually less likely to remember near-death experiences than those who hadn't had any drugs. Some scientists have speculated that lack of oxygen, changes in blood gases, altered brain functioning, or the release of neurotransmitters (messenger chemicals in the brain) may play a role in near-death experiences. However, there's little solid evidence that physiological events are responsible. There's also no proof that wishful thinking, cultural conditioning, posttraumatic stress, or other psychological mechanisms may be at work. For now, the most that scientists can say for sure about this medical mystery is that it needs further study.

Suicide

Suicide increases with age and is most common in persons aged 65 years and older. This age group accounts for 18 percent of all suicides in the United States. For every completed suicide, there are 10 to 40 unsuccessful attempts. (Chapter 4 presents a detailed discussion of the risk factors and warning signs of suicide.)

One of the main factors leading to suicide is illness, especially terminal illness. A great deal of debate centers on quality of life, yet there is no reliable or consistent way to measure this. Patients who are dying may feel some quality of life, even when others do not recognize it, or their evaluations of the quality of their lives may fluctuate. Dying patients who say their lives are not worth living may be suffering from depression; hopelessness is one of its characteristic symptoms.

"Rational" Suicide

An elderly widow suffering from advanced cancer takes a lethal overdose of sleeping pills. A young man with several AIDS-related illnesses shoots himself. A woman in her fifties, diagnosed as having Alzheimer's disease, asks a doctor to help her end her life. Are these suicides "rational" because these individuals used logical reasoning in deciding to end their lives?

The question is intensely controversial. Advocates of the right to "self-deliverance" argue that individuals in great pain or faced with the prospect of a debilitating, hopeless battle against an incurable disease can and should be able to decide to end their lives. As legislatures and the legal system tackle the thorny questions of an individual's right to die, mental health professionals worry that, even in those with fatal diseases, suicidal wishes often stem from undiagnosed depression.

Because depression may indeed warp the ability to make a rational decision about suicide, mental health professionals urge physicians and family members to make sure individuals with chronic or fatal illnesses are evaluated for depression and given medication, psychotherapy, or both. It is also important for everyone to allow enough time—an average of three to eight weeks—to see if treatment for depression will make a difference in their desire to keep living.

Physician-Assisted Suicide

According to U.S. surveys, there is greater support for physician-assisted suicide and euthanasia among patients and the general public than among physicians. More Caucasians support these practices than members of ethnic minority groups.

Oregon is the first state to legalize physician-assisted suicide for terminally ill patients. The Supreme Court has upheld the state's Death with Dignity Act, which bars suicide assistance for anyone whose judgment may be impaired by a mental disorder.

If patients have a right to die, should doctors help them end their lives? Physicians could stop any extraordinary efforts to sustain life (for example, by withholding oxygen or ending intravenous feedings); such actions are referred to as passive *euthanasia,* or *dyathanasia.* Euthanasia, the active form of so-called mercy killing, has generally been viewed as illegal and unethical. Euthanasia is tolerated and legally pardoned in the Netherlands but remains illegal in all European countries. The demand for physician-assisted death in the Netherlands has not risen; and patients and physicians have become more reluctant to ask for or offer this option over the past few years.

Some medical groups, such as the American Medical Association, oppose as unethical any physician's involvement in euthanasia. Others argue that individuals have the right to end their own lives and that physicians who provide prescriptions for lethal doses of certain drugs are acting out of compassion and respect for patients' wishes.

The Practicalities of Death

At a time of great emotional pain, grieving family members must cope with medical, legal, and practical concerns, including obtaining a medical certificate of the cause of death, registering the death, and making funeral arrangements. They also may want to arrange for organ donations and, in some circumstances, an autopsy.

Funeral Arrangements

A body can be either buried or cremated. Burial requires the purchase of a cemetery

autoscopy The sensation of one's self being outside its body, often experienced by individuals in near-death medical crises.

transcendence The sense of passing into a foreign region or dimension, often experienced by a person near death.

© Terry Vine/Stone/Getty Images

Funerals and memorial services help those in mourning to honor the deceased and to come to terms with their loss.

have two parts: a religious ceremony at a church or funeral home, and a burial ceremony at the grave site.

Alternatively, the body may be disposed of immediately, through burial, cremation, or bequeathal to a medical school, and a memorial service held later. In a memorial service, the body is not present, which may change the focus of the service from the person's death to his or her life.

Autopsies

An autopsy is a detailed examination of a body after death, also called a postmortem exam. There are two types:

- **Medicolegal.** This type of autopsy is performed to establish the cause of death and to gather information about the death for use as evidence in any legal proceedings. It is done to detect any crimes and to help identify the proper person for prosecution, to investigate possible industrial hazards or contagious diseases that may endanger the public health, or to establish the cause of death for insurance purposes.

- **Medical/educational.** This type of autopsy is performed, usually in the hospital where the person died, to increase medical knowledge and to determine a more exact cause of death. It may be requested by the attending physician or the family, but it cannot be performed without the family's permission.

Autopsies can be extremely valuable in establishing an accurate cause of death, revealing a different diagnosis that might have led to a change in therapy and prolonged survival in about 10 percent of cases. Thirty years ago about 50 percent of patients who died in hospitals were autopsied. However, the autopsy rate in the United States has been steadily declining, and today about 10 to 20 percent of deaths in teaching hospitals are autopsied.

plot, which many families do decades before death. A burial is typically the third most expensive purchase of a lifetime, behind the cost of a house and car. The average national costs range as high as $6,000, although they vary considerably. Memorial societies are voluntary groups that help people plan in advance for death. They obtain services at moderate cost, keep the arrangements simple and dignified, and—most important, perhaps—ease the emotional and financial burden on the rest of the family when death finally does come.

If the body is to be cremated, you must comply with some additional formalities, with which the funeral director can help you. After a *cremation* (incineration of the remains), you can either collect the ashes to keep, bury, or scatter yourself, or ask the crematorium to dispose of them.

The tradition of a funeral may help survivors come to terms with the death, enabling them to mourn their loss and to celebrate the dead person's life. Funerals are usually held two to four days after the death. Many

Grief

An estimated 8 million Americans lose a member of their immediate family each year. Each death leaves an average of five

people bereaved. Such loss may be the single most upsetting and feared event in a person's life. It produces a wide range of reactions, including anxiety, guilt, anger, and financial concern. Many may see the death of an old person as less tragic than the death of a child or young person. A sudden death is more of a shock than one following a long illness. A suicide can be particularly devastating, because family members may wonder whether they could have done anything to prevent it. The cause of death also can affect the reactions of friends and acquaintances. Some people express less sympathy and support when individuals are murdered or take their own lives.

According to the stage theory of grief, individuals respond to the loss of a loved one by progressing through several steps, just like people facing death. These consist of shock-numbness, yearning-searching, disorganization-despair, and reorganization. All these reactions can occur simultaneously, although most peak within six months. Acceptance continues to increase over time. The most common and one of the most painful experiences is the death of a parent. When both parents die, even adult individuals may feel like orphaned children. They mourn not just for the father and mother who are gone, but also for their lost role of being someone's child.

Bereavement is not a rare occurrence on college campuses, but it is largely an ignored problem. Counselors have called upon universities to help students who have lost a loved one through initiatives such as training nonbereaved students to provide peer support and raising consciousness about bereavement.

Grief's Effects on Health

Men and women who lose partners, parents, or children endure so much stress that they're at increased risk of serious physical and mental illness, and even of premature death. Studies of the health effects of grief have found the following:

- Grief produces changes in the respiratory, hormonal, and central nervous systems and may affect functions of the heart, blood, and immune systems.

- Grieving adults may experience mood swings between sadness and anger, guilt and anxiety.

- Grievers may feel physically sick, lose their appetite, sleep poorly, or fear that they're going crazy because they "see" the deceased person in different places.

- Friendships and remarriage offer the greatest protection against health problems.

- Some widows may have increased rates of depression, suicide, and death from cirrhosis of the liver. The greatest risk factors are poor previous mental and physical health and a lack of social support.

- Grieving parents, partners, and adult children are at increased risk of serious physical and mental illness, suicide, and premature death.

Sometimes grief progresses from an emotionally painful but normal experience to a more persistent problem, called *complicated grief*. Individuals who experience very long-lasting or severe symptoms, including inability to accept a loved one's death, persistent thoughts about the death, and preoccupation with the lost loved one, can benefit from professional treatment.

"Every man desires to live long," wrote Jonathan Swift, "but no man would be old." We all wish for long lives, yet we want to avoid the disease and disability that can tarnish our golden years. Here are the best ways to do so.

- **Exercise regularly.** By improving blood flow, staving off depression, warding off heart disease, and enhancing well-being, regular workouts help keep mind and body in top form.

- **Don't smoke.** Every cigarette you puff can snuff out seven minutes of your life, according to the Centers for Disease Control and Prevention.

- **Watch your weight and blood pressure.** Increases in these vital statistics can increase your risk of hypertension, cardiovascular disease, and other health problems.

- **Eat more fruits and vegetables.** These foods, rich in vitamins and protective antioxidants, can reduce your risk of cancer and damage from destructive free radicals.

- **Cut down on fat.** Fatty foods can clog the arteries and contribute to various cancers.

- **Limit drinking.** Alcohol can undermine physical health and sabotage mental acuity.

- **Cultivate stimulating interests.** Elderly individuals with complex and interesting lifestyles are most likely to retain sharp minds and memories beyond age 70.

- **Don't worry; be happy.** At any age, emotional turmoil can undermine well-being. Relaxation techniques, such as meditation, help by reducing stress.

- **Reach out.** Try to keep in contact with other people of all ages and experiences. Make the effort to invite them to your home or go out with them. On a regular basis, do something to help another person.

- **Make the most of your time.** Greet each day with a specific goal—to take a walk, write letters, visit a friend.

SELF SURVEY   What Is Your Aging IQ?

Answer True or False

T	F	1.	Everyone becomes "senile" sooner or later, if he or she lives long enough.
T	F	2.	American families have by and large abandoned their older members.
T	F	3.	Depression is a serious problem for older people.
T	F	4.	The numbers of older people are growing.
T	F	5.	The vast majority of older people are self-sufficient.
T	F	6.	Mental confusion is an inevitable, incurable consequence of old age.
T	F	7.	Intelligence declines with age.
T	F	8.	Sexual urges and activity normally cease around age 55–60.
T	F	9.	If a person has been smoking for 30 or 40 years, it does no good to quit.
T	F	10.	Older people should stop exercising and rest.
T	F	11.	As you grow older, you need more vitamins and minerals to stay healthy.
T	F	12.	Only children need to be concerned about calcium for strong bones and teeth.
T	F	13.	Extremes of heat and cold can be particularly dangerous to old people.
T	F	14.	Many older people are hurt in accidents that could have been prevented.
T	F	15.	More men than women survive to old age.
T	F	16.	Deaths from stroke and heart disease are declining.
T	F	17.	Older people on the average take more medications than younger people.
T	F	18.	Snake oil salesmen are as common today as they were on the frontier.
T	F	19.	Personality changes with age, just like hair color and skin texture.
T	F	20.	Sight declines with age.

Scoring

1. False. Even among those who live to be 80 or older, only 20–25 percent develop Alzheimer's disease or some other incurable form of brain disease. "Senility" is a meaningless term that should be discarded.

2. False. The American family is still the number-one caretaker of older Americans. Most older people live close to their children and see them often; many live with their spouses. In all, 8 out of 10 men and 6 out of 10 women live in family settings.

3. True. Depression, loss of self-esteem, loneliness, and anxiety can become more common as older people face retirement, along with the deaths of relatives and friends, and other such crises—often at the same time. Fortunately, depression is treatable.

4. True. By the year 2030, one in four people will be over 65 years of age.

5. True. Only a small percentage of the older population live in nursing homes. The rest live independently or with relatives or caregivers.

6. False. Mental confusion and serious forgetfulness in old age can be caused by Alzheimer's disease or other conditions that cause incurable damage to the brain, but some 100 other problems can cause the same symptoms. A minor head injury, a high fever, poor nutrition, adverse drug reactions, and depression can all be treated and the confusion will be cured.

7. False. Intelligence per se does not decline without reason. Most people maintain their intellect or improve as they grow older.

8. False. Most older people can lead an active, satisfying sex life.
9. False. Stopping smoking at any age not only reduces the risk of cancer and heart disease, it also leads to healthier lungs.
10. False. Many older people enjoy—and benefit from—exercises such as walking, swimming, and bicycle riding. Exercise at any age can help strengthen the heart and lungs, and lower blood pressure. See your physician before beginning a new exercise program.
11. False. Although certain requirements, such as that for "sunshine" vitamin D, may increase slightly with age, older people need the same amounts of most vitamins and minerals as younger people. Older people in particular should eat nutritious food and cut down on sweets, salty snack foods, high-calorie drinks, and alcohol.
12. False. Older people require fewer calories, but adequate intake of calcium for strong bones can become more important as you grow older. This is particularly true for women, whose risk of osteoporosis increases after menopause. Milk and cheese are rich in calcium as are cooked dried beans, collards, and broccoli. Some people need calcium supplements as well.
13. True. The body's thermostat tends to function less efficiently with age and the older person's body may be less able to adapt to heat or cold.

14. True. Falls are the most common cause of injuries among the elderly. Good safety habits, including proper lighting, nonskid carpets, and keeping living areas free of obstacles, can help prevent serious accidents.
15. False. Women tend to live 5 to 10 percent longer than men.
16. True. Fewer men and women are dying of stroke or heart disease.
17. True. The elderly consume 25 percent of all medications and, as a result, have many more problems with adverse drug reactions.
18. True. Medical quackery is a $10 billion business in the United States. People of all ages are commonly duped into "quick cures" for aging, arthritis, and cancer.
19. False. Personality doesn't change with age. Therefore, all old people can't be described as rigid and cantankerous. You are what you are for as long as you live. But you can change what you do to help yourself to good health.
20. False. Although changes in vision become more common with age, any change in vision, regardless of age, is related to a specific disease. If you are having problems with your vision, see your doctor.

Source: National Institute on Aging, www.counselingnotes.com/seniors/age/age_iq.htm.

Your Health Action Plan for Preparing for a Medical Crisis in an Aging Relative

"Medical crises are more common and more likely to lead to serious complications after age 60," says Kenneth Brummel-Smith, M.D., former president of the American Geriatrics Society. As your parents, grandparents, and other relatives get older, here is what you can do in advance:

- **Watch for warning signals.** If your relative begins stumbling or having near-misses on the highway, make sure he or she sees a doctor before a serious fall or accident occurs. There may be a cure or, if not a cure, a way to improve functioning.
- **Suggest a surrogate.** Even if a couple has been married for 40 years, neither has the legal right to make medical decisions for a spouse. The same is true for children and other relatives. The only way to get that right is to fill out a form, usually called an advance directive or medical power of attorney (discussed on page 635).
- **Talk to loved ones.** "Waiting for something bad to happen doesn't make it any easier to talk about," says Dr. Brummel-Smith, who suggests sitting down for a formal discussion at some point after a relative reaches age 65 "but definitely before age 75."
- **Focus on values.** "You don't have to discuss every possible drug or surgery or intervention," says Dr. Brummel-Smith. "What's important is that you understand the older person's values. What are fates worse than death? Independence may be more important than living a longer life." Many families use the "Five Wishes" form (available online at **www.agingwithdignity.org** and described on page 636) to discuss preferences for medical, personal, emotional, and spiritual care.
- **Involve the person's primary physician.** Often it's not a question of what doctors can do medically in a crisis, but of what they should do, which is the patient's decision. Encourage loved ones to discuss "what ifs" with their doctors and make their desires clear. For instance, a primary physician should know which treatments patients want (such as resuscitation during surgery) as well as those they don't want (such as remaining on a ventilator if unable to breathe on their own).
- **Investigate alternative living options.** Aging parents should visit retirement communities or nursing homes while they're still healthy, not with the idea of moving into them, but of knowing what's available. They also should find out if their health plan provides services for seniors after a medical crisis.
- **Make sure you know where to find key documents.** An easily accessible folder with copies of the latest lab reports, consultations, and advance directives helps to avoid unnecessary tests and get faster treatment when a crisis does occur.

MAKING THIS CHAPTER WORK FOR YOU

Review Questions

1. Steps for protecting against bone loss include
   a. having at least two drinks per day.
   b. getting moderate exposure to sunlight.
   c. avoiding heavy exercise.
   d. having a diet low in calcium.

2. When should concern change to intervention?
   a. Uncle Charlie is 85 and continues to drive himself to the grocery store and to the Senior Center during the daytime.
   b. Nana takes pills at breakfast, lunch, and dinner but sometimes mixes them up.

c. Mom's hot flashes have become a family joke.

d. Your older brother can never remember where he put his car keys.

3. You can best help a friend who is bereaved by
   a. encouraging him to have a few drinks to forget his pain.
   b. simply spending time with her.
   c. avoiding talking about his loss because it is awkward.
   d. reminding her about all she still has in her life.

4. Physically fit people over age 60
   a. have lower risk of dying from chronic heart disease.
   b. can regain the fitness level of a 25-year-old.
   c. show no difference in levels of anxiety and depression.
   d. have higher health-care expenses.

5. Which statement about aging is *false*?
   a. The most common nutritional disorder in the elderly is obesity.
   b. In men, sexual activity and longevity are linked.
   c. Hormone therapy reduces the risk of heart disease in menopausal women.
   d. Seniors who take up new hobbies late in life may slow aging within the brain.

6. The gender gap related to longevity
   a. is due to deficiencies in the Y chromosome.
   b. results from the presence of a mutant gene.
   c. may be due to the X chromosome and its hormonal influences on the immune system.
   d. is about 13 years in the United States.

7. Which of the following is a change associated with aging that is slowed by exercise?
   a. loss of connective tissue in skin
   b. decrease in certain hormone levels
   c. loss of lean muscle tissue
   d. decrease interest in food

8. Factors that contribute to staying healthy longer include all of the following *except*
   a. avoiding illness.
   b. moderate smoking.
   c. regular exercise.
   d. lifelong learning.

9. Which statement about the aging brain is *false?*
   a. When brain cells die, surrounding cells can fill the gaps to maintain cognitive function.
   b. Remembering names and recalling information may take longer.
   c. "Use it or lose it."
   d. Mental ability and physical ability both decline with age.

10. An advance directive
    a. indicates who should have your property in the event you die.
    b. may authorize which individuals may not participate in your health care if you are unable to care for yourself.

c. can specify your desires related to the use of medical treatments and technology to prolong your life.

d. should specify which physician you designate to be your health-care proxy.

Answers to these questions can be found on page 650.

Critical Thinking

1. How are your parents or other mentors staying fit and alert as they age? Do you think you might use similar strategies?

2. Do you think that coming to terms with mortality allows an individual to live each day to its fullest, rather than putting off what he or she would like to do until tomorrow? How does this concept affect your own life? Explain. Do you believe in a next life? How does this affect your view of life and death?

3. Have your living parents and grandparents written advanced directives or a living will? Have you discussed with them their preferences regarding treatment in the event of a medical crisis? If you haven't had this discussion with your family, how can you begin the process of helping your parents or grandparents communicate their wishes?

4. As many as 10,000 people in this country are chronically unconscious, kept alive by artificial respirators and feeding tubes. If you were in an accident that left you in a vegetative state, would you want doctors to do everything possible to fight for your life? Would you want to spend months or even years totally unaware of your surroundings? Should health-care professionals have the right to declare that anyone is too old, too ill, or too frail to try to save? Should they have the right to insist that someone live on even if that person isn't experiencing much of a life?

Media Menu

CENGAGENOW® Go to the CengageNOW for Health website at **www.cengage.com/sso** that will:

- Help you evaluate your knowledge of the material.
- Allow you to take an exam-prep quiz.
- Provide a Personalized Learning Plan targeting resources that address areas you should study.
- Coach you through identifying target goals for behavioral change and creating and monitoring your personal change plan throughout the semester.

Internet Connections

www.nia.nih.gov
This government site features a comprehensive array of resources on aging, including publications on a variety of geriatric health topics, current news events, and a resource directory for older people.

www.realage.com

This site features diet and exercise assessment tools—such as a BMI calculator, exercise estimator, and RealAge assessment quizzes on a variety of health topics—to help you determine your risk of disease and what you can do to reduce this risk. The main feature is an interactive, online personal lifestyle assessment that also gives you options for "growing younger."

http://aoa.gov

This site, part of the Department of Health and Human Services, has information for seniors and their families on promoting healthy lifestyles and general aging topics.

www.npr.org/programs/death/

This site, sponsored by National Public Radio, contains transcripts and resources from an *All Things Considered* series focusing on how Americans deal with death and dying. Features include personal stories, a place where you can tell your own story, and a comprehensive list of organizations that can help families who are coping with death, dying, and the diseases of old age.

Key Terms

The terms listed are used on the page indicated. Definitions of the terms are in the Glossary at the end of the book.

advance directives 635
aging 623
Alzheimer's disease 633
autoscopy 643
coma 639
dementia 633
do-not-resuscitate (DNR) 636
holographic will 636
hormone therapy (HT) 631
hospice 641
living will 635
menopause 629
perimenopause 629
persistent vegetative state 639
terminal illness 641
transcendence 643

Answers to Review Questions

Chapter 1
1. b; 2. c; 3. c; 4. c; 5. b; 6. b; 7. c; 8. d; 9. c; 10. c

Chapter 2
1. b; 2. b; 3. d; 4. b; 5. a; 6. b; 7. c; 8. c; 9. c; 10. a

Chapter 3
1. b; 2. c; 3. a; 4. d; 5. d; 6. d; 7. b; 8. a; 9. c; 10. a

Chapter 4
1. d; 2. a; 3. a; 4. b; 5. a; 6. b; 7. b; 8. c; 9. d; 10. d

Chapter 5
1. c; 2. d; 3. c; 4. b; 5. b; 6. b; 7. b; 8. c; 9. b; 10. a

Chapter 6
1. d; 2. c; 3. b; 4. c; 5. a; 6. d; 7. a; 8. a; 9. b; 10. d

Chapter 7
1. c; 2. a; 3. a; 4. a; 5. d; 6. b; 7. c; 8. d; 9. c; 10. b

Chapter 8
1. b; 2. b; 3. d; 4. d; 5. d; 6. d; 7. c; 8. c; 9. a; 10. a

Chapter 9
1. d; 2. d; 3. c; 4. b; 5. a; 6. d; 7. d; 8. b; 9. a; 10. c

Chapter 10
1. c; 2. d; 3. c; 4. b; 5. d; 6. b; 7. a; 8. c; 9. c; 10. a

Chapter 11
1. b; 2. a; 3. c; 4. a; 5. b; 6. d; 7. c; 8. d; 9. c; 10. d

Chapter 12
1. b; 2. b; 3. a; 4. d; 5. b; 6. d; 7. a; 8. d; 9. b; 10. c

Chapter 13
1. d; 2. c; 3. d; 4. b; 5. d; 6. c; 7. a; 8. b; 9. a; 10. c

Chapter 14
1. b; 2. d; 3. a; 4. d; 5. a; 6. d; 7. c; 8. b; 9. b; 10. a

Chapter 15
1. b; 2. b; 3. d; 4. c; 5. a; 6. d; 7. c; 8. a; 9. c; 10. a

Chapter 16
1. c; 2. d; 3. b; 4. c; 5. a; 6. d; 7. b; 8. b; 9. a; 10. c

Chapter 17
1. b; 2. a; 3. d; 4. c; 5. b; 6. d; 7. d; 8. b; 9. d; 10. a

Chapter 18
1. c; 2. c; 3. a; 4. b; 5. a; 6. b; 7. c; 8. c; 9. b; 10. b

Chapter 19
1. b; 2. c; 3. c; 4. a; 5. d; 6. c; 7. b; 8. b; 9. b; 10. a

Chapter 20
1. b; 2. b; 3. b; 4. a; 5. c; 6. c; 7. c; 8. b; 9. d; 10. c

GLOSSARY

abscess A localized accumulation of pus and disintegrating tissue.

Absorption The passage of substances into or across membranes or tissues.

abstinence Voluntary refrainment from sexual intercourse.

acquired immune deficiency virus (AIDS) The final stages of HIV infection, characterized by a variety of severe illnesses and decreased levels of certain immune cells.

active stretching A technique that involves stretching a muscle by contracting the opposing muscle.

acupuncture A Chinese medical practice of puncturing the body with needles inserted at specific points to relieve pain or cure disease.

acute injuries Physical injuries, such as sprains, bruises, and pulled muscles, which result from sudden traumas, such as falls or collisions.

adaptive response The body's attempt to reestablish homeostasis or stability.

addiction A behavioral pattern characterized by compulsion, loss of control, and continued repetition of a behavior or activity in spite of adverse consequences.

Adoption The legal process for becoming the parent to a child of other biological parents.

advance directives Documents that specify an individual's preferences regarding treatment in a medical crisis.

aerobic exercise Physical activity in which sufficient or excess oxygen is continually supplied to the body.

aging The characteristic pattern of normal life changes that occur as living things grow older.

alcohol abuse Continued use of alcohol despite awareness of social, occupational, psychological, or physical problems related to its use, or use of alcohol in dangerous ways or situations, such as before driving.

alcohol dependence Development of a strong craving for alcohol due to the pleasurable feelings or relief of stress or anxiety produced by drinking.

alcoholism A chronic, progressive, potentially fatal disease characterized by impaired control of drinking, a preoccupation with alcohol, continued use of alcohol despite adverse consequences, and distorted thinking, most notably denial.

allergy A hypersensitivity to a particular substance in one's environment or diet.

altruism Acts of helping or giving to others without thought of self-benefit.

Alzheimer's disease A progressive deterioration of intellectual powers due to physiological changes within the brain; symptoms include diminishing ability to concentrate and reason, disorientation, depression, apathy, and paranoia.

amenorrhea The absence or suppression of menstruation.

amino acids Organic compounds containing nitrogen, carbon, hydrogen, and oxygen; the essential building blocks of proteins.

amnion The innermost membrane of the sac enclosing the embryo or fetus.

amphetamine Any of a class of stimulants that trigger the release of epinephrine, which stimulates the central nervous system; users experience a state of hyper-alertness and energy, followed by a crash as the drug wears off.

anabolic steroids Drugs derived from testosterone and approved for medical use, but often used by athletes to increase their musculature and weight.

anaerobic exercise Physical activity in which the body develops an oxygen deficit.

androgyny The expression of both masculine and feminine traits.

angina pectoris A severe, suffocating chest pain caused by a brief lack of oxygen to the heart.

anorexia nervosa A psychological disorder in which refusal to eat and/or an extreme loss of appetite leads to malnutrition, severe weight loss, and possibly death.

antibiotics Substances produced by microorganisms, or synthetic agents, that are toxic to bacteria.

antidepressant Drug used primarily to treat symptoms of depression.

antioxidant Substances that prevent the damaging effects of oxidation in cells.

antiviral drug A substance that decreases the severity and duration of a viral infection if taken prior to or soon after onset of the infection.

anxiety disorders A group of psychological disorders involving episodes of apprehension, tension, or uneasiness, stemming from the anticipation of danger and sometimes accompanied by physical symptoms, which cause significant distress and impairment to an individual.

aorta The main artery of the body, arising from the left ventricle of the heart.

appetite A desire for food, stimulated by anticipated hunger, physiological changes within the brain and body, the availability of food, and other environmental and psychological factors.

arteriosclerosis Any of a number of chronic diseases characterized by degeneration of the arteries and hardening and thickening of arterial walls.

artificial insemination The introduction of viable sperm into the vagina by artificial means for the purpose of inducing conception.

assertive Behaving in a confident manner to make your needs and desires clear to others in a nonhostile way.

asthma A disease or allergic response characterized by bronchial spasms and difficult breathing.

atherosclerosis A form of arteriosclerosis in which fatty substances (plaque) are deposited on the inner walls of arteries.

atrium Either of the two upper chambers of the heart, which receive blood from the veins.

attention deficit/hyperactivity disorder (ADHD) A spectrum of difficulties in controlling motion and sustaining attention, including hyperactivity, impulsivity, and distractibility.

autoimmune disorder Resulting from the attack on body tissue by an immune system that fails to recognize the tissue as self.

autonomy The ability to draw on internal resources; independence from familial and societal influences.

autoscopy The sensation of one's self being outside its body, often experienced by individuals in near death medical crises.

aversion therapy A treatment that attempts to help a person overcome a dependence or bad habit by making the person feel disgusted or repulsed by that habit.

axon The long fiber that conducts impulses from the neuron's nucleus to its dendrites.

axon terminal The ending of an axon, from which impulses are transmitted to a dendrite of another neuron.

Ayurveda A traditional Indian medical treatment involving meditation, exercise, herbal medications, and nutrition.

bacteria (singular, **bacterium**) One-celled microscopic organisms; the most plentiful pathogens.

bacterial vaginosis A vaginal infection caused by overgrowth and depletion of various microorganisms living in the vagina, resulting in a malodorous white or gray vaginal discharge.

ballistic stretching Rapid bouncing movements.

barbiturates Antianxiety drugs that depress the central nervous system, reduce activity, and induce relaxation, drowsiness, or sleep; often prescribed to relieve tension and treat epileptic seizures or as a general anesthetic.

barrier contraceptives Birth control devices that block the meeting of egg and sperm, either by physical barriers, such as condoms, diaphragms, or cervical caps, or by chemical barriers, such as spermicide, or both.

basal metabolic rate (BMR) The number of calories required to sustain the body at rest.

behavioral therapy A technique that emphasizes application of the principles of learning to substitute desirable responses and behavior patterns for undesirable ones.

benzodiazepines Antianxiety drugs that depress the central nervous system, reduce activity, and induce relaxation, drowsiness, or sleep; often prescribed to relieve tension, muscular strain, sleep problems, anxiety, and panic attacks; also used as an anesthetic and in the treatment of alcohol withdrawal.

bidis Skinny, sweet-flavored cigarettes.

binge drinking For a man, having five or more alcoholic drinks at a single sitting; for a woman, having four drinks or more at a single sitting.

binge eating The rapid consumption of an abnormally large amount of food in a relatively short time.

biofeedback A technique of becoming aware, with the aid of external monitoring devices, of internal physiological activities in order to develop the capability of altering them.

bipolar disorder Severe depression alternating with periods of manic activity and elation.

bisexual Sexually oriented toward both sexes.

blastocyst In embryonic development, a ball of cells with a surface layer and an inner cell mass.

blended family A family formed when one or both of the partners bring children from a previous union to the new marriage.

blood-alcohol concentration (BAC) The amount of alcohol in the blood, expressed as a percentage.

body composition The relative amounts of fat and lean tissue (bone, muscle, organs, water) in the body.

body mass index (BMI) A mathematical formula that correlates with body fat; the ratio of weight to height squared.

botulism Possibly fatal food poisoning caused by a type of bacterium that grows and produces its toxin in the absence of air and is found in improperly canned food.

bulimia nervosa Episodic binge eating, often followed by forced vomiting or laxative abuse, and accompanied by a persistent preoccupation with body shape and weight.

burnout A state of physical, emotional, and mental exhaustion resulting from constant or repeated emotional pressure.

caesarean delivery The surgical procedure in which an infant is delivered through an incision made in the abdominal wall and uterus.

calorie The amount of energy required to raise the temperature of 1 gram of water by 1 degree Celsius. In everyday usage related to the energy content of foods and the energy expended in activities, a calorie is actually the equivalent of a thousand such calories, or a kilocalorie.

candidiasis An infection of the yeast *Candida albicans*, commonly occurring in the vagina, vulva, penis, and mouth and causing burning, itching, and a whitish discharge.

capillary A minute blood vessel that connects an artery to a vein.

carbon monoxide A colorless, odorless gas produced by the burning of gasoline or tobacco; displaces oxygen in the hemoglobin molecules of red blood cells.

carcinogen A substance or agent that causes cancer.

cardiometabolic Referring to the heart and to the biochemical processes involved in the body's functioning.

cardiorespiratory fitness The ability of the heart and blood vessels to circulate blood through the body efficiently.

celibacy Abstention from sexual activity; can be partial or complete, permanent or temporary.

certified social worker A person who has completed a two-year graduate program in counseling people with mental problems.

cervical cap A thimble-sized rubber or plastic cap that is inserted into the vagina to fit over the cervix and prevent the passage of sperm into the uterus during sexual intercourse; used with a spermicidal foam or jelly, it serves as both a chemical and a physical barrier to sperm.

cervix The narrow, lower end of the uterus that opens into the vagina.

chanchroid A soft, painful sore or localized infection usually acquired through sexual contact.

chiropractic A method of treating disease, primarily through manipulating the bones and joints to restore normal nerve function.

chlamydia A sexually transmitted infection caused by the bacterium *Chlamydia trachomatis*, often asymptomatic in women, but sometimes characterized by urinary pain; if undetected and untreated, may result in pelvic inflammatory disease (PID).

chlorinated hydrocarbons Highly toxic pesticides, such as DDT and chlordane, that are extremely resistant to breakdown; may cause cancer, birth defects, neurological disorders, and damage to wildlife and the environment.

cholesterol An organic substance found in animal fats; linked to cardiovascular disease, particularly atherosclerosis.

chronic fatigue syndrome (CFS) A cluster of symptoms whose cause is not yet known; a primary symptom is debilitating fatigue.

circumcision The surgical removal of the foreskin of the penis.

clitoris A small erectile structure on the female, corresponding to the penis on the male.

club drugs Illegally manufactured psychoactive drugs that have dangerous physical and psychological effects.

cocaine A white crystalline powder extracted from the leaves of the coca plant that stimulates the central nervous system and produces a brief period of euphoria followed by a depression.

codependency An emotional and psychological behavioral pattern in which the spouses, partners, parents, children, and friends of individuals with addictive behaviors allow or enable their loved ones to continue their self-destructive habits.

cognitive therapy A technique used to identify an individual's beliefs and attitudes, recognize negative thought patterns, and educate in alternative ways of thinking.

cohabitation Two people living together as a couple, without official ties such as marriage.

coitus interruptus The removal of the penis from the vagina before ejaculation.

coma A state of total unconsciousness.

complementary and alternative medicine (CAM) A term used to apply to all health-care approaches, practices, and treatments not widely taught in medical schools, not generally used in hospitals, and not usually reimbursed by medical insurance companies.

complete proteins Proteins that contain all the amino acids needed by the body for growth and maintenance.

complex carbohydrates Starches, including cereals, fruits, and vegetables.

computer vision syndrome A condition caused by computer use marked by tired, sore eyes, blurred vision, headaches, and neck, shoulder, and back pain.

conception The merging of a sperm and an ovum.

condom A latex sheath worn over the penis during sexual acts to prevent conception and/or the transmission of disease; the female condom lines the walls of the vagina.

contraception The prevention of conception; birth control.

corpus luteum A yellowish mass of tissue that is formed, immediately after ovulation, from the remaining cells of the follicle; it secretes estrogen and progesterone for the remainder of the menstrual cycle.

Cowper's gland Two small glands that discharge into the male urethra; also called bulbourethral glands.

culture The set of shared attitudes, values, goals, and practices of a group that are internalized by an individual within the group.

cunnilingus Sexual stimulation of a woman's genitals by means of oral manipulation.

cystitis Inflammation of the urinary bladder.

decibel A unit for measuring the intensity of sounds.

defense mechanism A psychological process that alleviates anxiety and eliminates mental conflict; includes denial, displacement, projection, rationalization, reaction formation, and repression.

delirium tremens (DTs) The delusions, hallucinations, and agitated behavior following withdrawal from long-term chronic alcohol abuse.

dementia Deterioration of mental capability.

dendrites Branching fibers of a neuron that receive impulses from axon terminals of other neurons and conduct these impulses toward the nucleus.

depression In general, feelings of unhappiness and despair; as a mental illness, also characterized by an inability to function normally.

detoxification The supervised removal of a poisonous or harmful substance (such as a drug) from the body; a therapy for alcoholics in which they are denied alcohol in a controlled environment.

diabetes mellitus A disease in which the inadequate production of insulin leads to failure of the body tissues to break down carbohydrates at a normal rate.

diagnostic related group (DRG) A category of conditions requiring hospitalization for which the cost of care has been determined prior to a client's hospitalization.

diaphragm A bowl-like rubber cup with a flexible rim that is inserted into the vagina to cover the cervix and prevent the passage of sperm into the uterus during sexual intercourse; used with a spermicidal foam or jelly, it serves as both a chemical and a physical barrier to sperm.

diastole The period between contractions in the cardiac cycle, during which the heart relaxes and dilates as it fills with blood.

diastolic blood pressure Lowest blood pressure between contractions of the heart.

dietary fiber The nondigestible form of carbohydrates found in plant foods, such as leaves, stems, skins, seeds, and hulls.

dilation and evacuation (D and E) A medical procedure in which the contents of the uterus are removed through the use of instruments.

distress A negative stress that may result in illness.

do-not-resuscitate (DNR) An advance directive expressing an individual's preference that resuscitation efforts not be made during a medical crisis.

drug Any substance, other than food, that affects bodily functions and structures when taken into the body.

drug abuse The excessive use of a drug in a manner inconsistent with accepted medical practice.

drug dependence Continued substance use even when its use causes cognitive, behavioral, and physical symptoms.

drug diversion The transfer of a drug from the person for whom it was prescribed to another individual.

drug misuse The use of a drug for a purpose (or person) other than that for which it was medically intended.

dynamic flexibility The ability to move a joint quickly and fluidly through its entire range of motion with little resistance.

dysfunctional Characterized by negative and destructive patterns of behavior between partners or between parents and children.

dysmenorrhea Painful menstruation.

dyspareunia A sexual difficulty in which a woman experiences pain during sexual intercourse.

dysthymia frequent, prolonged mild depression.

eating disorders Bizarre, often dangerous patterns of food consumption, including anorexia nervosa and bulimia nervosa.

ecosystem A community of organisms sharing a physical and chemical environment and interacting with each other.

ecstasy (MDMA) A synthetic compound, also known as methylenedioxymethamphetamine, that is similar in structure to methamphetamine and has both stimulant and hallucinogenic effects.

ectopic pregnancy A pregnancy in which the fertilized egg has implanted itself outside the uterine cavity, usually in the fallopian tube.

ejaculation The expulsion of semen from the penis.

ejaculatory duct The canal connecting the seminal vesicles and vas deferens.

electromagnetic fields (EMFs) The invisible electric and magnetic fields generated by an electrically charged conductor.

embryo An organism in its early stage of development; in humans, the embryonic period lasts from the second to the eighth week of pregnancy.

emergency contraception Types of oral contraceptive pills, usually taken within 72 hours after intercourse, that can prevent pregnancy.

emotional health The ability to express and acknowledge one's feelings and moods and exhibit adaptability and compassion for others.

emotional intelligence A term used by some psychologists to evaluate the capacity of people to understand themselves and relate well with others.

enabling To unwittingly contribute to a person's addictive or abusive behavior. Components of enabling include shielding or covering up for an abuser/addict; controlling them; taking over responsibilities; rationalizing addictive behavior; or cooperating with them.

enabling factors The skills, resources, and physical and mental capabilities that shape our behavior.

endocrine disruptors Synthetic chemicals that interfere with the ways that hormones work in humans and wildlife.

endocrine system The group of ductless glands that produce hormones and secrete them directly into the blood for transport to target organs.

endometrium The mucous membrane lining the uterus.

endorphins Mood-elevating, painkilling chemicals produced by the brain.

environmental tobacco smoke Secondhand cigarette smoke; the third leading preventable cause of death.

epididymis That portion of the male duct system in which sperm mature.

epilepsy A variety of neurological disorders characterized by sudden attacks (seizures) of violent muscle contractions and unconsciousness.

erectile dysfunction The consistent inability to maintain a penile erection sufficient for adequate sexual relations.

erogenous Sexually sensitive.

essential nutrients Nutrients that the body cannot manufacture for itself and must obtain from food.

estrogen The female sex hormone that stimulates female secondary sex characteristics.

ethyl alcohol The intoxicating agent in alcoholic beverages; also called ethanol.

eustress Positive stress, which stimulates a person to function properly.

evidence-based medicine A way of improving and evaluating patient care by combining the best research evidence with the patient's personal values.

failure rate The number of pregnancies that occur per year for every 100 women using a particular method of birth control.

fallopian tubes The pair of channels that transport ova from the ovaries to the uterus; the usual site of fertilization.

family A group of people united by marriage, blood, or adoption; residing in the same household; maintaining a common culture; and interacting with one another on the basis of their roles within the group.

fellatio Sexual stimulation of a man's genitals by means of oral manipulation.

fertilization The fusion of sperm and egg nucleus.

fetal alcohol effects (FAE) Milder forms of FAS, including low birthweight, irritability as newborns, and permanent mental impairment as a result of the mother's alcohol consumption during pregnancy.

fetal alcohol syndrome (FAS) A cluster of physical and mental defects in the newborn, including low birthweight, smaller-than-normal head circumference, intrauterine growth retardation, and permanent mental impairment caused by the mother's alcohol consumption during pregnancy.

fetus The human organism developing in the uterus from the ninth week until birth.

FITT A formula that describes the frequency, intensity, type, and length of time for physical activity.

flexibility The range of motion allowed by one's joints; determined by the length of muscles, tendons, and ligaments attached to the joints.

folic acid A form of folate used in vitamin supplements and fortified foods.

functional fiber Isolated, nondigestible carbohydrates with beneficial effects in humans.

functional fitness The ability to perform real-life activities, such as lifting a heavy suitcase.

fungi Organisms that reproduce by means of spores.

gamma globulin The antibodycontaining portion of the blood fluid (plasma).

GBL (gamma butyrollactone) The main ingredient in gamma hydroxybutyrate (GHB), also known as the "date rape drug"; once ingested, GBL converts to GHB and can cause the ingestor to lose consciousness.

gender Maleness or femaleness, as determined by a combination of anatomical and physiological factors, psychological factors, and learned behaviors.

general adaptation syndrome (GAS) An anxiety disorder characterized as chronic distress.

generalized anxiety disorder (GAD) An anxiety disorder characterized as chronic distress.

generic Refers to products without trade names that are equivalent to other products protected by trademark registration.

GHB (gamma hydroxbutyrate) A brain messenger chemical that stimulates the release of human growth hormone; commonly abused for its high and its alleged ability to trim fat and build muscles. Also known as "blue nitro" or the "date rape drug."

gingivitis Inflammation of the gums.

glia Support cells for neurons in the brain and spinal cord that separate the brain from the bloodstream, assist in the growth of neurons, speed transmission of nerve impulses, and eliminate damaged neurons.

gonadotropins Gonad-stimulating hormones produced by the pituitary gland.

gonorrhea A sexually transmitted infection caused by the bacterium *Neisseria gonorrhoeae*; symptoms include discharge from the penis; women are generally asymptomatic.

guided imagery An approach to stress control, self-healing, or motivating life changes by means of seeing oneself in the state of calmness, wellness, or change.

gum disease Inflammation of the gum and bones that hold teeth in place.

hallucinogen A drug that causes hallucinations.

hashish A concentrated form of a drug, derived from the cannabis plant, containing the psychoactive ingredient TCH, which causes a sense of euphoria when inhaled or eaten.

hazing Any activity that humiliates, degrades, or poses a risk of emotional or physical harm for the sake of joining a group or maintaining full status in that group.

health A state of complete well-being, including physical, psychological, spiritual, social, intellectual, and environmental components.

health belief model A model of behavioral change that focuses on the individual's attitudes and beliefs.

health literacy Ability to understand health information and use it to make good decisions about health and medical care.

health maintenance organization (HMO) An organization that provides health services on a fixed-contract basis.

health promotion An educational and informational process in which people are helped to change attitudes and behaviors in an effort to improve their health.

helminth A parasitic roundworm or flatworm.

hepatitis An inflammation and/or infection of the liver caused by a virus, often accompanied by jaundice.

herpes simplex A condition caused by one of the herpes viruses and characterized by lesions of the skin or mucous membranes; herpes simplex virus 2 is sexually transmitted and causes genital blisters or sores.

heterosexual Primary sexual orientation toward members of the other sex.

holistic An approach to medicine that takes into account body, mind, emotions, and spirit.

holographic will A will wholly in the handwriting of its author.

home health care Provision of medical services and equipment to patients in the home to restore or maintain comfort, function, and health.

homeopathy A system of medical practice that treats a disease by administering dosages of substances that would in healthy persons produce symptoms similar to those of the disease.

homeostasis The body's natural state of balance or stability.

homosexual Primary sexual orientation toward members of the same sex.

hormone Substance released in the blood that regulates specific bodily functions.

hormone therapy (HT) The use of supplemental hormones during and after menopause.

hospice A homelike health-care facility or program committed to supportive care for terminally ill people.

host A person or population that contracts one or more pathogenic agents in an environment.

human immunodeficiency virus (HIV) A type of virus that causes a spectrum of health problems, ranging from a symptomless infection to changes in the immune system, to the development of life-threatening diseases because of impaired immunity.

human papilloma virus (HPV) A pathogen that causes genital warts and increases the risk of cervical cancer.

hunger The physiological drive to consume food.

hypertension High blood pressure occurring when the blood exerts excessive pressure against the arterial walls.

hypothermia An abnormally low body temperature; if not treated appropriately, coma or death could result.

immune deficiency Partial or complete inability of the immune system to respond to pathogens.

immunity Protection from infectious diseases.

immunotherapy A series of injections of small but increasing doses of an allergen, used to treat allergies.

implantation The embedding of the fertilized ovum in the uterine lining.

incomplete proteins Proteins that lack one or more of the amino acids essential for protein synthesis.

incubation period The time between a pathogen's entrance into the body and the first symptom.

infertility The inability to conceive a child.

infiltration A gradual penetration or invasion.

inflammation A localized response by the body to tissue injury, characterized by swelling and the dilation of the blood vessels.

influenza Any type of fairly common, highly contagious viral diseases.

informed consent Permission (to undergo or receive a medical procedure or treatment) given voluntarily, with full knowledge and understanding of the procedure or treatment and its possible consequences.

inhalants Substances that produce vapors having psychoactive effects when sniffed.

integrative medicine An approach that combines traditional medicine with alternative/complementary therapies.

intercourse Sexual stimulation by means of entry of the penis into the vagina; coitus.

interpersonal therapy (IPT) A technique used to develop communication skills and relationships.

intimacy A state of closeness between two people, characterized by the desire and ability to share one's innermost thoughts and feelings with each other either verbally or nonverbally.

intoxication Maladaptive behavioral, psychological, and physiologic changes that occur as a result of substance abuse.

intramuscular Into or within a muscle.

intrauterine device A device inserted into the uterus through the cervix to prevent pregnancy by interfering with implantation.

intravenous Into a vein.

ionizing radiation A form of energy emitted from atoms as they undergo internal change.

irradiation Exposure to or treatment by some form of radiation.

isokinetic Having the same force; exercise with specialized equipment that provides resistance equal to the force applied by the user throughout the entire range of motion.

isometric Of the same length; exercise in which muscles increase their tension without shortening in length, such as when pushing an immovable object.

labia majora The fleshy outer folds that border the female genital area.

labia minora The fleshy inner folds that border the female genital area.

labor The process leading up to birth: effacement and dilation of the cervix; the movement of the baby into and through the birth canal, accompanied by strong contractions; and contraction of the uterus and expulsion of the placenta after birth.

lacto-vegetarians People who eat dairy products as well as fruits and vegetables (but not meat, poultry, or fish).

Lamaze method A method of childbirth preparation taught to expectant parents to help the woman cope with the discomfort of labor; combines breathing and psychological techniques.

laparoscopy A surgical sterilization procedure in which the fallopian tubes are observed, with a laparoscope inserted through a small incision, and then cut or blocked.

licensed clinical social worker (LCSW) See certified social worker.

lipoprotein A compound in blood that is made up of proteins and fat; a high-density lipoprotein (HDL) picks up excess cholesterol in the blood; a low-density lipoprotein (LDL) carries more cholesterol and deposits it on the walls of arteries.

living will An advance directive providing instructions for the use of life-sustaining procedures in the event of terminal illness or injury.

locus of control An individual's belief about the sources of power and influence over his or her life.

LSD (lysergic acid diethylamide) A synthetic psychoactive substance that produces hallucinations. It was originally developed to treat mental illness.

lumpectomy The surgical removal of a breast tumor and its surrounding tissue.

Lyme disease A disease caused by a bacterium carried by a tick; it may cause heart arrhythmias, neurological problems, and arthritis symptoms.

lymph nodes Small tissue masses in which some immune cells are stored.

macronutrients Nutrients required by the human body in the greatest amounts, including water, carbohydrates, proteins, and fats.

mainstream smoke The smoke inhaled directly by smoking a cigarette.

major depression Sadness that does not end; ongoing feelings of utter helplessness.

mammography A diagnostic X-ray exam used to detect breast cancer.

managed care Health-care services and reimbursement predetermined by third-party insurers.

marijuana The drug derived from the cannabis plant, containing the psychoactive ingredient THC, which causes a mild sense of euphoria when inhaled or eaten.

marriage and family therapist A psychiatrist, psychologist, or social worker who specializes in marriage and family counseling.

mastectomy The surgical removal of an entire breast.

masturbation Manual (or nonmanual) self-stimulation of the genitals, often resulting in orgasm.

medical abortion Method of ending a pregnancy within nine weeks of conception using hormonal medications that cause expulsion of the fertilized egg.

medical history The health-related information collected during the interview of a client by a health-care professional.

meditation A group of approaches that use quiet sitting, breathing techniques, and/or chanting to relax, improve concentration, and become attuned to one's inner self.

menarche The onset of menstruation at puberty.

meningitis An extremely serious, potentially fatal illness that attacks the membranes around the brain and spinal cord; caused by the bacterium Neisseria meningitis.

menopause The complete cessation of ovulation and menstruation for twelve consecutive months.

menstruation Discharge of blood from the vagina as a result of the shedding of the uterine lining at the end of the menstrual cycle.

mental disorder Behavioral or psychological syndrome associated with distress or disability or with a significantly increased risk of suffering death, pain, disability, or loss of freedom.

mental health The ability to perceive reality as it is, respond to its challenges, and develop rational strategies for living.

metabolic syndrome A cluster of disorders of the body's metabolism that make diabetes, heart disease, or stroke more likely.

metastasize To spread to other parts of the body via the bloodstream or lymphatic system.

micronutrients Vitamins and minerals needed by the body in very small amounts.

microwaves Extremely high frequency electromagnetic waves that increase the rate at which molecules vibrate, thereby generating heat.

mindfulness A method of stress reduction that involves experiencing the physical and mental sensations of the present moment.

minerals Naturally occurring inorganic substances, small amounts of some being essential in metabolism and nutrition.

minipill An oral contraceptive containing a small amount of progestin and no estrogen, which prevents contraception by making the mucus in the cervix so thick that sperm cannot enter the uterus.

miscarriage A pregnancy that terminates before the twentieth week of gestation; also called spontaneous abortion.

mononucleosis An infectious viral disease characterized by an excess of white blood cells in the blood, fever, bodily discomfort, a sore throat, and kidney and liver complications.

monophasic pill An oral contraceptive that releases synthetic estrogen and progestin at constant levels throughout the menstrual cycle.

mons pubis The rounded, fleshy area over the junction of the female pubic bones.

mood A sustained emotional state that colors one's view of the world for hours or days.

motivational enhancement A nonjudgmental but directive method for supporting motivation to change.

multiphasic pill An oral contraceptive that releases different levels of estrogen and progestin to mimic the hormonal fluctuations of the natural menstrual cycle.

multiple chemical sensitivity (MCS) A sensitivity to low-level chemical exposures from ordinary substances, such as perfumes and tobacco smoke, that results in physiological responses such as chest pain, depression, dizziness, fatigue, and nausea. Also known as environmentally triggered illness.

muscular endurance The ability to withstand the stress of continued physical exertion.

muscular strength Physical power; the maximum weight one can lift, push, or press in one effort.

mutagen An agent that causes alterations in the genetic material of living cells.

myocardial infarction A condition characterized by the dying of tissue areas in the myocardium, caused by interruption of the blood supply to those areas; the medical name for a heart attack.

naturopathy An alternative system of treatment of disease that emphasizes the use of natural remedies such as sun, water, heat, and air. Therapies may include dietary changes, steam baths, and exercise.

neuron A nerve cell; the basic working unit of the brain, which transmits information from the senses to the brain and from the brain to specific body parts; each neuron consists of a cell body, an axon terminal, and dendrites.

neuropsychiatry The study of the brain and mind.

neurotransmitters Chemicals released by neurons that stimulate or inhibit the action of other neurons.

nicotine The addictive substance in tobacco; one of the most toxic of all poisons.

nocturnal emissions Ejaculations while dreaming; wet dreams.

non exercise activity thermogenesis (NEAT) Nonvolitional movement that can be an effective way of burning calories.

nongonococcal urethritis (NGU) Inflammation of the urethra caused by organisms other than the Gonococcus bacterium.

nonvolitional sex Sexual behavior that violates a person's right to choose when and with whom to have sex and what behaviors to engage in.

nucleus The central part of a cell, contained in the cell body of a neuron.

obesity The excessive accumulation of fat in the body; class 1 obesity is defined by a BMI between 30 and 34.9; class 2 obesity is defined by a BMI between 35 and 39.9; class 3, or severe obesity, is a BMI of 40 or higher.

obsessive compulsive disorder An anxiety disorder characterized by obsessions and/or compulsions that impair one's ability to function and form relationships.

opioids Drugs that have sleepinducing and pain-relieving properties, including opium and its derivatives and nonopioid, synthetic drugs.

optimism The tendency to seek out, remember, and expect pleasurable experiences.

oral contraceptives Preparations of synthetic hormones that inhibit ovulation; also referred to as birth control pills or simply the pill.

organic Term designating food produced with, or production based on the use of, fertilizers originating from plants or animals, without the use of pesticides or chemically formulated fertilizers.

organophosphates Toxic pesticides that may cause cancer, birth defects, neurological disorders, and damage to wildlife and the environment.

osteoporosis A condition common in older people in which the bones become increasingly soft and porous, making them susceptible to injury.

outcomes The ultimate impacts of particular treatments or absence of treatment.

ovary The female sex organ that produces egg cells, estrogen, and progesterone.

overload principle Providing a greater stress or demand on the body than it is normally accustomed to handling.

overloading Method of physical training involving increasing the number of repetitions or the amount of resistance gradually to work the muscle to temporary fatigue.

over-the-counter (OTC) drugs Medications that can be obtained legally without a prescription from a medical professional.

overtrain Working muscles too intensely or too frequently, resulting in persistent muscle soreness, injuries, unintended weight loss, nervousness, and an inability to relax.

overuse injuries Physical injuries to joints or muscles, such as strains, fractures, and tendinitis, which result from overdoing a repetitive activity.

overweight A condition of having a BMI between 25.0 and 29.9.

ovo-lacto-vegetarians People who eat eggs, dairy products, and fruits and vegetables (but not meat, poultry, or fish).

ovulation The release of a mature ovum from an ovary approximately 14 days prior to the onset of menstruation.

ovum (plural, ova) The female gamete (egg cell).

ozone A form of oxygen that is a harmful component of air pollution.

panic attack A short episode characterized by physical sensations of lightheadedness, dizziness, hyperventilation, and numbness of extremities, accompanied by an inexplicable terror, usually of a physical disaster such as death.

panic disorder An anxiety disorder in which the apprehension or experience of recurring panic attacks is so intense that normal functioning is impaired.

Pap smear A test in which cells removed from the cervix are examined under a microscope for signs of cancer; also called a Pap test.

passive stretching A stretching technique in which an external force or resistance (your body, a partner, gravity, or a weight) helps the joints move through their range of motion.

pathogen A microorganism that produces disease.

PCP (phencyclidine) A synthetic psychoactive substance that produces effects similar to other psychoactive drugs when swallowed, smoked, sniffed, or injected, but also may trigger unpredictable behavioral changes.

pelvic inflammatory disease (PID) An inflammation of the internal female genital tract, characterized by abdominal pain, fever, and tenderness of the cervix.

penis The male organ of sex and urination.

perimenopause The period from a woman's first irregular cycles to her last menstruation.

perineum The area between the anus and vagina in the female and between the anus and scrotum in the male.

periodontis Severe gum disease in which the tooth root becomes infected.

persistent vegetative state A state of being awake and capable of reacting to physical stimuli, such as light, while being unaware of pain or other environmental stimuli.

phobia An anxiety disorder marked by an inordinate fear of an object, a class of objects, or a situation, resulting in extreme avoidance behaviors.

physical dependence The physiological attachment to, and need for, a drug.

physical fitness The ability to respond to routine physical demands, with enough reserve energy to cope with a sudden challenge.

phytochemicals Chemicals such as indoles, coumarins, and capsaicin, which exist naturally in plants and have disease-fighting properties.

placenta An organ that develops after implantation and to which the embryo attaches, via the umbilical cord, for nourishment and waste removal.

plaque The sticky film of bacteria that forms on teeth.

pollutant A substance or agent in the environment, usually the byproduct of human industry or activity, that is injurious to human, animal, or plant life.

polyabuse The misuse or abuse of more than one drug.

posttraumatic stress disorder (PTSD) The repeated reliving of a trauma through nightmares or recollection.

practice guidelines Recommendations for diagnosis and treatment of various health problems based on evidence from scientific research.

preconception care Health care to prepare for pregnancy.

precycling The use of products that are packaged in recycled or recyclable material.

predisposing factors The beliefs, values, attitudes, knowledge, and perceptions that influence our behavior.

preferred provider organization (PPO) A group of physicians contracted to provide health care to members at a discounted price.

prehypertension A condition of slightly elevated blood pressure, which is likely to worsen in time.

premature ejaculation A sexual difficulty in which a man ejaculates so rapidly that his partner's satisfaction is impaired.

premature labor Labor that occurs after the twentieth week but before the thirty-seventh week of pregnancy.

premenstrual dysphoric disorder (PMDD) A disorder that causes symptoms of psychological depression during the last week of the menstrual cycle.

premenstrual syndrome (PMS) A disorder that causes physical discomfort and psychological distress prior to a woman's menstrual period.

predrinking Consuming alcoholic beverages, usually with friends, before going out to bars or parties; also called pre-gaming, pre-loading, or front-loading.

prevention Information and support offered to help healthy people identify their health risks, reduce stressors, prevent potential medical problems, and enhance their well-being.

primary care Ambulatory or outpatient care provided by a physician in an office, emergency room, or clinic.

progesterone The female sex hormone that stimulates the uterus, preparing it for the arrival of a fertilized egg.

progestin-only pills See minipill.

progressive overloading Gradually increasing physical challenges once the body adapts to the stress placed upon it to produce maximum benefits.

progressive relaxation A method of reducing muscle tension by contracting, then relaxing, certain areas of the body.

proof The alcoholic strength of a distilled spirit, expressed as twice the percentage of alcohol present.

prostate gland A structure surrounding the male urethra that produces a secretion that helps liquefy the semen from the testes.

protein Organic compounds composed of amino acids; one of the essential nutrients.

protozoa Microscopic animals made up of one cell or a group of similar cells.

psychiatric drugs Medications that regulate a person's mental, emotional, and physical functions to facilitate normal functioning.

psychiatric nurse A nurse with special training and experience in mental health care.

psychiatrist Licensed medical doctor with additional training in psychotherapy, psychopharmacology, and treatment of mental disorders.

psychoactive Mind-affecting.

psychodynamic Interpreting behaviors in terms of early experiences and unconscious influences.

psychological dependence The emotional or mental attachment to the use of a drug.

psychologist Mental health-care professional who has completed doctoral or graduate program in psychology and is trained in psychotherapeutic techniques, but who is not medically trained and does not prescribe medications.

psychotherapy Treatment designed to produce a response by psychological rather than physical means, such as suggestion, persuasion, reassurance, and support.

quackery Medical fakery; unproven practices claiming to cure diseases or solve health problems.

range of motion The fullest extent of possible movement in a particular joint.

rape Sexual penetration of a female or a male by means of intimidation, force, or fraud.

rapid-eye-movement (REM) sleep Regularly occurring periods of sleep during which the most active dreaming takes place.

rating of perceived exertion (RPE) A self-assessment scale that rates symptoms of breathlessness and fatigue.

receptors Molecules on the surface of neurons on which neurotransmitters bind after their release from other neurons.

recycling The processing or reuse of manufactured materials to reduce consumption of raw materials.

refractory period The period of time following orgasm during which the male cannot experience another orgasm.

reinforcing factors Rewards, encouragement, and recognition that influence our behavior in the short run.

relapse prevention An alcohol recovery treatment method that focuses on social skills training to develop ways of preventing or minimizing a relapse.

relative risk The risk of developing cancer in persons with a certain exposure or trait compared to the risk in persons who do not have the same exposure or trait.

repetitive motion injury Inflammation of or damage to a part of the body due to repetition of the same movements.

rep (or repetition) In weight training, a single performance of a movement or exercise.

resting heart rate The number of heartbeats per minute during inactivity.

reversibility principle The physical benefits of exercise are lost through disuse or inactivity.

reuptake Reabsorption by the originating cell of neurotransmitters that have not connected with receptors and have been left in synapses.

rhythm method A birth control method in which sexual intercourse is avoided during those days of the menstrual cycle in which fertilization is most likely to occur.

rubella An infectious disease that may cause birth defects if contracted by a pregnant woman; also called German measles.

same-sex marriage Governmentally, socially, or religiously recognized marriage in which two people of the same sex live together as a family.

satiety A feeling of fullness after eating.

saturated fats A chemical term indicating that a fat molecule contains as many hydrogen atoms as its carbon skeleton can hold. These fats are normally solid at room temperature.

schizophrenia A general term for a group of mental disorders with characteristic psychotic symptoms, such as delusions, hallucinations, and disordered thought patterns during the active phase of the illness, and a duration of at least six months.

scrotum The external sac or pouch that holds the testes.

secondary sex characteristics Physical changes associated with maleness or femaleness, induced by the sex hormones.

self-actualization A state of wellness and fulfillment that can be achieved once certain human needs are satisfied; living to one's full potential.

self-disclosure Sharing personal information and experiences with another that he or she would not otherwise discover; self-disclosure involves risk and vulnerability.

self-efficacy Belief in one's ability to accomplish a goal or change a behavior.

self-esteem Confidence and satisfaction in oneself.

semen The viscous whitish fluid that is the complete male ejaculate; a combination of sperm and secretions from the prostate gland, seminal vesicles, and other glands.

seminal vesicles Glands in the male reproductive system that produce the major portion of the fluid of semen.

sets In weight training, the number of repetitions of the same movement or exercise.

sex Maleness or femaleness, resulting from genetic, structural, and functional factors.

sexual coercion Sexual activity forced upon a person by the exertion of psychological pressure by another person.

sexual dysfunction The inability to react emotionally and/or physically to sexual stimulation in a way expected of the average healthy person or according to one's own standards.

sexual harassment Uninvited and unwanted sexual attention.

sexual health The integration of the physical, emotional, intellectual, social, and spiritual aspects of sexual being in ways that are positively enriching and that enhance personality, communication, and love.

sexual orientation The direction of an individual's sexual interest, either to members of the opposite sex or to members of the same sex.

sexuality The behaviors, instincts, and attitudes associated with being sexual.

sexually transmitted disease (STD) A disease that is caused by a sexually transmitted infection that produces symptoms.

sexually transmitted infection (STI) The presence in the human body of an infectious agent that can be passed from one sexual partner to another.

sidestream smoke The smoke emitted by a burning cigarette and breathed by everyone in a closed room, including the smoker; contains more tar and nicotine than mainstream smoke.

simple carbohydrates Sugars; like all carbohydrates, they provide the body with glucose.

social isolation A feeling of unconnectedness with others caused by and reinforced by infrequency of social contacts.

social norms The unwritten rules regarding behavior and conduct expected or accepted by a group.

social phobia A severe form of social anxiety marked by extreme fears and avoidance of social situations.

specificity principle Each part of the body adapts to a particular type and amount of stress placed upon it.

sperm The male gamete produced by the testes and transported outside the body through ejaculation.

spermatogenesis The process by which sperm cells are produced.

spiritual health The ability to identify one's basic purpose in life and to achieve one's full potential.

spiritual intelligence The capacity to sense, understand, and tap into ourselves, others, and the world around us.

spirituality A belief in someone or something that transcends the boundaries of self.

stalking The willful, repeated, and malicious following of another person.

static flexibility The ability to assume and maintain an extended position at one end point in a joint's range of motion.

static stretching A gradual stretch held for a short time of 10 to 30 seconds.

sterilization A surgical procedure to end a person's reproductive capability.

stimulant An agent, such as a drug, that temporarily relieves drowsiness, helps in the performance of repetitive tasks, and improves capacity for work.

stress The nonspecific response of the body to any demands made upon it; may be characterized by muscle tension and acute anxiety, or may be a positive force for action.

stressor Specific or nonspecific agents or situations that cause the stress response in a body.

stroke A cerebrovascular event in which the blood supply to a portion of the brain is blocked.

subcutaneous Under the skin.

suction curettage A procedure in which the contents of the uterus are removed by means of suction and scraping.

sustainability A method of using a resource so that the resource is not depleted or permanently damaged.

synapse A specialized site at which electrical impulses are transmitted from the axon terminal of one neuron to a dendrite of another.

syphilis A sexually transmitted infection caused by the bacterium *Treponema pallidum* and characterized by early sores, a latent period, and a final period of life-threatening symptoms, including brain damage and heart failure.

systemic disease A pathologic condition that spreads throughout the body.

systole The contraction phase of the cardiac cycle.

systolic blood pressure Highest blood pressure when the heart contracts.

tar A thick, sticky dark fluid produced by the burning of tobacco, made up of several hundred different chemicals, many of them poisonous, some of them carcinogenic.

target heart rate Sixty to eighty-five percent of the maximum heart rate; the heart rate at which one derives maximum cardiovascular benefit from aerobic exercise.

terminal Illness An illness in which death is inevitable.

testes (singular, testis) The male sex organs that produce sperm and testosterone.

testosterone The male sex hormone that stimulates male secondary sex characteristics.

toxic shock syndrome (TSS) A disease characterized by fever, vomiting, diarrhea, and often shock, caused by a bacterium that releases toxic waste products into the bloodstream.

toxicity Poisonousness; the dosage level at which a drug becomes poisonous to the body, causing either temporary or permanent damage.

transcendence The sense of passing into a foreign region or dimension, often experienced by a person near death.

trans-fat Fat formed when liquid vegetable oils are processed to make table spreads or cooking fats; also found in dairy and beef products; considered to be especially dangerous dietary fats.

transgender Having a gender identity opposite one's biological sex.

transient ischemic attack (TIA) A cerebrovascular event in which the blood supply to a portion of the brain is blocked temporarily; repeated attacks are predictors of more severe strokes.

transtheoretical model of change A model of behavioral change that focuses on the individual's decision making; it states that an individual progresses through a sequence of six stages as he or she makes a change in behavior.

trichomoniasis An infection of the protozoan *Trichomonas vaginalis*; females experience vaginal burning, itching, and discharge, but male carriers may be asymptomatic.

triglyceride A blood fat that flows through the blood after meals and is linked to increased risk of coronary artery disease.

tubal ligation The suturing or tying shut of the fallopian tubes to prevent pregnancy.

tubal occlusion The blocking of the fallopian tubes to prevent pregnancy.

tuberculosis (TB) A highly infectious bacterial disease that primarily affects the lungs and is often fatal.

12-step programs Self-help group programs based on the principles of Alcoholics Anonymous.

ulcer A lesion in, or an erosion of, the mucous membrane of an organ.

unsaturated fats A chemical term indicating that a fat molecule contains fewer hydrogen atoms than its carbon skeleton can hold. These fats are normally liquid at room temperature.

urethra The canal through which urine from the bladder leaves the body; in the male, also serves as the channel for seminal fluid.

urethral opening The outer opening of the thin tube that carries urine from the bladder.

urethritis Infection of the urethra.

uterus The female organ that houses the developing fetus until birth.

vagina The canal leading from the exterior opening in the female genital area to the uterus.

vaginal contraceptive film (VCF) A small dissolvable sheet saturated with spermicide that can be inserted into the vagina and placed over the cervix.

vaginal spermicide A substance that kills or neutralizes sperm, inserted into the vagina in the form of a foam, cream, jelly, suppository, or film.

vaginismus A sexual difficulty in which a woman experiences painful spasms of the vagina during sexual intercourse.

values The criteria by which one makes choices about one's thoughts, actions, goals and ideals.

vas deferens Two tubes that carry sperm from the epididymis into the urethra.

vasectomy A surgical sterilization procedure in which each vas deferens is cut and tied shut to stop the passage of sperm to the urethra for ejaculation.

vector A biological or physical vehicle that carries the agent of infection to the host.

vegans People who eat only plant foods.

ventricle Either of the two lower chambers of the heart, which pump blood out of the heart and into the arteries.

virus A submicroscopic infectious agent; the most primitive form of life.

visualization An approach to stress control, self-healing, or motivating life changes by means of seeing oneself in the state of calmness, wellness, or change.

vital signs Measurements of physiological functioning; specifically, temperature, blood pressure, pulse rate, and respiration rate.

vitamins Organic substances that are needed in very small amounts by the body and carry out a variety of functions in metabolism and nutrition.

waist-to-hip ratio (WHR) The proportion of one's waist circumference to one's hip circumference.

wellness A deliberate lifestyle choice characterized by personal responsibility and optimal enhancement of physical, mental, and spiritual health.

withdrawal Development of symptoms that cause significant psychological and physical distress when an individual reduces or stops drug use.

zygote A fertilized egg.

REFERENCES

Chapter 1

1. "Constitution of the World Health Organization." *Chronicle of the World Health Organization*, Geneva, Switzerland: WHO, 1947.
2. Travis, John, and Regina Sara Ryan. *The Wellness Workbook*, 3rd ed. Berkeley, CA: Celestial Arts, 2004.
3. Travis, John. Personal interview.
4. Travis and Ryan, *The Wellness Workbook*.
5. Mitka, Mike. "Growth in Health Care Spending Slows, but Still Outpaces Rate of Inflation," *Journal of the American Medical Association*, Vol. 301, No. 8, February 25, 2009, p. 814.
6. CDC/NCHS. Health, United States, 2007 with Chartbook on Trends in the Health of Americans. Hyattsville, MD: NCHS, 2008.
7. http://wonder.cdc.gov/data2010.
8. CDC/NCHS. Health, United States, 2007 with Chartbook on Trends in the Health of Ameri9cans.
9. Pletcher, M. J., et al. "Trends in Opioid Prescribing by Race/Ethnicity for Patients Seeking Care in U.S. Emergency Departments." *Journal of the American Medical Association*, Vol. 299, No. 1, 2008, pp. 70–78.
10. CDC/NCHS. *Health*, United States, 2007 with Chartbook on Trends in the Health of Americans.
11. McKeever, Kevin. "Rheumatoid Arthritis Hits Women Harder," *HealthDay*, January 16, 2009. MedlinePlus.
12. Kulik, A., et al., "Gender Differences in the Long-Term Outcomes after Valve Replacement Surgery." *Heart*, Vol. 95, No. 4, April 2009, pp. 318–326.
13. American College Health Association. *American College Health Association National College Health Assessment: Reference Group Executive Summary Fall 2007*. Baltimore American College Health Association, 2008.
14. Reyna, Valerie F., and Frank Farley. "Risk and Rationality in Adolescent Decision Making: Implication for Theory, Practice, and Public Policy." *Psychological Science in the Public Interest*, Vol. 7, No. 1, pp. 1–44.
15. U.S. Department of Education, Higher Education Center, www.higheredcenter.org/socialnorms.
16. American College Health Association, *American College Health Association National College Health Assessment*.
17. Begsma, L. J., and M. E. Carney. "Effectiveness of Health-Promoting Media Literacy Education: A Systematic Review." *Health Education Research*, January 17, 2008, epub.
18. Baxter, Leslie, et al. "Everyday Health Communication Experiences of College Students." *Journal of American College Health*, Vol. 56, No. 4, pp. 427–434.
19. Torpy, Janet. "Evidence-Based Medicine." *Journal of the American Medical Association*, Vol. 301, No. 8, February 25, 2009, p. 900.
20. Khaw, K. T., et al. "Combined Impact of Health Behaviours and Mortality in Men and Women: The EPIC-Norfolk Prospective Population Study." *Public Library of Science Medicine*, Vol. 5, No. 1, e1t2 doi:10.1371/journal.pmed.0050012.
21. Hales, Dianne, and Kenneth W. Christian. *An Invitation to Personal Change*. Belmont: Cengage Publishing, 2009.
22. Griffith, Linda. "The Psychiatrist's Guide to Motivational Interviewing." *Psychiatry*, Vol. 5, No. 4, April 2008, pp. 42–47.
23. Prochaska, James, et al. *Changing for Good*. New York: Quill, 1994.
24. Horneffer-Ginter, Karen. "Stages of Change and Possible Selves: Two Tools for Promoting College Health." *Journal of American College Health*, Vol. 56, No. 4, pp. 351–358.

Chapter 2

1. Dubovsky, Steven. "Emotional Health = Heart Health." *Journal Watch: Psychiatry*, January 28, 2008.
2. "Positive Psychology in Practice." *Harvard Mental Health Letter*, Vol. 24, No. 11, May 28, pp. 1–3.
3. Craig, A., et al. "Psychological and Neural Correlates of Emotional Intelligence in a Large Sample of Adult Males and Females." *Intelligence*, Vol. 36, No. 5, September–October 2008, pp. 383–393.
4. Seligman, Martin. Personal interview.
5. Goodstein, Charles. Personal interview.
6. Flora, Carla. "The Pursuit of Happiness." *Psychology Today*, Vol. 42, No. 1, February 2009, pp. 61–69.
7. Roy-Byrne, Peter. "With a Little Help from My Friends: The Happiness Effect." *Journal Watch Psychiatry*, January 12, 2009 (online).
8. Weiss, Alexander, et al. "Happiness Is a Personal(ity) Thing: The Genetics of Personality and Well-Being in a Representative Sample." *Psychological Science*, Vol. 19, No. 3, March 2008, pp. 205–210.
9. Lyubomirsky, Sonja. *The How of Happiness: A Scientific Approach to Getting the Life You Want*. New York: Penguin Press, 2008.
10. "Experiences Bring More Joy Than Possessions Do." *HealthDay*, February 9, 2009, www.medlineplus.gov.
11. Lyubomirsky, Sonja. Personal interview.
12. Larsen, Jeff, and Arnie McKibban. "Is Happiness Having What You Want, Wanting What You Have, or Both?" *Psychological Science*, Vol. 19, No. 4, April 2008, pp. 371–377, doi: 10.1111/j.1467-9280.2008.02095.x
13. Fowler, J. H., and N. A. Christakis. "Dynamic Spread of Happiness in a Large Social Network: Longitudinal Analysis over 20 Years in the Framingham Heart Study." *British Medical Journal*, Vol. 337, December 4, 2008, p. a2338.
14. Steptoe, A., and A. V. Diez Roux. "Happiness, Social Networks, and Health." *British Medical Journal*, Vol. 337, December 4, 2008, p. a2781.
15. Larsen, Randy. Personal interview.
16. Schlundt, D. G., et al. "Religious Affiliation, Health Behaviors and Outcomes: Nashville REACH 2010," *British Journal of Nursing*, Vol. 17, No. 6, March 27–April 9, 2008, pp. 394–398.
17. Lawler-Row, K. A., and J. Elliott, "The Role of Religious Activity and Spirituality in the Health and Well-Being of Older Adults." *Journal of Health Psychology*, Vol. 14, No. 1, 2009, pp. 43–52.
18. Chida, Yoichi, et al. "Religiosity/Spirituality and Mortality: A Systematic Quantitative Review." *Psychotherapy and Psychosomatics*, Vol. 78, No. 2, January 2009, pp. 81–90.
19. Newberg, Andrew, and Mark Robert Waldman. *How God Changes Your Brain: Breakthrough Findings from a Leading Neuroscientist*. New York: Ballantine Books, 2009.
20. Edwards, Paul. Personal interview
21. Koenig, Harold. Personal interview
22. McCullough, Michael. Personal interview.
23. Mellor, et al. "Volunteering and Its Relationship with Personal and Neighborhood Well-Being." *Nonprofit and Voluntary Sector Quarterly*. 2008; 0: 0899764008317971v1.

24. Buysse, Daniel, et al. "Sleep Disorders." *Textbook of Psychiatry*, 5th ed., Robert Hales, Stuart Yudofsky, and Glen Gabbard (eds.). Washington, DC: American Psychiatric Pub, 2008, pp. 921–970.
25. "Sleep: Snooze or Lose." University of Michigan Health Services, www.uhs.umich.edu/wellness/other/sleep.html.
26. Thacher, Pamela. "University Students and the 'All Nighter': Correlates and Patterns of Students' Engagement in a Single Night of Total Sleep Deprivation." *Behavioral Sleep Medicine*, Vol. 6, 2008, pp. 16–31.
27. Brawn, T. P. et al. "Consolidation of Sensorimotor Learning During Sleep." *Learning and Memory*, Vol. 15, No. 11, October 30, 2008, pp. 815–819.
28. Pastiche, D. J., et al. "Effectiveness of Sleep Interventions on Sleep Amount and Quality," AAHE/RCB Student Poster Session, April 3, 2009.
29. Sin, C., et al. "Systematic Review on the Effectiveness of Caffeine Abstinence on the Quality of Sleep." *Journal of Clinical Nursing*, Vol. 18, No. 1, January 2009, pp. 13–21.
30. Paunio, T., et al. "Longitudinal Study on Poor Sleep and Life Dissatisfaction in a Nationwide Cohort of Twins." *American Journal of Epidemiology*, Vol. 169, No. 2, January 15, 2009.
31. Lauderdale, D., et al. "Short Sleep Duration and Incident Coronary Artery Calcification." *Journal of the American Medical Association*, Vol. 300, No. 24, December 24, 2008, pp. 2859–2866.
32. Cohen, S., et al. "Sleep Habits and Susceptibility to the Common Cold." *Archives of Internal Medicine*, Vol. 169, No. 1, 2009, pp. 62–67.
33. "The Importance of Sleep and Health: Six Reasons Not to Scrimp on Sleep." Harvard Health Publications, http://www.health.harvard.edu.
34. Glovinsky, P. B., et al. "Nonpharmacologic Strategies in the Management of Insomnia: Rationale and Implementation." *Sleep Medicine Clinics*, Vol. 3, No. 2, June 2008, pp. 189–204.
35. Morin, C. M., et al. "The Natural History of Insomnia: A Population-Based 3-Year Longitudinal Study." *Archives of Internal Medicine*, Vol. 169, No. 5, March 9, 2009, pp. 447–453.
36. Redolfi, S., et al. Relationship Between Overnight Rostral Fluid Shift and Obstructive Sleep Apnea in Nonobese Men." *American Journal of Respiratory and Critical Care Medicine*, Vol. 179, No. 3, February 1, 2009, pp. 241–246.

Chapter 3

1. American College Health Association. American College Health Association—National College Health Assessment (ACHA-NCHA) Web Summary. Updated August 2007, http://www.acha-ncha.org/data_highlights.html.
2. Lazarus, R., and R. Launier. "Stress-Related Transactions Between Person and Environment." *Perspectives in Interactional Psychology*. New York: Plenum, 1978.
3. Shirtcliff, E. A., et al. "Early Childhood Stress Is Associated with Elevated Antibody Levels to Herpes Simplex Virus Type 1." *Proceedings of the National Academy of Science*, February 2, 2009 (Epub ahead of print)
4. Rauscher, Mega. "Stressed Kids at Risk of Asthma in Adulthood." *HealthDay*, January 20, 2009. www.medlineplus.gov.

5. Hendry, Joene. "Family Stress May Make Kids Fat." *HealthDay*, January 21, 2009. www.medlineplus.gov.

6. Sgoifo, A., et al. "The Inevitable Link Between Heart and Behavior." *Neuroscience Biobehavior Review*, Vol. 33, No. 2, February 2009, pp. 61–62.

7. Hamer, Mark, et al. "Psychological Distress as a Risk Factor of Cardiovascular Events: Pathophysiological and Behavioral Mechanisms," *Journal of the American College of Cardiology*, Vol. 52, No. 25, December 16, 2008, pp. 2156–2162.

8. Grant, N., et al. "Social Isolation and Stress-Related Cardiovascular, Lipid, and Cortisol Responses." *Annals of Behavioral Medicine,* February 5, 2009. (Epub ahead of print)

9. Kimura, T., et al. "Perceived Stress, Severity of Asthma, and Quality of Life in Young Adults with Asthma." *Allergology International*, Vol. 58, No. 1, March 2009, pp. 71–79.

10. mtvU/Associated Press Survey, March 2008. Edison Media Research, www.edisonresearch.com.

11. Pryor, John, et al. *The American Freshman: National Norms for Fall 2008.* Los Angeles: University of California, Los Angeles Higher Education Research Institute, 2008.

12. mtvU/Associated Press Survey.

13. Walker, Rheeda, et al. "An Empirical Investigation of Acculturative Stress and Ethnic Identity as Moderators for Depression and Suicidal Ideation in College Students." *Cultural Diversity and Ethnic Minority Psychology*, Vol. 14, No. 1, 2008, pp. 75–82.

14. Goebert, Deborah. "Social Support, Mental Health, Minorities, and Acculturative Stress." In *Determinants of Minority Mental Health and Wellness.* New York: Springer, 2009.

15. Lindsey, Robert. "Sources of Stress for African American College Students." Poster Session, AAHPERD National Convention, March 31–April 4, 2009.

16. Thomas, S. A., and Gonzalez-Prendes, A. A. "Powerlessness, Anger, and Stress in African American Women: Implications for Physical and Emotional Health." *Health Care for Women International*, Vol. 30, No. 1-2, January 2009, pp. 93–113.

17. Pryor, *The American Freshman.*

18. "Job Losses Carry High 'Stress Tag'." *HealthDay,* February 12, 2009, www.medlineplus.gov.

19. "Managing Your Stress in Tough Economic Times." APA Help Center, http://www.apahelpcenter.org/articles/article.php?id5171.

20. Bushman, Brad. Personal interview.

21. Maslach, Christina. Personal interview.

22. Lutz, Antoine, et al. "Regulation of the Neural Circuitry of Emotion by Compassion Meditation: Effects of Meditative Expertise." *Public Library of Science One,* Vol. 3, No. 3: e1897.dol:10.1371/journal.pone.0001897.

23. Pace, T. W., et al. "Effect of Compassion Meditation on Neuroendocrine, Innate Immune and Behavioral Responses to Psychosocial Stress." *Psychoneuroendocrinology*, Vol. 34, No. 1, January 2009, pp. 87–98.

24. Barreira, T. V., et al. "Relationship Between Objectively Measured Physical Activity and Chronic Stress Level." Poster Session, AAHPERD National Convention, March 31–April 4, 2009.

25. Furong, Xu, et al. "Relations of Physical Activity and Mental Health in University Students." Poster Session, AAHPERD National Convention, March 31–April 4, 2009.

26. Zohar, Joseph, et al. "Post-traumatic Stress Disorder: Facts and Fiction." *Current Opinion in Psychiatry,* Vol. 21, 2008, pp. 74–77.

27. Bonanno, George, and Anthony Mancini. "The Human Capacity to Thrive in the Face of Potential Trauma." *Pediatrics*, Vol. 121, No. 2, February 2008, pp. 369–375.

28. Ursano, Robert, et al. "Posttraumatic Stress Disorder: Neurobiology, Psychology, and Public Health." *Psychiatric Times*, Vol. 25, No. 3, March 2008, pp. 16–20.

29. Vernon, L. L., et al. "Proactive Coping, Gratitude, and Posttraumatic Stress Disorder in College Women." *Anxiety, Stress & Coping.* Vol. 22, No. 1, January 2009, pp. 117–127.

30. Ursano, "Posttraumatic Stress Disorder: Neurobiology, Psychology, and Public Health."

31. Moore, S. A. "Cognitive Abnormalities in Posttraumatic Stress Disorder." *Current Opinion in Psychiatry,* Vol. 22, No. 1, January 2009, pp. 19–24.

32. "Posttraumatic Stress Disorder: A Growing Epidemic." *NIH Medlineplus: The Magazine*, Vol. 4, No. 1, Winter 2009, pp. 10–14.

33. Levin, Aaron. "Researchers Look for Link Between Brain Injury, Psychiatric Illness." *Psychiatric News,* Vol. 44, No. 1–2, January 2, 2009.

34. Heppner, P. S., et al. "The Association of Posttraumatic Stress Disorder and Metabolic Syndrome: A Study of Increased Health Risk in Veterans." *BMC Medicine*, Vol. 7, No. 1, January 9, 2009, p. 1.

35. Binder, E. B., et al. "Association of FKBP5 Polymorphisms and Childhood Abuse with Risk of Posttraumatic Stress Disorder Symptoms in Adults." *Journal of the American Medical Association,* Vol. 299, No. 11, March 19, 2008, pp. 1291–1305.

36. Zohar, "Post-Traumatic Stress Disorder."

37. Vernon, "Proactive Coping, Gratitude, and Posttraumatic Stress Disorder in College Women."

Chapter 4

1. Daly, Rich. "Depression Biggest Contributor to Global Disease Burden." *Psychiatric News*, Vol. 44, No. 1, January 2, 2009, p. 1.

2. Ibid.

3. Hales, Robert E., et al. (editors). *Textbook of Clinical Psychiatry*. Washington, D.C.: American Psychiatric Press, 2008.

4. Zivin, K., et al. "Persistence of Mental Health Problems and Needs in a College Student Population." *Journal of Affective Disorders*, January 27, 2009.

5. Ratcliffe, G. E., et al. "The Relationship Between Migraine and Mental Disorders in a Population-Based Sample." *General Hospital Psychiatry*, Vol. 31, No. 1, January–February 2009, pp. 14–19.

6. Khawaja, I. S., et al. "Depression and Coronary Artery Disease." *Psychiatry*, January 2009, pp. 38–51.

7. Marano, Giuseppe et al. "Depression and the Cardiovascular System: Increasing Evidence of a Link and Therapeutic Implications." *Expert Review of Cardiovascular Therapy*, Vol. 7, No. 9, September 2009, pp. 1123–1147.

8. Li, C., et al. "Prevalence of Depression Among U.S. Adults with Diabetes: Findings from the 2006 Behavioral Risk Factor Surveillance System." *Diabetes Care,* Vol. 31, 2008, pp. 105–107.

9. Hendry, Joene. "Teen Depression, Smoking Hard on the Bones." *HealthDay*, December 12, 2008. www.medlineplus.gov.

10. Arehart-Treichel, Joan. "Link Grows Stronger That Exercise Can Avert Depression." *Psychiatric News,* Vol. 44, No. 1, January 2, 2009, p. 12.

11. Tallaferro, L. A., et al. "Associations Between Physical Activity and Reduced Rates of Hopelessness, Depression, and Suicidal Behavior Among College Students." *Journal of American College Health,* Vol. 57, No. 4, January–February 2009, pp. 427–436.

12. Blanco, C., et al. "Mental Health of College Students and Their Non-College-Attending Peers: Results from the National Epidemiologic Study on Alcohol and Related Conditions." *Archives of General Psychiatry*, Vol. 65, No. 12, December 2008, pp. 1429–1437.

13. Moran, Mark. "Why Do College Students Shun Help for MH Problems?" *Psychiatric News*, Vol. 44, No. 1, January 2, 2009, p. 4.

14. Harrell, Z. A., et al. "Predictors of Alcohol Problems in College Women: The Role of Depressive Symptoms, Disordered Eating, and Family History of Alcoholism." *Addictive Behaviors*, Vol. 34, No. 3, March 2009, pp. 252–257.

15. Tallaferro. "Associations Between Physical Activity and Reduced Rates of Hopelessness, Depression, and Suicidal Behavior Among College Students."

16. Blanco, "Mental Health of College Students and Their Non-College-Attending Peers: Results from the National Epidemiological Study on Alcohol and Related Conditions."

17. Zivin, "Persistence of Mental Health Problems and Needs in a College Student Population."

18. Joska, John, and Dan Stein. "Mood Disorders." *Textbook of Psychiatry*, 5th ed., Robert Hales, Stuart Yudofsky, and Glen Gabbard (eds.). Washington, DC: American Psychiatric Pub. 2008, pp. 457–504.

19. American College Health Association. *American College Health Association National College Health Assessment: Reference Group Executive Summary Fall 2007.* Baltimore: American College Health Association, 2008.

20. Yoon, J., and A. S. Lau. "Maladaptive Perfectionism and Depressive Symptoms among Asian American College Students: Contributions of Interdependence and Parental Relations." *Cultural Diversity and Ethnic Minority Psychology*, Vol. 14, No. 2, April 2008, pp. 92–101.

21. Primack, B. A., et al. "Association Between Media Use in Adolescence and Depression in Young Adulthood: A Longitudinal Study." *Archives of General Psychiatry*, Vol. 66, No. 2, February 2009, pp. 181–188.

22. Cuijpers, P., et al. "Psychological Treatment of Depression in Primary Care: A Meta-analysis." *British Journal of General Psychiatry*, Vol. 59, No. 559, February 2009, pp. e51–60.

23. Barbui, C., et al. "Selective Serotonin Reuptake Inhibitors and Risk of Suicide: A Systematic Review of Observational Studies." *Canadian Medical Association Journal,* Vol. 180, No. 3, February 3, 2009, pp. 291–297.

24. Greden, John. Personal interview.

25. Kaplan, Arline. "Task Force Proposes New Bipolar Guidelines." *Psychiatric Times*, Vol. 25, No. 4, April 2008, p. 1.

26. Fountoulakis, K., et al. "Psychotherapeutic Intervention and Suicide Risk Reduction in Bipolar Disorder: A Review of the Evidence." *Journal of Affective Disorders,* Vol. 113, No. 1, pp. 21–29.

27. Hollander, Eric, and Daphne Simeon, "Anxiety Disorders," *Textbook of Psychiatry*, 5th ed., Robert Hales, Stuart Yudolfsky, and Glen Gabbard (eds.). Washington, DC, 2008, pp. 505–608.

28. Sexena, S., et al. "Rapid Effects of Brief Intensive Cognitive-Behavioral Therapy on Brain Glucose Metabolism in Obsessive-Compulsive Disorder." *Molecular Psychiatry*, January 8, 2008 [Epub ahead of print].

29. Ursano, Amy, et al. "Disorders Usually First Diagnosed in Infancy, Childhood, or Adolescence." *Textbook of Psychiatry*, 5th ed., Robert Hales, Stuart Yudofsky, and Glen Gabbard (eds.). Washington, DC: American Psychiatric Pub., 2008, pp. 505–608.

30. "Transcendental Meditation Seen Promising as ADHD Therapy," January 5, 2009, www.medlineplus.gov.

31. VA Press Release: 100,000 Calls to and 2,600 Rescues by VA's Suicide Prevention Hotline, Department of Veterans Affairs, February 7, 2009.

32. Kaplan, Arline. "A Rising Tide of Youth Suicide." *Psychiatric Times*, Vol. 25, No. 16, December 2008, pp. 1–9.

33. Bursztein, Cendrine, and Alan Apter. "Adolescent Suicide." *Current Opinion in Psychiatry*, Vol. 22, No. 1, January 2009, pp. 1–6.

34. Levin, Andrew. "SSRI Treatment of Children and Adolescents." *Psychiatric Times,* January 2009, pp. 26–28.

35. Horton, Leslie. "Social, Cultural, and Demographic Factors in Suicide." *Textbook of Suicide Assessment and Management*, Robert Simon, and Robert Hales, (eds.). Washington, DC: American Psychiatric Publishing, 2006, p. 107.

36. Tallaferro, "Associations Between Physical Activity and Reduced Rates of Hopelessness, Depression, and Suicidal Behavior Among College Students."

37. Schaffer, M., et al. "The Relationship Between Suicidal Behavior, Ideation and Binge Drinking among College Students." *Archives of Suicide Research,* Vol. 12, No. 2, April 2008, pp. 124–132.

38. Ibid.

39. Walker, R. L., et al. "An Empirical Investigation of Acculturative Stress and Ethnic Identity as Moderators for Depression and Suicidal Ideation in College Students." *Cultural Diversity and Ethnic Minority Psychology,* Vol. 14, No. 1, January 2008, pp. 75–82.

40. Valenstein, M., et al. "Higher-Risk Periods for Suicide Among VA Patients Receiving Depression Treatment: Prioritizing Suicide Prevention Efforts." *Journal of Affective Disorders,* Vol. 112, No. 1-3, January 2009, pp. 50–58.

41. Ursano, Robert, et al. "Psychodynamic Psychotherapy." *Textbook o Psychiatry,* 5th ed., Robert Hales, Stuart Yudofsky, and Glen Gabbard (eds.). Washington, DC: American Psychiatric Pub., 2008, pp. 1637–1654.

42. Shafranske, E. P. "Spiritually Oriented Psychodynamic Psychotherapy." *Journal of Clinical Psychology,* Vol. 65, No. 2, pp. 147–157.

43. Gabbard, Glen (editor). *Textbook of Psychotherapeutic Treatments.* Washington, DC: American Psychiatric Press, 2009.

44. Tengland, Per-Anders. *The Goals of Psychotherapy.* United Kingdom: PCCS Books, 2009.

45. Wright, Jesse, et al. "Cognitive Therapy." *Textbook of Psychiatry,* 5th ed., Robert Hales, Stuart Yudofsky, and Glen Gabbard (eds.). Washington, DC: American Psychiatric Pub., 2008, pp. 1211–1256.

46. Markowtiz, John. "Psychodynamic Psychotherapy." *Textbook of Psychiatry,* 5th ed., Robert Hales, Stuart Yudofsky, and Glen Gabbard (eds.). Washington, DC: American Psychiatric Pub., 2008, pp. 1171–1190.

Chapter 5

1. Godfrey, J. R., and M. E. Nelson. "Toward Optimal Health: Promoting Physical Activity in Women." *Journal of Women's Health* (Larchmt), Vol. 18, No. 3, March 2009, pp. 295–298.

2. Kokkinos, Peter, et al. "Exercise Capacity and Mortality in Black and White Men," *Circulation,* Vol. 117, No. 5, February 5, 2008, pp. 614–622.

3. Bungum, Tim. "Correlates of Physical Activity among Asian and African Americans." Presentation, 2009 AAHPERD National Convention, April 2009.

4. Kvaavik, E., et al. "Physical Fitness and Physical Activity at Age 13 Years as Predictors of Cardiovascular Disease Risk Factors at Ages 15, 25, 33, and 40 Years; Extended Follow-up of the Oslo Youth Study." *Pediatrics,* Vol. 123, No. 1, January 2009, pp. e80–86.

5. Preidt, Robert. "Neighborhood Influences Exercise Levels." *HealthDay,* March 25, 2008, www.medlineplus.gov.

6. Lee, Sukho, and Kyung-shin Park. "On Campus Living Increases Level of Physical Activity while Consuming More Calories." American Physiological Society Annual Meeting, April 1, 2008, www.the-APS.org/press.

7. Cherkas, L. F., et al. "The Association between Physical Activity in Leisure Time and Leukocyte Telomere Length." *Archives of Internal Medicine,* Vol. 168, No. 2, January 28, 2008, pp. 154–158.

8. Blanchard, Chris, et al. "Understanding Physical Activity Behavior in African American and Caucasian Students: An Application of the Theory of Planned Behavior." *Journal of American College Health,* Vol. 56, No. 4, January–February 2008, pp. 341–346.

9. Sabouri, Sharon, and Jennifer Irwin. "Prevalence of Sufficient Physical Activity among Parents Attending a University." *Journal of American College Health,* Vol. 56, No. 6, May–June 2008, pp. 680–685.

10. Sternfeld, B., et al. "Physical Activity and Risk of Recurrence and Mortality in Breast Cancer Survivors: Findings from the LACE Study." *Cancer Epidemiology, Biomarkers & Prevention,* Vol. 18, No. 1, January 2009, pp. 87–95.

11. Neilson, H. K., et al. "Physical Activity and Postmenopausal Breast Cancer: Proposed Biologic Mechanisms and Areas for Future Research." *Cancer Epidemiology, Biomarkers & Prevention,* Vol. 18, No. 1, January 2009, pp. 11–27.

12. American College of Sports Medicine. "Exercise Important in Shrinking Your Stress." March 26, 2008, www.acsm.org.

13. Rendi, M., et al. "Acute Psychological Benefits of Aerobic Exercise: A Field Study into the Effects of Exercise Characteristics." *Psychology, Health, and Medicine,* Vol. 13, No. 2, March 2008, pp. 180–184.

14. Broom, D. R., et al. "Exercise Dose and Quality of Life: A Randomized Controlled Trial." *Archives of Internal Medicine,* Vol. 169, No. 3, February 9, 2009, pp. 269–278.

15. Martin, C. K., et al.

16. http://www.health.gov/paguidelines.

17. Bell, Katie. "ACSM, AHA Support Federal Physical Activity Guidelines." *American College of Sports Medicine,* news release, October 7, 2008.

18. Donnelly, J. E., et al. "American College of Sports Medicine Position Stand: Appropriate Physical Activity Intervention Strategies for Weight Loss and Prevention of Weight Regain for Adults." *Medicine & Science in Sports & Exercise,* Vol. 41, No. 2, February 2009, pp. 459–471.

19. Nelson, M. E., and S. C. Folta. "Further Evidence for the Benefits of Walking." *American Journal of Clinical Nutrition,* Vol. 89, No. 1, January 2009, pp. 15–16.

20. Gray, S. R., et al. "The Effect of a 12 Week Walking Intervention on Markers of Insulin Resistance and Systemic Inflammation." *Preventative Medicine,* Vol. 48, No. 1, January 2009, pp. 39–44.

21. Boone-Heinonen, J., et al. "Walking for Prevention of Cardiovascular Disease in Men and Women: A Systematic Review of Observational Studies." *Obesity Review,* December 10, 2008.

22. Gordon-Larsen, P., et al. "Fifteen-Year Longitudinal Tends in Walking Patterns and Their Impact on Weight Change." *American Journal of Clinical Nutrition,* Vol. 89, No. 1, January 2009, pp. 19–26.

23. Richardson, C. R., et al. "A Meta-Analysis of Pedometer-Based Walking Interventions and Weight Loss." *Annals of Family Medicine,* Vol. 6, No. 1, January–February 2008, pp. 69–77.

24. Gwebu, Amukela. "College Students' Moral Reasoning about Performance-Enhancing Drugs in Sport." Presentation, 2009 AAHPERD National Convention, April 2009.

25. Pipe, Andrew. "Effects of Growth Hormone on Athletic Performance: A Review." *Clinical Journal of Sport Medicine,* Vol. 19, No. 1, January 2009, pp. 75–76.

26. Liu, Hau, et al. "Systematic Review: The Effects of Growth Hormone on Athletic Performance." *Annals of Internal Medicine,* Vol. 148, No. 10, May 20, 2008, p. 20.

27. Huang, Guoyan. "Supervised Yoga Exercise Training and Balance in College Students." Presentation, 2009 AAHPERD National Convention, April 2009.

28. Madigan, L. et al. "Management of Symptomatic Lumbar Degenerative Disk Disease." *Journal of the American Academy of Orthopedic Surgery,* Vol. 17, No. 2, February 2009, pp. 102–111.

29. Dore, G. A., et al. "Relation between Central Adiposity and Cognitive Function in the Maine-Syracuse Study: Attenuation by Physical Activity." *Annals of Behavioral Medicine,* June 27, 2008.

30. Brown, Theresa. "Perceptions of a Caring and Positive Climate in Exercise Classes." Presentation, 2009 AAHPERD National Convention, April 2009.

31. Preidt, Robert. "Winter Workouts Are Cool." *HealthyDay,* January 4, 2009. www.medlineplus.gov.

Chapter 6

1. Goldfarb, Stanley, "Just Add Water," *Journal of the American Society of Nephrology,* Vol. 26, No. 6, June 2008, pp. 655–566.

2. Sinha, R., et al. "Meat Intake and Mortality: A Prospective Study of Over Half a Million People." *Archives of Internal Medicine,* Vol. 169, No. 6, March 23, 2009, pp. 562–571

3. "Facts about Fructose." American Dietetic Association. www.eatright.org.

4. Gray, G. A. "Fructose: Should We Worry?" *International Journal of Obesity,* Vol. 32, Suppl. 7, December 2008, pp. S127–131.

5. Bachman, Jessica, et al. "Sources of Food Group Intakes among the US Population, 2001–2002." *Journal of the American Dietetic Association,* Vol. 108, No. 5, May 2008, pp. 804–814.

6. Grandjean, Ann, et al. "Popcorn Consumption and Dietary and Physiological Parameters of U.S. Children and Adults: Analysis of the National Health and Nutrition Examination Survey (NHANES) 1999–2002 Dietary Survey Data." *Journal of the American Dietetic Association,* Vol. 108, No. 5, May 2008, pp. 853–856.

7. Halton, T. L., et al. "Low-Carbohydrate-Diet Score and Risk of Type 2 Diabetes in Women." *American Journal of Clinical Nutrition,* Vol. 87, No. 2, February 2008, pp. 339–346.

8. Wei, M. Y., et al. "Vitamin D and Prevention of Colorectal Adenoma: A Meta-analysis." *Cancer Epidemiology, Biomarkers & Prevention,* Vol. 17, No. 11, November 2008, pp. 2958–2969.

9. Chiebowski, R. T., et al. "Calcium Plus Vitamin D Supplementation and the Risk of Breast Cancer." *Journal of the National Cancer Institute,* Vol. 100, No. 22, November 19, 2008, pp. 1581–1591.

10. Margolis, K. L., et al. "Effect of Calcium and Vitamin D Supplementation on Blood Pressure: The Women's Health Initiative Randomized Trial." *Hypertension,* Vol. 52, No. 5, November 2008, pp. 847–850.

11. Llewellyn, D. J., et al. "Serum 25-Hydroxyvitamin D Concentration and Cognitive Impairment." *Journal of Geriatric Psychiatry & Neurology,* February 4, 2009.

12. Wood, Heather. "Food for Thought." *Nature Clinical Practice Neurology,* Vol. 5, No. 1, January 2009.

13. Kremer, R., et al. "Vitamin D Status and Its Relationship to Body Fat, Final Height, and Peak Bone Mass in Young Women." *Journal of Clinical Endocrinology & Metabolism,* Vol. 94, No. 1, January 2009, pp. 67–73.

14. Ward, K., et al. "Vitamin D Status and Muscle Function in Post-Menarchal Adolescent Girls." *Journal of Clinical Endocrinology & Metabolism,* February 2009, epub.

15. Tang, B. M., et al. "Use of Calcium or Calcium in Combination with Vitamin D Supplementation to Prevent Fractures and Bone Loss in People Aged 50 Years and Older: A Meta-analysis." *Obstetrical & Gynecological Survey,* Vol. 63, No. 1, January 2008.

16. Lambert, H. L., et al. "Calcium Supplementation and Bone Mineral Accretion in Adolescent Girls: An 18-month Randomized Controlled Trial with 2-year Follow-up." *American Journal of Clinical Nutrition,* Vol. 87, No. 2, February 2008, pp. 455–462.

17. Visioli, F., et al. "Chocolate, Lifestyle, and Health." *Crit. Rev. Food Sci. Nutr.,* Vol. 49, No. 4, April 2009, pp. 299–312.

18. Nurk, E., et al. "Intake of flavonoid-rich Wine, Tea, and Chocolate by Elderly Men and Women Is Associated with Better Cognitive Test Performance." *Journal of Nutrition,* Vol. 139, No. 1, January 2009, pp. 120–127.

19. *Dietary Guidelines for Americans 2005,* USDHHS, USDA.

20. Albanes, Demetrius. "Vitamin Supplements and Cancer Prevention: Where Do Randomized Controlled Trials Stand?" *Journal of the National Cancer Institute,* Vol. 101, No. 1, January 2009, pp. 2–4.

21. Neuhouser, M. L., et al. "Multivitamin Use and Risk of Cancer and Cardiovascular Disease in the Women's Health Initiative Cohorts." *Archives of Internal Medicine,* Vol. 169, No. 3, February 9, 2009, pp. 294–304.

22. Lin, J., et al. "Vitamins C and E and Beta Carotene Supplementation and Cancer Risk: A Randomized Controlled Trial." *Journal of the National Cancer Institute,* Vol. 101, No. 1, January 2009, pp. 14–23.

23. Lippman, S. M. "Effect of Selenium and Vitamin E on Risk of Prostate Cancer and Other Cancers." *Journal of the American Medical Association,* Vol. 301, No. 1, January 7, 2009, pp. 39–51.

24. Christen, W. G., et al. "Folic Acid, Pyridoxine, and Cyanocobalamin Combination Treatment and Age-Related Macular Degeneration in Women." *Archives of Internal Medicine,* Vol. 169, No. 4, February 23, 2009, pp. 335–351.

25. "Slight Cut in Salt Intake Would Mean Fewer Heart Attacks, Deaths," *HealthDay,* March 11, 2009, www.medlineplus.gov.

26. Willett, W. C., and M. L. McCullough. "Dietary Pattern Analysis for the Evaluation of Dietary Guidelines." *Asia Pacific Journal of Clinical Nutrition,* Vol. 17, Suppl. 1, 2008, pp. 75–78.

27. www.hsph.harvard.edu/nutritionsource/what-should-you-eat.

28. Adams, Troy, and Willa Colner. "The Association of Multiple Risk Factors with Fruit and Vegetable Intake among a Nationwide Sample of College Students." *Journal of American College Health,* Vol. 56, No. 4, January–February 2008, pp. 455–461.

29. Ibid.

30. Larson, N. I., et al. "Making Time for Meals: Meal Structure and Associations with Dietary Intake in Young Adults." *Journal of the American Dietetic Association,* Vol. 109, No. 1, January 2009, pp. 72–79.

31. Gerend, M. A. "Does Calorie Information Promote Lower Calorie Fast Food Choices Among College Students?" *Journal of Adolescent Health,* Vol. 44, No. 1, January 2009, pp. 84–86.

32. Bleich, S. N., et al. "Increasing Consumption of Sugar-Sweetened Beverages Among U.S. Adults: 1988–1994 to 1999–2004." *American Journal of Clinical Nutrition,* Vol. 89, No. 1, January 2009, pp. 372–378.

33. Allison, D. B., and R. D. Mattes. "Nutritively Sweetened Beverage Consumption and Obesity." *Journal of the American Medical Association,* Vol. 301, No. 3, January 21, 2009, pp. 318–320.

34. Shoham, D. A., et al. "Sugary Soda Consumption and Albuminuria: Results from the National Health and Nutrition Examination Survey, 1999–2004." PLoS ONE, Vol. 3, No. 10, 2008, p. e3431.

35. Fung, T. T., et al. "Sweetened Beverage Consumption and Risk of Coronary Heart Disease in Women." *American Journal of Clinical Nutrition,* February 11, 2009.

36. Hattersley, L., et al. "Determinants and Patterns of Soft Drink Consumption in Young Adults: A Qualitative Analysis." *Public Health Nutrition,* February 2009, pp. 1–7.

37. Hardin-Fanning, F., et al. "The Effects of a Mediterranean-style Dietary Pattern on Cardiovascular Disease Risk." *Nursing Clinics of North America,* Vol. 43, No. 1, March 2008, pp. vii, 105–115.

38. Jenkins, D. J., et al. "Effect of a Low-Glycemic Index or a High-Cereal Fiber Diet on Type 2 Diabetes: A Randomized Trial." *Journal of the American Medical Association,* Vol. 300, No. 23, December 17, 2008, pp. 2742–2753.

39. Babio, N., et al. "Adherence to the Mediterranean Diet and Risk of Metabolic Syndrom and Its Components." *Nutrition, Metabolism and Cardiovascular Diseases,* January 26, 2009.

40. Sebastian, Rhonda, et al. "Effect of Snacking Frequency on Adolescents' Dietary Intakes and Meeting National Recommendations." *Journal of Adolescent Health,* Vol. 42, No. 5, May 2008, pp. 503–511.

41. Pooladi, Patricia. "Food Safety System Still Needs Overhaul." The Science Behind Today's News, National Academies Office of News and Public Information, February 20, 2009.

42. Harris, Gardner, and Pam Belluck. "New Look at Food Safety after Peanut Tainting." *New York Times,* January 30, 2009, p. 15.

Chapter 7

1. "Global Strategy on Diet, Physical Activity and Health." World Health Organization, www.who.int/dietphysicalactivity/publications/facts/obesity/en/.

2. http://www.cedc.gov/nchs/ressroom/07newsreleases/obesity.htm.

3. Katan, M. B. "Weight-Loss Diets for the Prevention and Treatment of Obesity." *New England Journal of Medicine,* Vol. 360, pp. 923–925.

4. Franco, M., et al. "Availability of Healthy Foods and Dietary Patterns: The Multi-Ethnic Study of Atherosclerosis." *American Journal of Clinical Nutrition,* Vol. 89, No. 3, March 2009, pp. 897–900.

5. Larson, N. I., et al. "Neighborhood Environments: Disparities in Access to Healthy Foods in the U.S." *American Journal of Preventive Medicine,* Vol. 36, No. 1, January 2009, pp. 74–81.

6. Morland, K. B., and K. R. Evenson. "Obesity Prevalence and the Local Food Environment." *Health Place,* Vol. 15, No. 2, June 2009, pp. 491–495.

7. Dittmarr, Helga. "How Do 'Body Perfect' Ideals in the Media Have a Negative Impact on Body Image and Behaviors? Factors and Processes Related to Self and Identity." *Journal of Social and Clinical Psychology,* Vol. 28, No. 1, pp. 1–8.

8. Lin, Linda, and Kathleen Reid. "The Relationship Between Media Exposure and Antifat Attitudes: The Role of Dysfunctional Appearance Beliefs." *Body Image,* Vol. 6, No. 1, January 2009, pp. 52–55.

9. Rasberry, Catherine, "Battling Body Image: Confessions of a Health Educator." *Journal of American College Health,* Vol. 56, No. 4, January–February 2008, pp. 423–426.

10. Pedersen, P. J., and P. L. Ketcham. "Exploring the Climate for Overweight and Obese Students in a Student Health Setting." *Journal of American College Health,* Vol. 57, No. 4, January–February, 2009, pp. 465–480.

11. Larson, N. I., et al. "Making Time for Meals: Meal Structure and Associations with Dietary Intake in Young Adults." *Journal of the American Dietetic Association,* Vol. 109, No. 1, January 2009, pp. 72–78.

12. Kasparek, Danella, et al. "Selected Health Behaviors That Influence college Freshman Weight Change." *Journal of American College Health,* Vol. 56, No. 4, January–February 2008, pp. 437–444.

13. Economos, C. D., et al. "College Freshman Stress and Weight Change: Differences by Gender." *American Journal of Health Behavior,* Vol. 32, No. 1, 2008, pp. 16–25.

14. Dawood, S., et al. "Prognostic Value of Body Mass Index in Locally Advanced Breast Cancer." *Clinical Cancer Research,* Vol. 56, No. 6, March 15, 2008, pp. 1718–1725.

15. Broom, D. R., et al. "Influence of Resistance and Aerobic Exercise on Hunger, Circulating Levels of Acylated Ghrelin, and Peptide YY in Healthy Males." *American Journal Physiol. Regul. Integr. Comp. Physiol.,* Vol. 296, No. 1, January 2009, pp. R29–35.

16. Sacks, F. M., et al. "Comparison of Weight-Loss Diets with Different Compositions of Fat, Protein, and Carbohydrates." *New England Journal of Medicine,* Vol. 360, No. 9, February 26, 2009, pp. 859–873.

17. D'Anci, K. E., et al. "Low-Carbohydrate Weight-Loss Diets: Effects on Cognition and Mood." *Appetite,* Vol. 52, No. 1, February 2009, pp. 96–103.

18. "FDA Warns about Weight Loss Products." *Health-Day,* December 23, 2008. www.medlineplus.gov.

19. Donnelly, J. E., et al. "American College of Sports Medicine Position Stand: Appropriate Physical Activity Intervention Strategies for Weight Loss and Prevention of Weight Regain for Adults." *Medicine & Science in Sports & Exercise,* Vol. 41, No. 2, February 2009, pp. 459–476.

20. Ibid.

21. Lee, D. C., et al. "Does Physical Activity Ameliorate the Health Hazards of Obesity?" *British Journal of Sports Medicine,* Vol. 43, No. 1, January 2009, pp. 49–51.

22. Timlin, M. T., et al. "Breakfast Eating and Weight Change in a 5-year Prospective Analysis of Adolescents: Project EAT." *Pediatrics,* Vol. 121, March 2008, p. e638.

23. Dixon, J. B., et al. "Adjustable Gastric Banding and Conventional Therapy for Type 2 Diabetics." *Journal of the American Medical Association,* Vol. 299, No. 3, January 23, 2008, pp. 316–323.

24. Inge, T. H., et al. "Reversal of Type 2 Diabetes Mellitus and Improvements in Cardiovascular Risk Factors after Surgical Weight Loss in Adolescents." *Pediatrics,* Vol. 123, No. 1, January 209, pp. 214–222.

25. Zeller, M. H., et al. "Psychosocial Functioning Improves Following Adolescent Bariatric Surgery." *Obesity* (Silver Spring). January 22, 2009. (Epub ahead of print)

26. Chang, E. C., et al. "Complexities of Measuring Perfectionism: Three Popular Perfectionism Measures and Their Relations with Eating Disturbances and Health Behaviors in a Female College Student Sample." *Eating Behaviors,* Vol. 9, 2008, pp. 102–110.

27. Pritchard, Mary, and Kyra Yaich. "Relationships among Loneliness, Interpersonal Dependency, and Disordered Eating in Young Adults." *Personality and Individual Differences,* Vol. 46, No. 3, February 2009, pp. 341–346.

28. Yager, Zali, and Jennifer O'Dea. "Prevention Programs for Body Image and Eating Disorders on University Campuses: A Review of Large Controlled Interventions." *Health Promotion International,* February 8, 2008.

29. Hardine, Anne. "Eating Disorders May Be Rising among Male Athletes." *HealthDay,* January 8, 2009. www.medlineplus.gov.

30. Greenleaf, C., et al. "Female Collegiate Athletes: Prevalence of Eating Disorders and Disordered Eating Behaviors." *Journal of American College Health,* Vol. 57, No. 5, March–April 2009, pp. 489–496.

31. "Binges Take about One Third of Food Budgets." *HealthDay,* December 31, 2008. www.medlineplus.gov.

32. Marsh, Rachel, et al. "Deficient Activity in the Neural Systems That Mediate Self-Regulatory Control in Bulimia Nervosa." *Archives of General Psychiatry,* Vol. 66, No. 1, January 2009, pp. 51–63.

Chapter 8

1. Fowler, J. H., and N. A. Christakis. "Dynamic Spread of Happiness in a Large Social Network: Longitudinal Analysis over 20 Years in the Framingham Heart Study." *British Medical Journal,* Vol. 337, December 4, 2008, p. a2338.

2. Graham, L. K. "What Is Social Networking? And How Do I Get Clued in to LinkedIn?" *Journal of the American Dietetic Association,* Vol. 109, No. 1, January 2009, p. 184.

3. Mitchell, K. J., and M. Ybarra. "Social Networking Sites: Finding a Balance Between Their Risks and Benefits," *Archives of Pediatric and Adolescent Medicine,* Vol. 163, No. 1, January 2009, pp. 87–89.

4. Fogel, Joshua, and Elham Nehmad. "Internet Social Network Communities: Risk Taking, Trust, and Privacy Concerns." *Computers in Human Behavior,* Vol. 25, No. 1, January 2009, pp. 153–160.

5. Versteeg, K. M., et al. "Teenagers Wanting Medical Advice: Is MySpace the Answer?" *Archives of Pediatric and Adolescent Medicine*, Vol. 163, No. 1, January 2009, pp. 91–92.

6. Moreno, M. A., et al. "Reducing At-Risk Adolescents' Display of Risk Behavior on a Social Networking Web Site: A Randomized Controlled Pilot Intervention Trial." *Archives of Pediatric and Adolescent Medicine,* Vol. 163, No. 1, January 2009, pp. 35–41.

7. Moreno, M. A., et al. "Display of Health Risk Behaviors on MySpace by Adolescents: Prevalence and Associations." *Archives of Pediatric and Adolescent Medicine*, Vol. 163, No. 1, January 2009, pp. 27–34.

8. Maple, Marilyn. Personal interview.

9. Goulston, Mark. Personal interview.

10. Lu, H. P., and K. L. Hsiao. "Gender Differences in Reasons for Frequent Blog Posting," *Online Information Review*, Vol. 33, No. 1, January 2009, pp. 135–156.

11. Ibid.

12. Morrison, R. L., "Are Women Tending and Befriending in the Workplace? Gender Differences in the Relationship between Workplace Friendships and Organizational Outcomes." *Sex Roles*, Vol. 60, No. 1–2, January 2009, pp. 1–13.

13. Carroll, Janell C. *Sexuality Now: Embracing Diversity*, 3rd ed. Belmont, CA: Cengage-Wadsworth, 2010.

14. Laumann, Edward. Personal interview.

15. Buss, David. *The Evolution of Desire.* New York: Basic Books, 1994.

16. Fisher, Helen. Personal interview.

17. American College Health Association. *American College Health Association-National College Health Assessment II: Reference Group Executive Summary Fall 2008.* Baltimore: American College Health Association, 2009.

18. Billingham, Robert. Personal interview.

19. Yager, Jan. Personal interview.

20. Rhoades, G. K., et al. "Couples' Reasons for Cohabitation: Associations with Individual Well-Being and Relationship Quality." *Journal of Family Issues,* Vol. 30, No. 2, February 2009, pp. 233–258.

21. Rhoades, G. K., et al. "The Pre-engagement Cohabitation Effect: A Replication and Extension of Previous Findings." *Journal of Family Psychology*, Vol. 23, No. 1, February 2009, pp. 107–111.

22. Sternberg, Robert. Personal interview.

23. National Center for Health Statistics, Washington, DC, www.cdc.gov/nchs.

24. Wienke, Chris, and Gretchen Hill. "Does the 'Marriage Benefit' Extend to Partners in Gay and Lesbian Relationships?" *Journal of Family Issues,* Vol. 30, No. 2, February 2009, pp. 259–289.

25. Frisch, M., and H. Bronnum-Hansen. "Morality among Men and Women in Same-Sex Marriage: A National Cohort Study of 8333 Danes," *American Journal of Public Health*, Vol. 99, No. 1, January 2009, pp. 133–137.

26. Crooks, Robert L., and Karla Baur. *Our Sexuality*, 10th ed. Belmont, CA: Cengage-Wadsworth, 2008.

27. Doss, D. B., et al. "Marital Therapy, Retreats and Books: The Who, What, When, and Why of Relationship Help-Seeking." *Journal of Marital and Family Therapy*, Vol. 35, No. 1, pp. 18–29.

28. "Bad Marriages Harder on Women's Health." *HealthDay*, March 5, 2009. www.medlineplus.gov.

29. U.S. Census Bureau, Washington, DC, www.census.gov.

Chapter 9

1. Herman-Gidens, Marcia. Personal interview.

2. László, K. D., and M. S. Kopp. "Effort-Reward Imbalance and Overcommitment at Work Are Associated with Painful Menstruation: Results from the Hungarostudy Epidemiological Panel 2006." *Journal of Occupational and Environmental Medicine*, Vol. 51, No. 2, February 2009, pp. 157-163.

3. Fontenot, Holly, and Allyssa Harris. "The Latest Advances in Hormonal Contraception." *Journal of Obstetric, Gynecologic, & Neonatal Nursing*, Vol. 37, No. 3, 2008, pp. 369–374, doi:10.1111/j.1552-6909.2008.00248.x.

4. Khajehei, M., et al. "Effect of Treatment with Dydrogesterone or Calcium plus Vitamin D on the Severity of Premenstrual Syndromes." *International Journal of Gynecology & Obstetrics*, Vol. 105, No. 2, May 2009, pp. 158–161.

5. Busse, J. W., et al. "Psychological Intervention for Premenstrual Syndrome: A Meta-analysis of Randomized Controlled Trials." *Psychotherapeutic Psychosomatics*, Vol. 78, No. 1, 2009, pp,. 6–15.

6. Jing, Z., et al. "Chinese Herbal Medicine for Premenstrual Syndrome." *Cochrane Database System Review*, January 21 2009, CD006414.Review.

7. Weisz, G., and L. Knaapen. "Diagnosing and Treating Premenstrual Syndrome in Five Western Nations." *Social Science Medicine*, Vol. 68, No. 8, April 2009, pp. 1498–1505

8. Liebowitz, A. A., et al. "Determinants and Policy Implications of Male Circumcision in the United States." *American Journal of Public Health*, Vol. 99, No. 1, pp. 138–145.

9. National Youth Risk Survey, http://www.cdc.gov/ Healthy Youth/yrbs/trends.htm.

10. Bleakley, A., et al. "How Sources of Sexual Information Relate to Adolescents' Beliefs about Sex." *American Journal of Health Behavior*, Vol. 33, No. 1, pp. 37–48.

11. Rosenbaum, J. E. "Patient Teenagers? A Comparison of the Sexual Behavior of Virginity Pledgers and Matched Nonpledgers." *Journal of Adolescent Research*, Vol. 24, No. 1, January 2009, pp. 91–113.

12. Parker-Pope, Tara. "The Myth of Rampant Teenage Promiscuity." *New York Times*, January 27, 2009, p. D6.

13. American College Health Association. *American College Health Association-National College Health Assessment II: Reference Group Executive Summary Fall 2008.* Baltimore: American College Health Association, 2009.

14. Laumann, E. O. et al. "A Population-Based Survey of Sexual Activity, Sexual Problems and Associated Help-Seeking Behavior Patterns in Mature Adults in the United States of America." *International Journal of Impotence Research*, Vol. 21, No. 3, May–June 2009, pp. 171–178.

15. Chandler, S. B. "Heterosexual Attitudes Toward Homosexuality among African American College Students." Presentation, 2009 AAHPERD meeting, April 2009.

16. Caroll, Janell C. *Sexuality Now: Embracing Diversity*, 3rd ed. Belmont, CA: Cengage-Wadsworth, 2010.

17. Hampton, Tracy. "Abstinence-Only Programs Under Fire." *Journal of the American Medical Association*, Vol. 299, No. 17, May 7, 2008, pp. 2013–2014.

18. Henderson, A. W., et al. "Ecological Models of Sexual Satisfaction among Lesbian/Bisexual and Heterosexual Women," *Archives of Sexual Behavior*, Vol. 38, No. 1, February 2009, pp. 50-65.

19. Laumann, "A Population-Based Survey of Sexual Activity."

20. Lamaire, A., et al. "Why Is It That Patients with Sexual Difficulties Do Not Consult a Doctor More Frequently?" *Sexologies*, Vol. 18, No. 1, January–March 2009, pp. 14–18.

21. Bonierbale, M. "From Sexual Difficulties to Sexual Dysfunctions." *Sexologies*, Vol. 18, No. 1, January–March 2009, pp. 10–13.

22. Cordell, W. H., et al. "Retinal Effects of Six Months of Daily Use of Tadalafil and Sildenafil." *Archives of Ophthalmology*, Vol. 127, No. 4, April 2009, pp. 367–373.

23. Kaminetsky, J. C., et al. "In Men with Erectile Dysfunction, Satisfaction with Quality of Erections Correlates with Erection Hardness, Treatment Satisfaction, and Emotional Well-Being." *Journal of Sexual Medicine*, Vol. 6, No. 3, January 2009, pp. 800–808.

24. Chevret-Measson, M., et al. "Improvement in Quality of Sexual Life in Female Partners of Men with Erective Dysfunction Treated with Sildenafil Citrate." *Journal of Sexual Medicine*, Vol. 6, No. 3, January 2009, pp. 761–769.

Chapter 10

1. "Facts on Publicly Funded Contraceptive Services in the United States." Guttmacher Institute, February 2009.

2. Ibid.

3. Carroll, Janell. *Sexuality Now*, 3rd ed. Belmont, CA: Cengage-Wadsworth, 2010.

4. Ibid.

5. Williamson, L. M., et al. "Limits to Modern Contraceptive Use among Young Women in Developing Countries: A Systematic Review of Qualitative Research." *Reproductive Health*, Vol. 6, No. 3, February 19, 2009.

6. Ibid.

7. Nearns J. "Health Insurance Coverage and Prescription Contraceptive Use among Young Women at Risk for Unintended Pregnancy," *Contraception*, Vol. 79, No. 2, pp. 105–110.

8. American College Health Association. *American College Health Association National College Health Assessment II: Reference Group Executive Summary Fall 2008.* Baltimore: American College Health Association, 2009.

9. Callahan, Bryan. "Female Health Company Receives FDA Approval for FC2 Female Condom." Media Release, March 11, 2009.

10. Macaluso, M., et al. "Efficacy of the Male Latex Condom and of the Female Polyurethane Condom as Barriers to Semen during Intercourse: A Randomized Clinical Trial." *American Journal of Epidemiology.*, Vol. 166, No. 1, July 2007, pp. 88–96.

11. Rose, E., et al. "The Validity of Teens' and Young Adults' Self-Reported Condom Use." *Archives of Pediatric and Adolescent Medicine*, Vol. 163, No. 1, January 2009, pp. 61–64.

12. "Newer Contraceptives Don't Increase Heart Risk." *HealthDay*, January 15, 2009. www.Medlineplus.gov.

13. Rosenberg, L., et al. "A Case-Control Study of Oral Contraceptive Use and Incident Breast Cancer." *American Journal of Epidemiology*, Vol. 169, February 15, 2009, pp. 473–479.

14. Shufelt, Chrisandra L., and C. Noel Bairey Merz. "Contraceptive Hormone Use and Cardiovascular Disease." *Journal of the American College of Cardiology*, Vol. 53, January 20, 2009, pp. 221–231.

15. Fontenot, Holly, and Allyssa Harris. "The Latest Advances in Hormonal Contraception." *Journal of Obstetric, Gynecologic, & Neonatal Nursing*, Vol. 37, No. 3, 2008, pp. 369–374, doi:10.1111/j.1552-6909.2008.00248.x.

16. Bitzer, J. and A. M. Paoletti. "Added Benefits and User Satisfaction with a Low-Dose Oral Contraceptive Containing Drospirenone: Results of Three Multicentre Trials." *Clinical Drug Investigations*, Vol. 29, No.1, 2009, pp. 73–78.

17. Fontenot and Harris, "Latest Advances in Hormonal Contraception."

18. Jones, David. "Why Emergency Contraception Remains Controversial." *Southern Medical Journal*, Vol. 102, No. 1, January 2009, pp. 5–7.

19. Black, K. "Developments and Challenges in Emergency Contraception." *Best Practice & Research Clinical Obstetrics & Gynecology*, Vol. 23, No. 2, pp. 221–231.

20. Galvin, S. L., et al. "Knowledge, Attitudes, and Use of Emergency Contraception among Hispanic Women

of North Carolina." *Southern Medical Journal*, Vol. 102, No. 1, January 2009, pp. 17–20.

21. Novikova, N., et al. "Does Readily Available Emergency Contraception Increase Women's Awareness and Use?" *The European Journal of Contraception & Reproductive Health Care*, Vol. 14, No. 1, February 2009, pp. 39–45.

22. Moreau, C., et al. "The Effect of Access to Emergency Contraceptive Pills on Women's Use of Highly Effective Contraceptives: Results from a French National Cohort Study." *American Journal of Public Health*, Vol. 99, March 2009, pp. 441–442.

23. Miller, Laura. "College Student Knowledge and Attitudes Toward Emergency Contraception." Presentation, AAHPERD National Convention, April 2009.

24. Vahratian, Anjel, et al. "College Students' Perceptions of Emergency Contraception Provision." *Journal of Women's Health*, Vol. 17, No. 1, January 1, 2008, pp. 103–111, doi:10.1089/jwh.2007.0391.

25. Cheng, L., et al. "Interventions for Emergency Contraception Provision." *Cochrane Database of Systematic Reviews*, No. 2, 2008, Art. No. CD001324. doi:10.1002/14651858.CD001324.pub3.

26. Wind, Rebecca. "U.S. Abortion Rate Continues Long-Term Decline, Falling to Lowest Level since 1974; More Effort Still Needed to Reduce Unintended Pregnancy." News Release, Guttmacher Institute, January 17, 2008, www.guttmacher.org/.

27. Steinberg, J. R., and N. F. Russo. "Abortion and Anxiety: What's the Relationship?" *Social Science Medicine*, Vol. 67, No. 2, July 2008, pp. 238–252.

28. Pedersen, Willy. "Abortion and Depression: A Population-Based Longitudinal Study of Young Women." *Scandinavian Journal of Public Health*, Vol. 36, No. 4, July 2008, pp. 424–428.

29. "An Overview of Abortion Laws." Guttmacher Institute State Center, June 1, 2008, www.guttmacher.org/statecenter.

30. Hamilton, B. E., et al. "Births: Preliminary Data for 2007." *National Vital Statistics Reports*, Vol. 57, No. 12, March 18, 2009.

31. Kahn, E. B., et al. "Cesarean Delivery among Women with Low-Risk Pregnancies: A Comparison of Birth Certificates and Hospital Discharge Data." *Obstetrics & Gynecology*, Vol. 113, No. 1, January 2009, pp. 33–40.

32. American Society of Reproductive Medicine, www.asrm.org.

Chapter 11

1. Zald, D. H., et al. "Midbrain Dopamine Receptor Availability Is Inversely Associated with Novelty-Seeking Traits in Humans." *Journal of Neuroscience*, Vol. 28, No. 53, December 31, 2008, pp. 14372–14378.

2. National Council on Problem Gambling, www.ncpgambling.org/.

3. Weinstock, J., et al. "College Students' Gambling Behavior: When Does It Become Harmful?" *Journal of American College Health*, Vol. 56, No. 5, March/April 2008, pp. 513–521.

4. Ibid.

5. Ibid.

6. Ford, Jason A., and Ryan D. Schroeder. "Academic Strain and Non-Medical Use of Prescription Stimulants among College Students." *Deviant Behavior*, Vol. 30, No. 1, January 2009, pp. 26–53.

7. Ibid.

8. Ibid.

9. *Wasting the Best and the Brightest: Substance Abuse at America's Colleges and Universities.* New York: National Center on Addiction and Substance Abuse at Columbia University, March 2007.

10. Ibid.

11. Ming, D., and M. B. Li. "New Insights into the Genetics of Addiction." *Nature Reviews Genetics*, Vol. 10, April 1, 2009, pp. 225–231.

12. *Wasting the Best and the Brightest: Substance Abuse at America's Colleges and Universities.*

13. Bukstein, O. G., and C. Nguyen. "New Agents of Abuse." *Psychiatric Times*, January 2009, pp. 35–37.

14. American College Health Association. *American College Health Association-National College Health Assessment II: Reference Group Executive Summary Fall 2008* Baltimore: American College Health Association, 2009.

15. Elbogen, E. B., and S. C. Johnson. "The Intricate Link Between Violence and Mental Disorder: Results from the National Epidemiologic Survey on Alcohol and Related Conditions." *Archives of General Psychiatry*, Vol. 66, No. 2, February 2009, pp 152–161.

16. Bukstein. "New Agents of Abuse."

17. Zhang, W., et al. "Coffee Consumption and Risk of Cardiovascular Diseases and All-Cause Mortality among Men with Type 2 Diabetes." *Diabetes Care*, February 19, 2009.

18. Rosso, A., et al. "Caffeine: Neuroprotective Functions in Cognition and Alzheimer's Disease." *American Journal of Alzheimer Disease and Other Dementias*, Vol. 23, No. 5, October–November 2008, pp. 417–422.

19. Ganmaa, D., et al. "Coffee, Tea, Caffeine and Risk of Breast Cancer: A 22-Year Follow-up." *International Journal of Cancer*, Vol. 122, No. 9, May 1, 2008, pp. 2071–2076.

20. Weng, X., et al. "Maternal Caffeine Consumption During Pregnancy and the Risk of Miscarriage: A Prospective Cohort Study." *American Journal of Obstetrics and Gynecology*, Vol. 198, No. 3, March 2008, pp. 279.e1–279.e8.

21. Substance Abuse and Mental Health Services Administration, Office of Applied Studies. "Trends in Nonmedical Use of Prescription Pain Relievers: 2002 to 2007." *The National Survey on Drug Use and Health Report*, Rockville, MD, February 5, 2009.

22. Judson, Rachel, and Susan W. Langdon. "Illicit Use of Prescription Stimulants among College Students: Prescription Status, Motives, Theory of Planned Behaviour, Knowledge and Self-Diagnostic Tendencies." *Psychology, Health & Medicine*, Vol. 14, No. 1, 2009, pp. 97–104.

23. Ford, "Academic Strain and Non-Medical Use of Prescription Stimulants among College Students."

24. Judson, "Illicit Use of Prescription Stimulants among College Students: Prescription Status, Motives, Theory of Planned Behaviour, Knowledge and Self-Diagnostic Tendencies."

25. Ibid.

26. Ibid.

27. Bukstein. "New Agents of Abuse."

28. Wilens, T. E., et al. "Misuse and Diversion of Stimulants Prescribed for ADHD: A Systematic Review of the Literature." *Journal of the American Academy of Child and Adolescent Psychiatry*, Vol. 47, No 1, January 2008, pp. 21–31.

29. Advocat, C. D., et al. "Licit and Illicit Use of Medications for Attention-Deficit Hyperactivity Disorder in Undergraduate College Students." *Journal of American College Health*, Vol. 56, No. 6, May/June 2008, pp. 601–606.

30. Leamon, Martin, et al. "Substance-Related Disorders." *Textbook of Clinical Psychiatry.* Washington, DC: American Psychiatric Press, 2008.

31. Ashtari, M., et al. "Diffusion Abnormalities in Adolescents and Young Adults with a History of Heavy Cannabis Use." *Journal of Psychiatric Research*, Vol. 43, No. 3, January 2009, pp. 189–204.

32. Daling, J. R., et al. "Association of Marijuana Use and the Incidence of Testicular Germ Cell Tumors." *Cancer*, Vol. 115, No. 6, March 15, 2009, pp. 1215–1223.

33. Hall, W., and M. Lynskey. "The Challenges in Developing a Rational Cannabis Policy." *Current Opinion in Psychiatry*, March 16, 2009.

34. Yücel, M., et al. "Regional Brain Abnormalities Associated with Long-Term Heavy Cannabis Use." *Archives of General Psychi9atry*, Vol. 65, No. 6, June 2008, pp. 694–701.

35. Bolla, K., et al. "Sleep Disturbance in Heavy Marijuana Users." *Sleep*, Vol. 21, No. 6, June 1, 2008, pp. 901–908.

36. Budney, A., et al. "Comparison of Cannabis and Tobacco Withdrawal: Severity and Contribution to Relapse." *Journal of Substance Abuse Treatment.* March 12, 2008.

37. "The Economic Costs of Methamphetamine Use in the United States." www.rand.org.

38. Day, Jeremy, and Regina Carelli. "Methamphetamine Induces Chronic Corticostriatal Depression: Too Much of a Bad Thing." *Neuron*, Vol. 58, No. 1, April 10, 2008, pp. 6–7.

39. McCord, James, et al. "Management of Cocaine-Associated Chest Pain and Myocardial Infarction." *Circulation*, Vol. 117, No. 14, April 8, 2008, pp. 1897–1907.

40. "Overcoming Cocaine or Stimulant Addiction." *Harvard Mental Health Letter*, March 2009, www.health.harvard.edu/mentalextra.

Chapter 12

1. Boekeloo, Bradley O., et al. "Perceptions about Residence Hall Wingmates and Alcohol-Related Secondhand Effects among College Freshmen. *Journal of American College Health*, Vol. 57, No. 6, May/June 2009, pp. 619–628.

2. National Institute on Alcohol Abuse and Alcoholism, www.niaa.nih.gov.

3. Ibid.

4. *Wasting the Best and the Brightest: Substance Abuse at America's Colleges and Universities.* New York: National Center on Addiction and Substance Abuse at Columbia University, March 2007.

5. Labrie, J. W., et al. "What Men Want: The Role of Reflective Opposite-Sex Normative Preferences in Alcohol Use among College Women." *Psychology of Addictive Behavior*, Vol. 23, No. 1, March 2009, pp. 157–162.

6. Moore, M. J., et al. "Relationship between Vigorous Exercise Frequency and Substance Use among First-Year Drinking College Students." *Journal of American College Health*, Vol. 56, No. 6, May/June 2088, pp. 686–690.

7. American College Health Association, *American College Health Association National College Health Assessment II. Reference Group Executive Summary Fall 2008.* Baltimore: American College Health Association, 2009.

8. Ham, L. S., et al. "Drinking Motives as Mediators of Social Anxiety and Hazardous Drinking among College Students." *Cognitive Behavioral Therapy*, March 18, 2009, pp. 1–13.

9. Labrie. "What Men Want: The Role of Reflective Opposite-Sex Normative Preferences in Alcohol Use among Women."

10. Ibid.

11. Parks, K. A., et al. "Risky Drinking in College Changes as Fraternity/Sorority Affiliation Changes: A Person-Environment Perspective." *Psychology of Addictive Behaviors*, Vol. 22, No. 2, June 2008, pp. 219–229.

12. Lewis, M. A., et al. "Examining the Relationship Between Typical Drinking Behavior and 21st Birthday Drinking Behavior among College Students: Implications for Event-Specific Prevention." *Addiction*, March 13, 2009.

13. *Wasting the Best and the Brightest.*

14. College Drinking Prevention, www.collegedrinking-prevention.gov.

15. Reingle, Jennifer, et al. "An Exploratory Study of Bar and Nightclub Expectancies." *Journal of American College Health*, Vol. 57, No. 6, May/June 2009, pp. 629–638.

16. Mohr, C. D., et al. "Evidence for Positive Mood Buffering among College Student Drinkers." *Personality and Social Psychology Bulletin*, June 12, 2008.

17. Wills, T. A., et al. "Movie Exposure to Alcohol Cues and Adolescent Alcohol Problems: A Longitudinal Analysis in a National Sample." *Psychology of Addictive Behavior,* Vol. 23, No. 1, March 2009, pp. 23–35.

18. McClure, A. C., et al. "Alcohol-Branded Merchandise and Its Association with Drinking Attitudes and Outcomes in U.S. Adolescents." *Archives of Pediatric Adolescent Medicine,* Vol. 163, No. 3, March 2009, pp. 211–217.

19. "Binge Drinking on College Campuses." Center for Science in the Public Interest, http://www.cspinet.org/.

20. Nelson, M. C., et al. "Alcohol Use, Eating Patterns, and Weight Behaviors in a University Population." *American Journal of Health Behavior,* Vol. 33, No. 3, May–June 2009, pp. 227–237.

21. Wells, S., et al. "Policy Implications of the Widespread Practice of 'Pre-Drinking' or 'Pre-Gaming' before Going to Public Drinking Establishments—Are Current Prevention Strategies Backfiring?" *Addiction,* Vol. 104, No. 1, January 2009, pp. 4–9.

22. Ibid.

23. Martin, Barbara Alvarez, et al. "The Role of Monthly Spending in College Student Drinking Behaviors and Their Consequences." *Journal of American College Health,* Vol. 57, No. 6, May/June 2009, pp. 587–596.

24. Wells, S., et al. "Policy Implications of the Widespread Practice of 'Pre-Drinking' or 'Pre-Gaming' before Going to Public Drinking Establishments—Are Current Prevention Strategies Backfiring?"

25. American College Health Association, *American College Health Association-National College Health Assessment.*

26. Krebs, Christopher P., et al. "College Women's Experiences with Physically Forced, Alcohol- or Other Drug-Enabled, and Drug-Facilitated Sexual Assault Before and Since Entering College." *Journal of American College Health,* Vol. 57, No. 6, May/June 2009, pp. 639–649.

27. Core Drug and Alcohol Survey, www.med.unc.edu/alcohol/prevention/coresurvey.html.

28. Mothers Against Drunk Driving, www.madd.org.

29. NIAAA, College Drinking Prevention, www.collegedrinkingprevention.gov/NIAAACollegeMaterials/TaskForce/CallToAction_02.aspx#CallToAction_02_a.

30. Elliott, C., et al. "Computer-Based Interventions for College Drinking: A Qualitative Review." *Addictive Behavior,* Vol. 33, No. 8, August 2008, pp. 994–1005.

31. LaBrie, Joseph W., et al. "A Night to Remember: A Harm-Reduction Birthday Card Intervention Reduces High-Risk Drinking During 21st Birthday Celebrations." *Journal of American College Health,* Vol. 57, No. 6, May/June 2009, pp. 659–663.

32. Caetano, R., et al. "The Hispanic Americans Baseline Alcohol Survey: Alcoholic Beverage Preference across Hispanic National Groups." *Alcoholism: Clinical and Experimental Research,* Vol. 33, No. 1, January 2009, pp. 150–159.

33. Barnett, N. P., et al. "Measured Alcohol Content in College Party Mixed Drinks." *Psychology of Addictive Behavior,* Vol. 23, No. 1, March 2009, pp. 152–156.

34. Gilbertson, R., et al. "Effects of Acute Alcohol Consumption in Older and Younger Adults: Perceived Impairment versus Psychomotor Performance." *Journal of Studies on Alcohol and Drugs,* Vol. 70, No. 2, March 2009, pp. 242–252.

35. American Heart Association, www.amerianheart.org.

36. Heinen, M. M., et al. "Alcohol Consumption and Risk of Pancreatic Cancer in the Netherlands Cohort Study." *American Journal of Epidemiology,* March 24, 2009.

37. Allen, N. E., et al. "Moderate Alcohol Intake and Cancer Incidence in Women." *Journal of the National Cancer Institute,* Vol. 101, No. 5, March 4, 2009, pp. 296–305.

38. Newcomb, P. A., et al. "No Difference Between Red Wine or White Wine Consumption and Breast Cancer Risk." *Cancer Epidemiol, Biomarkers & Prevention,* Vol. 18, No. 3, March 2009, pp. 1007–1010.

39. Leaman, Martin, et al. "Substance Abuse Disorders." *The American Psychiatric Publishing Textbook of Clinical Psychiatry,* 5th ed. Washington, DC: American Psychiatric Press, 2008.

40. Sayal, K., et al. "Binge Pattern of Alcohol Consumption during Pregnancy and Childhood Mental Health Outcomes: Longitudinal Population-Based Study." *Pediatrics,* Vol. 123, No. 2, February 2009, pp. e289–296.

41. Kirkpatrick, Jean. Personal interview.

Chapter 13

1. Tobacco Atlas, www.tobaccoatlas.org.

2. Ibid.

3. National Center for Health Statistics. *Health, United States, 2008, with Chartbook.* Hyattsville, MD: 2009.

4. Leischow, Scott. "Setting the National Tobacco Control Agenda," *Journal of the American Medical Association,* Vol. 301, No. 10, March 11, 2009, pp. 1058–1060.

5. "State-Specific Prevalence and Trends in Adult Smoking." *Morbidity & Mortality Weekly Report,* Vol. 58, No. 9, March 13, 2009, pp. 221–226.

6. *Wasting the Best and the Brightest: Substance Abuse at America's Colleges and Universities.* New York: National Center on Addiction and Substance Abuse at Columbia University, March 15, 2007.

7. Ibid.

8. Ibid.

9. Kenny, Brent, and Charles Holahan. "Depressive Symptoms and Cigarette Smoking in a College Sample." *Journal of American College Health,* Vol. 56, No. 4, March/April 2008, pp. 409–413.

10. *Wasting the Best and the Brightest.*

11. Julian, Maite. "More Colleges Stamp Out Smoking." *USA Today,* October 13, 2008, online.

12. Song, A. V., et al. "Perceptions of Smoking-Related Risks and Benefits as Predictors of Adolescent Smoking Initiation." *American Journal of Public Health,* Vol. 99, No. 3, March 2009, pp. 487–492.

13. Tobacco Atlas.

14. Ibid.

15. *Wasting the Best and the Brightest.*

16. Tobacco Atlas.

17. Young, E., et al. "Age of Smoking Initiation and Risk of Breast Cancer in a Sample of Ontario Women." *Tobacco Induced Diseases,* Vol. 5, No. 1, February 17, 2009, p. 4.

18. Andersen, M. R., "Smoking Cessation Early in Pregnancy and Birth Weight, Length, Head Circumference, and Endothelial Nitric Oxide Synthase Activity in Umbilical and Chorionic Vessels: An Observational Study of Healthy Singleton Pregnancies." *Circulation,* Vol. 119, No., 6, February 17, 2009, pp. 857–864.

19. Knott, V., et al. "Nicotine and Attention: Event-Related Potential Investigations in Nonsmokers," *Clinical EEG Neuroscience,* Vol. 40, No. 1, January 2009, pp. 11-20.

20. Kenfield, S. A., et al. "Smoking and Smoking Cessation in Relation to Mortality in Women." *Journal of the American Medical Association,* Vol. 299, No. 17, May 7, 2008, pp. 2037–2047.

21. Heeringa, J., et al. "Cigarette Smoking and Risk of Atrial Fibrillation: the Rotterdam Study." *American Heart Journal,* Vol. 156, No. 6, December 2008, pp. 1163–1169.

22. *Wasting the Best and the Brightest.*

23. "Smokeless Tobacco." Smoking & Tobacco Use Fact Sheet, CDC, www.cdc.gov.

24. Dunham, Will. "Chewing Tobacco Use Surges among Boys." *HealthDay,* March 5, 2009. www.medlineplus.gov.

25. *Wasting the Best and the Brightest.*

26. *Clinical Practice Guideline: Treating Tobacco Use and Dependence, 2008 Update.* Washington, DC: U.S. Department of Health and Human Services Public Health Service, May 2008.

27. Ibid.

28. Kenfield et al., "Smoking and Smoking Cessation in Relation to Mortality in Women."

29. Prokhorov, A. V., et al. "'Look at Your Health: Outcomes Associated with a Computer-Assisted Smoking Cessation Counseling Intervention for Community College Students." *Addictive Behaviors,* Vol. 33, No. 6, June 2008, pp. 757–771.

30. Deruiter, W. K., et al. "Characteristics of Physically Active Smokers and Implications for Harm Reduction." *American Journal of Public Health,* Vol. 98, No. 5, May 2008, pp. 925–931.

31. Sussman, Steve, and Ping Sun. "Youth Tobacco Use Cessation: 2008 Update," *Tobacco Induced Diseases* 2009, 5:3doi:10.1186/1617-9625-5-3.

32. Kuehn, B. M. "Studies Linking Smoking-Cessation Drug with Suicide Risk Spark Concerns." *Journal of the American Medical Association,* Vol. 301, No. 10, March 11, 2009, pp. 1007–1008.

33. National Cancer Institute, US National Institutes of Health. NCI Fact Sheet. www.cancer.gov/cancertopics/factsheet.

34. Llewellyn, D. J., et al. "Exposure to Secondhand Smoke and Cognitive Impairment in Non-Smokers: National Cross Sectional Study with Cotinine Measurement." *British Medical Journal,* Vol. 338, February 12, 2009, p. b462.

35. Salvi, C. M., et al. "Environmental Tobacco Smoke (ETS) and Respiratory Health in Children." *Journal of Allergy and Clinical Immunology,* Vol. 123, No. 3, March 2009, pp. 575–578.

36. Pierce, J., and M. León. "Effectiveness of Smoke-Free Policies." *The Lancet Oncology,* Vol. 9, No. 7, pp. 614–615.

37. Kelly, B. C. "Smoke-Free Air Policy: Subcultural Shifts and Secondary Health Effects among Club-Going Young Adults." *Sociology of Health and Illness,* February 9, 2009.

Chapter 14

1. Paez, K. A., et al. "Rising Out-of-Pocket Spending for Chronic Conditions: A Ten-Year Trend." *Health Affairs* (Millwood), Vol. 28, No. 1, January–February 2009, pp. 15–25.

2. Ford, Earl, et al. "Explaining the Decrease in U.S. Deaths from Coronary Disease, 1980–2000" *New England Journal of Medicine,* Vol. 356, June 7, 2007, pp. 2388–2398.

3. Preidt, Robert. "Increased Heart Risk Seen for Retired NFL Players." HealthDay, National Library of Medicine, March 30, 2008.

4. Hendry, Joene. "'Bulking Up' May Raise Athletes' Heart Disease Risk." HealthDay, National Library of Medicine, May 26, 2008.

5. Gregg, E. W. "The Public Health Response to Diabetes." *Journal of the American Medical Association,* Vol. 301, No. 15, April 15, 2009, pp. 1596–1598.

6. Yaffe, K. et al. "The Metabolic Syndrome and Development of Cognitive Impairment among Older Women." *Archives of Neurology,* Vol. 66, No. 3, March 2009, pp. 324–328.

7. Torpy, J. M. "Diabetes." *Journal of the American Medical Association,* Vol. 301, No. 15, April 15, 2009, p. 1620.

8. Ibid.

9. Kahn, S. E. "Glucose Control in Type 2 Diabetes." *Journal of the American Medical Association,* Vol. 301, No. 15, April 15, 2009, pp. 1590–1592.

10. Saudek, C. D. "Can Diabetes Be Cured?" *Journal of the American Medical Association,* Vol. 301, No. 15, April 15, 2009, pp. 1588–1590.

11. Purnell, J. Q., and D. R. Flum, "Bariatric Surgery and Diabetes: Who Should Be Offered the Option of Remission?" *Journal of the American Medical Association*, Vol. 301, No. 15, April 15, 2009, pp. 1593–1595.

12. Nathan, D. N. "Progress in Diabetes Research—What's Next?" *Journal of the American Medical Association*, Vol. 301, No. 15, April 15, 2009, pp. 1599–1601.

13. Robertson, Rose Marie. Personal interview.

14. "Top 10 Things to Know about Resistant Hypertension." American Heart Association, http://hyper.ahajournals.org/cgi/reprint/HYPERTENSIONAHA.108.189141.

15. Michos, E. D., and R. S. Blumenthal. "Prevalence of Low Low-Density Lipoprotein Cholesterol with Elevated High Sensitivity C-Reactive Protein in the U.S.: Implications of the JUPITER (Justification for the Use of Statins in Primary Prevention: An Intervention Trial Evaluating Rosuvastatin) Study." *Journal of the American College of Cardiology*, Vol. 53, No. 11, March 17, 2009, pp. 931–935.

16. Allin, K. H., et al. "Baseline C-Reactive Protein Is Associated with Incident Cancer and Survival in Patients with Cancer." *Journal of Clinical Oncology*, Vol. 27, No. 13, May 1, 2009, pp. 2217–2224.

17. Wolff, T., et al. "Aspirin for the Primary Prevention of Cardiovascular Events: An Update of the Evidence for the U.S. Preventive Services Task Force." *Annals of Internal Medicine*, Vol. 150, No. 6, March 17, 2009, pp. 405–410.

18. "One Pill Might Prevent Heart Disease." *HealthDay*, March 30, 2009. www.medlineplus.gov.

19. "Coffee or Tea Consumption May Lower Stroke Risk.*" HealthDay*, February20, 2009. www.medlineplus.gov.

20. Lisabeth, L. D., et al. "Age at Natural Menopause and Risk of Ischemic Stroke: The Framingham Heart Study." *Stroke*, Vol. 40, No. 4, April 2009, pp. 1044–1049.

21. Lisabeth, L. D. "Acute Stroke Symptoms: Comparing Women and Men." *Stroke*, February 19, 2009.

22. Romero, J. R., et al. "Carotid Artery Atherosclerosis, MRI Indices of Brain Ischemia, Aging, and Cognitive Impairment: The Framingham Study." *Stroke*, Vol. 40, No. 5, May 2009, pp. 1590–1596.

23. "Even Mild Strokes Can Do Harm." *HealthDay*, February 27, 2009. www.medlineplus.gov.

24. "Fast Arrival at Hospital After Stroke Pays Off." *HealthDay*, February 19, 2009. www.medlineplus.gov.

25. Reeves, M., et al. "Sex Differences in the Use of Intravenous rt-PA Thrombolysis Treatment for Acute Ischemic Stroke: A Meta-Analysis." *Stroke*, Vol. 40, No. 5, May 2009, pp. 1743–1749.

26. Stephenson, Joan. "Cancer No. 1 Killer by 2010." *Journal of the American Medical Association*, Vol. 301, No. 3, January 21, 2009, p. 263.

27. Frank, R. C. *Fighting Cancer with Knowledge and Hope.* New Haven, CT: Yale University Press, 2009.

28. American Cancer Society. *Cancer Facts & Figures 2008.* Atlanta: American Cancer Society, 2008.

29. Blanchard, C. M., et al. "Cancer Survivors' Adherence to Lifestyle Behavior Recommendations and Associations with Health-Related Quality of Life: Results from the American Cancer Society's SCS-II." *Journal of Clinical Oncology*, Vol. 26, No. 13, May 1, 2009, pp. 2198–2204.

30. American Cancer Society. *Cancer Facts & Figures 2008.* Atlanta: American Cancer Society, 2008.

31. Robinson, June, et al. "Indoor Tanning Knowledge, Attitudes, and Behavior among Young Adults from 1988–2007." *Archives of Dermatology*, Vol. 144, No. 4, April 2008, pp. 484–488.

32. Lachiewicz, Anne, et al. "Survival Differences between Patients with Scalp or Neck Melanoma and Those with Melanoma of Other sites in the Surveillance, Epidemiology, and End Results (SEER) Program." *Archives of Dermatology*, Vol. 144, No. 4, April 2008, pp. 515–521.

33. Voelker, R. "Breast Cancer Probed in Hispanic Women." *Journal of the American Medical Association*, Vol. 301, No. 13, April 1, 2009, p. 1325.

34. Voelker, R. "Promising Test Flags BRCA Mutations in Populations of Hispanic Women." *Journal of the American Medical Association*, Vol. 301, No. 13, April 1, 2009, p. 1326.

35. Wu, A. H., et al. "Dietary Patterns and Breast Cancer Risk in Asian American Women." *American Journal of Clinical Nutrition*, Vol. 89, No. 4, April 2009, p. 1145–1154.

36. Heiss, Gerardo, et al. "Health Risks and Benefits 3 Years after Stopping Randomized Treatment with Estrogen and Progestin." *Journal of the American Medical Association*, Vol. 299, No. 9, March 5, 2008, pp. 1036–1045.

37. Smith, P. D., et al. "American College Health Association Annual Pap Test and Sexually Transmitted Infection Survey: 2006." *Journal of American College Health*, Vol. 57, No. 4, January–February 2009, pp. 389–394.

38. Datta, S. D., et al. "Human Papillomavirus Infection and Cervical Cytology in Women Screened for Cervical Cancer in the United States, 2003–2005." *Annals of Internal Medicine*, Vol. 148, April 1, 2008, pp. 493–500.

39. Naucler, P., et al. "Efficacy of HPV DNA Testing with Cytology Triage and/or Repeat HPV DNA Testing in Primary Cervical Cancer Screening." *Journal of the National Cancer Institute Advance Access*, Vol. 101, January 13, 2009, pp. 88–99.

40. Frincu-Mallos, C. "Combined Colposcopy, HPV Testing, Cytology Improves Management of Women with Dysplasia." *Medscape Medical News*, October 21, 2008, online.

41. Daling, J. R., et al. "Association of Marijuana Use and the Incidence of Testicular Germ Cell Tumors." *Cancer*, Vol. 115, March 15, 2009, pp. 1215–1223.

42. Cole, B. F., et al. "Aspirin for the Chemoprevention of Colorectal Adenomas: Meta-Analysis of the Randomized Trials." *Journal of the National Cancer Institute*, Vol. 101, No. 4, February 18, 2009, pp. 256–266.

43. Andriole, G. L., et al. "Mortality Results from a Randomized Prostate-Cancer Screening Trial." *New England Journal of Medicine*, Vol. 360, No. 13, March 26, 2009, pp. 1310–1319.

44. Macsali, F., et al. "Oral Contraception, Body Mass Index, and Asthma: A Cross-Sectional Nordic-Baltic Population Survey." *The Journal of Allergy and Clinical Immunology*, Vol. 123, No. 2, February 2009, pp. 391–397.

45. "New Treatments Improve Control for Severe Asthma." *HealthDay*, March 16, 2009. www.medlineplus.gov.

Chapter 15

1. Dinan, T. G. "Inflammatory Markers in Depression." *Current Opinion in Psychiatry*, Vol. 22, No. 1, 2009, pp. 32–36.

2. Shirtcliff E. A., et al. "Early Childhood Stress Is Associated with Elevated Antibody Levels to Herpes Simplex Virus Type 1." *Proceedings of the National Academy of Science*, Vol. 106, No. 8, February 24, 2009, pp. 2963–2967.

3. Adams, Troy, et al. "The Association between Mental Health and Acute Infectious Illness among a National Sample of 18- to 24-Year-Old College Students." *Journal of American College Health*, Vol. 56, No. 6, pp. 657–663.

4. Hampton, Tracy. "Research Reveals Low Immunization Rates and Vaccination Awareness among Adults." *Journal of the American Medical Association*, Vol. 299, No. 9, March 3, 2008, p. 1007.

5. Cohen, S., et al. "Sleep Habits and Susceptibility to the Common Cold." *Archives of Internal Medicine*, Vol. 169, No. 1, January 12, 2009, pp. 62–67.

6. Nichol, K. L., et al. "Burden of Influenza-like Illness and Effectiveness of Influenza Vaccination among Working Adults Aged 50–64 Years." *Clinical Infectious Diseases: An Official Publication of the Infectious Diseases Society of America*, Vol. 48, No. 3, February 1, 2009, pp. 292–298.

7. "Inactivated Flu Vaccine Linked to Fewer Medical Visits Than Intranasal Vaccine." Medindia.net, March 4, 2009.

8. Bennett, N., et al. "Meningitis Vaccine Seems to Work Like a Charm." *HealthDay*, January 14, 2009. www.medlineplus.gov.

9. "Miningococcal Vaccines: What You Need to Know." www.cdc.gov.

10. Wu, H. M., et al. "Emergence of Ciprofloxacin-Resistant Neisseria Meningitidis in North America." *New England Journal of Medicine*, Vol. 360, No. 9, February 26, 2009, pp. 886–892.

11. El-Serag, H. B., et al. "Risk of Hepatobiliary and Pancreatic Cancers after Hepatitis C Virus Infection: A Population-based Study of U.S. Veterans." *Hepatology*, Vol. 49, No. 1, January 2009, pp. 116–123.

12. "Epstein-Barr Virus and Infectious Mononucleosis." National Center for Infectious Diseases, http://www.cdc.gov/ncidod/diseases/ebv/htm.

13. http://www.health.state.pa.us/sportshealth.

14. Hugonnet, J. E., et al. "Meropenem-Clavulanate Is Effective Against Extensively Drug-Resistant Mycobacterium Tuberculosis." *Science*, Vol. 323, No. 5918, February 27, 2009, pp. 1215–1218.

15. Gerber, M. A., et al. "Prevention of Rheumatic Fever and Diagnosis and Treatment of Acute Streptococcal Pharyngitis." *Circulation*, Vol. 119, No. 11, March 24, 2009, pp. 1541–1551.

16. Harbarth, S., et al. "Universal screening for Methicillin-Resistant *Staphylococcus aureus* at Hospital Admission and Nosocomial Infection in Surgical Patients." *Journal of the American Medical Association*, Vol. 299, No. 12, March 3, 2008, pp. 1149–1157.

17. Weiner, H. Richard. "Methicillin-Resistant *Staphylococcus aureus* on Campus: A New Challenge to College Health." *Journal of American College Health*, Vol. 56, No. 4, January/February 2008, pp. 347–350.

18. Fox, Maggie. "Simple Techniques Slash Hospital Infections." *Healthday*, March 21, 2009. www.medlineplus.gov.

19. Burton, D. C., et al. "Methicillin-Resistant Staphylococcus aureus Central Line-Associated Bloodstream Infections in U.S. Intensive Care Units, 1997–2007." *Journal of the American Medical Association*, Vol. 301, No. 7, February 18, 2009, pp. 727–736.

20. "3 Steps Might Help Stop MRSA's Spread." *Healthday*, March 20, 2009. www.medlineplus.gov.

21. "H1N1 Flu (Swine Flu) and You." www.cdc.gov.

22. "Advice on the Use of Masks in the Community Setting in Influenza A (H1Na) Outbreaks." World Health Organization, http://www.who.int/en/.

23. www.pandemicflu.gov.

Chapter 16

1. Genuis, Stephen. "Are Condoms the Answer to Rising Rates of Non-HIV Sexually Transmitted Infection? No." *British Medical Journal*, Vol. 336, January 26, 2008, p. 185, doi:10.1136/bmj.39402.527766.AD.

2. *Sexually Transmitted Disease Surveillance 2007 Supplement.* Atlanta, GA: CDC Division of STD Prevention, March 2009.

3. Ibid.

4. Frohan, S. E., et al. "Prevalence of Sexually Transmitted Infections and Bacterial Vaginosis among Female Adolescents in the United States." March 13, 2008, http://cdc.confex.com/cdc/std2008/techprogram/P14888.htm.

5. Crosby, Richard, et al. "Adolescents' Sexually Transmitted Disease Protective Attitudes Predict Sexually Transmitted Disease Acquisition in Early Adulthood." *Journal of School Health*, Vol. 78, No. 6, 2008, pp. 310–313, doi:10.1111/j.1746-1561.2008.00307.x.

6. U.S. Department of Health and Human Services, 2008 National STD Prevention Conference, Chicago, March 10–13, 2008, http://www.cdc.gov/stdconference/.

7. Hampton, Tracy. "Researchers Seek Ways to Stem STDs." *Journal of the American Medical Association*, Vol. 299, No. 16, April 23–30, 2008, pp. 1888–1889.

8. American College Health Association. *American College Health Association-National College Health Assessment II: Reference Group Executive Summary Fall 2008.* Baltimore: American College Health Association, 2009.

9. James. A. B., et al. "Chlamydia Prevalence among College Students: Reproductive and Public Health Implications." *Sexually Transmitted Diseases*, Vol. 35, No. 6, June 2008, pp. 529–532.

10. Crosby, R., et al. "Two Heads Are Better than One: The Association between Condom Decision-Making and Condom Use Errors and Problems." *Sexually Transmitted Infections*, Vol. 84, No. 3, June 2008, pp. 198–201.

11. Lu, B., et al. "Factors Associated with Acquisition and Clearance of Human Papillomavirus Infection in a Cohort of U.S. Men: A Prospective Study. *Journal of Infectious Disease*, Vol. 199, No. 3, February 1, 2009, pp. 362–371.

12. Huang, C. M., et al, "Human Papillomavirus and Vaccination." *Mayo Clinic Proceedings*, Vol. 83, No. 6, June 2008, pp. 701–707.

13. Datta, S. D., et al. "Human Papillomavirus Infection and Cervical Cytology in Women Screened for Cervical Cancer in the United States, 2003–2005." *Annals of Internal Medicine*, Vol. 148, No. 7, April 2008, pp. 493–500.

14. Winer, P. L., et al. "Risk of Female Human Papillomavirus Acquisition Associated with First Male Sex Partner." *Journal of Infectious Diseases*, Vol. 197, 2008, pp. 279–282.

15. Huang, et al., "Human Papillomavirus and Vaccination."

16. Gerend, M. A., and J. Barley. "HPV Vaccine Acceptability among Young Adult Males." *Sexually Transmitted Diseases*, Vol. 36, 2009, pp. 58–62.

17. "Genital Herpes." CDC Fact Sheet, www.cdc.gov.

18. Ibid.

19. *Sexually Transmitted Disease Surveillance 2007 Supplement: Chlamydia Prevalence Monitoring Project.* Atlanta, GA: CDC Division of STD Prevention, January 2009.

20. James, et al. "Chlamydia Prevalence among College Students."

21. *Sexually Transmitted Disease Surveillance 2007 Supplement: Chlamydia Prevalence Monitoring Project.*

22. Ibid.

23. James, et al. "Chlamydia Prevalence Among College Students."

24. "PID (Pelvic Inflammatory Disease)." CDC Fact Sheet, www.cdc.gov.

25. *Sexually Transmitted Disease Surveillance 2007 Supplement: Gonococcal Isolate Surveillance Project.* Atlanta, GA: CDC Division of STD Prevention, March 2009.

26. *Sexually Transmitted Disease Surveillance 2007 Supplement: Syphilis Surveillance Report.* Atlanta, GA: CDC Division of STD Prevention, March 2009.

27. http://www.cdc.gov/std/trichomonas/default.htm.

28. Holtgrave, D. R., et al. "Updated Annual HIV Transmission Rates in the United States." *Journal of Acquired Immune Deficiency Syndrome*, January 7, 2009.

29. Tanne, J. H. "HIV Prevalence in U.S. Capital Is at Epidemic Level." *British Medical Journal*, Vol. 338, March 23, 2009, p. b1205.

30. Lesserman, J. "Role of Depression, Stress, and Trauma in HIV Disease Progression." *Psychosomatic Medicine*, Vol. 70, No. 5, June 2008, pp. 539–545.

31. "The HIV/AIDS Epidemic in the United States." *HIV/AIDS Policy Fact Sheet*, Kaiser Family Foundation, February 2009. www.kff.org.

32. Kitahata, M. M., et al. "Effect of Early versus Deferred Antiretroviral Therapy for HIV on Survival." *New England Journal of Medicine*, Vol. 360, No. 18, April 30, 2009, pp. 1815–1826.

Chapter 17

1. Berenson, R. A., and C. A. Cassel. "Consumer-Driven Health Care May Not Be What Patients Need—Caveat Emptor." *Journal of the American Medical Association*, Vol. 301, No. 3, January 21, 2009, pp. 321–323.

2. "20 Tips to Help Prevent Medical Errors." Agency for Healthcare Research and Quality, www.ahrq.gov.

3. "Questions Are the Answer." Agency for Healthcare Research and Quality, http://www.ahra.gov/quetionsaretheanswer/.

4. American Society of Plastic Surgeons, www.plastic-surgery.org.

5. Barnes, P. M., et al. "Complementary and Alternative Medicine Use Among Adults and Children: United States, 2007," *National Health Statistics Reports (NHSR)*, No. 12, 2009, pp. 1–23.

6. Tilburt, J. C., et al. "Alternative Medicine Research in Clinical Practice: A U.S. National Survey." *Archives of Internal Medicine*, Vol. 169, No. 7, 2009, pp. 670–677.

7. Caspi, O., et al. "Informed Consent in Complementary and Alternative Medicine," *Evidence-Based Complementary and Alternative Medicine*, April 17, 2009.

8. "Hypnosis Helps Reduce Hot Flashes in breast Cancer Survivors." *Harvard Women's Health Watch*, Vol. 16, No. 6, 2009, p. 3.

9. Barnes, et al. "Complementary and Alternative Medicine Use Among Adults and Children."

10. Ibid.

11. Ibid.

12. Lorenc, A., et al. "How Parents Choose to Use CAM: A Systematic Review of Theoretical Models." *BMC Complementary and Alternative Medicine*, Vol. 9, No. 1, April 22, 2009, p. 9.

13. Barnes, P. M. "Complementary and Alternative Medicine Use Among Adults and Children."

14. Gaul, C., and R. Eismann. "Use of Complementary and Alternative Medicine in Patients Suffering from Primary Headache Disorders." *Cephalalgia*, April 2, 2009.

15. "Acupuncture: From Ancient Practice to Modern Science." *NIH MedlinePlus Magazine*, Winter 2009. http://www.nlm.nih.gov/medlineplus/magazine/.

16. "Hypnosis Helps Reduce Hot Flashes in Breast Cancer Survivors."

17. Mitka, Mike. "Growth in Health Care Spending Slows but Still Outpaces Rate of Inflation." *Journal of the American Medical Association*, Vol. 301, No. 8, February 25, 2009, pp. 815–816.

Chapter 18

1. National Center for Health Statistics, www.cdc.gov/nchs.

2. Ripley, Amanda. *The Unthinkable: Who Survives When Disaster Strikes—and Why*, New York: Crown, 2008.

3. Hyer, A. A., et al. "World Report on Child Injury Prevention." *The Lancet*, Vol. 373, No. 9658, January 10, 2009–January 16, 2009, pp. 102–103.

4. National Highway Traffic Safety Administration, www.nhtsa.dot.gov.

5. www.nhtsa.dot.gov.

6. Tator, Charles. "Recognition and Management of Spinal Cord Injuries in Sports and Recreation." *Physical Medicine Rehabilitation Clinics of North America*, Vol. 20, No. 1, February 2009, pp. 69–76.

7. Nerenberg, Arnold. Personal interview.

8. www.nhtsa.dot.gov.

9. Charlton, S. G., et al. "Driving While Conversing: Cell Phones That Distract and Passengers Who React." *Accident Analysis & Prevention*, Vol. 41, No. 1, January 2009, pp. 160–173.

10. Loeb, P. D., and W. A. Clarke. "The Cell Phone Effect on Pedestrian Fatalities." *Transportation Research Part E: Logistics and Transportation Review*, Vol. 45, No. 1, January 2009, pp. 284–290.

11. Lu, B. C., et al. "Helmets for Preventing Injury in Motorcycle Riders." *Cochrane Reviews*, www.cochrane.org/review/en/ab004333.html.

12. Rivera, F. P. "The Global Problem of Injuries to Children and Adolescents." *Pediatrics*, Vol. 123, No. 1, January 2009, pp. 168–169.

13. Schwebel, David, et al. "Physical Environment of the Home and Adolescent Injury Risk." *International Emergency Nursing*, Vol. 17, No. 1, January 2009, pp. 47–51.

14. Franklin, C. A., and T. W. Franklin. "Predicting Fear of Crime: Considering Differences Across Gender." *Feminist Criminology*, Vol. 4, No. 1, pp. 83–106.

15. Prothrow-Stith, Deborah. "Keynote Address: Making Campuses Safer Communities for Students." *Journal of American College Health*, Vol. 55, No. 5, March/April 2007, pp. 261–266.

16. "School Associated Violent Deaths." Centers for Disease Control and Prevention, www.cdc.gov/ncipc/sch-shooting-htm.

17. Carr, Joetta, et al. "Campus Violence White Paper." *Journal of American College Health*, Vol. 55, No. 5, March/April 2007, pp. 304–319.

18. Ibid.

19. Ibid.

20. Reed, Elizabeth, et al. "The Relation Between Interpersonal Violence and Substance Use Among a Sample of University Students: Examination of the Role of Victim and Perpetrator Substance." *Addictive Behaviors*, Vol. 34, No. 3, March 2009, pp. 316–318.

21. Thompson, Marie, et al. "Reasons for Not Reporting Victimizations to the Police: Do They Vary for Physical and Sexual Incidents?" *Journal of American College Health*, Vol. 55, No. 5, March/April 2007, pp. 277–282.

22. Boba, Rachel, and David Lilley. "Violence Against Women Act (VAWA) Funding a Nationwide Assessment of Effects on Rape and Assault." *Violence Against Women*, Vol. 15, No. 2, February 1, 2009, pp. 168–185.

23. Potter, S. J,. et al. "Empowering Bystanders to Prevent Campus Violence Against Women: A Preliminary Evaluation of a Poster Campaign." *Violence Against Women*, Vol. 15, No. 1, 2009, pp. 106–121.

24. McMahon, P. P., et al. "Sexual Violence on the College Campus: A Template for Compliance with Federal Policy." *Journal of American College Health*, Vol. 57, No. 3, November–December 2008, pp. 361–366.

25. Langford, Linda. "Preventing Violence and Promoting Safety in Higher Education Settings: Overview of a Comprehensive Approach." U.S. Department of Education's Higher Education Center for Alcohol and Other Drug Abuse and Violence Prevention, http://www.edc.org/hec/pubs/violence.pdf.

26. Carr, et al. "Campus Violence White Paper."

27. Rutherford, I. G., and S. A. DeVaney. "The Effect of Campus Shootings on the Quality of Graduate Students' College Experiences." *Consumer Interests Annual*, Vol. 54, 2008.

28. Carr, et al. "Campus Violence White Paper."

29. Buhl, E. R., et al. "Stalking Victimization Among College Women and Subsequent Help-Seeking

Behaviors." *Journal of American College Health*, Vol. 57, No 4, January–February 2009, pp. 419–426.

30. Chan, K. I., et al. "Prevalence of Dating Partner Violence and Suicidal Ideation Among Male and Female University Students Worldwide." *Journal of Midwifery & Women's Health*, Vol. 53, No. 6, 2008, pp. 529–537.

31. Wolitzky-Taylor, K. B., et al. "Prevalence and Correlates of Dating Violence in a National Sample of Adolescents." *Journal of the American Academy of Child and Adolescent Psychiatry*, Vol. 47, No. 7, July 2008, p. 755–762.

32. Woo, Samantha C. "Patterns of Relationships and Dating Violence Among African-American and Latino Adolescents." Presentation, American Public Health Association meeting, San Diego, October 2008.

33. Kimble, Matthew, et al. "Risk of Unwanted Sex for College Women: Evidence for a Red Zone." *Journal of American College Health*, Vol. 57, No. 3, November–December 2008, pp. 331–337.

34. Littleton, H. and C. E. Henderson, "If She Is Not a Victim, Does That Mean She Was Not Traumatized? Evaluation of Predictors of PTSD Symptomatology Among College Rape Victims." *Violence Against Women*, Vol. 15, No. 2, 2009, pp. 148–167.

35. Crawford, Emily, et al. "Drug-Facilitated Sexual Assault: College Women's Risk Perception and Behavioral Choices." *Journal of American College Health*, Vol. 57, No. 3, November–December 2008, pp. 261–272.

Chapter 19

1. Belli, Britti. "Cleaner, Greener U." *E. The Environmental Magazine*, Vol. 19, No. 2, March/April 2008, pp. 26–36.

2. Prüss-Ustün, A., et al. "The Impact of the Environment on Health by Country: A Meta-synthesis." *Environmental Health*, Vol. 7, February 25, 2008, p. 7.

3. Pope, C. A., et al. "Fine-Particulate Air Pollution and Life Expectancy in the United States." *New England Journal of Medicine*, Vol. 360, No. 4, January 22, 2009, pp. 376–386.

4. Musil, Robert. *Hope for a Heated Planet: How Americans Are Fighting Global Warming and Building a Better Future.* Rutgers, NJ: Rutgers University Press, 2009.

5. American Association for the Advancement of Science, www.aaas.org/climate.

6. Musil, *Hope for a Heated Planet.*

7. Fenger, Jes. "Air Pollution in the Last 50 Years—From Local to Global." *Atmospheric Environment*, Vol. 43, January 2009, pp. 13–22.

8. Greer, A., et al. "Climate Change and Infectious Diseases in North America: The Road Ahead." *Canadian Medical Association Journal*, Vol. 178, No. 6, March 11, 2008, pp. 715–722.

9. Piro, F. N., et al. "A Comparison of Self-Reported Air Pollution Problems and GIS-Modeled Levels of Air Pollution in People with and without Chronic Diseases." *Environmental Health*, Vol. 7, No. 1, February 28, 2008, p. 9.

10. Halonen, Jaana. "Particulate Air Pollution and Acute Cardiorespiratory Hospital Admissions and Mortality Among the Elderly." *Epidemiology*, Vol. 20, No. 1, 2009, pp. 143–153.

11. Piro, "A Comparison of Self-Reported Air Pollution Problems and GIS-Modeled Levels of Air Pollution in People with and without Chronic Diseases."

12. Pope, "Fine-Particulate Air Pollution and Life Expectancy in the United States."

13. Napier, G. L., and C. M. Kodner. "Health Risks and Benefits of Bottled Water." *Primary Care*, Vol. 35, No. 4, December 2008, pp. 789–802.

14. Ibid.

15. Ibid.

16. Ibid.

17. Krachler, Michael, and William Shotyk. "Trace and Ultratrace Metals in Bottled Waters: Survey of Sources Worldwide and Comparison with Refillable Metal Bottles." *Science of the Total Environment*, Vol. 407, No. 3, January 15, 2009, pp. 1089–1096.

18. Environmental Protection Agency, http://www.epa.gov/iaq/pubs/insidest.html.

19. "Environmental Cancer Risks." *Cancer Facts & Figures 2008.* American Cancer Society 2008.

20. Djeridane, Y., et al. "Influence of Electromagnetic Fields Emitted by GSM-900 Cellular Telephones on the Circadian Patterns of Gonadal, Adrenal and Pituitary Hormones in Men." *Radiation Research*, Vol. 169, No. 3, March 2008, pp. 337–343.

21. Loeb, P. D., and W. A. Clarke. "The Cell Phone Effect on Pedestrian Fatalities." *Transportation Research Part E: Logistics and Transportation Review*, Vol. 45, No. 1, January 2009, pp. 284–290.

22. Shah, Samit, et al. "Hear Today, Gone Tomorrow: An Assessment of Portable Entertainment Player Use and Hearing Acuity in a Community Sample." *Journal of the American Board of Family Medicine*, Vol. 22, No. 1, 2009, pp. 17–23.

23. Vogel, I., et al. "MP3 Players and Hearing Loss: Adolescents' Perceptions of Loud Music and Hearing Conservation." *Journal of Pediatrics*, Vol. 152. No. 3, March 2008, pp. 400–404.

Chapter 20

1. Federal Interagency Forum on Aging-Related Statistics. *Older Americans 2008: Key Indicators of Well-Being.* Washington, DC:P U.S. Government Printing Office, March 2008.

2. Ibid.

3. Ibid.

4. Ibid.

5. Guralnik, Jack. "Successful Aging: Is It in Our Future?" *Archives of Internal Medicine*, Vol. 168, No. 2, January 28, 2008, pp. 131–132.

6. Yates, Laurel, et al. "Exceptional Longevity in Men." *Archives of Internal Medicine*, Vol. 168, No. 3, February 11, 2008, pp. 284–290.

7. Terry, Dellara, et al. "Disentangling the Roles of Disability and Morbidity in Survival to Exceptional Old Age." *Archives of Internal Medicine*, Vol. 168, No. 3, February 11, 2008, pp. 277–283.

8. "Activity Benefits the Aging Mind and Body." *Mayo Clinic Health Letter*, online edition, February 2009.

9. Martin, C. K., et al. "Exercise Dose and Quality of Life: A Randomized Controlled Trial." *Archives of Internal Medicine*, Vol. 169, No. 3, February 9, 2009, pp. 269–271.

10. Brown, A. D., et al. "Effects of Cardiorespiratory Fitness and Cerebral Blood Flow on Cognitive Outcomes in Older Women," *Neurobiology of Aging*, January 2009.

11. Davidson, L. E., et al. "Effects of Exercise Modality on Insulin Resistance and Functional Limitation in Older Adults: A Randomized Controlled Trial." *Archives of Internal Medicine*, Vol. 169, No. 2, 2009, pp. 122–131.

12. Hughes, S. L., et al. "Best-Practice Physical Activity Programs for Older Adults: Findings from the National Impact Study," *American Journal of Public Health*, Vol. 99, No. 2, 2009, pp. 362–368.

13. Schonfeld, Amy. "More Data Show Positive Effects of Aspirin on Brain Matter." *Clinical Psychiatry News*, Vol. 35, No. 3, March 2007, p. 21.

14. Kang, Jae Hee, et al. "Low Dose Aspirin and Cognitive Function in the Women's Health Study Cognitive Cohort." *British Medical Journal*, April 27, 2007, ONLINE First, doi: 10.1136/bmj.39166.597836.BE.

15. ADAPT Research Group. "Naproxen and Celebcoxib Do Not Prevent AD in Early Results from a Randomized Controlled Trial." *Neurology*, April 2007.

16. Dodge, H. H., et al. "A Randomized Placebo-Controlled Trial of Ginkgo Biloba for the Prevention of Cognitive Decline." *Neurology*, February 27, 2008.

17. Plassman, B. L., et al. "Prevalence of Cognitive Impairment without Dementia in the United States." *Annals of Internal Medicine*, Vol. 148, No. 6, March 18, 2008, pp. 50–58.

18. Wilson, R. S., et al. "Educational Attainment and Cognitive Decline in Old Age." *Neurology*, Vol. 72, No. 5, 2009, pp. 460–465.

19. Geda, Yonas, et al. "Can Exercising Your Brain Prevent Memory Loss?" Presentation, American Academy of Neurology, April 2009.

20. Sherman, Sherry. Personal interview.

21. Speller, Marsha. Personal interview.

22. Pinkerton, JoAnn. Personal interview.

23. Nelson, Deborah, et al. "Effect of Physical Activity on Menopausal Symptoms among Urban Women." *Medicine & Science in Sports & Exercise*, Vol. 40, No. 1, January 2008, pp. 1–53.

24. Prentice, R. L., et al. "Estrogen Plus Progestin Therapy and Breast Cancer in Recently Postmenopausal Women." *Journal of Epidemiology*, March 27, 2008.

25. Lowe, Gordon. "Hormone Therapy and Risk of Myocardial Infarction." *Women's Health*, Vol. 5, No. 1, January 2009, pp. 29–31.

26. Lyytinen, Heli, et al. "Breast Cancer Risk in Postmenopausal Women Using Estradiol-Progestogen Therapy." *Obstetrics & Gynecology*, Vol. 113, No. 1, January 2009, pp. 65–73.

27. Holmberg, Lars, et al. "Increased Risk of Recurrence After Hormone Replacement Therapy in Breast Cancer Survivors." *Journal of the National Cancer Institute*, Vol. 100, April 2, 2008, pp. 475–482, doi:20.1093/jnci/djn115.

28. Gooren, L. "Advances in Testosterone Replacement Therapy." *Advances in the Management of Testosterone Deficiency*, T. H. Jones (ed.), Front Horm Res. Basel, Karger, Vol. 37, 2009, pp. 32–51.

29. Beecham, G. W., et al. "Genome-wide Association Study Implicates a Chromosome 12 Risk Locus for Late-Onset Alzheimer Disease." *American Journal of Human Genetics*, Vol. 84, No. 1, January 2009, pp. 35–43.

30. "Drinking, Smoking Up Early Alzheimer's." News Release, American Academy of Neurology 60th Anniversary Annual Conference, *Chicago*, April 12–19, 2008.

31. Whitmer, R. A., et al. "Central Obesity and Increased Risk of Dementia More Than Three Decades Later." *Neurology*, April 2009, doi:10.1212/01. wnl.0000306313.89165.ef.

32. Wang, H. X., et al. "Personality and Lifestyle in Relation to Dementia Incidence." *Neurology*, Vol. 72, No. 3, January 2009, pp. 253–259.

33. Eskelinen, M. H., et al. "Midlife Coffee and Tea Drinking and the Risk of Late-Life Dementia: A Population-Based CAIDE Study." *Journal of Alzheimer's Disease*, Vol. 16, No. 1, January 2009, pp. 85–91.

34. Huss, A., et al. "Residence Near Power Lines and Mortality from Neurodegenerative Diseases: Longitudinal Study of the Swiss Population." *American Journal of Epidemiology*, Vol. 169, No. 2, January 2009, pp. 167–175.

35. Haag, M. D. M., et al. "Statins Are Associated with a Reduced Risk of Alzheimer Disease Regardless of Lipophilicity: The Rotterdam Study." *Journal of Neurosurgical Psychiatry*, Vol. 80, 2009, pp. 13–17.

36. Gray, Shelly, et al. "Antioxidant Vitamin Supplement Use and Risk of Dementia or Alzheimer's Disease in Older Adults." *Journal of the American Geriatrics Society*, Vol. 56, No. 2, February 2008, pp. 291–295.

37. Qassem, Amir, et al. "Current Pharmacologic Treatment of Dementia: A Clinical Practice Guideline from the American College of Physicians and the American Academy of Family Physicians." *Annals of Internal Medicine,* Vol. 148, No. 5, March 4, 2008, pp. 370–378.

38. Bliuc, D., et al. "Mortality Risk Associated with Low-Trauma Osteoporotic Fracture and Subsequent Fracture in Men and Women." *Journal of the American Medical Association,* Vol. 301, No. 5, February 4, 2009, pp. 513–521.

39. Kaldjian, L. C., et al. "Goals of Care Toward the End of Life: A Structured Literature Review." *American Journal of Hospice and Palliative Medicine*®, Vol. 25, No. 6, 2009, pp. 501–511.

40. Kübler-Ross, Elisabeth. *Death: The Final Stage of Growth.* Englewood Cliffs, NJ: Prentice-Hall, 1975.

41. Renz, Monica, et al. "When the Tumor Is Not the Target: Between Utter Despair and Essential Hope," *Journal of Clinical Oncology,* Vol. 27, No. 1, January 1, 2009, pp. 146–149.

42. Smith, A. K., et al. "Racial and Ethnic Differences in End-of-Life Care in Fee-for-Service Medicare Beneficiaries with Advanced Cancer." *Journal of the American Geriatrics Society,* Vol. 57, No. 1, pp. 153–158.

INDEX

Oral health, 548–50. See also Dental health
Oral sex, 283–84, 520, 538
Organ donation, 638
Organic foods, 197
Organophosphates, 613
Orgasm, 284–86, 288–89
Orlistat, 218, 223
Ornish, Dean, 50, 461–62
Ornish diet, 216, 461–62
Ortho Evra patch, 314–16
Osteoporosis
    and alcohol use, 398
    and calcium, 178, 185, 635
    defined, 129
    exercise for prevention of, 129–30, 630
    risk factors, 634–35
    screening, 551
    and smoking, 418
OTC (over-the-counter) drugs, 59–60, 218, 348–49, 350
Outcomes, 553–54
Outercourse, 282, 301
Outpatient treatment, 403–4
Outpatient treatment centers, 564–65
Ova (ovum), 266, 267, 298
Ovarian cancer, 469, 476
Ovaries, 264, 266, 298
Over-the-counter (OTC) drugs, 59–60, 218, 348–49, 350
Overeaters Anonymous (OA), 225
Overeating, 215–16, 225
Overload principle, 132
Overloading, 140
Overtraining, 159
Overuse injuries, 159
Overweight. See Obesity/overweight
Ovo-lacto-vegetarians, 192
Ovulation, 266, 298
OxyContin, 352
Oxytocin, 246
Ozone, 603–4

P
Pain killers, 348, 352
Pain management, 147, 641
Pancreas, 168
Pancreatic cancer, 394, 469, 549
Pandemics, 509–10
Panic attacks, 104–5, 421
Panic disorder, 104–5, 421
Pantothenic acid, 176
Pap smear, 476, 528, 551, 553
Parasitic worms, 487
Parental influence. See also Genetic factors
    alcohol use, 382
    alcoholism, 405
    drug use, 355
    smoking, 415
Parkinson's disease, 191, 347
Partial-birth abortions, 324
Particle pollution, 604
Passionate love, 247
Passive stretching, 146
Patch (contraceptive), 314–16
Patch (nicotine), 428
Pathogens, 486
Patients' rights, 554–55
PCB, 612
PCP (phencyclidine), 369
Pedometers, 136
Peer pressure, 355
Peer-reviewed journals, 19
Pelvic examinations, 552–53
Pelvic inflammatory disease (PID), 430, 523, 531–32
Penis, 270, 284
Pennsylvania State University, 274–75
Perceived stress, 68
Percent daily values (%DVs), 196
Percutaneous transluminal coronary angioplasty (PTCA), 463
Performance-boosting drugs, 142–45

Performance-related fitness, 122–23
Pericardium, 455
Perimenopause, 629
Perinatology, 326
Perineum, 266
Periodontal disease, 549–50
Periodontitis, 549
Persistent vegetative state, 638
Personality, 70, 457
"Personalized" medicine, 546–47
Pessimism, 46
Pesticides, 199, 610–11, 613
PET (polyethylene terephthalate), 607
Peyote, 369
Phobias, 104
Phosphorus, 177
Physical activity
    and breast cancer risk, 474
    exercise (See Exercise)
    gender differences, 123
    and health, 127–31
    inactivity epidemic, 123, 124–27, 208, 441, 474
    NEAT (nonexercise activity thermogenesis), 219
    racial-ethnic differences, 123
Physical attraction, 244–45
Physical dependence, 353
Physical fitness, 121–63
    of Americans, 6
    for athletic performance, 122–23
    body composition, 149–52
    and cardiometabolic risk, 441
    cardiorespiratory endurance, 122, 133–38
    of college students, 124, 125–27, 130
    defined, 122
    and dimensions of health, 123
    exercise (See Exercise)
    "fat and fit," 220
    flexibility, 122, 145–48
    gender differences, 123–24
    for health, 122
    Internet sites, 163
    muscular endurance and strength, 122, 138–42
    product/program evaluation, 143, 152–54
    racial-ethnic differences, 123–24, 126
    of young adults, 11
Physical health
    and addictive behaviors, 338
    and alcohol use/abuse, 387, 393, 394–97
    defined, 4–5
    and fitness, 123
    and grief, 645
    and marriage, 253
    and obesity, 212–14
    and sexuality, 262
    and smoking, 413, 429–30
    and spirituality, 50–51
    and stress, 69–71
Physician-assisted suicide, 643
Physicians, 550–52, 555, 563, 641
Physician's directives, 635–36, 637
Phytochemicals, 178–80
PID (pelvic inflammatory disease), 430, 523, 531–32
Pilates, 147–48
The pill, 311–14, 319, 418, 464, 492
Pima Indians, 8, 443
Pinkerton, JoAnn, 630
Pipe smoking, 424
Pituitary gland, 264
Placebo effect, 20
Placenta, 326, 327
Plan B, 319
Plaque (arteries), 461
Plaque (dental), 549
Plastic surgery, 556–57
Plastics, 607, 615
PMDD (premenstrual dysphoric disorder), 269, 312

PMS (premenstrual syndrome), 267, 269
Pneumococcal vaccine, 495
Podiatrists, 564
Point-of-service (POS) plans, 567–68
Poisonings, 580
Polio vaccine, 495
Political issues
    abortion, 299, 321–24, 323
    euthanasia, 643
    sexual abstinence, 272–73, 274, 280–81, 300–301, 520
Pollutants, 602, 607–12
Pollution, 602–4, 607–12
Polyabuse, 353
Polyethylene terephthalate (PET), 607
Population Reference Bureau, 298
Pornography, 291–92
Portion control, 193–94, 207
Positive addictions, 338
Positive psychology, 40–41
Positive thinking, 43
Posttraumatic stress disorder (PTSD), 82–83, 586
Posture, 145
Pot (marijuana), 343, 344, 355, 357–60, 459
Potassium, 176, 179, 452
Potentiating interaction, 346
Poverty, 8, 187
Power, 123
PPOs (preferred provider organizations), 567–68
Practice guidelines, 20
Prayer, 5, 53
Preclinical trials, 19
Preconception care, 325
Precontemplation stage, 24
Precycling, 604
Prediabetes, 445
Predisposing factors, 21–22
Predrinking, 384–85
Preferred provider organizations (PPOs), 567–68
Pregnancy. See also Contraception; Fertility/infertility
    acupuncture for control of nausea, 558
    alcohol use during, 397–98
    body changes during, 325–26
    childbirth, 328–30
    cocaine use during, 366
    complications, 326–28
    and depression, 101
    and diabetes, 447
    Ecstasy use during, 361
    ectopic, 326–27, 523
    fetal development, 326
    flu shots, 498
    folic acid, 186
    food poisoning, 199
    genetic testing, 327–28
    and Group B streptococcus, 505
    home pregnancy tests, 325, 549
    hormones, 267
    and immunity, 492
    marijuana use during, 360
    miscarriage, 327, 614
    and obesity, 208
    opioid abuse during, 368
    pollution risks, 602
    preconception care, 325
    readiness for children, 300
    smoking during, 413, 418, 431–32
    strategies for healthy, 323
    teens, 274
    unintentional, 299, 303, 308
Prehypertension, 451
Premarital counseling, 252–53
Premature ejaculation, 288–89
Premature labor, 328
Premenstrual dysphoric disorder (PMDD), 269, 312
Premenstrual syndrome (PMS), 267, 269
Preparation stage, 25

Prescription drugs
    abuse of, 342, 351–52
    for ADHD, 106
    for alcoholism, 402
    anti-addiction, 370
    antianxiety, 355, 402
    antibiotics (See Antibiotics)
    antidepressants, 94, 102, 108, 114, 402
    antipsychotic, 107
    antiretroviral, 540
    antiviral, 487, 498, 529–30
    for bipolar disorder, 103
    for breast cancer, 475
    cholesterol-lowering, 454
    for erectile dysfunction, 288
    generic, 350–51
    for herpes simplex, 529–30
    for hypertension, 452
    improper use of, 350
    interactions, 346, 350, 396
    online sources, 351
    for panic attacks, 105
    for PMS treatment, 269
    for schizophrenia, 107
    side effects, 350
    sleep aids, 59, 60
    smoking cessation, 429
    for strokes, 465–66
    for weight loss, 223
Prevention
    defined, 14–15
    power of, 440
    strategies for, 15, 17, 480
PRICE prescription, 159
Primary care, 564
Pro-choice groups, 324
Pro-life groups, 324
Prochaska, James, 23–24
Procrastination, 85–86
Prodromal period, 488
Progesterone, 264, 267, 322, 325
Progestin, 311–12, 314–15
Progestin-only pills, 312
Progressive overloading, 132
Progressive relaxation, 80
Projection, 80
Proof (alcoholic beverages), 390
Propoxyphene, 367
Prospective studies, 19
Prostaglandins, 269
Prostate cancer, 129, 418, 469, 477–78, 481, 551
Prostate gland, 271
Prostate hypertrophy, 631
Prostate-specific antigen (PSA), 478
Prostitution, 291
Protection, defined, 15
Proteins
    and athletic performance, 155
    defined, 169
    dietary sources, 166
    functions of, 166
    recommended amount, 169
    for vegetarians, 192–93
Protozoa, 487
Psilocybin, 459
Psoriasis, 71
Psychiatric drugs, 114
Psychiatric nurses, 113
Psychiatrists, 112, 564
Psychoactive drugs, 347
Psychoactive substance abuse disorder, 353
Psychodynamic psychotherapy, 113
Psychological dependence, 353
Psychological health, 40–50. See also
    Emotional health/emotions; Mental
    health; Spiritual health
    and abortion, 323
    and addictive behaviors, 338
    and cardiovascular disease, 456–57
    components of, 40
    defined, 5